McGraw-Hill's
I.V. DRUG
Handbook

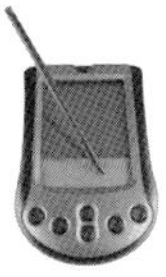

PDA DOWNLOAD

McGraw-Hill's

I.V. DRUG HANDBOOK

FOLLOW THESE INSTRUCTIONS TO DOWNLOAD YOUR PDA SOFTWARE

1) Use your Web browser to go to:
http://www.mcgraw-hillmedical.com/ivdh/

2) Register now

3) Fill in the required fields

4) Enter your unique registration code below

5) Download the software and sync into your handheld device

Scratch here to reveal your access code

NOTE: Book is not returnable once scratch-off is removed

Use this code to register and receive your PDA software. See above for complete directions.

If you have any problems accessing your download, please email: techsolutions@mhedu.com

ISBN 978-0-07-154862-5
MHID 0-07-154862-9
part of set
ISBN 978-0-07-154863-2
MHID 0-07-154863-7
and
ISBN 978-0-07-164014-5
MHID 0-07-164014-2

McGraw Hill Medical

mcgraw-hillmedical.com

McGraw-Hill's I.V. DRUG Handbook

Patricia Dwyer Schull, MSN, RN

McGraw-Hill Medical

New York Chicago San Francisco Lisbon London Madrid Mexico City
Milan New Delhi San Juan Seoul Singapore Sydney Toronto

The McGraw·Hill Companies

McGraw-Hill's I.V. Drug Handbook

1 2 3 4 5 6 7 8 9 0 DOC/DOC 12 11 10 9 8

Set ISBN 978-0-07-154863-2; MHID 0-07-154863-7
Book ISBN 978-0-07-154861-8; MHID 0-07-154861-0
Card ISBN 978-0-07-154862-5; MHID 0-07-154862-9

This book was set in Minion by International Typesetting and Composition; the Editor was Quincy McDonald; the Production Supervisor was Phil Galea; the Director of Editing, Design, and Production was John Williams; project management was provided by Arushi Chawla, International Typesetting and Composition.

This book was developed by MedVantage Publishing, LLC; the Director was Patricia Dwyer Schull, RN, MSN; the Clinical Manager was Minnie Bowen Rose, RN, BSN, MEd; the Editorial Manager was Kathy E. Goldberg; the Designers were Stephanie Peters and Joseph John Clark; the Copyeditor and Indexer was Karen Comerford; and the Editorial Supervisor was Julia S. Knipe.

RR Donnelley was printer and binder.

This book is printed on acid-free paper.

Library of Congress Cataloging-in-Publication Data

Schull, Patricia Dwyer.
Mcgraw-Hill's I.V. drug handbook / Patricia Dwyer Schull.
p. ; cm.
Includes bibliographical references and index.
ISBN-13: 978-0-07-154863-2 (pbk. : alk. paper)
ISBN-10: 0-07-154863-7
1. Intravenous therapy—Handbooks, manuals, etc. 2. Drugs—Administration—Handbooks, manuals, etc. 3. Nursing—Handbooks, manuals, etc. I. Title. II. Title: I.V. drug handbook.
[DNLM: 1. Pharmaceutical Preparations—administration & dosage—Handbooks. 2. Infusions, Intravenous—Handbooks. 3. Injections, Intravenous—Handbooks. QV 735 S386m 2009]
RM170.S38 2009
615'.6—dc22

2008028899

International Edition
Set ISBN 978-0-07-164014-5; MHID 0-07-164014-2
Book ISBN 978-0-07-164022-0; MHID 0-07-164022-3
Card ISBN 978-0-07-154862-5; MHID 0-07-154862-9

Contents

Foreword vii
Advisors ix
Contributors and reviewers x
Preface and user's guide xi

Part 1
Drugs A to Z 3
Safe I.V. drug administration
- I.V. drug compatibilities S2
- Conversions and calculations S6
- Drug infusion rates S7
- Venipuncture and peripheral venous access S10
- Preventing and treating extravasation S16
- High-alert drugs S17
- Hazardous I.V. drugs S18
- Guidelines for administering hazardous drugs S19
- Avoiding dangerous abbreviations S23
- Common abbreviations S24
- I.V. drugs and drug names that look or sound alike S26
- Monitoring blood levels S28
- Anaphylaxis: Treatment guidelines S30
- Adult cardiac arrest: Treatment guidelines S31
- Pediatric cardiac arrest: Treatment guidelines S32

Part 2
Less commonly used drugs 661

Part 3
Appendix
- Common laboratory values 692
- Body surface area in adults 695
- Body surface area in children 696

I.V. drug and solution compatibilities 697
Effects of dialysis on drug therapy 700
Identifying life-threatening adverse reactions 703

Selected references 710
Index 712

Foreword

Not so long ago, when I was an ICU nurse, the pharmacy printed pocket cards to serve as handy references for intravenous (I.V.) drugs. The concept of giving hospital staff a fast, easy-to-use guide to I.V. drugs is still a good one. In fact, the need for such a guide is greater than ever—considering the number of I.V. drugs given today, the complexity of I.V. therapy, increasing patient acuity, and our growing responsibilities surrounding drug administration.

Many I.V. drugs are powerful medications. Not only are more patients receiving them today; a significant number receive multiple I.V. drugs at the same time. Frequently, these patients are the sickest—and the most susceptible to life-threatening consequences of a medication error.

As you're undoubtedly aware, patient safety recently has taken center stage—to a degree we've never seen before. Over the last decade, numerous studies have explored the problem of medication errors, including which drugs are most often involved, how the errors come about, and what the consequences are. Of particular significance for I.V. drugs, a 2007 study in the *Archives of Internal Medicine* found that from 1998 to 2005, the number of serious adverse drug events (ADEs) reported to the Food and Drug Administration (FDA) increased 260% and ADE-related deaths rose 270%. Of the nearly 1,500 drugs linked to ADEs, a subset of 51 (most of which are administered I.V. and designated high-alert or hazardous) accounted for 43% of total ADEs. In every year studied, the FDA received 500 or more reports on each of these 51 drugs.

Furthermore, not only are those drugs commonly involved in errors, but they pose an increased risk of causing significant harm when used in error. Although mistakes may or may not be more common with these drugs, the *consequences* of these mistakes are more devastating. Of the drugs deemed high-alert by the Institute for Safe Medication Practices, the majority are given I.V. The same is true of hazardous drugs (those that can cause cancer, genetic mutations, reproductive or developmental problems, and certain other harmful effects).

Studies have found that multiple factors contribute to medication errors. So no matter how hard an individual healthcare provider tries to prevent medication errors, trying harder isn't the answer—or at least, not the only answer. To meet the challenge of administering I.V. drugs safely, healthcare providers require reliable, updated, easily accessible information on the drugs they give.

The *McGraw-Hill's I.V. Drug Handbook* is the 21st-century version of the old pharmacy pocket card. It's compact, so you can carry it with you just about anywhere, including on your PDA. But don't let its compact size fool you: this book is comprehensive. You'll be impressed by the number of drugs covered and the depth of coverage, as well as the vital supplementary information it contains. The handbook provides full, detailed monographs on more than 300 I.V. drugs.

Of course, each drug monograph covers the essentials—generic and trade drug names, mechanism of action, pharmacokinetics, available forms, approved indications, contraindications, precautions, adverse effects, and patient teaching.

Above and beyond these basics, you'll find additional crucial data:

- the latest FDA boxed warnings
- actions to take before you administer the drug (including supportive therapy to give)
- detailed instructions on preparing admixtures, which solutions to dilute, which to avoid, and correct administration rates
- dosing schedules and critical dosage adjustments
- essential patient monitoring.

The book's benefits don't stop there. Each high-alert or hazardous drug is specially marked for easy identification, and crucial warnings and instructions are highlighted with "Clinical alert" icons. A special 32-page full color insert includes sanctioned guidelines on treating cardiac arrest and stroke and administering hazardous I.V. drugs, a step-by-step illustrated procedure for starting an I.V. line, I.V. drug compatibility charts—and more. And you can download the full text to your PDA at no extra cost.

Like me, you'll appreciate the thought and planning that went into creating this impressive book. The writing (concise and jargon-free) and the design (customized for busy healthcare workers) make for easy reading and allow you to instantly find the information you seek. I'm certain that within the pages of the *McGraw-Hill's I.V. Drug Handbook,* you'll find all the information you need to administer I.V. drugs with confidence.

Vicki L. Buchda, MS, RN, CNAA
Vice-Chair, Division of Nursing Services
Mayo Clinic
Phoenix, Arizona

Advisors

Gloria F. Donnelly, RN, PhD, FAAN
Dean and Professor
College of Nursing and Health Professions
Drexel University
Philadelphia, Pa.

Maureen Duff, RGN, SCM, Dip HV, MSc, FFNMRCSI
Teaching Fellow
Department of Nursing and Midwifery
University of Stirling
Scotland, UK

Harriet R. Feldman, RN, PhD, FAAN
Dean and Professor
Lienhard School of Nursing
Interim Dean, School of Education
Pace University
Pleasantville and New York, N.Y.

Joyce E. Johnson, RN, PhD, CNAA, FAAN
Senior Vice President of Operations/Chief Nursing Officer
Georgetown University Hospital
Washington, D.C.

Peggy Kalowes, RN, PhD, CNS
Director
Center for Women's Cardiac Health and Research
Heart and Vascular Institute
Long Beach Memorial Hospital
Long Beach, Calif.

James A. Koestner, BS, PharmD
Critical Care Pharmacist
Vanderbilt University Medical Center
Nashville, Tenn.

Contributors and reviewers

Cathy L. Bartels, PharmD, FAAIM
Associate Professor
Creighton University Medical Center
Omaha, Neb.

Vicky Borders-Hemphill, PharmD
Medical Writer
Clinton, Md.

Julie M. Gerhart, MS, RPh
Pharmacy Affairs Manager
Merck & Co., Inc.
West Point, Pa.

Cheryl A. Grandinetti, PharmD
Senior Clinical Research Pharmacist
Pharmaceutical Management Branch
Cancer Therapy Evaluation Program
Division of Cancer Treatment and Diagnosis
National Cancer Institute
Rockville, Md.

Kathleen E. Jones, RN, CPN
Freelance Author
Westerville, Ohio

Sue Masoorli, RN
President, Chief Executive Officer
Perivascular Nurse Consultants, Inc.
Philadelphia, PA

Joan M. Menuchi, MSN, RN-BC
Former Clinical Educator
Philadelphia (Pa.) VA Medical Center
Medical Center Education Department
Philadelphia, Pa.

Keith M. Olsen, PharmD, FCCP, FCCM
Professor and Chair
Department of Pharmacy Practice
University of Nebraska Medical Center
Omaha, Nebraska

Dennis D. Pezzani, BS, RPh
Developer and Former Instructor
Pharmacy Technician Course
St. Charles Community College
Cottleville, Mo.
Expert Panel Member, 2006-2007
Institute for Certification of Pharmacy Technicians

Martha Polovich, MN, RN, AOCN
Associate Director, Clinical Practice
Duke Oncology Network
Durham, N.C.

Christine Price, PharmD
Pharmacy Clinical Coordinator
Morton Plant Mease Health Care
Clearwater, Fla.

Barbara Putrycus, RN, MSN, CCRN
Director Surgical Quality/Infection Control/Risk Management/Regulatory Compliance
Oakwood Hospital & Medical Center
Dearborn, Mich.

Mary E. Stassi, RN, C
Health Occupations Coordinator
St. Charles Community College
Cottleville, Mo.

Margaret A. Tiemann, RN, BS
Instructor
Health Information Technology
St. Charles Community College
Cottleville, Mo.

Preface and user's guide

I.V. drugs are the double-edged sword of pharmacology: potent, fast-acting, and life-saving-yet more apt to cause severe harm or even death when used in error. Not surprisingly, they've been called "the best of drugs and the worst of drugs."

Undeniably, I.V. drugs are indispensable for many patients. Their near-instant onset of action is crucial in cardiac emergencies, trauma, and other life-or-death situations that demand rapid drug infusion.

But mistakes with I.V. drugs can be catastrophic. Of all medication errors, those involving I.V. drugs carry the greatest potential for injury or death. Unsafe I.V. drug administration practices include failing to dilute the drug properly, failing to administer it properly, using the wrong I.V. bolus technique, overriding the proper administration rate, and calculating patient weights or dosages incorrectly.

A review of drug errors reported to the Food and Drug Administration (FDA) from 1993 to 1998 found that:

- 35% of errors resulted from I.V. pump errors
- 40% of deaths resulted from administration of the wrong I.V. dosage
- 16% of deaths stemmed from administration of the wrong I.V. drug.

With so much room for error and so much at risk when an error occurs, it's an understatement to say that administering I.V. drugs is a challenge. Witness this fact: Of the Joint Commission's eight nursing practice-related national patient safety goals for 2008, seven pertain to safe drug administration.

To give I.V. drugs safely and effectively, nurses must have expert skills. But skills alone aren't enough. You also need a specialized, reliable, and comprehensive I.V. drug database. This book is precisely the tool you've been seeking.

Responding to your need

We developed the *McGraw-Hill's I.V. Drug Handbook* to ensure that you have access, whenever and wherever you need it, to the vital facts you need to keep your patients safe. Assembled by pharmacology and nursing experts, it has been reviewed meticulously to ensure accuracy.

Don't let its small size fool you. Within its pages, you'll find all the essentials on I.V. drugs, plus many helpful extras and special features. The book's streamlined design steers you easily to the information you want. Clear, jargon-free writing guarantees that you'll grasp the information immediately. Special icons call your attention to crucial warnings and instructions.

You'll also find prominent icons identifying high-alert or hazardous drugs. Why is this important? When you know you're giving a high-alert drug, you can take extra steps to protect your patient. And when you know you're giving a hazardous drug, you can take extra steps to protect *yourself*. Healthcare workers who prepare and give hazardous drugs are at risk for serious adverse effects when exposed inadvertently. Consequences may include rashes, infertility, miscarriages, leukemia or other cancers, and birth defects in offspring. A 2007 study found a 20% higher rate of breast cancer and miscarriages and a 50% higher asthma rate in nurses who'd been exposed to hazardous drugs, compared to nurses who'd had little or no exposure.

Outstanding features

The *McGraw-Hill's I.V. Drug Handbook* provides full monographs for 275 commonly used I.V. drugs, as well as 40 condensed monographs for less commonly used I.V. agents. Each monograph lists the drug's generic and trade names, mechanism of action, pharmacokinetics, available forms, indications and dosages, contraindications and precautions, adverse effects, and patient teaching.

Above and beyond these basic facts, we provide additional information to deepen and broaden your understanding of the drug:

- latest FDA boxed warnings
- actions you must take before giving the drug (including supportive therapy to give before administering chemotherapy or certain other drugs)
- detailed instructions on preparing admixtures, including which solutions to dilute the drug (if needed) and which solutions to avoid
- drug administration rates
- dosing schedules and levels
- critical dosage adjustments
- essential patient monitoring.

A special 32-page, color insert titled "Safe I.V. drug administration" provides sanctioned guidelines on preparing and administering hazardous I.V. drugs, a step-by-step illustrated procedure for starting a peripheral I.V. line, I.V. drug compatibility charts—and more.

Understanding your responsibilities

As a nurse, you're legally responsible for ensuring the "five rights" of drug administration (right patient, drug, dosage, time, and rate). Also make sure you're familiar with the Joint Commission's 2008 National Patient Safety Goals, which mandate that healthcare facilities (and by extension, nurses) implement practices to improve or bring about:

- better communication among caregivers
- creation of a standardized list of abbreviations, symbols, and dosage designations *not* to be used
- improved safety of drug use
- verification of all labels both verbally and visually by two qualified individuals, if the person preparing the drug is not the same person who will administer it
- accurate and complete medication reconciliation across the continuum of care
- reduction of the risk of patient harm stemming from falls caused by medications
- active involvement of patients in their own care (including teaching them about their drugs).

User's guide to the *McGraw-Hill's I.V. Drug Handbook*

This book is organized in three main parts.

Part 1: A to Z drug monographs

Part 1 presents individual I.V. drug monographs in alphabetical order by generic name. Where applicable, the top banner above the drug name includes an icon indicating that the drug is a high-alert drug or a hazardous drug. *High-alert* drugs deserve special attention and safeguards.

Drugs designated as *hazardous* by the National Institute for Occupational Safety and Health, American Society of Health-System Pharmacists, and the Centers for Disease Control and Prevention include cancer chemotherapy agents; certain antivirals, hormones, and bioengineered drugs; and selected miscellaneous drugs. They must be handled within an established safety program.

Below the banner, each monograph presents essential information in the following order:

Generic name. A drug's generic name is the nonproprietary name, typically assigned by the manufacturer. When more than one therapeutic form of the drug is available, generic names of these forms are listed alphabetically.

Trade names. A drug's common trade, or brand, name is the proprietary, trademarked name under which it's marketed. This section lists *only* those trade-name drugs given by the I.V. route. Trade-name and generic drugs are therapeutically equivalent in strength, quality, performance, and use; when interchanged, they have the same effects and no differences. However, they may vary in preservatives, labeling, and possibly certain other attributes. Trade-name I.V. drugs available in Canada ♣ and the United Kingdom ❈ are marked with a special icon for easy identification.

Pharmacologic and therapeutic classes. This section specifies the drug's pharmacologic class (based on its pharmacologic properties and action—for example, vasodilator or fluoroquinolone) and therapeutic class (based on approved therapeutic uses of the drug—for instance, antineoplastic or antihypertensive). Many drugs fall into multiple therapeutic classes.

Controlled substance schedule. Opioids, stimulants, and certain other drugs come under the Controlled Substances Act. The Drug Enforcement Agency assigns each of these drugs a category, or schedule, based on its abuse potential and other factors. (See *Schedules of controlled substances,* page xiv.) When applicable, this section lists the drug's assigned schedule.

Pregnancy risk category. This section lists the category assigned by the FDA to indicate the drug's potential danger to the fetus when taken during pregnancy. (See *Understanding pregnancy risk categories,* page xiv).

FDA boxed warning. The FDA assigns a boxed warning if:

- the drug may cause an adverse reaction so serious (relative to the drug's potential benefit) that prescribers must carefully weigh risk against benefit
- a serious adverse reaction can be prevented or reduced through careful patient selection, rigorous monitoring, avoiding certain concomitant therapy, adding another drug, managing the patient in a specific way, or avoiding use in a specific clinical situation
- the FDA approved the drug with restrictions to assure its safe use because it concluded that the drug can be used safely only if its distribution or use is restricted.
- In this book, boxed warnings have been condensed and edited for space reasons. Be sure to review the complete package insert before administering a drug with a boxed warning.

Pharmacokinetics. This section summarizes how the drug achieves its therapeutic effect—the action that takes place when it reaches its target site and combines with cellular drug receptors to cause certain physiologic responses. When a drug's action isn't known or when researchers have proposed theories for the action but haven't clarified it definitively, we state this fact.

Below this summary, you'll find a pharmacokinetic profile in table form—onset of action, peak blood level, and duration of action-specific to I.V. administration.

How supplied. This section lists the physical forms in which the I.V. drug is produced and dispensed, along with available strengths (the amount of active ingredient present).

Indications and dosages. This section details FDA-approved indications for adults, children, infants, and neonates (when appropriate), along with recommended dosages and dosing frequency for each indication. The indications and dosages shown reflect current clinical trends, not unequivocal standards, and must be considered in light of the patient's condition and diagnosis. (Although we've made every effort to ensure the accuracy of all dosages, we urge you

Schedules of controlled substances

The Controlled Substances Act of 1970 regulates the production and distribution of stimulants, narcotics, depressants, hallucinogens, and anabolic steroids. Drugs regulated by this law fall into five categories, or schedules, based on their abuse potential, medicinal value, and harmfulness. Schedule I drugs are the most hazardous; schedule V drugs, the least hazardous.

Schedule I: High potential for abuse; no currently accepted medical use in the United States. Using the drug even under medical supervision is thought to be unsafe.

Schedule II: High potential for abuse; currently accepted medical use in the United States (or currently accepted medical use with severe restrictions). Abuse may lead to severe psychological or physical dependence. Emergency telephone orders for limited quantities may be authorized, but the prescriber must provide a written, signed prescription order.

Schedule III: Lower abuse potential than schedule I and II drugs; currently accepted medical use in the United States. Abuse may lead to a moderate or low degree of physical dependence or high psychological dependence. Telephone orders are permitted.

Schedule IV: Lower abuse potential than schedule I, II, or III drugs; currently accepted medical use in the United States. Abuse may lead to limited physical dependence or psychological dependence. Telephone orders are permitted.

Schedule V: Low abuse potential compared to drugs in other schedules; currently accepted medical use in the United States. Abuse may lead to limited physical dependence or to psychological dependence. Some schedule V drugs may be available in limited quantities without a prescription (if state law permits).

Understanding pregnancy risk categories

Whenever possible, pregnant women should avoid drug therapy. The risks of taking drugs during pregnancy range from relatively minor fetal defects (such as ear tags or extra digits) to fetal death.

When drug therapy is considered, the drug's benefits to the mother must be weighed against the risk to the fetus. Ideally, the drug should provide clear benefits to the mother without harming the fetus. To help prescribers and pregnant patients assess a drug's risk-to-benefit ratio, the Food and Drug Administration assigns one of five pregnancy risk categories to each drug. In addition, certain drugs are not rated.

Category A: No evidence of risk exists. Adequate, well-controlled studies in pregnant women don't show an increased risk of fetal abnormalities during any trimester.

Category B: The risk of fetal harm is possible but remote. Animal studies show no fetal risk; however, controlled studies haven't been done in humans. Or animal studies do show a risk to the fetus, but adequate studies in pregnant women haven't shown such a risk.

Category C: Fetal risk can't be ruled out. Although animal studies show risks, adequate, well-controlled human studies are lacking. Despite the potential fetal risks, use of the drug may be acceptable because of benefits to the mother.

Category D: Positive evidence of fetal risk exists. Nevertheless, potential benefits from the drug may outweigh the risk. For example, the drug may be acceptable in a life-threatening situation or serious disease if safer drugs can't be used or are ineffective.

Category X: Contraindicated during pregnancy. Studies in animals or humans or reports of adverse reactions show evidence of fetal risk that clearly outweighs any possible benefit to the patient.

Category NR: Not rated.

to review the official package insert for each drug you administer.)

Dosage adjustment. This section tells you which patient groups (such as children or elderly patients) and which diseases or disorders (such as renal or hepatic dysfunction) may necessitate dosage adjustment. When dosage adjustment is multifaceted or complex, we provide this information in table format.

Off-label uses. Here you'll find a list of off-label (unlabeled or unapproved) uses of the drug, when applicable. Off-label drug use has become increasingly common as clinical research moves ahead of the FDA's approval process. In some cases, off-label use has become the standard of care.

Administration. This section is subdivided into several categories, as applicable:

• ***Preparation*** describes the tests and assessments that should precede drug administration, as well as warnings to heed before giving the first dose and supportive therapies to administer (for instance, premedication with antiemetics for chemotherapy drugs).

• ***Dilution and compatibility*** details how to mix the drug properly, tells which solutions are compatible and incompatible for dilution, and lists any other solutions needed to prepare the drug for continuous or intermittent I.V. infusion.

• ***Infusion considerations*** specifies the flow rate to use when giving the drug by direct I.V. injection or intermittent or continuous I.V. infusion, what type of adminstration set or filter to use (or to avoid using), whether to flush the I.V. line before or after administration, and other crucial information.

• ***Monitoring*** describes essential patient monitoring to perform during drug therapy (and in some cases, after therapy ends) to help evaluate whether the drug is effective and to detect untoward reactions or interactions. Examples include monitoring blood drug levels to determine the correct dosage and prevent toxicity and checking the infusion site for local effects and extravasation.

• ***Storage*** lists the temperature range at which the drug (before or after reconstitution) should be stored, correct storage conditions (for example, refrigerated and protected from light), and the maximum number of hours or days for which it can be stored.

Contraindications and precautions. Here you'll find conditions that contraindicate use of the drug (such as preexisting diseases), followed by conditions that warrant cautious use. As a rule, never give a drug to a patient with a history of hypersensitivity to that drug. Drugs commonly implicated in hypersensitivity reactions include antibiotics, histamines, iodides, phenothiazines, tranquilizers, anesthetics, diagnostic agents (such as iodinated contrast media), and biologic agents (such as insulin, vaccines, and antitoxins).

For some patients, a specific drug may pose an increased risk of untoward effects—yet the physician prescribes it in the belief that potential benefits outweigh the risks for a particular patient. For instance, many drugs can be dangerous in elderly patients, pregnant or breastfeeding women, young children, and patients with renal or hepatic dysfunction. When administering a high-alert drug, precautions can be especially important.

Adverse reactions. Occurring in roughly 30% of hospital patients, adverse reactions are undesirable and unintended drug effects, which can range from mild to life-threatening. They may arise immediately and suddenly, or may take weeks or even months to develop. Adverse reactions can be particularly dangerous if a medication error occurs with a high-alert drug. Keep in mind that the sickest patients—those in intensive care—are the most vulnerable to adverse reactions and drug interactions. In this section, we list the most commonly reported adverse reactions by body system. Life-threatening reactions appear in **boldface.**

Interactions. With Americans taking more prescription and nonprescription drugs than ever, you're likely to encounter patients experiencing the effects of drug interactions. Many people also take herbal and nutritional supplements that can interact with drugs to cause dangerous effects or to impede a drug's intended effect. This section presents documented and clinically significant interactions that may occur if the drug is used concurrently with other drugs, specific foods, and certain herbs or supplements, or if it's combined with certain behaviors (for instance, smoking or alcohol use). It also describes the drug's effects on diagnostic test results, which can be especially important for hospital patients.

Toxicity and overdose. This section lists the clinical effects of an overdose, followed by immediate interventions to take and specific antidotes (if available).

Patient teaching. The nurse's responsibility for teaching patients about their care is greater than ever; also, today's patients are demanding more information about their treatment. This section describes key teaching points to cover with a patient who's receiving the drug, including essential information needed to protect your patient even after discharge. Topics include which symptoms to report immediately and which drugs, foods, herbs, or behaviors the patient should avoid during drug therapy.

Part 2: Less commonly used I.V. drugs

Part 2 presents abbreviated monographs on infrequently given I.V. drugs. These monographs list the drug's generic and trade names (along with high-alert or hazardous icons where aplicable), FDA boxed warnings (where applicable), indications and dosages, and essential administration and monitoring points.

Part 3: Appendices, references, and index

Appendices serve as handy guides on important drug topics and related issues, including normal laboratory values (to help you monitor your patient's response to drugs), I.V. drug and solution admixture compatibility chart (to help you avoid dangerous physical or chemical incompatibilities), effects of dialysis on drug therapy (to guide overdose interventions or ensure supplemental dosing). We've also included a guide to life-threatening adverse reactions, to help you quickly detect these reactions and intervene appropriately.

Website and PDA download bonuses

Visit our website, www.mcgraw-hillmedical.com for access to drug monographs, patient teaching aids to customize and give to your patients, the safe drug administration insert of this book, plus drug news and other crucial information to help you give I.V. drugs safely. From this website, you can access the full text of the *McGraw-Hill's I.V. Drug Handbook*—and even download it free to your personal digital assistant.

I'm confident this book will enhance your practice and help you continue to make I.V. drug therapy safer and more effective for your patients. No matter how complex the drug or the drug regimen, this book will serve as a reliable resource that will help you master the demands of I.V. drug administration.

Acknowledgments

I wish to thank the talented MedVantage Publishing team—Minnie Rose (clinical director), Julia Knipe (administrator), Kathy Goldberg (editorial manager), Karen Comerford (copyedit supervisor), and Stephanie Peters (design manager), as well as the clinical editors, text editors, copy editors, and designers whose skill and knowledge have helped to ensure that this book meets high standards of quality.

Thanks also to the entire McGraw-Hill team, including Scott Grillo, Quincy McDonald, John Williams, and Phil Galea.

I'm indebted as well to all of our advisors, contributors, and reviewers for their guidance, support, and willingness to share their knowledge with our readers.

Special thanks to my wonderful family-husband, children, grandchildren, extended family, and friends—for their support, understanding, and patience.

As always, I'm privileged to support the nursing community, whose members work tirelessly and selflessly to serve their patients with the best possible care and to protect them from harm. Know that I appreciate your enthusiastic support and will continue to work hard to bring you the tools you need to safeguard your patients.

Patricia Dwyer Schull, MSN, RN

Part 1

Drugs A to Z

Safe I.V. drug administration

abatacept

Orencia

Pharmacologic class: Selective costimulation modulator

Therapeutic class: Antirheumatic

Pregnancy risk category C

Action

Inhibits T cell (T lymphocyte) activation by binding to CD80 and CD86, blocking interaction with CD28. (This interaction provides costimulatory signal needed for full activation of T cells, implicated in rheumatoid arthritis pathogenesis.)

Pharmacokinetics

No systemic drug accumulation occurs on continued repeated treatment with 10 mg/kg at monthly intervals in rheumatic arthritis patients. Clearance may increase with body weight.

Onset	Peak	Duration
Unknown	Unknown	Unknown

How supplied

Powder for injection (lyophilized, white): 250 mg/15 mL in single-use vial

Indications and dosages

To reduce signs and symptoms, slow progression of structural damage, and improve physical function in patients with moderately to severely active rheumatoid arthritis who have not responded adequately to one or more disease-modifying antirheumatic drugs or tumor necrosis factor (TNF) antagonists (such as adalimumab, etanercept, or infliximab)

Adults weighing less than 60 kg (132 lb): 500 mg I.V. over 30 minutes at weeks 0, 2, and 4; thereafter, give every 4 weeks.

Adults weighing 60 to 100 kg (132 to 220 lb): 750 mg I.V. over 30 minutes at weeks 0, 2, and 4; thereafter, give every 4 weeks.

Adults weighing more than 100 kg: 1 g I.V. over 30 minutes at weeks 0, 2, and 4; thereafter, give every 4 weeks.

Administration

Dilution and compatibility

- Reconstitute each vial with 10 mL sterile water for injection, using only silicone-free disposable syringe included with product.
- When reconstituting, rotate vial by swirling gently. Avoid prolonged or vigorous agitation. Do not shake.
- Further dilute reconstituted solution to volume of 100 mL with normal saline solution.
- Use silicone-free syringe to add drug to infusion bag or bottle, and mix gently. Resulting drug concentration should be 5 mg/mL for two vials, 7.5 mg/mL for three vials, or 10 mg/mL for four vials.

Infusion considerations

- Give infusion over 30 minutes, using infusion set and nonpyogenic, low-protein-binding filter.
- Complete infusion within 24 hours of vial reconstitution.
- Do not infuse other drugs concurrently through same I.V. line.

Monitoring

- Watch for infusion-related reactions (hypotension or hypertension, dyspnea, nausea, dizziness, headache, flushing, urticaria, pruritus, rash, cough, or wheezing), which usually arise within 1 hour of administration. Be prepared to intervene appropriately.
- Assess patient's overall health at each visit to evaluate infection status.

• Closely monitor patient with chronic obstructive pulmonary disease (COPD) because of increased risk of adverse events.

Storage

• Store fully diluted solution at room temperature, or refrigerate at 2° to 8°C (36° to 46°F), if needed.

Contraindications and precautions

Contraindicated in hypersensitivity to drug or its components.

Use cautiously in increased risk of infection, history of recurrent infections, immunocompromised state, COPD, concurrent use of TNF antagonists, patients older than age 65, pregnant or breastfeeding patients, and ***children*** (safety and efficacy not established).

Adverse reactions

CNS: headache, dizziness
CV: hypertension, hypotension
EENT: nasopharyngitis, rhinitis
GI: nausea, dyspepsia, diverticulitis
GU: urinary tract infection, acute pyelonephritis
Musculoskeletal: back pain, extremity pain
Respiratory: cough, upper respiratory tract infection, pneumonia, wheezing, bronchitis, dyspnea
Skin: rash, flushing, urticaria, pruritus
Other: herpes simplex and herpes zoster infections, infusion-related reactions, hypersensitivity reaction, cancers

Interactions

Drug-drug. *Immunizations:* possible decrease in immunization efficacy

Toxicity and overdose

• Doses up to 50 mg/kg have been given without apparent toxic effect.

• In overdose, monitor for signs or symptoms of adverse reactions and provide appropriate symptomatic treatment.

Patient teaching

Instruct patient to promptly report signs and symptoms of cancer (such as unusual lumps or other unexplained symptoms).

• Advise patient to report signs and symptoms of infection.

• Caution patient to avoid immunizations during therapy and for 3 months afterward.

• Tell female of childbearing potential that pregnancy and breastfeeding are not recommended during therapy.

• As appropriate, review all other significant adverse reactions and interactions, especially those related to the drugs mentioned above.

abciximab

ReoPro, ReoPro ♣ ❋

Pharmacologic class: Platelet aggregation inhibitor

Therapeutic class: Antithrombotic, antiplatelet drug

Pregnancy risk category C

Action

Inhibits platelet aggregation and binding of fibrinogen and other adhesive molecules to platelet receptors, thereby inhibiting and prolonging bleeding time.

Pharmacokinetics

After I.V. bolus, free plasma concentrations fall rapidly. Initial half-life is less than 10 minutes; second-phase half-life, about 30 minutes. Platelet function generally recovers within 48 hours, although drug stays in circulation for 15 days or more in platelet-bound state. At end of infusion period, free plasma concentrations fall rapidly for approximately 6 hours, then decline more slowly.

Onset	Peak	Duration
Rapid	Unknown	48 hr

How supplied

Solution for injection (clear, colorless, nonpyrogenic): 2 mg/mL (5-mL vials containing 10 mg)

Indications and dosages

➤ Adjunct to aspirin and heparin to prevent acute cardiac ischemic complications in patients undergoing percutaneous coronary intervention (PCI)
Adults: 0.25 mg/kg I.V. bolus given 10 to 60 minutes before start of PCI, followed by infusion of 0.125 mcg/kg/minute (to a maximum of 10 mcg/minute) for 12 hours

➤ Adjunct to aspirin and heparin in patients with unstable angina who have not responded to conventional medical therapy and will undergo PCI within 24 hours
Adults: 0.25 mg/kg I.V. bolus, followed by 18- to 24-hour infusion of 10 mcg/minute, ending 1 hour after PCI

Administration

Preparation

• Obtain baseline CBC, platelet count, prothrombin time (PT), partial thromboplastin time, and International Normalized Ratio.
• Avoid noncompressible I.V. sites, such as subclavian and jugular veins.

Dilution and compatibility

• Give bolus injection undiluted.
• For I.V. infusion, dilute desired dose with 250 mL normal saline solution or D_5W, to yield 40 mcg/mL. Do not shake.
• Use low-protein-binding, 0.2- to 0.22-micron filter.
• Do not mix with other drugs (although no incompatibilities are known).
• Discard unused portion.

Infusion considerations

• For I.V. infusion, use continuous infusion pump and administer at a maximum rate of 10 mcg/minute.
• Give through separate I.V. line.

Monitoring

🔈 Stop continuous infusion after failed PCI.

🔈 Monitor for anaphylaxis, and keep emergency drugs and equipment available.

• Monitor platelet count 2 to 4 hours after bolus dose, and again at 24 hours or before discharge (whichever comes first).
• During femoral sheath insertion and for 6 hours after removal, frequently monitor digital pulse in leg where sheath was inserted.
• While femoral sheath is in place, patient must be on strict bed rest with head of bed elevated less than 30 degrees.
• Restrict patient to bed rest for 6 to 8 hours after drug withdrawal.
• After sheath removal, apply pressure to femoral artery for at least 30 minutes; then apply pressure dressing.

🔈 Monitor insertion site frequently for bleeding.

• Minimize arterial or venous punctures, automatic blood-pressure cuff use, I.M. injections, nasotracheal intubation, nasogastric tube placement, and urinary catheterization.
• Use indwelling venipuncture device, such as heparin lock, to withdraw blood.

Storage

• Refrigerate vials at 2° to 8°C (36° to 46°F).

Contraindications and precautions

Contraindicated in hypersensitivity to drug or murine proteins; active internal bleeding; bleeding diathesis; severe, uncontrolled hypertension; thrombo cytopenia (<100,000 platelets/mm^3); aneurysm; arteriovenous malformation;

history of cerebrovascular accident (CVA); oral anticoagulant therapy within past 7 days (unless PT is less than 1.2 times control); history of vasculitis or intracranial tumor; use of I.V. dextran before PCI or planned use of dextran during an intervention; or major surgery or trauma within past 6 weeks.

Use cautiously in patients receiving drugs that affect hemostasis (such as thrombolytics, anticoagulants, and antiplatelet drugs); within 12 hours of onset of acute myocardial infarction and prolonged PCI procedure (due to increased risk of bleeding); pregnant or breastfeeding patients; and ***children*** (safety and efficacy not established).

Adverse reactions

CNS: dizziness, headache, anxiety, agitation, abnormal thinking, hypoesthesia, difficulty speaking, confusion, weakness, **intracranial hemorrhage, cerebral ischemia, CVA, coma**
CV: pseudoaneurysm, palpitations, vascular disorders, arteriovenous fistula, hypotension, peripheral edema, weak pulse, chest pain, intermittent claudication, bradycardia, **ventricular or supraventricular tachycardia, atrial fibrillation or flutter, atrioventricular block, nodal arrhythmias, pericardial effusion, embolism, thrombophlebitis**
EENT: abnormal or double vision
GI: nausea, vomiting, diarrhea, constipation, abdominal pain, dyspepsia, ileus, gastroesophageal reflux, enlarged abdomen, dry mouth
GU: urine retention or urinary incontinence, painful or frequent urination, abnormal renal function, cystalgia, prostatitis
Hematologic: anemia, **leukocytosis, thrombocytopenia, bleeding**
Metabolic: diabetes mellitus, **hyperkalemia**
Musculoskeletal: myopathy, myalgia, increased muscle tension, muscle contractions, reduced muscle stretching ability
Respiratory: pneumonia, crackles, rhonchi, bronchitis, pleurisy, **pleural effusion, bronchospasm, pulmonary edema, pulmonary embolism**
Skin: pallor, cellulitis, petechiae, pruritus, bullous eruptions, diaphoresis
Other: abscess, peripheral coldness, back pain, incisional pain, development of human antichimeric antibodies, **anaphylaxis**

Interactions

Drug-drug. *Drugs that affect hemostasis (such as aspirin, dextran, dipyridamole, heparin, nonsteroidal anti-inflammatory drugs, oral anticoagulants, thrombolytics, ticlopidine):* increased bleeding risk
Drug-diagnostic tests. *Activated partial thromboplastin time, clotting time, PT:* increased values *Hemoglobin, platelets:* decreased values

Toxicity and overdose

- Although no overdose has been reported, expect such signs and symptoms as decreased platelet count and bleeding.
- If platelet count falls below 100,000 platelets/mm^3 or at least 25% below pretreatment value, obtain additional platelet samples in separate tubes containing EDTA, citrate, or heparin (to exclude pseudothrombocytopenia caused by anticoagulant interaction). If true thrombocytopenia is verified, stop drug immediately and transfuse platelets, as ordered and appropriate.

Patient teaching

- Tell patient what to expect during and after drug administration.
- Instruct patient to immediately report unusual bleeding or bruising.

- Caution patient to avoid activities that may cause injury, and to use soft toothbrush and electric razor to avoid gum and skin injury.
- Inform patient about importance of regular blood tests during therapy.
- As appropriate, review all other significant and life-threatening adverse reactions and interactions, especially those related to the drugs and tests mentioned above.

acetylcysteine (*N*-acetylcysteine)

Acetadote, Parvolex❄

Pharmacologic class: *N*-acetyl derivative of naturally occurring amino acid (L-cysteine)
Therapeutic class: Antidote
Pregnancy risk category B

Action

Maintains and restores hepatic glutathione (needed to inactivate toxic metabolites in acetaminophen overdose), thereby reducing extent of hepatic injury

Pharmacokinetics

Steady-state volume of distribution is 0.47 L/kg; drug is 83% bound to proteins. After single I.V. dose, plasma level of total acetylcysteine falls, with mean terminal half-life of 5.6 hours. Mean clearance is 0.11 L/kg/hour; with renal clearance at about 30% of total clearance.

Onset	Peak	Duration
Unknown	Unknown	Unknown

How supplied

Solution for injection (colorless): 200 mg/mL

Indications and dosages

➤ Acetaminophen overdose
Adults, elderly patients, and children: Loading dose or first dose, 150 mg/kg I.V. infusion in 200 mL D_5W over 60 minutes. Second dose or second maintenance dose, 50 mg/kg I.V. infusion in 500 mL D_5W over 4 hours. Third dose or third maintenance dose, 100 mg/kg I.V. infusion in 1,000 mL D_5W over 16 hours.

Off-label uses

- Distal intestinal obstruction syndrome
- Malaria
- Prevention of radiocontrast-induced renal dysfunction

Administration

Preparation
- Assess hepatotoxicity risk by measuring acetaminophen blood level as soon as possible, but no sooner than 4 hours after acute overdose (as results may be misleading).
- Empty stomach by lavage or emesis induction; have patient drink copious amounts of water. If activated charcoal has been given, perform lavage before giving acetylcysteine. Draw blood for acetaminophen plasma assay and baseline alanine aminotransferase (ALT), aspartate aminotransferase (AST), bilirubin, blood glucose, electrolytes, blood urea nitrogen, and creatinine clearance levels and prothrombin time.

Dilution and compatibility
- Do not use previously opened vials.
- Dilute in prescribed amount of D_5W to reduce drug's irritating or sclerosing properties.
- Be aware that drug is not compatible with rubber and metals—particularly iron, copper, and nickel.
- Know that drug may turn from essentially colorless to slightly pink or purple after stopper is punctured. Color change does not affect product quality.

Infusion considerations

- Give immediately if 24 hours or less have elapsed since acetaminophen ingestion or if ingestion time is unknown.
- Administer loading dose at a constant rate over 60 minutes. Give second dose by infusion at a constant rate over 4 hours; give third dose by infusion at a constant rate over 16 hours.
- Separate administration times of this drug and antibiotics.

Monitoring

Watch for infusion reactions occurring within 60 minutes after infusion begins. Such reactions start with acute flushing and erythema; they may resolve spontaneously or progress to acute hypersensitivity reaction (including anaphylaxis).

Monitor carefully for signs and symptoms of hypersensitivity reaction (such as shortness of breath, wheezing, rash, and hypotension).

- Continue to monitor acetaminophen blood levels and hepatic function.

Storage

- Store unopened vials at controlled room temperature.
- Know that diluted solution is stable for 24 hours at controlled room temperature.

Contraindications and precautions

Contraindicated in hypersensitivity to drug and status asthmaticus (except with antidotal use).

Use cautiously in brain tumor, bronchospasm, asthma, seizure disorders, hypothyroidism, respiratory insufficiency, alcoholism, patients weighing less than 88 lb (40 kg), fluid-restricted patients, and pregnant or breastfeeding patients.

Adverse reactions

CNS: dizziness
CV: hypotension, hypertension, tachycardia
EENT: pharyngitis, rhinorrhea
GI: nausea, vomiting
Skin: urticaria, rash, clamminess, pruritus, **angioedema**
Other: dysphoria, chills, fever, infusion reaction, hypersensitivity reactions (including shortness of breath, dyspnea, chest or throat tightness), **anaphylaxis.**

Interactions

Drug-drug. *Nitroglycerin:* increased nitroglycerin effects, causing hypotension and headache

Drug-diagnostic tests. *ALT, AST:* increased

Toxicity and overdose

- Status epilepticus, cerebral edema, and anoxic encephalopathy may occur in overdose.
- Discontinue drug promptly and provide supportive and symptomatic interventions.

Patient teaching

- Instruct patient to immediately report signs or symptoms of hypersensitivity reaction (such as flushing, shortness of breath, or feeling of faintness).
- As appropriate, review all other significant and life-threatening adverse reactions and interactions, especially those related to the drugs and tests mentioned above.

acyclovir sodium

Alti-Acyclovir✦, Avirax✦, Zovirax

Pharmacologic class: Acycloguanosine nucleoside analogue
Therapeutic class: Antiviral
Pregnancy risk category B

Action

Inhibits viral DNA polymerase, thereby inhibiting replication of viral DNA.

Specific for herpes simplex type 1 (HSV-1), herpes simplex type 2 (HSV-2), and varicella-zoster virus.

Pharmacokinetics

Drug is widely distributed in body fluids; in cerebrospinal fluid, concentration reaches approximately 50% of plasma values. Plasma protein-binding is relatively low. Renal excretion of unchanged drug is major elimination route, accounting for 62% to 91% of dose. Half-life and total body clearance hinge on renal function.

Onset	Peak	Duration
Immediate	Unknown	Unknown

How supplied

Powder for reconstitution for injection (white): 500 mg/10-mL vial, 1,000 mg/20-mL vial

Indications and dosages

➢ Mucosal and cutaneous HSV-1 and HSV-2 in immunocompromised patients

Adults and children older than age 12: 5 mg/kg I.V. infusion over 1 hour, given q 8 hours for 7 days

Children younger than age 12: 10 mg/kg I.V. infusion over 1 hour, given q 8 hours for 7 days

➢ Initial episode of severe genital herpes

Adults and children older than age 12: 5 mg/kg I.V. over 1 hour, given q 8 hours for 5 days

➢ Herpes simplex encephalitis

Adults and children older than age 12: 10 mg/kg I.V. over 1 hour, given q 8 hours for 10 days

Children ages 3 months to 12 years: 20 mg/kg I.V. over 1 hour, given q 8 hours for 10 days

Children from birth to 3 months: 10 mg/kg I.V. over 1 hour, given q 8 hours for 10 days

➢ Neonatal HSV infection

Children from birth to 3 months: 10 mg/kg I.V. over 1 hour, given q 8 hours for 10 days

➢ Varicella zoster infections in immunocompromised patients

Adults and adolescents older than age 12: 10 mg/kg I.V. over 1 hour, given q 8 hours for 7 days

Children younger than age 12: 20 mg/kg I.V. over 1 hour, given q 8 hours for 7 days

Dosage adjustment

- For patients with acute or chronic renal impairment, adjust dosing intervals as indicated below:

Dosage adjustments in renal impairment

Creatinine clearance (mL/min/1.73 m^2)	Percentage of recommended dose	Dosing interval (hr)
Greater than 50	100%	8
25 to 50	100%	12
10 to 25	100%	24
0 to 10	50%	24

- In hemodialysis patients, mean plasma half-life is approximately 5 hours; this results in 60% decrease in plasma levels after 6-hour dialysis period. Therefore, adjust dosing schedule so patient receives an additional dose each dialysis session.
- For obese adults, base dosage on ideal weight.
- Know that elderly patients have higher drug plasma levels, most likely from age-related renal function changes.

Off-label uses (selected)

- Cytomegalovirus and HSV infection after bone marrow or kidney transplantation
- Herpes zoster encephalitis
- Varicella pneumonia

Administration

Preparation

• Make sure patient is adequately hydrated before starting therapy.

Dilution and compatibility

• Know that drug is compatible with most electrolyte and glucose solutions for I.V. infusion.

• Be aware that drug is not compatible with bacteriostatic water for injection (causes precipitation).

• Know that use with biologic or colloidal fluids (such as blood products or protein solutions) is not recommended.

• Dissolve each 500 mg with 10 mL sterile water for injection, or each 1,000 mg with 20 mL sterile water for injection. Resulting concentration is 50 mg/mL.

• Shake vial well to ensure complete dissolution before transferring each individual dose.

• Use reconstituted solution within 12 hours.

• Withdraw prescribed dose and add to appropriate I.V. solution at volume selected for each 1-hour infusion. Infusion concentrations of approximately 7 mg/mL or lower are recommended. Higher concentrations (such as 10 mg/mL) may cause phlebitis or inflammation at injection site if extravasation occurs.

• Use fully diluted solution within 24 hours.

Infusion considerations

Do not give by I.V. bolus or by I.M. or subcutaneous route.

• Administer I.V. infusion at a constant rate over at least 1 hour using infusion pump or microdrip.

Be aware that too-rapid infusion may damage renal tubules.

• Continue to monitor fluid intake and output to maintain adequate urine flow during therapy.

Monitoring

• Assess for signs and symptoms of encephalopathy.

• Evaluate patient frequently for adverse reactions, especially bleeding tendency.

• Monitor CBC with differential and kidney function test results.

Storage

• Store unopened vials at 15° to 25°C (59° to 77°F).

• Be aware that refrigerating reconstituted solution may cause precipitation (which redissolves at room temperature).

Contraindications and precautions

Contraindicated in hypersensitivity to drug or valacyclovir.

Use cautiously in preexisting serious neurologic, hepatic, pulmonary, or fluid or electrolyte abnormalities; renal impairment; obesity; and pregnant or breastfeeding patients.

Adverse reactions

CNS: aggressive behavior, dizziness, malaise, weakness, fatigue, paresthesia, headache, ataxia, somnolence, delirium, **encephalopathic changes** (lethargy, tremors, obtundation, confusion, hallucinations, agitation, seizures, coma)
CV: peripheral edema, hypotension, phlebitis
EENT: vision abnormalities
GI: nausea, vomiting, diarrhea, anorexia, abdominal pain
GU: proteinuria, hematuria, oliguria, **renal failure, glomerulonephritis**
Hematologic: anemia, lymphadenopathy, thrombocytopenia, thrombocytosis, leukocytosis, neutrophilia, **thrombotic thrombocytopenic purpura/hemolytic uremic syndrome** (in immunocompromised patients), **disseminated intravascular coagulation, hemolysis, leukopenia, leukocytoclastic vasculitis, neutropenia**

Hepatic: jaundice, **hepatitis, hyperbilirubinemia**
Musculoskeletal: myalgia
Skin: photosensitivity rash, pruritus, angioedema, alopecia, urticaria, severe local inflammatory reactions (with extravasation), **toxic epidermal necrolysis, erythema multiforme**
Other: fever, excessive thirst, pain at injection site, **anaphylaxis, Stevens-Johnson syndrome**

Interactions

Drug-drug. *Interferon:* increased effect of acyclovir
Nephrotoxic drugs: increased nephrotoxicity risk
Probenecid: increased acyclovir blood level
Zidovudine: increased CNS effects, especially drowsiness
Drug-diagnostic tests. *Alanine aminotransferase, aspartate aminotransferase (after rapid I.V. infusion), bilirubin, blood urea nitrogen (BUN), creatinine:* increased

Toxicity and overdose

- Overdoses involving ingestion of up to 20 g have occurred. Adverse reactions may include agitation, coma, seizures, and lethargy. Drug may precipitate in renal tubules when solubility (2.5 mg/mL) is exceeded in intratubular fluid. Overdose may follow bolus injection or inappropriately high doses, and may occur in patients whose fluid and electrolyte balance were not properly monitored, leading to elevated BUN and serum creatinine levels and subsequent renal failure.
- Discontinue drug with onset of CNS adverse reactions. Until renal function is restored, patients with acute renal failure or anuria may need hemodialysis.

Patient teaching

Instruct patient to immediately report unusual bleeding or bruising and signs and symptoms of liver dysfunction (unusual fatigue, flulike symptoms, appetite loss, nausea, yellowing of skin or eyes, dark urine or pale stools, and right-side abdominal pain).

- Advise patient to drink enough fluids to ensure adequate urine output.
- Teach patient to monitor urine output and report significant changes.
- Caution patient to avoid injuring skin and gums by using a soft toothbrush and electric razor.
- Advise patient to minimize GI upset by eating small, frequent servings of food and drinking plenty of fluids.
- Caution patient to avoid driving and other hazardous activities until drug's effects on concentration and alertness are known.
- Advise patient to avoid sexual intercourse when visible herpes lesions are present.
- Inform patient about need for regular blood testing during therapy.
- As appropriate, review all other significant and life-threatening adverse reactions and interactions, especially those related to the drugs and tests mentioned above.

[redacted]

adenosine

Adenocard, Adenocor❋, Adenoscan

Pharmacologic class: Endogenous nucleoside
Therapeutic class: Antiarrhythmic, diagnostic agent
Pregnancy risk category C

Action

Converts paroxysmal supraventricular tachycardia (PSVT) to normal sinus rhythm by slowing conduction through atrioventricular (AV) node and interrupting reentry pathway. Also used as diagnostic agent in thallium scanning.

Pharmacokinetics

Drug is metabolized rapidly either by phosphorylation to adenosine monophosphate by adenosine kinase or by deamination to inosine by adenosine deaminase in cytosol. Inosine may leave cell intact or may degrade to hypoxanthine, xanthine, and ultimately uric acid. Drug clears rapidly from circulation by cellular uptake, primarily by erythrocytes and vascular endothelial cells. Extracellular adenosine is cleared mainly by cellular uptake, with half-life of less than 10 seconds in whole blood; excessive amounts may be deaminated by ectoform of adenosine deaminase.

Onset	Peak	Duration
Immediate	Unknown	Unknown

How supplied

Solution for injection (in normal saline): 3 mg/mL

Indications and dosages

Adenocard—

➢ PSVT, including that associated with Wolff-Parkinson-White syndrome (after attempting vagal maneuvers when appropriate)

Adults and children weighing more than 50 kg (110 lb): Initially, 6 mg by rapid peripheral I.V. bolus over 1 to 2 seconds. If desired effect does not occur within 1 to 2 minutes, give 12 mg by rapid I.V. bolus; may repeat 12-mg I.V. bolus dose a second time if required. Maximum single dosage is 12 mg.

Children weighing less than 50 kg: 0.05 to 0.1 mg/kg by rapid I.V. bolus. If this dosage proves ineffective, in 1 to 2 minutes increase dose by 0.05 mg/kg to 0.1 mg/kg q 2 minutes, to a maximum dosage of 0.3 mg/kg or 12 mg.

Adenoscan—

➢ Diagnosis of coronary artery disease in conjunction with thallium-201 myocardial perfusion scintigraphy in patients unable to exercise adequately during testing

Adults: 140 mcg/kg/minute by peripheral I.V. infusion over 6 minutes, for a total dosage of 0.84 mg/kg. Required thallium-201 dose is injected at midpoint (after first 3 minutes) of Adenoscan infusion.

Off-label uses

- Acute vasodilator testing in pulmonary artery hypertension
- Coronary artery bypass grafting procedure
- Diagnosis of supraventricular arrhythmias
- Myocardial imaging (using ^{99m}technetium)
- Percutaneous transluminal angioplasty
- Pulmonary hypertension
- Stress echocardiography

Administration

Preparation

- Ask patient about recent use of aloe, buckthorn, cascara sagrada, guarana, rhubarb root, or senna. If recently used, notify prescriber.

Check label carefully to confirm that preparation is for I.V. use (bolus or infusion).

Make sure emergency resuscitation drugs and equipment are available before starting drug.

Dilution and compatibility

- Do not dilute Adenocard.

A

• Dilute single dose of Adenoscan in sufficient normal saline solution to distribute over 6 minutes.
• Discard unused portion of drug.

Infusion considerations

Adenocard—

Be aware that drug is intended for peripheral I.V. bolus only.
• Do not administer through central line (may cause prolonged asystole).
• Give by rapid I.V. bolus undiluted directly into vein, or give through I.V. line in port closest to insertion site over 1 to 2 seconds.
• Do not give more than 12 mg as a single dose.
• Flush I.V. line immediately and rapidly with normal saline solution to drive drug into bloodstream.

Adenoscan—

Be aware that drug is intended for continuous I.V. infusion only.
• Give by continuous I.V. infusion only over 6 minutes.
• Use the following table to determine appropriate infusion rate:

Patient weight		Infusion rate
kg	lb	(mL/min)
45	99	2.1
50	110	2.3
55	121	2.6
60	132	2.8
65	143	3.0
70	154	3.3
75	165	3.5
80	176	3.8
85	187	4.0
90	198	4.2

Monitoring

Monitor heart rhythm for new arrhythmias after giving dose.

Watch for bronchoconstriction in patients with asthma, emphysema, or bronchitis. Discontinue drug if severe respiratory distress occurs.
• Check vital signs; assess for chest pain or pressure, dyspnea, and sweating.

Storage

• Store at room temperature (refrigeration causes crystallization).

Contraindications and precautions

Contraindicated in hypersensitivity to drug, second- or third-degree AV block or sinus node disease (except in patients with functioning artificial pacemakers), and bronchoconstrictive lung disease.

Use cautiously in asthma, angina, pregnant patients, ***elderly patients***, and ***children.***

Adverse reactions

CNS: light-headedness, dizziness, apprehension, headache, tingling in arms, numbness
CV: chest pain, palpitations, hypotension, ST-segment depression, **first- or second-degree AV block, atrial tachyarrhythmias, prolonged asystole, other arrhythmias**
EENT: blurred vision, tightness in throat
GI: nausea
Musculoskeletal: discomfort in neck, jaw, and arms
Respiratory: chest pressure, dyspnea and urge to breathe deeply, hyperventilation, **bronchospasm**
Skin: burning sensation, facial flushing, sweating
Other: pressure in groin, metallic taste

Interactions

Drug-drug. *Carbamazepine:* worsening of progressive heart block
Digoxin, verapamil: increased risk of ventricular fibrillation
Dipyridamole: increased adenosine effect
Theophylline: decreased adenosine effect

Drug-food. *Caffeine-containing substances:* decreased adenosine effect

Toxicity and overdose

- Short half-life generally precludes overdose problems, and adverse reactions usually are self-limiting. If overdose occurs, expect bradycardia.
- If adverse reactions persist, give competitive antagonist (such as theophylline or caffeine), as prescribed, and resuscitate as necessary.

Patient teaching

- Advise patient to report problems at infusion site.
- When giving Adenoscan to diagnose coronary artery disease in conjunction with thallium-201 myocardial perfusion scintigraphy, instruct patient not to consume caffeine-containing foods or beverages (including decaffeinated coffee and chocolate) for 24 hours before test and not to smoke on test day.
- Inform patient that 1 to 2 minutes of flushing, chest pain, chest pressure, and breathing difficulty may occur during administration. Assure patient these effects will subside quickly.

Instruct patient to immediately report difficulty breathing.

- As appropriate, review all other significant and life-threatening adverse reactions and interactions, especially those related to the drugs and food mentioned above.

[redacted]

albumin (human normal serum)

Pharmacologic class: Blood product, colloid
Therapeutic class: Volume expander
Pregnancy risk category C

Action

Expands blood volume, thereby reducing hemoconcentration and blood viscosity, regulating circulatory blood volume, providing colloidal oncotic pressure, and regulating fluid balance. Also acts as a carrier for intermediate metabolites in transport.

Pharmacokinetics

Drug is distributed throughout extracellular water; extravascular fluid compartment contains more than 60% of body's albumin pool. Total body albumin in 154-lb (70-kg) male is approximately 320 g. Albumin accounts for 70% to 80% of colloid osmotic pressure of plasma; binds naturally to therapeutic and toxic materials in circulation. Drug has circulating life span of 15 to 20 days, with turnover of approximately 15 g/day.

Onset	Peak	Duration
15 min	Variable*	Variable*

*Varies with initial blood volume

How supplied

Albumin (50 mg/mL) 5% solution for injection: 50-mL, 250-mL, 500-mL, and 1,000-mL vials
Albumin (250 mg/mL) 25% solution for injection: 20-mL, 50-mL, and 100-mL vials

Indications and dosages

➤ Hypovolemia with shock

Adults: Initially, 500 mL of 5% solution by rapid I.V. infusion, repeated in 30 minutes if desired effect does not occur. Or 100 to 200 mL of 25% solution; may repeat in 15 to 30 minutes.
Children: 10 to 20 mL/kg of 5% solution by I.V. infusion, repeated in 30 minutes if desired effect does not occur, to a maximum of 6 g/kg/day. Or 2.5 to 5 mL of 25% solution; may repeat in 15 to 30 minutes.

➢ Severe burns to maintain plasma volume and prevent intravascular hemoconcentration

Adults: For initial therapy, give large crystalloid volumes and lesser amounts of albumin I.V. to maintain plasma volume. After 24 hours, may increase albumin I.V. to maintain plasma albumin level of about 2.5 to 3 g/dL.

➢ Acute hypoproteinemia

Adults: 50 to 70 g/day (200 to 280 mL) of 25% solution by I.V. infusion (if edema is present or considerable albumin has been lost), not to exceed 2 mL/minute

Children: 25 g/day (100 mL) of 25% solution by I.V. infusion (if edema is present or considerable albumin has been lost), not to exceed 2 mL/minute

➢ Erythrocyte resuspension

Adults: Usual dosage is 25 g of 25% solution I.V. per liter of erythrocytes.

➢ Hyperbilirubinemia/erythroblastosis fetalis

Infants: 1 g/kg (4 mL/kg of 25% solution) I.V. 1 to 2 hours before exchange transfusion

➢ Acute nephrosis

Adults: Initially, 100 mL of 25% solution I.V., repeated daily for 7 days if needed (given concurrently with loop diuretic)

Administration

Preparation

• Make sure patient is well hydrated before administering.

• Withhold angiotensin-converting enzyme (ACE) inhibitors 24-hours before giving albumin, if possible.

Dilution and compatibility

• Be aware that 5% solution requires no further dilution.

• Know that 25% solution may be given undiluted or diluted with D_5W or normal saline solution.

Do not use sterile water for injection, because of risk of fatal hemolysis and acute renal failure.

Do not infuse solutions containing protein hydrolysates or alcohol through same administration set as albumin, as this may cause proteins to precipitate.

• For erythrocyte resuspension, add albumin 25% to isotonic suspension of washed red blood cells immediately before transfusion.

• Do not use if solution is turbid.

• Use within 4 hours after opening. Discard unused portion.

Infusion considerations

• Give by I.V. infusion according to prescribed infusion rate, which varies with patient's age, clinical condition, and diagnosis.

Do not administer too rapidly. Generally, after initial volume replacement with 5% solution, do not exceed administration rate of 5 to10 mL/minute in patients with hypoproteinemia, because vascular overload leading to pulmonary edema may occur. For 25% solution, do not exceed 2 to 3 mL/minute. However, when used to treat patients in shock with greatly reduced blood volume, give as rapidly as needed to improve clinical condition and restore normal blood volume.

In patients with slightly low or normal blood volume, do not infuse faster than 1 mL/minute.

Know that in children, usual administration rate is 25% of adult rate.

Monitoring

• Check vital signs and fluid intake and output frequently; maintain adequate hydration.

Monitor for hemorrhage and shock after injury or surgery; rapid postinfusion blood pressure rise may cause bleeding from severed vessels.

Monitor for signs and symptoms of circulatory overload and pulmonary

edema, especially in patients with heart failure.
- Monitor hemoglobin, hematocrit, protein, and electrolyte levels.

Storage
- Store at controlled room temperature. Do not freeze.

Contraindications and precautions
Contraindicated in hypersensitivity to drug, heart failure, hypervolemia, pulmonary edema, and severe anemia.

Use cautiously in dehydration, renal insufficiency, hepatic disease, pulmonary disease, hypertension, low cardiac reserve, and pregnant patients.

Adverse reactions
CNS: headache, light-headedness, dizziness
CV: tachycardia, hypotension, hypertension, **fluid overload**
EENT: blurred vision, throat tightness
GI: nausea, vomiting, increased salivation
Musculoskeletal: back pain
Respiratory: respiratory changes, hyperventilation, dyspnea, chest pressure, **pulmonary edema**
Skin: rash, urticaria, flushing, pruritus
Other: metallic taste, groin pressure, infection, allergic reactions including chills, fever, and **anaphylaxis**

Interactions
Drug-drug. *ACE inhibitors:* increased risk of atypical reactions
Drug-diagnostic tests. *Alkaline phosphatase:* false increase

Toxicity and overdose
- In overdose, expect extension of adverse reactions, especially respiratory difficulty.

Discontinue drug and provide symptomatic interventions, as necessary.

Patient teaching
Instruct patient to report signs and symptoms of pulmonary edema, such as difficulty breathing.
- Inform patient about need for regular blood testing during therapy.
- As appropriate, review all other significant and life-threatening adverse reactions and interactions, especially those related to the drugs and tests mentioned above.

aldesleukin (interleukin-2, IL-2)
Proleukin

Pharmacologic class: Interleukin-2 (IL-2), human recombinant (lymphokine)
Therapeutic class: Antineoplastic (miscellaneous)
Pregnancy risk category C

FDA BOXED WARNING

- Give only to patients with normal cardiac and pulmonary function, as shown by thallium stress testing and pulmonary function tests (PFTs). Use extreme caution when giving to patients with normal thallium stress test and normal PFTs who have a history of cardiac or pulmonary disease.
- Give under supervision of physician experienced in cancer chemotherapy, in setting where intensive care facilities and cardiopulmonary or intensive care specialists are available.
- Drug is linked to capillary leak syndrome, which causes hypotension and reduced organ perfusion (possibly severe and resulting in death).
- Before starting drug, preexisting bacterial infections must be treated, because drug may impair neutrophil function and increase disseminated infection risk. Patients with indwelling central

lines are at special risk for infection with gram-positive microorganisms. Prophylactic antibiotics can help prevent staphylococcal infections.

- Withhold drug in patients who develop moderate to severe lethargy or somnolence; continued administration may cause coma.

Action

Activates cellular immunity and inhibits tumor growth by increasing lymphocytes and cytokines, which lyse tumor cells

Pharmacokinetics

Drug distributes rapidly into extravascular space and reaches high plasma concentrations after short I.V. infusion. It is eliminated by renal metabolism, with little or no bioactive protein excreted in urine.

Onset	Peak	Duration
Rapid	Unknown	Unknown

How supplied

Powder for injection for reconstitution (white to off-white, preservative-free, lyophilized): 22 million international units/single-use vial

Indications and dosages

➢ Metastatic renal-cell carcinoma, metastatic melanoma

Adults older than age 18: 600,000 international units/kg given I.V. over 15 minutes q 8 hours for a maximum of 14 doses, followed by 9 days of rest. Repeat for another 14 doses, for a maximum of 28 doses per course.

Dosage adjustment

- If adverse reactions necessitate dosage adjustment, withhold dose entirely rather than reduce dosage. Give subsequent doses according to these guidelines:

Cardiovascular adverse reactions

Withhold dose for:

atrial fibrillation, supraventricular tachycardia (SVT), or bradycardia that requires treatment, recurs, or persists.

systolic blood pressure (BP) below 90 mm Hg with increasing pressor requirements.

any ECG change consistent with myocardial infarction (MI), ischemia, or myocarditis with or without chest pain; suspected cardiac ischemia.

May give subsequent doses if:

patient is asymptomatic and recovers fully to normal sinus rhythm.

systolic BP is 90 mm Hg or higher, and pressor requirements are stable or improving.

patient is asymptomatic, MI and myocarditis have been ruled out, clinical suspicion of angina is low, and no evidence of ventricular hypokinesia exists.

Central nervous system adverse reactions

Withhold dose for:

mental status changes, including moderate confusion or agitation.

May give subsequent doses if:

mental status changes resolve completely.

Gastrointestinal adverse reactions

Withhold dose for:

signs and symptoms of hepatic failure, including encephalopathy, increasing ascites, hypoglycemia, and liver pain.

stool guaiac repeatedly above 4+.

May give subsequent doses if:

all signs of hepatic failure resolve. Discontinue all further treatment for that course. Begin new course (if warranted) no sooner than 7 weeks after adverse event has ended and patient is discharged.

stool guaiac test is negative.

Genitourinary adverse reactions

Withhold dose for:

serum creatinine above 4.5 mg/dL, or 4 mg/dL or higher in patients with severe volume overload, acidosis, or hyperkalemia.

persistent oliguria, urine output below 10 mL/hour for 16 to 24 hours with rising serum creatinine.

May give subsequent doses if:
serum creatinine is below 4 mg/dL fluid and electrolyte status is stable.
urine output exceeds 10 mL/hour with decrease of serum creatinine above 1.5 mg/dL or serum creatinine normalization.

Respiratory adverse reactions

Withhold dose for:
oxygen (O_2) saturation below 90%.

May give subsequent doses if:
O_2 saturation exceeds 90%.

Skin adverse reactions

Withhold dose for:
bullous dermatitis, marked worsening of preexisting skin condition.

May give subsequent doses if:
bullous dermatitis resolves.

Body as a whole adverse reactions

Withhold dose for:
sepsis syndrome with clinical instability.

May give subsequent doses if:
sepsis syndrome resolves, patient is clinically stable, and infection is being treated.

Off-label uses

- Acute myeloid leukemia
- AIDS and HIV infection
- Kaposi's sarcoma
- Multiple myeloma
- Non-Hodgkin's lymphoma

Administration

Preparation

Follow hazardous drug guidelines on page S19 for handling, preparation, and administration.

- Before starting drug, obtain weight, chest X-ray, ECG, cardiac enzymes, CBC with differential, platelet count, triiodothyronine and thyroxine levels, prothrombin time, partial thromboplastin time, and urinalysis.
- Know that serum creatinine level should be 1.5 mg/dL or lower before therapy starts.

Do not give drug if patient is drowsy or severely lethargic; contact prescriber immediately.

- Know that continuous cardiac monitoring is usually indicated.
- Be aware that at least two I.V. lines are usually required (one for aldesleukin and a keep-open line for other fluids and drugs).

Dilution and compatibility

Avoid reconstituting or diluting with bacteriostatic water for injection or normal saline solution because of increased aggregation.

- Reconstitute according to label directions with 1.2 mL sterile water for injection by injecting diluent against side of vial to prevent excessive foaming.
- Gently swirl contents to avoid excess foaming. Do not shake.
- When reconstituted as directed, each milliliter contains 18 million international units (1.1 mg) of drug.
- For intermittent or continuous infusion, further dilute reconstituted dose with 50 mL of D_5W; resulting solution should be a clear and colorless to slightly yellow liquid.
- Do not mix with other drugs in same container.
- Bring solution to room temperature before administering.
- Give within 48 hours of reconstitution.
- Discard unused portion.

Infusion considerations

- Before and after each dose, flush I.V. line with D_5W.
- Administer I.V. infusion over 15 minutes.

Do not use inline filter, as filter may absorb drug.

Monitoring

Assess frequently for hypovolemia with central venous monitoring.

A

• Monitor heart rate and rhythm, vital signs, and fluid intake and output.
• Assess for signs and symptoms of hypersensitivity reaction and infection.
Monitor for adverse CNS effects; report these immediately.
• Continue to evaluate chest X-rays, CBC, electrolyte levels, PFTs, arterial blood gases, and liver and kidney function test results.
• Evaluate patient response 4 weeks after treatment course ends and immediately before scheduled start of next course. Give additional courses only if tumor has shrunk since last course and retreatment is not contraindicated.
• Separate each treatment course by at least 7 weeks from discharge date.

Storage

• Until use, refrigerate vials in carton at 2° to 8°C (36° to 46°F). Protect from light.
• Know that reconstituted or diluted drug is stable for up to 48 hours at refrigerated and room temperatures of 2° to 25° C (36° to 77° F). However, refrigerate reconstituted and diluted solutions, as product contains no preservative.

Contraindications and precautions

Contraindicated in hypersensitivity to drug or its components, arrhythmias, cardiac tamponade, seizures, severe GI bleeding, coma or toxic psychosis lasting more than 48 hours, organ allograft, and abnormal thallium stress test or PFT results. Retreatment is contraindicated permanently in patients who previously experienced drug-related toxicities including sustained ventricular tachycardia of five or more beats, arrhythmias not controlled or unresponsive to treatment, chest pain with ECG changes consistent with angina or myocardial infarction (MI), cardiac tamponade, renal failure requiring dialysis for more than 72 hours, coma or toxic psychosis lasting more than 48 hours, repetitive or hard-to-control seizures, bowel ischemia or perforation, or GI bleeding requiring surgery.

Use cautiously in anemia, bacterial infections, cardiac disease, CNS metastases, hepatic disease, pulmonary disease, renal disease, thrombocytopenia, pregnant or breastfeeding patients, and ***children.***

Adverse reactions

CNS: dizziness, mental status changes, syncope, sensory or motor dysfunction, headache, fatigue, rigors, weakness, malaise, asthenia, poor memory, depression, sleep disturbances, hallucinations, confusion, anxiety, coma, stupor, psychosis, lethargy, somnolence
CV: bradycardia, sinus tachycardia, premature atrial complexes, premature ventricular contractions, vasodilation, supraventricular tachycardia, angina, **bacterial endocarditis, MI, myocardial ischemia, cardiac arrest, capillary leak syndrome, severe hypotension**
EENT: reversible visual changes, conjunctivitis, rhinitis
GI: nausea, vomiting, diarrhea, constipation, dyspepsia, abdominal pain, stomatitis, enlarged abdomen, anorexia, **intestinal perforation, ileus, GI bleeding**
GU: hematuria, proteinuria, dysuria, **renal failure, oliguria, anuria**
Hematologic: anemia, purpura, eosinophilia, **thrombocytopenia, coagulation disorders, leukopenia, leukocytosis**
Hepatic: jaundice, ascites
Metabolic: hyperglycemia, **hypoglycemia, acidosis, alkalosis**
Musculoskeletal: joint and back pain, myalgia
Respiratory: cough, chest pain, tachypnea, wheezing, dyspnea, pulmonary congestion, crackles, rhonchi, **pulmonary**

edema, respiratory failure, apnea, pleural effusion
Skin: erythema, pruritus, rash, dry skin, petechiae, urticaria, exfoliative dermatitis
Other: weight gain or loss, fever, chills, edema, infection, sepsis pain or reaction at injection site, hypersensitivity reaction

Interactions

Drug-drug. *Aminoglycosides, asparaginase, doxorubicin, indomethacin, methotrexate:* increased aldesleukin toxicity
Antihypertensives: increased hypotensive effect
Glucocorticoids: reduced antitumor effects
Interferon alfa: increased risk of hypersensitivity reaction, myocardial injury, exacerbation of autoimmune and inflammatory disorders
Psychotropic drugs: altered CNS function
Drug-diagnostic tests. *Bilirubin, glucose, blood urea nitrogen, creatinine, potassium, transaminases:* increased
Calcium, magnesium, phosphorus, potassium, protein sodium, uric acid: decreased

Toxicity and overdose

- Exceeding recommended dosage may hasten onset of expected dose-limiting toxicities.
- Monitor for signs and symptoms that persist after drug cessation; provide supportive interventions. Life-threatening toxicities may be treated with I.V. dexamethasone (although this drug may negate therapeutic effects of aldesleukin).

Patient education

Inform patient that drug lowers resistance to infections. Advise patient to immediately report fever, cough, breathing problems, and other signs or symptoms.

Instruct patient to immediately report chest pain, irregular or fast heart beats, easy bruising or bleeding, and abdominal pain.

- Refer patient to dietitian if adverse GI effects significantly limit food intake.
- Inform patient of importance of regular blood testing and chest X-rays during therapy.
- As appropriate, review all other significant and life-threatening adverse reactions and interactions, especially those related to the drugs and tests mentioned above.

alfentanil hydrochloride

Alfenta

Pharmacologic class: Opioid agonist
Therapeutic class: Opioid analgesic
Controlled substance schedule II
Pregnancy risk category C

Action

Binds to and depresses opiate receptors in CNS, altering perception of and response to pain

Pharmacokinetics

Liver is a major biotransformation site. Repeated or continuous administration increases plasma concentrations and causes drug to accumulate, particularly in patients with reduced plasma clearance. Drug is 92% plasma-protein bound. Only 1% of dose is excreted unchanged; urinary excretion is a major elimination route for metabolites. Pharmacokinetics can be described as a three-compartment model with sequential distribution half-lives of 1 and 14 minutes; and a terminal elimination half-life of 90 to 111 minutes.

Onset	Peak	Duration
Immediate	Variable	30-60 min

How supplied

Solution for injection (clear, colorless): 500 mcg in 2 mL-, 5 mL-, 10 mL-, and 20-mL ampules

Indications and dosages

➢ Analgesic adjunct in maintenance of balanced anesthesia given in combination with a barbiturate, nitrous oxide, oxygen, or other analgesic; as primary anesthetic for anesthesia induction in patients undergoing general surgery requiring endotracheal intubation and mechanical ventilation; or as analgesic component for monitored anesthesia care (MAC)

Adults: Individualize dosage and titrate to desired effect based on patient's weight, physical status, underlying condition, use of other drugs, and type and duration of surgery and anesthesia. Give by continuous I.V. infusion in incremental doses.

Dosage adjustment

- In obese patients (more than 20% above ideal weight), determine dosage on basis of lean weight.
- Reduce dosage in elderly or debilitated patients.

Administration

Preparation

🔊 In patients receiving anesthesia induction dosages, ensure that qualified personnel, opioid antagonist, resuscitative and intubation equipment, and adequate facilities are available to manage intraoperative and postoperative respiratory depression.

- Consider fluid replacement before induction anesthesia.
- Monitor vital signs before administering.

🔊 When giving drug within 14 days of monoamine oxidase (MAO) inhibitors, monitor patient appropriately and keep vasodilators and beta-adrenergic blockers readily available to treat hypertension.

- Be aware that neuromuscular blocker given before anesthesia induction may reduce skeletal muscle rigidity.

Dilution and compatibility

- Know that drug is compatible with normal saline solution, 5% dextrose in normal saline solution, D_5W, and lactated Ringer's solution.
- Add 230 mL diluent to 20 mL alfentanil to yield 40 mcg/mL alfentanil solution for infusion. Recommended concentration is 25 to 80 mcg/mL.
- Do not use if solution is discolored.

Infusion considerations

- Give induction dose slowly, over at least 3 minutes and titrate rate to patient response.
- When administering for MAC, continue infusion to end of procedure.
- Be aware that tuberculin syringe or equivalent is recommended for accurate administration of undiluted small volumes.

Monitoring

- Continue to monitor vital signs and ECG frequently, especially for hypotension and delayed respiratory depression.

🔊 During MAC, stay alert for respiratory effects, such as decreased oxygen saturation, apnea, slowed respiratory rate, and upper airway obstruction.

- Be aware that skeletal muscle rigidity, which may immediately follow anesthetic induction doses, relates to dosage and administration rate. It may be decreased by giving neuromuscular blockers just before alfentanil administration with dosages according to patient response.

🔊 Be prepared to give atropine if bradycardia occurs.
• Monitor hepatic and renal function tests results.

Storage
• Store at controlled room temperature of 15° to 25°C (59° to77°F); protect from light.

Contraindications and precautions
Contraindicated in hypersensitivity to drug and in patients intolerant of other opioid agonists.

Use cautiously in pulmonary disease, including decreased respiratory reserve or potentially compromised respiration; head injury; hepatic or renal dysfunction; obesity; concurrent MAO inhibitor use; labor and delivery (use not recommended); ***elderly patients;*** pregnant or breastfeeding patients; and ***children younger than age 12*** (safety and efficacy not established).

Adverse reactions
CNS: dizziness, headache, confusion, somnolence, agitation, drowsiness
CV: hypertension, hypotension, bradycardia, tachycardia, irregular pulse rate, chest tightness, arrhythmias, **asystole**
EENT: blurred vision, laryngospasm
GI: nausea, vomiting
Musculoskeletal: skeletal muscle rigidity, myoclonic movements
Respiratory: bronchospasm, hypercarbia, **respiratory depression, hypoxia, apnea**
Skin: pruritus, urticaria
Other: shivering, drug dependence, pain at injection site, hypersensitivity reaction including **anaphylaxis** (rare)

Interactions
Drug-drug. *Antihistamines (including many cough and cold agents):* increased drowsiness
Cimetidine: reduced alfentanil clearance
CNS depressants (such as barbiturates, inhalation general anesthetics, opioids, and tranquilizers): increased effects and duration of these drugs
Diazepam: increased risk of vasodilation, hypotension, and delayed recovery
Erythromycin: significant inhibition of alfentanil clearance and increased risk of respiratory depression
MAO inhibitors (such as phenelzine, selegiline, tranylcypromine): unpredictable reactions (rare)
Drug-behaviors. *Alcohol use:* increased CNS effects

Toxicity and overdose
• In overdose, expect extension of pharmacologic actions, such as respiratory depression and muscular rigidity.
• Establish patent airway. As ordered, give opioid antagonist (such as naloxone) to manage respiratory depression, initiate oxygen or assisted or controlled ventilation for hypoventilation or apnea, give I.V. fluids and vasoactive agents to manage hemodynamic instability, and administer neuromuscular blocker for muscular rigidity. Do not give opioid antagonist in absence of clinically significant respiratory or cardiovascular depression.

Patient teaching
• Inform patient that drug causes drowsiness.
• Instruct patient not to drive or perform other hazardous tasks until drug effects dissipate.
• As appropriate, review all other significant and life-threatening adverse reactions and interactions, especially those related to the drugs and behaviors mentioned above.

allopurinol sodium
Aloprim, Rimapurinol ❋

Pharmacologic class: Xanthine oxidase inhibitor
Therapeutic class: Antigout drug
Pregnancy risk category C

Action
Inhibits conversion of xanthine to uric acid and increases reutilization of hypoxanthine and xanthine for nucleic acid synthesis, thereby decreasing uric acid levels in serum and urine

Pharmacokinetics
After I.V dose, drug is eliminated rapidly from systemic circulation, primarily by oxidative metabolism to oxypurinol, with no detectable allopurinol plasma level 5 hours later. Approximately 12% of I.V. dose is excreted unchanged, 76% is excreted as oxypurinol, and remainder is excreted as riboside conjugates in urine.

Onset	Peak	Duration
Unknown	0.5 hr	Unknown

How supplied
Powder for reconstitution for injection: 500 mg/30-mL vial

Indications and dosages
➣ Management of patients with leukemia, lymphoma, or solid-tumor cancers who are receiving cancer therapy that elevates serum and urinary uric acid levels and who cannot tolerate oral therapy
Adults: 200 to 400 mg/m^2/day I.V. as a single infusion, using serum uric acid levels as index for dosing frequency. Total dosage should not exceed 600 mg/day.
Children: 200 mg/m^2/day I.V. starting 24 to 48 hours before chemotherapy begins, as a single infusion or in equally divided infusions at 6-, 8-, or 12-hour intervals

Dosage adjustment
• Reduce dosage in renal impairment to avoid drug and metabolite accumulation; use lowest effective dosage. With creatinine clearance between 3 and 10 mL/minute, recommended dosage is 100 mg/day; with clearance between 10 and 20 mL/minute, 200 mg/day. With extreme renal impairment (creatinine clearance less than 3 mL/minute), dosing intervals may need to extend beyond 24 hours.

Off-label uses
• Hematemesis caused by gastritis secondary to nonsteroidal anti-inflammatory drugs
• Pain from acute pancreatitis
• Seizures refractory to standard therapy

Administration
Preparation
• Obtain serum uric acid and electrolyte levels before starting drug.
• Begin drug 24 to 48 hours before initiation of chemotherapy known to cause tumor-cell lysis.

Dilution and compatibility
• Do not mix with other drugs.
• Do not use with solutions containing sodium bicarbonate.
• Dissolve contents of each 30-mL vial in 25 mL sterile water for injection, to yield 20 mg/mL. Swirl until completely dissolved. Reconstitution yields clear, almost colorless solution with no more than slight opalescence.
• Dilute further with normal saline solution or D_5W.

• Know that maximum concentration for administration is 6 mg/mL.
• Start administration within 10 hours of reconstitution.

Infusion considerations

• Do not give through same I.V. port with other drugs.
• Flush I.V. line before and after administration.
• Give by I.V. infusion over 30 minutes to 1 hour or more, based on diluent volume and patient comfort.
• Divide doses larger than 300 mg.

Monitoring

Observe for signs and symptoms of hypersensitivity reaction; discontinue drug at first sign of rash.
• Assess fluid intake and output; intake should be sufficient to yield daily output of at least 2 L of slightly alkaline urine.
• Continue to monitor uric acid levels to help evaluate drug efficacy.
• In patients with decreased renal function and concurrent illnesses that can affect renal function (such as hypertension or diabetes mellitus), perform renal function tests—particularly blood urea nitrogen (BUN) and serum creatinine or creatinine clearance.
• In patients with preexisting hepatic disease, monitor periodic liver function tests, especially during early stage of therapy.
• Watch for signs and symptoms of tumor lysis syndrome (such as hyperuricemia, hyperkalemia, hyperphosphatemia, and hypocalcemia), and be prepared to correct electrolyte deficiencies.
• Monitor prothrombin time, CBC with differential, and serum electrolyte levels.

Storage

• Do not refrigerate reconstituted or diluted solution.
• Store at controlled room temperature of 20° to 25°C (68° to 77°F).

Contraindications and precautions

Contraindicated in hypersensitivity to drug and idiopathic hemochromatosis.

Use cautiously in acute gout attack, renal insufficiency, dehydration, and pregnant or breastfeeding patients.

Adverse reactions

CNS: agitation, dystonia, headache, mental status changes, myoclonus, tremor, twitching, **paralysis, seizure, status epilepticus, cerebral infarction, coma, cerebrovascular accident**
CV: bradycardia, cardiovascular disorder, decreased venous pressure, ECG abnormality, flushing, hypertension, hypotension, thrombophlebitis, **septic shock, heart failure, hemorrhage, ventricular fibrillation, cardiorespiratory arrest**
EENT: pharyngitis
GI: nausea, vomiting, diarrhea, constipation, enlarged abdomen, GI bleeding, splenomegaly, intestinal obstruction, flatulence, proctitis
GU: renal failure or insufficiency, hematuria, abnormal renal function, oliguria, urinary tract infection
Hematologic: anemia, bone marrow suppression, eosinophilia, **leukopenia, neutropenia, pancytopenia, thrombocytopenia, disseminated intravascular coagulation, bone marrow aplasia**
Hepatic: hepatomegaly, hyperbilirubinemia, jaundice, **hepatic failure**
Metabolic: electrolyte abnormalities, glycosuria, hypercalcemia, hyperglycemia, hyperkalemia, hypernatremia, hyperphosphatemia, hyperuricemia, hypervolemia, hypocalcemia, hypokalemia, hypomagnesemia, hyponatremia, **lactic acidosis, metabolic acidosis, water intoxication**
Musculoskeletal: arthralgia, hypotonia
Respiratory: increased respiration rate, **acute respiratory distress syndrome,**

respiratory failure or insufficiency, apnea, pulmonary embolus
Skin: rash, pruritus, urticaria, ecchymosis, cellulitis, alopecia
Other: edema, fever, chills, diaphoresis, infection, mucositis, pain, local injection site reaction, hypersensitivity, **sepsis, tumor lysis syndrome**

Interactions

Drug-drug. *Amoxicillin, ampicillin, bacampicillin:* increased risk of rash
Anticoagulants (except warfarin): increased anticoagulant effect
Antineoplastics: increased risk of myelosuppression
Azathioprine, mercaptopurine: inhibition of allopurinol metabolism
Chlorpropamide: increased hypoglycemic effects
Diazoxide, diuretics, mecamylamine, pyrazinamide: increased uric acid levels
Ethacrynic acid, thiazide diuretics: increased risk of allopurinol toxicity
Uricosurics: increased uric acid excretion
Urine-acidifying drugs (ammonium chloride, ascorbic acid, potassium or sodium phosphate): increased risk of renal calculi
Xanthines: increased theophylline levels
Drug-diagnostic tests. *Alanine aminotransferase, alanine phosphatase, aspartate aminotransferase, bilirubin, BUN, creatinine, eosinophils:* increased
Granulocytes, hemoglobin, platelets, white blood cells: decreased
Drug-behaviors. *Alcohol use:* increased uric acid level

Toxicity and overdose

• Massive overdose or acute poisoning has not been reported. In overdose, expect signs and symptoms to include extension of pharmacologic effects and adverse reactions.
• No antidote exists; however, drug is dialyzable. Provide supportive and symptomatic interventions.

Patient teaching

Instruct patient to promptly report painful urination, bloody urine, rash, eye irritation, or swelling of lips and mouth.
• Caution patient to avoid driving and other hazardous tasks until drug effects are known.
• Advise patient to avoid alcohol during therapy.
• As appropriate, review all other significant and life-threatening adverse reactions and interactions, especially those related to the drugs, tests, and behaviors mentioned above.

alprostadil

Prostin VR Pediatric

Pharmacologic class: Prostaglandin E_1
Therapeutic class: Ductus arteriosus patency adjunct
Pregnancy risk category NR

FDA BOXED WARNING

• Give drug only where ventilatory assistance is available immediately. About 10% to 12% of neonates with congenital heart defects who receive drug experience apnea. Apnea is most common in neonates who weighed less than 2 kg (4.4 lb) at birth, and usually appears during first hour of drug infusion. Monitor respiratory status throughout treatment.

Action

Relaxes smooth muscle of ductus arteriosus

Pharmacokinetics

Drug is rapidly converted to compounds that are metabolized further before excretion. Approximately 80% of circulating drug is metabolized rapidly in one pass through lungs, primarily by beta- and omega-oxidation. Drug is 81% bound to albumin in plasma. Metabolites are excreted primarily by the kidneys, with almost 90% of I.V. dose excreted in urine within 24 hours. Remainder of dose is excreted in feces.

Onset	Peak	Duration
Rapid	1-2 hr	Length of infusion

How supplied

Solution for intravascular infusion: 500 mcg/mL in dehydrated alcohol

Indications and dosages

➤ Palliative therapy for infants to temporarily maintain a patent ductus arteriosus

Infants: 0.05 to 0.1 mcg/kg/minute by continuous I.V. infusion. Once therapeutic response occurs, reduce infusion to lowest dosage required to maintain response (as reducing it from 0.1 to 0.05 to 0.025 to 0.01 mcg/kg/minute). If response to 0.05 mcg/kg/minute is inadequate, increase dosage to a maximum of 0.4 mcg/kg/minute. (However, higher infusion rates generally do not produce greater effects.)

Administration

Dilution and compatibility

- To prepare infusion solution, dilute 1 mL (500 mcg) of drug solution with sodium chloride injection or dextrose injection. Undiluted drug solution may interact with plastic sidewalls of volumetric infusion chambers, changing appearance of chamber and creating hazy solution. In this case, replace solution and infusion chamber.
- Prepare fresh solution for administration every 24 hours. Discard solution that is more than 24 hours old.

Infusion considerations

Do not give by direct injection or intermittent infusion.

- Administer into large peripheral vein or central vein, or give through umbilical artery catheter at ductal opening.
- Use infusion pump for continuous infusion.
- Start infusion at 0.05 to 0.1 mcg/kg/minute. When therapeutic response occurs, reduce to lowest dosage that maintains adequate response.

Do not give at a rate faster than 0.4 mcg/kg/minute.

- Be aware that drug must be infused continuously because it is metabolized rapidly.

Monitoring

Evaluate for adverse cardiovascular effects (especially bradycardia) and adverse CNS reactions (especially seizures), which are more common in smaller infants and after 48 hours of infusion.

Monitor arterial pressure with umbilical artery catheter, auscultation, or Doppler transducer.

Assess for signs of sepsis and for bleeding caused by disseminated intravascular coagulation (DIC).

- Monitor blood oxygenation, systemic blood pressure, and blood pH to evaluate drug efficacy.
- Monitor clotting studies and serum electrolyte levels.

Storage

- Refrigerate at 2° to 8°C (36° to 46°F).

Contraindications and precautions

Contraindicated in hypersensitivity to drug and respiratory distress syndrome.

Use cautiously in bleeding tendencies and ***neonates.***

Adverse reactions

CNS: seizures

CV: tachycardia, hypotension, partial atrioventricular block, supraventricular tachycardia, **congestive heart failure, ventricular fibrillation, bradycardia, cardiac arrest**

GI: diarrhea, **gastric outlet obstruction**
Hematologic: DIC, inhibited platelet aggregation
Metabolic: hypokalemia
Musculoskeletal: cortical proliferation of long bones (with long-term infusions)
Respiratory: apnea
Skin: flushing
Other: edema, fever, **sepsis**

Interactions

Drug-drug. *Anticoagulants:* increased bleeding risk

Toxicity and overdose

- In overdose, expect extension of adverse reactions, including tachycardia, hypotension, flushing, bradycardia, and apnea.
- Discontinue infusion and provide supportive and symptomatic interventions, such as mechanical ventilation for apnea, if ordered.

Patient teaching

- Explain reason for drug use to parents or caregivers. Provide updates on drug efficacy.
- Inform parents about adverse effects and subsequent nursing interventions, as appropriate.

alteplase (tissue plasminogen activator, recombinant)

Actilyse❁, Activase, Activase rt-PA♣, Cathflo Activase, Lysatec rt-PA♣

Pharmacologic class: Plasminogen activator
Therapeutic class: Thrombolytic
Pregnancy risk category C

Action

Causes fibrin-enhanced conversion of plasminogen to plasmin, which in turn breaks down local fibrin and fibrinogen, thereby dissolving thrombus

Pharmacokinetics

Initial volume of distribution approximates plasma volume. Drug is cleared from plasma by liver within 5 minutes (50%) to 10 minutes (80%) after infusion ends.

Onset	Peak	Duration
Prompt	Unknown	Unknown

How supplied

Powder for reconstitution for injection (white, lyophilized): 2-mg single-patient vials (Cathflo Activase); 50- and 100-mg vials (Activase)

Indications and dosages

➢ Management of acute myocardial infarction (MI) to improve ventricular function, reduce incidence of congestive heart failure, and decrease mortality associated with acute MI; given as soon as possible after symptom onset (Activase only)

3-hour infusion—
Adults: 100 mg (total) I.V. over 3 hours as follows: 60 mg over first hour (6- to 10-mg I.V. bolus over first 1 to 2 minutes), 20 mg I.V. over second hour, and 20 mg I.V. over third hour.
Adults weighing less than 65 kg (143 lb): 1.25 mg/kg I.V. in divided doses over 3 hours. Total dosage should not exceed 100 mg.
Accelerated infusion—
Adults weighing more than 67 kg (148 lb): 100 mg (total) I.V. as follows: 15-mg I.V. bolus over 1 to 2 minutes, 50 mg I.V. over next 30 minutes, and 35 mg I.V. over next 60 minutes.
Adults weighing 67 kg or less: 15 mg I.V. bolus given over 1 to 2 minutes, followed by 0.75 mg/kg I.V. over next 30 minutes (not to exceed 50 mg), followed by

0.5 mg/kg I.V. over next 60 minutes (not to exceed 35 mg). Total dosage should not exceed 100 mg.

➤ Management of acute ischemic cerebrovascular accident (CVA) in adults to improve neurologic recovery and help prevent disability (Activase only).

Adults: Start therapy within 3 hours after onset of CVA symptoms, after intracranial hemorrhage has been excluded by diagnostic imaging methods sensitive for hemorrhage. Administer 0.9 mg/kg Activase I.V. over 1 hour to a maximum dosage of 90 mg, with 10% of total dosage given as I.V. bolus in first minute.

➤ Management of acute massive pulmonary embolism (PE); lysis of acute PE with or without accompanied unstable hemodynamics (Activase only).

Adults: 100 mg I.V. Activase over 2 hours, followed by heparin near end or immediately after Activase infusion when partial thromboplastin time (PTT) or prothrombin time (PT) returns to twice normal or less.

➤ To restore function to central venous access device (CVAD), as assessed by ability to withdraw blood (Cathflo Activase only).

Adults weighing 30 kg (66 lb) or more: 2 mg in 2 mL instilled into dysfunctional catheter at a concentration of 1 mg/mL. If catheter function is not restored within 120 minutes after first dose, second dose may be instilled.

Adults weighing 10 to 30 kg (22 to 66 lb): Instill 110% of volume of internal lumen of dysfunctional catheter (not to exceed 2 mg in 2 mL) at a concentration of 1 mg/mL. If catheter function is not restored within 120 minutes after first dose, may instill second dose.

Off-label uses

- Blocked venous catheter (2-mg bolus injected into catheter for adults and children age 2 and older)
- Peripheral arterial thromboembolism
- Small-vessel occlusion by microthrombi

Administration

Preparation

- Obtain PT, PTT, activated PTT, CBC, fibrinogen levels, platelets, and (if ordered) blood type and crossmatch.
- Before giving drug for MI management, obtain ECG and creatine kinase (CK) level.
- Before giving drug for CVA, obtain noncontrast computed tomography brain scan.
- Before giving drug for PE, obtain lung scan or pulmonary angiography.

Be aware that intracranial hemorrhage must be ruled out before therapy begins.

Dilution and compatibility

- Know that drug is *not* compatible with bacteriostatic water for injection.
- Do not reconstitute or dilute with solutions other than those recommended.
- Do not mix with other drugs.

Activase 100-mg vials—

- Insert one end of transfer device into upright vial of diluent supplied by manufacturer. Holding vial upside down, push center of vial down onto piercing pin. Invert vial and allow diluent to flow into drug.
- Mix by swirling gently for a few minutes. Do not shake.
- Insert infusion set into drug vial, and infuse.
- After infusion, flush tubing with normal saline solution to ensure delivery of total dose.

Activase 50-mg vials—

- Reconstitute only with unpreserved sterile water for injection supplied by manufacturer.
- Using large-bore needle, shoot diluent stream directly into powder.

A

• Wait a few minutes for foam to settle; then draw up dose and administer right away.
• If necessary, further dilute to 0.5 mg/mL immediately before administration with equal volume of normal saline solution or D_5W. Be aware that dilution with less-than-recommended volume to a concentration greater than 1 mg/mL results in hypertonic solution, and dilution beyond 5 mg/mL may cause precipitation.
• Mix by swirling or slow inversion. Do not shake.
• Administer right away.
• After infusion, flush tubing with at least 30 mL normal saline solution to ensure delivery of total dose.

2-mg single-patient vials (Cathflo for CVAD occlusion)—
• Reconstitute with 2.2 mL unpreserved sterile water for injection to a final concentration of 1 mg/mL. Direct diluent stream into powder. Allow to stand undisturbed until large bubbles dissipate.
• Mix by swirling gently for about 3 minutes. Do not shake.
• Infuse right away.
• After infusion, flush tubing with normal saline solution to ensure delivery of total dose. Avoid excessive pressure when attempting to clear catheter.

Infusion considerations

Activase—
• Start a second and separate I.V. line, as prescribed, for administration of other drugs.
• Do not use filter, because protein absorption may occur, causing drug loss.
• Give only by I.V. bolus or infusion using controlled-infusion device.
• Administer at rate prescribed for selected indication.
If uncontrolled bleeding occurs, stop infusion and notify prescriber immediately.

Cathflo Activase—
• Instruct patient to exhale and hold breath any time catheter is not connected to I.V. tubing or syringe, to prevent air from entering open catheter.
• Know that Cathflo dosages above 2 mg are not recommended.

Monitoring
• Monitor vital signs, ECG, and neurologic status.
• Maintain strict bed rest.
Watch for signs and symptoms of bleeding tendency and hemorrhage.
Monitor patient on Cathflo Activase for GI bleeding, venous thrombosis, and sepsis.
• Evaluate results of clotting studies.

Storage
• Store Activase at controlled room temperature before and after reconstitution (if needed); protect from light.
• Refrigerate Cathflo Activase at 2° to 30°C (36° to 86°F) for 8 hours after reconstitution (if needed).

Contraindications and precautions

Contraindicated in hypersensitivity to drug or its components. *When Activase is used for acute MI or PE*—contraindicated in active internal bleeding, previous CVA, recent intracranial or intraspinal surgery or trauma, intracranial neoplasm, arteriovenous malformation, or aneurysm; bleeding diathesis; and severe uncontrolled hypertension. *When Activase is used for acute ischemic CVA*—contraindicated in history or evidence of intracranial hemorrhage on pretreatment evaluation; suspicion of subarachnoid hemorrhage; recent (within 3 months) intracranial or intraspinal surgery, serious head trauma, or previous CVA; uncontrolled hypertension at time of treatment; seizure at CVA onset; active internal bleeding; intracranial neoplasm; arteriovenous malformation; aneurysm; and bleeding diathesis.

Use cautiously in hypersensitivity to anistreplase or streptokinase, GI or genitourinary bleeding, ophthalmic hemorrhage, organ biopsy, severe hepatic or renal disease, ***elderly patients***, pregnant or breastfeeding patients, and ***children.***

Adverse reactions

CNS: cerebral hemorrhage, intracranial bleeding, cerebral edema, cerebral herniation, seizure, CVA (with accelerated infusion)
CV: hypotension, bradycardia, recurrent ischemia, **pericardial effusion, pericarditis, mitral regurgitation, electromechanical dissociation, arrhythmias, cardiogenic shock, heart failure, cardiac arrest, cardiac tamponade, myocardial rupture, embolization, venous thrombosis**
GI: nausea, vomiting, **GI bleeding**
GU: GU tract bleeding
Hematologic: spontaneous bleeding, bone marrow depression
Musculoskeletal: musculoskeletal pain
Respiratory: pulmonary edema, pulmonary re-embolism, pleural effusion
Skin: bruising, flushing
Other: fever, edema, phlebitis or bleeding at I.V. site, hypersensitivity reaction (including rash, **anaphylaxis, laryngeal edema**), **sepsis**

Interactions

Drug-drug. *Aspirin, drugs affecting platelet activity (such as abciximab, dipyridamole, heparin, oral anticoagulants, and vitamin K antagonists):* increased risk of bleeding
Nitroglycerin: decreased alteplase blood level
Drug-diagnostic tests. *Coagulation tests:* unreliable results
Blood urea nitrogen: elevated

Toxicity and overdose

- If overdose occurs, expect severe bleeding.
- Discontinue alteplase and anticoagulants immediately. Obtain blood for coagulation tests and blood type and crossmatch. Administer platelets, packed red blood cells, fresh-frozen plasma, desmopressin, or aminocaproic acid, as ordered. Be prepared to give protamine if heparin also has been given. As ordered, give atropine for bradycardia and lidocaine or procainamide for reperfusion arrhythmias. For ventricular tachycardia and ventricular fibrillation, expect to assist with cardioversion. If bleeding does not resolve, give vasopressor or a suitable plasma expander (such as albumin, plasma protein fraction, or hetastarch) or use Trendelenburg position, as ordered. *Do not give dextran.*
- In accidental administration of 2-mg Cathflo Activase dose directly into systemic circulation, serious bleeding (such as intracranial or GI bleeding) may occur. Discontinue Cathflo Activase and withdraw it from catheter. Expect concentration of circulating alteplase levels to return to exogenous levels of 5 to 10 mg/mL within 30 minutes.

Patient teaching

Instruct patient to immediately report adverse reactions, especially unusual bleeding or bruising.
- Stress importance of strict bed rest.
- Advise patient to avoid activities that can cause injury, and to use soft toothbrush and electric razor to avoid gum and skin injury.
- Inform patient about the need for frequent blood testing during therapy.
- As appropriate, review all other significant and life-threatening adverse reactions and interactions, especially those related to the drugs and tests mentioned above.

amifostine

Ethyol

Pharmacologic class: Organic thiophosphate cytoprotective agent
Therapeutic class: Antineoplastic
Pregnancy risk category C

Action

Undergoes rapid conversion to free thiol, an active metabolite that reduces toxic effects of cisplatin on renal tissue and reduces toxic effects of radiation on normal oral tissues

Pharmacokinetics

Drug clears rapidly from plasma, with distribution half-life of less than 1 minute and elimination half-life of 8 minutes. It is metabolized by alkaline phosphatase in tissues to its active metabolite, which occurs in greater amounts in normal tissues than tumor tissues and is available to bind to and detoxify reactive metabolites of cisplatin and radiation. Measurable metabolite levels have been found in bone marrow. Drug is excreted minimally in urine.

Onset	Peak	Duration
Rapid	Unknown	Unknown

How supplied

Powder for reconstitution for injection (white, lyophilized): 500-mg anhydrous base and 500 mg mannitol in 10-mL single-use vials

Indications and dosages

➢ To reduce cumulative renal toxicity of cisplatin in patients with ovarian cancer
Adults: 910 mg/m² I.V. daily as a 15-minute infusion, starting 30 minutes before chemotherapy. If previous treatment cycle was interrupted due to hypotension, give 740 mg/m² I.V. daily as a 15-minute infusion, starting 30 minutes before chemotherapy.

➢ To reduce moderate to severe xerostomia in patients undergoing postoperative radiation treatment for head or neck cancer, where radiation port includes substantial portion of parotid glands
Adults: 200 mg/m² I.V. daily as a 3-minute infusion, starting 15 to 30 minutes before standard fraction radiation therapy

Off-label uses

- Adverse effects of radiation therapy (mucositis, myelosuppression, proctitis, radioiodine-disturbance of salivary secretion, respiratory disease)
- Antineoplastic adverse reactions (myelosuppression, nephrotoxicity, neurotoxicity prophylaxis)
- Malignant melanoma (adjunct)
- Myelodysplastic syndrome
- Non-small-cell lung cancer (adjunct)
- To protect lung fibroblasts from damaging effects of paclitaxel

Administration

Preparation

- Obtain baseline blood pressure and ensure that patient is adequately hydrated before starting drug.
- Be aware that hypotensive or dehydrated patients should not receive drug.
- Know that antihypertensive therapy should be interrupted 24 hours before amifostine therapy begins in patients receiving drug at doses recommended for chemotherapy.
- Before each dose and during therapy, give antiemetics, including dexamethasone I.V. and serotonin 5-HT_3 receptor antagonist, as prescribed.

Dilution and compatibility
• Reconstitute single-dose vial with 9.7 mL sterile normal saline solution.
• Know that drug may be further diluted and can be prepared in polyvinyl chloride (PVC) bags at concentrations ranging from 5 to 40 mg/mL.
• Do not mix with other drugs or with solutions other than normal saline solution.
• After reconstitution, drug should be clear. Do not use if cloudy.
Infusion considerations
• Do not infuse longer than 15 minutes, as this increases risk of adverse reactions.
Keep patient supine during administration.
• Stop infusion temporarily if blood pressure decreases significantly from baseline.
Discontinue infusion immediately and permanently if acute allergic or cutaneous reaction occurs.
Monitoring
• Monitor blood pressure every 5 minutes during infusion and thereafter as indicated.
If hypotension occurs, place patient in Trendelenburg position and give normal saline solution through separate I.V. line, as ordered.
• Assess for severe nausea and vomiting and xerostomia resolution.
• Monitor fluid intake and output.
• Monitor blood calcium level; give calcium supplements as needed and prescribed.
Storage
• Store powder at controlled room temperature of 20° to 25°C (68° to 77°F).
• Reconstituted or diluted solution prepared in PVC infusion bags may be stored for 5 hours at room temperature or refrigerated for 24 hours.

Contraindications and precautions

Contraindicated in hypersensitivity to drug, aminothiol compounds or mannitol, concurrent antihypertensive therapy that cannot be discontinued for 24 hours before amifostine treatment, and definitive radiotherapy.

Use cautiously in hypocalcemia, dehydration, nausea, vomiting, hypotension, obesity, arrhythmias, heart failure, ischemic heart disease, renal impairment, history of cerebrovascular accident or transient ischemic attacks, ***elderly patients,*** pregnant patients (safety and efficacy not established), breastfeeding patients, and ***children*** (safety and efficacy not established).

Adverse reactions

CNS: dizziness, drowsiness, rigors, somnolence, **loss of consciousness**
CV: hypotension, syncope, tachycardia, bradycardia, chest pain, extrasystoles, **myocardial ischemia**
EENT: laryngeal edema
GI: nausea, vomiting, diarrhea
Metabolic: hypocalcemia
Respiratory: dyspnea, sneezing, hypoxia
Skin: flushing, rash, urticaria, erythroderma, **Stevens-Johnson syndrome, toxic epidermal necrolysis, erythema multiforme**
Other: chills, warm sensation, hiccups, allergic reactions

Interactions

Drug-drug. *Antihypertensives:* increased risk of hypotension
Drug-diagnostic tests. *Calcium:* decreased

Toxicity and overdose

• If overdose occurs, expect hypotension and possibly anxiety and reversible urine retention.
• Discontinue infusion. Administer I.V. normal saline solution, as ordered, and implement supportive measures as indicated.

Patient teaching

- Emphasize importance of staying supine during administration to prevent hypotension.
- Caution patient to avoid driving and other hazardous activities until drug's effects on concentration and alertness are known.
- Advise patient to minimize GI upset by eating small, frequent servings of food and drinking plenty of fluids.
- Provide dietary counseling. Refer patient to dietitian if adverse GI effects significantly limit food intake.
- Inform patient that sneezing is a normal drug effect.
- As appropriate, review all other significant and life-threatening adverse reactions and interactions, especially those related to the drugs and tests mentioned above.

amikacin sulfate

Amikin

Pharmacologic class: Aminoglycoside
Therapeutic class: Anti-infective
Pregnancy risk category D

Action

Interferes with protein synthesis in bacterial cells by binding to 30S ribosomal subunit, leading to bacterial cell death

Pharmacokinetics

Mean total apparent volume of distribution is 24 L. Serum protein binding ranges from 0% to 11%. Mean peak serum concentration occurs at end of infusion; mean serum half-life is slightly more than 2 hours. Mean serum clearance rate is about 100 mL/minute; renal clearance is 94 mL/minute in patients with normal renal function. Of I.V. dose, 84% is excreted in urine in 9 hours and about 94% within 24 hours.

Onset	Peak	Duration
Immediate	30 min	8-12 hr

How supplied

Solution for injection (light straw-colored): 50 mg/mL, 250 mg/mL

Indications and dosages

➢ Severe systemic infections caused by sensitive strains of *Pseudomonas aeruginosa, Escherichia coli,* or *Proteus, Klebsiella, Serratia, Enterobacter, Actinobactor, Providencia, Citrobactor,* and *Staphylococcus* species
Adults, children, and older infants: 15 mg/kg/day I.V. in two to three divided doses q 8 to 12 hours in 100 to 200 mL of D_5W given over 30 to 60 minutes. Maximum daily dosage is 1.5 g.

➢ Uncomplicated urinary tract infections caused by susceptible organisms
Adults, children, and older infants: 250 mg I.V. twice daily

Dosage adjustment

- In renal impairment, reduce dosage or dosing intervals by giving normal dosage at prolonged intervals based on creatinine clearance or by multiplying patient's serum creatinine by 9 and giving recommended single dose every 18 hours.
- Alternatively in renal impairment, give reduced dosages at fixed intervals based on serum creatinine levels, serum amikacin levels, and creatinine clearance values, and determine amount of maintenance dosage to give every 12 hours by reducing loading dose in proportion to creatinine clearance reduction.
- Be aware that approximately half of normal mg/kg dose can be given after hemodialysis.
- Know that in peritoneal dialysis, parenteral dose of 7.5 mg/kg may be given;

then drug should be instilled in peritoneal dialysate at desired serum concentration.

Off-label uses

- *Mycobacterium avium-intracellulare* infection

Administration

Preparation

- Ensure adequate fluid intake to avoid dehydration.

Dilution and compatibility

- Dilute in 100 to 200 mL of normal saline solution or D_5W.
- Do not mix with other drugs. Administer separately.

Infusion considerations

- Give over 30 to 60 minutes in adults.
- Know that infants should receive a 1- to 2-hour infusion.

Monitoring

- Monitor kidney function test results, urine cultures, urine output, urine protein, and urine specific gravity.
- Draw peak blood levels 30 to 60 minutes after I.V. infusion.
- Monitor results of peak and trough drug blood levels to avoid peak levels above 30 mcg/mL and trough levels above 10 mcg/mL.
- Evaluate for signs and symptoms of ototoxicity (hearing loss, tinnitus, ataxia, and vertigo).
- Assess for secondary superinfections, particularly upper respiratory tract infections.

Storage

- Drug may be stored for 24 hours at room temperature at concentrations of 0.25 mg/mL and 5 mg/mL in compatible solutions.

Contraindications and precautions

Contraindicated in hypersensitivity to aminoglycosides, sulfite sensitivity, renal or hepatic disease, myasthenia gravis, parkinsonism, and breastfeeding patients.

Use cautiously in decreased renal function, neuromuscular disorders, ***elderly patients,*** and pregnant patients.

Adverse reactions

CNS: dizziness, vertigo, tremor, numbness, depression, confusion, lethargy, headache, paresthesia, ataxia, **neuromuscular blockade, seizures, neurotoxicity**
CV: hypotension, hypertension, palpitations
EENT: nystagmus and other visual disturbances, ototoxicity, hearing loss, tinnitus
GI: nausea, vomiting, splenomegaly, stomatitis, increased salivation, anorexia
GU: azotemia, increased urinary casts, polyuria, painful urination, sexual dysfunction, **oliguria, nephrotoxicity**
Hematologic: purpura, eosinophilia, **leukemoid reaction, aplastic anemia, neutropenia, agranulocytosis, leukopenia, thrombocytopenia, pancytopenia, hemolytic anemia**
Hepatic: hepatomegaly, hepatic necrosis, hepatotoxicity
Musculoskeletal: joint pain, muscle twitching, **acute muscular paralysis**
Respiratory: apnea
Skin: rash, alopecia, urticaria, itching, exfoliative dermatitis
Other: weight loss, superinfection

Interactions

Drug-drug. *Acyclovir, amphotericin B, cephalosporin, cisplatin, diuretics, vancomycin:* increased risk of ototoxicity and nephrotoxicity
Depolarizing and nondepolarizing neuromuscular junction blockers, general anesthetics: increased amikacin effect, possibly leading to respiratory depression
Dimenhydrinate: masking of ototoxicity signs and symptoms

Indomethacin: increased amikacin peak and trough levels
Penicillin (parenteral): amikacin inactivation
Drug-diagnostic tests. *Alanine aminotransferase, alkaline phosphatase, aspartate aminotransferase, bilirubin, blood urea nitrogen, creatinine, lactate dehydrogenase, nonprotein nitrogen:* increased
Calcium, potassium, magnesium, sodium: decreased
Reticulocytes: increased or decreased

Toxicity and overdose

- In overdose, expect extension of adverse reactions.
- Monitor fluid balance, creatinine clearance, and plasma levels carefully. Hemodialysis or complexation with ticarcillin may be indicated. Calcium salts or neostigmine may reverse neuromuscular blockade.

Patient teaching

Inform patient that drug may cause hearing loss, seizures, and other neurologic problems. Tell patient to report these symptoms immediately.

Advise patient to immediately report fever, cough, breathing problems, sore throat, and other signs and symptoms of infection.

Instruct patient to notify prescriber promptly if urine volume is much more or much less than normal.

- Caution patient to avoid driving and other hazardous activities until drug's effects on concentration and alertness are known.
- Advise patient to minimize GI upset by eating small, frequent servings of food and drinking plenty of fluids.
- Inform patient about the need for regular blood and urine testing during therapy.
- As appropriate, review all other significant and life-threatening adverse reactions and interactions, especially those related to the drugs and tests mentioned above.

amino acids

amino acid injection

FreAmine, HepatAmine

crystalline amino acid infusions

Aminosyn, FreAmine III, Novamine, Travasol, TrophAmine

crystalline amino acid infusions with dextrose

Aminosyn (various strengths), Travasol (various strengths)

crystalline amino acid infusions with electrolytes

Aminosyn (various strengths), FreAmine (various strengths), ProcalAmine, Travasol (various strengths)

crystalline amino acid infusions with electrolytes in dextrose

Aminosyn (various strengths)

hepatic failure or hepatic encephalopathy formulations

HepatAmine

high metabolic stress formulations

Aminosyn-HBC, BranchAmin 4%, FreAmine-HBC

renal failure formulations

Aminosyn-RF 5.2%, RenAmin

Pharmacologic class: Protein substrate
Therapeutic class: Caloric drug, nitrogen product
Pregnancy risk category C

Action

Provide protein in parenteral nutrition needed to prevent nitrogen loss or correct negative nitrogen balance. Also provide substrate for protein synthesis (anabolism) or help conserve existing body protein (protein-sparing effect) by reducing protein breakdown rate. Promote wound healing and act as buffers in extracellular and intracellular fluids.

Pharmacokinetics

The mean terminal elimination half-life is 17.4 hours after a single I.V. dose. Drug is excreted in urine and feces.

Onset	Peak	Duration
Immediate	Immediate	Unknown

How supplied

Solution for injection (sterile, nonpyrogenic hypertonic solution of essential and nonessential amino acids): many strengths and concentrations available

Indications and dosages

➢ Recommended dietary allowance for protein and calories in patients on I.V. nutrition

Note: **Recommended dietary allowance for protein is approximately 0.9 g/kg for healthy adults and 1.4 to 2.2 g/kg for healthy growing infants and children. Traumatized or malnourished patients may have substantially increased protein and calorie requirements.**

Adults: Daily doses of approximately 1 to 1.5 g/kg I.V. for adults are generally sufficient to promote positive nitrogen balance. However, severely catabolic states may necessitate higher doses (which warrant frequent laboratory evaluation).

Children and infants: Daily doses of approximately 2 to 3 g/kg I.V. for infants are generally sufficient to promote positive nitrogen balance. However, severely catabolic states may necessitate higher doses (which warrant frequent laboratory evaluation). In children, parenteral nutrition requirements are constrained by greater relative fluid requirements and greater caloric requirements per kg. Amino acids probably are best given in 2.5% concentration. For most pediatric patients on I.V. nutrition, recommended dosage is 2.5 g/kg/day amino acids with dextrose alone or with I.V. lipid calories of 100 to 130 kcal/kg/day. In malnutrition or stress, requirements may rise. May start with half-strength nutritional solution at a rate of about 60 to 70 mL/kg/day; within 24 to 48 hours, may increase solution volume and concentration until full-strength pediatric solution (amino acids and dextrose) is given at a rate of 125 to 150 mL/kg/day.

Note: **Indications and dosages given below are limited to those used in some common nutritional therapies.**

➢ Total parenteral nutrition (TPN) supplement for patients with negative nitrogen balance secondary to inability of GI tract to absorb protein, patients unable to receive adequate nutrition through tube feedings, and patients requiring bowel rest

Adults: 1 to 1.7 g/kg/day I.V. (by peripheral vein) with low concentration of dextrose solution as required, or 500 mL amino acids by I.V. injection (through central vein), mixed with 500 mL concentrated dextrose solution, electrolytes, and vitamins, given over 8 hours

Children: Follow manufacturer's directions and use with caution.

➢ Nutritional supplement for patients with high metabolic stress

Adults: With adequate calories, 1.5 g/kg/day I.V. may be mixed with other solutions, as directed, and given by peripheral vein if amino acid solution contains minimal calories and central route is not indicated.

➢ Nutritional supplement for patients with renal failure

Adults: Follow manufacturer's directions; if needed, mix formulations with other solutions before infusing.

Children: Initially, start with low dosage, following manufacturer's directions. Increase to maximum daily dosage of 0.5 to 1g/kg I.V. If needed, mix formulations with other solutions before infusing.

➢ Nutritional supplement in patients with hepatic failure; or in patients with hepatic encephalopathy (such as cirrhosis or hepatitis)

Adults: (HepatAmine) 80 to 120 g amino acids (12 to 18 g nitrogen) mixed with other solutions as required (typically, 500 mL HepatAmine with 500 mL 50% dextrose, electrolytes, and vitamins) I.V. daily given over 8 to 12 hours. Use slow infusion rate initially; increase gradually to 60 to 125 mL/hour. May give by peripheral vein if central route is not indicated.

Administration

Preparation

Be aware that specific formulation to use depends on patient's status, underlying disease or disorder, and duration of therapy.

Know that not all amino acid products are approved for use in children.

- When starting therapy, monitor blood glucose level frequently until it stabilizes.
- Be aware that if central route is not indicated, amino acid solutions diluted with low dextrose concentrations may be infused by peripheral vein.

Dilution and compatibility

Use strict aseptic technique when mixing and preparing solution. Replace all I.V. equipment every 24 hours.

Be aware that some amino acid products are highly concentrated and intended for compounding only—not for direct infusion.

- Do not add antibiotics, steroids, or pressor agents to amino acid solutions.
- Know that bleomycin is incompatible with amino acids.
- Do not give solutions through same administration set as blood, because pseudoagglutination may occur.
- Do not add multivitamins to solution until ready to administer.
- Consult with pharmacist before mixing with other drugs.
- Use 0.22-micron inline microfilter for dextrose and amino acid solutions.
- Use 1.2-micron inline microfilter for lipid solutions.
- Discard remaining solution after 24 hours.

Infusion considerations

Do not give by I.V. push or bolus.

Do not give hypertonic solution via peripheral vein.

- Do not give crystalline amino acids unless solution is clear and seal is intact; however, slight yellowish color does not alter product quality and efficacy.

Begin I.V. infusion at a slow rate (1 to 2 mL/minute). Control rate carefully with infusion pump; monitor rate closely and distribute daily dosage evenly over 24 hours by constant drip.

Do not stop therapy abruptly, as rebound hypoglycemia may occur.

- For subclavian administration, infuse drug into midsuperior vena cava.

Monitoring

- Check infusion site often for signs of infection, phlebitis, and tissue damage.
- Change I.V. set every 24 hours.
- Monitor blood glucose level daily.
- Evaluate fractional urine regularly for glycosuria, which may signal glucose intolerance and sepsis onset.

• Monitor serum electrolyte levels; report unusual electrolyte losses (for instance, from nasogastric tube, vomiting, drainage, or diarrhea).
• Monitor blood urea nitrogen (BUN) level.
• Evaluate patient's nutritional status regularly.
Watch for circulatory overload in patients with cardiac insufficiency.
Assess for sepsis continually, such as by checking temperature every 4 hours.
Storage
• Follow manufacturer's directions for storing specific products.

Contraindications

Contraindicated in hypersensitivity to amino acids, intracranial or intraspinal hemorrhage, severe renal or hepatic disease, and metabolic disorders involving impaired nitrogen utilization (all formulations); severe electrolyte and acid-base imbalance and hyperammonemia (renal failure formulations); anuria (hepatic failure and hepatic encephalopathy formulations); and anuria, hyperammonemia, hepatic coma, and severe electrolyte or acid-base imbalance (high metabolic stress formulations).

Use cautiously in heart failure, hypertension, diabetes mellitus, hepatic or renal impairment, ***elderly patients,*** pregnant patients, and ***children.***

Adverse reactions

CNS: headache, dizziness, confusion, **loss of consciousness**
CV: hypertension, tachycardia, **heart failure, venous thrombosis, circulatory overload**
GI: nausea, vomiting, abdominal pain
GU: osmotic diuresis, glycosuria
Hepatic: jaundice, **fatty liver, hepatic impairment**
Metabolic: rebound hypoglycemia (with abrupt cessation of long-term infusion), hyperglycemia, excessive urea buildup, fatty-acid deficiency, electrolyte imbalances, hyperammonemia, hypophosphatemia, hypocalcemia, hyperchloremia, dehydration, **metabolic acidosis or alkalosis, uremia, hyperosmolar hyperglycemic nonketotic syndrome**
Musculoskeletal: osteoporosis
Respiratory: pulmonary edema
Skin: rash, generalized flushing, warm sensation, papular eruptions, urticaria, extravasation necrosis, phlebitis or tissue sloughing at injection site
Other: fever, chills, pain, hypersensitivity reaction, **catheter sepsis**

Interactions

Drug-drug. *Tetracycline:* reduced protein-sparing effect of amino acids
Drug-diagnostic tests. *Blood glucose, BUN, chlorides:* increased
Calcium, phosphates: decreased

Toxicity and overdose

• In overdose, expect exaggerated adverse reactions.
• Provide supportive and symptomatic interventions.

Patient teaching

Tell patient TPN infusion may increase infection risk. Advise patient to immediately report fever, chills, and other signs and symptoms of infection.
• Instruct patient to report unusual pain, redness, swelling, and other changes at infusion site.
• Advise patient to notify prescriber of vomiting or diarrhea.
• Caution patient to avoid driving and other hazardous activities until drug's effects on concentration and alertness are known.
• As appropriate, review all other significant and life-threatening adverse reactions and interactions, especially those related to the drugs and tests mentioned above.

aminocaproic acid

Amicar

Pharmacologic class: Carboxylic acid derivative
Therapeutic class: Hemostatic
Pregnancy risk category C

Action

Interferes with plasminogen activator substances and blocks action of fibrinolysin (plasmin)

Pharmacokinetics

After prolonged administration, drug distributes throughout extravascular and intravascular compartments, penetrating red blood cells and other tissue cells. It is not protein-bound. Primary elimination route is renal. About 65% of dose is recovered in urine unchanged, and 11% appears as the metabolite adipic acid. Terminal elimination half-life is approximately 2 hours.

Onset	Peak	Duration
1 hr	Unknown	Less than 3 hr

How supplied

Solution for injection (with benzyl alcohol): 250 mg/mL

Indications and dosages

➤ Excessive bleeding caused by fibrinolysis

Adults: 4 to 5 g I.V. in 250 mL compatible I.V. solution over 1 hour, followed by continuous infusion of 1 g/hour in 50 mL diluent. Continue for 8 hours or until bleeding stops. Maximum daily dosage is 30 g.

Off-label uses

- Acute promyelocytic leukemia in patients who develop coagulopathy associated with low levels of alpha-2-plasmin inhibitor
- Amegakaryocytic thrombocytopenia
- Dental extractions
- Subarachnoid hemorrhage
- To prevent and abort attacks of hereditary angioneurotic edema
- To reduce postsurgical bleeding complications in patients undergoing cardiopulmonary bypass procedures

Administration

Dilution and compatibility

- Dilute each 1 g of drug in 50 mL of compatible solution.
- Dilute 4 to 5 g in 250 mL compatible I.V. solution, such as normal saline solution, D_5W, or Ringer's solution.
- Be aware that although sterile water for injection is compatible, resulting solution is hypo-osmolar.

Infusion considerations

- Give at prescribed rate using infusion pump to ensure accurate dosing.
- Five grams or less (in 250 mL of solution) may be infused over first hour; but then each succeeding gram should be infused over 1 hour in at least 50 mL/g solution.

Do not administer rapidly.

Be aware that rapid administration or insufficient dilution may cause hypotension, bradycardia, or arrhythmia.

Monitoring

- Monitor vital signs, fluid intake and output, and ECG.

Assess for signs and symptoms of thrombophlebitis and pulmonary embolism.

Monitor neurologic status, especially for indications of impending seizure.

Evaluate for blood dyscrasias, particularly bleeding tendencies.

- Monitor kidney and liver function test results, serum electrolyte levels, and CBC with differential.

Discontinue therapy if creatine kinase (CK) level increases.

Storage

• Store at controlled room temperature. Do not freeze.

Contraindications

Contraindicated in hypersensitivity to drug, evidence of active intravascular clotting, upper urinary tract bleeding, disseminated intravascular coagulation, pregnancy, and ***neonates.***

Use cautiously in cardiac, hepatic, or renal failure.

Adverse reactions

CNS: dizziness, malaise, headache, delirium, hallucinations, weakness, **seizures, intracranial hypertension, cerebrovascular accident**

CV: hypotension, ischemia, syncope, **thrombosis, thrombophlebitis, cardiomyopathy, bradycardia, arrhythmias**

EENT: conjunctival suffusion, decreased vision, tinnitus, nasal congestion

GI: nausea, vomiting, diarrhea, abdominal pain, dyspepsia

GU: intrarenal obstruction, renal failure

Hematologic: bleeding tendencies, generalized thrombosis, agranulocytosis, leukopenia, thrombocytopenia, coagulation disorder

Musculoskeletal: myopathy, muscle weakness, myalgia, myositis, **rhabdomyolysis**

Respiratory: dyspnea, **pulmonary embolism**

Skin: rash, pruritus, necrosis

Other: edema, injection site reaction, pain, allergic reaction including **anaphylactoid reactions**

Interactions

Drug-drug. *Activated prothrombin, prothrombin complex concentrates:* increased signs of active intravascular clotting

Estrogens, hormonal contraceptives: increased risk of hypercoagulation

Drug-diagnostic tests. *Alanine aminotransferase, aldolase, aspartate aminotransferase, blood urea nitrogen, CK, creatinine, potassium:* increased

Drug-herb. *Alfalfa, anise, arnica, astragalus, bilberry, black currant seed oil, capsaicin, cat's claw, celery, chaparral, clove oil, dandelion, dong quai, evening primrose oil, feverfew, garlic, ginger, ginkgo, papaya extract, rhubarb, safflower oil, skullcap:* increased anticoagulant effect

Coenzyme Q10, St. John's wort: decreased anticoagulant effect

Toxicity and overdose

• Several cases of acute overdose have occurred, with signs and symptoms ranging from none to transient hypotension to severe acute renal failure leading to death. Seizures also may occur.

• No known treatment for overdose exists, although some evidence suggests that drug is removed by hemodialysis and possibly by peritoneal dialysis. Discontinue drug and provide supportive and symptomatic interventions.

Patient teaching

• Inform patient that drug may significantly affect many body systems. Provide reassurance that patient will be monitored closely through observation and tests.

Instruct patient to immediately report such signs and symptoms as calf pain, shortness of breath, and unusual bleeding.

• Inform patient about the need for frequent blood testing during therapy.

• As appropriate, review all other significant and life-threatening adverse reactions and interactions, especially those related to the drugs, tests, and herbs mentioned above.

aminophylline (theophylline, ethylenediamine)

Norphyl, Phyllocontin, Phyllocontin❉, Truphylline

Pharmacologic class: Xanthine
Therapeutic class: Bronchodilator
Pregnancy risk category C

Action

Unclear. Thought to directly relax smooth muscle of bronchial airways and increase pulmonary blood flow by inhibiting phosphodiesterase.

Pharmacokinetics

Drug distributes rapidly into body fluids but poorly into body fat. It is metabolized in the liver. Steady-state serum theophylline level depends on infusion rate and theophylline clearance rate. Half-life varies; it may be prolonged in chronic alcoholic abusers and patients who have heart failure or who take certain interacting drugs. Newborns and neonates have extremely slow clearance rates compared to infants and children older than age 1; older children have rapid clearance rates.

Onset	Peak	Duration
Immediate	Variable	Variable

How supplied

Solution for injection (clear): 25 mg/mL in 10- and 20 mL ampules and vials

Indications and dosages

***Note:* Aminophylline dosage equals the theophylline dosage divided by 0.8. Dosages below are provided as theophylline.**

➢ Symptomatic relief of bronchospasm in patients with acute exacerbation of asthma and other chronic lung diseases (such as emphysema and bronchitis)

Loading dose (theophylline-naive patients): 4.6 mg/kg (calculated using ideal body weight) I.V. over 30 minutes. For subsequent doses, see below:

Adults ages 16 to 60 (nonsmokers): After loading dose of 4.6 mg/kg (as above), 0.4 mg/kg/hour I.V. for first 12 hours; adjust dosage according to serum level during first 12-hour period for target serum level of 10 mcg/mL.

Adults ages 16 to 60 (smokers): After loading dose of 4.6 mg/kg (as above), 0.8 mg/kg/hour I.V. for first 12 hours; then adjust dosage based on serum level.

Children and adolescents ages 12 to 16 (nonsmokers): After loading dose of 4.6 mg/kg (as above), 0.5 mg/kg/hour I.V. for first 12 hours; then adjust dosage based on serum level.

Children and adolescents ages 12 to 16 (smokers): After loading dose of 4.6 mg/kg (as above), 0.7 mg/kg/hour I.V. for first 12 hours; then adjust dosage based on serum level.

Children ages 9 to 12: After loading dose of 4.6 mg/kg (as above), 0.7 mg/kg/hour I.V. for first 12 hours; then adjust dosage based on serum level.

Children ages 1 to 9: After loading dose of 4.6 mg/kg (as above), 0.8 mg/kg/hour I.V.; then adjust dosage based on serum level.

Infants 6 to 52 weeks: After loading dose, give dosage as mg/kg/hour calculated by multiplying 0.008 by age in weeks + 0.21.

➢ Neonatal apnea

Loading dose (theophylline-naive patients): 4.6 mg/kg (calculated using ideal body weight) I.V. over 30 minutes. For subsequent doses, see below:

Neonates (more than 24 days old): After loading dose of 4.6 mg/kg (as above), 1.5 mg/kg I.V q 12 hours to achieve a serum concentration of 7.5 mcg/mL

Neonates (24 days old or younger): After loading dose of 4.6 mg/kg (as above), 1 mg/kg I.V q 12 hours to achieve a serum concentration of 7.5 mcg/mL

Dosage adjustment

- Decrease dosage in heart failure or hepatic disease, elderly patients, and smokers based on drug blood levels.
- Know that patients with cardiac decompensation, shock, cor pulmonale, hepatic dysfunction, or sepsis with multiorgan failure should receive 0.2 mg/kg/hour, not to exceed 400 mg/day, unless serum levels indicate the need for a higher dosage.

Off-label uses (selected)

- Dyspnea in patients with chronic obstructive pulmonary disease (COPD)

Administration

Preparation

- Individualize dosage based on serum theophylline level to provide maximum benefit with minimal risk of adverse reactions.
- Once loading dose achieves a serum level of 10 to 15 mcg/mL, start constant I.V. infusion. Base administration rate on pharmacokinetic parameters for the specific patient population and calculated to achieve a target serum level of 10 mcg/mL.
- If patient who has already received theophylline needs a loading dose, do not estimate serum level based on history; instead, use immediate serum level determination.

If patient has received theophylline within previous 24 hours, obtain serum theophylline level before giving loading dose.

Dilution and compatibility

Check drug label carefully to make sure it states, "For I.V. use."

- Dilute according to label directions.
- Give maintenance dose in large volume of fluid for infusion.

Do not give in I.V. solution containing invert sugar, fructose, or fat emulsions.

Avoid alkali-labile drugs in admixtures with aminophylline.

- Do not mix in syringe with other drugs.
- Do not administer unless solution is clear.
- Do not use if crystals have separated from infusion.

Infusion considerations

- Infuse at a rate no faster than 25 mg/minute.

Be aware that rapid administration may cause arrhythmia.

In patients with cor pulmonale, cardiac decompensation, or hepatic dysfunction and in those taking drugs that markedly reduce theophylline clearance (such as cimetidine), do not exceed initial infusion rate of 17 mg/hour (21 mg/hour as aminophylline) unless serum levels can be monitored at 24-hour intervals. These patients may require 5 days to reach steady state.

Monitoring

Assess for arrhythmias, especially after loading dose.

- Obtain serum drug level 20 to 30 minutes after starting continuous infusion.
- Know that serum level obtained 30 minutes after I.V. loading dose (once distribution is complete) can be used to assess need for and amount of subsequent loading doses, if clinically indicated, and to guide continuing therapy.

Adjust dosage if patient experiences signs or symptoms of toxicity (tachycardia, headache, anorexia, nausea, vomiting, diarrhea, restlessness, and irritability).

- Continue to check vital signs and fluid intake and output.
- Monitor patient's response to drug and assess pulmonary function test results.

Storage
- Protect from light and freezing.
- Store between 15° and 30°C (59° and 86°F).

Contraindications
Contraindicated in hypersensitivity to xanthine compounds or ethylenediamine, GI disease, and seizure disorders.

Use cautiously in COPD, diabetes mellitus, glaucoma, renal or hepatic disease, heart failure or other cardiac or circulatory impairment, hypertension, hyperthyroidism, peptic ulcer, severe hypoxemia, fever, sepsis with multiorgan failure, pulmonary edema, ***elderly patients, neonates, infants,*** and ***young children.***

Adverse reactions
CNS: irritability, dizziness, nervousness, restlessness, headache, insomnia, stammering speech, abnormal behavior, mutism, unresponsiveness alternating with hyperactivity, **seizures**
CV: palpitations, sinus tachycardia, extrasystoles, **marked hypotension, arrhythmias, circulatory failure**
GI: nausea, vomiting, diarrhea, epigastric pain, hematemesis, gastroesophageal reflux, anorexia
GU: urine retention (in males with enlarged prostate), diuresis, increased excretion of renal tubular cells and red blood cells, proteinuria
Metabolic: hyperglycemia
Musculoskeletal: muscle twitching
Respiratory: tachypnea, **respiratory arrest**
Skin: flushing
Other: fever, hypersensitivity reactions (including exfoliative dermatitis and urticaria)

Interactions
Drug-drug. *Adenosine:* decreased antiarrhythmic effect
Barbiturates, nicotine, phenytoin, rifampin: decreased aminophylline blood level
Beta-adrenergic blockers: antagonism of aminophylline effects
Calcium channel blockers, cimetidine, ciprofloxacin, disulfiram, erythromycin, fluvoxamine, hormonal contraceptives, influenza vaccine, interferon, ketoconazole, methotrexate, norfloxacin, ofloxacin: elevated aminophylline blood level
Carbamazepine, isoniazid, loop diuretics (such as furosemide): increased or decreased aminophylline blood level
Ephedrine, other sympathomimetics: arrhythmias
Lithium: increased lithium excretion
Drug-diagnostic tests. *Aspartate aminotransferase, glucose:* increased
Drug-herb. *Cayenne:* increased risk of aminophylline toxicity
Drug-behaviors. *Smoking:* decreased aminophylline effects

Toxicity and overdose
- Toxic serum levels range from above 80 to 100 mcg/mL in acute ingestion and above 40 mcg/mL in chronic ingestion. Signs and symptoms include nausea, vomiting, seizures, abdominal pain, metabolic acidosis, electrolyte imbalance, leukocytosis, tachycardia, hypotension, and arrhythmias.
- Stop I.V. infusion and obtain serum theophylline level immediately. Maintain adequate ventilation and hydration. Expect to give diazepam for grand mal seizures, verapamil for atrial arrhythmias, lidocaine or procainamide for ventricular arrhythmias, and dopamine for hypotension. Do not give stimulants. Enhance elimination with hemoperfusion or hemodialysis if serum drug level 100 mcg/mL. Resuscitate as necessary.

Patient teaching
- Caution patient to avoid driving and other hazardous activities until drug's

effects on concentration and alertness are known.

- Teach patient to minimize GI upset by eating small, frequent servings of food and drinking plenty of fluids.
- Advise patient to establish effective bedtime routine to minimize insomnia.
- Instruct patients who smoke to notify prescriber if they stop smoking; dosage adjustment may be needed.
- As appropriate, review all other significant and life-threatening adverse reactions and interactions, especially those related to the drugs, tests, herbs, and behaviors mentioned above.

amiodarone hydrochloride

Cordarone

Pharmacologic class: Adrenergic blocker

Therapeutic class: Antiarrhythmic (class III)

Pregnancy risk category D

FDA BOXED WARNING

- Because of substantial toxicity, drug is indicated only in patients with life-threatening arrhythmias.
- Drug may cause potentially fatal pulmonary toxicities, including hypersensitivity pneumonitis and interstitial/alveolar pneumonitis. Pulmonary toxicity is fatal about 10% of time.
- Hepatic injury is common but usually mild, manifesting only as abnormal liver enzyme levels. However, overt hepatic disease can occur and, in rare cases, is fatal.
- Drug may exacerbate arrhythmias by reducing tolerance for them or making them harder to reverse. Arrhythmias and significant heart block or sinus bradycardia occur in 2% to 5% of patients.
- Even in patients at high risk for arrhythmic death in whom toxicity is an acceptable risk, drug poses major management problems. Therefore, other agents should be tried first whenever possible.
- Difficulty of using drug effectively and safely poses significant risk. Patients with indicated arrhythmias must be hospitalized to receive loading dose; response generally takes at least 1 week, but usually 2 or more.

Action

Prolongs duration and refractory period of action potential. Slows electrical conduction, electrical impulse generation from sinoatrial node (SA), and conduction through accessory pathways; also dilates blood vessels.

Pharmacokinetics

Drug disposition after I.V. dose is complex. Peak serum levels vary after single 15-minute I.V. infusion of 5 mg/kg in healthy patients and after 10-minute infusion of 150 mg in patients with ventricular fibrillation or hemodynamically unstable ventricular tachycardia. Due to rapid distribution, serum levels fall to 10% of peak values within 30 to 45 minutes after infusion ends. With short-term I.V. use, no established relationship exists between drug concentration and therapeutic response. Drug is eliminated mainly by hepatic metabolism and biliary excretion; negligible excretion of amiodarone or desethylamiodarone occurs in urine.

Onset	Peak	Duration
Variable	Unknown	Variable

How supplied

Solution for injection: 50 mg/mL in 3-mL ampules

Indications and dosages

➤ Treatment and prophylaxis of life-threatening ventricular arrhythmias

Adults: 150 mg in 100 mL D_5W by rapid I.V. infusion over 10 minutes; then dilute 900 mg in 500 mL D_5W and give 360 mg by slow I.V. infusion over next 6 hours at 1 mg/minute; then give 540-mg I.V. maintenance infusion over next 18 hours at 0.5 mg/minute, followed by oral therapy

Off-label uses

- Atrioventricular (AV) nodal reentry tachycardia
- To convert atrial fibrillation and atrial flutter to normal sinus rhythm
- To prevent recurrence of symptomatic paroxysmal and persistent atrial fibrillation after cardioversion

Administration

Preparation

🔊 Follow hazardous drug guidelines on page S19 for handling, preparation, and administration.

🔊 Know that because of drug's pharmacokinetic properties, difficult dosing schedule, and severity of adverse effects unless patient is monitored properly, drug should be given only by clinicians who are experienced in treating life-threatening arrhythmias, are thoroughly familiar with drug's risks and benefits, and have access to facilities capable of adequately monitoring drug efficacy and adverse effects.

🔊 Be aware that antiarrhythmics may be ineffective or arrhythmogenic in patients with hypokalemia. Before giving amiodarone, correct hypokalemia and hypomagnesemia that may exaggerate prolonged QTc interval and cause arrhythmias.

- Obtain baseline chest X-ray and pulmonary, liver, and thyroid function test results.

Dilution and compatibility

- Dilute with D_5W.
- Know that drug is not compatible with normal saline solution.

Infusion considerations

🔊 Give loading dose in hospital setting with continuous ECG monitoring.

- Use central venous catheter (CVC) when giving repeated doses; if possible, use dedicated catheter for drug.
- Use volumetric pump and 0.2-micron inline filter.
- Know that drug levels above 3 mg/mL in D_5W have been linked to high incidence of peripheral vein phlebitis; levels of 2.5 mg/mL or lower are less irritating. Therefore, for infusions longer than 1 hour, do not exceed concentrations of more than 2 mg/mL, unless using CVC.

Monitoring

🔊 Monitor patient closely; drug may cause serious or life-threatening adverse reactions.

🔊 Watch for slow onset of life-threatening arrhythmias, especially after giving loading dose.

🔊 Monitor ECG continuously after dosage changes.

- Continue to monitor for and correct hypokalemia and hypomagnesemia, as needed.
- Check blood pressure, pulse, and heart rhythm regularly.
- Assess for signs and symptoms of lung inflammation.
- Continue to monitor chest X-ray and pulmonary, liver, and thyroid function test results.
- Closely monitor patient receiving concurrent drugs, because amiodarone can interact with many drugs. Monitor digoxin blood levels if patient is receiving digoxin; monitor prothrombin time (PT) or International Normalized Ratio in patient receiving anticoagulants.

Storage

- Until use, store in carton at controlled room temperature of 20° to 25°C (68° to 77°F); protect from light.

Contraindications

Contraindicated in hypersensitivity to drug, cardiogenic shock, second- or third-degree AV block, marked sinus bradycardia, breastfeeding, and ***neonates.***

Use cautiously in electrolyte imbalances (especially hypokalemia and hypomagnesemia), severe pulmonary or hepatic disease, thyroid disorders, history of heart failure, ***elderly patients,*** pregnant patients, and ***children.***

Adverse reactions

CNS: dizziness, fatigue, headache, insomnia, paresthesia, peripheral neuropathy, poor coordination, abnormal gait, malaise, involuntary movements, tremor, sleep disturbances

CV: hypotension, **heart failure, worsening arrhythmia, AV block, SA node dysfunction, bradycardia, asystole, cardiac arrest, cardiogenic shock, electromechanical dissociation, ventricular tachycardia**

EENT: corneal microdeposits, corneal or macular degeneration, visual disturbances, dry eyes, eye discomfort, optic neuritis or neuropathy, scotoma, lens opacities, photophobia, visual halos, **papilledema**

GI: nausea, vomiting, constipation, abdominal pain, abnormal salivation, anorexia

GU: decreased libido

Hematologic: coagulation abnormalities, thrombocytopenia

Hepatic: nonspecific hepatic disorders, **hepatic dysfunction**

Metabolic: hypothyroidism, hyperthyroidism

Respiratory: cough, dyspnea, hemoptysis, hypoxia, wheezing, **bronchospasms, acute respiratory distress syndrome, pulmonary inflammation or fibrosis, pulmonary edema**

Skin: flushing, photosensitivity, cellulitis, **toxic epidermal necrolysis**

Other: abnormal taste and smell, edema, fever, **Stevens-Johnson syndrome**

Interactions

Drug-drug. *Anticoagulants:* increased PT

Azole antifungals, fluoroquinolones, macrolide antibiotics: increased risk of life-threatening arrhythmias

Beta-adrenergic blockers: increased risk of bradycardia, hypotension, and sinus arrest

Calcium channel blockers: increased risk of AV block (verapamil, diltiazem) or hypotension (any calcium channel blocker), sinus arrest, and bradycardia

Cholestyramine: decreased amiodarone blood level

Cimetidine, ritonavir: increased amiodarone blood level

Class I antiarrhythmics (disopyramide, flecainide, lidocaine, mexiletine, procainamide, quinidine): increased blood levels of these drugs, leading to toxicity

Cyclosporine: elevated cyclosporine and creatinine levels

Dextromethorphan: impaired dextromethorphan metabolism (with amiodarone use of 2 weeks or longer)

Digoxin: increased digoxin blood level, leading to toxicity

Fentanyl: increased risk of bradycardia, hypotension, sinus arrest, and decreased cardiac output

Methotrexate: impaired methotrexate metabolism, possibly causing toxicity (with amiodarone use longer than 2 weeks)

Phenytoin: decreased amiodarone blood level or increased phenytoin

blood level (with amiodarone use longer than 2 weeks)
Theophylline: increased theophylline blood level (with amiodarone use longer than 1 week)
Drug-diagnostic tests. *Kidney function tests:* abnormal results
Liver function tests: elevated
Drug-herb. *St. John's wort:* possibly reduced amiodarone blood level

Toxicity and overdose

- Some cases of overdose (including fatal ones) have occurred. Signs and symptoms include bradycardia, hypotension, AV block, cardiogenic shock, and hepatotoxicity.
- Provide supportive interventions; monitor heart rhythm and blood pressure. If bradycardia continues, expect patient to receive beta-adrenergic agonist and pacemaker. For hypotension accompanied by inadequate tissue perfusion, give positive inotropic or vasopressor agents and volume expander, as prescribed. Neither amiodarone nor its metabolite is dialyzable.

Patient teaching

- Inform patient that drug may cause serious adverse reactions (such as a feeling of faintness or difficulty breathing). Instruct patient to report these immediately.
- Tell patient that adverse reactions are most common with high doses and may become more frequent after 6 months.
- Inform patient that regular blood tests, chest X-rays, and pulmonary function tests are required during therapy.
- As appropriate, review all other significant and life-threatening adverse reactions and interactions, especially those related to the drugs, tests, and herbs mentioned above.

A

amphotericin B cholesteryl sulfate

Amphotec, Amphocil

amphotericin B desoxycholate

Amphocin, Fungilin, Fungizone Intravenous

amphotericin B lipid complex

Abelcet

amphotericin B liposome

AmBisome

Pharmacologic class: Systemic polyene antifungal
Therapeutic class: Antifungal
Pregnancy risk category B

FDA BOXED WARNING

- Amphotericin B desoxycholate should be used mainly to treat progressive and potentially life-threatening fungal infections. It should not be used to treat noninvasive forms of fungal disease (such as oral thrush, vaginal candidiasis, or esophageal candidiasis) in patients with normal neutrophil counts.

Action

Binds to sterols in fungal cell membrane, which increases permeability and allows potassium to exit cell. Depending on concentrations achieved and susceptibility of organism, fungal death or impairment results.

Pharmacokinetics

Depending on formulation, steady-state volume of distribution and total plasma clearance increase with escalating doses, resulting in less-than-proportional increases in plasma concentration. Half-lives and excretion time also vary with formulation. Liposomal encapsulation or lipid complex formulation may substantially affect functional properties relative to those of unencapsulated or nonlipid-associated drug. These formulations stay in the vasculature longer and can localize and reach greater concentrations in regions with increased capillary permeability (compared with regions of normal tissue, which are impermeable to lipid-complexed drugs).

Onset	Peak	Duration
Rapid	End of infusion	Variable

How supplied

Amphotericin B cholesteryl sulfate—
Injection: 50 mg, 100 mg
Amphotericin B desoxycholate—
Injection: 50-mg vial
Amphotericin B lipid complex—
Suspension for injection: 100 mg/20-mL vials
Amphotericin B liposome—
Injection: 50 mg

Indications and dosages

➢ Invasive aspergillosis
Adults: *Amphotericin B desoxycholate—* For patients with good cardiorenal function who tolerate test dose, 0.25 to 0.3 mg/kg daily by slow I.V. infusion (0.1 mg/mL over 2 to 6 hours); increase gradually to 0.5 to 0.7 mg/kg daily. Patients with neutropenia or rapidly progressing, potentially fatal infections may require higher dosages (1 to 1.5 mg/kg daily).
Adults and children age 1 month and older: *Amphotericin B liposome—*3 to 5 mg/kg I.V. daily
➢ Invasive aspergillosis in patients with renal impairment or unacceptable toxicity who cannot tolerate or do not respond to amphotericin B desoxycholate in effective doses
Adults and children: *Amphotericin B cholesteryl sulfate—*If patient tolerates test dose, 3 to 4 mg/kg I.V. daily in D_5W by continuous infusion at 1 mg/kg/hour. *Amphotericin B lipid complex—*5 mg/kg I.V. daily, prepared as 1-mg/mL infusion and given at a rate of 2.5 mg/kg/hour.
➢ Blastomycosis
Adults: *Amphotericin B desoxycholate—* 0.25 to 1 mg/kg/day I.V.
➢ Blastomycosis in patients who cannot tolerate or do not respond to conventional amphotericin B
Adults and children: *Amphotericin B lipid complex—*5 mg/kg/day I.V. for average duration of approximately 4 weeks
➢ Systemic histoplasmosis
Adults: *Amphotericin B desoxycholate—* If patient tolerates test dose, gradually increase from initial recommended dosage of 0.25 to 0.3 mg/kg daily by slow I.V. infusion (0.1 mg/mL over 2 to 6 hours) to usual dosage of 0.5 to 0.7 mg/kg daily I.V. for 4 to 8 weeks. Higher dosages (0.7 to 1 mg) may be needed in rapidly progressing, potentially fatal infections.
➢ Systemic coccidioidomycosis
Adults: *Amphotericin B desoxycholate—* If patient tolerates test dose, gradually increase from initial recommended dosage of 0.25 to 0.3 mg/kg daily by slow I.V. infusion (0.1 mg/mL over 2 to 6 hours) to usual dosage of 0.5 to 1 mg/kg I.V. daily.
➢ Systemic cryptococcosis
Adults: *Amphotericin B desoxycholate—* If patient tolerates test dose, gradually increase from initial recommended dosage of 0.25 to 0.3 mg/kg daily by slow I.V. infusion (0.1 mg/mL over 2 to 6 hours) to usual dosage of 0.3 to 1 mg/kg I.V. daily (with or without flucytosine) for 2 weeks to several months.

Adults and children ages 1 month and older: *Amphotericin B liposome*—3 to 5 mg/kg I.V. daily

➤ Cryptococcal meningitis in HIV-infected patients

Adults: *Amphotericin B desoxycholate*—If patient tolerates test dose, gradually increase from initial recommended dosage of 0.25 to 0.3 mg/kg daily by slow I.V. infusion (0.1 mg/mL over 2 to 6 hours) to usual dosage of 0.3 to 1 mg/kg I.V. daily (with or without flucytosine) for 2 weeks to several months.

Adults and children: *Amphotericin B lipid complex*—5 mg/kg I.V. infusion daily for 6 weeks, followed by 12 weeks of oral fluconazole therapy. *Amphotericin B liposome*—6 mg/kg I.V. infusion daily.

➤ Disseminated candidiasis

Adults: *Amphotericin B desoxycholate*—If patient tolerates test dose, gradually increase from initial recommended dosage of 0.25 to 0.3 mg/kg daily by slow I.V. infusion (0.1 mg/mL over 2 to 6 hours) to usual dosage of 0.5 to 0.7 mg/kg daily by slow I.V. infusion for 7 to 14 days in low-risk patients or 6 weeks in high-risk patients.

Adults and children ages 1 month and older: *Amphotericin B liposome*—3 to 5 mg/kg I.V. daily for 5 to 7 days

➤ Disseminated candidiasis in patients who cannot tolerate or do not respond to conventional amphotericin B

Adults and children: *Amphotericin B lipid complex*—5 mg/kg/day I.V. for average duration of approximately 4 weeks

➤ Systemic zygomycosis, including mucormycosis

Adults: *Amphotericin B desoxycholate*—If patient tolerates test dose, gradually increase from initial recommended dosage of 0.25 to 0.3 mg/kg daily by slow I.V. infusion (0.1 mg/mL over 2 to 6 hours) to usual dosage of 1 to 1.5 mg/kg I.V. daily for 2 to 3 months.

➤ Subcutaneous zygomycosis, including *Conidiobolus* and *Basidiobolus*

Adults: *Amphotericin B desoxycholate*—If patient tolerates test dose, gradually increase from initial recommended dosage of 0.25 to 0.3 mg/kg daily by slow I.V. infusion (0.1 mg/mL over 2 to 6 hours) to usual dosage of 0.5 to 0.7 mg/kg daily by slow I.V. infusion.

➤ Systemic disseminated sporotrichosis

Adults: *Amphotericin B desoxycholate*—If patient tolerates test dose, gradually increase from initial recommended dosage of 0.25 to 0.3 mg/kg daily by slow I.V. infusion (0.1 mg/mL over 2 to 6 hours) to usual dosage of 0.5 to 0.7 mg/kg daily by slow I.V. infusion to maximum dosage of 1 mg/kg I.V. daily for up to 9 months.

➤ Cutaneous leishmaniasis

Adults: *Amphotericin B desoxycholate*—If patient tolerates test dose, gradually increase from initial recommended dosage of 0.25 to 0.3 mg/kg daily by slow I.V. infusion (0.1 mg/mL over 2 to 6 hours) until 0.5 to 1 mg/kg daily is reached.

➤ Cutaneous leishmaniasis in patients who cannot tolerate or do not respond to conventional amphotericin B

Adults and children: *Amphotericin B lipid complex*—5 mg/kg/day I.V. for an average duration of approximately 4 weeks

➤ Visceral leishmaniasis in immunocompetent patients

Adults and children ages 1 month and older: *Amphotericin B liposome*—3 mg/kg I.V. over 2 hours on days 1 through 5, 14, and 21. Repeat course if initial treatment fails to clear parasites.

➤ Visceral leishmaniasis in immunocompromised patients

Adults and children ages 1 month and older: *Amphotericin B liposome*—4 mg/kg I.V. over 2 hours on days 1 through 5, 10, 17, 24, 31, and 38

➢ Empiric therapy for presumed fungal infection in febrile neutropenic patients
Adults: *Amphotericin B desoxycholate*—If patient tolerates test dose, gradually increase from initial recommended dosage of 0.25 to 0.3 mg/kg daily by slow I.V. infusion (0.1 mg/mL over 2 to 6 hours) to usual dosage of 0.25 to 1 mg/kg I.V. daily. *Amphotericin B liposome*—3 mg/kg daily given I.V. over 120 minutes for 2 weeks.

Off-label uses

- Chemoprophylaxis in immunocompromised patients
- Coccidioidal arthritis
- *Penicillium marneffei* infection
- Prophylaxis of fungal infections in bone-marrow transplant recipients, primary amoebic meningoencephalitis caused by *Naegleria fowleri*, and ocular aspergillosis

Administration

Preparation

Follow hazardous drug guidelines on page S19 for handling, preparation, and administration of amphotericin B desoxycholate.

- Before starting therapy, stabilize patient's condition, including correcting electrolyte deficiencies. In some patients, hydration and sodium repletion may reduce nephrotoxicity risk and supplemental alkali drugs may decrease renal tubular acidosis.
- Pretreat with antihistamines, antipyretics, or corticosteroids, as prescribed. However, minimize corticosteroid dosages and duration due to risk of increased potassium depletion.

Know that drug should be given only by clinicians thoroughly familiar with drug, its administration, and adverse reactions.

Be aware that drug is used mainly to treat progressive, potentially life-threatening fungal infections. Do not use for noninvasive fungal infections, such as oral thrush, vaginal candidiasis, or esophageal candidiasis in patients with normal neutrophil counts.

Due to widely varying tolerance and clinical status, test dose may be ordered before first dose is given. For conventional amphotericin B (desoxycholate form), test dose is 1 mg in 20 mL D_5W given over 20 to 30 minutes; monitor vital signs every 30 minutes for 2 hours. For amphotericin B cholesteryl sulfate, test dose is 10 mL of final preparation containing 1.6 to 8.3 mg, infused I.V. over 15 to 30 minutes.

Be aware that amphotericin B desoxycholate is the traditional form and that the various amphotericin B forms are not exchangeable from dose to dose or between forms.

Dilution and compatibility

Do not mix any amphotericin B form with sodium chloride, other electrolytes, or bacteriostatic products.

Amphotericin B cholesteryl sulfate—

- Do not filter drug or use inline filter.
- Use 20G needle to reconstitute by rapidly adding 10 mL sterile water for injection to each 50 mg of drug, to achieve 5 mg/mL.
- Shake gently and rotate vial until all solids dissolve. Solution may be opalescent or clear.

• Further dilute with D_5W to achieve final concentration of approximately 0.6 mg/mL, using these guidelines:

Amphotericin B dosage (mg)	Diluent volume (mL)	D_5W solution (mL)
10 to 35	2 to 7	50
35 to 70	7 to 14	100
70 to 175	14 to 35	250
175 to 350	35 to 70	500
350 to 1,000	70 to 200	1,000

Amphotericin B desoxycholate—
• Use inline filter with pores larger than 1 micron.
• To reconstitute initial concentrate of 5 mg/mL, rapidly express 10 mL sterile water for injection without bacteriostatic agent directly into lyophilized cake, using sterile needle (at least 20G) and syringe.
• Shake vial immediately until colloidal solution is clear.
• To obtain infusion solution providing 0.1 mg/mL amphotericin B, dilute further (1:50) with D_5W (with pH above 4.2). Most commercial D_5W injections have pH above 4.2.
Amphotericin B lipid complex—
• Shake vial gently until yellow sediment at bottom is not visible.
• Withdraw exact total daily dose from one or more vials using one or more syringes and 18G needles.
• Replace needle on syringe with 5-micron filter supplied with each vial. Use new filter for each 400 mg (80 mL).
• Empty syringe contents through filter into infusion of D_5W.
• Use 4 mL D_5W for each 1 mL (5 mg) of drug, to achieve final concentration of 1 mg/mL.
• Dilute to final concentration of 2 mg/mL for fluid-restricted patients and children.
• Use clear solution only.
• Discard unused portion.
• Shake diluted solution every 2 hours during administration to ensure even drug distribution.
Amphotericin B liposome—
• Administer with infusion pump and inline filter with pores larger than 1 micron.
• Reconstitute each 50-mg vial with 12 mL sterile water for injection (without bacteriostatic agent), to yield 4 mg/mL.
Do not reconstitute with normal saline solution, add normal saline solution to reconstituted concentration, or mix with other drugs.
• Shake vial vigorously for 30 seconds (yellow translucent suspension will form).
• Withdraw exact total daily dose from one or more vials using one or more 20-mL syringes and needles.
• Replace needle with 5-micron filter supplied with each vial. Use new needle for each 50-mg vial.
• Empty syringe contents through filter into infusion of D_5W.
• Use sufficient diluent to achieve final concentration of 1 to 2 mg/mL.
• Dilute further to a concentration of 0.2 to 0.5 mg/mL for infants and small children, to provide adequate volume for infusion.

Infusion considerations
• Choose distal vein for I.V. site.
• Give through separate I.V. line.
• Flush I.V. line with D_5W before and after infusion.
• Give by slow I.V. infusion as directed for drug form, condition being treated, and patient's clinical status.
• Administer amphotericin B cholesteryl sulfate by I.V. infusion at a rate of 1 mg/kg/hour; if tolerated, may shorten infusion time to 2 hours.

• Give amphotericin B desoxycholate by I.V. infusion over 2 to 6 hours.
• Give amphotericin B lipid complex by I.V. infusion at a rate of 2.5 mg/kg/hour.
• Give amphotericin B liposome by I.V. infusion over 2 hours; if previous infusions were well tolerated, may reduce infusion time to 60 minutes.
Be aware that rapid infusion may cause hypotension, hypokalemia, arrhythmia, and shock.
• If amphotericin B desoxycholate is discontinued for 1 week or longer, restart drug at 0.25 mg/kg daily, and increase dosage gradually.
Know that total daily dosage of amphotericin B desoxycholate should never exceed 1.5 mg/kg.

Monitoring

Monitor for signs and symptoms of infusion-related reactions (fever, chills, hypotension, GI symptoms, breathing difficulties, and headache). If these occur, stop infusion and notify prescriber immediately.
• Know that infusion-related reactions are common within 1 to 3 hours after infusion begins. Usually, they are more severe with first few doses and diminish with subsequent doses.
• Obtain vital signs and temperature every 30 minutes for at least 4 hours after giving test dose.
• Assess fluid intake and output.
• Monitor kidney and liver function test results, hematopoietic function, and serum electrolyte levels.
• Evaluate for signs and symptoms of ototoxicity (hearing loss, tinnitus, ataxia, and vertigo).
• Be aware that giving desoxycholate form on alternate days may decrease anorexia and phlebitis.
• Alternate I.V. sites regularly.

Storage

Amphotericin B cholesteryl sulfate—
• Refrigerate at 2° to 8°C (36° to 46°F) after reconstitution and use within 24 hours. After dilution, refrigerate at 2° to 8°C and use within 24 hours. Discard partially used vials. Store unopened vials at 15 ° to 30°C (59° to 86°F).
Amphotericin B desoxycholate—
• Refrigerate at 2° to 8°C (36° to 46°F), protected from light; keep in carton until use. Concentrate (5 mg/mL after reconstitution with 10 mL sterile water for injection) may be stored in dark at room temperature for 24 hours or refrigerated for 1 week with minimal loss of potency and clarity; discard unused material. Use solutions prepared for I.V. infusion (0.1 mg/mL or less) promptly after preparation, and protect from light during administration.
Amphotericin B lipid complex—
• Before admixture, store at 2° to 8°C (36° to 46°F) and protect from light. Do not freeze. Keep in carton until use. After mixing with D_5W, store for up to 48 hours at 2° to 8°C and for an additional 6 hours at room temperature. Discard any unused drug.
Amphotericin B liposome—
• Store unopened vials at temperatures up to 25°C (77°F). Store reconstituted drug at 2° to 8°C (36° to 46°F) for up to 24 hours. Use within 6 hours after dilution with D_5W. Do not freeze.

Contraindications and precautions

Contraindicated in hypersensitivity to drug, renal dysfunction, and breastfeeding.

Use cautiously in renal impairment, electrolyte abnormalities, pregnant patients, and ***children.***

A

Adverse reactions

CNS: anxiety, confusion, headache, insomnia, weakness, depression, dizziness, drowsiness, hallucinations, speech difficulty, ataxia, vertigo, stupor, psychosis, insomnia, dystonia, myalgia, rigors, asthenia, **seizures**
CV: hypotension, hypertension, tachycardia, phlebitis, chest pain, orthostatic hypotension, vasodilation, arrhythmia, valvular heart disease, **cardiomegaly, systole, atrial fibrillation, bradycardia, cardiac arrest, shock, supraventricular tachycardia**
EENT: double or blurred vision, amblyopia, eye hemorrhage, hearing loss, tinnitus, rhinitis, sinusitis, epistaxis, hemoptysis, pharyngitis
GI: nausea, vomiting, diarrhea, constipation, dyspepsia, flatulence, melena, abdominal pain, abdominal distention, dry mouth, oral inflammation, oral candidiasis, anorexia, gingivitis, stomatitis, **ileus, GI hemorrhage**
GU: painful urination, hematuria, albuminuria, glycosuria, excessive urea buildup, urine of low specific gravity, nephrocalcinosis, **renal failure, renal tubular acidosis, oliguria, anuria**
Hematologic: eosinophilia, normochromic or hypochromic anemia, phlebitis, purpura, **blood transition reaction, hemorrhage, leukocytosis, thrombocytopenia, leukopenia, agranulocytosis, coagulation disorders**
Hepatic: jaundice, **acute hepatic failure, hepatitis, hepatomegaly**
Metabolic: hypomagnesemia, hypokalemia, hypocalcemia, hypernatremia, hyperglycemia, dehydration, hypoproteinemia, hypervolemia, **acidosis**
Musculoskeletal: muscle, joint, neck, back, or bone pain
Respiratory: increased cough, hypoxia, lung disorders, hyperventilation, wheezing, dyspnea, tachypnea, atelectasis, **asthma, bronchospasm, respiratory failure, respiratory alkalosis, pulmonary edema, pleural effusion**
Skin: discoloration, bruising, flushing, pruritus, urticaria, acne, rash, sweating, nodules, skin ulcers, alopecia, dry skin, maculopapular rash
Other: hiccup, chills, fever, infection, peripheral or facial edema, weight changes, herpes simplex, graft vs. host disease, pain or reaction at injection site, tissue damage with extravasation, hypersensitivity reactions including **anaphylaxis, infusion-related reactions, sepsis**

Interactions

Drug-drug. *Antineoplastics (such as mechlorethamine):* renal toxicity, bronchospasm, hypotension
Cardiac glycosides: increased risk of digitalis toxicity (in potassium-depleted patients)
Corticosteroids: increased potassium depletion
Cyclosporine, tacrolimus: increased creatinine levels
Flucytosine: increased flucytosine toxicity
Imidazoles (clotrimazole, fluconazole, ketoconazole, miconazole): antagonism of amphotericin B effects
Leukocyte transfusion: pulmonary reactions
Nephrotoxic drugs (such as aminoglycoside antibiotics, pentamidine): increased risk of renal toxicity
Skeletal muscle relaxants: increased skeletal muscle relaxation
Thiazides: increased electrolyte depletion
Zidovudine: increased myelotoxicity and nephrotoxicity
Drug-diagnostic tests. *Alanine aminotransferase, alkaline phosphatase, amylase, aspartate aminotransferase, bilirubin,*

blood urea nitrogen, creatinine, gamma-glutamyltransferase, lactate dehydrogenase, nitrogenous compounds (urea), uric acid: increased
Calcium, hemoglobin, magnesium, platelets, potassium, protein: decreased
Eosinophils, glucose, white blood cells: increased or decreased
Liver function tests: abnormal results
Prothrombin time: prolonged or decreased
Drug-herb. *Gossypol:* increased risk of renal toxicity

Toxicity and overdose

• Overdose can lead to cardiorespiratory arrest.
• Discontinue therapy and monitor patient's clinical status (cardiorespiratory, renal, and liver function; hematologic status; and serum electrolytes). Provide supportive interventions as indicated. Drug is not hemodialyzable.

Patient teaching

Advise patient to contact prescriber immediately if fever, chills, headache, vomiting, diarrhea, cough, or breathing problems occur.
• Instruct patient to report hearing loss, dizziness, or unsteady gait.
• Caution patient to avoid driving and other hazardous activities until drug's effects on concentration, alertness, and vision are known.
• Instruct patient to drink plenty of fluids.
• Tell patient to monitor urine output and notify prescriber of significant changes.
• Advise patient to minimize GI upset by eating small, frequent servings of food.
• Inform patient about the need for frequent laboratory and other testing during therapy.
• As appropriate, review all other significant and life-threatening adverse reactions and interactions, especially those related to the drugs, tests, and herbs mentioned above.

ampicillin sodium

Ampicin ✤, Penbritin ✤ ❉, Rimacillin ❉

Pharmacologic class: Aminopenicillin
Therapeutic class: Anti-infective
Pregnancy risk category B

Action

Destroys bacteria by inhibiting bacterial cell-wall synthesis during microbial multiplication

Pharmacokinetics

Drug is distributed into cerebrospinal fluid (in presence of inflamed meninges) and into peritoneal fluid, tissue fluid, and intestinal mucosa. It is approximately 20% reversibly protein-bound. Approximately 75% to 85% of dose is excreted unchanged in urine.

Onset	Peak	Duration
Immediate	Unknown	Variable

How supplied

Powder for reconstitution for injection: 125 mg, 250 mg, 500 mg, 1 g, 2 g, 10 g

Indications and dosages

➤ Respiratory tract, skin, and soft-tissue infections caused by *Haemophilus influenzae,* staphylococci, and streptococci
Adults and children weighing 40 kg (88 lb) or more: 250 to 500 mg I.V. q 6 hours
Adults and children weighing less than 40 kg: 25 to 50 mg/kg/day I.V. in divided doses q 6 to 8 hours

A

➢ Bacterial meningitis caused by *Neisseria meningitidis, Escherichia coli,* group B streptococci, or *Listeria monocytogenes*; septicemia caused by *Streptococcus* species, penicillin G-susceptible staphylococci, enterococci, *E. coli, Proteus mirabilis,* or *Salmonella* species
Adults: 150 to 200 mg/kg/day by continuous I.V. infusion in equally divided doses q 3 to 4 hours, to a maximum dosage of 14 g
Children: 100 to 200 mg/kg/day I.V. in divided doses q 3 to 4 hours
➢ GI or urinary tract infections, including *Neisseria gonorrhoeae* infection in women
Adults and children weighing more than 40 kg (88 lb): 500 mg I.V. q 6 hours
Adults and children weighing 40 kg or less: 50 to 100 mg/kg/day I.V. in equally divided doses q 6 to 8 hours
➢ Endocarditis prophylaxis for dental, oral, or upper respiratory tract procedures
Adults: 2 g I.V. within 30 minutes before procedure
Children: 50 mg/kg I.V. within 30 minutes before procedure
➢ To prevent bacterial endocarditis before GI or genitourinary surgery or instrumentation
High-risk adults: 2 g I.V. with gentamicin 1.5 mg/kg I.V. within 30 minutes before procedure, followed 6 hours later by 1 g I.V.
High-risk children: 50 mg/kg I.V. with 1.5 mg/kg gentamicin I.V. within 30 minutes before procedure, followed 6 hours later by 25 mg/kg I.V.
Moderate-risk adults: 2 g I.V. within 30 minutes before procedure
Moderate-risk children: 50 mg/kg I.V. within 30 minutes before procedure
➢ Prophylaxis for neonatal group B streptococcal disease
Adult females: During labor, loading dose of 2 g I.V.; then 1 g I.V. every 4 hours until delivery
➢ *N. gonorrhoeae* infections
Adult males: 1,000 mg I.V. in two divided doses given at 8- to 12-hour intervals
Adult females and children weighing 40 kg (88 lb) or more: 500 mg I.V. q 6 hours
Children weighing less than 40 kg: 50 mg/kg/day I.V. in divided doses q 6 to 8 hours
➢ Urethritis caused by *N. gonorrhoeae* (in males)
Adults and children weighing 40 kg (88 lb) or more: 500 mg I.V., repeated 8 to 12 hours later

Dosage adjustment

- Change dosing interval to every 6 to 12 hours if creatinine clearance is 10 to 50 mL/minute or to every 12 hours if clearance is less than 10 mL/minute.

Administration

Preparation

- Ask patient about penicillin allergy before giving drug.

Dilution and compatibility

- Mix powder with at least 5 mL of bacteriostatic water for injection.
- For intermittent I.V. infusion, mix with 50 to 100 mL normal saline solution.
- Do not mix or give through same line with aminoglycosides, as this inactivates ampicillin.

Infusion considerations

- For direct I.V. injection, give over 3 to 5 minutes (250 to 500 mg) or over 10 to 15 minutes (1 to 2 g). Do not exceed 100 mg/minute.
- For intermittent I.V. infusion, give over 15 to 30 minutes.

🔈 Be aware that too-rapid infusion may cause seizures.

Monitoring

- Watch for signs and symptoms of hypersensitivity reaction.

🔈 Monitor for seizures when giving high doses.

- Frequently obtain patient's temperature and check for other signs and symptoms of superinfection, especially oral or rectal candidiasis.

Monitor for bruising and other signs of bleeding.

- Monitor CBC and liver function test results.
- Change I.V. site every 48 hours.

Storage

- Drug is stable for 8 hours at concentrations up to 30 mg/mL in bacteriostatic water for injection or normal saline solution.

Contraindications and precautions

Contraindicated in hypersensitivity to penicillin, cephalosporins, imipenem, or other beta-lactamase inhibitors.

Use cautiously in severe renal insufficiency, infectious mononucleosis, and pregnant or breastfeeding patients.

Adverse reactions

CNS: lethargy, hallucinations, anxiety, confusion, agitation, depression, fatigue, dizziness, **seizures**
CV: vein irritation, **thrombophlebitis, heart failure**
EENT: blurred vision, itchy eyes
GI: nausea, vomiting, diarrhea, abdominal pain, enterocolitis, gastritis, stomatitis, glossitis, black "hairy" tongue, furry tongue, oral or rectal candidiasis, **pseudomembranous colitis**
GU: vaginitis, nephropathy, **interstitial nephritis**
Hematologic: anemia, eosinophilia, **agranulocytosis, hemolytic anemia, leukopenia, thrombocytopenic purpura, thrombocytopenia, neutropenia**
Hepatic: nonspecific hepatitis
Musculoskeletal: arthritis exacerbation
Respiratory: wheezing, dyspnea, hypoxia, **apnea**
Skin: rashes, urticaria, fever, diaphoresis
Other: pain at injection site, superinfections, hyperthermia, hypersensitivity reaction, **anaphylaxis, serum sickness**

Interactions

Drug-drug. *Allopurinol:* increased risk of rashes
Chloramphenicol: synergistic or antagonistic effects
Hormonal contraceptives: decreased contraceptive efficacy, increased risk of breakthrough bleeding
Probenecid: decreased renal excretion of ampicillin, increased ampicillin blood level
Tetracyclines: reduced bactericidal effect
Drug-diagnostic tests. *Conjugated estrone, estradiol, estriol-glucuronide, total conjugated estriols:* increased levels in pregnant patients
Coombs' test, urine glucose: false-positive
Eosinophils: increased
Granulocytes, hemoglobin, platelets, white blood cells: decreased

Toxicity and overdose

- In serious overdose, expect extension of adverse reactions affecting neurologic, cardiovascular, genitourinary, hematologic, hepatic, and respiratory systems.
- Discontinue drug. In hypersensitivity reaction, expect to give antihistamines, epinephrine, and corticosteroids if necessary. Know that ampicillin may be removed from circulation by hemodialysis.

Patient teaching

Instruct patient to immediately report signs and symptoms of hypersensitivity reaction, such as rash, fever, or chills.

Advise patient to promptly report unusual bleeding or bruising.

- Teach patient to avoid activities that can cause injury. Advise patient to use soft toothbrush and electric razor to avoid gum and skin injury.

- Inform patient that drug lowers resistance to certain other infections. Tell patient to report new signs or symptoms of infection, especially in mouth or rectum.
- Advise patient to minimize GI upset by eating small, frequent servings of food and drinking plenty of fluids.
- Inform patient about the need for regular blood testing during therapy.
- Teach patient taking hormonal contraceptives that drug may reduce contraceptive efficacy; advise her to use alternative birth control method.
- As appropriate, review all other significant and life-threatening adverse reactions and interactions, especially those related to the drugs and tests mentioned above.

ampicillin sodium and sulbactam sodium

Unasyn

Pharmacologic class: Aminopenicillin/beta-lactamase inhibitor
Therapeutic class: Anti-infective
Pregnancy risk category B

Action

Destroys bacteria by inhibiting bacterial cell-wall synthesis during microbial multiplication. Addition of sulbactam enhances drug's resistance to beta-lactamase, an enzyme that can inactivate ampicillin.

Pharmacokinetics

Both drugs are distributed to peritoneal, blister, and tissue fluid and to intestinal mucosa and inflamed meninges. Ampicillin is approximately 28% reversibly protein-bound; sulbactam, 38% reversibly protein-bound. Both drugs have a mean half-life of approximately 1 hour. Higher and more prolonged serum levels occur with concurrent probenecid administration. Approximately 75% to 85% of dose of both drugs is excreted unchanged in urine during first 8 hours in patients with normal renal function.

Onset	Peak	Duration
Rapid	End of infusion	Variable

How supplied

Powder for reconstitution for injection (white to off-white): Vials, piggyback vials containing 1.5 g (1 g ampicillin sodium and 0.5 g sulbactam sodium), 3 g (2 g ampicillin sodium and 1 g sulbactam sodium), and 15 g (10 g ampicillin sodium and 5 g sulbactam sodium)

Indications and dosages

➤ Intra-abdominal, gynecologic, and skin-structure infections caused by susceptible beta-lactamase-producing strains

Adults and children weighing 40 kg (88 lb) or more: 1.5 to 3 g (1 g ampicillin and 0.5 g sulbactam to 2 g ampicillin and 1 g sulbactam) I.V. q 6 hours. Maximum dosage is 4 g sulbactam daily.
Children age 1 year and older: 75 mg (50 mg ampicillin and 25 mg sulbactam)/kg I.V. q 6 hours

Dosage adjustment

- In renal impairment, give doses less frequently, as shown below. (Ratio of one drug to the other remains constant regardless of renal function).

Dosages In Renal Impairment

Creatinine clearance (mL/min/1.73 m^2)	Recommended dosage
30 or greater	1.5 to 3 g q 6 to 8 hr
15 to 29	1.5 to 3 g q 12 hr
5 to 14	1.5 to 3 g q 24 hr

Administration

Preparation

- Ask patient about penicillin allergy before giving.
- In children, do not routinely exceed 14 days of I.V. therapy.

Dilution and compatibility

- Do not mix with other drugs.
- Know that dry powder is freely soluble in aqueous diluent to yield pale yellow to yellow solution.
- Reconstitute powder with at least 3.2 mL of sterile water for injection.
- Before administering, let vial stand several minutes until foam evaporates, to permit visual inspection for complete solubilization.
- Do not mix or give through same I.V. line with aminoglycosides, as this inactivates ampicillin/sulbactam.
- Must be further diluted for direct or intermittent infusion in D_5W, normal saline solution, lactated Ringer's solution, or D_5W in one-half normal saline solution to a concentration of 5 to 45 mg/mL
- Give final diluted solution within time prescribed to ensure proper potency.

Infusion considerations

- Administer direct I.V. dose over 10 to 15 minutes.
- Give intermittent I.V. infusion in 50 to 100 mL of compatible solution over 15 to 30 minutes.

Be aware that too-rapid infusion may cause seizures.

Monitoring

- Monitor for signs and symptoms of hypersensitivity reaction.
- Check for signs of infection at injection site.

Monitor for seizures when giving high doses.

Monitor for bruising and other signs of bleeding.

- Check patient's temperature and watch for other signs and symptoms of superinfection, especially oral or rectal candidiasis.
- Monitor CBC and liver function test results.
- Change I.V. site every 48 hours.

Storage

- Store at or below 30°C (86°F) before reconstitution.

Contraindications and precautions

Contraindicated in hypersensitivity to penicillins, cephalosporins, imipenem, or other beta-lactamase inhibitors.

Use cautiously in severe renal insufficiency, infectious mononucleosis, and pregnant or breastfeeding patients.

Adverse reactions

CNS: lethargy, hallucinations, anxiety, confusion, agitation, depression, fatigue, dizziness, **seizures**

CV: vein irritation, **thrombophlebitis, heart failure**

EENT: blurred vision, itchy eyes

GI: nausea, vomiting, diarrhea, abdominal pain, enterocolitis, gastritis, stomatitis, glossitis, black "hairy" tongue, furry tongue, oral and rectal candidiasis, **pseudomembranous colitis**

GU: hematuria, hyaline casts in urine, vaginitis, nephropathy, **interstitial nephritis**

Hematologic: anemia, eosinophilia, **agranulocytosis, hemolytic anemia, leukopenia, thrombocytopenic purpura, thrombocytopenia, neutropenia**

Hepatic: nonspecific hepatitis

Musculoskeletal: arthritis exacerbation

Respiratory: wheezing, dyspnea, hypoxia, **apnea**

Skin: rash, urticaria, diaphoresis

Other: pain at injection site, fever, hyperthermia, superinfections, hypersensitivity reactions, **anaphylaxis, serum sickness**

Interactions

Drug-drug. *Allopurinol:* increased risk of rashes
Chloramphenicol: synergistic or antagonistic effects
Hormonal contraceptives: decreased contraceptive efficacy, increased risk of breakthrough bleeding
Probenecid: decreased renal excretion and increased blood level of ampicillin
Tetracyclines: reduced bactericidal effects
Drug-diagnostic tests. *Alanine aminotransferase, alkaline phosphatase, aspartate aminotransferase, bilirubin, blood urea nitrogen, creatine kinase, creatinine, gamma-glutamyltransferase, eosinophils, lactate dehydrogenase:* increased
Estradiol, estriol-glucuronide, granulocytes, hemoglobin, lymphocytes, neutrophils, platelets, white blood cells: decreased
Coombs' test: false-positive
Urinalysis: red blood cells, hyaline casts

Toxicity and overdose

- In serious overdose, expect extension of adverse reactions affecting neurologic, cardiovascular, genitourinary, hematologic, hepatic, and respiratory systems. If cerebrospinal fluid reaches high levels of beta-lactams, expect neurologic adverse reactions, including seizures.
- Discontinue drug. For hypersensitivity reaction, expect to give antihistamines, epinephrine, and corticosteroids as necessary. Know that ampicillin and possibly sulbactam may be removed by hemodialysis.

Patient teaching

(Clinical alert) Instruct patient to immediately report signs and symptoms of hypersensitivity reaction, such as rash, fever, or chills.
(Clinical alert) Tell patient to report unusual bleeding or bruising.
- Instruct patient to avoid activities that can cause injury, and to use soft toothbrush and electric razor to avoid gum and skin injury.
- Inform patient that drug lowers resistance to certain infections. Instruct patient to report new signs or symptoms of infection, especially in mouth or rectum.
- Tell patient to report signs and symptoms of infection or other problems at injection site.
- Advise patient to minimize GI upset by eating small, frequent servings of food and drinking plenty of fluids.
- Inform patient taking hormonal contraceptives that drug may reduce contraceptive efficacy. Advise her to use alternative birth control method.
- Inform patient about the need for regular blood testing during therapy.
- As appropriate, review all other significant and life-threatening adverse reactions and interactions, especially those related to the drugs and tests mentioned above.

anidulafungin

Eraxis

Pharmacologic class: Semisynthetic echinocandin
Therapeutic class: Antifungal
Pregnancy risk category C

Action

Inhibits glucan synthase, an enzyme present in fungal (but not mammalian) cells; this action inhibits formation of 1,3-beta-D-glucan, an essential component of fungal cell wall.

Pharmacokinetics

After I.V. administration, drug has short distribution half-life (0.5 to 1 hour) and a volume of distribution (30 to 50 L) similar to total body fluid volume. It is moderately bound (84%) to plasma proteins. Clearance is approximately 1 L/hour, with terminal elimination half-life of 40 to 50 hours. Drug is excreted in feces and, to a lesser extent, in urine.

Onset	Peak	Duration
Unknown	Unknown	Unknown

How supplied

Powder for reconstitution for injection (lyophilized, preservative-free, white to off-white): 50-mg single-use vial

Indications and dosages

➢ Candidemia and other *Candida* infections (intra-abdominal abscess, peritonitis)

Adults: Single 200-mg loading dose by I.V. infusion on day 1, followed by 100 mg I.V. daily thereafter. Treatment duration depends on clinical response; generally, therapy continues for at least 14 days after last positive culture.

➢ Esophageal candidiasis

Adults: Single 100-mg loading dose by I.V. infusion on day 1, followed by 50 mg I.V. daily thereafter. Treatment should continue for at least 14 days, and for at least 7 days after symptoms resolve; duration depends on clinical response. Due to risk of esophageal candidiasis relapse in patients with HIV, suppressive antifungal therapy may be considered after treatment ends.

Administration

Dilution and compatibility

- Reconstitute only with supplied diluent (20% dehydrated alcohol in water for injection).
- Further dilute only with 5% dextrose or normal saline solution, to yield infusion solution concentration of 0.5 mg/mL.
- Give by I.V. infusion within 24 hours of reconstitution.
- Do not dilute with other solutions or infuse through same I.V. line with other drugs or electrolytes.

Infusion considerations

Do not give by I.V. bolus.

Do not infuse at a rate exceeding 1.1 mg/minute.

Monitoring

If patient has abnormal liver function tests during therapy, monitor for evidence of worsening hepatic function, and weigh risks and benefits of continuing therapy.

- Monitor for rash, urticaria, flushing, dyspnea, and hypotension. (However, these are rare when drug is given slowly).

Storage

- Store unreconstituted vials, reconstituted solution, diluted solution, and infusion solution at 25°C (77°F); excursions permitted to 15° to 30°C (59° to 86°F). Do not freeze.

Contraindications and precautions

Contraindicated in hypersensitivity to drug, its components, or other echinocandins.

Use cautiously in hepatic impairment, pregnant or breastfeeding patients, and ***children*** (safety and efficacy not established).

Adverse reactions

CNS: headache
CV: hypotension, phlebitis
GI: aggravated dyspepsia, nausea, vomiting, diarrhea
Hematologic: neutropenia, leukopenia
Respiratory: dyspnea
Skin: rash, urticaria, pruritus, flushing
Other: fever

A

Interactions

Drug-diagnostic tests. *Alanine aminotransferase, alkaline phosphatase, aspartate aminotransferase, gamma-glutamyltransferase:* increased
Potassium: decreased

Toxicity and overdose

- No overdoses have been reported. Expect signs and symptoms to include transaminase elevations.
- Provide symptomatic interventions. Know that drug is not dialyzable.

Patient teaching

Instruct patient to report rash, itching, unusual bruising or bleeding, unusual tiredness, or yellowing of skin or eyes.

- Advise patient to report troublesome adverse effects, such as GI upset.
- As appropriate, review all other significant adverse reactions and interactions, especially those related to the tests mentioned above.

antihemophilic factor (AHF, factor VIII)

Advate, Alphanate, Bioclate, HelixateFS, Hemofil M, Hyate:C, Koate-DVI, Kogenate FS, Monarc-M, Monoclate-P, Recombinate, ReFacto

Pharmacologic class: Blood product derivative
Therapeutic class: Antihemophilic
Pregnancy risk category C

FDA BOXED WARNING

- Drug is made from human plasma and may contain infectious agents. Plasma donor screening, testing, and inactivation or removal methods reduce this risk.

Action

Promotes conversion of prothrombin to thrombin (needed for hemostasis and blood clotting); also replaces missing or deficient clotting factors, thereby controlling or preventing bleeding

Pharmacokinetics

Drug clears rapidly from plasma. Half-life is approximately 10 to 18 hours.

Onset	Peak	Duration
Immediate	Unknown	Unknown

How supplied

Powder for reconstitution for injection (nonpyrogenic, concentrated or lyophilized): 250, 500, 1,000, 1,500, 2,000, and 3,000 units/vial in numerous preparations

Indications and dosages

➤ Spontaneous hemorrhage in patients with hemophilia A (factor VIII deficiency)

Adults and children: Dosage is highly individualized, depending on patient's weight, severity of deficiency and hemorrhage, presence of inhibitors, and factor VIII level desired. Dosage is calculated as follows: AHF required (units) equals weight (kg) multiplied by desired factor VIII increase (% of normal) multiplied by 0.5.

To control bleeding, desired factor VIII level is 20% to 40% of normal for minor hemorrhage (early hemarthrosis, muscle bleed, or oral bleed), 30% to 60% of normal for moderate hemorrhage (more extensive hemarthrosis, muscle bleed, or hematoma), or 60% to 100% of normal for severe hemorrhage (head injury, throat bleed, severe abdominal pain).

To prevent spontaneous hemorrhage, desired factor VIII level is 5% of normal; for minor surgery (tooth extraction) desired level is 60% to 80% (60% to 100% for Advate only) of normal, accomplished by a single infusion plus oral antifibrinolytic within 1 hour; 80% to 100% (80% to 120% for Advate only) before and after surgery, repeated q 8 to 24 hours depending on healing state for major surgery.

Administration

Preparation

- Before giving, verify that patient does not have history of hypersensitivity to drug or mouse, hamster, or bovine protein.
- Follow prescriber's instructions regarding hepatitis B prophylaxis before starting therapy.
- Keep in mind that although infusion dosage and frequency can be calculated, preferably appropriate laboratory tests (including serial AHF assays) should be performed on plasma at suitable intervals to ensure adequate AHF levels have been reached and are maintained.
- Monitor pulse rate before administration; notify prescriber if it is rapid.

Dilution and compatibility

- Warm bottles of concentrate and diluent to room temperature before mixing.
- Roll bottle gently between hands until drug is well mixed.
- Follow manufacturer's directions for dilution. Use only diluent provided with specific product.
- After drug is reconstituted, do not shake.
- Do not mix with other I.V. solutions.
- Use filter and plastic syringe; do not allow drug to contact glass (to prevent binding to glass surfaces).
- Administer within 3 hours of reconstitution.

Infusion considerations

- Initiate at a rate of approximately 2 mL/minute; can increase gradually to 10 mL/minute, as tolerated.
- Give total dose over 5 to 10 minutes.

Monitoring

Monitor for signs and symptoms of anaphylaxis; be prepared to intervene appropriately.

Be aware that intravascular hemolysis may occur in patients with blood group A, B, or AB who receive large or frequently repeated doses; monitor hematocrit and direct Coombs' test results. Correct hemolytic anemia with compatible group O red blood cells or AHF from group-specific plasma.

Watch for bleeding tendency and hemorrhage.

Assess for severe headache, which may indicate intracranial hemorrhage.

- Monitor CBC and coagulation studies.
- Continue to monitor vital signs, especially pulse rate, during administration. If pulse rate increases significantly, slow administration rate or temporarily halt injection to allow symptoms to disappear.

Storage

- Refrigerate concentrate until ready to reconstitute drug.
- After drug is reconstituted, do not refrigerate or store near heat.
- For all products except Hyate:C, refrigerate at 2° to 8°C (36° to 46°F) or at room temperature, not to exceed 30°C (86°F). Store Hyate:C at –20° to –15°C (–4° to 5°F).

Contraindications and precautions

Contraindicated in hypersensitivity to drug or mouse, hamster, or bovine protein.

Use cautiously in hepatic disease; blood types A, B, and AB; patients receiving factor VIII inhibitors; pregnant patients; and ***neonates*** and ***infants***.

Adverse reactions

CNS: headache; lethargy; fatigue; dizziness; jitteriness; drowsiness; depersonalization; tingling in arms, ears, and face; intracranial hemorrhage

CV: chest tightness, angina pectoris, tachycardia, slight hypotension, thrombosis
EENT: blurred or abnormal vision, eye disorder, otitis media, epistaxis, rhinitis, sore throat
GI: nausea, vomiting, diarrhea, constipation, stomachache, abdominal pain, gastroenteritis, anorexia
Hematologic: increased bleeding tendency, thrombocytopenia, hemolytic anemia, intravascular hemolysis, hyperfibrinogenemia
Musculoskeletal: myalgia, muscle weakness, bone pain, finger pain
Respiratory: dyspnea, coughing, wheezing, **bronchospasm**
Skin: rash, acne, flushing, diaphoresis, urticaria
Other: taste changes, fever, chills, cold feet, cold sensations, infected hematoma, stinging or bleeding at injection site, allergic reactions (including **anaphylaxis), risk of viral transmission (including hepatitis B and HIV)**

Interactions

Drug-diagnostic tests. *Bilirubin, creatine kinase:* increased *Hemoglobin, platelets:* decreased

Toxicity and overdose

- No information on overdose is available.
- If overdose occurs, discontinue drug immediately and provide symptomatic and supportive interventions.

Patient teaching

- [Clinical alert] Instruct patient to immediately report signs and symptoms of allergic response (such as rash, tightness in chest, respiratory difficulty, hives, itching, low-grade fever), bleeding tendency, and sudden-onset headache.
- [Clinical alert] Advise patient to immediately report signs and symptoms of hepatitis (such as low-grade fever, anorexia, nausea, vomiting, fatigue, dark urine, or yellowing of skin or eyes).
- Caution patient not to take aspirin during therapy.
- Instruct patient to contact prescriber if drug becomes less effective.
- Advise patient to avoid driving and other hazardous activities until drug's effects on concentration, alertness, and vision are known.
- Notify patient about the need for regular blood testing during therapy.
- As appropriate, review all other significant and life-threatening adverse reactions and interactions, especially those related to the tests mentioned above.

[redacted]

antihemophilic factor/von Willebrand factor complex (human), dried, pasteurized

Humate-P

Pharmacologic class: Blood product derivative
Therapeutic class: Antihemophilic
Pregnancy risk category C

Action

Of the two noncovalently bound proteins (factor VIII and von Willebrand factor) that drug contains, factor VIII is crucial in inactivating factor X, ultimately leading to formation of thrombin and fibrin (needed for hemostasis and blood clotting); von Willebrand factor promotes platelet aggregation and adhesion on vascular endothelium and serves as a stabilizing carrier protein for procoagulant protein factor VIII.

Pharmacokinetics

Drug clears rapidly from plasma; other pharmacokinetic factors vary widely. Median terminal half-life of von Willebrand factor is 11 hours (range, 3.5 to 33.6 hours); in hemophilia A, mean half-life is 12.2 hours (range, 8.4 to 17.4 hours).

Onset	Peak	Duration
Immediate	Unknown	Unknown

How supplied

Powder for reconstitution for I.V. infusion (human-derived; contains albumin; dried, pasteurized preparation): 250 international units factor VIII (factor VIII:C) and 600 international units von Willebrand factor (VWF:RCo)/single-dose vial with 5 mL diluent; 500 international units factor VIII:C and 1,200 international units VWF:RCo/single-dose vial with 10 mL diluent; 1,000 international units factor VIII:C and 2,400 international units VWF:RCo/single-dose vial with 15 mL diluent

Indications and dosages

➢ Prevention and treatment of hemorrhagic episodes in patients with hemophilia A

Adults: Dosage is highly individualized, based on patient weight, hemorrhage severity, plasma factor VIII activity, and presence of factor VIII inhibitors. For dosage recommendations, see table below:

Minor hemorrhage

- Early joint or muscle bleed
- Severe epistaxis

Loading dose (international units of factor VIII:C/kg)

15 international units/kg I.V. infusion to achieve factor VIII:C plasma level of approximately 30% of normal. One infusion may be sufficient. If needed, may give half of loading dose once or twice daily for 1 to 2 days.

Moderate hemorrhage

- Advanced joint or muscle bleed
- Neck, tongue, or pharyngeal hematoma (without airway compromise)
- Tooth extraction
- Severe abdominal pain

Loading dose (international units of factor VIII:C/kg)

25 international units//kg I.V. infusion to achieve factor VIII:C plasma level of approximately 50% of normal, followed by 15 international units/kg q 8 to 12 hours for 1 to 2 days to maintain factor VIII:C plasma level at 30% of normal. Repeat same dose once or twice daily for up to 7 days or until adequate wound healing occurs.

Life-threatening hemorrhage

- Major surgery
- GI hemorrhage
- Neck, tongue, or pharyngeal hematoma (with risk of airway compromise)
- Intracranial, intra-abdominal, or intrathoracic bleeding
- Fracture

Loading dose (international units of factor VIII:C/kg)

40 to 50 international units/kg I.V. infusion, followed by 20 to 25 international units/kg q 8 hours to maintain factor VIII:C plasma level at 80% to 100% of normal for 7 days. Continue same dose once or twice daily for another 7 days to maintain factor VIII:C level at 30% to 50% of normal.

➢ Spontaneous or trauma-induced hemorrhage and prevention of excessive bleeding during and after surgery in patients with severe von Willebrand disease (VWD) and in mild or moderate VWD where desmopressin use is known or suspected to be inadequate

Adults and children: Dosage is highly individualized based on extent and location of bleeding and coagulation studies. As a rule, 40 to 80 international units VWF:RCo (corresponding to 17 to 33

international units factor VIII:C in Humate-P)/kg by I.V. infusion q 8 to 12 hours. Repeat doses for as long as needed. Recommended dosages are as follows:
Type 1, mild (if desmopressin is not appropriate)—For major hemorrhage, loading dose of 40 to 60 international units/kg by I.V. infusion and maintenance dose of 40 to 50 international units/kg q 8 to 12 hours for 3 days, keeping VWF:RCo nadir above 50%; follow with 40 to 50 international units/kg daily for up to 7 days.
Type 1, moderate or severe—For minor hemorrhage, 40 to 50 international units/kg for one or two doses. For major hemorrhage, loading dose of 50 to 75 international units/kg by I.V. infusion and maintenance dose of 40 to 60 international units/kg q 8 to12 hours for 3 days, keeping VWF:RCo nadir above 50%; then 40 to 60 international units/kg daily for a maximum of 7 days.
Types 2 and 3—For minor hemorrhage, 40 to 50 international units/kg for one or two doses. For major hemorrhage, loading dose of 60 to 80 international units/kg by I.V. infusion and maintenance dose of 40 to 60 international units/kg every 8 to 12 hours for 3 days, keeping VWF:RCo nadir above 50%; then 40 to 60 international units/kg daily for maximum of 7 days.

Dosage adjustment

• Adjust dosage as needed based on drug trough levels.

Administration

Preparation

• Know that prescriber must determine if coagulation disorder is caused by factor VIII or von Willebrand factor (VWF), because drug yields no benefit in other coagulation disorders.
• Be aware that dosage must always be adjusted individually based on clinical judgment of potential for compromise of vital structures and by frequent monitoring of plasma factor VIII activity.
• Know that in general, 1 international unit/kg factor VIII should raise factor VIII level by approximately 2 units/dL.
• Strongly consider giving hepatitis A and B vaccine before administering this drug, if indicated and ordered.
• Obtain coagulation studies before starting therapy.

Dilution and compatibility

• Know that drug is packaged with diluent and Mix2Vial filter transfer set. Use only diluent supplied.
• Warm drug and diluent in unopened vials to room temperature no higher than 37° C (98° F).
• Open Mix2Vial package by peeling away lid. Grip Mix2Vial together with clear packaging, and firmly snap blue end onto diluent stopper.
• While holding onto diluent vial, carefully remove clear outer packaging from Mix2Vial set while making sure only clear outer packaging (not Mix2Vial) is pulled up.
• With drug vial firmly on a surface, invert diluent vial with set attached, and firmly snap transparent adaptor onto drug vial stopper. Diluent will automatically transfer by vacuum into drug vial.
• With drug and diluent vials still attached, gently swirl drug vial to ensure drug dissolves fully. Do not shake.
• With one hand, grasp drug side of Mix2Vial set; with other hand, grasp blue diluent side of Mix2Vial set and unscrew set into two pieces.
• Inject air into drug vial. While keeping syringe plunger pressed, invert system upside down and draw concentrate into syringe by pulling plunger back slowly.
• Firmly grasp syringe barrel while keeping plunger facing down, and unscrew syringe from Mix2Vial. Attach syringe to venipuncture set.

• Be aware that a few small flakes may remain, but these should be removed by Mix2Vial set filter.
• Administer within 3 hours of reconstitution.

Infusion considerations
• Infuse I.V. slowly at a maximum rate of 4 mL/minute.

Monitoring
Monitor for allergic reactions, including anaphylaxis; intervene appropriately.
Watch for bleeding tendency and hemorrhage.
Assess for severe headache (may indicate intracranial hemorrhage).
Closely monitor patient with VWD who has other thrombotic risk factors.
Because drug contains blood group isoagglutinins (anti-A and anti-B), monitor for signs of intravascular hemolysis and decreasing hematocrit in patients with type A, B, or AB who are receiving large or frequent doses.
• Monitor CBC and coagulation studies.
• Continue to monitor vital signs during administration.
• Monitor trough levels for both factors. For either factor, level should not exceed 100 international units/dL when drug is given for excessive bleeding during surgery.

Storage
• Refrigerate at 2° to 8°C (36° to 46°F). Avoid freezing.
• Know that drug also may be stored at room temperature not exceeding 30°C (86°F) for up to 6 months.
• Do not refrigerate after reconstitution, as precipitation may occur.

Contraindications and precautions

Contraindicated in patients with history of anaphylactic or severe systemic response to antihemophilic factor or VWF and in patients with hypersensitivity to any drug component.

Use cautiously in patients with VWD who have other thrombotic risk factors, pregnant or breastfeeding patients, and in ***children*** with hemophilia A (safety and efficacy not established).

Adverse reactions

CNS: paresthesia, **cerebral hemorrhage, subdural hematoma**
CV: phlebitis, vasodilation, **thrombosis**
EENT: epistaxis, ear bleeding
GI: nausea, **GI hemorrhage**
GU: hematuria, menorrhagia
Hematologic: increased bleeding tendency, thrombocytopenia, hemolytic anemia, intravascular hemolysis, hyperfibrinogenemia, postoperative hemorrhage
Musculoskeletal: extremity pain
Respiratory: hemoptysis
Other: pain; chills; peripheral edema; postoperative wound or injection-site bleeding; groin or shoulder bleeding; allergic reactions, including urticaria, chest tightness, rash, pruritus, edema, **shock,** and **anaphylaxis; risk of viral transmission (including parvovirus, hepatitis B, HIV, and possibly Creutzfeldt-Jakob disease)**

Interactions

Drug-diagnostic tests. *Bilirubin, creatine kinase:* increased
Hematocrit, hemoglobin, platelets: decreased

Toxicity and overdose

• If overdose occurs, monitor for signs of intravascular hemolysis and decreasing hematocrit.
• Discontinue drug and provide symptomatic and supportive interventions.

Patient teaching

Instruct patient to immediately report signs and symptoms of allergic response (such as rash, tightness in chest, respiratory difficulty, hives, itching, low-grade fever), bleeding tendency, or sudden-onset headache.

Advise patient to immediately report signs and symptoms of parvovirus (such as low-grade fever, rash, arthralgia, or arthritis).

Instruct patient to immediately report signs and symptoms of hepatitis A or B (such as low-grade fever, anorexia, nausea, vomiting, fatigue, dark urine, or yellowing of skin or eyes).

- Caution patient not to use aspirin during therapy.
- Notify patient about the need for regular blood testing during therapy.
- As appropriate, review all other significant and life-threatening adverse reactions and interactions, especially those related to the tests mentioned above.

anti-inhibitor coagulant complex

Autoplex-T, Feiba VH

Pharmacologic class: Blood product derivative, hemostatic

Therapeutic class: Antihemophilic

Pregnancy risk category C

Action

Contains factors II, IX, and X mainly in nonactive form, and factor VII, mainly in active form in approximately equal units of factor VIII inhibitor-bypassing activity. Also contains prothrombin complex factors and factor VIII coagulant antigen. Drug shortens activated partial thromboplastin time (APTT) of plasma containing factor VIII inhibitor, correcting clotting time to normal levels.

Pharmacokinetics

Product is prepared from pooled human plasma.

Onset	Peak	Duration
Unknown	Unknown	Unknown

How supplied

Powder for reconstitution for I.V. injection or infusion (vapor-heated): 500 units/vial, 1,000 units/vial, and 2,500 units/vial in single-dose vials

Indications and dosages

➤ To control spontaneous bleeding in hemophilia A and B patients with factor VIII inhibitors undergoing surgery

Adults and children: Generally, recommended dosage ranges from 50 to 100 units/kg. However, be sure to distinguish between the following four indications:

Joint hemorrhage—50 units/kg at 12-hour intervals; may increase to 100 units/kg at 12-hour intervals

Mucous-membrane bleeding—50 units/kg at 6-hour intervals under careful monitoring; if hemorrhage continues, increase dosage to 100 units/kg at 6-hour intervals. Do not exceed dosage of 200 units/kg daily.

Soft-tissue hemorrhage (such as retroperitoneal bleeding)—100 units/kg at 12-hour intervals. Do not exceed dosage of 200 units/kg.

Other severe hemorrhage (such as CNS bleeding)—100 units/kg at 12-hour intervals (or in some cases, 6-hour intervals) until clear clinical improvement occurs

Off-label uses (selected)

- Nonhemophiliac patients with acquired inhibitors to factors VIII, XI, and XII
- Patients with von Willebrand's disease with a factor VIII inhibitor

Administration

Preparation

- Be aware that patients with preexisting abnormal platelet counts or impaired platelet function may respond inadequately.

• Know that drug must be used only in patients with circulating inhibitors to one or more coagulation factors, and ***not*** to treat bleeding episodes caused by coagulation-factor deficiencies. Do not give to patients with significant signs of disseminated intravascular coagulation (DIC) or fibrinolysis.

Unless absolutely necessary, do not give a single dose exceeding 100 units/kg or daily doses exceeding 200 units/kg.

Do not give antifibrinolytics until 12 hours after administration of this drug.

Dilution and compatibility

• Use filter and plastic syringe; do not let drug contact glass (to prevent binding to glass surfaces).

• Know that drug is packaged with 20 or 50 mL sterile water for injection as diluent and one needleless transfer device.

• Warm unopened vial containing sterile water for injection to room temperature no higher than 37°C (98°F).

• Open package with needleless transfer device by peeling away lid without touching the inside. Do not remove device from package. Turn package over and insert plastic spike through diluent stopper.

• Grip package at edge and pull package off device. Turn system over so bottle is on top. Quickly insert other plastic spike into drug vial stopper. Diluent will transfer automatically by vacuum into drug vial. Connect the two vials quickly to close the open fluid pathway created by first insertion of spike to diluent vial.

• Swirl drug vial gently to ensure that drug dissolves fully.

• Turn needleless transfer device handle down toward drug concentrate vial, and remove cap attached to syringe connection of transfer device. Draw air into syringe and connect syringe to transfer device. Inject air into concentrate vial. While keeping syringe plunger in place, turn system upside down with concentrate vial on top. Draw concentrate into syringe by pulling plunger back slowly.

• Turn handle of transfer device to original position (facing sideways). Disconnect syringe and attach suitable needle for I.V. injection or infusion.

Infusion considerations

• Know that drug injection or infusion must be completed within 3 hours of reconstitution.

• Do not exceed injection or infusion rate of 2 units/kg/minute.

Monitoring

Monitor for allergic reactions, including anaphylactoid reactions. If such a reaction occurs, discontinue therapy immediately and intervene as appropriate and ordered, such as by giving glucocorticoids and antihistamines.

If patient experiences signs or symptoms of intravascular coagulation (such as blood pressure or pulse rate changes, respiratory distress, chest pain, or cough), stop drug immediately and initiate appropriate diagnostic and therapeutic measures.

Monitor laboratory results for signs of DIC (such as decreased fibrinogen, decreased platelet count, fibrin-fibrinogen degradation products, and significantly prolonged thrombin time, prothrombin time [PT] or partial thromboplastin time [PTT]), especially in patients receiving high doses.

Be aware that nonhemophiliac patients with acquired inhibitors against factors VIII, IX, or XII may have bleeding tendency and increased thrombosis risk simultaneously.

Know that tests used to monitor drug efficacy, such as APTT, do not correlate with clinical improvement; therefore, attempts to normalize these values by increasing dosage may fail and are strongly discouraged, due to risk of causing DIC through overdose.

Monitor for signs and symptoms of myocardial infarction (MI) in patients receiving high doses or prolonged administration or who have MI risk factors.

- In joint hemorrhage, monitor for drug efficacy, as shown by clinical improvement (such as pain relief, reduced swelling, and joint mobilization).
- In mucous-membrane bleeding, give drug under careful monitoring of visible bleeding site and repeated hematocrit measurements.

Storage

- Before reconstituting, refrigerate at 2° to 8°C (36° to 46°F). Do not freeze.
- Do not refrigerate after reconstitution.

Contraindications and precautions

Contraindicated in patients with normal coagulation mechanism.

Use cautiously in patients with other thrombotic risk factors, pregnant patients, and ***newborns*** (safety and efficacy not established).

Adverse reactions

CNS: headache, dizziness, drowsiness, fatigue, weakness
CV: chest pain, hypertension, hypotension, bradycardia, tachycardia, **thrombosis, thromboembolism, MI**
EENT: rhinorrhea
GI: nausea, vomiting, abdominal pain
Hematologic: decreased fibrinogen, thrombocytopenia, shock, DIC
Hepatic: non-A, non-B hepatitis
Musculoskeletal: joint pain
Respiratory: cough, **respiratory distress**
Other: chills; fever; flushing; poor appetite; allergic reactions ranging from mild, short-term urticarial rashes and hives to **severe anaphylactoid reactions; risk of viral transmission (including non-A and non-B hepatitis and HIV)**

Interactions

Drug-diagnostic tests. *Fibrin, platelets:* decreased
Fibrin split products: increased
PT, PTT: increased or decreased

Toxicity and overdose

- No information on overdose is available.

In overdose, watch for signs and symptoms of DIC. Discontinue administration and treat symptomatically and supportively.

Patient teaching

Instruct patient to immediately report signs and symptoms of allergic response (such as rash, tightness in chest, respiratory difficulty, hives, or itching).

Advise patient to immediately report signs and symptoms of hepatitis (such as low-grade fever, anorexia, nausea, vomiting, fatigue, dark urine, or yellowing of skin or eyes).

- Inform patient of need for regular blood testing during therapy.
- As appropriate, review all other significant and life-threatening adverse reactions and interactions, especially those related to the tests mentioned above.

antithrombin III, human (AT-III, heparin cofactor 1)

Thrombate III

Pharmacologic class: Blood derivative, alpha$_2$-glycoprotein
Therapeutic class: Antithrombin, anticoagulant
Pregnancy risk category B

Action

Inactivates thrombin and activated forms of factors IXa, Xa, XIa, and XIIa, and plasmin, thereby inhibiting coagulation and thromboembolism formation

Pharmacokinetics

In asymptomatic patients with hereditary antithrombin III (AT-III) deficiency, mean 50% disappearance time (time needed to fall to 50% of peak plasma level after initial administration) is approximately 22 hours, and biologic half-life is 2.5 days based on immunologic assays and 3.8 days based on functional assays of AT-III. Half-life for radiolabeled AT-III is 2.8 to 4.8 days.

Onset	Peak	Duration
Immediate	Unknown	Variable

How supplied

Powder for reconstitution for I.V. infusion (lyophilized): 500 and 1,000 international units in single-use vials

Indications and dosages

➢ Treatment of hereditary AT-III deficiency to prevent thrombosis during surgical or obstetric procedures or during acute thrombotic episodes
Adults: Individualize initial dosage to amount required to increase AT-III activity to 120% of normal (determined 20 minutes after administration). Base dosage calculation on anticipated 1.4% increase in plasma AT-III activity produced by 1 international unit/kg. Use this formula to calculate dosage: Required dosage (international units) equals desired activity (%) minus baseline AT-III activity (%) multiplied by weight (kg) divided by 1.4 (international units/kg).

Individualize maintenance dosage to amount required to maintain AT-III activity at 80% of normal.

Administration

Preparation

- Know that diagnosis of hereditary AT-III deficiency should be based on clear family history of venous thrombosis, decreased plasma AT-III levels, and exclusion of acquired deficiency.
- Be aware that goal is to raise AT-III level to normal and maintain this level for 2 to 8 days, depending on indication, type and extent of surgery, patient's medical condition, medical history, and prescriber's judgment.
- Reduce heparin dosage when giving this drug, as ordered.

Dilution and compatibility

- Know that drug is packaged with suitable volume of sterile water for injection, sterile double-ended transfer needle, and sterile filter needle.
- Warm diluent in unopened vial to room temperature no higher than 25°C (77°F).
- Mix powder with 10 to 20 mL sterile water for injection (depending on desired dosage) by directing diluent stream against wall of concentrate vial to minimize foaming.
- When diluent transfer is complete, remove diluent vial and transfer needle, and immediately swirl continuously (do not shake) until completely dissolved. Some foaming may occur, but avoid excessive foaming.
- Attach filter needle to sterile syringe and withdraw drug syringe through filter needle. Remove filter needle from syringe and replace with appropriate injection or butterfly needle for administration.
- Do not mix with other solutions.
- Administer within 3 hours of reconstitution.

Infusion considerations

- Know that usual I.V. infusion rate is 50 to a maximum of 100 international units/minute.
- Infuse over 10 to 20 minutes.

A

If adverse reactions occur, decrease infusion rate or, if indicated, stop infusion until symptoms disappear.

Monitoring

- Monitor AT III activity levels at least every 12 hours and before next infusion to maintain plasma AT III activity level above 80%. In some situations, such as after surgery, hemorrhage or acute thrombosis, and during I.V. heparin therapy, AT III half-life may decrease. In such conditions, monitor plasma AT III activity levels and give AT III as necessary.

Watch for signs and symptoms of too-rapid infusion, such as dyspnea and hypertension.

- Monitor vital signs and temperature frequently.
- Monitor fluid intake and output to detect dehydration.

Storage

- Before reconstitution, refrigerate at 2° to 8°C (36° to 46°F). Avoid freezing.
- Do not refrigerate after reconstitution, as precipitation may occur.

Contraindications and precautions

Use cautiously in pregnant or breast-feeding patients and in ***children*** (safety and efficacy not established).

Adverse reactions

CNS: dizziness, light-headedness, headache
CV: vasodilation, reduced blood pressure, chest pain or tightness
EENT: perception of film over eyes
GI: nausea, sensation of intestinal fullness
GU: diuresis
Musculoskeletal: muscle cramps
Respiratory: dyspnea, shortness of breath
Skin: urticaria, oozing lesions, hives, hematoma
Other: foul taste, chills, fever, **risk of viral transmission (including hepatitis C and possibly Creutzfeldt-Jakob disease)**

Interactions

Drug-drug. *Heparin:* increased anticoagulant effect

Toxicity and overdose

- In overdose, expect extension of pharmacologic action and adverse reactions.
- Stop administration and provide symptomatic and supportive interventions.

Patient teaching

Instruct patient to immediately report chest tightness, dizziness, and fever.

- Caution patient to avoid driving and other hazardous activities until drug's effects on concentration and alertness are known.
- Advise patient to minimize GI upset and unpleasant taste by eating small, frequent servings of healthy food and drinking plenty of fluids.
- Instruct patient about the need for regular blood testing during therapy.
- As appropriate, review all other significant and life-threatening adverse reactions and interactions, especially those related to the drugs mentioned above.

argatroban

Novastan

Pharmacologic class: L-arginine–derived thrombin inhibitor
Therapeutic class: Anticoagulant
Pregnancy risk category B

Action

Binds rapidly to site of thrombi, neutralizing conversion of fibrinogen to fibrin, activation of coagulation factors, and platelet aggregation (processes crucial to thrombus formation)

Pharmacokinetics

Drug is distributed mainly in extracellular fluid. It is metabolized by hydroxylation and aromatization of 3-methyltetrahydroquinoline ring in liver, with 54% protein binding. It is excreted primarily in feces; terminal elimination half-life is 39 to 51 minutes.

Onset	Peak	Duration
Rapid	1-3 hr	Unknown

How supplied

Solution for injection (clear, colorless to pale yellow, slightly viscous): 100 mg/mL in 2.5-mL single-use vials

Indications and dosages

➤ Treatment or prophylaxis of thrombosis in patients with heparin-induced thrombocytopenia

Adults: 2 mcg/kg/minute as a continuous I.V. infusion, to a maximum dosage of 10 mcg/kg/minute

➤ Anticoagulation during percutaneous coronary intervention (PCI) in patients who have or are at risk for heparin-induced thrombocytopenia

Adults: Start continuous I.V. infusion at 25 mcg/kg/minute and a loading dose of 350 mcg/kg by I.V. bolus over 3 to 5 minutes. Check activated clotting time (ACT) 5 to 10 minutes after bolus dose is given; adjust dosage until ACT is between 300 and 450 seconds.

Dosage adjustment

- Adjust dosage as needed to maintain activated partial thromboplastin time (APTT) at 1.5 to 3 times initial baseline value (not to exceed 100 seconds) to treat or prevent thrombosis in patients with heparin-induced thrombocytopenia.
- If ACT is less than 300 seconds, give additional I.V. bolus dose of 150 mcg/kg, then increase infusion rate to 30 mcg/kg/minute and check ACT after 5 to 10 minutes. If ACT exceeds 450 seconds, decrease infusion rate to 15 mcg/kg/minute and check ACT after 5 to 10 minutes. Maintain adjusted infusion dosage once therapeutic ACT has been achieved in patients receiving anticoagulation during PCI.
- In patients with hepatic impairment, start at lower dosage and titrate carefully until desired anticoagulation level occurs.

Administration

Preparation

- Stop all parenteral anticoagulants before starting argatroban.
- Before administering, obtain baseline APTT.

Dilution and compatibility

Know that each 2.5-mL vial contains 250 mg and is a concentrated drug (100 mg/mL) that must be diluted 100-fold before infusion.

- Do not mix with other drugs before diluting.
- Dilute in normal saline solution for injection, D_5W for injection, or lactated Ringer's solution for injection to a concentration of 1 mg/mL.
- Further dilute by injecting contents of 2.5-mL vial into 250-mL bag of diluent.
- Use 250 mg (2.5 mL) per 250 mL diluent or 500 mg (5 mL) per 500 mL diluent.
- After preparation, solution may show slight transient haziness due to microprecipitates, which dissolve rapidly on mixing.
- Mix constituted solution by inverting diluent bag repeatedly for 1 minute.

Infusion considerations

• For patients with heparin-induced thrombocytopenia, recommended dosages and infusion rates for a dose of 2 mcg/kg/minute are as follows:

Patient weight (kg)	Dosage (mcg/min)	Infusion rate (mL/hr)
50	100	6
60	120	7
70	140	8
80	160	10
90	180	11
100	200	12
110	220	13
120	240	14
130	260	16
140	280	17

• For patients receiving drug for anticoagulation during PCI, follow prescribed infusion rate, as above.

Monitoring

Monitor for signs and symptoms of anaphylaxis; be prepared to intervene appropriately.

Monitor for bleeding tendency and hemorrhage. Know that unexplained drop in hematocrit or blood pressure or other unexplained signs or symptoms may indicate hemorrhage, which can occur at any site.

• Assess neurologic status and vital signs frequently.

• Monitor CBC and coagulation studies.

• Check for signs and symptoms of arrhythmias and hypotension.

• When discontinuing argatroban and starting oral anticoagulants, do not give loading dose of warfarin; begin oral therapy with expected daily dose.

Storage

• Store in original carton at room temperature 25°C (77°F), with excursions permitted to 15° to 30°C (59° to 86°F). Protect from light.

• Do not freeze.

Contraindications and precautions

Contraindicated in hypersensitivity to drug or its components and in overt major bleeding.

Use with extreme caution in diseases and other circumstances marked by increased hemorrhage risk, including severe hypertension; immediately after lumbar puncture; spinal anesthesia; major surgery (especially involving brain, spinal cord, or eye); hematologic conditions linked to increased bleeding tendencies (such as congenital or acquired bleeding disorders); and GI lesions (such as ulcers). Avoid high doses in PCI patients with clinically significant hepatic disease or aspartate aminotransferase or alanine aminotransferase levels that are three times upper limit of normal or higher. Use cautiously in patients with hepatic impairment or disease, pregnant or breastfeeding patients, and *children and adolescents* younger than age 18.

Adverse reactions

CNS: headache, **intracranial hemorrhage**

CV: hypotension, angina pectoris, **coronary occlusion, bradycardia, atrial fibrillation, cardiac arrest, ventricular tachycardia, cerebrovascular disorders, myocardial infarction, myocardial ischemia, aortic stenosis, coronary thrombosis, arterial thrombosis**

GI: nausea, vomiting, diarrhea, abdominal pain, **GI bleeding**

GU: urinary tract infection, minor GU tract bleeding and hematuria, **renal dysfunction**

Hematologic: groin bleeding, brachial bleeding, **retroperitoneal hemorrhage, bleeding or hemorrhage**
Musculoskeletal: back pain
Respiratory: cough, dyspnea, pneumonia, hemoptysis
Skin: rash
Other: pain, infection, chest pain, fever, allergic reaction including **anaphylaxis, sepsis**

Interactions

Drug-drug. *Oral anticoagulants:* prolonged prothrombin time, increased International Normalized Ratio, increased risk of bleeding
Thrombolytics: increased risk of bleeding
Drug-diagnostic tests. *Hematocrit, hemoglobin:* decreased

Toxicity and overdose

- In overdose, expect overt bleeding or other indicators of bleeding, including unexplained hematocrit or blood pressure decrease, weakness, or confusion.
- No specific antidote exists. Excessive anticoagulation with or without bleeding may be controlled by discontinuing drug or decreasing infusion dosage. Know that anticoagulation parameters generally return to baseline within 2 to 4 hours after drug discontinuation, but reversal of anticoagulant effect may take longer in patients with hepatic impairment. If life-threatening bleeding occurs and excessive plasma drug levels are suspected, discontinue drug immediately and obtain APTT and other coagulation parameters. Provide symptomatic and supportive interventions as appropriate. Know that dialysis may partially clear drug.

Patient teaching

Instruct patient to immediately report hypersensitivity reactions and unusual bleeding or bruising.

- Advise patient to avoid activities that can cause injury, and to use a soft toothbrush and electric razor to avoid gum and skin injury.
- Explain that patient will need to undergo regular blood testing during therapy.
- As appropriate, review all other significant or life-threatening adverse reactions and interactions, especially those related to the drugs and tests mentioned above.

arsenic trioxide

Trisenox

Pharmacologic class: Nonmetallic element, white arsenic
Therapeutic class: Antineoplastic
Pregnancy risk category D

FDA BOXED WARNING

- Give under supervision of physician experienced in managing patients with acute leukemia.
- Some patients with acute promyelocytic leukemia (APL) treated with drug have had symptoms similar to retinoic acid–acute promyelocytic leukemia (RA-APL) or APL differentiation syndrome, marked by fever, dyspnea, weight gain, pulmonary infiltrates, and pleural or pericardial effusions. Syndrome can be fatal; at first sign, give high-dose steroids immediately as ordered, regardless of patient's white blood cell count; continue steroids for at least 3 days or longer until signs and symptoms abate. Most patients do not require arsenic trioxide termination during treatment of APL differentiation syndrome.
- Drug may prolong QT interval and cause complete atrioventricular block. QT interval prolongation may lead to torsades de pointes–type ventricular arrhythmia, which can be fatal.

• Before starting therapy, obtain 12-lead ECG and assess serum electrolyte (potassium, calcium, and magnesium) and creatinine levels. Correct electrolyte abnormalities and, if possible, discontinue drugs known to cause QT interval prolongation. During therapy, maintain potassium level above 4 mEq/L and magnesium level above 1.8 mg/dL. If absolute QT interval value exceeds 500 msec, reassess and take immediate action to correct concomitant risk factors.

Action

Unclear. May cause morphologic changes and DNA fragmentation in promyelocytic leukemia cells, causing cell death and degradation of or damage to PML/RAR-alpha (a fusion protein).

Pharmacokinetics

Metabolism involves reduction of pentavalent arsenic to trivalent arsenic by arsenate reductase and methylation of trivalent arsenic to monomethylarsonic acid and monomethylarsonic acid to dimethylarsinic acid by methyltransferases. Liver is main site of methylation reactions. Drug is stored mainly in liver, kidneys, heart, lungs, hair, and nails; it is excreted in urine.

Onset	Peak	Duration
Unknown	Unknown	Unknown

Availability

Solution for injection (clear, colorless, preservative-free): 1 mg/mL in 10 mg/ 10-mL single-use ampules

Indications and dosages

➢ APL in patients who have relapsed or are refractory to retinoid and anthracycline chemotherapy and whose APL is characterized by presence of T(15:17) translocation or PML/RAR-alpha gene expression

Adults and children age 5 and older: *Induction phase*—0.15 mg/kg I.V. daily until bone marrow remission occurs, to a maximum of 60 doses. *Consolidation phase*—0.15 mg/kg I.V. daily for 25 doses over 5 weeks, starting 3 to 6 weeks after induction phase ends.

Administration

Preparation

Know that drug is carcinogenic; follow facility hazardous drug policy for preparing and handling antineoplastics.

Before starting therapy, obtain baseline 12-lead ECG and assess serum electrolyte (potassium, calcium, and magnesium) and creatinine levels for abnormalities and correct as needed.

• If possible, discontinue drugs known to prolong the QT interval. For QTc greater than 500 msec, complete corrective measures and reassess QTc with serial ECGs before giving arsenic trioxide.

Dilution and compatibility

• Dilute in 100 to 250 mL D_5W for injection or normal saline solution for injection.

• Do not mix with other drugs.

• Discard unused drug.

Infusion considerations

• Infuse over 1 to 2 hours; may infuse over 4 hours if patient has a vasomotor reaction.

Monitoring

• Evaluate vital signs and neurologic status.

• Assess for hypoglycemia and hyperglycemia if patient is diabetic.

• Monitor CBC and coagulation studies throughout therapy.

Storage

• Store at 25°C (77°F), with excursions permitted to 15° to 30°C (59° to 86°F). Do not freeze.

• After dilution, drug may be stored for 24 hours at room temperature and 48 hours when refrigerated.

Contraindications and precautions

Contraindicated in hypersensitivity to drug.

Use cautiously in renal impairment, cardiac abnormalities, ***elderly patients,*** pregnant patients, breastfeeding patients (use not recommended), and ***children younger than age 5*** (safety and efficacy not established).

Adverse reactions

CNS: headache, insomnia, paresthesia, dizziness, tremor, drowsiness, anxiety, confusion, agitation, rigors, weakness, depression, fatigue, **seizures, coma**
CV: ECG abnormalities, chest pain, hypotension, hypertension, tachycardia, **prolonged QT interval, torsades de pointes**
EENT: blurred vision, painful red eye, dry eyes, eye irritation, swollen eyelids, tinnitus, earache, nasopharyngitis, postnasal drip, epistaxis, sinusitis, sore throat
GI: nausea, vomiting, constipation, diarrhea, fecal incontinence, loose stools, abdominal pain, abdominal tenderness, abdominal distention, dyspepsia, dry mouth, oral candidiasis, anorexia, hemorrhagic diarrhea, **GI hemorrhage**
GU: urinary incontinence, intermenstrual bleeding, renal impairment, **oliguria, renal failure, vaginal hemorrhage**
Hematologic: anemia, lymphadenopathy, **leukocytosis, thrombocytopenia, neutropenia, febrile neutropenia, disseminated intravascular coagulation, hemorrhage**
Metabolic: hypokalemia, hypomagnesemia, hyperglycemia, hypocalcemia, acidosis, **hypoglycemia, hyperkalemia**
Musculoskeletal: joint, muscle, bone, back, neck, or limb pain
Respiratory: dyspnea, cough, hypoxia, wheezing, crackles, tachypnea, decreased breath sounds, crepitation, hemoptysis, rhonchi, upper respiratory tract infection, **pleural effusion**
Skin: flushing, erythema, pallor, bruising, petechiae, pruritus, dermatitis, dry skin, hyperpigmentation, urticaria, skin lesions, local exfoliation, diaphoresis, night sweats
Other: weight gain or loss, fever, facial edema, herpes simplex or herpes zoster infection, bacterial infection, pain and edema at injection site, **hypersensitivity reaction, sepsis, APL differentiation syndrome**

Interactions

Drug-drug. *Drugs that can cause electrolyte abnormalities (such as amphotericin B, diuretics):* increased risk of electrolyte abnormalities
Drugs that can prolong QT interval (antiarrhythmics, thioridazines, some quinolones): increased QT interval prolongation
Drug-diagnostic tests. *Alanine aminotransferase, aspartate aminotransferase, calcium, magnesium:* increased
Glucose, potassium: altered levels
Hemoglobin, neutrophils, platelets: decreased

Toxicity and overdose

• Overdose signs and symptoms may include confusion, muscle weakness, and seizures.
• Immediately discontinue drug and consider starting chelation therapy with dimercaprol 3 mg/kg I.M. every 4 hours until immediate life-threatening toxicity subsides. Thereafter, give penicillamine 250 mg P.O. up to four times daily (1 g/day or less maximum), as ordered. For APL differentiation syndrome, give high-dose steroids as ordered and monitor electrolyte levels. Correct serum potassium and magnesium levels to maintain these within prescribed

limits. For arrhythmias, intervene as appropriate and ordered.

Patient teaching

Instruct patient to immediately report signs and symptoms of allergic response, fever, breathing problems, and seizures.

Tell patient drug increases risk of serious infection. Instruct patient to immediately report signs or symptoms of infection.

Emphasize importance of avoiding pregnancy during therapy.

- Caution patient to avoid driving and other hazardous activities until drug's effects on concentration and alertness are known.
- Advise patient to minimize GI upset by eating small, frequent servings of food and drinking plenty of fluids.
- Encourage patient to establish effective bedtime routine to minimize insomnia.
- Inform patient about the need for regular blood testing during therapy.
- Advise breastfeeding patient not to breastfeed while taking this drug. Provide guidance to help her decide whether to discontinue breastfeeding or stop drug.
- As appropriate, review all other significant and life-threatening adverse reactions and interactions, especially those related to the drugs and tests mentioned above.

[redacted]

ascorbic acid (vitamin C)

Pharmacologic class: Vitamin
Therapeutic class: Nutritional supplement
Pregnancy risk category C

Action

Water-soluble vitamin with antioxidant properties; stimulates collagen formation and enhances tissue repair

Pharmacokinetics

Drug is distributed throughout water-soluble compartments—mostly in white blood cells, platelets, adrenal cortex, and pituitary gland. It is not stored in body. Excess is excreted in urine.

Onset	Peak	Duration
Unknown	Unknown	Unknown

How supplied

Solution for injection (clear, colorless to slightly yellow): 500 mg/mL in 50-mL vial

Indications and dosages

➤ Prevention of scurvy

Adults: Average dosage is 70 to 150 mg I.V. daily.

➤ Treatment of scurvy

Adults: 300 mg to 1 g I.V. daily

➤ To enhance wound healing

Adults: 300 to 500 mg I.V. daily for 7 to 10 days, before and after surgery

➤ Severe burns

Adults: 1 to 2 g I.V. daily

Off-label uses (selected)

- Idiopathic methemoglobinemia

Administration

Dilution and compatibility

- Dilute in large volume of normal saline solution for injection or D_5W for injection to minimize adverse reactions.
- Use within 4 hours after withdrawal from vial.
- Discard remaining contents after first withdrawal.

Infusion considerations

- Administer at prescribed rate and avoid rapid infusion.

Monitoring

Do not stop high-dose therapy abruptly, as bleeding gums and loosened teeth may occur.

Storage

• Until use, store in carton at controlled room temperature not exceeding 25°C (77°F); protect from light.

Contraindications and precautions

Use high-dose, long-term therapy cautiously in history of recurrent renal calculi; impaired renal function; concurrent anticoagulant therapy; sodium-restricted diet; diabetes mellitus; pregnant or breastfeeding patients; and *children* (safety and efficacy not established).

Adverse reactions

CNS: dizziness (with too-rapid administration)
CV: temporary faintness (with too-rapid administration)
GI: vomiting

Interactions

Drug-diagnostic tests. *Amine-dependent test for occult blood in stool*: false-negative
Urine glucose test: possible false reading (with high dose)

Toxicity and overdose

• Serious toxicity is rare. With doses above 1 g, expect nausea, vomiting, diarrhea, rebound scurvy, increased iron absorption, and precipitation of gout.
• Halt drug temporarily until signs and symptoms subside; if these persist, discontinue drug and provide supportive interventions.

Patient teaching

• Instruct patient to report vomiting, dizziness, or feeling of faintness.
• As appropriate, review all other significant adverse reactions and interactions, especially those related to the tests mentioned above.

atenolol

Tenormin I.V. Injection

Pharmacologic class: Beta-adrenergic blocker (selective)
Therapeutic class: Antianginal, antihypertensive
Pregnancy risk category D

FDA BOXED WARNING

• Caution patients with coronary artery disease (CAD) not to discontinue drug abruptly, as this may cause severe angina exacerbation, myocardial infarction (MI), and ventricular arrhythmias. (The last two complications may occur with or without preceding angina exacerbation.) With planned drug discontinuation, observe patients carefully and advise them to minimize physical activity; if angina worsens or acute coronary insufficiency develops, drug should be reinstituted promptly, at least temporarily. Because CAD is common and may go unrecognized, abrupt withdrawal may pose a risk even in patients treated only for hypertension.

Action

Selectively blocks $beta_1$-adrenergic (myocardial) receptors; decreases cardiac output, peripheral resistance, and myocardial oxygen consumption. At higher doses, also inhibits $beta_2$-adrenergic receptors, primarily located in bronchial and vascular musculature.

Pharmacokinetics

Only a small amount (6% to16%) is bound to plasma proteins. More than 85% of dose is excreted in urine within 24 hours With impaired renal function, elimination relates closely to glomerular filtration rate, with significant accumulation when creatinine clearance falls below 35 mL/minute/1.73 m^2.

Onset	Peak	Duration
Unknown	5 min	Unknown

How supplied

Solution for injection (aqueous): 5 mg/10-mL ampule

Indications and dosages

➤ Acute MI

Adults: Initially, 5 mg I.V. over 5 minutes, followed by 5 mg I.V. 10 minutes later. At 10 minutes after last I.V. dose, give oral dosage as prescribed, followed by oral dosages for 6 to 9 days.

Dosage adjustment

• In elderly patients, start at low end of dosage range because of greater likelihood of decreased hepatic, renal, or cardiac function and of concomitant disease and other drug therapy.

Administration

Preparation

🔊 In patients with known or suspected acute MI, start therapy as soon as possible after arrival in coronary care or similar unit, immediately after hemodynamic condition has stabilized.

• Assess renal function before therapy begins.

Dilution and compatibility

• Mix dose with dextrose or sodium chloride solution.

• Use I.V. solution within 48 hours of mixing.

Infusion considerations

🔊 Administer I.V. infusion slowly (no faster than 1 mg/minute).

Monitoring

🔊 If apical pulse is slower than 60 beats/minute, withhold dose and call prescriber.

• Watch for signs and symptoms of hypersensitivity reaction.

• Monitor vital signs (especially blood pressure), ECG, and exercise tolerance.

• Check closely for hypotension if patient is on hemodialysis.

• Monitor blood glucose level regularly if patient is diabetic; drug may mask signs and symptoms of hypoglycemia.

🔊 Do not discontinue drug suddenly. Instead, taper dosage over 2 weeks and observe patient carefully during withdrawal.

Storage

• Keep ampules in outer packaging until use. Store at controlled room temperature of 20° to 25°C (68° to 77°F), protected from light.

Contraindications and precautions

Contraindicated in hypersensitivity to drug or its components, cardiogenic shock, sinus bradycardia, greater than first-degree heart block, or overt congestive heart failure (CHF).

Use cautiously in CHF controlled by cardiac glycosides or diuretics, untreated pheochromocytoma, renal failure, hepatic impairment, pulmonary disease, diabetes mellitus, thyrotoxicosis, pregnant or breastfeeding patients, and ***children*** (safety and efficacy not established).

Adverse reactions

CNS: fatigue, lethargy, vertigo, drowsiness, dizziness, depression, disorientation, short-term memory loss, lightheadedness, abnormal dreams

CV: hypertension, hypotension, orthostatic hypotension, **bradycardia, arrhythmias, heart failure, cardiogenic shock, myocardial reinfarction**

EENT: dry eyes, **laryngospasm**

GI: nausea, diarrhea, **ischemic colitis, mesenteric arterial thrombosis**
GU: erectile dysfunction, Peyronie's disease, **renal failure**
Hematologic: agranulocytosis
Metabolic: hypoglycemia
Musculoskeletal: leg pain
Respiratory: dyspnea, wheezing, respiratory distress, **bronchospasm, pulmonary emboli**
Other: fever, cool extremities, development of antinuclear antibodies, hypersensitivity reaction

Interactions

Drug-drug. *Calcium channel blockers:* additive effect
Clonidine: life-threatening blood pressure rise after clonidine withdrawal or simultaneous withdrawal of both drugs
Dobutamine, dopamine, isoproterenol: decrease in beneficial beta-cardiovascular effects
Reserpine: increased hypotension, marked bradycardia
Drug-diagnostic tests. *Alanine aminotransferase, alkaline phosphatase, aspartate aminotransferase, antinuclear antibody titers, blood urea nitrogen, creatinine, lactate dehydrogenase, platelets, potassium, uric acid:* increased
Glucose: increased or decreased
Insulin tolerance test: false results
Drug-behaviors. *Alcohol use:* increased hypotension

Toxicity and overdose

- In overdose, expected signs and symptoms include lethargy, dyspnea, wheezing and other respiratory disorders, sinus pause and bradycardia, CHF, hypotension, bronchospasm, and hypoglycemia.
- Remove drug from general circulation by hemodialysis, as ordered. Other treatments may include atropine I.V. for bradycardia. If patient does not respond to vagal blockade, give isoproterenol cautiously, as ordered; in refractory cases, transvenous cardiac pacing may be indicated. Second- or third-degree heart block may warrant isoproterenol or transvenous cardiac pacing. As prescribed, give cardiac glycoside or similar drug and a diuretic for cardiac failure; give vasopressors, such as dopamine or norepinephrine, for hypotension and monitor blood pressure continuously. For bronchospasm, give a $beta_2$ stimulant, such as isoproterenol or terbutaline, and/or aminophylline. Administer glucose I.V. for hypoglycemia, as ordered. Resuscitate as necessary.

Patient teaching

Instruct patient to immediately report signs and symptoms of allergic response, breathing problems, and chest pain.
- Tell patient drug may cause temporary blood pressure drop on rising suddenly. Teach patient to rise slowly and carefully.

Inform females that drug cannot be taken during pregnancy; urge them to report planned or suspected pregnancy.
- Inform males that drug may cause erectile dysfunction (impotence); advise them to discuss this issue with prescriber.
- Advise patient to minimize physical activity during drug withdrawal.
- As appropriate, review all other significant and life-threatening adverse reactions and interactions, especially those related to the drugs, tests, and behaviors mentioned above.

atracurium besylate

Tracrium ❉

Pharmacologic class: Nondepolarizing neuromuscular blocker
Therapeutic class: Skeletal muscle relaxant, adjunct to anesthesia
Pregnancy risk category C

FDA BOXED WARNING

- Drug should be given only by trained personnel in a facility where respirations can be monitored, assisted, and controlled and where reversal agents, intubation, artificial respiration, and oxygen therapy are immediately available.

Action

Antagonizes neurotransmitter action of acetylcholine by binding competitively with cholinergic receptors on motor end-plate

Pharmacokinetics

Metabolites in bile and urine are similar. Duration of neuromuscular block produced by drug does not correlate with plasma pseudocholinesterase levels and is not affected by absence of renal function. Drug may undergo extensive degradation; neither the liver nor kidneys play a major role in elimination. Bile and urine are the major excretion routes (totaling more than 90% of labeled dose within 7 hours of dosing), of which atracurium represents only a minor fraction.

Onset	Peak	Duration
2 min	3-5 min	35-70 min

How supplied

Solution for injection (aqueous): 10 mg/mL in 5-mL single-dose vial, 10 mg/mL in 10-mL multidose vial with benzyl alcohol

Indications and dosages

➤ Adjunct to general anesthesia to facilitate endotracheal intubation and relax skeletal muscles during surgery or mechanical ventilation

Adults and children age 2 and older: Initially, 0.4 to 0.5 mg/kg by I.V. bolus under balanced anesthesia. With prolonged surgery, maintenance dosage of 0.08 to 0.1 mg/kg is given 20 to 45 minutes after initial dose; may repeat q 15 to 25 minutes under balanced anesthesia (slightly longer under isoflurane or enflurane), as needed. During long procedures, after bolus dose, continuous infusion may be initiated at a rate of 9 to 10 mcg/kg/minute to rapidly counteract spontaneous neuromuscular function; thereafter, 5 to 9 mcg/kg/minute (individualized for each patient) should maintain neuromuscular block; for use in intensive care unit (ICU), infusion rate of 11 to 13 mg/kg/minute should provide adequate neuromuscular block in adults.
Children ages 1 month to 2 years: 0.3 to 0.4 mg/kg I.V. under halothane anesthesia; repeat if needed.

Dosage adjustment

- Know that isoflurane or enflurane anesthesia potentiates atracurium. Same initial dosage of 0.4 to 0.5 mg/kg may be used for intubation before these inhalation agents are given; however, if first administered under steady state of isoflurane or enflurane, reduce initial dosage by approximately one-third (to 0.25 to 0.35 mg/kg) to adjust for potentiating effects of these agents. With halothane, consider smaller dosage reductions.
- Although drug is a less potent histamine releaser than d-tubocurarine or metocurine, consider possibility of substantial histamine release in sensitive patients. For these patients, recommended initial dosage is lower (0.3 to 0.4 mg/kg) than for others and should be given slowly or in divided doses.
- Be aware that burn patients may require increased dosages (depending on burn size and time elapsed since

burn) because of possible resistance to nondepolarizing neuromuscular blockers.

Administration

Preparation

Use only under direct supervision of trained medical staff who can maintain a patent airway and are familiar with drug's actions, characteristics, and hazards.

Before giving, make sure emergency respiratory equipment is at hand.

Do not give drug until patient recovers from succinylcholine-induced neuromuscular block.

- Know that with recommended dosages, good or excellent conditions for nonemergency intubation can be expected in 2 to 2.5 minutes in most patients, with maximum neuromuscular block occurring about 3 to 5 minutes after injection. Under balanced anesthesia, clinically required neuromuscular block generally lasts 20 to 35 minutes, recovery to 25% of control occurs approximately 35 to 45 minutes after injection, and recovery is usually 95% complete about 60 minutes after injection.

Be aware that 10-mL multiple-dose vial contains benzyl alcohol. In neonates, benzyl alcohol has been linked to increased incidence of neurologic and other complications, which can be fatal.

- Know that infants and children may need slightly more frequent maintenance doses than adults.
- Keep in mind that patient can hear while drug is in effect. Provide ongoing reassurance.

Ensure that patient receives sedative or general anesthetic before receiving atracurium.

Dilution and compatibility

- Prepare infusion solution by mixing drug with appropriate diluent, such as D_5W for injection, normal saline solution for injection, or 5% dextrose and normal saline solution for injection.

Do not use lactated Ringer's solution because of increased risk of spontaneous degradation.

- Use infusion solutions within 24 hours of preparation.

Do not mix or administer in same syringe with alkaline solutions, such as barbiturate solutions, because atracurium may be inactivated and free acid may be precipitated.

- Discard unused solutions.

Infusion considerations

Give I.V. only. Never administer I.M.

- Give initial doses by I.V. bolus at prescribed rate.
- Know that amount of infusion solution required per minute depends on drug concentration in solution, desired dosage, and patient's weight. Follow manufacturer's guidelines for delivery in mL/hour.
- When giving by infusion in operating room, initiate drug only after early evidence of spontaneous recovery from bolus dose. Initial infusion rate of 9 to 10 mcg/kg/minute may be needed to rapidly counteract spontaneous recovery of neuromuscular function. Thereafter, rate of 5 to 9 mcg/kg/minute should be sufficient to maintain continuous neuromuscular block in range of 89% to 99% in most adults and children under balanced anesthesia. Occasionally, patients may need infusion rates as low as 2 or as high as 15 mcg/kg/minute.
- In ICU patients, infusion rate of 11 to 13 mcg/kg/minute should provide adequate neuromuscular block in adults. Limited information suggests pediatric ICU patients may require faster infusion rates than adults.
- Know that enflurane or isoflurane (and to a lesser extent, halothane) potentiate drug's neuromuscular blocking

effect when given by infusion. Consider reducing infusion rate for patients receiving inhalation anesthesia. Reduce rate by approximately one-third in presence of steady-state enflurane or isoflurane anesthesia; consider smaller reductions in presence of halothane.

- Adjust rate of continuous I.V. infusion according to response, as determined by peripheral nerve stimulation.
- Give slowly or in divided doses over 1 minute in patients at risk for substantial histamine release.

Monitoring

- Be ready to reverse drug effects with anticholinesterase drug once spontaneous recovery begins.

Monitor patient for anaphylaxis and injection site reaction.

Because malignant hyperthermia can develop in absence of established triggering agents (such as halogenated anesthetics and succinylcholine), be prepared to recognize and intervene in this potentially fatal condition in any patient scheduled for general anesthesia.

- Check vital signs and airway patency until patient recovers completely from drug effects.
- Assess for pain, and give analgesics as needed and ordered. Be aware that patient may be unable to express pain while drug is in effect.
- Evaluate patient's recovery with muscle strength tests, nerve stimulation, and train-of-four monitoring.
- While drug is in effect, explain events to patient as they occur.

Storage

- Refrigerate at 2° to 8°C (36° to 46°F) after dilution to preserve potency. When removing drug from refrigeration to room temperature, store at 25°C (77°F).
- Use within 14 days, even if refrigerated.
- Do not freeze.
- Know that infusion solutions containing 0.2 or 0.5 mg/mL can be stored in recommended diluents in refrigerator or at room temperature for 24 hours without significant potency loss.

Contraindications and precautions

Contraindicated in hypersensitivity to drug or benzyl alcohol (multiple-dose vials only).

Use cautiously when substantial histamine release would be especially hazardous (as in patients with clinically significant cardiovascular disease), history of severe anaphylactoid reactions or asthma, myasthenia gravis, severe electrolyte imbalance, carcinomatosis, ***elderly patients,*** pregnant or breastfeeding patients, and ***infants younger than 1 month*** (safety and efficacy not established).

Adverse reactions

CNS: inadequate neuromuscular blockade, **malignant hypothermia** (rare), **prolonged neuromuscular blockade, seizures**

CV: hypotension, increased or decreased mean arterial pressure, **tachycardia, bradycardia**

Respiratory: wheezing, dyspnea, **bronchospasm, laryngospasm**

Skin: flushing, rash, urticaria, erythema, pruritus

Other: injection site reaction, allergic reactions including **anaphylaxis** (rare)

Interactions

Drug-drug. *Acetylcholinesterase inhibitors:* inhibition of muscle relaxation and reversal of neuromuscular blockade

Aminoglycosides, enflurane, halothane, isoflurane, lithium, procainamide, polymyxins, magnesium salts, quinidine: increased muscle relaxation

Corticosteroids: prolonged weakness

Edrophonium, neostigmine, pyridostigmine: atracurium inhibition, reversal of neuromuscular blockade

Succinylcholine: faster atracurium onset, increased depth of muscle relaxation

Toxicity and overdose

• Overdose may increase risk of histamine release and cardiovascular effects, especially hypotension.

• If cardiovascular support is necessary, position patient properly, administer fluids, and give vasopressors if necessary and ordered. Ensure patent airway by initiating manual or mechanical ventilation as necessary. If overdose causes longer duration of neuromuscular block, use peripheral nerve stimulator to monitor recovery. As ordered, give anticholinesterase-reversing agent (such as neostigmine, edrophonium, or pyridostigmine) in conjunction with anticholinergic (such as atropine or glycopyrrolate) to promote recovery.

Patient teaching

• Before giving, carefully describe drug effects to patient.

• Explain that patient will be able to hear but not move.

• As appropriate, review all other significant and life-threatening adverse reactions and interactions, especially those related to the drugs mentioned above.

atropine sulfate

Pharmacologic class: Antimuscarinic, belladonna alkaloid

Therapeutic class: Anticholinergic, antispasmodic

Pregnancy risk category C

Action

Inhibits smooth muscle and glands innervated by postganglionic cholinergic nerves; also exerts CNS activity, which may be stimulating or depressing, depending on dose

Pharmacokinetics

Drug crosses placental barrier and may be distributed in small amount in breast milk. It is metabolized in liver to several metabolites, including tropic acid, tropine (or similar compound), and possibly esters of tropic acid and glucuronic conjugates. From 30% to 50% of dose is excreted unchanged in urine.

Onset	Peak	Duration
Immediate	2-4 min	Unknown

How supplied

Solution for injection (clear): 1 mg/10-mL syringe, 4 mg/0.5-mL ampule, 0.4 mg/1-mL single-dose vial, 0.4 mg/mL in 20-mL multidose vial; 0.5 mg/1-mL vial; 1 mg/1-mL ampule and single-dose vial

Indications and dosages

➢ Preanesthetic to decrease salivation and bronchial secretions; treatment of parkinsonism; to reduce pylorospasm and hypertonicity of small intestine and colonic hypermotility; to relieve uterine hypertonicity; to relax spasm of biliary and ureteral colic and bronchial spasm; to reduce detrusor tone; treatment of urinary tract disorder; to stop crying or laughing episodes in patients with brain lesions; peptic ulcer management; closed head injuries causing acetylcholine release in cerebrospinal fluid, causing abnormal EEG, stupor, and other neurologic signs; antidote for pilocarpine, physostigmine, isoflurophate, choline esters, certain species of *Amanita,* and acetylcholinesterase insecticide poisoning

Adults: 0.4 to 0.6 mg I.V. Dosage may be much higher in some cases.

A

Children: Dosage depends on weight, as indicated below. (However, dosages may be much higher in some cases.)
Children weighing more than 40.8 kg (90 lb): 0.4 to 0.6 mg I.V.
Children weighing 29.5 kg to 40.8 kg (65 to 90 lb): 0.4 mg I.V.
Children weighing 18.1 kg to 29.5 kg (40 to 65 lb): 0.3 mg I.V.
Children weighing 10.9 kg to 18.1 kg (24 to 40 lb): 0.2 mg I.V.
Children weighing 7.7 kg to 10.9 kg (17 to 24 lb): 0.15 mg I.V.
Children weighing 3.2 to 7.3 kg (7 to 16 lb): 0.1 mg I.V.

Off-label uses

• Cholinergic-mediated bronchial asthma

Administration

Preparation

• Be aware that patients with Down syndrome may be unusually sensitive to drug.

Dilution and compatibility

• Do not add drug to I.V. solutions.
• Discard unused portion of single-dose vials or syringes.

Infusion considerations

• Do not administer unless solution is clear.
• Infuse directly into large vein or Y-tube or three-way stopcock of I.V. infusion set over at least 1 minute.
Be aware that slow I.V. infusion or adult dosages below 0.5 mg may slow the heart rate further.

Monitoring

Watch closely for signs and symptoms of anaphylaxis; be prepared to intervene appropriately.
• Monitor heart rate for bradycardia or tachycardia.
• Evaluate fluid intake and output.
• Assess for urine retention or urinary hesitancy.
• Monitor for signs and symptoms of glaucoma.

Storage

• Store at controlled room temperature of 15° to 30°C (59° to 86°F).

Contraindications and precautions

Contraindicated in hypersensitivity to drug, when inhibition of postganglionic cholinergic nerves is undesirable (as in glaucoma and tachycardia), and in asthma.

Use cautiously in chronic renal, hepatic, pulmonary, or cardiac disease; prostatic hypertrophy; ***elderly patients;*** pregnant or breastfeeding patients; and ***children.***

Adverse effects

CNS: headache, restlessness, ataxia, asthenia, disorientation, delirium, insomnia, dizziness, drowsiness, nervousness, excitement, **coma**
CV: palpitations, **bradycardia, tachycardia**
EENT: photophobia, blurred vision, nasal dryness, increased intraocular pressure, mydriasis, cycloplegia, nasal congestion
GI: nausea, vomiting, constipation, bloating, dysphagia, dry mouth
GU: urine retention, urinary hesitancy, erectile dysfunction
Skin: decreased sweating, flushing, urticaria, dry skin, hot skin, rash
Other: thirst, slurred speech, fever, anhidrosis, taste loss, **anaphylaxis, death**

Interactions

Drug-drug. *Amantadine, antiarrhythmics, anticholinergics, antihistamines, antiparkinsonians, glutethimide, meperidine, muscle relaxants, phenothiazines, tricyclic antidepressants:* increased atropine effects
Antimyasthenics: decreased intestinal motility
Cyclopropane: ventricular arrhythmias

Haloperidol: decreased antipsychotic effect
Metoclopramide: decreased effect of atropine on GI motility
Potassium chloride wax-matrix tablets: increased severity of mucosal lesions
Drug-herb. *Jaborandi tree, pill-bearing spurge:* decreased drug effects
Jimsonweed: cardiovascular changes
Squaw vine: reduced metabolic breakdown of drug
Drug-behaviors. *Sun exposure:* increased photophobia risk

Toxicity and overdose

- Overdose signs and symptoms include fever, delirium, coma, tachycardia, and excitement.
- Give short-acting barbiturate or diazepam, as ordered, to control marked excitement and seizures. Use ice bags and alcohol sponges to help reduce fever, especially in children. As ordered, give physostigmine as atropine antidote (slow I.V. injection of 1 to 5 mL of 1 mg/5-mL solution) to rapidly abolish delirium and coma caused by large atropine doses; may repeat physostigmine dose every 5 minutes for a total of 2 mg in children and every 30 minutes for a total of 6 mg in adults.

Patient teaching

Instruct patient to immediately report allergic response.
Inform patient that headache, eye pain, and blurred vision may signal glaucoma; encourage patient to report these symptoms at once.
- Caution patient to avoid driving and other hazardous activities until drug's effects on concentration, alertness, and vision are known.
- As appropriate, review all other significant and life-threatening adverse reactions and interactions, especially those related to the drugs, herbs, and behaviors mentioned above.

azithromycin

Zithromax

Pharmacologic class: Macrolide
Therapeutic class: Anti-infective
Pregnancy risk category B

Action

Inhibits protein synthesis after binding with 50S ribosomal subunit of susceptible organisms; demonstrates cross-resistance to erythromycin-resistant gram-positive strains and resistance to most strains of *Enterococcus faecalis* and methicillin-resistant *Staphylococcus aureus*

Pharmacokinetics

Serum protein binding varies. After I.V. dose, plasma concentration declines, with mean apparent plasma clearance of 630 mL/minute and terminal elimination half-life of 68 hours. Prolonged terminal half-life presumably results from extensive uptake and subsequent release of drug from tissues. Drug is excreted largely in bile, with some excretion in urine.

Onset	Peak	Duration
Unknown	Dependent on plasma level	Unknown

How supplied

Powder for reconstitution for injection (lyophilized): 500 mg in 10-mL vials

Indications and dosages

➤ Community-acquired pneumonia caused by *Chlamydia pneumoniae, Haemophilus influenzae, Legionella*

pneumophila, Moraxella catarrhalis, Mycoplasma pneumoniae, Streptococcus pneumoniae, and *S. aureus* in patients requiring initial I.V. therapy
Adults and adolescents age 16 and older: 500 mg I.V. daily for at least two doses, followed by daily oral doses for a total of 7 to 10 days
➢ Pelvic inflammatory disease caused by *Chlamydia trachomatis, Neisseria gonorrhoeae,* or *Mycoplasma hominis* in patients requiring initial I.V. therapy
Adults: 500 mg I.V. daily on days 1 and 2, followed by daily oral doses for a total of 7 days. If anaerobes are suspected, give with appropriate anaerobicidal antibiotic, as prescribed.

Administration

Preparation

- Obtain specimens for culture and sensitivity testing before starting therapy.

Dilution and compatibility

- Reconstitute 500-mg vial with 4.8 mL sterile water for injection, to yield concentration of 100 mg/mL.
- Shake vial until drug dissolves completely.
- As appropriate, dilute solution further to provide drug concentration of 1 to 2 mg/mL by transferring 5 mL of 100 mg/mL azithromycin solution into appropriate amount of normal or half-normal saline solution for injection, D_5W for injection, or lactated Ringer's solution for injection.
- Do not mix with or infuse through same I.V. line as other additives or drugs.

Infusion considerations

Do not administer as I.V. bolus or by I.M. injection.
- Give by I.V. infusion only at 1 mg/mL over 3 hours or 2 mg/2 mL over 1 hour.
- Infuse over no less than 60 minutes.

Monitoring

Assess for signs and symptoms of allergic reaction; if such a reaction occurs, discontinue drug immediately and intervene appropriately.
Monitor for signs and symptoms of pseudomembranous colitis.
- Monitor temperature, white blood cell count, and culture and sensitivity results.

Storage

- After dilution, drug may be stored for 24 hours at or below room temperature of 30°C (86°F) or for 7 days if refrigerated at 5°C (41°F).

Contraindications and precautions

Contraindicated in hypersensitivity to drug, erythromycin, or other macrolide or ketolide anti-infectives.

Use cautiously in severe hepatic impairment, severe renal insufficiency, risk of prolonged QT interval, breastfeeding patients, and ***children younger than age 16*** (safety and efficacy not established).

Adverse reactions

CNS: dizziness, drowsiness, fatigue, headache, vertigo
GI: nausea, diarrhea, abdominal pain, vomiting, stomatitis, anorexia, cholestatic jaundice, dyspepsia, gastritis, flatulence, **pseudomembranous colitis**
GU: nephritis, vaginitis, candidiasis
Respiratory: dyspnea
Skin: rash, pruritus
Other: pain and local inflammation at injection site, oral moniliasis, taste changes, serious allergic reactions including **angioedema, Stevens-Johnson syndrome, toxic necrolysis,** and **anaphylaxis** (rare)

Interactions

Drug-drug. *Carbamazepine, cyclosporine, digoxin, dihydroergotamine, ergotamine, hexobarbital, phenytoin,*

theophylline, triazolam: increased blood levels of these drugs
Warfarin: increased International Normalized Ratio
Drug-diagnostic tests. *Alanine aminotransferase, alkaline phosphatase, aspartate aminotransferase, bilirubin, creatinine:* increased
Drug-behaviors. *Sun exposure:* photosensitivity

Toxicity and overdose

- No information on overdose is available. If it occurs, expect extension of adverse reactions.
- Provide symptomatic interventions.

Patient teaching

Instruct patient to immediately report signs and symptoms of allergic reaction, such as rash.

- Tell patient to report diarrhea.
- As appropriate, review all other significant and life-threatening adverse reactions and interactions, especially those related to the drugs, tests, and behaviors mentioned above.

aztreonam

Azactam Injection

Pharmacologic class: Monobactam
Therapeutic class: Anti-infective
Pregnancy risk category B

Action

Inhibits bacterial cell-wall synthesis during active multiplication by binding with penicillin-binding protein 3

Pharmacokinetics

Apparent mean volume of distribution at steady-state averages 12.6 L (roughly equivalent to extracellular fluid volume). Serum half-life averages 1.7 hours (1.5 to 2) in patients with normal renal function, independent of dosage and administration route. For healthy patient weighing 154 lb (70 kg), serum clearance is 91 mL/minute and renal clearance is 56 mL/minute. Mean serum half-life increases and renal clearance decreases in elderly patients. Half-life is prolonged in impaired renal function and prolonged slightly in hepatic impairment.

Onset	Peak	Duration
Dose-dependent	1 hr	Unknown

How supplied

Powder for reconstitution for injection (lyophilized): 1-g and 2-g vials
Solution for injection (frozen): 1 g/50 mL and 2 g/50 mL in single-dose plastic containers

Indications and dosages

➤ Infections caused by susceptible gram-negative organisms

Adults: For urinary tract infections, 500 mg or 1 g I.V. q 8 or 12 hours. For moderately severe systemic infections, 1 or 2 g I.V. q 8 or 12 hours. For severe or life-threatening infections, 2 g I.V. q 6 or 8 hours. Maximum dosage is 8 g/day.
Children: For mild to moderate infections 30 mg/kg I.V. q 8 hours. For moderate to severe infections, 30 mg/kg I.V. q 6 or 8 hours. Maximum dosage is 120 mg/kg/day.

Dosage adjustment

- Because of prolonged serum half-life in renal impairment, give half of recommended dosage in patients with estimated creatinine clearance of 10 to 30 mL/minute/ 1.73 m^2 after initial loading dose of 1 or 2 g. In patients with severe renal failure (creatinine clearance less than 10 mL/minute/1.73 m^2), such as those on hemodialysis, initially give usual dose of 500 mg, 1 g, or 2 g; maintenance dose should be one-fourth of usual initial dosage given at usual fixed interval of 6, 8, or 12 hours. For serious or life-threatening infections, in addition to maintenance dose, give one-eighth of initial dosage after each hemodialysis session.

- Obtain creatinine clearance in elderly patients, as serum creatinine may not accurately reflect renal status. Adjust dosage as necessary.

Administration

Preparation

- Know that duration of therapy depends on infection severity. However, drug generally should be continued for at least 48 hours after symptoms disappear or evidence of bacterial eradication is obtained. Persistent infections may require several weeks of treatment.

Dilution and compatibility

- Drug is compatible with normal saline solution for injection, 5% or 10% dextrose injection, Ringer's or lactated Ringer's solution, 5% dextrose and normal saline solution for injection, 5% dextrose and 0.45% sodium chloride injection, 5% dextrose and 0.2% sodium chloride injection, sodium lactate injection, Ionosol B and 5% dextrose, Isolyte E, Isolyte E with 5% dextrose, Isolyte M with 5% dextrose, Normosol-R, Normosol-R and 5% dextrose, Normosol-M and 5% dextrose, Mannitol injection 5% or 10%, lactated Ringer's and 5% dextrose injection, Plasma-Lyte M and 5% dextrose, 10% Travert injection, 10% Travert and Electrolyte No. 1 injection, 10% Travert and Electrolyte No. 2 injection, 10% Travert and Electrolyte No. 3 injection.
- Drug is compatible with I.V. infusion solutions prepared with normal saline solution for injection or dextrose 5% injection to which clindamycin phosphate, gentamicin sulfate, tobramycin sulfate, or cefazolin sodium has been added at recommended concentrations. It remains stable for up to 48 hours at room temperature and up to 7 days when refrigerated.
- Ampicillin sodium admixtures with aztreonam in normal saline solution are stable for 24 hours at room temperature and for 48 hours when refrigerated; admixtures with dextrose 5% injection are stable for 2 hours at room temperature and for 8 hours when refrigerated.
- Aztreonam–cloxacillin sodium and aztreonam–vancomycin hydrochloride admixtures are stable in Dianeal 137 (peritoneal dialysis solution) with 4.25% dextrose for up to 24 hours at room temperature.
- Be aware that admixtures other than those listed above are not recommended.
- Know that aztreonam is incompatible with nafcillin sodium, cephradine, and metronidazole.
- Thaw commercially available frozen drug at room temperature, and use within 24 to 72 hours. Do not refreeze.
- Reconstitute powder for bolus injection by adding 6 to 10 mL sterile water for injection.
- Reconstitute powder for intermittent I.V. infusion by adding compatible I.V. solution to provide a concentration not exceeding 20 mg/mL.
- After adding diluent to vial, shake immediately and vigorously.
- Know that reconstituted solutions are colorless to light straw yellow; they may develop a slight pinkish tint on standing, but this does not affect potency.
- Be aware that reconstituted solutions are not for multiple-dose use. Discard unused solution after reconstitution.

Infusion considerations
• Flush I.V. tubing with compatible solution before and after giving drug.
• Be aware that drug is given by intermittent I.V. infusion, but initial dose may be given by slow I.V. bolus injection over 3 to 5 minutes into tubing of compatible I.V. solution.
• Give prescribed intermittent I.V. infusion dose over 20 to 60 minutes.
Do not use plastic containers in series connections. Such use could cause air embolism due to residual air being drawn from primary container before administration of fluid from secondary container ends.
Monitoring
Monitor carefully for hypersensitivity reactions, especially in patients allergic to penicillin, carbapenems, or cephalosporins. Be prepared to provide emergency interventions as appropriate.
Monitor patient closely for signs and symptoms of pseudomembranous colitis.
• Monitor CBC with differential, alanine aminotransferase (ALT), aspartate aminotransferase (AST), prothrombin time (PT), partial thromboplastin time (PTT), and serum creatinine.
• Monitor renal function regularly if prolonged aminoglycoside therapy or high aminoglycoside doses are used concurrently, due to increased risk of nephrotoxicity and ototoxicity.
• Drug occasionally causes hepatobiliary dysfunction; monitor liver function tests periodically.
Storage
• Store original package at room temperature; avoid excessive heat.
• After reconstitution, solutions for I.V. infusion prepared with sterile water for injection or sodium chloride injection at recommended concentrations may be kept at controlled room temperature of 15° to 30°C (59° to 86°F) for 48 hours, or refrigerated at 2° to 8°C (36° to 46°F) for 7 days.
• Store frozen plastic containers at or below –20°C (–4°F).

Contraindications
Contraindicated in hypersensitivity to drug or its components.

Use cautiously in hypersensitivity to beta-lactams (such as penicillins, cephalosporins, and other carbapenems), renal or hepatic impairment, ***elderly patients***, pregnant or breastfeeding patients, and ***children younger than 9 months*** (safety and efficacy not established).

Adverse reactions
CV: phlebitis, thrombophlebitis, hypotension, transient ECG changes, chest pain
GI: diarrhea, nausea, vomiting, abdominal cramps, diarrhea associated with *Clostridium difficile*, **pseudomembranous colitis**
Hematologic: neutropenia, pancytopenia, anemia, eosinophilia, leukocytosis, thrombocytosis, **thrombocytopenia**
Hepatic: jaundice, **hepatitis**
Respiratory: wheezing, dyspnea
Skin: rash, urticaria, petechiae, pruritus, purpura, erythema multiforme, diaphoresis, **toxic epidermal necrolysis** (rare)
Other: superinfection, hypersensitivity reactions including **bronchospasm, angioedema,** and **anaphylaxis** (rare)

Interactions
Drug-drug. *Aminoglycosides (high doses or prolonged therapy):* increased risk of nephrotoxicity and ototoxicity
Drug-diagnostic tests. *Coombs' test:* positive
ALT, AST, eosinophils, platelets, PT, PTT, serum creatinine: increased
Neutrophils: decreased

Toxicity and overdose
- Overdose signs and symptoms are extensions of adverse reactions.
- Discontinue drug and provide symptomatic interventions. If necessary, use hemodialysis or peritoneal dialysis, as ordered.

Patient monitoring
Instruct patient to immediately report signs or symptoms of hypersensitivity reactions (such as rash or difficulty breathing) or liver impairment (such as unusual tiredness, weakness, nausea, yellowing of skin or eyes, tenderness on right upper side of abdomen, or flulike symptoms).
- As appropriate, review all other significant and life-threatening adverse reactions and interactions, especially those related to the drugs and tests mentioned above.

benztropine mesylate
Cogentin

Pharmacologic class: Anticholinergic, belladonna alkaloid
Therapeutic class: Antiparkinsonian
Pregnancy risk category C

Action
Inhibits cholinergic excitatory pathways and restores balance of neurotransmitters (dopamine and acetylcholine) in CNS, thereby decreasing such parkinsonism symptoms as excess salivation, rigidity, and tremors

Pharmacokinetics
Little pharmacokinetic information is available on anticholinergic drugs, although effects are known to be cumulative and long-lasting.

Onset	Peak	Duration
Rapid	Unknown	Unknown

How supplied
Solution for injection (clear, colorless): 1 mg/mL in 2-mL ampules

Indications and dosages
➢ Postencephalitic parkinsonism

Adults: 2 mg I.V. daily in one or more doses; may increase dosage as necessary. In highly sensitive patients, initial dosage may be as low as 0.5 mg I.V. at bedtime, increased as necessary.

➢ Idiopathic parkinsonism

Adults: Initially, 0.5 to 1 mg I.V. at bedtime; may increase to 4 to 6 mg as needed. Usual dosage is 1 to 2 mg.

➢ Drug-induced extrapyramidal disorders

Adults: 1 to 4 mg I.V. once or twice daily. In acute dystonic reactions, 1 to 2 mg may relieve symptoms quickly. When extrapyramidal disorder develops soon after neuroleptic therapy starts, 1 to 2 mg benztropine I.V. two or three times daily usually provides relief within 1 or 2 days. After 2 weeks, withdraw drug, as ordered, to determine continued need.

Dosage adjustment
- Reduce dosage in patients at risk for hyperthermia.

Administration
Preparation
- Know that I.V. route is seldom used, as drug onset is essentially the same as with I.M administration.
- Be aware that therapy should start with lowest effective dosage because of cumulative drug action.

Know that drug is not recommended for tardive dyskinesia, as it does not relieve symptoms and in some cases may aggravate them.

Infusion considerations
• Administer at prescribed rate.
Monitoring
Be aware that severe anhidrosis and fatal hyperthermia have occurred.
Assess for signs and symptoms of ileus, including constipation and abdominal distention.
• Monitor blood pressure closely, especially in elderly patients.
• Monitor fluid intake and output; check for urine retention.
Storage
• Store in well-ventilated area at controlled room temperature..

Contraindications and precautions

Contraindicated in hypersensitivity to drug, tardive dyskinesia, and ***children younger than age 3.***

Use cautiously in seizure disorders, arrhythmias, tachycardia, hypertension, hypotension, hepatic or renal dysfunction, mental disorders, alcoholism, patients at risk for hyperthermia, ***elderly patients,*** pregnant or breastfeeding patients, and ***children older than age 3.***

Adverse reactions

CNS: confusion, depression, hallucinations, memory impairment, nervousness, disorientation, exacerbation of psychotic symptoms, listlessness, numbness in fingers, **toxic psychosis**
CV: tachycardia
EENT: blurred vision, dilated pupils
GI: nausea, constipation, vomiting, dry mouth, **paralytic ileus**
GU: urine retention, dysuria
Skin: rash, urticaria, decreased sweating, dermatoses
Other: fever, **heat stroke, hyperthermia**

Interactions

Drug-drug. *Antihistamines, bethanechol, disopyramide, phenothiazines, quinidine, tricyclic antidepressants:* additive anticholinergic effects
Drug-herb. *Angel's trumpet, jimsonweed, scopolia:* increased anticholinergic effects
Drug-behaviors. *Alcohol use:* increased sedation

Toxicity and overdose

• In overdose, expect signs and symptoms similar to those of atropine poisoning or antihistamine overdose (such as CNS depression), confusion, nervousness, and listlessness. Other effects may include intensification of mental symptoms or toxic psychosis in patients with mental illness who are receiving neuroleptics (such as phenothiazines), hallucinations (especially visual), dizziness, muscle weakness, ataxia, mydriasis, blurred vision, palpitations, tachycardia, hypertension, nausea, vomiting, dry mouth, constipation, dysphagia, dysuria, numbness of fingers, and hot, dry, flushed skin. Allergic reactions, headache, delirium, anhidrosis, hyperthermia, glaucoma, coma, shock, seizures, and respiratory arrest also are possible.
• Give physostigmine salicylate 1 to 2 mg subcutaneously or I.V. as ordered; may give a second injection after 2 hours if required. Otherwise, provide symptomatic and supportive interventions. As ordered, administer local miotic for mydriasis and cycloplegia; use ice bags or other cold applications and alcohol sponges for hyperpyrexia. Short-acting barbiturates may be prescribed to counter CNS excitement, but use caution to avoid subsequent depression. Provide supportive care for depression; avoid convulsant stimulants, such as picrotoxin, pentylenetetrazol, and bemegride. As ordered, give vasopressors and fluids for circulatory collapse. For severe respiratory depression, maintain respiration and provide artificial respiration, if indicated.

Patient teaching

Instruct patient to immediately report GI complaints.

- Advise patient to use caution during activities that require physical or mental alertness, as drug causes sedation.
- Teach patient to avoid increased heat exposure.
- Caution patient not to stop therapy abruptly.
- As appropriate, review all other significant and life-threatening adverse reactions and interactions, especially those related to the drugs, herbs, and behaviors mentioned above.

bevacizumab

Avastin

Pharmacologic class: Monoclonal antibody
Therapeutic class: Immunologic agent
Pregnancy risk category C

FDA BOXED WARNING

- Drug may cause potentially fatal GI perforation and wound dehiscence. GI perforation sometimes is associated with intra-abdominal abscess and does not correlate to duration of therapy. Typically, it presents as abdominal pain, constipation, and vomiting. GI perforation should be included in differential diagnosis of patients who develop abdominal pain when receiving bevacizumab. Discontinue therapy permanently in patients with GI perforation or wound dehiscence requiring medical intervention.
- Appropriate interval between termination of bevacizumab and subsequent elective surgery to avoid risks of impaired wound healing and wound dehiscence has not been determined.
- Serious and in some cases fatal hemoptysis has occurred in patients with non-small-cell lung cancer treated with chemotherapy and bevacizumab. Patients with recent hemoptysis should not receive bevacizumab.

Action

Binds to vascular endothelial growth factor, preventing or reducing microvascular formation and growth and inhibiting metastatic disease progression

Pharmacokinetics

Predicted time to reach steady state is 100 days. Estimated half-life is approximately 20 days (range, 11 to 50 days). Clearance varies with weight, gender, and tumor burden.

Onset	Peak	Duration
Unknown	Unknown	Unknown

How supplied

Solution for injection (clear to slightly opalescent, colorless to pale brown): 25 mg/mL in 4-mL and 16-mL vials

Indications and dosages

➢ First-line or second-line treatment of metastatic carcinoma of colon or rectum
Adults: When used with FOLFOX4 (oxaliplatin, leucovorin, and fluorouracil), 10 mg/kg by I.V. infusion q 14 days

➢ First-line treatment with carboplatin and paclitaxel for unresectable, locally advanced, recurrent, or metastatic non-squamous or non-small-cell lung cancer
Adults: 15 mg/kg by I.V. infusion q 3 weeks

Administration

Preparation

- Know that drug is usually given in combination with 5-fluorouracil-based chemotherapy.

• Do not administer within 28 days after major surgery. Suspend therapy several weeks before patient undergoes elective surgery.

Dilution and compatibility

• Withdraw necessary amount for 5-mg/kg dose, and dilute in 100 mL normal saline solution for injection.

Do not mix or administer with dextrose solutions.

• Do not shake solution.

Infusion considerations

Do not administer by I.V. push or bolus.

• Initially, infuse drug over 90 minutes. If patient tolerates infusion well, infuse second dose over 60 minutes. If patient continues to tolerate drug well, infuse each dose over 30 minutes thereafter.

Withhold dose if hypertension occurs.

Stop infusion if patient develops hypertensive crisis, severe bleeding, wound dehiscence, urinary problems, or abdominal pain (which may signal intra-abdominal abscess or GI perforation).

Monitoring

Although infusion reactions rarely follow first dose, stay alert for hypertension, hypertensive crisis with neurologic signs and symptoms, wheezing, oxygen desaturation, chest pain, headache, rigors, and diaphoresis. If reaction is severe, interrupt infusion and provide appropriate interventions. (No data exist regarding the most appropriate way to identify patients who may safely receive bevacizumab after having a severe infusion reaction.)

Monitor patient closely for signs and symptoms of thromboembolism, GI perforation (such as abdominal pain, vomiting, and constipation), hemorrhage, and hypertensive crisis.

Stay alert for delayed wound healing and wound dehiscence.

Monitor for reversible posterior leukoencephalopathy syndrome (RPLS), which may present as headache, seizure, lethargy, confusion, blindness, and other visual and neurologic disturbances. Mild to severe hypertension may occur, but is not crucial for RPLS diagnosis. Magnetic resonance imaging is needed to confirm RPLS. Symptoms may begin from 16 hours to 1 year after bevacizumab initiation; they usually resolve or improve within days, although some patients have ongoing neurologic sequelae. Safety of reinitiating drug in patients who previously experienced RPLS is unknown.

Discontinue drug permanently in patients who develop GI perforation, wound dehiscence, serious bleeding, severe arterial thromboembolic event, nephrotic syndrome, hypertensive crisis, or hypertensive encephalopathy.

Discontinue drug if patient develops RPLS. As indicated and ordered, initiate treatment for hypertension.

Temporarily suspend therapy in moderate to severe proteinuria and in severe hypertension not controlled with medical management.

• Assess blood pressure frequently, especially in patients with hypertension induced or exacerbated by bevacizumab in whom drug has been stopped.

• Monitor CBC with differential, as well as urine protein and serum electrolyte levels.

Storage

• Refrigerate at 2° to 8°C (36° to 46°F) in original carton until use. Protect from light.

• Do not freeze.

Contraindications and precautions

Use cautiously in hypersensitivity to drug, cardiovascular disease, patients recovering from major surgery, ***elderly patients***, pregnant or breastfeeding patients, and ***children*** (safety and efficacy not established).

Adverse reactions

CNS: asthenia, dizziness, headache, confusion, syncope, fatigue, sensory neuropathy
CV: hypotension, hypertension, **hypertensive crisis, heart failure, thromboembolism, deep vein thrombosis, intra-abdominal thrombosis, RPLS**
EENT: epistaxis
GI: nausea, vomiting, diarrhea, constipation, abdominal pain, stomatitis, dyspepsia, flatulence, colitis, dry mouth, anorexia, **GI perforation, intra-abdominal abscess**
GU: proteinuria, **nephrotic syndrome**
Hematologic: leukopenia, neutropenia, hemorrhage, thrombocytopenia
Metabolic: hypokalemia
Respiratory: upper respiratory tract infection, dyspnea, pneumonitis, pulmonary infiltrates, **massive hemoptysis**
Skin: exfoliative dermatitis, alopecia, skin ulcer, wound-healing complications, **wound dehiscence**
Other: abnormal taste, altered voice, pain, weight loss, non-GI fistula formation, **infusion reaction**

Interactions

Drug-drug. *Irinotecan:* increased concentration of irinotecan metabolite
Drug-diagnostic tests. *Potassium, white blood cells:* decreased
Urine protein: increased

Toxicity and overdose

- Maximum tolerated dosage has not been determined. Highest dosage tested in humans (20 mg/kg I.V.) caused headache in 9 of 16 patients and severe headache in three.
- Provide supportive interventions.

Patient teaching

Instruct patient to immediately report dizziness, severe bleeding, stomach pain, headache, seizure, lethargy, confusion, blindness or other visual problems, urinary problems, or wound opening.
- Instruct patient to tell prescriber if he has been exposed to chickenpox or if he has gout, heart disease, viral infection, urinary problems, hepatic disease, or another form of cancer.
- Advise patient to tell prescriber if surgery is planned; drug may delay wound healing.
- Caution patient not to get immunizations unless prescriber approves.
- Instruct female patient to tell prescriber if she is pregnant, plans to become pregnant, or is breastfeeding.
- As appropriate, review all other significant and life-threatening adverse reactions and interactions, especially those related to the drugs and tests mentioned above.

[redacted]

bivalirudin

Angiomax

Pharmacologic class: Thrombin inhibitor
Therapeutic class: Anticoagulant
Pregnancy risk category B

Action

Selectively inhibits thrombin by binding to its catalytic site and anion-binding exosite of circulating and clot-bound thrombin, thereby preventing conversion of fibrinogen to fibrin and subsequent clot formation

Pharmacokinetics

Drug does not bind to plasma proteins (other than thrombin) or to red blood cells. It exhibits linear pharmacokinetics after I.V. administration in patients undergoing percutaneous transluminal coronary angioplasty (PTCA); in these patients, mean steady-state concentration is 12.3 ± 1.7 mcg/mL after I.V. bolus of 1 mg/kg and a 4-hour 2.5 mg/kg/hour I.V. infusion. Drug clears from plasma by combination of renal mechanisms and proteolytic cleavage, with half-life of 25 minutes in patients with normal renal function. Elimination relates to glomerular filtration rate. Total body clearance is similar for patients with normal renal function and mild renal impairment (60 to 89 mL/minute). Clearance falls approximately 20% in moderate and severe renal impairment and approximately 80% in dialysis-dependent patients.

Onset	Peak	Duration
Immediate	Immediate	1 hr

How supplied

Powder for reconstitution for injection (white, lyophilized cake): 250 mg in single-use vial

Indications and dosages

➢ Patients with unstable angina who are undergoing PCTA

Adults: 0.75 mg/kg I.V. bolus just before PCTA. Five minutes after bolus dose, activated clotting time (ACT) should be performed and an additional bolus of 0.3 mg/kg given, if necessary. Follow this with infusion of 1.75 mg/kg/hour for duration of procedure. As an option, infusion may continue for up to 4 hours after procedure. After 4-hour infusion, may give an additional I.V. infusion at 0.2 mg/kg/hour for up to 20 hours, along with aspirin as prescribed.

Dosage adjustment

• Reduce infusion dosage in renal impairment, as follows: Give 1.75 mg/kg/hour I.V. in moderate renal impairment (30 to 59 mL/minute). With creatinine clearance less than 30 mL/minute, consider reducing infusion rate to 1 mg/ kg/hour. If patient is on hemodialysis, reduce infusion rate to 0.25 mg/kg/hour. No reduction in bolus dose is needed.

Administration

Preparation

• Know that drug is intended to be given with aspirin.

Dilution and compatibility

• For I.V. bolus injection and infusion, add 5 mL sterile water for injection to each 250-mg vial; mix gently until dissolved. Dilute further in 50 mL D_5W or normal saline solution to a final concentration of 5 mg/mL.

• If a low-rate infusion is used after initial infusion, prepare a solution with a lower concentration of bivalirudin by reconstituting a 250-mg vial with 5 mL sterile water for injection. Gently swirl until all material dissolves. Further dilute each reconstituted vial in 500 mL D_5W or normal saline solution, to yield a final concentration of 0.5 mg/mL.

• Be aware that when reconstituted with sterile water for injection, drug is a clear to opalescent, colorless to slightly yellow solution.

• Do not mix with other drugs.

Infusion considerations

Give by bolus injection or I.V. infusion as directed.

Never give I.M.

Monitoring

Monitor blood pressure, hemoglobin, and hematocrit. Be aware that blood pressure or hematocrit decrease may signal hemorrhagic event.

• Monitor venipuncture site closely for bleeding.

• Monitor ACT in patients with renal impairment.

Storage
• Store at 20° to 25°C (68° to 77°F); excursions are permitted to 15° to 30°C (59° to 86°F).
• Reconstituted solution may be stored at 2° to 8°C (36° to 46°F) for up to 24 hours. Diluted solution with concentration between 0.5 and 5 mg/mL is stable at room temperature for up to 24 hours.

Contraindications and precautions
Contraindicated in hypersensitivity to drug or its components and in active major bleeding.

Use cautiously in renal impairment, cerebrovascular accident, diseases linked to increased bleeding risk, concurrent use of other platelet-aggregation inhibitors, pregnant or breastfeeding patients, and ***children.***

Adverse reactions
CNS: headache, anxiety, nervousness, insomnia
CV: hypotension, hypertension, angina, **bradycardia, ventricular fibrillation**
GI: nausea, vomiting, abdominal pain, dyspepsia
GU: urine retention
Hematologic: severe spontaneous bleeding, minor or major hemorrhage, retroperitoneal bleeding, thrombocytopenia
Musculoskeletal: pelvic or back pain
Other: pain, fever, pain at injection site

Interactions
Drug-drug. *Abciximab, anticoagulants (including heparin, heparinoids, and low-molecular-weight heparin), thrombolytics, ticlopidine:* increased bleeding risk
Drug-diagnostic tests. *Activated partial thromboplastin time, prothrombin time:* increased
Drug-herb. *Ginkgo biloba:* increased bleeding risk

Toxicity and overdose
• Single bolus doses of up to 7.5 mg/kg have been given without associated bleeding or other adverse events.
• In overdose, discontinue drug immediately and monitor patient closely for bleeding. No known antidote exists; however, drug is hemodialyzable.

Patient teaching
Instruct patient to immediately report bleeding, bruising, or tarry stools.
• Tell patient to avoid activities that can cause injury and to use soft toothbrush and electric razor to avoid gum and skin injury.
• Advise family members to consider taking classes in cardiopulmonary resuscitation.
• As appropriate, review all other significant and life-threatening adverse reactions and interactions, especially those related to the drugs, tests, and herbs mentioned above.

bleomycin sulfate
Blenoxane

Pharmacologic class: Antitumor antibiotic
Therapeutic class: Antineoplastic
Pregnancy risk category D

FDA BOXED WARNING

• Give under supervision of physician in facility with adequate diagnostic and treatment resources.
• Know that pulmonary fibrosis is most severe toxicity, and most often presents as pneumonitis progressing to pulmonary fibrosis. Occurrence is highest in patients who are elderly or are receiving total dose exceeding 400 units.

Action

Unclear. Appears to inhibit DNA synthesis and, to a lesser degree, RNA and protein synthesis. Binds to DNA, causing severing of single and double DNA strands.

Pharmacokinetics

When creatinine clearance exceeds 35 mL/minute, serum or plasma terminal elimination half-life is approximately 115 minutes; when it is below 35 mL/minute, serum or plasma terminal elimination half-life increases exponentially as creatinine clearance decreases. In patients with normal renal function, 60% to 70% of dose is recovered in urine as active bleomycin. Patients with moderately severe renal failure may excrete less than 20% of dose in urine, suggesting that severe renal impairment can cause drug accumulation in blood.

Onset	Peak	Duration
Unknown	10-20 min	Unknown

How supplied

Powder for reconstitution for injection: 15-unit vials, 30-unit vials

Indications and dosages

➢ Hodgkin's lymphoma

Adults: 10 to 20 units/m^2 I.V. once or twice weekly. After 50% response, give maintenance dose of 1 unit/m^2 I.V. daily or 5 units/m^2 I.V. weekly.

➢ Squamous-cell carcinoma of head, neck, skin, penis, cervix, or vulva; non-Hodgkin's lymphoma; testicular carcinoma

Adults and adolescents: 10 to 20 units/m^2 I.V. once or twice weekly

Dosage adjustment

- Some patients (especially those with severe renal impairment) may require dosage reduction.
- Because of possibile anaphylactoid reaction, lymphoma patients should receive 2 units or less for first two doses. If no acute reaction occurs, follow regular dosage schedule.

Off-label uses

- AIDS-related Kaposi's sarcoma
- Esophageal carcinoma
- Hemangioma
- Osteosarcoma
- Verrucous carcinoma
- Warts

Administration

Preparation

Follow hazardous drug guidelines on page S19 for handling, preparation, and administration.

- Assess baseline pulmonary function status before starting therapy.
- Premedicate patient with acetaminophen, corticosteroids, and diphenhydramine, as prescribed, to reduce anaphylaxis risk.

Administer test dose, as ordered, to patients with lymphoma.

- Be aware that improvement of Hodgkin's disease and testicular tumors usually is prompt and occurs within 2 weeks; improvement is unlikely if it is not seen by this time. Squamous-cell cancers respond more slowly, sometimes taking up to 3 weeks before improvement appears.

Dilution and compatibility

- For I.V. injection, dissolve contents of 15- or 30-unit vial in 5 or 10 mL, respectively, of normal saline solution for injection.
- For intermittent infusion, further dilute in 50 to 100 mL normal saline solution.

Do not reconstitute or dilute with D_5W or other dextrose-containing diluent, as drug potency may decrease.

Infusion considerations

Clinical alert: Give cumulative doses above 400 units with extreme caution due to increased risk of pulmonary toxicity.

- For I.V. bolus injection, administer slowly over 10 minutes.
- For intermittent I.V. infusion, give over 15 minutes or longer.

Monitoring

Clinical alert: Monitor closely for severe idiosyncratic reactions (hypotension, fever, chills, wheezing, and mental confusion), which may follow the first or second dose. Intervene symptomatically by giving volume expanders, pressors, antihistamines, and corticosteroids, as ordered and indicated.

Clinical alert: Monitor pulmonary function, including chest X-rays, every 1 to 2 weeks. Assess breath sounds and monitor pulmonary diffusion capacity for carbon monoxide (DLco) monthly (if indicated) to detect pulmonary toxicity. Earliest symptom is dyspnea; earliest sign is fine crackles.

Clinical alert: Know that when drug is used with other antineoplastics, pulmonary toxicity may occur at lower dosages. Discontinue drug if DLco falls below 30% of pretreatment value or overt signs and symptoms of pulmonary toxicity occur.

Clinical alert: Be aware that patient may experience sudden onset of acute chest pain syndrome (suggesting pleuropericarditis) during infusion.

- Monitor renal and hepatic function tests (although renal and hepatic toxicity are rare).
- Assess mouth for sores, ulcers, pain, and bleeding.

Storage

- Refrigerate powder at 2° to 8°C (36° to 46°F).
- After reconstitution with normal saline solution, drug is stable for 24 hours at room temperature.

Contraindications and precautions

Contraindicated in hypersensitivity to drug and in patients who have experienced idiosyncratic reactions to it.

Use with extreme caution in significant renal or pulmonary impairment. Use cautiously in patients undergoing radiation therapy, ***elderly patients,*** pregnant or breastfeeding patients, females of childbearing age, and ***children*** (safety and efficacy not established).

Adverse reactions

CNS: malaise
CV: hypotension, phlebitis, **acute chest pain syndrome** (rare), **Raynaud's phenomenon, myocardial infarction, cerebrovascular accident, thrombocytic microangiopathy, cerebral arteritis**
GI: vomiting, diarrhea, anorexia, stomatitis
Hepatic: hepatotoxicity
Respiratory: dyspnea, crackles, **pulmonary fibrosis, pneumonitis**
Skin: alopecia, erythema, rash, vesicles, striae, hyperpigmentation, mucocutaneous toxicity, "radiation recall," skin tenderness, hyperkeratosis, nail changes
Other: fever, chills, weight loss, tumor site pain, **idiosyncratic reactions, anaphylaxis**

Interactions

Drug-drug. *Nephrotoxic drugs:* decreased bleomycin clearance
Drug-diagnostic tests. *Uric acid:* increased

Toxicity and overdose

- No cases of overdose have been reported.
- If overdose occurs, provide symptomatic and supportive interventions.

Patient teaching

- Advise patient to avoid spicy, hot, or rough food, as these may cause GI upset.

- Instruct patient to avoid activities that can cause injury and to use soft toothbrush and electric razor to avoid gum and skin injury.
- Inform patient that drug may cause hair loss, but that hair will grow back once treatment ends.
- Tell patient about the need for frequent laboratory and other testing during therapy.
- Urge female patient to use reliable contraceptive method during therapy.
- Advise breastfeeding patient to discontinue breastfeeding during therapy.
- As appropriate, review all other significant and life-threatening adverse reactions and interactions, especially those related to the drugs and tests mentioned above.

bortezomib

Velcade

Pharmacologic class: Proteasome inhibitor

Therapeutic class: Antineoplastic

Pregnancy risk category D

Action

Inhibits proteasomes (enzyme complexes that regulate protein homeostasis within cells). Reversibly inhibits chymotrypsin-like activity at 26S proteasome, leading to activation of signaling cascades, cell-cycle arrest, and apoptosis.

Pharmacokinetics

Drug is distributed widely to peripheral tissues. It is metabolized in the liver; average protein binding is 83%. With twice-weekly doses, mean maximum plasma levels range from 89 to 120 ng/mL for 1.3-mg/m² dose. With multiple dosages, mean elimination half-life ranges from 76 to 108 hours after 1.3-mg/m² dose.

Onset	Peak	Duration
Unknown	Unknown	Unknown

How supplied

Cake or powder for reconstitution for injection (white to off-white, preservative-free): 3.5 mg (contains 35 mg mannitol)

Indications and dosages

➤ Multiple myeloma in patients who have received at least one previous therapy; mantle-cell lymphoma in patients who have received at least one previous therapy

Adults: 1.3 mg/m² I.V. bolus twice weekly for 2 weeks (days 1, 4, 8, and 11), followed by 10-day rest period (days 12 to 21). Let at least 72 hours elapse between doses. One treatment cycle equals 21 days (3 weeks). For extended therapy of more than eight cycles, may administer on standard schedule of once weekly for 4 weeks (days 1, 8, 15, 22), followed by 13-day rest period (days 23 to 35).

Dosage adjustment

- Withhold dose if platelet count falls below 25,000/mm³; reinitiate at decreased dosage.
- Be aware that patients with new or worsening peripheral neuropathy may require dosage adjustment or dosing schedule changes.

Administration

Preparation

- Obtain baseline CBC with white cell differential and platelet count.

Dilution and compatibility

- Reconstitute drug in vial with 3.5 mL normal saline solution for injection.

Infusion considerations

- Give by I.V. push over 3 to 5 seconds.

Monitoring

Monitor vital signs and temperature. Especially watch for tachycardia, fever, and hypertension.

Stay alert for reversible posterior leukoencephalopathy syndrome (RPLS), which can present as headache, seizure, lethargy, confusion, blindness, and other visual and neurologic disturbances. Mild to severe hypertension may occur but is not necessary for RPLS diagnosis. Magnetic resonance imaging is needed to confirm diagnosis. Safety of reinitiating drug in patients who previously experienced RPLS is unknown.

Discontinue drug in patients with RPLS, and intervene for hypertension (if present), as ordered.

Monitor CBC with white cell differential; watch for signs and symptoms of blood dyscrasias, and be prepared to intervene for anemia.

Obtain platelet count before each dose. Be prepared to give transfusions if GI or intracerebral hemorrhage occurs.

Watch for tumor lysis syndrome, especially in patients with high pretreatment tumor burden. Check for hyperphosphatemia, hyperkalemia, and renal dysfunction.

- Monitor respiratory status, watching for dyspnea, cough, and other signs and symptoms of upper respiratory tract infection.
- Closely monitor patients who have heart disease or risk factors for it.
- Because drug is metabolized by liver enzymes and clearance may decrease in hepatic impairment, closely monitor for hepatic toxicities.
- Watch closely for toxicities in patients with renal impairment.
- Monitor nutritional and hydration status for changes caused by adverse GI effects; as indicated, give antiemetics, antidiarrheals, and fluid and electrolyte replacement. Also observe patient for hypotension.
- Monitor for signs and symptoms of peripheral neuropathy, such as burning sensation, hyperesthesia, hypoesthesia, paresthesia, discomfort, and neuropathic pain or weakness.

Storage

- Store unopened vials at controlled room temperature 25°C (77°F); excursions permitted to 15° to 30°C (59° to 86°F).
- Keep in original package to protect from light.
- Reconstituted solution may be stored for up to 8 hours after preparation when exposed to normal indoor lighting.

Contraindications and precautions

Contraindicated in hypersensitivity to drug, mannitol, or boron.

Use cautiously in history of syncope; hepatic or renal impairment; peripheral neuropathy; dehydration; patients receiving drugs that can cause hypotension; patients at risk for heart disease; females of childbearing age; and ***children*** (safety and efficacy not established).

Adverse reactions

CNS: headache, insomnia, dizziness, anxiety, peripheral neuropathy, paresthesia, dysesthesia, fatigue, malaise, weakness, rigors, asthenia, psychiatric disorders, **RPLS** (rare)
CV: tachycardia, hypertension
GI: nausea, vomiting, diarrhea, constipation, abdominal pain, anorexia
Hematologic: eosinophilia, anemia, **thrombocytopenia, neutropenia**
Metabolic: dehydration
Musculoskeletal: bone pain, limb pain, back pain, arthralgia, muscle cramps, myalgia
Respiratory: cough, dyspnea, upper respiratory tract infection, lower respiratory tract or lung infection
Skin: rash, pruritus, urticaria
Other: decreased appetite, fever, herpes zoster, lower limb edema, **tumor lysis syndrome**

Interactions

Drug-drug. *CYP3A4 inducers (including carbamazepine, nevirapine, phenobarbital, phenytoin, and rifampin):* possible decrease in bortezomib serum level and efficacy

CYP3A4 inhibitors (including amiodarone, cimetidine, clarithromycin, delavirdine, diltiazem, disulfiram, erythromycin, fluoxetine, fluvoxamine, nefazodone, nevirapine, propoxyphene, quinupristin, verapamil, zafirlukast, and zileuton): possible increase in bortezomib serum level and efficacy

Drug-food. *Grapefruit juice:* increased risk of toxicity or reduced efficacy

Toxicity and overdose

- Deaths have occurred in patients receiving more than twice the recommended therapeutic dosage. Acute onset of symptomatic hypotension and thrombocytopenia occurred.
- No known antidote exists. In overdose, monitor vital signs and provide appropriate supportive care.

Patient teaching

- Inform patient that drug can cause serious blood disorders. Tell patient which signs and symptoms to report right away.
- Tell patient that drug may cause significant adverse reactions. Provide reassurance that he will be monitored closely; tell him to report significant problems.
- Instruct patient to avoid driving and other hazardous activities until drug's effects on concentration and alertness are known.
- Advise patient to minimize adverse GI effects by eating small, frequent servings of healthy food and drinking plenty of fluids.
- Tell patient to immediately report signs and symptoms of upper respiratory tract infection.
- Inform patient about the need for frequent laboratory and other testing during therapy.
- As appropriate, review all other significant and life-threatening adverse reactions and interactions, especially those related to the drugs and food mentioned above.

bumetanide

Bumetanide Injection

Pharmacologic class: Loop diuretic
Therapeutic class: Antihypertensive
Pregnancy risk category C

FDA BOXED WARNING

- Drug is a potent diuretic; excessive amounts may cause profound diuresis, with fluid and electrolyte depletion. Give only under careful medical supervision; adjust dosage and dosing schedule to patient's needs.

Action

Inhibits reabsorption of sodium and chloride in ascending limb of loop of Henle; increases renal excretion of water, sodium, chloride, and magnesium

Pharmacokinetics

Drug is metabolized by the liver and is 94% to 96% bound to protein. Maximum plasma concentrations are higher in elderly patients. Drug is eliminated rapidly, with half-life of 1 to 1.5 hours in adults. It is excreted largely in urine, with some excretion in feces.

Onset	Peak	Duration
Several min	15-30 min	Unknown

B

How supplied

Solution for injection: 0.25-mg/mL vial

Indications and dosages

➢ Edema caused by heart failure or hepatic or renal disease

Adults: 0.5 to 1 mg I.V., repeated q 2 to 3 hours as needed, up to 10 mg/day

Dosage adjustment

- Because drug is largely excreted by the kidneys, use caution in selecting dosages for patients with renal impairment.
- For elderly patients, start dosage selection at low end of recommended range.

Off-label uses (selected)

- Drug-related edema
- Hypercalcemia

Administration

Preparation

- Weigh patient at start of therapy.
- Be aware that drug may be given alone or with other antihypertensives.
- Know that sulfonamide-sensitive patients may have bumetanide sensitivity.
- Individualize dosages through careful monitoring of patient response.
- Be aware that parenteral administration should be switched to oral administration as soon as possible.

Dilution and compatibility

- Dilute with D_5W for injection, normal saline solution for injection, or lactated Ringer's solution for injection.
- Administer solutions freshly prepared or within 24 hours.

Infusion considerations

- Give by I.V. BOLUS injection slowly over 2 minutes.

Monitoring

- Monitor blood pressure regularly.
- Monitor serum electrolytes, especially potassium. If needed, add supplemental potassium or potassium-sparing diuretics to regimen, as ordered.
- Monitor uric acid, urine glucose, and blood urea nitrogen (BUN) levels.
- Assess for ototoxicity when giving high or frequent doses, especially in patients with renal impairment.

🔊 Observe for signs and symptoms of thrombocytopenia (rare).

🔊 Monitor elderly patients closely for extreme blood pressure changes, orthostatic hypotension, and dehydration.

Storage

- Store at controlled room temperature of 15° to 30°C (59° to 86°F).

Contraindications and precautions

Contraindicated in hypersensitivity to drug, uncorrected electrolyte imbalances, hepatic coma, anuria, and oliguria.

Use cautiously in sulfonamide sensitivity, severe hepatic disease accompanied by cirrhosis or ascites, renal impairment, electrolyte depletion, diabetes mellitus, worsening azotemia, ***elderly patients***, pregnant or breastfeeding patients, and ***children younger than age 18***.

Adverse reactions

CNS: dizziness, headache, weakness, **encephalopathy**

CV: hypotension, ECG changes

EENT: impaired hearing

GI: nausea, abdominal pain

Hematologic: thrombocytopenia (rare)

Metabolic: dehydration, hyperglycemia, hyperuricemia, hypokalemia, hypomagnesemia, hyponatremia, **hypochloremic alkalosis**

Musculoskeletal: arthralgia, muscle cramps

Skin: rash, hives, pruritus

Interactions

Drug-drug. *Aminoglycosides, cisplatin:* increased risk of ototoxicity

Amphotericin B, corticosteroids, mezlocillin, other diuretics, piperacillin, stimulant laxatives: additive hypokalemia

Antihypertensives, nitrates: additive hypotension
Indomethacin: blunting of increase in urine volume and sodium excretion; inhibition of bumetanide-induced increase in plasma renin activity
Lithium: decreased lithium excretion, possible lithium toxicity
Nonsteroidal anti-inflammatory drugs, probenecid: inhibition of diuretic response
Drug-diagnostic tests. *BUN, cholesterol, creatinine, glucose, nitrogenous compounds:* increased *Calcium, magnesium, platelets, potassium, sodium:* decreased
Drug-herb. *Dandelion:* interference with diuretic activity
Ginseng: resistance to diuresis
Licorice: rapid potassium loss
Drug-behaviors. *Acute alcohol ingestion:* additive hypotension

Toxicity and overdose

- Overdose may cause profound water loss and electrolyte depletion manifested by weakness, dizziness, mental confusion, anorexia, lethargy, vomiting, and muscle cramps. With dehydration and reduced blood volume, patient may suffer circulatory collapse with possible vascular thrombosis and embolism.
- Administer fluid and electrolyte replacement, as ordered, and carefully monitor urine output and serum electrolyte levels.

Patient teaching

- Instruct patient to move slowly when rising to avoid dizziness or light-headedness from sudden blood pressure drop.
- Caution patient to avoid alcohol because of increased risk of hypotension.
- Advise patient to eat food high in potassium. Provide other dietary counseling as appropriate to help prevent or minimize electrolyte imbalances.
- As appropriate, review all other significant and life-threatening adverse reactions and interactions, especially those related to the drugs, tests, herbs, and behaviors mentioned above.

[redacted]

buprenorphine hydrochloride

Buprenex

Pharmacologic class: Opioid agonist-antagonist
Therapeutic class: Opioid analgesic
Controlled substance schedule III
Pregnancy risk category C

Action

Unclear. May bind to opiate receptors in CNS, altering perception of and response to painful stimuli while causing generalized CNS depression. Also has partial antagonist properties, which may lead to opioid withdrawal in patients with physical drug dependence. Approximately 0.3 mg is equivalent to 10 mg morphine sulfate in analgesic and respiratory depressant effects.

Pharmacokinetics

Drug is metabolized by the liver and is largely protein-bound. Clearance relates to hepatic blood flow; it may be higher in children than adults. Drug is excreted primarily in feces unchanged, with some excretion in urine.

Onset	Peak	Duration
Immediate	2 min	Unknown

How supplied

Solution for injection (clear): 300-mcg (0.3-mg)/mL ampule

B

Indications and dosages

➢ Moderate to severe pain

Adults: 0.3 mg by slow I.V. q 6 hours as needed. Repeat initial dose after 30 to 60 minutes, if needed.

Children ages 2 to 12: 2 to 6 mcg (0.002 to 0.006 mg)/kg by slow I.V. q 4 to 6 hours

Dosage adjustment

- Patients with respiratory disease or impaired hepatic function, debilitated patients, elderly patients, and those receiving other drugs that decrease hepatic clearance may require reduced dosages.

Administration

Preparation

Use with extreme caution. Drug may cause respiratory depression (especially initial dose).

- Be aware that some children may not need to be remedicated for 6 to 8 hours.

Dilution and compatibility

- Mix with lactated Ringer's solution for injection, D_5W for injection, or normal saline solution for injection.

Infusion considerations

- Give by slow I.V. injection over at least 2 minutes using a controlled infusion pump.

Monitoring

- Reposition immobilized patient frequently; keep head of bed elevated.
- Monitor respiratory status throughout therapy. Respiratory rate of 12 breaths/minute or slower may warrant withholding of dose or decreasing dosage.

Storage

- Store at 20° to 25°C (68° to 77°F). Avoid excessive heat (over 40°C [104°F]).
- Protect from prolonged exposure to light.

Contraindications and precautions

Contraindicated in hypersensitivity to drug.

Use cautiously in monoamine oxidase (MAO) inhibitor use within past 14 days; concurrent use of centrally acting agents; increased intracranial pressure (ICP); respiratory impairment; severe renal, hepatic, or respiratory disease; hepatic coma; myxedema; hypothyroidism; adrenal cortical insufficiency; prostatic hypertrophy; kyphoscoliosis; urethral stricture; acute alcoholism; delirium tremens; CNS depression; coma; toxic psychosis; debilitated patients; ***elderly patients;*** pregnant or breastfeeding patients; and ***children younger than age 2.***

Adverse reactions

CNS: confusion, malaise, hallucinations, dizziness, euphoria, headache, unusual dreams, psychosis, slurred speech, paresthesia, depression, tremor, agitation, weakness, fatigue, nervousness, depersonalization, **seizures, coma, increased ICP**

CV: hypertension, hypotension, tachycardia, Wenckebach block (Mobitz type 1), **bradycardia**

EENT: blurred vision, diplopia, amblyopia, miosis, conjunctivitis, other visual abnormalities, tinnitus

GI: nausea, vomiting, constipation, flatulence, dyspepsia, ileus, dry mouth

GU: urine retention

Respiratory: hypoventilation, dyspnea, cyanosis, **apnea, respiratory depression**

Skin: diaphoresis, pruritus, rash

Other: physical or psychological drug dependence, drug tolerance, flushing or warmth, chills, pallor, injection-site reaction

Interactions

Drug-drug. *Antihistamines, sedative-hypnotics, other CNS depressants:* additive CNS depression

MAO inhibitors: increased CNS and respiratory depression, increased hypotension
Drug-herb. *Chamomile, hops, kava, skullcap, valerian:* increased CNS depression
Drug-behaviors. *Alcohol use:* increased CNS depression

Toxicity and overdose

• Overdose signs and symptoms are unknown. Drug's antagonist activity may manifest at dosages somewhat above recommended therapeutic range; however, dosages within this range may cause clinically significant respiratory depression in some circumstances.
• Carefully monitor patient's respiratory and cardiac status. Reestablish adequate respiratory exchange through providing a patent airway and using assisted or controlled ventilation. Give oxygen, I.V. fluids, vasopressors, and other supportive measures, as indicated and ordered. Doxapram, a respiratory stimulant, may be used. Be aware that naloxone may be ineffective in reversing respiratory depression; therefore, primary management should be reestablishing adequate ventilation with mechanical assistance, if required.

Patient teaching

• Instruct patient to move slowly when sitting up or standing to avoid dizziness or light-headedness from sudden blood pressure drop.
• Caution patient to avoid driving and other hazardous activities until drug's effects on concentration and alertness are known.
• Advise patient to increase daily fluid intake to help prevent or minimize constipation.
• As appropriate, review all other significant and life-threatening adverse reactions and interactions, especially those related to the drugs, herbs, and behaviors mentioned above.

busulfan

Busilvex ❋, Busulfex

Pharmacologic class: Alkylating agent
Therapeutic class: Antineoplastic
Pregnancy risk category D

FDA BOXED WARNING

• Drug causes profound myelosuppression at recommended dosages. Give under supervision of physician experienced in allogeneic hematopoietic stem-cell transplantation, cancer chemotherapy, and management of severe pancytopenia, in facility with adequate diagnostic and treatment resources.

Action

Unclear. Drug hydrolyzes in aqueous media to reduce methanesulfonate groups, producing carbonium ions that alkylate DNA. DNA damage may account for much of drug's cytotoxicity.

Pharmacokinetics

Drug is metabolized predominantly by conjugation with glutathione, and undergoes further oxidative metabolism in the liver. It binds irreversibly to plasma elements (mainly albumin). It achieves cerebrospinal fluid concentrations approximately equal to those in plasma. Elimination half-life is 2.5 hours. Drug is excreted in urine, with negligible amounts excreted in feces.

Onset	Peak	Duration
Unknown	Unknown	Unknown

How supplied

Solution for injection (clear, colorless): 6 mg/mL in 10-mL vials

Indications and dosages

➤ Allogeneic hematopoietic progenitor stem-cell transplantation in chronic myelogenous leukemia, given in combination with cyclophosphamide as a conditioning regimen

Adults: 0.8 mg/kg of ideal body weight (IBW) or actual weight (whichever is lower) I.V. q 6 hours for 4 days. Starting 6 hours after 16th busulfan dose, give cyclophosphamide 60 mg/kg/day I.V. over 1 hour for 2 days.

Dosage adjustment

- Determine dosage based on IBW, as follows: IBW (kg, men) = 50 + 0.91 times (height in cm minus 152). IBW (kg, women) = 45 + 0.91 times (height in cm minus 152). For obese or severely obese patients, use adjusted IBW (AIBW), as follows: AIBW = IBW + 0.25 times (actual weight minus IBW).

Off-label uses

- Adjunctive therapy in ovarian cancer
- Bone marrow transplantation

Administration

Preparation

🔈 Follow hazardous drug guidelines on page S19 for handling, preparation, and administration.

🔈 Be aware that drug is highly toxic and has a narrow therapeutic index.

- Hydrate patient vigorously to reduce risk of renal toxicity.
- Premedicate with phenytoin, as busulfan crosses blood-brain barrier and can cause seizures.
- Give antiemetic before first dose; continue on fixed schedule throughout administration.

Dilution and compatibility

🔈 Dilute drug before use.

- Withdraw dose from ampule using 5-micron filter needle that comes with package.
- Remove filter needle, and use new needle to add drug to diluent.
- Dilute for injection using D_5W for injection or normal saline solution for injection. Volume should be 10 times the busulfan volume, ensuring a final drug concentration of approximately 0.5 mg/mL. For example, calculate dosage for 70-kg (154-lb) patient as follows: (70 kg) times (0.8 mg/kg) divided by (6 mg/mL) = 9.3 mL busulfan (56 mg total dose).
- To prepare final solution for infusion, add 9.3 mL busulfan to 93 mL diluent (normal saline for injection or D_5W for injection), calculated as follows: (9.3 mL busulfan) times 10 = 93 mL diluent plus 9.3 mL of drug, to yield final busulfan concentration of 0.54 mg/mL (9.3 mL times 6 mg/mL divided by 102.3 mL = 0.54 mg/mL).
- Remove needle and filter. Replace with new needle and dispense syringe contents into I.V. bag or syringe already containing calculated amount of normal saline solution for injection or D_5W for injection. Ensure that drug flows into and through solution.

🔈 Do not put busulfan into I.V. bag that does not contain normal saline solution or D_5W.

🔈 Always add busulfan to diluent, rather than adding diluent to busulfan.

- Mix thoroughly by inverting bag or syringe several times.

Infusion considerations

- Use infusion pump to administer diluted solution. Set flow rate to deliver entire prescribed dose over 2 hours.
- Administer through central venous catheter. Before and after each infusion, flush catheter line with approximately 5 mL normal saline solution or D_5W.

• Do not infuse together with another I.V. solution of unknown compatibility.
• Know that when diluted in D_5W or normal saline solution, drug is stable at room temperature (25°C [77°F]) for up to 8 hours; however, infusion must be completed within that time. If diluted in normal saline solution, drug is stable when refrigerated at 2° to 8°C (36° to 46°F) for up to 12 hours; however, infusion must be completed within that time.
Be aware that rapid infusion is not recommended.

Monitoring

Assess for bleeding and excessive bruising. handle patient gently to avoid bruising.
• Continue antiemetic on fixed schedule throughout therapy.
• Continue to monitor patient closely for adequate hydration and renal function.
• Check for signs and symptoms of local or systemic infection.
• Monitor CBC and white blood cell (WBC) and platelet counts daily.
To detect hepatotoxicity (which may indicate hepatic veno-occlusive disease), monitor serum transaminases, alkaline phosphatase (ALP), and bilirubin levels daily through transplant day 28.
Know that diffuse pulmonary fibrosis ("busulfan lung") is a rare but potentially life-threatening complication, with symptom onset as late as 10 years after therapy.
• Evaluate oral hygiene regularly.

Storage

• Refrigerate unopened vials between 2° and 8°C (36° and 46°F).

Contraindications and precautions

Contraindicated in hypersensitivity to drug or its components.

Use cautiously in active infection, decreased bone marrow reserve, chronic debilitating disease, depressed neutrophil and platelet counts, seizure disorders, obesity, patients receiving concurrent myelosuppressive or radiation therapy, and females of childbearing potential.

Adverse reactions

CNS: anxiety, confusion, depression, dizziness, headache, weakness, insomnia, **encephalopathy, seizures, cerebral hemorrhage, coma**
CV: chest pain, hypotension, hypertension, tachycardia, vasodilation, ECG changes, **heart block, left-sided heart failure, thrombosis, pericardial effusion, ventricular extrasystole, atrial fibrillation, arrhythmias, cardiac tamponade, cardiomegaly**
EENT: cataract, ear disorders, epistaxis, rhinitis, pharyngitis
GI: nausea, vomiting, diarrhea, constipation, abdominal pain, dyspepsia, abdominal enlargement, pancreatitis, rectal disorder, hematemesis, dry mouth, stomatitis, anorexia
GU: dysuria, hematuria, sterility, **hemorrhagic cystitis, oliguria**
Hematologic: myelosuppression
Hepatic: hepatitis, hepatomegaly
Metabolic: hypokalemia, hypomagnesemia, hypophosphatemia, hyperglycemia
Musculoskeletal: arthralgia, myalgia, back pain
Respiratory: hyperventilation, dyspnea, lung disorder, cough, **pulmonary fibrosis**
Skin: pruritus, rash, acne, alopecia, erythema nodosum, exfoliative dermatitis, skin discoloration
Other: allergic reactions, chills, fever, injection site infection or inflammation, edema, pain, **secondary cancers**

Interactions

Drug-drug. *Acetaminophen:* decreased busulfan clearance

Live-virus vaccines: decreased antibody response to vaccine, increased risk of adverse reactions
Myelosuppressants: additive bone marrow depression
Nephrotoxic and ototoxic drugs (such as aminoglycosides, loop diuretics): additive nephrotoxicity and ototoxicity
Phenytoin: increased busulfan clearance
Drug-diagnostic tests. *ALP, aspartate aminotransferase, bilirubin, blood glucose, nitrogenous compounds (urea):* increased
Calcium, magnesium, potassium: decreased
Hemoglobin, WBCs: decreased

Toxicity and overdose

- In absence of hematopoietic progenitor stem-cell transplantation, recommended dosage would constitute overdose. Principal toxic effects are profound bone marrow hypoplasia and aplasia and pancytopenia, but CNS, liver, lungs, and GI tract also may be affected.
- No known antidote exists other than hematopoietic progenitor stem-cell transplantation. Closely monitor hematologic status and provide vigorous supportive measures, as indicated. Dialysis and glutathione administration also may be considered.

Patient teaching

- Inform patient that drug does not cure leukemia but may induce remission.
- Advise patient to drink plenty of fluids to avoid dehydration.
- Instruct patient to immediately report inability to eat or drink; prescriber may add another drug to boost appetite.
- Inform patient that drug may heighten risk of secondary cancers.
- Tell patient drug may increase risk of infection. Advise patient to avoid contact with people who have known illnesses and to avoid public transportation, if possible.
- Advise patient that drug increases risk of bleeding and bruising.
- Instruct patient to avoid activities that can cause injury and to use soft toothbrush and electric razor to avoid gum and skin injury.
- Inform patient about the need for frequent blood testing to monitor drug effects.
- Instruct females of childbearing potential to avoid becoming pregnant during therapy.
- Provide guidance to help breastfeeding patient decide whether to stop breastfeeding or discontinue drug.
- As appropriate, review all other significant and life-threatening adverse reactions and interactions, especially those related to the drugs and tests mentioned above.

butorphanol tartrate

Apo-Butorphanol🍁, PMS-Butorphanol🍁, Stadol

Pharmacologic class: Opioid agonist-antagonist
Therapeutic class: Opioid analgesic
Controlled substance schedule IV
Pregnancy risk category C

Action

Interacts with mu opioid receptor as mixed agonist-antagonist and at K receptor as agonist to produce analgesia

Pharmacokinetics

Drug is metabolized extensively in the liver to two metabolites (hydroxybutorphanol and norbutorphanol). It is approximately 80% bound to plasma proteins. Elimination half-life of hydroxybutorphanol is about 18 hours, leading to considerable accumulation, especially in elderly patients and patients with decreased creatinine clearance. Drug is eliminated primarily through urine and feces as metabolites.

Onset	Peak	Duration
2-3 min	30-60 min	3-4 hr

How supplied

Solution for injection (clear): 1 mg/mL, 2 mg/mL

Indications and dosages

➢ Moderate to severe pain

Adults: 0.5 to 2 mg I.V. q 3 to 4 hours as needed

➢ Labor pains

Adults: 1 to 2 mg I.V., repeated after 4 hours as needed

➢ Balanced anesthesia

Adults: 2 mg I.V. shortly before anesthesia induction, and/or 0.5 to 1 mg I.V. in increments during anesthesia. Increment may be higher, up to 0.6 mg/kg (4 mg/70 kg), depending on previous sedative, sedative-hypnotics, and analgesia

Dosage adjustment

- Reduce dosage by approximately half of recommended dosage in hepatic or renal impairment and in elderly patients. Determine subsequent dosages by patient's response rather than fixed dosage interval; generally, however, do not give doses at intervals of less than 6 hours.

Administration

Preparation

- Be aware that I.V. route is preferred for severe pain.

Dilution and compatibility

- Drug may be given undiluted.

Infusion considerations

- Give 2 mg or less over 3 to 5 minutes.
- Titrate often according to patient response.

Monitoring

🔈 Know that drug may cause infant respiratory distress in neonates, especially if given within 2 hours of delivery.

🔈 Monitor respiratory status closely.

- Watch for signs and symptoms of withdrawal in long-term use and in opioid-dependent patients.
- Assess elderly patients closely for drug sensitivity.

Storage

- Store at room temperature of 15° to 30°C (59° to 86°F).

Contraindications and precautions

Contraindicated in hypersensitivity to drug or its components.

Use cautiously in head injury, ventricular dysfunction, coronary insufficiency, respiratory disease or depression, renal or hepatic dysfunction, history of drug abuse, ***elderly patients,*** pregnant or breastfeeding patients, and ***children younger than age 18.***

Adverse reactions

CNS: drowsiness, sedation, dizziness, tremor, syncope, euphoria, floating feeling, stimulation, lethargy, asthenia, headache, anxiety, confusion, insomnia, nervousness, paresthesia

CV: hypertension, hypotension, palpitations, tachycardia, vasodilation, chest pain, **arrhythmias**

EENT: blurred vision, nasal congestion

GI: nausea, vomiting, constipation, epigastric distress, dry mouth

GU: impaired urination

Respiratory: bronchitis, cough, dyspnea, upper respiratory tract infection

Skin: pruritus

Other: unpleasant taste, local stinging, heat sensation, drug abuse or dependence, withdrawal symptoms, hypersensitivity reactions including **anaphylactic shock**

Interactions

Drug-drug. *CNS depressants:* additive CNS effects

Drug-behaviors. *Alcohol use:* additive CNS effects

Toxicity and overdose

- Overdose signs and symptoms are those of opioids in general, including hypoventilation, cardiovascular insufficiency, coma, and death.
- Maintain adequate ventilation, peripheral perfusion, normal body temperature, and patent airway. Continually observe vital signs, level of consciousness, and mental status. Provide oxygen, ventilation, and I.V. therapy, as indicated and ordered.

Patient teaching

- Inform patient that drug may be habit-forming.
- Advise patient to avoid driving and other hazardous activities until drug's effects on concentration and alertness are known.
- Instruct patient to avoid alcohol use during therapy.
- As appropriate, review all other significant and life-threatening adverse reactions and interactions, especially those related to the drugs and behaviors mentioned above.

[redacted]

caffeine citrate

Cafcit

Pharmacologic class: Methylxanthine

Therapeutic class: CNS stimulant

Pregnancy risk category C

Action

Relaxes bronchial smooth muscles, causes CNS and cardiac muscle stimulation, and acts as a diuretic. In apnea of prematurity, theories regarding drug action include stimulation of respiratory center, increased minute ventilation, decreased hypercapnia threshold, increased response to hypercapnia, increased skeletal muscle tone, decreased diaphragmatic fatigue, faster metabolic rate, and greater oxygen consumption. Most of these effects stem from antagonism of adenosine receptors.

Pharmacokinetics

In preterm neonates, drug metabolism is limited by immature hepatic enzyme system. Drug distributes rapidly to the brain. Cerebrospinal fluid levels in preterm neonates approximate plasma levels. Mean volume of distribution in infants (0.8 to 0.9 L/kg) is slightly higher than in adults. Mean half-life and fraction excreted unchanged in urine (A_e) in infants relate inversely to gestational or postconceptional age. In neonates, mean half-life is approximately 3 to 4 days and A_e is approximately 86%.

Onset	Peak	Duration
Unknown	Unknown	Unknown

How supplied

Solution for injection (clear, colorless, preservative-free): 20 mg (equal to 10 mg caffeine base)/mL in 3-mL single-dose vial

Indications and dosages

➤ Short-term treatment of apnea of prematurity in infants of gestational ages 28 weeks to less than 33 weeks

Neonates: Loading dose: 1 mL/kg (20 mg/kg) I.V. over 30 minutes. Maintenance dose (starting 24 hours after loading dose):

0.25 mL/kg (5 mg/kg) I.V. over 10 minutes q 24 hours.

Administration

Preparation

Check prescribed dosage carefully. Be aware that dosage expressed as caffeine base (caffeine B.S.) is half the dosage when expressed as caffeine citrate. (Twenty milligrams citrate is equivalent to 10 mg base.)

- Before starting drug, obtain baseline serum caffeine level in infants previously treated with theophylline. (Preterm infants metabolize theophylline to caffeine.) Likewise, measure baseline serum caffeine levels in infants of mothers who consumed caffeine before delivery, as caffeine readily crosses placenta.

Be aware that serum levels above 50 mg/L are linked to serious toxicity.

Dilution and compatibility

- Know that drug is chemically stable for 24 hours at room temperature when combined with the following: D_5W; intralipid 20% I.V. fat emulsion; Aminosyn 8.5% crystalline amino acid solution; dopamine hydrochloride injection 40 mg/mL diluted to 0.6 mg/mL with D_5W; calcium gluconate injection 10% (0.465 mEq/Ca^{+2}/mL); heparin sodium injection 1,000 units/mL diluted to 1 unit/mL with D_5W; fentanyl citrate injection 50 mcg/mL diluted to 10 mcg/mL with D_5W.

Do not mix with medications or solutions other than those listed above.

Infusion considerations

- Use syringe infusion pump.
- Infuse I.V. loading dose over 30 minutes. Infuse I.V. maintenance dose over 10 minutes.
- Discard unused portion of solution.

Monitoring

Continue to monitor serum caffeine citrate level. Adjust dosages as needed to avoid toxicity in patients with hepatic or renal impairment.

Monitor for signs and symptoms of necrotizing enterocolitis (abdominal distention, vomiting, bloody stools, and lethargy).

Monitor for signs and symptoms of bleeding and disseminated intravascular coagulation (DIC).

- Monitor hepatic and renal function.
- Monitor serum glucose level.

Storage

- Store at controlled room temperature of 15° to 30°C (59° to 86°F).

Contraindications and precautions

Contraindicated in hypersensitivity to drug or components.

Use cautiously in hepatic or renal disorders, seizure disorders, cardiovascular disease, and pregnant or breastfeeding patients.

Adverse reactions

CNS: insomnia, excitement, irritability, jitteriness, muscle tremor, headache, **cerebral hemorrhage**
CV: tachycardia, extrasystoles, palpitations, increased left ventricular output, increased stroke volume
EENT: retinopathy of prematurity
GI: nausea, vomiting, abdominal pain, gastritis, **GI hemorrhage, necrotizing enterocolitis**
GU: diuresis, **renal failure**
Hematologic: hemorrhage, DIC
Metabolic: hyperglycemia, hypoglycemia, **acidosis**
Respiratory: dyspnea, pulmonary edema
Skin: rash, dry skin, skin breakdown
Other: accidental injury, abnormal healing, feeding intolerance, hypersensitivity, **sepsis**

Interactions

Drug-drug. *Phenytoin:* decreased caffeine half-life and increased clearance

Theophylline: increased theophylline serum level

Drug-diagnostic tests. *Serum urate (Bittner measurement method):* false-positive elevation

Urine vanillylmandelic acid: increased

Toxicity and overdose

- Overdose signs and symptoms include fever, tachypnea, jitteriness, insomnia, fine tremor of extremities, hypertonia, opisthotonus, tonic-clonic movements, nonpurposeful jaw and lip movements, seizures, renal failure, hyperglycemia, acidosis, and elevated blood urea nitrogen level and white blood cell count.
- Provide symptomatic and supportive interventions, as ordered, including control of seizures with diazepam or barbiturate and exchange transfusions.

Patient teaching

- Explain use of drug to parents or caregivers.

calcitriol

Calcijex

Pharmacologic class: Vitamin D analogue

Therapeutic class: Hypocalcemic agent

Pregnancy risk category C

Action

Stimulates intestinal calcium transport; known sites of action are intestine, bone, kidney, and parathyroid gland. In bone, calcitriol stimulates calcium resorption (in conjunction with parathyroid); in the kidneys, it increases tubular reabsorption of calcium.

Pharmacokinetics

Drug must be metabolically activated in the liver and kidneys before it acts fully on target tissues. When given by bolus injection, it is rapidly available in bloodstream. Vitamin D metabolites are transported in blood, bound to specific plasma proteins, and eliminated in bile and urine.

Onset	Peak	Duration
Rapid	Unknown	3-5 days

How supplied

Solution for injection (clear, colorless to yellow): 1 mcg/1 mL in 1-mL ampules

Indications and dosages

➤ Hypocalcemia management in patients undergoing chronic renal dialysis

Adults: Recommended initial dosage (depending on severity of hypocalcemia or secondary hyperparathyroidism)—1 mcg (0.02 mcg/kg) to 2 mcg three times weekly, approximately every other day. Initial dosages as small as 0.5 mcg and as large as 4 mcg three times weekly have been used. If response is unsatisfactory, dosage may be increased by 0.5 to 1 mcg at 2- to 4-week intervals.

Dosage adjustment

- During titration period, obtain serum calcium and phosphorus levels at least twice weekly. If hypercalcemia occurs or serum calcium times phosphate product exceeds 70, discontinue drug immediately until these parameters are appropriate; then reinitiate at lower dosage. Dosage may need to be decreased as parathyroid hormone (PTH) level falls in response to therapy. Thus, incremental dosing must be individualized and commensurate with PTH and serum calcium and phosphorus levels. See the following table for suggested dosage titration:

PTH level	Dosage
Same or increasing	Increase
Decreasing less than 30%	Increase
Decreasing 31% to 59%	Maintain
Decreasing 61% or more	Decrease
1.5 to 3 × upper limit of normal (ULN)	Maintain
Below recommended target range (1.5 to 3 × ULN)	Reduce or discontinue drug

• For elderly patients, start dosage at low end of recommended range.

Administration

Preparation

• Know that optimal dosage must be determined carefully for each patient.
• Be aware that drug efficacy assumes patient is receiving adequate and appropriate daily calcium intake (adult recommended dietary allowance is 800 mg). To ensure adequate calcium intake, give calcium supplements as ordered, or instruct patient in proper dietary measures.
• In dialysis patients, give nonaluminum phosphate-binding compound, as ordered, to control serum phosphorus levels.
• Withhold vitamin D and its other derivatives during calcitriol therapy.

Dilution and compatibility

• Drug may be given undiluted.
• Discard unused portion.

Infusion considerations

• Give as bolus I.V. injection into I.V. line at end of dialysis.

Monitoring

• Be aware that drug withdrawal may lead to rebound effect; titrate downward to maintenance dosage as appropriate.
Closely monitor patients receiving digitalis preparations, as hypercalcemia may trigger arrhythmias in these patients.
• During initial phase of therapy, monitor serum calcium and phosphorus levels at least twice weekly. Then periodically monitor serum calcium, phosphorus, magnesium, alkaline phosphatase, and 24-hour urinary calcium and phosphorus levels.
Discontinue drug immediately if hypercalcemia develops.
• Be aware that adynamic bone disease may occur if PTH is suppressed to abnormal level. Monitor PTH level for indication of bone turnover rate.

Storage

• Store at controlled room temperature of 15° to 30°C (59° to 86°F). Protect from light.

Contraindications and precautions

Contraindicated in hypersensitivity to drug, hypercalcemia, and evidence of vitamin D toxicity.

Use cautiously in patients receiving concurrent digitalis preparations, ***elderly patients,*** pregnant or breastfeeding patients, and ***children.***

Adverse reactions

CNS: weakness, headache, somnolence, **overt psychosis** (rare)
CV: hypertension, **arrhythmias**
EENT: conjunctivitis, photophobia, rhinorrhea
GI: nausea, vomiting, anorexia, constipation, dry mouth, **pancreatitis**
GU: polyuria, polydipsia, nocturia, albuminuria, hypercalciuria, decreased libido
Musculoskeletal: muscle pain, bone pain
Skin: pruritus
Other: ectopic calcifications, metallic taste, weight loss, hyperthermia, mild pain on injection, hypersensitivity reactions

Interactions

Drug-drug. *Magnesium-containing antacids:* increased serum magnesium level

Drug-diagnostic tests. *Alanine aminotransferase, aspartate aminotransferase, blood urea nitrogen:* increased
PTH: decreased
Total cholesterol: increased

Toxicity and overdose

- Overdose may cause hypercalcemia, hypercalciuria, and hyperphosphatemia. Progressive hypercalcemia from overdose of vitamin D and its metabolites may be severe enough to warrant emergency attention.
- For acute accidental overdose, provide general supportive measures. Obtain serial serum electrolyte measurements (especially calcium) and urinary calcium excretion rate; check for hypercalcemia-related ECG abnormalities. (Such monitoring is critical in patients receiving digitalis preparations.) Discontinue supplemental calcium as ordered, and begin low-calcium diet. Given drug's relatively short duration of action, further measures probably are unnecessary. Correct persistent or markedly elevated serum calcium level by giving such drugs as phosphates and corticosteroids as ordered; take measures to induce appropriate forced diuresis. Peritoneal dialysis using calcium-free dialysate may be ordered.

Patient teaching

- Instruct patient to adhere to prescribed diet and calcium supplementation and to avoid using unapproved nonprescription drugs (including magnesium-containing antacids).
- Teach patient about signs and symptoms of hypercalcemia.
- Provide guidance to breastfeeding patient to help her decide whether to stop breastfeeding or discontinue drug.
- As appropriate, review all other significant and life-threatening adverse reactions and interactions, especially those related to the drugs and tests mentioned above.

calcium chloride

Calciject🍁

Pharmacologic class: Mineral
Therapeutic class: Dietary supplement, electrolyte replacement agent
Pregnancy risk category C

Action

Essential for functional integrity of nervous and musculoskeletal systems, normal cardiac contractility, and coagulation; also functions as enzyme cofactor and affects secretory activity of endocrine and exocrine glands

Pharmacokinetics

Drug is rapidly incorporated into skeletal tissue, crosses placenta, and reaches higher concentration in fetal blood than maternal blood; it is also distributed in breast milk. Approximately 80% of body calcium is excreted in feces as insoluble salts; urinary excretion accounts for remaining 20%, with small amount excreted by sweat glands.

Onset	Peak	Duration
Immediate	Immediate	Unknown

How supplied

Solution for injection (clear, hypertonic, preservative-free): 10% solution in single-dose 10-mL syringes

Indications and dosages

➤ Hypocalcemic emergency
Adults: 5 to 10 mL I.V. at rate of 0.5 to 1 mL/minute, preferably in a central or deep vein

➢ Hypocalcemic disorders in children
Children: 0.027 to 0.05 mL I.V. at rate not exceeding 0.5 to 1 mL/minute

Administration

Preparation

• Be aware that drug is used for cardiac resuscitation when weak or inadequate contractions return after defibrillation or when epinephrine injection fails to strengthen myocardial contractions.

• Know that drug is used to combat deleterious effects of hyperkalemia, pending correction of increased extracellular potassium level.

Do not give by I.M. or subcutaneous injection.

Dilution and compatibility

Do not mix with carbonates, phosphates, sulfates, or tartrates.

• Know that drug may chelate tetracyclines.

• If time permits, warm solution to body temperature.

• Dilute in equal amount of normal saline solution for injection or sterile water for injection.

• Further dilute as prescribed in compatible solution.

Infusion considerations

Give by slow I.V. infusion only, at a rate no faster than 0.5 to 1 mL/minute.

Be aware that rapid I.V. administration may cause bradycardia, sense of oppression, tingling, heat wave sensation, or chalky taste.

• Give through large vein using small needle or central line to prevent vein irritation.

• Halt infusion if patient complains of discomfort; resume when symptoms disappear.

Monitoring

• Keep patient supine for 15 minutes after administration to prevent orthostatic hypotension.

Check I.V. site frequently to avoid tissue damage caused by extravasation. If infiltration occurs, immediately discontinue I.V. administration at that site and infiltrate affected area locally with 1% procaine hydrochloride (to which hyaluronidase may be added, as prescribed). Local heat application may be helpful.

• Know that drug may cause peripheral vasodilation, local burning sensation, and possibly a moderate blood pressure drop.

• Monitor calcium level frequently, especially in elderly patients.

Storage

• Store at controlled room temperature of 15° to 30°C (59° to 86°F).

Contraindications and precautions

Contraindicated for cardiac resuscitation in patients with ventricular fibrillation and hypercalcemia.

Use cautiously in renal insufficiency, pernicious anemia, cardiac disease, sarcoidosis, hyperparathyroidism, hypoparathyroidism, history of renal calculi, ***children,*** and ***premature neonates.***

Adverse reactions

CV: arrhythmia, blood pressure decrease, **ventricular fibrillation, bradycardia** (with rapid I.V. injection)
Skin: rash, severe tissue sloughing or necrosis with extravasation
Other: altered or chalky taste, tingling sensation, sense of oppression or heat wave

Interactions

Drug-drug. *Cardiac glycosides:* increased risk of cardiac glycoside toxicity
Fluoroquinolones, tetracyclines: formation of complexes that render these drugs inactive
Iron salts: decreased iron absorption
Drug-diagnostic tests. *Calcium:* increased

Toxicity and overdose

- Too-rapid injection may lower blood pressure and cause cardiac syncope. Inadvertent systemic calcium overloading may lead to acute hypercalcemic syndrome (markedly elevated calcium level, lethargy, weakness, intractable nausea and vomiting, coma, and death). However, because of rapid drug excretion, persistent hypercalcemia from calcium overdose is unlikely.
- If excessive calcium administration causes adverse reactions, discontinue drug promptly. Reevaluate patient and provide appropriate interventions, if necessary.

Patient teaching

- As appropriate, review all other significant and life-threatening adverse reactions and interactions, especially those related to the drugs and tests mentioned above.

carboplatin

Paraplatin, Paraplatin-AQ♣

Pharmacologic class: Alkylating agent
Therapeutic class: Antineoplastic
Pregnancy risk category D

FDA BOXED WARNING

- Give under supervision of physician experienced in cancer chemotherapy, in facility with adequate diagnostic and treatment resources.
- Bone marrow suppression is dose-related and may be severe, leading to infection and bleeding. Anemia may be cumulative and warrant transfusions.
- Vomiting is a common adverse effect.
- Anaphylactic-like reactions may occur within minutes of administration.

Action

In apparently cell-cycle-phase nonspecific manner, causes predominantly interstrand DNA cross-links, leading to cell death

Pharmacokinetics

When creatinine clearance is about 60 mL/minute or greater, plasma levels of intact drug decay after 30-minute I.V. infusion of 300 to 500 mg/m². Initial plasma half-life is 1.1 to 2 hours; postdistribution plasma half-life, 2.6 to 5.9 hours. Total body clearance, apparent volume of distribution, and mean residence time are 4.4 L/hour, 16 L/hour, and 3.5 L/hour, respectively. Although drug is not bound to plasma proteins, platinum from drug becomes irreversibly bound to plasma proteins and is eliminated slowly, with minimum half-life of 5 days. Major elimination route is renal. Patients with creatinine clearances of 60 mL/minute or greater excrete 65% of dose in urine within 12 hours and 71% of dose within 24 hours. With creatinine clearance below 60 mL/minute, total body and renal clearance decreases as creatinine clearance falls.

Onset	Peak	Duration
Rapid	Unknown	Unknown

How supplied

Solution for injection (aqueous): 50 mg/5-mL, 150 mg/15-mL, 450 mg/45-mL, and 600 mg/60-mL multidose vials

Indications and dosages

➤ Single-agent therapy for recurrent ovarian carcinoma

Adults: 360 mg/m² I.V. on day 1, repeated q 4 weeks depending on response. However, do not repeat single dose until neutrophil count is at least 2,000/mm³ and platelet count at least 100,000/mm³. Base subsequent dosages on blood counts.

➤ Previously untreated advanced ovarian carcinoma, in combination with cyclophosphamide

Adults: 300 mg/m² I.V. on day 1 q 4 weeks, with cyclophosphamide 600 mg/m² on day 1 q 4 weeks. Give both drugs for six cycles.

Dosage adjustment

- Reduce dosage in impaired renal function. If baseline creatinine clearance is 41 to 59 mL/minute, give 250 mg/m² on day 1; if it is 16 to 40 mL/minute, give 200 mg/m² on day 1. Data are too limited to allow recommendation for treatment when creatinine clearance is below 15 mL/minute.
- Adjust subsequent doses based on degree of bone marrow suppression.
- To minimize toxicity risk, use dosing formulas incorporating glomerular filtration rate with elderly patients.

Off-label uses

- Advanced endometrial cancer
- Advanced or recurrent squamous-cell carcinoma of head and neck
- Brain tumor
- Cervical cancer
- Esophageal cancer
- Neuroblastoma
- Relapsed and refractory acute leukemia
- Small-cell lung cancer
- Testicular cancer
- Wilms' tumor

Administration

Preparation

Follow hazardous drug guidelines on page S19 for handling, preparation, and administration.

- Obtain baseline creatinine clearance to evaluate renal function.
- Premedicate with antiemetics, as prescribed.

Dilution and compatibility

- Drug is a premixed aqueous solution that can be diluted to a concentration as low as 0.5 mg/mL with appropriate amounts of sterile water for injection, normal saline solution for injection, or D_5W for injection.
- Do not use with needles or I.V. sets containing aluminum, as such contact may cause precipitate to form.
- Know that reconstituted solution is stable at room temperature for 8 hours. After that time, discard.

Infusion considerations

- Administer I.V. infusion over at least 15 minutes.

Monitoring

- Evaluate fluid and electrolyte balance, and make sure patient maintains adequate fluid intake.

Check I.V. site frequently to avoid tissue damage resulting from extravasation.

- Assess for signs and symptoms of hypersensitivity reactions.

Closely monitor CBC to help detect drug-induced anemia and other hematologic problems.

- Monitor alkaline phosphatase (ALP), aspartate aminotransferase (AST), and total bilirubin levels.

Storage

- Store unopened vials at 25°C (77°F), with excursions permitted from 15° to 30°C (59° to 86°F).
- Protect from light.

Contraindications and precautions

Contraindicated in history of severe allergic reaction to cisplatin or platinum-containing compounds, severe bone marrow depression, and significant bleeding.

Use cautiously in hearing loss, electrolyte imbalances, renal impairment, active infection, diminished bone marrow reserve, ***elderly patients,*** females of childbearing potential, pregnant or breastfeeding patients, and ***children*** (safety and efficacy not established).

Adverse reactions

CNS: weakness, peripheral neuropathy, central neurotoxicity, **cerebrovascular accident**
CV: hypotension, **heart failure, embolism**
EENT: visual disturbances, ototoxicity
GI: nausea, vomiting, constipation, diarrhea, abdominal pain
GU: nephrotoxicity
Hematologic: anemia, bleeding, transfusion, **leukopenia, thrombocytopenia, neutropenia**
Hepatic: hepatotoxicity
Metabolic: hypocalcemia, hypokalemia, hypomagnesemia, hyponatremia
Respiratory: bronchospasm
Skin: alopecia, rash, urticaria, erythema, pruritus, necrosis with extravasation
Other: altered taste, infection, injection-site reaction, pain, hypersensitivity reactions including **anaphylaxis**

Interactions

Drug-drug. *Live-virus vaccines:* decreased antibody response to vaccine, increased risk of adverse reactions
Myelosuppressants: additive bone marrow depression
Nephrotoxic or ototoxic drugs (such as aminoglycosides, loop diuretics): additive nephrotoxicity or ototoxicity
Drug-diagnostic tests. *ALP, AST, blood urea nitrogen, creatinine:* increased
Electrolytes, hematocrit, hemoglobin. neutrophils, platelets, red blood cells, white blood cells: decreased

Toxicity and overdose

- Anticipated complications of overdose result from bone marrow suppression or hepatic toxicity.
- No known antidote for carboplatin overdose exists.

Patient teaching

- Instruct patient to report signs and symptoms of allergic response and other adverse reactions, such as breathing problems, mouth sores, rash, itching, and reddened skin.
- Advise patient to immediately report unusual bleeding or bruising.
- Caution patient to avoid driving and other hazardous activities until drug's effects on concentration and alertness are known.
- Urge patient to avoid activities that can cause injury, and to use soft toothbrush and electric razor to avoid gum and skin injury.
- Instruct patient to drink plenty of fluids to ensure adequate urine output.
- Provide dietary counseling; if GI adverse effects significantly limit food intake, refer patient to dietitian.
- Advise females of childbearing potential to avoid pregnancy.
- Provide guidance to breastfeeding patient to help her decide whether to stop breastfeeding or discontinue drug.
- As appropriate, review all other significant and life-threatening adverse reactions and interactions, especially those related to the drugs and tests mentioned above.

carmustine

BCNU, BiCNU

Pharmacologic class: Alkylating agent
Therapeutic class: Antineoplastic
Pregnancy risk category D

FDA BOXED WARNING

• Give under supervision of physician experienced in cancer chemotherapy.
• Most common and severe toxic effect is bone marrow suppression—notably thrombocytopenia and leukopenia, which may contribute to bleeding and overwhelming infections in already compromised patients. Monitor blood counts weekly for at least 6 weeks after dose. Do not give courses more often than every 6 weeks.

Action

Unclear. Thought to alkylate DNA and RNA and to inhibit several key enzymatic processes by carbamoylation of amino acids in proteins.

Pharmacokinetics

After I.V. administration, drug degrades rapidly, with no intact drug detectable after 15 minutes. It is metabolized in the liver. Because of high lipid solubility and relative lack of ionization at physiologic pH, metabolites readily cross blood-brain barrier. Approximately 60% to 70% of total dose is excreted in urine in 96 hours and about 10% as respiratory carbon dioxide. Fate of remainder is unknown.

Onset	Peak	Duration
Unknown	Unknown	Unknown

How supplied

Powder for reconstitution for injection (lyophilized, pale-yellow flakes or congealed mass): 100-mg vials

Indications and dosages

➤ Brain tumor; multiple myeloma in combination with prednisone; secondary therapy in Hodgkin's disease; secondary therapy in other lymphomas (used alone or with other treatments, such as surgery or radiation)

Adults: When given as a single agent in previously untreated patients, 150 to 200 mg/m^2 I.V. as a single dose q 6 weeks, or 75 to 100 mg/m^2/day for 2 days q 6 weeks. Repeat dose q 6 weeks if platelet count exceeds 100,000/mm^3 and white blood cell (WBC) count exceeds 4,000/mm^3.

Dosage adjustment

• When used in conjunction with other myelosuppressants in patients with depleted bone marrow reserve, adjust dosage accordingly.
• After initial dose, adjust dosage according to hematologic response (white blood cell and platelets) to preceding dose, as shown below:

WBC nadir (per mm^3)	Platelet nadir (per mm^3)	% of previous dosage
Above 4,000	Above 100,000	100%
3,000 to 3,999	75,000 to 99,999	100%
2,000 to 2,999	25,000 to 74,999	70%
Below 2,000	Below 25,000	50%

Off-label uses

• Mycosis fungoides

Administration

Preparation

Follow hazardous drug guidelines on page S19 for handling, preparation, and administration.

Accidental skin contact with reconstituted drug can cause transient hyperpigmentation of affected areas. Use gloves during preparation. If lyophilized material or solution contacts skin or mucosa, immediately wash area thoroughly with soap and water.

- Know that pulmonary function tests (PFTs) should be performed before therapy begins.
- Assess baseline kidney and liver function tests.
- Use caution when selecting dosages for elderly patients, as they are more likely to have decreased renal function. (Carmustine and its metabolites are excreted substantially by the kidneys.)
- Premedicate with antiemetic, as ordered, 30 to 60 minutes before administering drug.

Dilution and compatibility

- Reconstitute by dissolving 100-mg vial with 3 mL sterile dehydrated alcohol (provided with drug), followed by 27 mL sterile water for injection; this yields a concentration of 3.3 mg/mL.
- Further dilute with D_5W.

Infusion considerations

- Infuse over 1 to 2 hours.
- Know that infusion lasting less than 1 hour causes intense pain and burning at I.V. site.

Infuse solution in glass containers only; drug is unstable in plastic I.V. bags.

Monitoring

Continue to monitor PFTs regularly throughout therapy to check for pulmonary toxicity. Be aware that pulmonary toxicity is dose-related; patients receiving cumulative doses above 1,400 mg/m^2 are at significantly higher risk. Some patients who received drug in childhood and early adolescence developed delayed-onset pulmonary fibrosis up to 17 years after treatment.

- Continue to assess kidney and liver function tests regularly.
- Monitor CBC for up to 6 weeks after dose, to detect delayed bone marrow toxicity.

Storage

- Refrigerate unopened vial of dry drug at 2° to 8°C (36° to 46°F).
- Store diluent ampules at controlled room temperature of 15° to 30°C (59° to 86°F), or refrigerate at 2° to 8°C (36° to 46°F).
- If vial has been reconstituted as directed and further diluted to a concentration of 0.2 mg/mL in D_5W, store at room temperature. Protect from light and use within 8 hours.

Contraindications and precautions

Contraindicated in hypersensitivity to drug or its components.

Use cautiously in infection; depressed bone marrow reserve; respiratory, hepatic, or renal impairment; recent radiation therapy or chemotherapy, ***elderly patients,*** females of childbearing potential, pregnant or breastfeeding patients, and ***children*** (safety and efficacy not established).

Adverse reactions

CNS: headache
CV: hypotension, tachycardia
EENT: neuroretinitis, conjunctival suffusion
GI: nausea, vomiting, esophagitis
GU: azotemia, decreased kidney size, **renal failure, nephrotoxicity**
Hematologic: anemia, **leukopenia, thrombocytopenia, cumulative bone marrow depression, bone marrow dysplasia**
Hepatic: hepatotoxicity

Respiratory: pulmonary fibrosis, pulmonary infiltrates
Skin: alopecia, hyperpigmentation (with accidental skin exposure), facial flushing
Other: I.V. site pain, allergic reactions, **secondary cancers** (with long-term use)

Interactions

Drug-drug. *Anticoagulants, aspirin, nonsteroidal anti-inflammatory drugs:* increased risk of bleeding
Antineoplastics: additive bone marrow depression
Cimetidine: potentiation of bone marrow depression
Digoxin, phenytoin: decreased blood levels of these drugs
Live-virus vaccines: decreased antibody response to vaccines, increased risk of adverse reactions
Drug-diagnostic tests. *Alkaline phosphatase, aspartate aminotransferase, bilirubin, nitrogenous compounds (urea):* increased
Hemoglobin, WBCs: decreased
Drug-behaviors. *Smoking:* increased risk of respiratory toxicity

Toxicity and overdose

- Overdose may manifest as bone marrow depression, renal and hepatic toxicity, and respiratory abnormalities.
- No proven antidote has been established. Withhold drug and provide supportive interventions.

Patient teaching

Instruct patient to promptly report signs and symptoms of infection (sore throat, fever) and other adverse reactions, such as mouth sores, difficulty breathing, urinary problems, unusual tiredness, yellowing of skin or eyes, and abnormal bruising or bleeding.
- Inform patient that severe flushing may follow I.V. dose but should subside in 2 to 4 hours.
- Advise patient to avoid activities that can cause injury, and to use soft toothbrush and electric razor to avoid gum and skin injury.
- Instruct patient to minimize GI upset by eating small, frequent servings of healthy food and drinking plenty of fluids.
- Teach patient to monitor urine output and report significant changes.
- Inform patient that drug may cause hair loss.
- Advise patient that he'll undergo regular blood testing during therapy.
- As appropriate, review all other significant and life-threatening adverse reactions and interactions, especially those related to the drugs, tests, and behaviors mentioned above.

caspofungin acetate

Cancidas

Pharmacologic class: Glucan synthesis inhibitor
Therapeutic class: Antifungal
Pregnancy risk category C

Action

Inhibits synthesis of beta (1, 3)-D-glucan, an important component of cell wall in susceptible *Aspergillus* and other fungal cells. This inhibition leads to cell rupture and death.

Pharmacokinetics

Distribution is the primary mechanism affecting plasma clearance; drug is minimally distributed into red blood cells. It is metabolized slowly by hydrolysis and N-acetylation; additional metabolism involves hydrolysis into constitutive amino acids and their degradates. Drug is 97% bound to albumin. After a single 1-hour I.V. infusion, plasma levels fall in at least three phases with differing half-lives. Little excretion or biotransformation takes place during first 30 hours after administration.

Onset	Peak	Duration
Immediate	9-11 hr	40-50 hr

How supplied

Powder for reconstitution for injection (lyophilized, white to off-white): 50 mg and 75 mg in single-use vials

Indications and dosages

➤ Invasive aspergillosis in patients refractory to or intolerant of other therapies
Adults: 70 mg I.V. as a single loading dose on first day, followed by 50 mg/day thereafter
➤ Esophageal candidiasis
Adults: 50 mg/day by slow I.V. infusion

Dosage adjustment

- Reduce dosage to 35 mg/day in patients being treated for invasive aspergillosis who have moderate hepatic insufficiency (Child-Pugh score 7 to 9).
- Know that patients being treated for invasive aspergillosis who also are receiving carbamazepine, dexamethasone, efavirenz, nevirapine, or phenytoin may require a dosage increase to 70 mg/day.

Administration

Preparation
- Be aware that patients with HIV infection may receive suppressive oral therapy to help prevent oropharyngeal candidiasis relapse.

Dilution and compatibility
🔊 Do not mix with other drugs or with diluents containing dextrose.
- Reconstitute powder using normal saline solution for injection or bacteriostatic water for injection. Mix gently until solution is clear.
- Further dilute with sodium chloride or lactated Ringer's solution.
- Do not use if solution is cloudy.

Infusion considerations
- Administer by slow I.V. infusion over 1 hour.

Monitoring
🔊 Monitor I.V. site carefully for phlebitis and other complications.
- Monitor CBC and serum electrolyte levels; watch for signs and symptoms of hypokalemia.
- Stay alert for histamine-mediated signs and symptoms (rash, facial swelling, pruritus, and warm sensation).
- Monitor vital signs, especially for tachycardia and tachypnea.
- Monitor nutritional and hydration status.

Storage
- Store vials at 2° to 8°C (36° to 46°F).
- Know that reconstituted drug may be stored at approximately 25°C (77°F) for 1 hour before preparation of infusion solution.
- Know that final infusion solution may be stored in I.V. bag or bottle at approximately 25°C (77°F) for 24 hours or at 2° to 8°C (36° to 46°F) for 48 hours.

Contraindications and precautions

Contraindicated in hypersensitivity to drug.

Use cautiously in concurrent therapy with cyclosporine (use not recommended) or inducers of drug clearance (such as carbamazepine, dexamethasone, efavirenz, nevirapine, or phenytoin—but not rifampin), hepatic impairment, bone marrow depression, renal insufficiency, pregnant or breastfeeding patients, and ***children younger than age 18*** (safety and efficacy not established).

Adverse reactions

CNS: headache, paresthesia
CV: tachycardia, phlebitis

GI: nausea, vomiting, diarrhea, abdominal pain, anorexia
Hematologic: eosinophilia, anemia
Metabolic: hypokalemia
Musculoskeletal: pain, myalgia
Respiratory: tachypnea
Skin: histamine-mediated symptoms (including rash, facial swelling, pruritus, and warm sensation)

Interactions

Drug-drug. *Cyclosporine:* markedly increased caspofungin blood level
Inducers of drug clearance, mixed inducers-inhibitors (carbamazepine, dexamethasone, efavirenz, nelfinavir, nevirapine, phenytoin): reduced caspofungin blood level
Tacrolimus: possible alteration in tacrolimus blood level
Drug-diagnostic tests. *Alkaline phosphatase, eosinophils:* increased
Hemoglobin, potassium: decreased

Toxicity and overdose

- In overdose, expect extension of adverse reactions.
- Provide symptomatic and supportive interventions. Monitor for histamine-mediated symptoms, abnormal liver function tests, and other adverse reactions. Drug is not dialyzable.

Patient teaching

- Teach patient about signs and symptoms of histamine-mediated symptoms; tell patient when to notify prescriber.
- Advise patient to minimize GI adverse effects by eating small, frequent servings of healthy food and ensuring adequate fluid intake.
- As appropriate, review all other significant adverse reactions and interactions, especially those related to the drugs and tests mentioned above.

[redacted]

cefazolin sodium

Ancef

Pharmacologic class: First-generation cephalosporin
Therapeutic class: Anti-infective
Pregnancy risk category B

Action

Structurally and pharmacologically related to penicillin; interferes with bacterial cell-wall synthesis, causing cell to rupture and die. Active against gram-negative and gram-positive bacteria, with expanded activity against gram-negative bacteria. Shows minimal immunosuppressive activity.

Pharmacokinetics

Drug distributes widely to most tissues and fluids, but does not readily enter cerebrospinal fluid. Serum half-life is approximately 1.8 hours. Drug promptly crosses placental barrier, is present in low concentrations in breast milk, and is excreted rapidly in urine.

Onset	Peak	Duration
Rapid	End of infusion	6-12 hr

How supplied

Powder for reconstitution for injection: 250 mg, 500 mg, 1 g, 5 g, 10 g, 20 g
Solution for injection: 500 mg/50 mL in D_5W, 1 g/50 mL in D_5W in premixed containers

Indications and dosages

➤ Respiratory tract infections caused by group A beta-hemolytic streptococci, *Klebsiella* species, *Haemophilus influenzae, Staphylococcus aureus,* and *Streptococcus pneumoniae;* skin infections caused by *S. aureus* and beta-hemolytic streptococci; biliary tract infections caused by *Escherichia coli, Klebsiella* species, *Proteus mirabilis,* and *S. aureus;* bone and joint infections caused by *S. aureus;* genital infections caused by *E. coli, Klebsiella* species, *P. mirabilis,* and strains of enterococci; septicemia caused by *E. coli, Klebsiella* species, *P. mirabilis, S. aureus,* and *S. pneumoniae;* endocarditis caused by *S. aureus* or beta-hemolytic streptococci

Adults: For mild infections, 250 to 500 mg q 8 hours I.V. For moderate to severe infections, 500 to 1,000 mg I.V. q 6 to 8 hours. For life-threatening infections, 1,000 to 1,500 mg I.V. q 6 hours, to a maximum dosage of 6 g/day.

Children: For mild to moderate infections, 25 to 50 mg/kg/day I.V. in divided doses t.i.d. or q.i.d. For severe infections, 100 mg/kg/day I.V. in divided doses t.i.d. or q.i.d.

➢ Acute uncomplicated urinary tract infections caused by *E. coli, Klebsiella* species, *P. mirabilis,* and strains of *Enterococcus* and *Enterobacter* species

Adults: 1 g I.V. q 12 hours

➢ Surgical prophylaxis

Adults: 1g I.V. 30 to 60 minutes before surgery, then 0.5 to 1 g I.V. q 6 to 8 hours for 24 hours. If surgery exceeds 2 hours, another 0.5- to 1-g dose I.V. may be given intraoperatively.

➢ Pneumococcal pneumonia

Adults: 500-mg I.V. infusion q 12 hours

Dosage adjustment

- In renal impairment, after initial loading dose, reduce dosage as follows: For creatinine clearance of 40 to 70 mL/minute, give 60% of normal daily dosage every 12 hours. For clearance of 20 to 40 mL/minute, give 25% of normal daily dosage every 12 hours. For clearance of 5 to 20 mL/minute, give 10% of normal daily dosage every 24 hours.

Administration

Preparation

🔊 Before starting therapy, determine if patient has had previous hypersensitivity reactions to cefazolin, other cephalosporins, penicillins, or other drugs.

- Obtain specimens for culture and sensitivity tests as needed before starting therapy.
- Assess baseline CBC and kidney and liver function test results.
- Do not exceed adult recommended dosage in children.

Dilution and compatibility

- Reconstitute each 500-mg or 1-g dose with at least 10 mL sterile water for injection. Shake well.
- For direct I.V. injection, further dilute 500-mg or 1-g dose in 5 mL sterile water for injection.
- For intermittent I.V. infusion, further dilute 500-mg or 1-g dose in 50 to 100 mL normal saline solution; D_5W; dextrose 10% in water; 5% dextrose in lactated Ringer's solution; 5% dextrose in 0.2%, 0.45%, or 0.9% sodium chloride solution; lactated Ringer's solution; or other compatible infusion solutions.
- Do not mix in same infusion with aminoglycoside, because both drugs may be inactivated.
- Know that reconstituted solution may range from pale yellow to yellow.
- Be aware that powder and solution tend to darken depending on storage conditions. However, when stored as recommended, product potency is unchanged.
- Thaw premixed drug at room temperature.
- Do not add other drugs to premixed containers. Discard unused solution.

Infusion considerations

- For direct I.V. injection, administer slowly over 3 to 5 minutes.
- For intermittent I.V. infusion, administer in volume-control set or in separate,

secondary I.V. container over 30 to 60 minutes.

Do not use plastic containers in series connections. Such use could result in air embolism due to residual air being drawn from primary container before administration of fluid from secondary container ends.

Monitoring

In patients receiving high doses, monitor closely for seizures; be prepared to intervene appropriately.

Be aware that cross-sensitivity to penicillins and other cephalosporins may occur. If allergic reaction occurs, discontinue treatment. In acute hypersensitivity reaction, be prepared to give epinephrine and provide other emergency measures, including oxygen, I.V. fluids, I.V. antihistamines, corticosteroids, pressor amines, and airway management, as indicated.

Monitor for signs and symptoms of pseudomembranous colitis; institute therapeutic measures as indicated. Mild cases usually respond to drug withdrawal alone. In moderate to severe cases, be prepared to give fluids and electrolytes, protein supplements, and oral antibiotic effective against Clostridium difficile colitis.

- Monitor CBC, prothrombin time, and kidney and liver function test results.
- Watch for signs and symptoms of superinfection and other serious adverse reactions.

Storage

- Before reconstitution, protect drug from light and store at controlled room temperature of 20° to 25°C (68° to 77°F). Reconstituted solution is stable for 24 hours at controlled room temperature and for 96 hours if refrigerated at 5°C (41°F).
- Store frozen premixed containers at or below –20°C (–4°F). After thawing, solution remains potent for 48 hours at 25°C (77°F) and for 30 days if refrigerated at 5°C (41°F). Do not refreeze.

Contraindications and precautions

Contraindicated in hypersensitivity to cephalosporins.

Use cautiously in hypersensitivity to penicillins, renal impairment, phenylketonuria, history of GI disease (especially colitis), emaciated patients, ***elderly patients,*** pregnant or breastfeeding patients, and ***children younger than 1 month*** (safety and efficacy not established).

Adverse reactions

CNS: headache, lethargy, confusion, hemiparesis, paresthesia, syncope, **seizures**
CV: hypotension, palpitations, chest pain, vasodilation
EENT: hearing loss
GI: nausea, vomiting, diarrhea, abdominal cramps, oral candidiasis, **pseudomembranous colitis**
GU: vaginal candidiasis, **nephrotoxicity**
Hematologic: lymphocytosis, eosinophilia, **bleeding tendency, hemolytic anemia, hypoprothrombinemia, neutropenia, thrombocytopenia, agranulocytosis, bone marrow depression**
Hepatic: hepatic failure, hepatomegaly
Musculoskeletal: arthralgia
Respiratory: dyspnea
Skin: urticaria, maculopapular or erythematous rash
Other: chills, fever, superinfection, **anaphylaxis, serum sickness**

Interactions

Drug-drug. *Aminoglycosides, loop diuretics:* increased risk of nephrotoxicity
Anticoagulants: increased anticoagulant effect
Chloramphenicol: antagonistic effect
Probenecid: decreased excretion and increased blood level of cefazolin

Drug-diagnostic tests. *Alanine aminotransferase, alkaline phosphatase, aspartate aminotransferase, bilirubin, blood urea nitrogen, creatinine, eosinophils, gamma-glutamyltransferase, lactate dehydrogenase:* increased
Coombs' test, nonenzyme-based urine glucose tests (such as Clinitest), urinary 17-ketosteroids: false-positive results
Hemoglobin, platelets, prothrombin time, white blood cells: decreased
Drug-behaviors. *Alcohol consumption within 72 hours of administration:* acute alcohol intolerance (disulfiram-like reaction)

Toxicity and overdose

- With inappropriately large doses (especially in renal impairment), expect signs and symptoms to include neuromuscular hypersensitivity (such as seizures).
- If seizures occur, immediately discontinue drug and give anticonvulsant, as ordered. In overwhelming overdose, hemodialysis should be considered to remove drug. Provide supportive therapy.

Patient teaching

Instruct patient to immediately report signs and symptoms of allergic reaction, reduced urine output, persistent diarrhea, bruising, and bleeding.
- Advise patient to maintain adequate fluid intake during therapy.
- Teach patient to avoid alcohol while taking drug.
- Advise patient with diabetes mellitus to use enzyme-based test (Clinistix, Testape) to monitor urine glucose, as drug may cause false results with other tests.
- As appropriate, review all other significant and life-threatening adverse reactions and interactions, especially those related to the drugs, tests, and behaviors mentioned above.

cefepime hydrochloride

Maxipime

Pharmacologic class: Fourth-generation cephalosporin
Therapeutic class: Anti-infective
Pregnancy risk category B

Action

Structurally and pharmacologically related to penicillin; interferes with bacterial cell-wall synthesis and division by binding to cell wall, causing cell death. Active against gram-negative and gram-positive bacteria, with expanded activity against gram-negative bacteria. Shows minimal immunosuppressive activity.

Pharmacokinetics

Drug distributes widely to most tissues and fluids, and enters cerebrospinal fluid of patients with inflamed meninges. It is partially metabolized; protein binding is approximately 20% (independent of serum level). Drug crosses placental barrier, is secreted in breast milk, and is excreted in urine mostly as unchanged drug.

Onset	Peak	Duration
Rapid	End of infusion	12 hr

How supplied

Powder for reconstitution for injection (white to pale yellow): 500-mg vial, 1-g vial, 2-g vial; 1-g and 2-g piggyback bottles; 1 g/15-mL vial

Indications and dosages

➤ Urinary tract infections (UTIs) caused by *Escherichia coli, Klebsiella pneumoniae,* and *Proteus mirabilis*
Adults: 500 mg to 1g by I.V. infusion q 12 hours for 7 to 10 days

➢ Severe UTIs caused by *E. coli* or *K. pneumoniae*, moderate to severe skin infections caused by *Staphylococcus aureus* or *Streptococcus pyogenes*
Adults: 2 g by I.V. infusion q 12 hours for 10 days

➢ Febrile neutropenia
Adults and children ages 2 months to 16 years: 2 g by I.V. infusion q 8 hours for 7 days

➢ Complicated intra-abdominal infections caused by alpha-hemolytic streptococci, *E. coli, K. pneumoniae, Pseudomonas aeruginosa, Enterobacter* species, and *Bacteroides fragilis*
Adults: 2 g by I.V. infusion q 12 hours for 7 to 10 days (given with metronidazole)

➢ Moderate to severe pneumonia caused by *K. pneumoniae, P. aeruginosa, Enterobacter* species, and *Streptococcus pneumoniae*
Adults: 1 to 2 g by I.V. infusion q 12 hours for 10 days

Dosage adjustment

- In renal impairment (creatinine clearance of 60 mL/minute or less), adjust dosage after initial dose.
- In patients undergoing hemodialysis, give repeat dosage equivalent to initial dosage at end of each dialysis session.
- In patients undergoing continuous ambulatory peritoneal dialysis, give normal recommended dosage, but at intervals of every 48 hours.
- In elderly patients with creatinine clearance of 60 mL/minute or less, adjust dosage as appropriate.

Administration

Preparation

Before starting therapy, determine if patient has had previous hypersensitivity reactions to cefepime, other cephalosporins, penicillins, or other drugs.

- Do not exceed adult recommended dosage in children.
- Obtain specimens for culture and sensitivity tests as needed before starting therapy.
- Assess baseline CBC and kidney and liver function test results.

Dilution and compatibility

- Reconstitute with 50 or 100 mL of compatible I.V. infusion solution.
- Be aware that drug is compatible at concentrations of 1 to 40 mg/mL when mixed with normal saline solution, D_5W, dextrose 10% in water, M/6 sodium lactate solution, dextrose 5% in normal saline solution, lactated Ringer's solution, Normosol-M in dextrose 5%, and Normosol-R in dextrose 5%.
- Do not mix with ampicillin (at concentrations above 40 mg/mL), metronidazole, aminoglycosides, or aminophylline if prescribed concurrently. Give each drug separately.
- Know that freshly reconstituted solution ranges in color from colorless to amber.
- Be aware that powder and solution tend to darken depending on storage conditions; however, when stored as recommended, product potency is unaffected.

Infusion considerations

- For I.V. infusion, use small I.V. needle and infuse into large vein over 30 to 60 minutes.

Monitoring

In patients receiving high doses, monitor closely for seizures; be prepared to intervene appropriately.

Be aware that cross-sensitivity to penicillins and other cephalosporins may occur. If allergic reaction occurs, discontinue treatment. In acute hypersensitivity reaction, be prepared to give epinephrine and provide other emergency measures, including oxygen, I.V. fluids, I.V. antihistamines, corticosteroids, pressor amines, and airway management, as indicated.

Monitor for signs and symptoms of pseudomembranous colitis; institute therapeutic measures as indicated. Mild cases usually respond to drug withdrawal alone. In moderate to severe cases, be prepared to give fluids and electrolytes, protein supplements, and oral antibiotic effective against Clostridium difficile colitis.

- Monitor CBC, prothrombin time, and kidney and liver function test results.
- Monitor for signs and symptoms of superinfection and other serious adverse reactions.

Storage

- Store dry powder between 2° and 25°C (36° and 77°F); protect from light. Reconstituted or diluted solution is stable for 24 hours at controlled room temperature and for 7 days if refrigerated at 5°C (41°F); however, if mixed with ampicillin, stability time decreases significantly.

Contraindications and precautions

Contraindicated in hypersensitivity to cephalosporins, penicillins, or other beta-lactams.

Use cautiously in hypersensitivity to penicillin, renal impairment, phenylketonuria, history of GI disease (especially colitis), emaciated patients, ***elderly patients,*** pregnant or breastfeeding patients, and ***children younger than 2 months*** (safety and efficacy not established).

Adverse reactions

CNS: headache, lethargy, paresthesia, syncope, **seizures**
CV: phlebitis, hypotension, palpitations, chest pain, vasodilation, **thrombophlebitis**
EENT: hearing loss
GI: nausea, vomiting, diarrhea, abdominal cramps, oral candidiasis, **pseudomembranous colitis**
GU: vaginal candidiasis, **nephrotoxicity**
Hematologic: lymphocytosis, eosinophilia, **bleeding tendency, hemolytic anemia, hypoprothrombinemia, neutropenia, thrombocytopenia, agranulocytosis, bone marrow depression**
Hepatic: hepatic failure, hepatomegaly
Musculoskeletal: arthralgia
Respiratory: dyspnea
Skin: urticaria, maculopapular or erythematous rash, redness, swelling, induration
Other: chills, fever, superinfection, phlebitis at I.V. site, **anaphylaxis, serum sickness**

Interactions

Drug-drug. *Aminoglycosides, loop diuretics:* increased risk of nephrotoxicity
Probenecid: decreased excretion and increased blood level of cefepime
Drug-diagnostic tests. *Alanine aminotransferase, alkaline phosphatase, aspartate aminotransferase, bilirubin, blood urea nitrogen, creatinine, eosinophils, gamma-glutamyltransferase, lactate dehydrogenase:* increased
Coombs' test, nonenzyme-based urine glucose tests (such as Clinitest), urinary 17-ketosteroids: false-positive results
Hemoglobin, platelets, prothrombin time, white blood cells: decreased
Drug-herb. *Angelica, anise, arnica, asafetida, bogbean, boldo, celery, chamomile, clove, danshen, fenugreek, feverfew, garlic, ginger, ginkgo, ginseng, horse chestnut, horseradish, licorice, meadowsweet, onion, papain, passionflower, poplar, prickly ash, quassia, red clover, turmeric, wild carrot, wild lettuce, willow:* increased risk of bleeding

Toxicity and overdose

- In overdose, expect extension of adverse reactions, including seizures.
- If seizures occur, immediately discontinue drug and give anticonvulsant, as ordered. In overwhelming overdose,

hemodialysis should be considered to remove drug. Provide supportive and symptomatic interventions.

Patient teaching

Instruct patient to immediately report signs and symptoms of allergic reaction, reduced urine output, persistent diarrhea, bruising, or bleeding.

- Caution patient not to take herbs without consulting prescriber.
- Advise patient to maintain adequate fluid intake during therapy.
- Instruct patient with diabetes mellitus to use enzyme-based test (Clinistix, Testape) to monitor urine glucose, because drug may cause false results with other tests.
- As appropriate, review all other significant and life-threatening adverse reactions and interactions, especially those related to the drugs, tests, and herbs mentioned above.

cefotaxime sodium

Claforan

Pharmacologic class: Third-generation cephalosporin

Therapeutic class: Anti-infective

Pregnancy risk category B

Action

Structurally and pharmacologically related to penicillin; interferes with bacterial cell-wall synthesis and division by binding to cell wall, causing cell death. Active against gram-negative and gram-positive bacteria, with expanded activity against gram-negative bacteria. Shows minimal immunosuppressive activity.

Pharmacokinetics

Drug distributes widely to most tissues and fluids; it achieves adequate penetration into inflamed meninges and crosses placental barrier. It is partially metabolized to active metabolite; protein binding is about 38%. About 20% to 36% of dose is excreted in urine unchanged; 15% to 25% is excreted as major metabolite, with some excretion into breast milk.

Onset	Peak	Duration
Rapid	End of infusion	4-12 hr

How supplied

Powder for reconstitution for injection (off-white to pale yellow): 1 g, 2 g, 10 g
Solution for injection: 1 g/50 mL and 2 g/50 mL in premixed containers

Indications and dosages

➤ Perioperative prophylaxis

Adults and children weighing more than 50 kg (110 lb): 1 g I.V. 30 to 90 minutes before surgery

➤ Prophylaxis in patients undergoing cesarean delivery

Adults: 1 g I.V. as soon as umbilical cord is clamped

➤ Disseminated gonorrhea

Adults and children weighing 50 kg or more: 1 g by I.V. infusion q 8 hours

➤ Uncomplicated infections caused by susceptible organisms

Adults and children weighing 50 kg or more: 1 g I.V. q 12 hours

Children ages 1 month to 12 years weighing less than 50 kg: 50 to 180 mg/kg/day I.V. in four to six divided doses

➤ Moderate to severe infections caused by susceptible organisms

Adults and children weighing 50 kg or more: 1 to 2 g I.V. q 8 hours

➤ Life-threatening infections caused by susceptible organisms

Adults and children weighing 50 kg or more: 2 g I.V. q 4 hours; maximum dosage is 12 g/day.

➢ Septicemia and other infections that commonly require antibiotics in higher doses

Adults and children weighing 50 kg or more: 2 g I.V. q 6 to 8 hours

Dosage adjustment

- In renal impairment, determine dosage by degree of impairment, severity of infection, and susceptibility of causative organism. Reduce dosage by 50% in creatinine clearance less than 20 mL/minute.

Administration

Preparation

Before starting therapy, determine if patient has had previous hypersensitivity reactions to cefotaxime, other cephalosporins, penicillins, or other drugs.

- Obtain specimens for culture and sensitivity tests as needed before starting therapy.
- Assess baseline CBC and kidney and liver function test results.

Dilution and compatibility

- Reconstitute powder for I.V. injection with at least 10 mL sterile water, and give over 3 to 5 minutes. For intermittent infusion, may further dilute drug with 50 or 100 mL normal saline solution or D_5W.
- Know that reconstituted drug may be diluted further for continuous I.V. infusion of up to 1,000 mL with compatible solution, such as normal saline solution, D_5W or dextrose 10% in water, D_5W and normal saline solution, half-normal saline solution, or lactated Ringer's solution.
- Do not use diluents with pH above 7.5 (such as sodium bicarbonate).
- Do not mix in same infusion with aminoglycoside, as both drugs may be inactivated.
- Know that reconstituted solution may range from very pale yellow to amber, depending on concentration and diluent used.
- Be aware that powder and solution tend to darken depending on storage conditions; however, when stored as recommended, product potency is unaffected.
- Thaw premixed drug at room temperature.
- Do not add other drugs to premixed containers. Discard unused solution.

Infusion considerations

- For I.V. bolus injection, give single dose over 3 to 5 minutes. Doses given over less then 1 minute have caused life-threatening arrythmias.
- For intermittent infusion, give a single dose over 30 minutes.
- For continuous I.V. infusion, give over 6 to 24 hours, depending on concentration.
- Rotate infusion sites.

Do not use plastic containers in series connections. Such use could result in air embolism due to residual air being drawn from primary container before administration of fluid from secondary container ends.

Monitoring

In patients receiving high doses, monitor closely for seizures; be prepared to intervene appropriately.

Be aware that cross-sensitivity to penicillins and other cephalosporins may occur. If allergic reaction develops, discontinue treatment. In acute hypersensitivity reaction, be prepared to give epinephrine and provide other emergency measures, including oxygen, I.V. fluids, I.V. antihistamines, corticosteroids, pressor amines, and airway management, as indicated.

Monitor for signs and symptoms of pseudomembranous colitis; institute therapeutic measures as indicated. Mild cases usually respond to drug withdrawal alone. In moderate to severe cases, be prepared to give fluids and electrolytes, protein supplements, and oral antibiotic effective against Clostridium difficile colitis.
• Monitor CBC, prothrombin time, and kidney and liver function test results.
• Monitor for signs and symptoms of superinfection and other serious adverse reactions.

Storage

• When reconstituted as described above, solution is stable for 24 hours at controlled room temperature and 10 days if refrigerated at 5°C (41°F).
• Store frozen premixed containers at or below –20°C (–4°F). After thawing, solution maintains potency for 24 hours at room temperature at or below 22°C (72°F) and for 10 days if refrigerated at or below 5°C (41°F). Do not refreeze.

Contraindications and precautions

Contraindicated in hypersensitivity to cephalosporins.

Use cautiously in hypersensitivity to penicillins, renal impairment, phenylketonuria, history of GI disease (especially colitis), emaciated patients, ***elderly patients,*** pregnant or breastfeeding patients, and ***children younger than 1 month*** (safety and efficacy not established).

Adverse reactions

CNS: headache, lethargy, paresthesia, syncope, **seizures**
CV: hypotension, palpitations, chest pain, vasodilation
EENT: hearing loss
GI: nausea, vomiting, diarrhea, abdominal cramps, oral candidiasis, **pseudomembranous colitis**
GU: vaginal candidiasis, **nephrotoxicity**
Hematologic: lymphocytosis, eosinophilia, **bleeding tendency, hemolytic anemia, hypoprothrombinemia, neutropenia, thrombocytopenia, agranulocytosis, bone marrow depression**
Hepatic: hepatic failure, hepatomegaly
Musculoskeletal: arthralgia
Respiratory: dyspnea
Skin: urticaria, maculopapular or erythematous rash
Other: chills, fever, superinfection, injection site inflammation, **anaphylaxis, serum sickness**

Interactions

Drug-drug. *Aminoglycosides, loop diuretics:* increased risk of nephrotoxicity
Probenecid: decreased excretion and increased blood level of cefotaxime
Drug-diagnostic tests. *Alanine aminotransferase, alkaline phosphatase, aspartate aminotransferase, bilirubin, blood urea nitrogen, creatinine, eosinophils, gamma-glutamyltransferase, lactate dehydrogenase:* increased
Coombs' test, nonenzyme-based urine glucose tests (such as Clinitest), urinary 17-ketosteroids: false-positive results
Hemoglobin, platelets, prothrombin time, white blood cells: decreased
Drug-herb. *Angelica, anise, arnica, asafetida, bogbean, boldo, celery, chamomile, clove, danshen, fenugreek, feverfew, garlic, ginger, ginkgo, ginseng, horse chestnut, horseradish, licorice, meadowsweet, onion, papain, passionflower, poplar, prickly ash, quassia, red clover, turmeric, wild carrot, wild lettuce, willow:* increased risk of bleeding

Toxicity and overdose

• In overdose, expect signs and symptoms to include dyspnea, hypothermia, cyanosis, and tonic-clonic seizures.
• If seizures occur, immediately discontinue drug and administer anticonvulsant,

as ordered. Provide supportive and symptomatic therapy.

Patient teaching

🔈 Instruct patient to immediately report signs and symptoms of allergic reaction, reduced urine output, persistent diarrhea, bruising, and bleeding.

- Advise patient to maintain adequate fluid intake during therapy.
- Caution patient not to take herbs without consulting prescriber.
- Instruct patient with diabetes mellitus to use enzyme-based test (Clinistix, Testape) to monitor urine glucose, because drug may cause false results with other tests.
- As appropriate, review all other significant and life-threatening adverse reactions and interactions, especially those related to the drugs, tests, and herbs mentioned above.

cefoxitin sodium

Apo-Cefoxitin🍁, Mefoxin

Pharmacologic class: Second-generation cephalosporin
Therapeutic class: Anti-infective
Pregnancy risk category B

Action

Structurally and pharmacologically related to penicillin; interferes with bacterial cell-wall synthesis and division by binding to cell wall, causing cell death. Active against gram-negative and gram-positive bacteria, with expanded activity against gram-negative bacteria. Shows minimal immunosuppressive activity.

Pharmacokinetics

Drug distributes widely to most tissues and fluids; it crosses placental barrier but has poor penetration into cerebrospinal fluid. Only small percentage of dose is metabolized. Drug is largely protein-bound. It is excreted mainly in urine as unchanged drug, with small amount excreted in breast milk.

Onset	Peak	Duration
Rapid	End of infusion	4-8 hr

How supplied

Powder for reconstitution for injection (off-white): 1 g, 2 g
Solution for injection (colorless to light amber): 1 g/50 mL in D_5W, 2 g/50 mL in D_5W in premixed containers

Indications and dosages

➢ Respiratory tract infections, skin infections, bone and joint infections, urinary tract infections, gynecologic infections, septicemia

Adults: For most infections, 1 g I.V. q 6 to 8 hours. For severe infections, 1 g I.V. q 4 hours or 2 g I.V. q 6 to 8 hours. For life-threatening infections, 2 g I.V. q 4 hours or 3 g I.V. q 6 hours.
Children age 3 months and older: For most infections, 13.3 to 26.7 mg/kg I.V. q 4 hours or 20 to 40 mg/kg q 6 hours

➢ Preoperative prophylaxis

Adults: 1 to 2 g I.V. within 60 minutes of incision, then q 6 hours for up to 24 hours

Dosage adjustment

- In renal impairment, give initial loading dose of 1 to 2 g, followed by maintenance dosages shown on the next page.

Renal function	CrCl (mL/min)	Dosage (g)	Frequency (hr)
Mild impairment	50 to 30	1 to 2	8 to 12
Moderate impairment	29 to 10	1 to 2	12 to 24
Severe impairment	9 to 5	0.5 to 1	12 to 24
Renal failure	Below 5	0.5 to 1	24 to 48

• In patients undergoing hemodialysis, give loading dose of 1 to 2 g after each dialysis session. Give maintenance dosages listed in above table.

Administration

Preparation

Before starting therapy, determine if patient has had previous hypersensitivity reactions to cefoxitin, other cephalosporins, penicillins, or other drugs.

• Obtain specimens for culture and sensitivity tests as needed before starting therapy.

• Assess baseline CBC and kidney and liver function test results.

Dilution and compatibility

• Reconstitute 1-g dose with 10 mL sterile water for injection; reconstitute 2-g dose with 20 mL.

• For intermittent or continuous I.V. infusion, add reconstituted drug to compatible solution, such as D_5W, normal saline solution, or D_5W in normal saline solution.

• Do not mix in same infusion with aminoglycoside, because both drugs may be inactivated.

• Be aware that powder and solution may darken depending on storage conditions; however, when stored as recommended, product potency is unaffected.

• Thaw premixed drug at room temperature.

• Do not add other drugs to premixed containers. Discard unused solution.

Infusion considerations

• For direct I.V. injection, give 10 mL sterile water with each gram of cefoxitin over 3 to 5 minutes. Inject into large vein and rotate sites, or give through existing I.V. tubing.

• For intermittent or continuous I.V. infusion, infuse as prescribed.

Do not use plastic containers in series connections. Such use could result in air embolism due to residual air being drawn from primary container before administration of fluid from secondary container ends.

Monitoring

In patients receiving high doses, monitor closely for seizures; be prepared to intervene appropriately.

Be aware that cross-sensitivity to penicillins and other cephalosporins may occur. If allergic reaction occurs, discontinue treatment. In acute hypersensitivity reaction, be prepared to give epinephrine and provide other emergency measures, including oxygen, I.V. fluids, I.V. antihistamines, corticosteroids, pressor amines, and airway management, as indicated.

Monitor for signs and symptoms of pseudomembranous colitis; institute therapeutic measures as indicated. Mild cases usually respond to drug withdrawal alone. In moderate to severe cases, be prepared to give fluids and electrolytes, protein supplements, and oral antibiotic effective against *Clostridium difficile* colitis.

• Monitor CBC, prothrombin time, and kidney and liver function test results.

• Monitor for signs and symptoms of superinfection and other serious adverse reactions.

Storage

• Store powder at 2° to 25°C (36° to 77°F). Store reconstituted solution at controlled room temperature for 6 hours, or for 7 days if refrigerated at 5°C (41°F).

• Store frozen premixed containers at or below –20°C (–4°F). After thawing, solution maintains potency for 24 hours at room temperature and for 21 days if refrigerated at 2° to 8°C (36° to 46°F). Do not refreeze.

Contraindications and precautions

Contraindicated in hypersensitivity to cephalosporins or penicillins.

Use cautiously in renal impairment, hepatic disease, biliary obstruction, history of GI disease, ***elderly patients,*** pregnant or breastfeeding patients, and ***children younger than 3 months*** (safety and efficacy not established).

Adverse reactions

CNS: headache, lethargy, paresthesia, syncope, **seizures**
CV: hypotension, palpitations, chest pain, vasodilation, thrombophlebitis
EENT: hearing loss
GI: nausea, vomiting, diarrhea, abdominal cramps, oral candidiasis, **pseudomembranous colitis**
GU: vaginal candidiasis, **nephrotoxicity**
Hematologic: lymphocytosis, eosinophilia, **bleeding tendency, hemolytic anemia, hypoprothrombinemia, neutropenia, thrombocytopenia, agranulocytosis, bone marrow depression**
Hepatic: hepatic failure, hepatomegaly
Musculoskeletal: arthralgia
Respiratory: dyspnea
Skin: urticaria, maculopapular or erythematous rash
Other: chills, fever, superinfection, inflammation at injection site, **anaphylaxis, serum sickness**

Interactions

Drug-drug. *Aminoglycosides, loop diuretics:* increased risk of nephrotoxicity
Probenecid: decreased excretion and increased blood level of cefoxitin
Drug-diagnostic tests. *Alanine aminotransferase, alkaline phosphatase, aspartate aminotransferase, bilirubin, blood urea nitrogen, creatinine, eosinophils, gamma-glutamyltransferase, lactate dehydrogenase:* increased
Coombs' test, nonenzyme-based urine glucose tests (such as Clinitest), urinary 17-ketosteroids: false-positive results
Hemoglobin, platelets, prothrombin time, white blood cells: decreased

Toxicity and overdose

• In overdose, expect extension of adverse reactions, including seizures.

• If seizures occur, immediately discontinue drug and give anticonvulsant, as ordered. In overwhelming overdose, hemodialysis may be considered to remove drug. Provide supportive and symptomatic therapy.

Patient teaching

Instruct patient to immediately report signs and symptoms of allergic reaction, reduced urine output, persistent diarrhea, bruising, and bleeding.

• Advise patient to maintain adequate fluid intake during therapy.

• Instruct patient with diabetes mellitus to use enzyme-based test (Clinistix, Testape) to monitor urine glucose, because drug may cause false results with other tests.

• As appropriate, review all other significant and life-threatening adverse reactions and interactions, especially those related to the drugs and tests mentioned above.

[redacted]

ceftazidime

Fortaz, Fortum, Kefadim, Tazicef

Pharmacologic class: Third-generation cephalosporin
Therapeutic class: Anti-infective
Pregnancy risk category B

Action

Structurally and pharmacologically related to penicillin; interferes with bacterial cell-wall synthesis and division by binding to cell wall, causing cell death. Active against gram-negative and gram-positive bacteria, with expanded activity against gram-negative bacteria. Shows minimal immunosuppressive activity.

Pharmacokinetics

Drug distributes widely to most tissues and fluids, achieves good penetration into cerebrospinal fluid, and crosses placental barrier. It is not metabolized and is excreted largely by the kidneys (almost exclusively by glomerular filtration) as unchanged drug, with small amount excreted in breast milk.

Onset	Peak	Duration
Rapid	End of infusion	6-12 hr

How supplied

Powder for reconstitution for injection (white to off-white): 500 mg, 1 g, 2 g, 6 g, 10 g
Solution for injection: 1 g/50 mL, 2 g/50 mL in premixed containers

Indications and dosages

➤ Skin infections; bone and joint infections; urinary tract and gynecologic infections, including gonorrhea; respiratory tract infections; intra-abdominal infections; septicemia

Adults and children age 12 and older: For most infections, 500 mg to 2 g I.V. q 8 to 12 hours. For pneumonia and skin infections, 0.5 to 1 g I.V. q 8 to 12 hours. For bone and joint infections, 2 g I.V. q 12 hours. For severe and life-threatening infections, 2 g I.V. q 8 hours. For complicated urinary tract infections (UTIs), 500 mg q 8 to 12 hours. For uncomplicated UTIs, 250 mg I.V. q 12 hours.

Children ages 1 month to 12 years: 30 to 50 mg/kg I.V. q 8 hours

Infants younger than 4 weeks: 30 mg/kg I.V. q 12 hours

Dosage adjustment

- In renal impairment (glomerular filtration rate less than 50 mL/minute), reduce dosage to compensate for slower excretion. In suspected renal insufficiency, give 1 g as initial loading dose, followed by maintenance dosages as shown below.

Renal function	CrCl (mL/min)	Dosage (g)	Frequency (hr)
Mild impairment	31 to 50	1	12
Moderate impairment	16 to 30	1	24
Severe impairment	6 to 15	0.5	24
Renal failure	Below 5	0.5	48

- In patients undergoing hemodialysis, give 1-g loading dose, followed by 1 g after each dialysis session.
- In patients undergoing intraperitoneal dialysis or continuous ambulatory peritoneal dialysis, give 1-g loading dose, followed by 0.5 g every 24 hours.

Off-label uses

- Febrile neutropenia
- Prophylaxis of perinatal infections

Administration

Preparation

Before starting therapy, determine if patient has had previous hypersensitivity reactions to ceftazidime, other cephalosporins, penicillins, or other drugs.

- Obtain specimens for culture and sensitivity tests as needed before starting therapy.
- Assess baseline CBC and kidney and liver function test results.

Dilution and compatibility

- Reconstitute powder for injection with sterile water for injection.
- For I.V. bolus injection, dilute each gram in at least 10 mL sterile water for injection.
- For intermittent I.V. infusion, dilute further with 100 mL sterile water or another compatible fluid, such as normal saline solution or D_5W.
- Do not dilute with sodium bicarbonate.
- Do not mix in same infusion with aminoglycoside, because both drugs may be inactivated.
- Be aware that solutions range in color from light yellow to amber, depending on diluent and volume used.
- Be aware that powder and solution tend to darken depending on storage conditions; however, when stored as recommended, product potency is unaffected.
- Thaw premixed drug at room temperature.
- Do not add other drugs to premixed containers. Discard unused solution.

Infusion considerations

- For I.V. bolus injection, give single dose over 3 to 5 minutes. Inject into large vein; rotate injection sites.
- For intermittent I.V. infusion, infuse over 30 minutes.

Do not use plastic containers in series connections. Such use could result in air embolism due to residual air being drawn from primary container before administration of fluid from secondary container ends.

Monitoring

In patients receiving high doses, monitor closely for seizures; be prepared to intervene appropriately.

Be aware that cross-sensitivity to penicillins and other cephalosporins may occur. If allergic reaction occurs, discontinue treatment. In acute hypersensitivity reaction, be prepared to give epinephrine and provide other emergency measures, including oxygen, I.V. fluids, I.V. antihistamines, corticosteroids, pressor amines, and airway management, as indicated.

Monitor for signs and symptoms of pseudomembranous colitis; institute therapeutic measures as indicated. Mild cases usually respond to drug withdrawal alone. In moderate to severe cases, be prepared to give fluids and electrolytes, protein supplements, and oral antibiotic effective against *Clostridium difficile* colitis.

- Monitor CBC, prothrombin time, and kidney and liver function test results.
- Monitor for signs and symptoms of superinfection and other serious adverse reactions.

Storage

- Store powder at 15° to 30°C (59° to 86°F); protect from light. When reconstituted with sterile water for injection, solution is stable for 24 hours at controlled room temperature or for 7 days if refrigerated. Do not refreeze.
- Store frozen premixed containers at or below –20°C (–4°F). Do not refreeze.

Contraindications and precautions

Contraindicated in hypersensitivity to cephalosporins.

Use cautiously in hypersensitivity to penicillin, renal impairment, hepatic disease, biliary obstruction, phenylketonuria, history of GI disease, ***elderly patients,*** pregnant or breastfeeding patients, and ***children.***

Adverse reactions

CNS: headache, confusion, hemiparesis, lethargy, paresthesia, syncope, asterixis, neuromuscular excitability (with increased drug blood levels in renally impaired patients), **seizures, encephalopathy**
CV: hypotension, palpitations, chest pain, vasodilation
EENT: hearing loss
GI: nausea, vomiting, diarrhea, abdominal cramps, oral candidiasis, **pseudomembranous colitis**
GU: vaginal candidiasis, **nephrotoxicity**
Hematologic: lymphocytosis, eosinophilia, **bleeding tendency, hemolytic anemia, hypoprothrombinemia, neutropenia, thrombocytopenia, agranulocytosis, bone marrow depression**
Hepatic: hepatic failure, hepatomegaly
Musculoskeletal: arthralgia
Respiratory: dyspnea
Skin: urticaria, maculopapular or erythematous rash
Other: chills, fever, superinfection, phlebitis and injection site inflammation, **anaphylaxis, serum sickness**

Interactions

Drug-drug. *Aminoglycosides, loop diuretics:* increased risk of nephrotoxicity
Chloramphenicol: antagonism of ceftazidime's effects
Probenecid: decreased excretion and increased blood level of ceftazidime
Drug-diagnostic tests. *Alanine aminotransferase, alkaline phosphatase, aspartate aminotransferase, bilirubin, blood urea nitrogen, creatinine, eosinophils, gamma-glutamyltransferase, lactate dehydrogenase:* increased
Hemoglobin, platelets, prothrombin time, white blood cells: decreased
Coombs' test, nonenzyme-based urine glucose tests (such as Clinitest), urinary 17-ketosteroids: false-positive results
Drug-herb. *Angelica, anise, arnica, asafetida, bogbean, boldo, celery, chamomile, clove, danshen, fenugreek, feverfew, garlic, ginger, ginkgo, ginseng, horse chestnut, horseradish, licorice, meadowsweet, onion, papain, passionflower, poplar, prickly ash, quassia, red clover, turmeric, wild carrot, wild lettuce, willow:* increased risk of bleeding

Toxicity and overdose

- In overdose, expect signs and symptoms to include neuromuscular excitability, seizures, and coma.
- If seizures occur, immediately discontinue drug and administer anticonvulsant, as ordered. In overwhelming overdose in patients with renal insufficiency, peritoneal dialysis or hemodialysis should be considered to remove drug. Provide supportive and symptomatic therapy.

Patient teaching

Instruct patient to immediately report signs and symptoms of allergic reaction, reduced urine output, persistent diarrhea, bruising, and bleeding.
- Advise patient to maintain adequate fluid intake during therapy.
- Caution patient not to take herbs without consulting prescriber.
- Instruct patient with diabetes mellitus to use enzyme-based test (Clinistix, Testape) to monitor urine glucose, because drug may give false results with other tests.
- As appropriate, review all other significant and life-threatening adverse reactions and interactions, especially those related to the drugs, tests, and herbs mentioned above.

ceftizoxime sodium

Cefizox

Pharmacologic class: Third-generation cephalosporin

Therapeutic class: Anti-infective

Pregnancy risk category B

Action

Structurally and pharmacologically related to penicillin; interferes with bacterial cell-wall synthesis and division by binding to cell wall, causing cell death. Active against gram-negative and gram-positive bacteria, with expanded activity against gram-negative bacteria. Shows minimal immunosuppressive activity.

Pharmacokinetics

Drug distributes widely to most tissues and fluids, has good penetration into cerebrospinal fluid, and crosses placental barrier. It is not metabolized; protein binding is approximately 30%; serum half-life is 1.7 hours. It is excreted largely by the kidneys (by glomerular filtration and renal tubular secretion) as unchanged drug, with small amount excreted in breast milk.

Onset	Peak	Duration
Rapid	End of infusion	6-12 hr

How supplied

Powder for reconstitution for injection (white to pale yellow): 500-mg, 1-g, and 2-g vials

Solution for injection: 1 g/50 mL and 2 g/50 mL in premixed containers

Indications and dosages

➤ Skin infections; bone and joint infections; urinary tract infections (UTIs) and gynecologic infections (including gonorrhea); respiratory tract infections; intra-abdominal infections; septicemia

Adults: For mild or moderate infections, 1 g I.V. q 8 to 12 hours. For uncomplicated UTIs, 500 mg I.V. q 12 hours. For severe infections, 2 g I.V. q 8 to 12 hours. For life-threatening infections, 4 g I.V. q 8 hours.

Children age 6 months and older: 50 mg/kg I.V. q 6 to 8 hours

Dosage adjustment

- After loading dose of 500 mg or 1 g, give maintenance dosages listed below. (Also give these dosages to patients on hemodialysis at end of each session.)

Renal function	CrCl (mL/min)	Less severe infections	Life-threatening infections
Mild impairment	79 to 50	500 mg q 8 hr	750 mg to 1.5 g q 8 hr
Moderate to severe impairment	49 to 5	250 to 500 mg q 12 hr	500 mg to 1 g q 12 hr
Patients on dialysis	4 to 0	500 mg q 48 hr or 250 mg q 24 hr	500 mg to 1 g q 48 hr or 500 mg q 24 hr

Administration

Preparation

Before starting therapy, determine if patient has had previous hypersensitivity reactions to ceftizoxime, other cephalosporins, penicillins, or other drugs.

- Do not exceed adult recommended dosage in children.
- Obtain specimens for culture and sensitivity tests as needed before starting therapy.
- Assess baseline CBC and kidney and liver function test results.

Dilution and compatibility

• Reconstitute powder with sterile water for injection in at least 10 mL solution per gram, as shown below. Shake reconstituted solution well to dissolve powder.

Vial	Dose	Diluent	Concentration
500 mg	15 mL	5.3 mL	95 mg/mL
1 g	10 mL	10.7 mL	95 mg/mL
2 g	20 mL	21.4 mL	95 mg/mL

• For intermittent, piggyback, or continuous I.V. administration, dilute reconstituted drug further in 50 to 100 mL of compatible solution, such as normal saline solution, D_5W, dextrose 10% in water, dextrose 5% and normal saline solution, dextrose 5% and half-normal saline solution, dextrose 5% and 0.2% sodium chloride solution, or lactated Ringer's solution.

• Do not mix in same infusion with aminoglycoside, because both drugs may be inactivated.

• Be aware that powder and solution may darken depending on storage conditions; however, when stored as recommended, product potency is unaffected.

• Thaw premixed drug at room temperature.

• Do not add other drugs to premixed containers. Discard unused solution.

Infusion considerations

• Administer single I.V. injection over 3 to 5 minutes. Use large vein; rotate injection sites.

• For intermittent, piggyback, or continuous I.V. administration, infuse over at least 30 minutes.

Do not use plastic containers in series connections. Such use could result in air embolism, due to residual air being drawn from primary container before administration of fluid from secondary container ends.

Monitoring

In patients receiving high doses, monitor closely for seizures; be prepared to intervene appropriately.

Be aware that cross-sensitivity to penicillins and other cephalosporins may occur. If allergic reaction occurs, discontinue treatment. In acute hypersensitivity reactions, be prepared to give epinephrine and provide other emergency measures, including oxygen, I.V. fluids, I.V. antihistamines, corticosteroids, pressor amines, and airway management, as indicated.

Monitor for signs and symptoms of pseudomembranous colitis; institute therapeutic measures as indicated. Mild cases usually respond to drug withdrawal alone. In moderate to severe cases, be prepared to give fluids and electrolytes, protein supplements, and oral antibiotic effective against *Clostridium difficile* colitis.

• Monitor CBC, prothrombin time, and kidney and liver function test results.

• Monitor for signs and symptoms of superinfection and other serious adverse reactions.

Storage

• Before reconstituting powder, store at controlled room temperature of 15° to 30°C (59° to 86°F) in original package; protect from light. When reconstituted or diluted with sterile water for injection or mixed with compatible infusion solution, drug is stable for 24 hours at controlled room temperature, or for 96 hours if refrigerated at 5°C (41°F).

• Store frozen premixed containers at or below –20°C (–4°F). Do not refreeze.

Contraindications and precautions

Contraindicated in hypersensitivity to cephalosporins.

Use cautiously in hypersensitivity to penicillin, renal impairment, hepatic disease, biliary obstruction, phenylketonuria, history of GI disease, ***elderly patients,*** pregnant or breastfeeding patients, and ***children younger than 6 months*** (safety and efficacy not established).

Adverse reactions

CNS: headache, confusion, hemiparesis, lethargy, paresthesia, syncope, **seizures**
CV: hypotension, palpitations, chest pain, vasodilation
EENT: hearing loss
GI: nausea, vomiting, diarrhea, abdominal cramps, oral candidiasis, **pseudomembranous colitis**
GU: vaginal candidiasis, **nephrotoxicity**
Hematologic: lymphocytosis, eosinophilia, **bleeding tendency, hemolytic anemia, hypoprothrombinemia, neutropenia, thrombocytopenia, agranulocytosis, bone marrow depression**
Hepatic: hepatic failure, hepatomegaly
Musculoskeletal: arthralgia
Respiratory: dyspnea
Skin: urticaria, maculopapular or erythematous rash
Other: chills, fever, superinfection, pain at injection site, **anaphylaxis, serum sickness**

Interactions

Drug-drug. *Aminoglycosides, loop diuretics:* increased risk of nephrotoxicity
Probenecid: decreased excretion and increased blood level of ceftizoxime
Drug-diagnostic tests. *Alanine aminotransferase, alkaline phosphatase, aspartate aminotransferase, bilirubin, blood urea nitrogen, creatinine, eosinophils, gamma-glutamyltransferase, lactate dehydrogenase:* increased
Coombs' test, nonenzyme-based urine glucose tests (such as Clinitest), urinary 17-ketosteroids: false-positive results
Hemoglobin, platelets, prothrombin time, white blood cells: decreased
Drug-herb. *Angelica, anise, arnica, asafetida, bogbean, boldo, celery, chamomile, clove, danshen, fenugreek, feverfew, garlic, ginger, ginkgo, ginseng, horse chestnut, horseradish, licorice, meadowsweet, onion, papain, passionflower, poplar, prickly ash, quassia, red clover, turmeric, wild carrot, wild lettuce, willow:* increased risk of bleeding.

Toxicity and overdose

- In overdose, expect extension of adverse reactions, including seizures.
- If seizures occur, immediately discontinue drug and give anticonvulsant, as ordered. In overwhelming overdose, peritoneal dialysis or hemodialysis should be considered to remove drug. Provide supportive and symptomatic therapy.

Patient teaching

Instruct patient to immediately report signs and symptoms of allergic reaction, reduced urine output, persistent diarrhea, bruising, and bleeding.
- Advise patient to maintain adequate fluid intake during therapy.
- Caution patient not to take herbs without consulting prescriber.
- Instruct patient with diabetes mellitus to use enzyme-based test (Clinistix, Testape) to monitor urine glucose, because drug may cause false results with other tests.
- As appropriate, review all other significant and life-threatening adverse reactions and interactions, especially those related to the drugs, tests, and herbs mentioned above.

ceftriaxone sodium

Rocephin

Pharmacologic class: Third-generation cephalosporin
Therapeutic class: Anti-infective
Pregnancy risk category B

Action

Structurally and pharmacologically related to penicillin; interferes with bacterial cell-wall synthesis and division by binding to cell wall, causing cell death. Active against gram-negative and gram-positive bacteria, with expanded activity against gram-negative bacteria. Shows minimal immunosuppressive activity.

Pharmacokinetics

Drug distributes widely to most tissues and fluids, has good penetration into cerebrospinal fluid, and crosses placental barrier. It is partially metabolized; protein binding is dose-dependent. Drug has a long half-life. It is excreted largely in urine as unchanged drug, with some excretion of inactive metabolites in bile and a small amount in breast milk. Pharmacokinetics are slightly altered in elderly patients and in renal or hepatic impairment.

Onset	Peak	Duration
Rapid	End of infusion	12-24 hr

How supplied

Powder for reconstitution for injection (white to yellowish orange): 250 mg, 500 mg, 1 g, 2 g
Solution for injection: 1 g/50 mL and 2 g/50 mL in premixed containers

Indications and dosages

➤ Infections of respiratory system, bones, joints, and skin; septicemia caused by susceptible organisms
Adults: 1 to 2 g I.V. once daily or in equally divided doses q 12 hours. Maximum daily dosage is 4 g.
➤ Surgical prophylaxis
Adults: 1 g I.V. as a single dose within 1 hour before start of surgical procedure
➤ Meningitis
Adults: 1 to 2 g I.V. q 12 hours for 10 to 14 days
Children: Initially, 100 mg/kg/day I.V. (not to exceed 4 g). Then, 100 mg/kg/day I.V. once daily or in equally divided doses q 12 hours (not to exceed 4 g) for 7 to 14 days.
➤ Skin and skin-structure infections
Children: 50 to 75 mg/kg/day I.V. once or twice daily. Maximum dosage is 2 g/day.
➤ Other serious infections
Children: 50 to 75 mg/kg/day I.V. once or twice daily

Dosage adjustment

- In hepatic dysfunction or significant renal disease, do not exceed 2 g/day.

Off-label uses

- Disseminated gonorrhea
- Endocarditis
- Epididymitis
- Gonorrhea-associated meningitis
- Lyme disease
- *Neisseria meningitidis* carriers
- Pelvic inflammatory disease

Administration

Preparation

Before starting therapy, determine if patient has had previous hypersensitivity reactions to ceftriaxone, other cephalosporins, penicillins, or other drugs.

Do not give to hyperbilirubinemic neonates, especially preterm neonates.
- Obtain specimens for culture and sensitivity tests as needed before starting therapy.
- Assess baseline CBC and kidney and liver function test results.

Dilution and compatibility
- Reconstitute drug with sterile water for injection, normal saline solution, D_5W, half-normal saline solution, or D_5W and normal saline solution.
- After initial reconstitution, further dilute to desired concentration for intermittent I.V. infusion.
- Do not mix in same infusion with other drugs; be aware that aminoglycosides may inactivate ceftriaxone.
- Know that solution color ranges from light yellow to amber, depending on length of storage, concentration, and diluent used.
- Be aware that powder and solution may darken depending on storage conditions; however, when stored as recommended, product potency is unaffected.
- Thaw premixed drug at room temperature.
- Do not add other drugs to premixed containers. Discard unused solution.

Infusion considerations
- Administer by I. V. infusion over 30 minutes.

Do not use plastic containers in series connections. Such use could result in air embolism due to residual air being drawn from primary container before administration of fluid from secondary container ends.

Monitoring

In patients receiving high doses, monitor closely for seizures; be prepared to intervene appropriately.

Be aware that cross-sensitivity to penicillin and other cephalosporins may occur. If allergic reaction arises, discontinue treatment. In acute hypersensitivity reaction, be prepared to give epinephrine and provide other emergency measures, including oxygen, I.V. fluids, I.V. antihistamines, corticosteroids, pressor amines, and airway management, as indicated.

C

Monitor for signs and symptoms of pseudomembranous colitis; institute therapeutic measures as indicated. Mild cases usually respond to drug withdrawal alone. In moderate to severe cases, be prepared to give fluids and electrolytes, protein supplements, and oral antibiotic effective against *Clostridium difficile* colitis.
- Monitor CBC, prothrombin time, and kidney and liver function test results.
- Monitor for signs and symptoms of superinfection and other serious adverse reactions.
- Discontinue drug if patient develops signs or symptoms suggesting gallbladder disease or has sonographic findings of "sludge" (ceftriaxone-calcium salt) or echo with acoustic shadowing, which may be misinterpreted as gallstones.

Storage
- Store powder at room temperature, protected from light until reconstitution. When reconstituted or diluted with compatible solution, drug is stable from 3 to 10 days depending on solution used.
- Store frozen premixed containers at or below –20°C (–4°F). Do not refreeze.

Contraindications and precautions

Contraindicated in hypersensitivity to cephalosporins.

Use cautiously in hypersensitivity to penicillin, renal impairment, hepatic disease, biliary obstruction, phenylketonuria, history of GI disease, ***elderly patients,*** and pregnant or breastfeeding patients.

Adverse reactions

CNS: headache, confusion, hemiparesis, lethargy, paresthesia, syncope, **seizures**
CV: hypotension, palpitations, chest pain, vasodilation
EENT: hearing loss
GI: nausea, vomiting, diarrhea, abdominal cramps, oral candidiasis, gallbladder abnormalities, **pseudomembranous colitis**
GU: vaginal candidiasis
Hematologic: lymphocytosis, eosinophilia, **bleeding tendency, hemolytic anemia, hypoprothrombinemia, neutropenia, thrombocytopenia, agranulocytosis, bone marrow depression**
Hepatic: jaundice, **hepatomegaly**
Musculoskeletal: arthralgia
Respiratory: dyspnea
Skin: urticaria, maculopapular or erythematous rash
Other: chills, fever, superinfection, **anaphylaxis, serum sickness**

Interactions

Drug-drug. *Aminoglycosides, loop diuretics:* increased risk of nephrotoxicity
Probenecid: decreased excretion and increased blood level of ceftriaxone
Drug-diagnostic tests. *Alanine aminotransferase, alkaline phosphatase, aspartate aminotransferase, bilirubin, blood urea nitrogen, creatinine, eosinophils, gamma-glutamyltransferase, lactate dehydrogenase:* increased
Coombs' test, nonenzyme-based urine glucose tests (such as Clinitest), urinary 17-ketosteroids: false-positive results
Hemoglobin, platelets, prothrombin time, white blood cells: decreased
Drug-herb. *Angelica, anise, arnica, asafetida, bogbean, boldo, celery, chamomile, clove, danshen, fenugreek, feverfew, garlic, ginger, ginkgo, ginseng, horse chestnut, horseradish, licorice, meadowsweet, onion, papain, passionflower, poplar, prickly ash, quassia, red clover, turmeric, wild carrot, wild lettuce, willow:* increased risk of bleeding.

Toxicity and overdose

- In overdose, expect extension of adverse reactions, including seizures.
- If seizures occur, immediately discontinue drug and give anticonvulsant, as ordered. Be aware that neither peritoneal dialysis nor hemodialysis will remove drug. Provide supportive and symptomatic therapy.

Patient teaching

- Instruct patient to immediately report signs and symptoms of allergic reaction, persistent diarrhea, bruising, and bleeding.
- Caution patient not to use herbs without consulting prescriber.
- Instruct patient with diabetes mellitus to use enzyme-based test (Clinistix, Testape) to monitor urine glucose, because drug may cause false results with other tests.
- As appropriate, review all other significant and life-threatening adverse reactions and interactions, especially those related to the drugs, tests, and herbs mentioned above.

cefuroxime sodium

Zinacef, Zinnat ❋

Pharmacologic class: Second-generation cephalosporin
Therapeutic class: Anti-infective
Pregnancy risk category B

Action

Structurally and pharmacologically related to penicillin; interferes with bacterial cell-wall synthesis and division by binding to cell wall, causing instability and death. Active against gram-negative and gram-positive bacteria, with expanded spectrum of activity against gram-negative bacteria. Shows minimal immunosuppressive activity.

Pharmacokinetics

Drug distributes widely to most tissues, penetrates cerebrospinal fluid and inflamed meninges better than most first- and second-generation cephalosporins, and crosses placental barrier. It is not metabolized; approximately 50% is protein-bound. Serum half-life is 80 minutes. Approximately 89% of dose is excreted by the kidneys (by glomerular filtration and renal tubular secretion) as unchanged drug, with some excreted in breast milk.

Onset	Peak	Duration
Rapid	End of infusion	6-12 hr

How supplied

Powder for reconstitution for injection (white to off-white): 750 mg, 1.5 g, 7.5 g
Solution for injection (light yellow to amber): 750 mg/50 mL and 1.5 g/50 mL in premixed containers

Indications and dosages

➢ Moderate to severe infections, including those of urinary tract, respiratory tract, skin, bone, and joints; gynecologic infections; and septicemia
Adults and children age 12 and older: 750 mg to 1.5 g I.V. q 8 hours for 5 to 10 days
Children ages 3 months to 12 years: 50 to 100 mg/kg/day I.V. in divided doses q 6 to 8 hours
➢ Gonorrhea
Adults: 750 mg to 1.5 g I.V. as a single dose
➢ Bacterial meningitis
Adults and children age 12 and older: Up to 3 g I.V. q 8 hours
Children ages 3 months to 12 years: 200 to 240 mg/kg I.V. daily in divided doses q 6 to 8 hours

Dosage adjustment

• In renal impairment, use dosages and frequency shown below:

CrCl (mL/min)	Dosage (mg)	Frequency (hr)
Less than 20	750	8
10 to 20	750	12
Less than 10	750	24

Administration

Preparation

Before starting therapy, determine if patient has had previous hypersensitivity reactions to cefuroxime, other cephalosporins, penicillins, or other drugs.
• Do not exceed adult recommended dosage in children.
• Obtain specimens for culture and sensitivity tests as needed before starting therapy.
• Assess baseline CBC and kidney and liver function test results.

Dilution and compatibility

• Reconstitute drug in vial with at least 20 mL sterile water for injection per gram of drug. Shake well.
• For intermittent I.V. infusion, further dilute with 100 mL D_5W or normal saline solution.
• Do not mix with sodium bicarbonate.
• Do not mix in same infusion with aminoglycoside, because both drugs may be inactivated.
• Know that drug is also available as premixed piggyback vials and infusion packs.
• Thaw premixed drug at room temperature.

• Know that solutions range in color from light yellow to amber, depending on concentration and diluent used.
• Be aware that powder and solution tend to darken depending on storage conditions; however, when stored as recommended, product potency is unaffected.
• Do not add other drugs to premixed containers. Discard unused solution.
• Give reconstituted solutions within 24 hours, or within 48 hours if refrigerated.

Infusion considerations
• Give slowly by direct I.V. injection over 3 to 5 minutes into large vein or flowing I.V. line.
• For intermittent infusion, give over 15 minutes to 1 hour through Y-tube administration set of a flowing I.V. line; temporarily discontinue other solutions until cefuroxime administration ends.
• For continuous infusion, add diluted solution to I.V. bottle or bag containing normal saline solution, 5% or 10% dextrose injection, 5% dextrose in half-normal saline solution, 5% dextrose in normal saline solution, or 1/6 M sodium lactate injection.
Do not use plastic containers in series connections. Such use could result in air embolism due to residual air being drawn from primary container before administration of fluid from secondary container ends.

Monitoring
In patients receiving high doses, monitor closely for seizures; be prepared to intervene appropriately.
Be aware that cross-sensitivity to penicillin and other cephalosporins may occur. If allergic reaction arises, discontinue treatment. In acute hypersensitivity reaction, be prepared to give epinephrine and provide other emergency measures, including oxygen, I.V. fluids, I.V. antihistamines, corticosteroids, pressor amines, and airway management, as indicated.
Monitor for signs and symptoms of pseudomembranous colitis; institute therapeutic measures as indicated. Mild cases usually respond to drug withdrawal alone. In moderate to severe cases, be prepared to give fluids and electrolytes, protein supplements, and oral antibiotic effective against *Clostridium difficile* colitis.
• Monitor CBC, prothrombin time, and kidney and liver function test results.
• Monitor for signs and symptoms of superinfection and other serious adverse reactions.

Storage
• Store dry powder at 15° to 30°C (59° to 86°F); protect from light.
• Store frozen premixed containers at or below –20°C (–4°F). Thawed premixed drug is stable for 28 days when refrigerated at 5°C (41°F). Do not refreeze.

Contraindications and precautions

Contraindicated in hypersensitivity to cephalosporins.

Use cautiously in hypersensitivity to penicillins, carnitine deficiency, renal or hepatic impairment, ***elderly patients,*** pregnant or breastfeeding patients, and ***children younger than 3 months*** (safety and efficacy not established).

Adverse reactions

CNS: headache, hyperactivity, hypertonia, **seizures**
GI: nausea, vomiting, diarrhea, abdominal pain, dyspepsia, **pseudomembranous colitis**
GU: hematuria, vaginal candidiasis, **renal dysfunction, acute renal failure**
Hematologic: hemolytic anemia, aplastic anemia, hemorrhage
Hepatic: hepatic failure, hepatomegaly
Metabolic: hyperglycemia

Skin: toxic epidermal necrolysis, **erythema multiforme, Stevens-Johnson syndrome**
Other: allergic reaction, drug fever, superinfection, **anaphylaxis**

Interactions

Drug-drug. *Probenecid:* decreased excretion and increased blood level of cefuroxime
Drug-diagnostic tests. *Blood glucose, Coombs' test, urine glucose test using Benedict's solution:* false-positive results
Glucose, hematocrit, hemoglobin, platelets, prothrombin time, white blood cells: decreased
White blood cells in urine: increased

Toxicity and overdose

- In overdose, expect extension of adverse reactions, including seizures.
- If seizures occur, immediately discontinue drug and give anticonvulsant, as ordered. In overwhelming overdose, peritoneal dialysis or hemodialysis should be considered to remove drug. Provide supportive and symptomatic therapy.

Patient teaching

Instruct patient to immediately report signs and symptoms of allergic reaction, severe diarrhea, reduced urine output, persistent diarrhea, bruising, and bleeding.
- Advise patient to maintain adequate fluid intake during therapy.
- Teach patient with diabetes mellitus to use enzyme-based test (Clinistix, Testape) to monitor urine glucose, because drug may cause false results with other tests.
- As appropriate, review all other significant and life-threatening adverse reactions and interactions, especially those related to the drugs and tests mentioned above.

cetuximab

Erbitux

Pharmacologic class: Epidermal growth factor receptor (EGFR) inhibitor
Therapeutic class: Antineoplastic
Pregnancy risk category C

FDA BOXED WARNING

- Drug may cause severe infusion reactions (rarely fatal). Approximately 90% of such reactions occur with first infusion. If severe reaction occurs, stop infusion immediately and discontinue therapy permanently.
- Cardiopulmonary arrest, sudden death, or both occurred in 2% of patients with squamous-cell carcinoma of head and neck who received drug plus radiation therapy (compared to none of 212 patients treated with radiation therapy alone). Fatal events occurred within 1 to 43 days after last drug administration. When combined with radiation therapy, drug should be used cautiously in head and neck cancer patients with known coronary artery disease, congestive heart failure, and arrhythmias. Monitor serum electrolyte levels closely during and after therapy.

Action

Binds to EGFR, competitively inhibiting binding of epidermal growth factor and other ligands and blocking phosphorylation and activation of receptor-associated kinases. These actions cause cell-growth inhibition, apoptosis induction, and decreased matrix metalloproteinases and vascular endothelial growth factor.

Pharmacokinetics

Volume of distribution is independent of dose and approximates vascular space volume. At recommended dosages, steady-state concentrations occur by third weekly infusion, with mean peak and trough levels across studies ranging from 168 to 235 mcg/mL and 41 to 85 mcg/mL, respectively. Mean half-life is approximately 112 hours (range, 63 to 230 hours).

Onset	Peak	Duration
Unknown	Unknown	Unknown

How supplied

Solution for injection (clear, colorless): 50-mL single-use vial containing 100 mg

Indications and dosages

➢ EGFR-expressing metastatic colorectal carcinoma, used alone in patients intolerant to irinotecan-based chemotherapy or in combination with irinotecan in patients refractory to irinotecan-based therapy

Adults: 400 mg/m² initial loading dose given as 120-minute I.V. infusion, followed by maintenance dosage of 250 mg/m² infused I.V. over 60 minutes

➢ Locally or regionally advanced squamous-cell carcinoma of head and neck, in combination with radiation therapy

Adults: 400 mg/m² as initial loading dose (first infusion) given as 120-minute I.V. infusion 1 week before radiation therapy begins. For recommended weekly maintenance dosage (all other infusions), 250 mg/m² infused I.V. over 60 minutes weekly for duration of radiation therapy (6 to 7 weeks), given 1 hour before radiation therapy.

➢ Recurrent or metastatic squamous-cell carcinoma of head and neck (used alone) in patients for whom platinum-based therapy has failed

Adults: Initially, 400-mg/m² I.V. infusion followed by 250 mg/m² I.V. weekly until disease progresses or unacceptable toxicity occurs

Off-label uses

- Cancers that overexpress EGFR

Dosage adjustment

- Permanently reduce dosage 50% in patients who experience mild to moderate (grade 1 or 2) infusion reaction.
- Interrupt therapy if patient develops acute onset or worsening of pulmonary symptoms.
- On first occurrence of severe acneiform rash, delay infusion 1 to 2 weeks. If condition improves, continue therapy at 250 mg/m²; if no improvement occurs, withdraw drug. On second occurrence, delay infusion 1 to 2 weeks; if condition improves, reduce dosage to 200 mg/m²; if no improvement occurs, withdraw drug. On third occurrence, delay infusion for 1 to 2 weeks; if condition improves, reduce dosage to 150 mg/m²; if no improvement occurs, withdraw drug. On fourth occurrence, withdraw drug.

Administration

Preparation

- Expect patients with colorectal cancer to undergo immunohistochemical testing for EGFR expression using DakoCytomation EGFR pharmDx test kit.

🔊 Make sure appropriate medical resources are available to treat severe infusion reactions during infusion.

- Premedicate with histamine$_1$-antagonist (such as 50 mg diphenhydramine I.V.), as ordered.

Dilution and compatibility

🔊 Do not shake or dilute vial.

- Be aware that drug is clear and colorless, but may contain small amount of easily visible white, amorphous particulates.

Infusion considerations
Do not give by I.V. push or bolus.
- Use low-protein-binding, 0.22-micron inline filter, placed as close as possible to patient.
- Administer by I.V. infusion pump or syringe pump.
- Piggyback drug to patient's infusion line.
- Give initial dose over 2 hours at a rate of 5 mL/minute; give subsequent weekly doses over 1 hour. Maximum infusion rate should not exceed 5 mL/minute.
- At end of infusion, flush I.V. lines with normal saline solution.

Monitoring
Observe patient closely for 1 hour after infusion (or longer in patients who experience infusion reactions). Severe and life-threatening infusion reactions have occurred, including rapid-onset airway obstruction (bronchospasm, stridor, hoarseness), urticaria, and hypotension. Immediately and permanently discontinue drug in patients who experience severe (grade 3 or 4) infusion reaction.
Watch for pulmonary toxicities in patients with history of interstitial pneumonitis or pulmonary fibrosis. Be prepared to interrupt or discontinue therapy and intervene appropriately.
In patient with dermatologic toxicities, monitor for inflammatory or infectious sequelae; be prepared to modify dosage or discontinue drug, if indicated.
Stay alert for potentially serious cardiotoxicity if patient is receiving drug in combination with radiation therapy and cisplatin.
- Closely monitor serum electrolyte levels (including serum magnesium, potassium, and calcium) during therapy and after combination drug and radiation therapy in patients with history of coronary artery disease, arrhythmias, or heart failure.
- Monitor for hypomagnesemia and hypocalcemia during therapy and for 8 weeks afterward.
- Stay alert for severe diarrhea and electrolyte depletion.

Storage
- Refrigerate vials at 2° to 8°C (36° to 46°F). Discard unused portion of vial. Do not freeze.
- Know that preparations in infusion containers are chemically and physically stable for up to 12 hours at 2° to 8°C (36° to 46°F) and for up to 8 hours at controlled room temperature of 20° to 25°C (68° to 77°F). Discard remaining solution in infusion container after 8 hours at controlled room temperature, or after 12 hours at 2° to 8°C. Discard unused portion of vial.

Contraindications and precautions
Use cautiously in hypersensitivity to murine proteins or drug components; dermatologic or pulmonary toxicities; patients receiving concurrent radiation therapy and cisplatin; patients receiving concurrent radiation therapy who have history of coronary artery disease, arrhythmias, or congestive heart failure; pregnant or breastfeeding patients; and ***children*** (safety and efficacy not established).

Adverse reactions
CNS: headache, insomnia, depression, malaise, asthenia
CV: cardiopulmonary arrest
EENT: conjunctivitis
GI: abdominal pain, diarrhea, nausea, vomiting, constipation, stomatitis, dyspepsia, anorexia
GU: renal failure
Hematologic: leukopenia, anemia
Metabolic: dehydration, electrolyte abnormalities
Musculoskeletal: back pain

Respiratory: dyspnea, increased cough, **interstitial lung disease, pulmonary embolus**
Skin: acneiform rash, alopecia, skin disorder, nail disorder, pruritus
Other: weight loss, fever, pain, infection, peripheral edema, **severe infusion reaction**

Interactions

Drug-diagnostic tests. *Calcium, magnesium:* decreased
Drug-behaviors. *Sun exposure:* exacerbated skin reactions

Toxicity and overdose

- In overdose, expect extension of adverse reactions.
- Provide symptomatic and supportive interventions.

Patient teaching

Advise patient to immediately report rash, which may indicate skin toxicity.

Instruct patient to immediately report new or worsening respiratory or cardiovascular symptoms.

- Teach patient to use sunscreen and wear a hat when outdoors and to limit sun exposure, which can exacerbate skin reactions.
- Caution female of childbearing potential that drug may cause pregnancy loss or harm fetus.
- Advise female to discontinue breastfeeding during therapy and for 60 days after last dose.
- As appropriate, review all other significant and life-threatening adverse reactions and interactions, especially those related to the tests and behaviors mentioned above.

chloramphenicol

Chloromycetin, Kemicetine

Pharmacologic class: Dichloroacetic acid derivative
Therapeutic class: Anti-infective
Pregnancy risk category C

FDA BOXED WARNING

- Bone marrow hypoplasia (including aplastic anemia and death) has been reported after topical use. Do not give drug when less potentially dangerous agents could be effective.

Action

Exerts bacteriostatic activity by binding with 50S subunit of ribosome and inhibiting protein synthesis

Pharmacokinetics

Drug diffuses rapidly, but distribution is not uniform. After infusion, it must be hydrolyzed to active form, and reaches adequate blood levels slowly. Most of drug detectable in blood is in microbiologically active free form. Highest concentrations occur in the liver and kidneys; lowest, in brain and cerebrospinal fluid (CSF). Drug enters CSF even without meningeal inflammation; CSF levels are roughly half those found in blood. Drug also crosses placental barrier. Metabolite is excreted rapidly in urine; small amounts of active drug are found in bile, feces, and breast milk.

Onset	Peak	Duration
Immediate	1-2 hr	8 hr

How supplied

Powder for reconstitution for injection: 1-g vial

Indications and dosages

➢ Serious infections when less potentially dangerous drugs are ineffective or contraindicated

Adults: 50 to 100 mg/kg/day I.V. in divided doses q 6 hours, to a maximum dosage of 4 g/day

Children: 50 to 75 mg/kg/day I.V. in divided doses q 6 hours

➢ Bacteremia or meningitis

Children: 50 to 100 mg/kg/day I.V. in divided doses q 6 hours

Dosage adjustment

• Reduce dosage in hepatic and renal impairment.

• In preterm and term infants and in children with immature metabolic functions, reduce dosage to avoid "gray syndrome" (toxic reaction).

Administration

Preparation

Follow hazardous drug guidelines on page S19 for handling, preparation, and administration.

Know that because of its narrow therapeutic window, drug can cause serious reactions and should be used only when safer anti-infectives are ineffective or contraindicated.

• Be aware that I.V. chloramphenicol should be switched to oral therapy as soon as possible.

Dilution and compatibility

• Dilute with aqueous solution, including sterile water for injection or D_5W injection, to at least 100 mg/mL.

Infusion considerations

• Give by I.V. bolus injection over at least 1 minute.

• For intermittent infusion, drug may be further diluted in 50 to 100 mL D_5W and given over 10 to 30 minutes.

• Give within 24 hours of preparation.

Do not give I.M.

Monitoring

Monitor patient for signs and symptoms of aplastic anemia, which may arise weeks or months after therapy ends.

Closely monitor infants and children with immature metabolic functions for signs of gray syndrome, such as abdominal distention with or without emesis, progressive pallid cyanosis, vasomotor collapse (commonly accompanied by irregular respiration), and death within a few hours of onset. Other initial signs may include refusal to suck, loose green stools, flaccidity, ashen-gray skin, decreased temperature, and refractory lactic acidosis.

• Monitor CBC closely.

• Assess hepatic enzyme levels in patients with hepatic disease.

• Monitor creatinine levels in patients with renal insufficiency or failure.

• Watch for signs and symptoms of superinfection.

Storage

• Store at controlled room temperature of 15° to 30°C (59° to 86°F).

Contraindications and precautions

Contraindicated in hypersensitivity to drug, severe renal or hepatic impairment, prophylaxis for bacterial infections, or acute porphyria.

Use cautiously in hepatic disease, renal disease, bone marrow depression, pregnant or breastfeeding patients, and ***preterm and term infants and children with immature metabolic functions.***

Adverse reactions

CNS: confusion, delirium, depression, headache, peripheral neuropathy

EENT: optic neuritis, vision loss

GI: nausea, vomiting, diarrhea, abdominal pain, colitis, pruritus ani, dry mouth, glossitis
Hematologic: reticulocytopenia, aplastic anemia, bone marrow depression, granulocytopenia, hypoplastic anemia, leukopenia, thrombocytopenia
Skin: rash, itching, urticaria, contact dermatitis, **angioedema**
Other: fever, **anaphylaxis, gray syndrome in neonates**

Interactions

Drug-drug. *Aminoglycosides, penicillins:* decreased activity of these drugs
Barbiturates: increased barbiturate and decreased chloramphenicol blood levels
Hepatic enzyme inducers: decreased chloramphenicol blood level
Hydantoin, iron salts: increased blood levels of these drugs
Myelosuppressants, drugs that cause blood dyscrasias: increased bone marrow depression
Vitamin B_{12}*:* antagonism of hematopoietic response
Warfarin: enhanced warfarin action
Drug-diagnostic tests. *Alanine aminotransferase, aspartate aminotransferase, hemoglobin, platelets, red blood cells, white blood cells:* altered results

Toxicity and overdose

- In infants and children with immature metabolic functions, toxic reactions and deaths may occur.
- Immediately discontinue drug in infants with initial signs of toxicity. If this does not reverse the process, provide symptomatic and supportive therapy.

Patient teaching

Instruct patient to report bleeding or bruising, even if therapy ended several weeks or months earlier.
- Tell patient to report rash or itching.
- Caution patient to avoid pregnancy during therapy. Advise patients taking hormonal contraceptives to use additional birth control method, as drug may make these contraceptives ineffective.
- As appropriate, review all other significant and life-threatening adverse reactions and interactions, especially those related to the drugs and tests mentioned above.

chlordiazepoxide hydrochloride

Apo-Chlordiazepoxide✤, Librium

Pharmacologic class: Benzodiazepine
Therapeutic class: Anxiolytic, sedative-hypnotic
Controlled substance schedule IV
Pregnancy risk category D

Action

Unknown. May potentiate effects of gamma-aminobutyric acid (inhibitory neurotransmitter) by increasing neuronal membrane permeability; may depress CNS at limbic and subcortical levels of brain. Anxiolytic effect occurs at doses well below those that cause sedation or ataxia.

Pharmacokinetics

Drug is widely distributed and metabolized in the liver, with extensive plasma protein-binding. It has several active metabolites with long half-lives. It is excreted largely in urine as metabolites, with some excreted in breast milk.

Onset	Peak	Duration
1-5 min	Unknown	0.25-1 hr

How supplied

Powder for reconstitution for injection: 100-mg ampules

Indications and dosages

➢ Severe anxiety

Adults: Initially, 50 to 100 mg I.V.; then 25 to 50 mg P.O. three to four times daily as needed

➢ Acute alcohol withdrawal

Adults: Initially, 50 to 100 mg I.V.; repeat dose as needed, up to 300 mg/day.

Dosage adjustment

- Reduce dosage in patients age 65 and older, debilitated patients, and children.
- Be aware that dosage may need to be reduced in hepatic impairment.

Administration

Preparation

Administer with extreme care to elderly patients, seriously ill patients, and those with limited pulmonary reserve. Watch for apnea or cardiac arrest; be prepared to provide emergency interventions.

Do not give to patients with acute alcoholic intoxication or to those in shock or coma.

Dilution and compatibility

Be aware that diluents for I.M. and I.V. uses are distinctly different. Do not use diluent provided for I.M. use when giving drug I.V.; do not use I.V. diluent for I.M. injections. Read labels carefully.

- Dilute I.V. drug with 5 mL normal saline solution or sterile water for injection. Agitate gently until powder dissolves thoroughly.
- Prepare drug immediately before administration. Discard unused portion.

Infusion considerations

- Administer by I.V. bolus injection slowly over at least 1 minute.

Monitoring

- After administration, observe patient closely, and enforce bedrest for at least 3 hours.
- In prolonged therapy, monitor CBC and hepatic enzyme levels.
- Monitor renal and hepatic studies.

Storage

- Store powder at room temperature of 15° to 30°C (59° to 86°F); protect from light and heat.

Contraindications and precautions

Contraindicated in hypersensitivity to drug, other benzodiazepines, or tartrazine; CNS depression; uncontrolled severe pain; porphyria; pregnancy or breastfeeding, and ***children younger than age 12.***

Use cautiously in hepatic dysfunction, severe renal impairment, and debilitated or ***elderly patients.***

Adverse reactions

CNS: dizziness, drowsiness, hangover, headache, depression, paradoxical stimulation

CV: hypotension, tachycardia, **bradycardia**

EENT: blurred vision

GI: nausea, vomiting, constipation, diarrhea

Hematologic: agranulocytosis

Hepatic: jaundice

Skin: rash

Other: physical or psychological drug dependence, drug tolerance, phlebitis and thrombosis at I.V. site

Interactions

Drug-drug. *Antidepressants, antihistamines, opioids:* additive CNS depression

Barbiturates, rifampin: decreased chlordiazepoxide efficacy

Cimetidine, disulfiram, fluoxetine, hormonal contraceptives, isoniazid, ketoconazole, metoprolol, propoxyphene,

propranolol, valproic acid: enhanced chlordiazepoxide effect
Levodopa: decreased levodopa efficacy
Drug-diagnostic tests. *Alanine aminotransferase, aspartate aminotransferase, bilirubin:* increased
Granulocytes: decreased
Metyrapone test: decreased response
Radioactive iodine uptake test (^{123}I or ^{131}I): decreased uptake
Urine 17-ketogenic steroids, urine 17-ketosteroids: altered results
Drug-herb. *Chamomile, hops, kava, skullcap, valerian:* increased CNS depression
Drug-behaviors. *Alcohol use:* increased CNS depression

Toxicity and overdose

- When used alone, drug rarely causes significant circulatory or respiratory depression. Mild signs and symptoms of overdose include confusion, drowsiness, lethargy, somnolence, impaired coordination, and diminished reflexes. More serious signs and symptoms include hypotension, hypotonia, ataxia, coma, and rarely death.
- Closely monitor respirations, pulse, and blood pressure. Give I.V. fluids, as ordered, and maintain patent airway. For hypotension, expect to give pressors. If kidney function is normal, administer osmotic diuretics, I.V. fluids, and electrolytes, as ordered. Dialysis may not be helpful; however, in critical situations, renal dialysis and exchange transfusions may be indicated.

Patient teaching

- Instruct patient to avoid driving and other hazardous activities until drug's effects on concentration and alertness are known.
- Advise patient to avoid alcohol during therapy.
- Caution patient not to stop taking drug abruptly after several weeks or more of continuous use. Instruct patient to discuss dosage tapering with prescriber.
- Caution female not to take drug if she is pregnant or might become pregnant during therapy. Advise her to use reliable contraception.
- As appropriate, review all other significant and life-threatening adverse reactions and interactions, especially those related to the drugs, tests, herbs, and behaviors mentioned above.

[redacted]

chlorothiazide

Sodium Diuril

Pharmacologic class: Thiazide
Therapeutic class: Diuretic, antihypertensive
Pregnancy risk category C

Action

Increases sodium and water excretion and inhibits sodium reabsorption in distal tubule, thereby promoting excretion of chloride, potassium, magnesium, and bicarbonate

Pharmacokinetics

No metabolism occurs; drug is excreted unchanged in urine.

Onset	Peak	Duration
15 min	30 min	Unknown

How supplied

Powder for reconstitution for injection (white, lyophilized): 500-mg vials

Indications and dosages

➢ Edema associated with heart failure, renal dysfunction, cirrhosis, corticosteroid therapy, or estrogen therapy
Adults: In emergency use or for patients unable to receive oral form, 0.5 to 1 g I.V. as a single dose or in two divided doses

Administration

Preparation

- Assess electrolyte, bilirubin, creatinine, uric acid, magnesium, cholesterol, low-density lipoprotein (LDL), and triglyceride levels before starting therapy.

Clinical alert: Know that drug is not safe for I.M. or subcutaneous use, and that I.V. use in children is not recommended.

- Be aware that I.V. dosage is individualized. Use smallest dosage that achieves response; adjust dosage according to blood pressure response. Rarely, patients may require up to 2 g/day in divided doses.

Dilution and compatibility

- Add 18 mL sterile water for injection to vial to prepare isotonic solution for final concentration of 28 mg/mL.

Clinical alert: Never add less than 18 mL diluent.

- Know that drug is compatible with normal saline solution and dextrose injection for I.V. infusion.
- Prepare fresh solution immediately before each administration; discard unused portion after 24 hours.

Infusion considerations

- Give slowly by direct I.V. injection or by I.V. infusion at a rate not exceeding 0.5 g/5 minutes.
- Avoid concurrent administration with whole blood or blood derivatives.

Clinical alert: Use extreme caution to avoid extravasation.

Monitoring

- Monitor blood pressure regularly.
- Continue to assess levels of serum electrolytes, bilirubin, creatinine, uric acid, magnesium, cholesterol, LDL, and triglycerides.

Clinical alert: Closely monitor patient with hepatic impairment; be aware that minor changes in fluid and electrolyte balance may cause hepatic coma.

- Monitor urine calcium level.
- Evaluate blood and urine glucose levels in patients with diabetes.

Storage

- Store powder between 2° and 25°C (36° and 77°F).
- Store reconstituted solution at room temperature of 15° to 30°C (59° to 86°F).

Contraindications and precautions

Contraindicated in hypersensitivity to drug, other thiazides, benzodiazepines, sulfonamides, or tartrazine; anuria; gout; systemic lupus erythematosus; glucose tolerance abnormalities; hyperparathyroidism; bipolar disorder; and breastfeeding.

Use cautiously in renal or severe hepatic impairment and in pregnant patients.

Adverse reactions

CNS: dizziness, drowsiness, lethargy, weakness, headache, insomnia, nervousness, vertigo, weakness, paresthesia, confusion, fatigue, asterixis, **encephalopathy**
CV: hypotension, ECG changes, chest pain, **thrombophlebitis, arrhythmias**
EENT: nystagmus
GI: nausea, vomiting, abdominal cramps, pancreatitis, anorexia
GU: polyuria, nocturia, erectile dysfunction, libido loss
Hematologic: blood dyscrasias
Hepatic: jaundice, **hepatitis**
Metabolic: dehydration, hypovolemia, hyperglycemia, hypokalemia, hypocalcemia, hypomagnesemia, hyponatremia, hypophosphatemia, hyperuricemia, hyperlipidemia, gout attack, **hypochloremic alkalosis**
Musculoskeletal: muscle cramps or spasms

Skin: photosensitivity, rash, urticaria, flushing
Other: fever, weight loss, hypersensitivity reactions

Interactions

Drug-drug. *Allopurinol:* increased risk of hypersensitivity reaction
Amphotericin B, corticosteroids, mezlocillin, piperacillin, ticarcillin: additive hypokalemia
Antihypertensives, barbiturates, nitrates, opiates: increased hypotension
Digoxin: increased risk of hypokalemia
Lithium: decreased lithium excretion, lithium toxicity
Nonsteroidal anti-inflammatory drugs: decreased chlorothiazide efficacy
Drug-diagnostic tests. *Bilirubin, calcium, creatinine, serum and urine glucose (in diabetic patients), uric acid:* increased
Cholesterol, LDLs, magnesium, potassium, protein-bound iodine, sodium, triglycerides, urine calcium: decreased
Drug-herb. *Ginkgo:* reduced antihypertensive effect
Licorice, stimulant laxative herbs (aloe, cascara sagrada, senna): increased risk of hypokalemia
Drug-behaviors. *Acute alcohol ingestion:* additive hypotension
Sun exposure: increased risk of photosensitivity

Toxicity and overdose

- In overdose, expect extension of adverse reactions, including hypotension, electrolyte depletion (such as hypokalemia, hypochloremia, hyponatremia), dehydration, and possibly hepatic dysfunction.
- Correct hypotension, electrolyte imbalance, dehydration, and hepatic dysfunction as indicated and ordered. Role of hemodialysis is unknown.

Patient teaching

- Caution patient to use alcohol cautiously, if at all.
- Inform patient that drug increases risk of dehydration. Tell patient to stay indoors in hot weather and to increase fluid intake when sweating more than usual.
- Instruct patient about the need for follow-up kidney function tests, blood tests, and blood pressure monitoring.
- As appropriate, review all other significant and life-threatening adverse reactions and interactions, especially those related to the drugs, tests, herbs, and behaviors mentioned above.

chlorpromazine hydrochloride

Largactil🍁 ❋

Pharmacologic class: Phenothiazine
Therapeutic class: Antipsychotic, anxiolytic, antiemetic
Pregnancy risk category C

Action

Unknown. May block postsynaptic dopamine receptors in brain and depress areas involved in wakefulness and emesis. Also possesses anticholinergic, antihistaminic, and adrenergic-blocking properties.

Pharmacokinetics

Drug distributes widely (including to CNS). It is metabolized in the liver to several active metabolites with long half-lives, and is highly protein-bound. Excretion occurs in urine mostly as metabolites, with some excretion in bile, feces, and breast milk. Less than 1% is excreted as unchanged drug.

Onset	Peak	Duration
Rapid	Unknown	Unknown

How supplied

Injection (aqueous solution): 25-mg/mL ampules and multidose vials

Indications and dosages

➣ Acute nausea and vomiting during surgery
Adults: 2 mg I.V. (not to exceed 25 mg)
Children ages 6 months to 12 years: 1 mg I.V. at 2-minute intervals (not to exceed 0.25 mg/kg)
➣ Tetanus
Adults: 25 to 50 mg I.V.
Children ages 6 months to 12 years weighing 23 to 45 kg (50 to 100 lb): 0.5 mg/kg I.V. q 6 to 8 hours. Do not exceed 75 mg/day except in severe cases.
Children ages 6 months to 12 years weighing up to 23 kg (50 lb): 0.5 mg/kg I.V. q 6 to 8 hours. Do not exceed 40 mg/day except in severe cases.
➣ Intractable hiccups
Adults: If symptoms persist after oral or I.M. therapy, give 25 to 50 mg by slow I.V. infusion, with patient positioned flat in bed.

Dosage adjustment

- Reduce dosage in patients who are debilitated, emaciated, or older than age 60.

Off-label uses

- Anxiety disorders
- Migraine
- Phencyclidine psychosis

Administration

Preparation

🔊 Know that I.V. infusion is recommended only for severe hiccups.
🔊 Do not inject subcutaneously.

Dilution and compatibility

- When giving by direct I.V. injection, dilute to 1 mg/mL using normal saline solution.
- When giving by I.V. infusion, dilute in 500 to 1,000 mL normal saline solution and infuse at a rate not exceeding 1 mg/minute.

🔊 Do not mix with meperidine, morphine, or other products preserved with cresols, as solution may become discolored and precipitate may form.

Infusion considerations

- For direct I.V. injection, give at a rate of at least 1 mg/minute for adults or 2 mg/minute for children.
- For I.V. infusion, infuse slowly, with patient positioned flat in bed.

Monitoring

- Monitor blood pressure closely during I.V. infusion.

🔊 Stay alert for signs and symptoms of neuroleptic malignant syndrome (hyperpyrexia, muscle rigidity, altered mental status, irregular pulse or blood pressure, tachycardia, diaphoresis, and arrhythmias). Stop drug immediately if these occur.

- Assess for extrapyramidal symptoms; be prepared to intervene appropriately.
- Monitor CBC and liver function test results.

Storage

- Store at controlled room temperature of 15° to 30°C (59° to 86°F); protect from light.

Contraindications and precautions

Contraindicated in hypersensitivity to drug, other phenothiazines, or sulfites; angle-closure glaucoma; bone marrow depression; or severe hepatic or cardiovascular disease.

Use cautiously in cardiac disease, diabetes mellitus, respiratory disease, prostatic hypertrophy, CNS tumors, epilepsy, intestinal obstruction, ***elderly***

patients, pregnant or breastfeeding patients, and ***children*** (use not recommended in those younger than age 6).

Adverse reactions

CNS: sedation, drowsiness, extrapyramidal reactions, tardive dyskinesia, pseudoparkinsonism, **neuroleptic malignant syndrome, seizures**
CV: tachycardia, hypotension
EENT: blurred vision, dry eyes, lens opacities, nasal congestion
GI: constipation, ileus, anorexia, dry mouth
GU: urine retention, menstrual irregularities, galactorrhea, gynecomastia, inhibited ejaculation, priapism
Hematologic: eosinophilia, **agranulocytosis, leukopenia, hemolytic anemia, aplastic anemia, thrombocytopenia**
Hepatic: jaundice, **hepatitis**
Skin: rash, photosensitivity, pigmentation changes, sterile abscess
Other: allergic reactions, hyperthermia

Interactions

Drug-drug. *Antidepressants, antihistamines, general anesthetics, monoamine oxidase inhibitors, opioids, sedative-hypnotics:* additive CNS depression
Antihistamines, disopyramide, quinidine, tricyclic antidepressants (TCAs): increased anticholinergic effects
Antihypertensives: additive hypotension
Barbiturates: increased metabolism and decreased efficacy of chlorpromazine
Bromocriptine: decreased bromocriptine efficacy
Epinephrine: antagonism of peripheral vasoconstriction, epinephrine reversal
Guanethidine: inhibition of antihypertensive effects
Lithium: disorientation, loss of consciousness, extrapyramidal symptoms
Meperidine: excessive sedation and hypotension
Norepinephrine: reduced pressor effect
Phenytoin: altered phenytoin blood level, lowered seizure threshold
Pimozide: increased risk of potentially serious cardiovascular reactions
Propranolol: increased blood levels of both drugs
TCAs: increased TCA blood levels and effects
Valproic acid: decreased elimination and increased effects of valproic acid
Drug-diagnostic tests. *Alanine aminotransferase, alkaline phosphatase, aspartate aminotransferase, bilirubin:* increased
Granulocytes, hematocrit, hemoglobin, platelets, white blood cells: decreased
Pregnancy tests: false-positive or false-negative result
Urine bilirubin: false-positive result
Drug-herb. *Angel's trumpet, jimsonweed, scopolia:* increased anticholinergic effects
Chamomile, hops, kava, skullcap, valerian: increased CNS depression
St. John's wort: photosensitivity
Yohimbe: increased risk of toxicity
Drug-behaviors. *Alcohol use:* increased CNS depression
Sun exposure: increased risk of photosensitivity

Toxicity and overdose

- In overdose, expect signs and symptoms to include CNS and cardiovascular manifestations, such as sedation, drowsiness, and hypotension, and autonomic nervous system dysfunction.
- Stop drug and provide supportive and symptomatic interventions, including maintaining vital signs and airway. For hypotension, expect to give pressor (such as norepinephrine); do not give epinephrine because it may worsen hypotension. Know that dialysis will not remove drug. Resuscitate, as indicated.

Patient teaching

- Instruct patient to avoid driving and other hazardous activities until drug's effects on concentration and alertness are known.
- Teach patient to rise slowly from lying or sitting position to avoid sudden blood pressure decrease. Advise patient to report dizziness with position changes. Caution patient that hot tubs and hot showers or baths may make dizziness worse.
- As appropriate, review all other significant and life-threatening adverse reactions and interactions, especially those related to the drugs, tests, herbs, and behaviors mentioned above.

cidofovir

Vistide

Pharmacologic class: Purine nucleotide cytosine analogue

Therapeutic class: Antiviral

Pregnancy risk category C

FDA BOXED WARNING

- Drug is indicated only to treat cytomegalovirus (CMV) retinitis in patients with AIDS.
- Renal impairment is major toxicity. As few as one or two doses have caused acute renal failure resulting in dialysis or contributing to death. To reduce possible nephrotoxicity, prehydrate with I.V. normal saline solution and give probenecid with each drug infusion, as ordered. Monitor renal function within 48 hours before each dose, and modify dosage as indicated.
- Drug is contraindicated in patients receiving other nephrotoxic agents.
- Drug may cause neutropenia. Monitor neutrophil counts during therapy.
- In animal studies, drug was carcinogenic and teratogenic and caused hypospermia.

Action

Exerts antiviral effect by interfering with DNA synthesis of CMV, thereby inhibiting viral replication

Pharmacokinetics

Drug is less than 6% protein-bound. Elimination half-life is 2.6 hours. It is eliminated through renal tubular secretion in urine (with concurrent probenecid use).

Onset	Peak	Duration
Rapid	End of infusion	Unknown

How supplied

Solution for injection: 75 mg/mL in 5-mL single-use vial

Indications and dosages

➤ CMV retinitis in AIDS patients

Adults: 5 mg/kg I.V. infused over 1 hour q week for 2 continuous weeks; then 5 mg/kg I.V. once q 2 weeks as a maintenance dose

Dosage adjustment

- If serum creatinine clearance increases 0.3 to 0.4 mg/dL above baseline, reduce dosage from 5 mg to 3 mg.
- If serum creatinine clearance increases approximately 0.5 mg/dL above baseline or approximately 3+ proteinuria develops, discontinue drug.

Administration

Preparation

Follow hazardous drug guidelines on page S19 for handling, preparation, and administration.

Be aware that drug carries a high risk of nephrotoxicity. Follow administration instructions carefully, including preinfusion and postinfusion hydration with I.V. normal saline solution and premedication and postmedication with probenecid.
Premedicate with probenecid 2 g P.O. 3 hours before starting cidofovir infusion and as prescribed post-cidofovir infusion.
Before starting drug infusion, give 1 L normal saline solution over 1 to 2 hours.

Dilution and compatibility

Be aware that drug must be mixed in 100 mL normal saline solution for injection before I.V. administration.

- Discard partially used vial.

Infusion considerations

- Infuse over 1 hour using infusion pump.

Give 1 L normal saline solution during or immediately after infusion over 1 to 3 hours (unless contraindicated).

Monitoring

- Assess white blood cell count and creatinine and urine protein levels within 48 hours of each dose.
- Closely monitor intraocular pressure and visual acuity.
- Monitor hepatic enzyme levels in patients with hepatic disease.

Storage

- Store at controlled room temperature of 20° C to 25°C (68° to 77°F).
- Admixture may be refrigerated at 2° to 8°C (36° to 46°F) for approximately 24 hours. Bring to room temperature before administering.

Contraindications and precautions

Contraindicated in hypersensitivity to drug, probenecid, or other sulfa-containing agents; creatinine level above 1.5 mg/dL; calculated creatinine clearance of 55 mL/minute or less; urine protein level of 100 mg/dL or higher; or concurrent use of other nephrotoxic drugs.

Use cautiously in mild renal impairment, ***elderly patients,*** pregnant or breastfeeding patients, and ***children younger than age 12*** (safety and efficacy not established).

Adverse reactions

CNS: headache, asthenia, **seizures, coma**
EENT: decreased intraocular pressure
GI: nausea, vomiting, diarrhea, anorexia, oral candidiasis
GU: proteinuria, **nephrotoxicity**
Hematologic: neutropenia
Hepatic: hepatomegaly
Metabolic: metabolic acidosis
Musculoskeletal: muscle contractions
Respiratory: dyspnea, increased cough
Skin: rash, alopecia
Other: pain, fever, chills, infection, pain at I.V. site

Interactions

Drug-drug. *Other nephrotoxic drugs:* increased risk of nephrotoxicity
Drug-diagnostic tests. *Alanine aminotransferase, alkaline phosphatase, aspartate aminotransferase, blood urea nitrogen, creatinine, lactate dehydrogenase:* increased
Bicarbonate, creatinine clearance, hemoglobin, neutrophils, platelets: decreased

Toxicity and overdose

- In overdose, expect extension of adverse reactions, including nephrotoxicity.
- Give probenecid and hydration with I.V. normal saline solution, as ordered. Stop drug if significant renal impairment occurs.

Patient teaching

Instruct patient to immediately report postinfusion fever, vision changes, nausea, vomiting, rash, and urine output changes.

- Advise patient to take probenecid, as prescribed.

- Teach patient to have regular eye examinations.
- Urge female of childbearing potential to use effective contraception during therapy and for 1 month afterward.
- Instruct male to use barrier contraception during therapy and for 3 months afterward.
- As appropriate, review all other significant and life-threatening adverse reactions and interactions, especially those related to the drugs and tests mentioned above.

[redacted]

cimetidine

Apo-Cimetidine✤, Dyspamet❉, Galenamet❉, Zita❉

Pharmacologic class: Histamine$_2$ (H_2)-receptor antagonist
Therapeutic class: Antiulcer drug
Pregnancy risk category B

Action

Competitively inhibits histamine action at H_2-receptor sites of gastric parietal cells, thereby inhibiting gastric acid secretion

Pharmacokinetics

Drug distributes widely in body tissues, and crosses placental barrier. It is approximately 40% metabolized in the liver and about 20% protein-bound. Half-life is about 2 hours in patients with normal renal function, but lower with reduced renal function. It is excreted primarily in urine, with some excretion in feces and breast milk.

Onset	Peak	Duration
10 min	30 min	4-5 hr

How supplied

Solution for injection (clear): 300 mg/2-mL single-dose vials, 300 mg/50-mL single dose premixed in normal saline solution in plastic containers

Indications and dosages

➢ Gastric hypersecretory conditions (such as Zollinger-Ellison syndrome); intractable ulcers

Adults and children older than age 16: 300 mg I.V. q 6 hours in hospitalized patients or patients unable to take oral medications. May increase dosage as necessary, but do not exceed 2,400 mg/day.

➢ Prevention of stress-induced upper GI bleeding in critically ill patients

Adults and children older than age 16: 50 mg/hour as a continuous I.V. infusion

Dosage adjustment

- Because drug is excreted primarily by the kidneys, reduce dosage in renal impairment. In hepatic impairment, further dosage reduction may be necessary.

Off-label uses

- Acetaminophen overdose
- Adjunctive therapy in burns
- Anaphylaxis
- Barrett's esophagus
- Renal carcinoma

Administration

Dilution and compatibility

- For I.V. injection, dilute doses in normal saline solution or other compatible solution to a volume of 20 mL.
- Know that other compatible solutions include most saline solutions, lactated Ringer's solution, dextrose 5% or 10% in water, 5% sodium bicarbonate, and a few total parenteral nutrition admixtures.
- For intermittent I.V. infusion, dilute 300-mg dose in at least 50 mL of compatible solution.

• For continuous I.V. infusion, dilute 900-mg dose in 100 to 1,000 mL of compatible solution.
• Do not add solutions or other drugs to premixed containers.

Infusion considerations
• Administer I.V. injection over at least 5 minutes.
• Give intermittent infusion over 15 to 20 minutes.
• Give continuous infusion at a rate of 37.5 mg/hour over 24 hours, using infusion pump for volumes less than 250 mL.
• When giving drug to prevent stress ulcers, administer by continuous infusion at a rate of 50 mg/hour.

Do not use plastic containers in series connections. Such use could result in air embolism due to residual air being drawn from primary container before administration of fluid from secondary container ends.

Monitoring
• Monitor creatinine levels in patients with renal insufficiency or failure.
• Assess elderly or chronically ill patients for confusion (which usually resolves once therapy ends).

Storage
• Know that drug is stable at room temperature for 48 hours when mixed with compatible solution. When diluted in sterile water for injection, it may be stored in glass vial to a concentration of 15 mg/mL for 14 days at 22°C (77°F) or for 42 days at 4°C (39.2°F).
• Store premixed drug at controlled room temperature of 15° to 30°C (59° to 86°F).

Contraindications and precautions

Contraindicated in hypersensitivity to cimetidine or other H_2-receptor antagonists.

Use cautiously in renal impairment, ***elderly patients,*** pregnant or breastfeeding patients, and ***children younger than age 16*** (safety and efficacy not established).

Adverse reactions

CNS: confusion, dizziness, drowsiness, hallucinations, agitation, psychosis, depression, anxiety, headache
GI: diarrhea
GU: reversible erectile dysfunction, gynecomastia

Interactions

Drug-drug. *Calcium channel blockers, carbamazepine, chloroquine, lidocaine, metformin, metronidazole, moricizine, pentoxifylline, phenytoin, propafenone, quinidine, quinine, some benzodiazepines, some beta-adrenergic blockers (chlordiazepoxide, diazepam, midazolam), sulfonylureas, tacrine, theophylline, triamterene, tricyclic antidepressants, valproic acid, warfarin:* decreased metabolism of these drugs, possible toxicity
Drug-diagnostic tests. *Creatinine, transaminases, prolactin (after I.V. bolus of cimetidine):* increased
Parathyroid hormone: decreased
Skin tests using allergenic extracts: false-negative results (discontinue drug 24 hours before testing)
Drug-food. *Caffeine-containing foods and beverages (such as coffee, chocolate):* increased drug blood level, increased risk of toxicity
Drug-herb. *Pennyroyal:* change in rate at which herb's toxic metabolite forms
Yerba maté: decreased yerba maté clearance, possible toxicity
Drug-behaviors. *Alcohol use:* increased blood alcohol level
Smoking: reversal of cimetidine effects

Toxicity and overdose

• In overdose (rare), hypotension, tachycardia, arrhythmias, respiratory failure, and death may occur.
• Stop drug and provide symptomatic and supportive interventions and (if needed) assisted ventilation. Know that beta blocker may be given to control

tachycardia and that drug is not significantly removed by dialysis.

Patient teaching

- Inform patient with gastric ulcer that ulcer may take up to 2 months to heal.
- Advise patient not to discontinue therapy, even if he feels better, without first consulting prescriber. Ulcer may recur if therapy ends too soon.
- As appropriate, review all other significant adverse reactions and interactions, especially those related to the drugs, tests, foods, herbs, and behaviors mentioned above.

ciprofloxacin hydrochloride

Cipro I.V., Ciproxin

Pharmacologic class: Fluoroquinolone
Therapeutic class: Anti-infective
Pregnancy risk category C

Action

Inhibits bacterial DNA synthesis by inhibiting DNA gyrase in susceptible gram-negative and gram-positive organisms

Pharmacokinetics

Drug distributes widely to most body fluids and tissues, with less penetration into cerebrospinal fluid. It also crosses placental barrier. It may be metabolized in the liver to several metabolites. Drug is excreted primarily in urine, with some excreted in breast milk.

Onset	Peak	Duration
Rapid	End of infusion	12 hr

How supplied

Injection 1% (aqueous concentrate): 200 mg/20-mL, 400 mg/40-mL vials

Solution for injection 0.2% (clear, colorless to slightly yellow): 200 mg/100 mL and 400 mg/200 mL premixed in D_5W in flexible latex-free containers

Indications and dosages

➤ Acute sinusitis

Adults: 400 mg I.V. q 12 hours for 10 days

➤ Prostatitis

Adults: 400 mg I.V. q 12 hours for 28 days

➤ Intra-abdominal infections

Adults: 400 mg I.V. q 12 hours for 7 to 14 days

➤ Febrile neutropenic patients

Adults: 400 mg I.V. q 8 hours for 7 to 14 days

➤ Inhalation anthrax (postexposure)

Adults: 400 mg I.V. q 12 hours for 60 days

Children: 10 mg/kg I.V. q 12 hours for 60 days, not to exceed 400 mg/dose

➤ Infections of lower respiratory tract, skin and skin structures, bones, and joints

Adults: 400 mg I.V. q 8 hours for 7 to 14 days. Severe bone and joint infections may necessitate up to 6 weeks of therapy.

➤ Nosocomial pneumonia

Adults: 400 mg I.V. q 8 hours for 10 to 14 days

➤ Urinary tract infections

Adults: 200 to 400 mg I.V. q 12 hours for 3 days in acute uncomplicated infections, or for 7 to 14 days in mild to severe complicated infections

Dosage adjustment

- In renal impairment or insufficiency, reduce dosage based on creatinine clearance, but more reliably based on serum drug levels.

Off-label uses

- Chancroid
- Cystic fibrosis
- Pseudomembranous colitis associated with anti-infectives

Administration

Preparation

• In patients with renal insufficiency, assess creatinine level before giving first dose.

• Ensure that patient is adequately hydrated and has sufficient urine output to prevent crystalluria (rare).

Dilution and compatibility

• Using a compatible solution, dilute prescribed dose to a final concentration of 1 to 2 mg/mL.

• Know that compatible solutions include normal saline solution, sterile water for injection, lactated Ringer's solution, dextrose 5% or 10% in water, 5% dextrose and 0.225% sodium chloride for injection, or 5% dextrose in half-normal saline solution.

• Do not add other drugs or solutions to premixed containers.

Infusion considerations

• Infuse I.V. dose into large vein over at least 1 hour, using pump to ensure 1-hour duration, to minimize patient discomfort and reduce risk of vein irritation.

• Know that too-rapid I.V. infusion increases risk of anaphylaxis and other adverse reactions.

• Temporarily discontinue other solutions during ciprofloxacin administration.

Do not use plastic containers in series connections. Such use could result in air embolism due to residual air being drawn from primary container before administration of fluid from secondary container ends.

Monitoring

Watch for signs and symptoms of serious adverse reactions, including GI problems, jaundice, and hypersensitivity reactions.

• Continue adequate hydration throughout therapy.

• In patients with renal insufficiency, monitor creatinine level at least weekly during prolonged therapy; monitor blood drug level closely.

• Monitor hematopoietic and hepatic function and electrolyte levels, especially during prolonged therapy.

• Monitor blood glucose level, especially in patients with diabetes mellitus.

Storage

• Store vials between 5° and 30°C (41° and 86°F). After reconstitution, store admixture below 30°C, but protect from freezing.

• Store flexible containers between 5° and 25°C (41° and 77°F).

Contraindications and precautions

Contraindicated in hypersensitivity to drug or other fluoroquinolones.

Use cautiously in cirrhosis, renal impairment, underlying CNS disease, ***elderly patients,*** pregnant or breastfeeding patients, and ***children younger than age 18.***

Adverse reactions

CNS: agitation, headache, restlessness, confusion, delirium, **toxic psychosis**
CV: orthostatic hypotension, vasculitis
EENT: nystagmus
GI: nausea, vomiting, diarrhea, constipation, abdominal pain or discomfort, dyspepsia, dysphagia, flatulence, pancreatitis, **pseudomembranous colitis**
GU: albuminuria, candiduria, renal calculi
Hematologic: methemoglobinemia, agranulocytosis, hemolytic anemia
Hepatic: jaundice, **hepatic necrosis**
Metabolic: hyperglycemia, **hyperkalemia**
Musculoskeletal: myalgia, myoclonus, tendinitis, tendon rupture
Skin: rash, exfoliative dermatitis, toxic epidermal necrolysis, **erythema multiforme**
Other: altered taste, anosmia, myasthenia gravis exacerbation, overgrowth of

nonsusceptible organisms, hypersensitivity reactions including **anaphylaxis** and **Stevens-Johnson syndrome**

Interactions

Drug-drug. *Cyclosporine:* transient creatinine increase
Hormonal contraceptives: reduced contraceptive efficacy
Oral anticoagulants: increased anticoagulant effect
Phenytoin: increased or decreased phenytoin blood level
Probenecid: decreased renal elimination of ciprofloxacin, causing increased blood level
Theophylline: increased theophylline blood level, greater risk of toxicity
Drug-diagnostic tests. *Alanine aminotransferase, alkaline phosphatase, aspartate aminotransferase, bilirubin, cholesterol, glucose, lactate dehydrogenase, potassium, triglycerides:* increased
Prothrombin time: prolonged

Toxicity and overdose

- Overdose may cause renal dysfunction and other adverse reactions. Severe overdose may lead to oliguric acute renal failure.
- Provide supportive measures, including adequate hydration. In severe overdose, expect to give prednisone. Dialysis has limited value but may be used in patients with compromised renal function.

Patient teaching

- Advise patient to drink 8 oz of water every hour while awake to ensure adequate hydration.

Instruct patient to stop taking drug and notify prescriber at first sign of rash.

- Urge patients taking hormonal contraceptives to use supplemental birth control method such as condoms, because drug reduces contraceptive efficacy.
- Inform breastfeeding patient that drug is excreted in breast milk and can affect infant's bone growth. Advise her to consult prescriber before using drug.
- As appropriate, review all other significant and life-threatening adverse reactions and interactions, especially those related to the drugs and tests mentioned above.

cisatracurium besylate

Nimbex

Pharmacologic class: Neuromuscular blocker
Therapeutic class: Skeletal muscle relaxant
Pregnancy risk category B

Action

Competitively binds to cholinergic receptors on motor endplate, antagonizing the action of acetylcholine and blocking neuromuscular transmission (intermediate onset and intermediate duration)

Pharmacokinetics

Drug degrades into metabolites, independent of liver metabolism. Half-life of metabolites is longer in patients with renal or hepatic impairment. Drug is excreted largely in urine (mostly as metabolites), with less than 10% excreted as unchanged drug and about 4% excreted in feces.

Onset	Peak	Duration
1-2 min	2-5 min	25-44 min

How supplied

Solution for injection: 2 mg/mL in 5-mL single-use vials; 2 mg/mL in 10-mL multidose vials with benzyl alcohol; 10 mg/mL in 20-mL single-use vials

Indications and dosages

➢ Adjunct to general anesthesia; skeletal muscle relaxation during mechanical ventilation

Adults: Initially, 0.15 mg/kg I.V., then maintain on 0.03 mg/kg I.V. q 40 to 50 minutes; or initially, 0.2 mg/kg I.V., then maintain on 0.03 mg/kg I.V. q 50 to 60 minutes. Or initially, maintenance I.V. infusion of 3 mcg/kg/minute, titrated to 1 to 2 mcg/kg/minute p.r.n.

Children ages 2 to 12: 0.1 mg/kg I.V. over 5 to 10 seconds; then give maintenance infusion at 3 mcg/kg/minute, titrating to 1 to 2 mcg/kg/minute p.r.n.

Administration

Preparation

Give only under direct supervision of trained medical staff who are familiar with drug actions, characteristics, and hazards and can maintain patent airway.

Do not give drug unless mechanical ventilation support and emergency equipment are readily available.

- Be aware that 20-mL single-use vials containing 10 mg/mL are intended for use only in intensive care units.

Dilution and compatibility

- Know that drug is compatible with normal saline solution, D_5W, and 5% dextrose in normal saline solution.
- Be aware that drug is not compatible with lactated Ringer's solution.
- Dilute with compatible solution to 0.1 or 0.2 mg/mL.

Infusion considerations

- Always use volume infusion pump or microdrip (60 gtt/mL).
- Know that initial dose may be given as I.V. bolus over 5 to 10 seconds, followed by continuous infusion at prescribed rate.
- Start infusion only after early evidence of spontaneous recovery from initial bolus.
- Adjust administration rate to patient's response, as determined by peripheral nerve stimulator.

Monitoring

Monitor vital signs and ECG. Stay alert for respiratory depression, bradycardia, and hypotension.

- Continue to use peripheral nerve stimulator to monitor degree of neuromuscular blockade during administration and to monitor recovery from neuromuscular blockade after drug therapy ends.

Storage

- Refrigerate at 2° to 8°C (36° to 46°F). Do not freeze; protect from light.
- After removing drug from refrigeration to room temperature, store at 25°C (77°F).
- Use within 21 days, even if refrigerated.

Contraindications and precautions

Contraindicated in hypersensitivity to drug, other bis-benzylisoquinolinium agents, or benzyl alcohol (10-mL multidose vials only).

Use cautiously in neuromuscular disease, peripheral neuropathy, concurrent anticonvulsant therapy, and pregnant or breastfeeding patients.

Adverse reactions

CV: hypotension, flushing, **bradycardia**
Respiratory: bronchospasm, prolonged apnea
Skin: rash

Interactions

Drug-drug. *Aminoglycosides, bacitracin, clindamycin, colistimethate sodium, colistin, lincomycin, lithium, local anesthetics, magnesium salts, polymyxins, procainamide, quinidine, tetracyclines:* enhanced neuromuscular blockade

Carbamazepine, phenytoin: shortened duration of neuromuscular blockade
Enflurane or isoflurane given with nitrous oxide or oxygen: prolonged duration of cisatracurium action
Succinylcholine: faster onset of maximal neuromuscular blockade
Drug-herb. *St. John's wort:* increased risk of cardiovascular collapse, delayed emergence from anesthesia

Toxicity and overdose

- Overdose may prolong neuromuscular blockade beyond time needed. Watch for bradycardia and respiratory depression.
- Ensure patent airway with manual or mechanical ventilation. Once recovery from neuromuscular block begins, promote further recovery by giving anticholinesterase agent (such as edrophonium or neostigmine) in conjunction with anticholinergic (such as atropine or glycopyrrolate), as ordered.

Patient teaching

- Before giving, carefully describe drug effects. Explain that patient will be able to hear but not to move.
- Reassure patient, family, or caregiver that breathing will be closely monitored and supported during drug administration and that breathing and muscle function will return to normal after drug is discontinued.

cisplatin

Platinol, Platinex

Pharmacologic class: Alkylating agent, platinum coordination complex
Therapeutic class: Antineoplastic
Pregnancy risk category D

FDA BOXED WARNING

- Give under supervision of physician experienced in cancer chemotherapy, in facility with adequate diagnostic and treatment resources.
- Drug may cause severe cumulative renal toxicity. Other major dose-related toxicities are myelosuppression, nausea, and vomiting.
- Drug may lead to significant ototoxicity (which may be more pronounced in children), high-frequency hearing loss, and deafness.
- Anaphylactic-like reactions may occur within minutes of administration.
- Use caution to prevent inadvertent overdose. Dosages above 100 mg/m^2/cycle once every 3 to 4 weeks are rarely used. Avoid inadvertent overdose stemming from confusion with Paraplatin (carboplatin) or failure to differentiate daily doses from total dose per cycle.

Action

Inhibits DNA synthesis by causing intrastrand and interstrand cross-linking of DNA

Pharmacokinetics

Platinum (contained as central atom) distributes widely, with a half-life of 20 to 30 minutes. Although drug itself does not undergo protein binding, platinum is approximately 90% protein-bound. Resulting complexes undergo slow elimination, with minimum half-life of approximately 5 days. Parent drug is removed through renal metabolism and excreted in urine; about 10% is removed by biliary excretion.

Onset	Peak	Duration
Unknown	18-23 days	39 days

How supplied

Solution for injection: 1 mg/mL in 50-mg and 100-mg vials

Indications and dosages

➢ Metastatic testicular tumors

Adults: 10 to 20 mg/m² I.V. daily for 5 days per cycle, repeated q 3 to 4 weeks

➢ Metastatic ovarian cancer

Adults: 75 to 100 mg/m² I.V., repeated q 4 weeks in combination with cyclophosphamide, or 100 mg/m² q 4 weeks as a single agent

➢ Advanced bladder cancer

Adults: 50 to 70 mg/m² I.V. q 3 to 4 weeks as a single agent; dosage depends on whether patient has undergone radiation or chemotherapy.

Off-label uses

- Cervical carcinoma
- Squamous-cell carcinoma

Administration

Preparation

Follow hazardous drug guidelines on page S19 for handling, preparation, and administration.

- Before starting therapy, assess renal function tests and CBC with white cell differential.
- Do not give initial or repeat doses unless serum creatinine level is below 1.5 mg/100 mL, blood urea nitrogen (BUN) is below 25 mg/100 dL, and circulating blood elements are at acceptable levels (platelet count 100,000/mm³ or higher and white blood cell count 4,000/mm³ or higher).
- Know that patients who previously received radiation therapy or chemotherapy may need dosage modification.
- Give 2 L of I.V. fluids, as prescribed, 8 to 12 hours before drug infusion to help prevent toxicity.

Dilution and compatibility

- Prepare drug with equipment that does not contain aluminum.
- Initially dilute drug dose with 10 mL sterile water for injection.
- Dilute further in 2 L dextrose 5% in 0.22% or 0.45% normal saline solution or normal saline solution for injection.

Do not use D_5W.

Infusion considerations

Be aware that infusion rate must be sufficient to maintain hydration and adequate urine output. However, too-rapid infusion may increase risk of nephrotoxicity and ototoxicity.

- Infuse each liter over 3 to 4 hours to minimize toxicity.
- In well-hydrated patients with good renal function, 100 to 500 mL may be infused over 30 minutes, as tolerated.

Monitoring

- Continue to assess renal function tests and CBC with white cell differential before each dose.
- Monitor neurologic status, hepatic enzyme and uric acid levels, and audiogram results.
- Monitor urine output closely.
- Do not give subsequent doses until audiometric tests indicate that auditory acuity is normal. Be aware that ototoxicity may be more pronounced in children.

Storage

- Store at 15° to 25°C (59° to 77°F); protect from light. Do not refrigerate.

Contraindications and precautions

Contraindicated in hypersensitivity to drug or other platinum-containing compounds, severely impaired renal function, severe myelosuppression, hearing impairment, pregnancy, and breastfeeding.

Use cautiously in mild to moderate renal impairment, active infection, mild to moderate myelosuppression, chronic debilitating illness, heart failure, electrolyte abnormalities, and females of childbearing potential.

Adverse reactions

CNS: malaise, weakness, **seizures**
EENT: ototoxicity, tinnitus
GI: severe nausea, vomiting, diarrhea
GU: sterility, **nephrotoxicity**
Hematologic: anemia, **leukopenia, thrombocytopenia**
Hepatic: hepatotoxicity
Metabolic: hypocalcemia, hypokalemia, hypomagnesemia, hyperuricemia
Skin: alopecia
Other: phlebitis at I.V. site, **anaphylaxis**

Interactions

Drug-drug. *Amphotericin B, loop diuretics:* increased risk of hypokalemia and hypomagnesemia
Antineoplastics: additive bone marrow depression
Live-virus vaccines: decreased antibody response to vaccine, increased risk of adverse reactions
Nephrotoxic drugs (such as aminoglycosides): additive nephrotoxicity
Ototoxic drugs (such as loop diuretics): additive ototoxicity
Phenytoin: reduced phenytoin blood level
Drug-diagnostic tests. *Aspartate aminotransferase, bilirubin, BUN, creatinine, uric acid:* increased
Calcium, magnesium, phosphate, potassium, sodium: decreased
Coombs' test: positive result

Toxicity and overdose

- Acute overdose may cause intractable nausea and vomiting, neuritis, deafness, ocular toxicity (including retinal detachment), significant bone marrow depression, renal failure, and hepatic failure. Use extreme caution to avoid inadvertent overdose; notify prescriber immediately if a given dose exceeds 100 mg/m^2/cycle.
- Provide supportive and symptomatic therapy. No proven antidotes are known. Hemodialysis, even when started within 4 hours of overdose, has little benefit.

Patient teaching

- Instruct patient to drink 8 oz of water every hour while awake.
- (Clinical alert) Advise patient to promptly report bleeding, bruising, hearing loss, yellowing of skin or eyes, decreased urine output, and suspected infection.
- Inform patient that drug may cause hair loss.
- Instruct female patient to use reliable contraception; drug can harm fetus.
- As appropriate, review all other significant and life-threatening adverse reactions and interactions, especially those related to the drugs and tests mentioned above.

clindamycin phosphate

Apo-Clindamycin, Cleocin Phosphate, Dalacin

Pharmacologic class: Lincosamide
Therapeutic class: Anti-infective
Pregnancy risk category B

FDA BOXED WARNING

- To reduce development of bacterial resistance and maintain drug efficacy, use only to treat or prevent infections that are proven or strongly suspected to be caused by bacteria.
- Drug may cause pseudomembranous colitis, ranging from mild to life-threatening. Consider this diagnosis in patients who develop diarrhea after drug administration.
- If diagnosis of pseudomembranous colitis is established, initiate therapeutic

measures. Mild cases usually respond to drug withdrawal alone. In moderate to severe cases, consider giving fluids and electrolytes, protein supplements, and antibacterial drug effective against *Clostridium difficile* colitis, as ordered.
- Diarrhea, colitis, and pseudomembranous colitis may first appear up to several weeks after clindamycin therapy ends.
- Reserve drug for serious infections when less toxic antimicrobials are inappropriate. Do not use for nonbacterial infections, such as most upper respiratory tract infections.

Action

Inhibits protein synthesis in susceptible bacteria at level of 50S ribosome, thereby inhibiting peptide bond formation and causing cell death

Pharmacokinetics

Drug distributes widely to most body tissues and fluids (except cerebrospinal fluid) and crosses placental barrier. It is partially metabolized to inactive metabolites. Half-life is 2.4 to 3 hours, and increases slightly in reduced renal or hepatic function. About 10% of active drug is excreted in urine, with small amounts excreted in feces and breast milk. Most of urinary excretion consists of inactive metabolites.

Onset	Peak	Duration
Rapid	End of infusion	6-8 hr

How supplied

Solution for injection: 150-mg base/mL in 2-mL, 4-mL, and 6-mL vials containing benzyl alcohol; 4-mL and 6-mL ADD-Vantage vials; 300 mg, 600 mg, and 900 mg in 50-mL single-dose plastic containers with dextrose 5% injection

Indications and dosages

➢ Serious infections caused by aerobic gram-positive and sensitive anaerobes
Adults: 600 to 1,200 mg/day I.V. in two to four equally divided doses

➢ Severe infections caused by sensitive organisms (such as *Bacteroides fragilis, Fusobacterium* species, pneumococci, staphylococci, and streptococci)
Adults: 1.2 to 2.7 g/day I.V. in two to four equally divided doses

➢ Life-threatening infections caused by aerobic gram-positive and sensitive anaerobes
Adults: Up to 4.8 g/day I.V. in equally divided doses

➢ Acute pelvic inflammatory disease
Adults: 900 mg I.V. q 8 hours (given with gentamicin)

➢ Infections caused by aerobic gram-positive and sensitive anaerobes
Children older than age 1 month to age 16: Depending on severity of infection, 20 to 40 mg/kg/day I.V. or 350 to 450 mg/m^2/day I.V. in equally divided doses
Neonates younger than 1 month: 15 to 20 mg/kg/day I.V. in three to four equally divided doses

Off-label uses

- Bacterial vaginosis
- *Chlamydia trachomatis* infection in females
- CNS toxoplasmosis in AIDS patients (given with pyrimethamine)
- *Pneumocystis jiroveci* pneumonia (given with primaquine)

Administration

Preparation

Be aware that drug as 150-mg base/mL contains benzyl alcohol, which is linked to "gasping syndrome" in premature infants.

Dilution and compatibility

- Reconstitute each 18 mg of drug solution with at least 1 mL normal saline

solution, 5% dextrose in water (D_5W), or lactated Ringer's solution.
- Dilute further in a compatible solution such as, D_5W, normal saline solution, 5% dextrose in normal saline solution.
- Dilute 300-mg and 600-mg doses in 50 mL; dilute 900-mg dose in 50 to 100 mL; dilute 1,200-mg dose in 100 mL.
- Know that drug in plastic containers is supplied as a premixed solution.

Infusion considerations

Do not give undiluted or as I.V. bolus injection.

Do not administer dosages above 1,200 mg in less than a 1-hour infusion.

Do not use plastic containers in series connections. Such use could result in air embolism due to residual air being drawn from primary container before administration of fluid from secondary container ends.

Be aware that too-rapid infusion may cause severe hypotension and cardiac arrest. Use the following table for infusion rates.

Dosage (mg)	Infusion rate (min)
300	10
600	20
900	30
1,200	40

Monitoring
- Monitor creatinine level closely in patients with renal insufficiency.
- Monitor hepatic enzyme levels in patients with hepatic disease.
- Assess for signs and symptoms of hypersensitivity reactions.
- Assess for diarrhea and signs and symptoms of colitis.
- Monitor CBC with white cell differential regularly, especially in prolonged therapy.
- Monitor serum drug levels during high-dose therapy.
- Monitor for overgrowth of nonsusceptible organisms, particularly yeasts.

Storage
- Store solution from vials at controlled room temperature of 20° to 25°C (68° to 77°F) for 24 hours when mixed with compatible solution.

C

Contraindications and precautions

Contraindicated in hypersensitivity to drug or lincomycin.

Use cautiously in renal or hepatic impairment, GI disease, history of asthma or significant allergies, known alcohol intolerance, pregnant patients, and ***neonates.***

Adverse reactions

GI: nausea, vomiting, diarrhea, abdominal pain, esophagitis, **pseudomembranous colitis**

Hematologic: neutropenia, leukopenia, agranulocytosis, thrombocytopenia purpura

Hepatic: jaundice, **hepatic dysfunction**

Skin: maculopapular rash, generalized morbilliform-like rash

Other: bitter taste, phlebitis at I.V. site, superinfection, hypersensitivity reaction including **anaphylaxis**

Interactions

Drug-drug. *Erythromycin:* antagonistic effect

Kaolin/pectin: decreased GI absorption of clindamycin

Hormonal contraceptives: decreased contraceptive efficacy

Neuromuscular blockers: enhanced neuromuscular blockade

Drug-diagnostic tests. *Alanine aminotransferase, alkaline phosphatase, aspartate aminotransferase, bilirubin, creatine kinase:* increased

Platelets, white blood cells: transient decrease

Toxicity and overdose

- In overdose, expect extension of adverse reactions.
- Discontinue drug and provide symptomatic and supportive interventions.

Patient teaching

Urge patient to immediately report rash, unusual fatigue, or yellowing of skin or eyes, and to seek immediate attention if diarrhea occurs during or after treatment.

- Tell patient drug may have bitter taste but this effect will resolve on its own.
- Instruct patient using hormonal contraceptives to use supplemental birth control method such as condoms, because drug may reduce hormonal contraceptive efficacy.
- As appropriate, review all other significant and life-threatening adverse reactions and interactions, especially those related to the drugs and tests mentioned above.

clofarabine

Clolar, Evoltra

Pharmacologic class: Purine nucleoside antimetabolite
Therapeutic class: Antineoplastic
Pregnancy risk category D

Action

Inhibits DNA synthesis by decreasing cellular deoxynucleotide triphosphate pools through inhibitory action on ribonucleotide reductase, terminating DNA chain elongation, and inhibiting repair through incorporation into DNA chain by competitive inhibition of DNA polymerases. Drug is cytotoxic to rapidly proliferating and quiescent cancer cell types in vitro.

Pharmacokinetics

Drug is metabolized to active compound; hepatic metabolism is negligible. It is approximately 47% protein-bound, predominantly to albumin. Terminal half-life is about 5 hours for parent compound and 24 hours for active compound. Drug is excreted largely unchanged in urine.

Onset	Peak	Duration
Unknown	Unknown	Unknown

How supplied

Solution for injection (clear, colorless, preservative-free): 1 mg/mL (20 mg in 20-mL flint vials)

Indications and dosages

➤ Relapsed or refractory acute lymphoblastic leukemia after at least two previous regimens
Children and adults ages 1 to 21: 52 mg/ m^2/day by I.V. infusion over 2 hours for 5 consecutive days every 2 to 6 weeks, depending on toxicity and response

Administration

Preparation

Follow hazardous drug guidelines on page S19 for handling, preparation, and administration.

- Assess hepatic and renal function before starting drug.
- Be aware that giving corticosteroids on days 1 through 3 may help prevent systemic inflammatory response syndrome (SIRS) and capillary leak syndrome (CLS). If early signs or symptoms of these life-threatening syndromes occur, stop drug immediately and start appropriate supportive measures.
- Give continuous I.V. fluids throughout 5 days of therapy to reduce effects of tumor lysis and other adverse events.

• If hyperuricemia (caused by tumor lysis) is expected, give prophylactic allopurinol, as prescribed.

Dilution and compatibility

• Withdraw the required dose using a sterile 0.2-micron syringe filter and dilute with D_5W or normal saline solution to a concentration of approximately 0.36 mg/mL.

• Use drug within 24 hours of preparation.

Infusion considerations

• Administer by I.V. infusion over 2 hours.

• To prevent incompatibilities, do not give other drugs through same I.V. line.

Monitoring

Closely monitor respiratory status and blood pressure during infusion.

Monitor for signs and symptoms of tumor lysis syndrome or cytokine release (such as tachypnea, tachycardia, hypotension, and pulmonary edema), which could progress to SIRS, CLS, or organ dysfunction. Withdraw drug immediately if patient develops significant signs or symptoms of SIRS; or give corticosteroids, diuretics, and albumin, if prescribed. Drug may be reinstituted (generally at lower dosage) when patient is stable.

Discontinue drug if hypotension occurs. If hypotension is transient and resolves without drug intervention, reinstitute drug as ordered (generally at lower dosage).

Monitor renal and hepatic functions frequently. If creatinine or bilirubin level rises substantially, discontinue drug. Drug may be reinstituted (possibly at lower dosage) when patient is stable and organ function returns to baseline.

Monitor hematologic status carefully during therapy; drug may cause severe bone marrow depression.

• Monitor for signs and symptoms of infection.

• Closely monitor patients concurrently receiving drugs that affect blood pressure or cardiac function.

• Continue to assess hepatic function during therapy.

• Avoid concurrent administration of hepatotoxic or renotoxic drugs during therapy.

• Know that after recovery or return to baseline organ function, treatment cycles typically are repeated about every 2 to 6 weeks. Dosage is based on body surface area, calculated using actual height and weight before start of each cycle.

Storage

• Store vials before dilution at 25°C (77°F); excursions are permitted to 15° to 30°C (59° to 86°F). Store diluted drug at room temperature.

Contraindications and precautions

Use with extreme caution in patients with renal or hepatic impairment. Use cautiously in active infection, dehydration, hypotension, adults older than age 21, and pregnant or breastfeeding patients.

Adverse reactions

CNS: dizziness, headache, somnolence, tremor, anxiety, depression, lethargy, fatigue, irritability, rigors
CV: tachycardia, flushing, hypertension, hypotension
EENT: sore throat, epistaxis
GI: nausea, vomiting, diarrhea, constipation, abdominal pain, anorexia, gingival bleeding, oral candidiasis
GU: hematuria
Hematologic: febrile neutropenia, neutropenia, anemia, thrombocytopenia
Hepatic: hepatomegaly, jaundice
Musculoskeletal: arthralgia, back pain, myalgia, limb pain
Respiratory: pneumonia, cough, dyspnea, pleural effusion, **respiratory distress**

Skin: contusion, dermatitis, herpes simplex, dry skin, erythema, palmar-plantar erythrodysesthesia, petechiae, pruritus, cellulitis
Other: decreased appetite, weight loss, edema, injection-site pain, mucosal inflammation, pain, fever, bacteremia, sepsis, staphylococcal infection, transfusion reaction

Interactions

Drug-drug. *Hepatotoxic or renotoxic drugs:* additive toxicity
Drug-diagnostic tests. *Alanine aminotransferase, aspartate aminotransferase, bilirubin:* increased
Drug-herb. *Alpha-lipoic acid, coenzyme Q10:* decreased chemotherapeutic efficacy
Glutamine: possible increase in tumor growth

Toxicity and overdose

- In overdose, expect vomiting, maculopapular rash, hyperbilirubinemia, cardiotoxicity (tachycardia, peripheral perfusion), and bone marrow suppression.
- No specific antidote is known. Provide symptomatic and supportive therapy.

Patient teaching

- Teach patient about appropriate measures to avoid dehydration caused by vomiting and diarrhea. Tell patient to seek medical advice if signs and symptoms of dehydration (such as dizziness, light-headedness, fainting spells, or decreased urine output) arise.
- Advise females of childbearing potential to avoid pregnancy during therapy.
- Caution breastfeeding patient to discontinue breastfeeding during therapy.
- As appropriate, review all other significant and life-threatening adverse reactions and interactions, especially those related to the drugs, tests, and herbs mentioned above.

coagulation factor VIIa (recombinant)

NovoSeven, NiaStase ♣

Pharmacologic class: Coagulation factor VIIa
Therapeutic class: Antihemophilic agent
Pregnancy risk category C

Action

Promotes hemostasis by activating intrinsic pathway of coagulation cascade to form fibrin

Pharmacokinetics

Median volume of distribution is 103 mL/kg, half-life is 1.7 to 2.7 hours, and median clearance is 33 mL/kg/hour.

Onset	Peak	Duration
Unknown	Unknown	Unknown

How supplied

Powder for reconstitution for injection (white, lyophilized): 1.2 mg, 2.4 mg, and 4.8 mg in single-use vials

Indications and dosages

➢ Bleeding episodes in patients with hemophilia A or B who have inhibitors to factor VIII or IX
Adults: 90 mcg/kg I.V. bolus q 2 hours until hemostasis occurs or therapy is deemed ineffective

Administration

Dilution and compatibility

- Reconstitute only with sterile water for injection, as follows: 1.2-mg vial with 2.2 mL, 2.4-mg vial with 4.3 mL, and 4.8-mg vial with 8.5 mL, to yield 0.6 mg/mL concentration per vial.

Safe I.V. drug administration

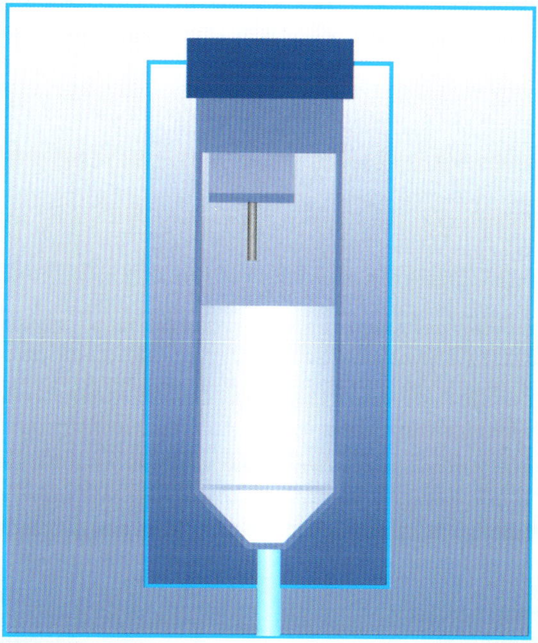

The following guidelines on preparing, administering, and monitoring I.V. drug therapy will help you ensure patient safety and drug effectiveness.

I.V. drug compatibilities

Use the table below to determine if you can safely mix two drugs together in the same syringe or administer them together through the same I.V. line.

KEY
C: compatible
I: incompatible
*: conflicting data exist
Blank space: no data available

	acyclovir sodium	amikacin	amiodarone	amphotericin B	aztreonam	calcium chloride	calcium gluconate	cefazolin	cefepime	ceftazidime	clindamycin	cyclosporine	dexamethasone	digoxin	diltiazem	diphenhydramine	dobutamine	dopamine	enalaprilat
acyclovir sodium															I		I	I	
amikacin			C	I	C	C	C	C	C	I	C	C	C	C	C	C			C
amiodarone		C		C		C	C	I		I	C			I			C	C	
amphotericin B		I	C		I										C	*		I	I
aztreonam		C		I		C	C			C	C		C		C	C	C	C	C
calcium chloride		C	C														*	C	
calcium gluconate		C	C		C			I			I		C			C	*		C
cefazolin		C	I		C		I				*	C	C		C				C
cefepime		C									C								
ceftazidime		I	I		C						C				C				C
clindamycin		C	C		C		I	*	C	C		C							C
cyclosporine		C						C			C							*	
dexamethasone		C			C		C	C								*			
digoxin			I														I		
diltiazem	I	C		C	C			C			C						C	C	
diphenhydramine		C		*	C		C						*						
dobutamine	I		C		C	*	*							I	C			C	C
dopamine	I		C	I	C	C						*			C		C		C
enalaprilat		C		I	C		C	C		C	C						C	C	
epinephrine		C	C			*	*										C		
esmolol		C	C			C		C		C	C			C			C	C	C
famotidine	C		C	C			C	C		C			C	C		C	C	C	C
fluconazole		C		C				C		C	C	C							
furosemide		*	*												I	I	I		

epinephrine		C	C			*	*										C					C		C
esmolol		C	C			C		C		C	C			C	C		C	C	C			C		I
famotidine	C		C	C			C	C		C			C	C		C	C	C	C	C	C		C	*
fluconazole		C	C				C			C	C											C		
furosemide		*	*													I	I			C	I	*		
heparin		I		I	C		C	*	C	*	C		C	C	*	*	*	C	C	C	C	C		C
hydrocortisone		C		I	C	C	C				C		C		*			C	C	C	C	C	C	C
hydromorphone hydrochloride																								
imipenem and cilastatin sodium					C										C							C		
insulin			C		C			C						I	*		*	I			C	C		
labetalol		C	C				C	C		C	C						C	C	C		C	C		I
levofloxacin		C									C		C				C	C		C				I
lorazepam		C	C		I								*		C	I						C		C
magnesium		C	*	*	C	I	*	C			I	*					*		C		C	C		
methylprednisolone			C	C	C		C	C			C					I		C	C			C		
metoprolol																								
metronidazole		C	C		I			*	C	C	C	C						*	C		C		C	
midazolam		C	C				C	C		I	C		*	C			*	C			C	C		I
milrinone		C	C			C	C	C			C		C	C			C	C		C				I
morphine		C	C		C	C		C		C	C		C	C		C	C	C	C		C	C	C	I
nitroglycerin			C														C	C			C	C		C
nitroprusside			*			C											C	C	C	C	C	C		C
norepinephrine															C		C	C				C		
ondansetron		C		I	C			C		C	C	*	*			C		C				C		I
phenylephrine			C				C									C	C					C		
potassium chloride		C	C				C	C	C	C			C	C		*	*	C	C	C	C	C	C	I
propofol		I		I	C	I	C	C		C	C	C	C	C		C	C	C	C	C	C	C		C
sodium bicarbonate		C	I	I	C	I	I			I							I	I						C
tobramycin			C		C		C	C	I	*	*	C							C		C			*
vancomycin		C	C		*		C	*	C	*		C	I			C			C		C	C		
vecuronium			C					C									C	C		C	C			

I.V. drug compatibilities (continued)

KEY
C: compatible
I: incompatible
*: conflicting data exist
Blank space: no data available

	acyclovir sodium	amikacin	amiodarone	amphotericin B	aztreonam	calcium chloride	calcium gluconate	cefazolin	cefepime	ceftazidime	clindamycin	cyclosporine	dexamethasone	digoxin	diltiazem	diphenhydramine	dobutamine	dopamine	enalaprilat
heparin		I		I	C		C	*	C	*	C		C	C	*	*	*	C	C
hydrocortisone		C		I	C	C	C				C		C		*	C		C	C
hydromorphone hydrochloride																			
imipenem and cilastatin sodium			I		C										C				
insulin			C		C			C						I	*		*	I	
labetalol		C	C				C	C		C	C						C	C	C
levofloxacin		C									C		C				C	C	
lorazepam		C	C		I								C		C	I			
magnesium		C	*	*	C	I	*	C			I	C					*		C
methylprednisolone			C	C	C		C				C				*	I		C	C
metoprolol																			
metronidazole		C	C		I			*	C	C	C	C						*	C
midazolam		C	C				C	C		I	C		*	C			*	C	
milrinone		C	C			C	C	C		C	C		C	C	C		C	C	
morphine		C	C		C	C		C		C	C		C	C		C	C	C	C
nitroglycerin			C												C		C	C	
nitroprusside			*			C											C	C	C
norepinephrine			C												C		C	C	
ondansetron		C		I	C			C		C	C	*	*			C		C	
phenylephrine			C				C									C	C		
potassium chloride		C	C		C		C	C	C	C				C	C		*	*	C
propofol		I		I	C	I	C	C		C	C	C	C	C		C	C	C	C
sodium bicarbonate		C	I		C	I	I			I					*		I	I	
tobramycin			C		C		C	C	I	*	*	C			C				C
vancomycin		C	C		*		C	*	C	*			I		C	C			C
vecuronium			C					C									C	C	

	epinephrine	esmolol	famotidine	fluconazole	furosemide	heparin	hydrocortisone	hydromorphone hydrochloride	imipenem and cilastatin sodium	insulin	labetalol	levofloxacin	lorazepam	magnesium	methylprednisolone	metoprolol	metronidazole	midazolam	milrinone	morphine	nitroglycerin	nitroprusside	norepinephrine	ondansetron	phenylephrine	potassium chloride	propofol	sodium bicarbonate	tobramycin	vancomycin	vecuronium
	C	C	C	C	C		*		C	I	*	I	C	C	*		C	C	C	I	*	C		C	C	C	C	C	I	*	C
	C	C	C		C	*				C			C	*			C	I		C				C			C	C			C
						C							C					C						C		C		I			
			C			C				C			I					I	I					C							
		C	C			I	C		C		I	I		C				C	C	C	C	C	I			C	C	*	C	C	
		C	C		I	*				I				C			C	C		C	C	C	C			C	C	*	C	C	
	C				I	I				I			C							C	I	I			C			C		C	
			C		C	C	C	C	I			C					C		C					*		C	C			C	C
		C	C			C	*			C	C						C		C	C		C		C		C	C	I	C	C	
			C			*											C	*	C	C				*		I	I				
																				C											
		C		C		C	C				C		C	C	C			C	C	C									C		
		C	C		I	C	I	C	I	C	C				*		C		C	C	C	C	C	C		C	*	I	C	C	C
	C				I	C			I	C			C	C	C		C	C		C	C	C	C			C	C	C	C	C	C
		C	C	C	I	I	C			C	C	C		C	C	C	C	C	C			C	C	C		C	C	I	C	C	C
		C	C		C	*				C	C	I						C	C			C					C				C
	C	C	C		C	C				C	C	I		C				C	C	C	C		C			C					C
			C							I	C							C	C	C		C					C				
			C		I	C	C	C	C				*		*			C		C						C	C	I		C	
			C			C						C															I			C	
	C	C	C	C	I	C		C	C		C	C		C	C				C	C	C		C		C		C	C			
	C	C	C		C	C	C			C	C		C	C	C			*	C	C	C		C	C	I			C	I	C	C
					C	C	C	I		*	*	C		I				I	C	I				I		C	C			I	
		C			*	I			C	C			C			C	C	C	C							I					
		C	C			*	I			C	C	C	C	C				C	C	C				C	C		C	I			C
		C				C	C						C					C	C	C	C	C					C			C	

Conversions and calculations

Accurate conversions and calculations are crucial to ensuring safe drug administration. Use the tables below when you need to convert one unit to another, find equivalent measures, convert temperatures between Celsius and Fahrenheit, or calculate dosages or administration rates.

Metric measures

Solids

1 milligram (mg) = 1,000 micrograms (mcg)
1 gram (g) = 1,000 mg
1 kilogram (kg) = 1,000 g

Liquids

1 milliliter (ml) = 1 cubic centimeter (cc)
1 ml = 1,000 microliters (mcl)
1 cc = 1,000 mcl
1 liter (L) = 1,000 ml
1 L = 1,000 cc

Household to metric equivalents

1 teaspoon (tsp) = 5 ml
1 tablespoon (tbs) = 15 ml
1 ounce (oz) = 30 ml
2 tbs = 30 ml
1 oz = 30 g
1 pound (lb) = 454 g
2.2 lb = 1 kg
1 inch = 2.54 centimeters (cm)

Temperature conversions

To convert Celsius (°C) to Fahrenheit (°F)

Use the following equation:

$(°C \times 9/5) + 32 = °F$

Example: 38 °C times 9/5 is 68.4; 68.4 plus 32 equals 100.4 °F.

To convert °F to °C

$(°F - 32) \times 5/9 = °C$

Example: 98.6 °F minus 32 is 66.8.; 66.8 times 5/9 equals 37 °C.

Calculating dosages and administration rates

$$\text{Concentration of solution in mg/ml} = \frac{\text{mg of drug}}{\text{ml of solution}}$$

$$\text{Infusion rate in mg/minute} = \frac{\text{mg of drug}}{\text{ml of solution}} \times \text{flow rate (ml/hour)} \div 60 \text{ minutes}$$

$$\text{Concentration of solution in mcg/ml} = \frac{\text{mg of drug} \times 1{,}000}{\text{ml of solution}}$$

Infusion rate in mcg/minute =

$$\frac{\text{mg of drug} \times 1{,}000}{\text{ml of solution}} \times \text{flow rate (ml/hour)} \div 60 \text{ minutes}$$

Infusion rate in mcg/kg/minute =

$$\frac{\text{mg of drug} \times 1{,}000}{\text{ml of solution}} \times \text{flow rate (ml/hour)} \div 60 \text{ minutes} \div \text{weight in kg}$$

Infusion rate in ml/hour = ml of solution ÷ 60 minutes

$$\text{Infusion rate in gtt/minute} = \frac{\text{ml of solution}}{\text{time in minutes}} \times \text{drip factor (gtt/ml)}$$

Drug infusion rates

The tables below show infusion rates for common drug infusions. Before using these tables as your administration guide, make sure the concentration of the prescribed infusion matches the concentration shown in the table.

Dobutamine infusion rates

Using this table, you can determine the infusion rate for an infusion containing dobutamine 250 mg mixed in 250 ml of dextrose 5% in water (1,000 mcg/ml).

Dosage (mcg/kg/minute)	Patient's weight (kg)														
	40	45	50	55	60	65	70	75	80	85	90	95	100	105	110
	Infusion rate (ml/hour)														
0.5	1	1	2	2	2	2	2	2	2	3	3	3	3	3	3
1.5	4	4	5	5	5	6	6	7	7	8	8	9	9	9	10
2.5	6	7	8	8	9	10	11	11	12	13	14	14	15	16	17
5.0	12	14	15	17	18	20	21	23	24	26	27	29	30	32	33
7.5	18	20	23	25	27	29	32	34	36	38	41	43	45	47	50
10.0	24	27	30	33	36	39	42	45	48	51	54	57	60	63	66
12.5	30	34	38	41	45	49	53	56	60	64	68	71	75	79	83
15.0	36	41	45	50	54	59	63	68	72	77	81	86	90	95	99
20.0	48	54	60	66	72	78	84	90	96	102	108	114	120	126	132
25.0	60	68	75	83	90	98	105	113	120	128	135	143	150	158	165
30.0	72	81	90	99	108	117	126	135	144	153	162	171	180	189	198
35.0	84	95	105	116	126	137	147	158	168	179	189	200	210	221	231
40.0	96	108	120	132	144	156	168	180	192	204	216	228	240	252	264

Nitroprusside infusion rates

Using this table, you can determine the infusion rate for an infusion containing nitroprusside 50 mg in 250 ml of dextrose 5% in water (200 mcg/ml).

Dosage (mcg/kg/minute)	Patient's weight (kg)														
	40	45	50	55	60	65	70	75	80	85	90	95	100	105	110
	Infusion rate (ml/hour)														
0.3	4	4	5	5	5	6	6	7	7	8	8	9	9	9	10
0.5	6	7	8	8	9	10	11	11	12	13	14	14	15	16	17
1.0	12	14	15	17	18	20	21	23	24	26	27	29	30	32	33
1.5	18	20	23	25	27	29	32	34	36	38	41	43	45	47	50
2.0	24	27	30	33	36	39	42	45	48	51	54	57	60	63	66
3.0	36	41	45	50	54	59	63	68	72	77	81	86	90	95	99
4.0	48	54	60	66	72	78	84	90	96	102	108	114	120	126	132
5.0	60	68	75	83	90	98	105	113	120	128	135	143	150	158	165
6.0	72	81	90	99	108	117	126	135	144	153	162	171	180	189	198
7.0	84	95	105	116	126	137	147	158	168	179	189	200	210	221	231
8.0	96	108	120	132	144	156	168	180	192	204	216	228	240	252	264
9.0	108	122	135	149	162	176	189	203	216	230	243	257	270	284	297
10.0	120	135	150	165	180	195	210	225	240	255	270	285	300	315	330

(continued)

Drug infusion rates (continued)

Dopamine infusion rates

Using this table, you can determine the infusion rate for an infusion containing dopamine 400 mg in 250 ml of dextrose 5% in water (1,600 mcg/ml).

Dosage (mcg/kg/minute)	Patient's weight (kg)													
	40	45	50	55	60	65	70	75	80	85	90	95	100	105
	Infusion rate (ml/hour)													
0.5	1	1	1	1	1	1	1	1	2	2	2	2	2	2
1.5	2	3	3	3	3	4	4	4	5	5	5	6	6	6
2.5	4	4	5	5	6	6	7	7	8	8	8	9	9	10
5.0	8	8	9	10	11	12	13	14	15	16	17	18	19	20
7.5	11	13	14	15	17	18	20	21	23	24	25	27	28	30
10.0	15	17	19	21	23	24	26	28	30	32	34	36	38	39
12.5	19	21	23	26	28	30	33	35	38	40	42	45	47	49
15.0	23	25	28	31	34	37	39	42	45	48	51	53	56	59
20.0	30	34	38	41	45	49	53	56	60	64	68	71	75	79
25.0	38	42	47	52	56	61	66	70	75	80	84	89	94	98
30.0	45	51	56	62	67	73	79	84	90	96	101	107	113	118
35.0	53	59	66	72	79	85	92	98	105	112	118	125	131	138
40.0	60	68	75	83	90	98	105	113	120	128	135	143	150	158
45.0	68	76	84	93	101	110	118	127	135	143	152	160	169	177
50.0	75	84	94	103	113	122	131	141	150	159	169	178	188	197

Nitroglycerin infusion rates

When infusing nitroglycerin, first find the prescribed concentration and then determine the infusion rate in ml/hour.

Dosage (mcg/minute)	Nitroglycerin 25 mg/250 ml D_5W (100 mcg/ml) Infusion rate (ml/hour)	Nitroglycerin 50 mg/250 ml D_5W (200 mcg/ml) Infusion rate (ml/hour)
5	3	2
10	6	3
15	9	5
20	12	6
25	15	8
30	18	9
40	24	12
50	30	15
60	36	18
70	42	21
80	48	24
90	54	27
100	60	30

KEY D_5W: dextrose 5% in water

Drug infusion rates (continued)

Epinephrine infusion rates

Use this table to determine the rate at which to infuse epinephrine 1 mg in 250 ml of dextrose 5% in water (4 mcg/ml).

Dosage (mcg/minute)	Infusion rate (ml/hour)
1	15
2	30
3	45
4	60
5	75
6	90
7	105
8	120
9	135
10	150
15	225

Phenylephrine infusion rates

Using this table, you can determine the infusion rate for an infusion containing phenylephrine 20 mg in 250 ml of dextrose 5% in water or normal saline solution (80 mcg/ml).

Dosage (mcg/minute)	Rate (ml/hour)
9	7
11	8
12	9
13	10
15	11
16	12
17	13
19	14
20	15
21	16
23	17
24	18
25	19
27	20
29	22
32	24
35	26
37	28
40	30
43	32
45	34
48	36
51	38
53	40

Venipuncture and peripheral venous access

More than 90% of all hospitalized patients have some type of I.V. access device. I.V. access can be obtained through a central or peripheral vein. The choice depends on the specific agent to be delivered, anticipated length of therapy, and condition of the patient's veins.

Central venous access is a better choice for administering agents that can irritate the vein's intimal lining, such as vesicants (drugs that can cause tissue necrosis when they leak outside the vein), vasopressors, concentrated electrolyte or glucose solutions, and some chemotherapy agents. The increased blood flow dilutes the irritating properties of these agents. Peripheral venous access is indicated for withdrawal of venous blood samples and delivery of many I.V. medications, fluid solutions, blood, and blood products.

Peripheral venous access devices include winged stainless steel needles (commonly called butterflies), catheter over-the-needle devices, and midline catheters. Stainless steel needles are used mainly for blood withdrawal and are considered unsafe for infusion therapy because of the increased risk of infiltration. Midline catheters, which are approximately 6" long, are inserted above the antecubital fossa; however, these catheters extend only to the axillary vein.

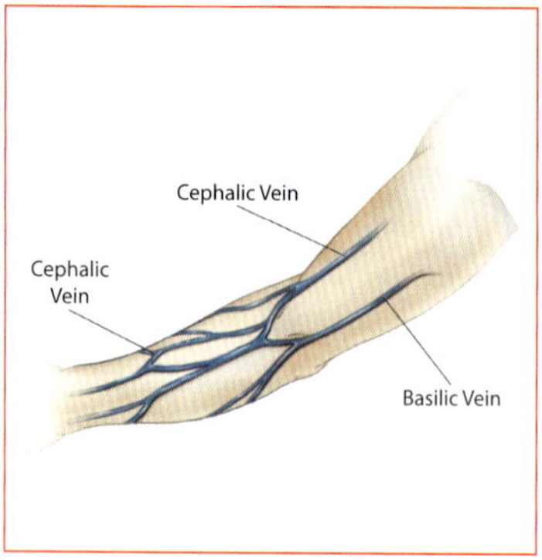

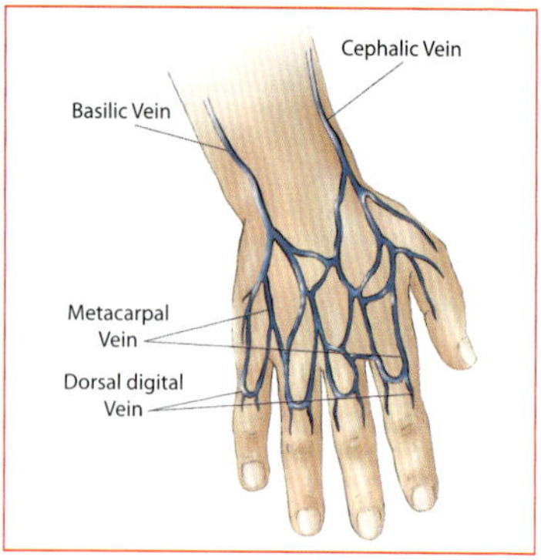

For peripheral I.V. access, the most commonly used veins, as shown above, are the:

- cephalic vein, which runs from the thumb side of the arm to the shoulder. The second largest forearm vein, it's appropriate for most I.V. therapies.
- basilic vein, which runs from the little finger to the shoulder. The largest vein in the arm, it's appropriate for all I.V. therapies.
- metacarpal veins, on the dorsum of the hand. These veins are painful to access and are used mostly in preoperative patients.
- dorsal venous arch, on the dorsum of the wrist. This short vein is comfortable to use for most patients.

The next few pages describe the procedure to use for inserting a peripheral I.V. catheter into an adult. The most important steps are highlighted below, including preparation; patient teaching; selecting, palpating, and dilating a vein; selecting the access device; inserting the catheter; applying a dressing; and providing monitoring and aftercare.

Preparing the equipment

After checking the physician's order, gather the required equipment: safety over-the-needle I.V. access device, tourniquet, chlorhexidine prep pad, nonsterile gloves, transparent dressing, needleless end-cap or I.V. tubing. *(Federal law requires that all I.V. catheters and needles have a safety needle protection system in all healthcare settings.)*

Patient teaching

Before you begin, explain the procedure to the patient to minimize fear and anxiety. *(In a fearful patient, an autonomic nervous system response may complicate vein visualization and cause vein constriction.)* Using terms the patient can understand, explain:

- why the I.V. line is required
- how long the infusion will last
- what type of drug will be infused
- possible complications, including infiltration, infection, nerve injury, and hematoma.

Then obtain verbal consent from the patient (except in an emergency).

Selecting the access device

An over-the-needle catheter device is most commonly used to deliver I.V. antibiotics and fluids. Use a catheter of the smallest size and shortest length capable of delivering the prescribed therapy; the catheter gauge should not exceed 50% of the vein's diameter. For most infusion therapies, a smaller-gauge catheter, such as 22G, is standard; it can deliver up to 2,000 ml/hour in a suitable vein. Blood in the vein acts as a cushion between the catheter and lining of the vein, preventing trauma. A 22G catheter can be used to infuse blood and blood products for patients with poor venous access.

A 24G catheter is used routinely for pediatric and geriatric patients; it can deliver more than 1,500 ml/hour in a suitable vein. A 20G catheter can be used to deliver more than 3,500 ml/hour. This catheter size is appropriate for administering whole blood or packed red blood cells, as well as for preoperative and obstetric patients; large-gauge catheters are preferred for these patients. Rapid I.V. fluid replacement, multiple simultaneous infusions, and blood transfusions may be needed in an emergency and require a large-bore access device.

Mechanical phlebitis can occur if the catheter is too large for the vein or if it isn't properly stabilized and moves within the vein. Chemical phlebitis can occur in small veins with minimal blood flow. If the patient complains of burning or discomfort at the I.V. site during the infusion, suspect that the I.V. agent is irritating the lining of the vein. Remove the catheter and consult the physician, who may order insertion of a central venous catheter.

Selecting a peripheral vein

Select a superficial vein in an upper extremity, if possible. Using lower-extremity veins increase the risk of embolism and thrombophlebitis. Also, remember that final catheter-tip placement should fall below the patient's shoulder.

Avoid inserting the I.V. catheter into the lower inner aspect of the wrist (approximately 3") above the palm or into the area 3" above the thumb. Incorrect I.V. insertion and drug infiltration into these areas can lead to permanent nerve injuries, such as wrist drop and carpal tunnel injury. Also avoid areas of joint flexure, such as the wrist and elbow. Instead, choose the dorsal surface of the arm for greater patient comfort. *(Keep in mind that the large, deeper veins are more comfortable for the patient because they have a better hemodilution rate and are supported by the long bones in the arm.)*

Once you've selected a vein, start the procedure distal to a previous I.V. site, and work proximally on the same vein. This way, you can move proximally for subsequent I.V. insertions.

Dilating and palpating the vein

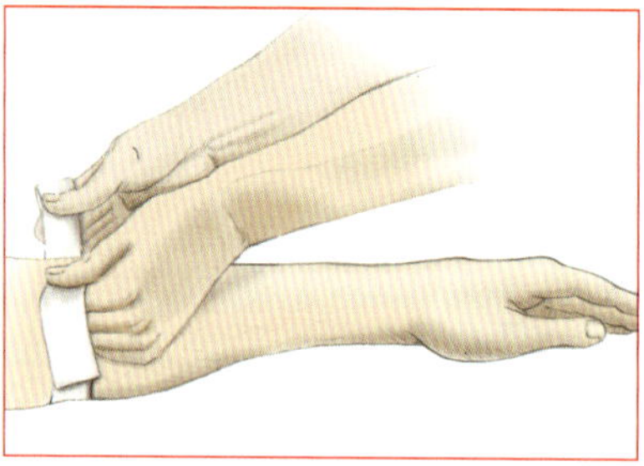

Apply a tourniquet, as shown, above the antecubital fossa to allow complete assessment of the veins of the hand and the dorsal and volar areas of the forearm. (*Remember that tourniquets are single-patient-use items.)* Lower the patient's arm below heart level, and gently tap the vein to cause distention. Ask the patient to open and close the fist so the vein engorges.

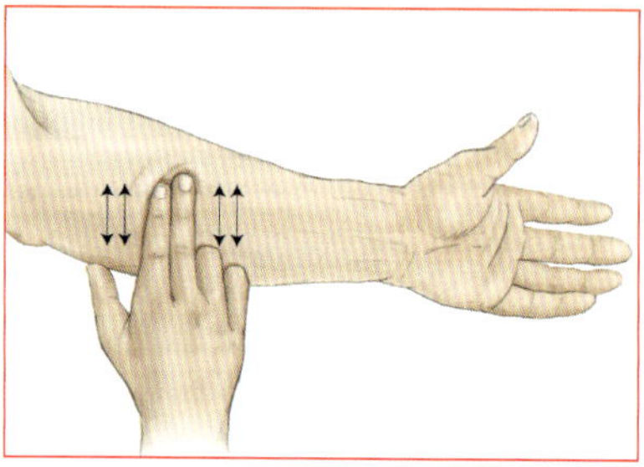

With your index finger, use a "press and release" motion to locate the desired vein. The vein should be soft, spongy, and straight for approximately 1". (*Repeatedly using your index finger to identify a vein increases the finger's sensitivity and ease in* locating *veins.)* Using your index and middle fingers, as shown, palpate the vein from side to side to assess it for scarred valves and previous injuries.

Preparing the site

Using hair clippers or scissors, remove excess hair from the I.V. access site. Then clean the skin at the site. Chlorhexidine, the agent preferred by the Infusion Nurses Society and the Centers for Disease Control and Prevention, kills *Staphylococcus epidermidis* organisms—the most common cause of I.V. site infections. Apply chlorhexidine using a side-to-side and up-and-down motion; *don't* move in concentric circles. Clean the skin vigorously for at least 30 seconds, and allow it to air dry.

Inserting the catheter

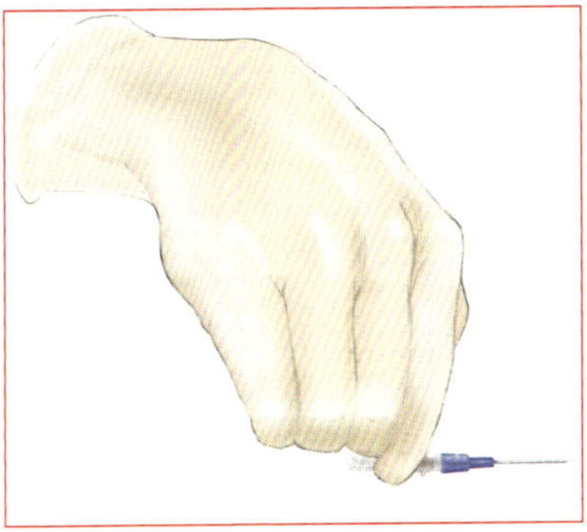

Don gloves. Hold the catheter horizontally, as shown, with your hand on top of the access device to ensure the proper entry angle and give your wrist maximum flexibility during insertion. Always keep the bevel of the stylet up, with your fingers on the flashback chamber (not on the color-coded hub). Your fingers should align with the catheter. Don't hold the catheter like a dart, because this may cause the inserter to go through the skin and the back wall of the vein.

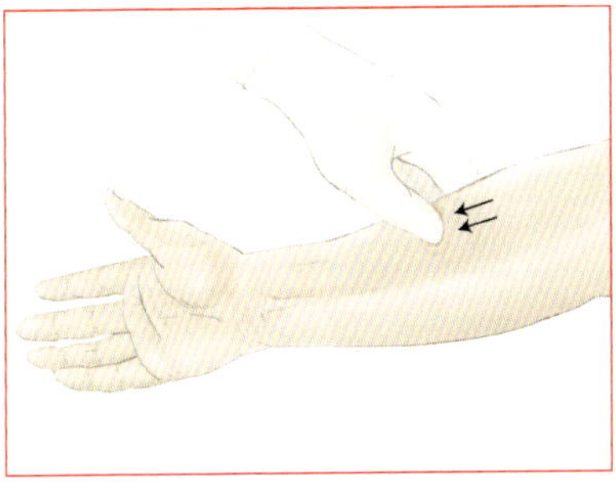

Next, retract the skin, which allows easier insertion by reducing needle drag on the skin and surrounding tissues. To retract, pull the skin downward tightly, with your thumb placed 3" below the chosen insertion site, as shown. Pulling downward also reduces pain and anchors the vein in place, allowing a quick, smooth entry and preventing the vein from rolling during venipuncture.

When entering a superficial vein (which is visible), insert the catheter through the skin at a 0- to 5-degree angle.

When entering a deep vein, insert the catheter through the skin at a 5- to 15-degree angle, as shown. Keep in mind that although you can palpate a deep vein, you can't visualize it because a layer of fascia or fat covers the vein under the skin.

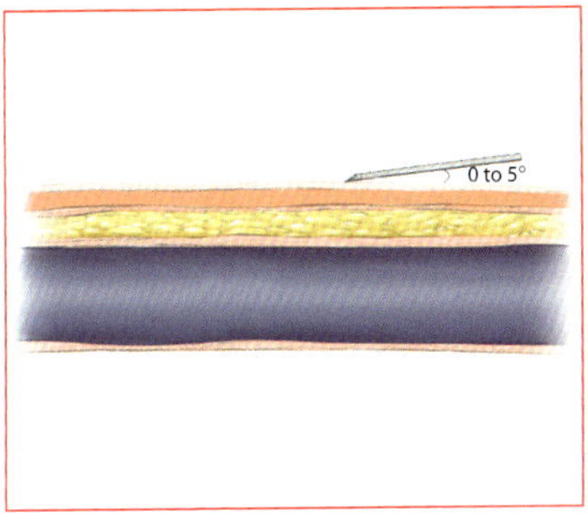

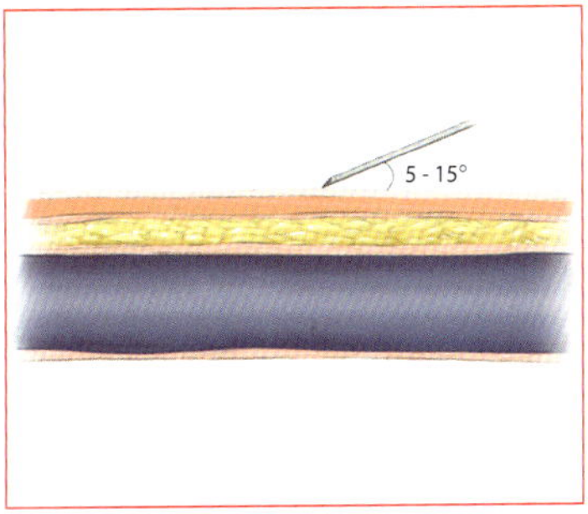

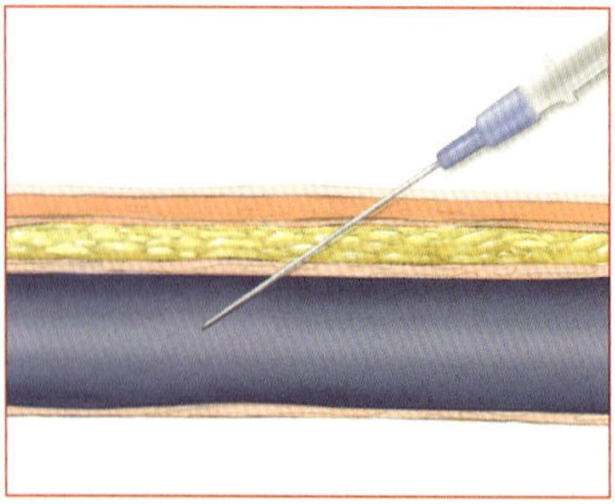

Still pulling tightly downward on the skin, use a quick stabbing motion to insert the catheter through the skin and into the vein. Be sure to insert the catheter directly on top of the vein, as shown—not on the side of the vein. When the catheter has entered the bloodstream, blood return will appear in the flashback chamber of the catheter.

Advancing the catheter

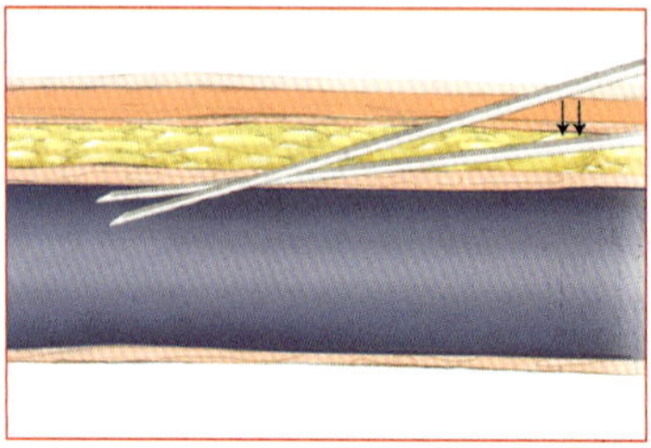

Once you see the blood return, level off the entry angle of the catheter by lowering the flashback chamber flat onto the skin, as shown. While retracting the skin, advance the catheter slightly until one-third of it is in the vein. Then remove the tourniquet to prevent blood from leaking through the catheter air vent.

Removing the stylet

Remove the stylet from the catheter by holding the color-coded hub with one hand and withdrawing the stylet with the other hand. Be sure to follow the manufacturer's directions. Discard the stylet into a sharps container. Never try to reinsert the stylet into the catheter while the catheter is in the vein, as this can cause shearing of the catheter tip and lead to a catheter emboli.

After removing the stylet, immediately connect the I.V. tubing or a needleless injection port to the catheter hub. Then retract the skin tightly and advance the catheter to the hub.

Applying a dressing

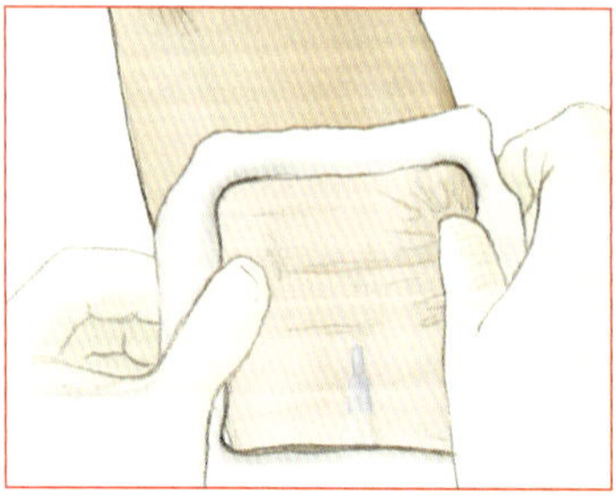

Cover the I.V. site with a transparent semipermeable membrane (TSM) dressing—the dressing of choice because it allows frequent visual assessment of the I.V. site without tampering. Position the dressing over the I.V. insertion site and smooth it from the center to the edges, as shown. Don't tape the edges or apply nonsterile tape under the dressing. The dressing should stabilize the catheter, preventing catheter movement. Change a TSM dressing when it becomes damp, loose, or soiled.

Use a gauze dressing only if the patient is allergic to transparent dressings. When using gauze, position it over the insertion site and seal all edges with tape. Change the dressing every 48 hours, or whenever it becomes moist or drainage appears.

Monitoring and aftercare

Flush saline locks every 8 hours with 2 to 3 ml of saline solution to maintain patency.

- Inspect the I.V. insertion site at least every 4 hours if the patient is receiving a nonvesicant infusion. If the patient's receiving a vasopressor, vesicant, or caustic solution, assess the I.V. site at least every 2 hours. Swelling and coolness at the I.V. site are the main signs of infiltration and extravasation which may cause extensive soft-tissue necrosis.
- Remove the I.V. catheter at the first sign of an I.V.-related complication. If extravasation occurs, stop the infusion and notify the physician immediately to obtain treatment orders; treatment delays can lead to severe injury. Also, check your facility's policy on treating infiltrations and extravasations.
- Monitor an infiltrated I.V. site for skin color changes and temperature changes; if either occurs, notify the physician immediately. Don't apply warm or cool compresses to the compromised site, and don't elevate the arm.
- Prolonged I.V. drug therapy requires multiple venipunctures. Rotate a peripheral I.V. catheter site every 72 hours. However, in some circumstances, less-frequent rotation is acceptable, depending on the catheter site, vein, length and type of prescribed I.V. therapy, and ease of venous access. (For instance, for a patient with poor veins, 72-hour rotation may be impractical.)
- Pediatric I.V. sites don't need to be rotated on a routine schedule. A midline catheter can stay in place for 2 to 4 weeks.

Removing the I.V. catheter

To remove the catheter, use aseptic technique. Carefully remove the dressing and tape. Then don gloves. While lightly applying two fingers of one hand above the insertion site, withdraw the catheter slowly. Apply pressure over the site for 30 seconds to 2 minutes, or until bleeding stops. Once the bleeding has stopped, an adhesive bandage can be applied.

Documentation

A nursing responsibility and legal requirement, documentation conveys pertinent information about the patient's venous status and I.V. site to all healthcare team members. Document the date, time, anatomical location of the accessed vein, type of insertion device used (including length and gauge), I.V. medications or solutions delivered and their administration rate, and patient tolerance of the procedure. The nurse who inserted the I.V. device should sign the documentation sheet.

Continue to document your ongoing assessment of the I.V. site. For instance, "No signs of I.V.-related complications observed" denotes that you saw no complications at the I.V. site. After removing the I.V. catheter, document the location of the I.V. site, reason for removal, and condition of the site.

Adapted with permission from Perivascular Nurse Consultants, Inc.

Preventing and treating extravasation

Extravasation—escape of a vesicant drug into surrounding tissues—can result from a damaged vein or from leakage around a venipuncture site. Vesicant drugs (such as daunorubicin and vincristine) can cause severe tissue damage if extravasation occurs.

To help prevent extravasation, make sure the existing I.V. line is patent before you administer a drug by the I.V. route. Check patency by:
- inspecting the site for edema or pain
- flushing the I.V. line with 0.9% sodium chloride solution
- gently aspirating blood from the catheter.

Alternatively, you may insert a new I.V. catheter to ensure correct catheter placement. For vesicant drugs, consider using a central venous catheter.

If extravasation occurs, stop the infusion at once. Aspirate the remaining drug from the catheter and remove the I.V. line (unless you need the catheter to administer an antidote). If the extravasated drug was daunorubicin or doxorubicin, apply a cold compress to the area; if it was vinblastine or vincristine, apply a warm compress. Then instill the appropriate antidote according to facility policy.

Administering antidotes

Antidotes for extravasation typically are either given through the existing I.V. line or injected subcutaneously around the infiltrated site using a 1-ml tuberculin syringe. Be sure to use a new needle for each antidote injection.

Extravasated drug	Antidote and dosage
• aminophylline • calcium solutions • contrast media • dextrose solutions (concentrations of 10% or more) • etoposide • nafcillin • potassium solutions • teniposide • total parenteral nutrition solutions • vinblastine • vincristine • vindesine	**hyaluronidase:** 15 units/ml, as 0.2 ml subcutaneous injection near extravasation site
• dactinomycin	**ascorbic acid injection:** 50 mg
• daunorubicin • doxorubicin	**hydrocortisone sodium succinate:** 100 mg/ml: 50 to 200 mg
• dopamine • epinephrine • metaraminol • norepinephrine	**phentolamine:** 5 to 10 mg diluted in 10 to 15 ml of normal saline solution, administered within 12 hours of extravasation
• mechlorethamine	**sodium thiosulfate 10%:** 10 ml

High-alert drugs

Certain drugs expose patients to an increased risk of significant harm when used in error. In 2007, the Institute for Safe Medication Practices (ISMP) updated its list of high-alert drugs based on voluntary medication error reports, harmful medication errors described in the literature, practitioner feedback, and expert reviews. The ISMP has identified both high-alert drug classes (or categories) and specific high-alert drugs.

High-alert drug classes and categories	Specific high-alert drugs
• adrenergic agonists, I.V. • adrenergic antagonists, I.V. • anesthetic agents, general, inhaled and I.V. • antiarrhythmics, I.V. • anticoagulants • cardioplegic solutions • chemotherapeutic agents • dextrose (20% or greater) • dialysis solutions • epidural and intrathecal drugs • glycoprotein IIb/IIIa inhibitors • hypoglycemics, oral • inotropic drugs, I.V. • liposomal drug forms • moderate sedation agents, I.V. (or oral agents for children) • narcotics and opioids • neuromuscular blocking agents • radiocontrast agents, I.V. • thrombolytics and fibrinolytics, I.V. • total parenteral nutrition solutions	• amiodarone, I.V. • colchicine, injection • epoprostenol • heparin, low molecular weight • heparin, unfractionated, I.V. • insulin, subcutaneous and I.V. • lidocaine, I.V. • magnesium sulfate injection • methotrexate, oral nononcologic use • oxytocin • potassium chloride for injection • potassium phosphates injection • promethazine, I.V. • sodium chloride injection • sodium nitroprusside for injection • sterile water for injection, inhalation, and irrigation in containers of 100 ml or more • warfarin

Hazardous I.V. drugs

The I.V. drugs listed below have been designated as hazardous by the National Institute for Occupational Safety and Health, Centers for Disease Control and Prevention, and/or the American Society of Health-System Pharmacists. The list doesn't include all hazardous I.V. drugs. The agents listed here meet one or more of the following criteria: carcinogenicity, teratogenicity or other developmental toxicity, reproductive toxicity, organ toxicity at low doses, genotoxicity, or structure and toxicity profiles that mimic existing drugs determined to be hazardous by the above criteria. All healthcare workers handling these drugs must follow appropriate precautions along with recommendations included in the manufacturer's complete package insert.

- Aldesleukin
- Alemtuzumab
- Amifostine
- Arsenic trioxide
- Asparaginase
- Azacitidine
- Bleomycin
- Bortezomib
- Busulfan
- Carboplatin
- Carmustine
- Chloramphenicol
- Cidofovir
- Cisplatin
- Cladribine
- Clofarabine
- Colchicine
- Cyclophosphamide
- Cytarabine
- Cyclosporine
- Dacarbazine
- Dactinomycin
- Daunorubicin HCl
- Denileukin
- Docetaxel
- Doxorubicin
- Epirubicin
- Estramustine phosphate sodium
- Estrogen-progestin combinations
- Estrogens, conjugated
- Etoposide
- Fluorouracil
- Ganciclovir
- Gemcitabine
- Gemtuzumab ozogamicin
- Goserelin
- Ibritumomab tiuxetan
- Idarubicin
- Ifosfamide
- Interferon alfa-2a
- Interferon alfa-2b
- Irinotecan HCl
- Mechlorethamine
- Melphalan
- Methotrexate
- Mitomycin
- Mitoxantrone HCl
- Mycophenolate mofetil
- Oxaliplatin
- Oxytocin
- Paclitaxel
- Pegaspargase
- Pentamidine isethionate
- Pentostatin
- Plicamycin
- Prednimustine
- Tacrolimus
- Teniposide
- Thiotepa
- Topotecan
- Tositumomab
- Vinblastine sulfate
- Vincristine sulfate
- Vinorelbine tartrate
- Zidovudine

Guidelines for handling, preparing, and administering hazardous drugs

Healthcare professionals who work with or near hazardous drugs may be exposed to these agents in the air; on work surfaces, clothing, or medical equipment; or through contact with patient urine or feces. Hazardous drugs include many cancer chemotherapy agents, antivirals, hormones, and certain miscellaneous drugs. (Follow these hazardous drug guidelines for handling, preparation, and administration of all drugs with the special "hazardous drug" icon [⊗] at the top of the monograph.)

The safety of healthcare workers who handle hazardous drugs is an ongoing concern. More than 5 million healthcare workers, including nurses, pharmacists, and physicians, are thought to be at risk. The greatest exposure occurs during preparation, administration, and disposal of these agents. In 2004, the National Institute for Occupational Safety and Health (NIOSH) issued an alert to inform workers of the possible risks of hazardous drugs. The alert included the following:

Warning! Working with or near hazardous drugs in healthcare settings may cause skin rashes, infertility, miscarriage, birth defects, and possibly leukemia or other cancers.

In 2006, the American Society of Health-System Pharmacists (ASHP) published revised guidelines on handling hazardous drugs. The following guidelines reflect the latest recommendations of ASHP, NIOSH, and the Centers for Disease Control and Prevention.

General preparation

- Read all material safety data sheets for each hazardous drug you handle.
- Prepare hazardous drugs in a controlled area designated for that purpose alone and restricted to authorized personnel. Identify these areas clearly with warning signs.
- Prepare hazardous drugs inside a ventilated cabinet with negative air pressure, to avoid spread of airborne drug contaminants and protect drugs that require sterile handling.
- Always work below eye level, within easy reach of a spill kit and a hazardous drug waste container.
- Wash hands with soap and water immediately before and after preparation.
- Use stringent sterile technique during any procedure in which sterile dosage forms are manipulated with needles and syringes.
- Whenever possible, use luer-lock syringes, I.V. administration sets, and connections, as these are less likely to separate during preparation.
- When supplemental protection is needed, use closed-system drug-transfer devices, glove bags, and needleless systems inside the ventilated cabinet.

(continued)

- Know that hazardous drugs must be clearly labeled or otherwise identified to prevent improper handling during preparation, transport, and use. Preparation and cleaning areas also need to be identified with warning signs or labels, and must be clear to non-English readers.

Personal protective equipment

Always wear personal protective equipment (PPE) during any activity involving hazardous drugs, including:
- reconstituting or admixing these drugs
- handling vials or finished products
- opening drug packaging
- assembling the delivery system
- administering these drugs
- labeling hazardous containers
- disposing of drug-related waste
- handling excretions from patients who have received hazardous drugs.

Gloves

- Wear two pairs of high-quality, powder-free gloves. Make sure the inner pair is beneath the cuff of your gown and the outer pair covers the outside cuff.
- Before donning gloves, inspect them for defects.
- Remove the outer gloves after wiping down the final drug preparation but before labeling or removing it from the designated area. Place these gloves in a containment bag.
- Use clean gloves (the inner pair) to wipe the surface of the container, put the label on the final drug preparation, and place the drug container into the pass-through.
- Don fresh gloves to complete the final check, place the container for transport, and remove it from the pass-through.
- Change gloves every 30 minutes during compounding, or immediately if they become damaged or contaminated.

Gown

Wear a disposable, nonabsorbent gown made of polypropylene material with a closed front, long sleeves, and elastic cuffs.

Face and eye shield

Wear a face or eye shield (as appropriate) if splashes, sprays, or aerosolizations to the eyes, nose, or mouth are possible during drug handling or administration.

Proper sequence for donning PPE

After washing your hands, don the first pair of gloves, then the gown and face shield (as appropriate), and then the second pair of gloves (which should extend beyond the cuff of your gown).

Dose reconstitution

- Avoid pressurizing vial contents, as this may cause the drug to spray out around or through the needle. To avoid pressurization, draw air into the syringe to create negative pressure in the vial.

- After drawing up the diluent, insert the needle into the syringe and pull back on the plunger.
- Transfer small amounts of diluent slowly as equal volumes of air are removed.
- Keeping the needle in the vial, swirl contents slowly until they dissolve.
- Make sure the syringe is no more than three-quarters full when it holds the final drug dosage.

Dose withdrawal and transfer

- Keeping the vial inverted, withdraw only the proper amount of drug solution.
- Remove the needle with the vial upright, making sure the needle hub is clear.
- To withdraw a dose from an ampule, gently tap the neck of the ampule. Then wipe the neck with alcohol and attach a 5-micron filter needle to a syringe. Draw the solution through the needle, clearing it from the needle and hub.
- If the drug will be dispensed in the syringe, draw back the plunger to clear fluid from the needle and hub. Replace the needle with a locking cap, and then wipe and lock the syringe.
- When using a needleless system, use gauze pads at connection points to contain leaks.
- If the drug will be transferred to an I.V. bag or bottle, prime the I.V. set before adding the drug. Puncture only the septum of the injection port. After injecting the drug solution into the bag, wipe the port, container, and I.V. set (if attached).
- Once drug preparation is complete, seal the final product in a plastic bag or other sealable container for transport before taking it out of the ventilated cabinet; then label it with a unique identifier. Seal and wipe all waste containers inside the ventilated cabinet before removal. Finally, remove your outer gloves and sleeve covers (if used) and bag them while still inside the ventilated cabinet.

Administration

- Wash your hands and don gloves and gown in the sequence described above. If spraying, splashing, or aerosolization could occur during administration, wear a face shield or goggles.
- Visually examine the drug dose while it's still in the transport bag. If it appears intact, remove it from the bag.
- Place an absorbent pad on the work or administration area to contain spills or contamination.

Oral (noninjectable or nonparenteral) administration

- Oral hazardous drugs should be dispensed in the final dosage and form whenever possible.
- Avoid crushing tablets or opening capsules; instead, use liquid forms whenever possible.
- Never crush or compound an oral drug in an unprotected environment.
- Be aware that liquid hazardous drugs should be dispensed and maintained in sealable plastic bags.
- If the dose appears intact, remove it from the transport bag and administer the drug to the patient.

(continued)

I.M. or subcutaneous administration

- If the dose appears intact, remove it from the transport bag.
- Remove the syringe cap and connect the appropriate safety needle.
- Don't expel air from the syringe or prime the safety needle.
- After administering the dose, discard the syringe (with safety needle attached) directly into an appropriate waste container.

I.V. administration

- If the dose appears intact, remove it from the transport bag.
- If priming is necessary at the administration site, prime the I.V. tubing with an I.V. solution that doesn't contain a hazardous drug, or by using the backflow method.
- Place gauze pads under the connections at injection ports to catch leaks during administration.
- Use the transport bag as a containment bag for contaminated materials. Discard hazardous drug bags and bottles with their administration sets attached.

Disposal and clean-up

- Handle hazardous wastes and contaminated materials separately from other trash.
- Wash surfaces contaminated with hazardous drugs with detergent, hypochlorite solution, and neutralizer, as appropriate.
- Clean and decontaminate work areas before and after each hazardous drug-handling activity and at the end of each shift. Clean up small spills immediately.
- Dispose of drug-contaminated syringes and needles in puncture-proof containers labeled "Chemotherapy waste" or "Hazardous waste."
- Never push or force materials contaminated with hazardous drugs into waste containers.

After exposure to a hazardous drug

- In case of skin contact with a cytotoxic drug, immediately remove contaminated clothing and wash the affected area with soap and water. Don't scrub, because this will abrade the skin. Rinse the area thoroughly, and consult a physician for further treatment and monitoring.
- In case of eye contact, flush the affected eye with water or normal saline solution continuously for 15 minutes. Consult a physician for further treatment and monitoring.
- Document the exposure incident in your employee record and your facility's medical surveillance log.
- Know that facilities should routinely monitor all workers who handle hazardous drugs (including symptom complaints, physical findings, and laboratory values) to identify abnormalities. Also, workers who handle or administer hazardous drugs should inform their primary healthcare providers of their occupation and potential exposure.

Avoiding dangerous abbreviations

To help reduce medication errors, all healthcare team members must use abbreviations correctly. The Joint Commission mandates that healthcare organizations standardize a list of abbreviations, acronyms, and symbols that should not be used. Organizations must approve a minimum required list of prohibited abbreviations, which includes the first five items shown below. The Joint Commission also advises organizations to consider adding the remaining items to their "Do not use" list.

Abbreviation	Potential problem	Solution
U (for "unit")	Mistaken as "0," "4," or "cc"	Write "unit."
IU (for "international unit")	Mistaken as "IV" ("intravenous") or 10 ("ten")	Write "international unit."
Q.D., Q.O.D. (for "once daily," "every other day")	Mistaken for each other. Period after "Q" may be mistaken for "I"; "O" may be mistaken for "I."	Write "daily" or "every other day."
Trailing zero (X.0 mg) (prohibited only for drug-related notations); lack of leading zero (.X mg)	Decimal point is missed.	Never write a zero by itself after decimal point (X mg); always use a zero before decimal point (0.X mg).
MS MSO_4 $MgSO_4$	Confused for one another. May mean "morphine sulfate" or "magnesium sulfate."	Write "morphine sulfate" or "magnesium sulfate."
µg (for "microgram")	Mistaken for "mg" (milligrams), resulting in 1,000-fold overdose	Write "mcg."
H.S. (for "half-strength" or "at bedtime")	Mistaken for "half-strength" or "hour of sleep" ("at bedtime")	Write "half-strength" or "at bedtime."
q.H.S. (for "at bedtime")	Mistaken for "every hour"	Write "at bedtime."
T.I.W. (for "3 times a week")	Mistaken for "3 times a day" or "twice weekly"	Write "3 times weekly" or "three times weekly."
S.C. or S.Q. (for "subcutaneous")	Mistaken for "S.L." (sublingual) or "5 every"	Write "Sub-Q," "subQ," or "subcutaneously."
D/C (for "discharge")	Misinterpreted as "discontinue"	Write "discharge."
cc (for "cubic centimeters")	Mistaken for "U" (units) if poorly written	Write "ml" for milliliters.
AS, AD, AU (for "left ear," "right ear," "both ears")	Mistaken for OS, OD, or OU	Write "left ear," "right ear," or "both ears."

Common abbreviations

The abbreviations below are commonly used by nurses. Not all of them, however, are acceptable. Those in red marked with a Clinical Alert logo were identified as contributing to medication errors in the National Patient Safety Goals of the Joint Commission and by the Institute for Safe Medication Practices. To avoid mistakes and to ensure Joint Commission compliancy, spell out the entire term.

ABG	arterial blood gas
a.c.	before meals
ACE	angiotensin-converting enzyme
ACLS	advanced cardiac life support
ACTH	adrenocorticotropic hormone
AD	right ear
ADH	antidiuretic hormone
ADLs	activities of daily living
AICD	automatic implantable cardiac defibrillator
AIDS	acquired immunodeficiency syndrome
ALP	alkaline phosphatase
ALT	alanine aminotransferase
APTT	activated partial thrombo-plastin time
AS	left ear
AST	aspartate aminotransferase
AU	each ear
AV	atrioventricular
B_1	$beta_1$
B_2	$beta_2$
BCLS	basic cardiac life support
b.i.d.	twice daily
BP	blood pressure
BSA	body surface area
B.T.	bedtime
BUN	blood urea nitrogen
c̄	with
C	Celsius
cAMP	cyclic 3', 5' adenosine monophosphate
CBC	complete blood count
cc	cubic centimeter
CI	cardiac index
CK	creatine kinase
cm	centimeter
CMV	cytomegalovirus
CNS	central nervous system
COPD	chronic obstructive pulmonary disease
CR	controlled release
CV	cardiovascular
CVA	cerebrovascular accident
CYP	cytochrome
D_5W	dextrose 5% in water
DIC	disseminated intravascular coagulation
D/C	discharge, discontinue
dl	deciliter
DNA	deoxyribonucleic acid
ECG	electrocardiogram
EEG	electroencephalogram
EENT	eyes, ears, nose, and throat
F	Fahrenheit
FDA	Food and Drug Administration
g	gram
G	gauge
GABA	gamma-aminobutyric acid
GFR	glomerular filtration rate
GGT	gamma-glutamyltransferase
GI	gastrointestinal
GnRH	gonadotropin-releasing hormone
gr	grain
gtt	drops
G6PD	glucose-6-phosphate dehydrogenase
GU	genitourinary
H_1	$histamine_1$
H_2	$histamine_2$
HCL	hydrochloride

Clinical alert. **Do not use.**

HCT	hematocrit
HDL	high-density lipoprotein
Hg	mercury
Hgb	hemoglobin
HIV	human immunodeficiency virus
HMG-CoA	3-hydroxy-3-methylglutaryl coenzyme A
HR	heart rate
🔊 h.s.	at bedtime
🔊 H.S.	half-strength
🔊 I.J.	injection
I.M.	intramuscular
🔊 I.N.	intranasal
INR	International Normalized Ratio
IPPB	intermittent positive-pressure breathing
🔊 IU	international unit
I.V.	intravenous
K	potassium
kg	kilogram
KVO	keep vein open
L	liter
lb	pound
LD	lactate dehydrogenase
LDL	low-density lipoprotein
m	meter
m^2	square meters
🔊 µg	microgram
MAO	monoamine oxidase
mcg	microgram
MDI	metered-dose inhaler
mEq	milliequivalent
mg	milligram
🔊 $MgSO_4$	magnesium sulfate
ml	milliliter
mm	millimeter
mm^3	cubic millimeters
mm Hg	millimeters of mercury
mmol	millimole
🔊 MS	morphine sulfate
🔊 MSO_4	morphine sulfate
Na	sodium
NA	not applicable
NaCl	sodium chloride
ng	nanogram
NG	nasogastric
N.P.O.	nothing by mouth
NSAID	nonsteroidal anti-inflammatory drug
🔊 O.D.	right eye
🔊 O.S.	left eye
OTC	over the counter
🔊 O.U.	each eye
oz	ounce
p.c.	after meals
PCA	patient-controlled analgesia
per	through, by
P.O.	by mouth
P.R.	by rectum
p.r.n.	as needed
PT	prothrombin time
PTT	partial thromboplastin time
PVC	premature ventricular contraction
q	every
🔊 Q.D.	every day
🔊 q.h.s.	at bedtime
q.i.d.	four times daily
🔊 Q.O.D.	every other day
RBC	red blood cell
RDA	recommended dietary allowance
RNA	ribonucleic acid
RSV	respiratory syncytial virus
SA	sinoatrial
🔊 S.C.	subcutaneous
SI	International System of Units
SIADH	syndrome of inappropriate antidiuretic hormone secretion
S.L.	sublingual
🔊 S.Q.	subcutaneous
SSRI	selective serotonin reuptake inhibitor
T_3	triiodothyronine
T_4	thyroxine
TCA	tricyclic antidepressant
t.i.d.	three times daily
🔊 T.I.W.	three times a week
tRNA	transfer ribonucleic acid
tsp	teaspoon
🔊 U	unit
USP	United States Pharmacopeia
VMA	vanillylmandelic acid
WBC	white blood cell

🔊 Clinical alert. **Do not use.**

I.V. drugs and drug names that look or sound alike

The drug names below can easily be confused, verbally or in writing, because they either sound alike or have similar spellings. Drug names can be confused regardless of the route by which they're administered. Some of the groupings below include drugs that aren't given I.V.—but all groupings include at least one I.V. drug. Generic drug names appear in regular type; trade names are capitalized and in boldface.

acetazolamide, acetohexamide
Adderall, **Inderal**
albuterol, atenolol
Aldactazide, Aldactone
Aldomet, Aldoril
Aldoril, Elavil
alfentanil, fentanyl, **Sufenta, sufetanil**
alprazolam, diazepam, lorazepam, midazolam
Altace, alteplase
Amicar, Amikin
amiloride, amiodarone, amlodipine
Anafranil, enalapril
Apresazide, Apresoline
Asacol, Os-Cal, Oxytrol
Atarax, **Ativan**
atenolol, timolol
Avinza, Invanz
azithromycin, erythromycin
Benadryl, Bentyl, Benylin, Betalin
Bumex, Buprenex
bupivacaine, ropivacaine
Calan, **Colace**
Cardene, Cardizem
Cardene, codeine
cefazolin, cefprozil
cefotaxime, ceftizoxime
cefuroximine, deferoxamine
Cefzil, Kefzol
Celexa, Cerebyx
chlorpromazine, chlorpropamide, promethazine
Ciloxan, Cytoxan
ciprofloxacin, ofloxacin
clonidine, quinidine
cycloserine, cyclosporine
dacarbazine, procarbazine
dactinomycin, daunorubicin
danazol, **Dantrium**
dapsone, **Diprosone**
daunorubicin, idarubicin
Decadron, **Percodan**
desoximetasone, dexamethasone
Desoxyn, digitoxin, digoxin
diazepam, **Ditropan**
diazoxide, **Dyazide**
dimenhydrinate, diphenhydramine
Diprivan, Ditropan
dipyridamole, disopyramide
dobutamine, dopamine
doxapram, doxazosin, doxepin, doxycycline
Doxil, Paxil, **Plavix**
dronabinol, droperidol
dyclonine, dicyclomine
Echogen, Epogen
Eldepryl, enalapril
eloxatin, **Exelon**
enalapril, ramipril
ephedrine, epinephrine
esmolol, **Osmitrol**
etidronate, etretinate
folic acid, folinic acid
Foradil, Toradol

fosinopril, lisinopril, **Risperdal**
fosphenytoin, phenytoin
furosemide, torsemide
guaifenesin, guanfacine
Haldol, Stadol
heparin, **Hepsera, Hespan**
hydralazine, hydroxyzine
hydromorphone, morphine
Hyperstat, Nitrostat
imipenem, **Omnipen**
Inderal, Inderide, Isordil
Intropin, Isoptin
Lanoxin, Lasix, Lonox
Levbid, Lithobid
Librax, Librium
Loniten, Lotensin, lovastatin
melphalan, **Mephyton**
meperidine, meprobamate
Mesantoin, Mestinon
metaproterenol, metoprolol
methotrexate, metolazone
metoprolol, misoprostol
mithramycin, mitomycin
naloxone, naltrexone
Navane, Nubain
niacinamide, nicardipine
nicardipine, nifedipine, nimodipine
Norpace, Norpramin
Ocufen, Ocuflox
paclitaxel, paroxetine
pancuronium, pipecuronium
paroxetine, pralidoxime, pyridoxine
pentobarbital, phenobarbital
pentosan, pentostatin
Phenaphen, Phenergan
phentermine, phentolamine
Pitocin, Pitressin
Pravachol, Prevacid
Pravachol, propranolol
Premarin, Primaxin
ProAmatine, protamine
probenecid, **Procanbid**
promazine, promethazine
protamine, **Protopam, Protropin**
quinidine, quinine
ranitidine, rimantadine
Relpax, Revex, Revia
Reminyl, Robinul
Retrovir, ritonavir
rifabutin, rifampin
Rifadin, Rifamate, Rifater
Rifadin, Ritalin, ritodrine
Septa, Septra
Solu-Cortef, Solu-Medrol
Sufenta, Survanta
tegaserod, **Tegretol, Toradol**
terbutaline, tolbutamide
thiamine, **Thorazine**
Ticar, Tigan
Tobradex, Tobrex
tolazamide, tolbutamide
Trandate, Tridate
VePesid, Versed
verapamil, **Verelan**
Verelan, Virilon
vinblastine, vincristine, vindesine, vinorelbine
Xanax, Zantac
Zantac, Zyrtec
Zofran, Zosyn

Monitoring blood levels

The table below shows therapeutic and toxic blood levels for selected drugs. Keep in mind that such levels may vary slightly among laboratories.

Drug	Therapeutic blood level	Toxic blood level
acetaminophen	10 to 20 mcg/ml	> 150 mcg/ml
alprazolam	0.025 to 0.102 mcg/ml	Not defined
amikacin	Peak: 25 to 35 mcg/ml	> 35 mcg/ml
	Trough: 5 to 10 mcg/ml	> 10 mcg/ml
aminophylline	10 to 20 mcg/ml	> 20 mcg/ml
amiodarone	1 to 2.5 mcg/ml	> 2.5 mcg/ml
amitriptyline	120 to 250 ng/ml	> 500 ng/ml
amobarbital	1 to 5 mcg/ml	> 10 mcg/ml
atenolol	0.2 to 0.7 mcg/ml	35 mcg/ml
bepridil	1 to 2 ng/ml	> 2 ng/ml
calcium	9 to 10.5 mg/dl	> 12 mg/dl
carbamazepine	4 to 14 mcg/ml	> 15 mcg/ml
clonazepam	10 to 80 ng/ml	> 100 ng/ml
creatinine	0.6 to 1.2 mg/dl	> 4 mg/dl
cyclosporine	50 to 300 ng/ml	> 400 ng/ml
desipramine	115 to 300 ng/ml	> 400 ng/ml
diazepam	0.5 to 2 mcg/ml	> 3 mcg/ml
digoxin	0.8 to 2 ng/ml	Adults: > 2.5 ng/ml
	Trough (> 12 hours after dose):	Children: > 3 ng/ml
	Heart failure: 0.8 to 1.5 ng/ml	
	Arrhythmias: 1.5 to 2 ng/ml	
diltiazem	0.05 to .40 mcg/ml	3.7 to 6.1 mcg/ml
diphenylhydantoin	10 to 20 mcg/ml	20 to 50 mcg/ml
disopyramide	2 to 8 mcg/ml	> 8 mcg/ml
ethchlorvynol	2 to 8 mcg/ml	> 20 mcg/ml
ethosuximide	40 to 100 mcg/ml	> 100 mcg/ml
flecainide	0.2 to 1 mcg/ml	> 1 mcg/ml
fluconazole	5 to 15 mcg/ml	Not defined
fluoxetine	0.09 to 0.40 mcg/ml	Not defined
gentamicin	Peak: 4 to 12 mcg/ml	> 12 mcg/ml
	Trough: 1 to 2 mcg/ml	> 2 mcg/ml
glucose	70 to 110 mg/dl	> 300 mg/dl
glutethimide	2 to 6 mcg/ml	> 5 mcg/ml
haloperidol	5 to 20 ng/ml	> 20 ng/ml
hydromorphone	0.008 to 0.049 mcg/ml	Not defined

Drug	Therapeutic blood level	Toxic blood level
imipramine	225 to 300 ng/ml	> 500 ng/ml
kanamycin	Peak: 25 to 35 mcg/ml	> 35 to 40 mcg/ml
	Trough (mild to moderate infection): 1 to 4 mcg/ml	> 10 to 15 mcg/ml
	Trough (severe infection): 4 to 8 mcg/ml	> 10 to 15 mcg/ml
lidocaine	1.5 to 6 mcg/ml	> 6 mcg/ml
lithium	0.6 to 1.2 mEq/L	> 1.5 mEq/L
lorazepam	50 to 240 ng/ml	300 to 600 ng/ml
magnesium	12 to 32 mcg/ml	80 to 120 mcg/ml
meperidine	100 to 550 ng/ml	> 1,000 ng/ml
meprobamate	6 to 12 mcg/ml	> 60 mcg/ml
methsuximide	10 to 40 mcg/ml	> 44 mcg/ml
metoprolol	0.03 to 0.27 mcg/ml	Not defined
mezlocillin	35 to 45 mcg/ml	> 45 mcg/ml
milrinone	150 to 250 ng/ml	> 250 ng/ml
nifedipine	0.025 to 0.1 mcg/ml	> 0.1 mcg/ml
nortriptyline	50 to 140 ng/ml	> 300 ng/ml
oxazepam	0.2 to 1.4 mcg/ml	> 2 mcg/ml
paroxetine	0.031 to 0.062 mcg/ml	Not defined
phenobarbital	10 to 40 mcg/ml	> 40 mcg/ml
phenytoin	10 to 20 mcg/ml	> 20 mcg/ml
potassium	3.5 to 5.0 mEq/L	> 6 mEq/L
primidone	4 to 12 mcg/ml	> 12 mcg/ml
procainamide	4 to 8 mcg/ml	> 10 mcg/ml
propofol	2 to 16 mcg/ml	Not defined
propranolol	50 to 200 ng/ml	> 200 ng/ml
quinidine	2 to 5 mcg/ml	> 5 mcg/ml
salicylates	100 to 300 mcg/ml	> 300 mcg/ml
sertraline	0.055 to 0.25 mcg/ml	Not defined
sodium	135 to 145 mEq/L	> 160 mEq/L
streptomycin	25 mcg/ml	> 25 mcg/ml
theophylline	10 to 20 mcg/ml	> 20 mcg/ml
tobramycin	Peak: 4 to 12 mcg/ml	> 12 mcg/ml
	Trough: 1 to 2 mcg/ml	> 2 mcg/ml
tocainide	4 to 10 mcg/ml	Not defined
valproic acid	50 to 100 mcg/ml	> 100 mcg/ml
vancomycin	Peak: 20 to 40 mcg/ml	> 40 mcg/ml
	Trough: 5 to 15 mcg/ml	> 15 mcg/ml
verapamil	0.08 to 0.3 mcg/ml	Not defined
zolpidem	0.003 to 0.018 mcg/ml	Not defined

Anaphylaxis: Treatment guidelines

A hypersensitivity reaction may occur when a patient comes in contact with a certain agent, such as a drug, food, or other foreign protein. In some patients, this reaction progresses to life-threatening anaphylaxis, marked by sudden development of urticaria and respiratory distress. If this reaction continues, it may precipitate vascular collapse, leading to shock and, occasionally, death.

Hypersensitivity reaction

Adults: Epinephrine 0.2 to 0.5 ml of 1:1,000 solution subcutaneously or intramuscularly; repeat q 10 to 15 minutes to maximum dosage of 1 mg.
Children: Epinephrine 10 mcg/kg of 1:1,000 solution subcutaneously or intramuscularly, to maximum of 500 mcg/dose; may repeat q 15 minutes for 2 doses, then q 4 hours p.r.n.

↓

Adults or children: Diphenhydramine 1 to 2 mg/kg I.V.or I.M.

↓

Adults: Hydrocortisone 100 mg I.V. initially; then administer as indicated.
Children: Hydrocortisone 0.16 to 1 mg/kg I.V. given once or twice daily

↓

If poor response, use anaphylaxis algorithm.

Anaphylaxis

Administer CPR if patient loses circulation or breathing; follow Advanced Cardiac Life Support guidelines.

↓

If hypotension occurs, give vasopressors (such as dopamine, norepinephrine, or neosynephrine). Provide fluid resuscitation with large volumes of normal saline or lactated Ringer's solution.

↓

Adults and children: If bronchospasm occurs, give 1 to 2 nebulized treatments of inhaled bronchodilator and consider loading dose of 6 mg/kg theophylline I.V., followed by maintenance dose as indicated.

↓

Adults: Epinephrine 0.2 to 0.5 ml of 1:1,000 solution subcutaneously or intramuscularly; repeat q 10 to 15 minutes to maximum dosage of 1 mg.
Children: Epinephrine 10 mcg/kg of 1:1,000 solution subcutaneously or intramuscularly; to maximum of 500 mcg/dose; may repeat dose q 15 minutes for 2 doses, then q 4 hours as needed

↓

If patient doesn't respond, dilute epinephrine to yield 1:10,000 solution. For adults, infuse at 1 mcg/minute; may titrate to 2 to 10 mcg/minute. For children, infuse at 0.1 mcg/kg/minute.

KEY:
CPR: cardiopulmonary resuscitation

Adult cardiac arrest: Treatment guidelines

If you suspect your patient is in cardiac arrest, take appropriate steps, as described below.

Assess responsiveness.

Unresponsive

Begin primary survey. Activate emergency response system. Call for defibrillator. Assess breathing (open airway; look, listen, and feel for breathing).

Not breathing

Give two breaths. Assess pulse, if pulseless, start chest compressions. Continue CPR for 2 minutes (5 cycles of 30 compressions to 2 breaths). Assess pulse and cardiac rhythm. Attach monitor or defibrillator.

No pulse

Initiate CPR (5 cycles of 30 compressions to 2 breaths) for 2 minutes. Assess cardiac rhythm.

VF or VT on monitor

Administer CPR until defibrillator charged: Give 1 shock (360j for monophasic defibrillator; 200j for biphasic defibrillator). Immediately restart CPR for 2 minutes. After 2 minutes, check cardiac rhythm and pulse; if VF or VT, give 1 shock (360j for monophasic defribrillator or 200 to 300j for biphasic defibrillator). Start CPR immediately after the shock is delivered. Continue CPR for 2 minutes. Assess pulse and cardiac rhythm.

Asystole or PEA on monitor

Administer CPR for 2 minutes. After 2 minutes of CPR, check cardiac rhythm and pulse, then immediately restart CPR if PEA and asystole persist. Always verify asystole in 2 leads.

Conduct secondary ABCD survey

Airway: Attempt to insert airway device. Once an advanced airway is in place, give 8 to 10 breaths/minute and continuous chest compressions at 100 per minute.

Breathing: Confirm and secure airway device; provide ventilation and oxygenation.

Circulation: Obtain I.V. or I.O. access, administer adrenergic drug; consider antiarrhythmics, buffer agents, and pacing. For asystole or PEA, give epinephrine 1 mg I.V.; repeat every 3 to 5 minutes. Give vasopressin 40 units to replace the first or second dose of epinephrine. For PEA with a rate less than 60/minute, consider atropine 1 mg every 3 to 5 minutes for a total dose of 3 mg. For VF/VT, give Epinephrine 1 mg I.V or I.O.; repeat every 3 to 5 minutes. May use vasopressin 40 units to replace the first or second dose of epinephrine.

Differential diagnosis: Search for and treat reversible causes.

KEY
ABCD: airway, breathing, circulation, differential diagnosis
CPR: cardiopulmonary resuscitation
I.O.: intraosseous
PEA: pulseless electrical activity
VF: ventricular fibrillation
VT: ventricular tachycardia

Pediatric cardiac arrest: Treatment guidelines

For a pediatric patient in suspected cardiac arrest, take the following steps.

Assess responsiveness.

Unresponsive
Begin primary survey. Activate emergency response system.
Attach monitor/defibrillator as soon as available.
Assess breathing (open airway; look, listen, and feel for breathing).

Not breathing
Give two breaths that make the chest rise.
Assess pulse. Start chest compressions (5 cycles of 30 compressions to 2 breaths) if patient is pulseless.

No pulse
Continue CPR. Assess heart rhythm.

VF or VT on monitor
Attempt defibrillation
Deliver 1 shock at 2 J/kg. Resume CPR immediately for 2 minutes.
After 2 minutes, if VF or pulseless VT continues. Deliver 1 shock at 4 J/kg. Give epinephrine I.V. or I.O. at 0.01 mg/kg.
Resume CPR immediately for 2 minutes.
After 2 minutes, if VF or pulseless VT continues. Deliver 1 shock at 4 J/kg.

Asystole or PEA on monitor
Give epinephrine 0.01 mg/kg I.V. or I.O. Continue CPR for 2 minutes then reassess; pulse and cardiac rythm. Always verify asystole in 2 leads.

Conduct secondary ABCD survey
Airway: Attempt to insert airway device.
Breathing: Confirm and secure airway device; ventilate and oxygenate.
Circulation: Obtain I.V. access; defibrillate and give drugs as appropriate.
*For VF/VT, give epinephrine 0.01 mg/kg (0.1 ml/kg of 1:10,000 solution) I.V. or I.O.; repeat q 3 to 5 minutes; then consider amiodarone or lidocaine.
For asystole, give epinephrine 0.01 mg/kg (0.1 ml/kg of 1:10,000 solution) I.V. or I.O.; repeat q 3 to 5 minutes.
Differential diagnosis: Search for and treat reversible causes, including hypoxemia, hypovolemia, metabolic disorders, and thromboembolism.

KEY
ABDC: airway, breathing, circulation, differential diagnosis
CPR: cardiopulmonary resuscitation
I.O.: intraosseus
J: joules
PEA: pulseless electrical activity
VF: ventricular fibrillation
VT: ventricular tachycardia

• Aim diluent stream so it runs down side of vial—not directly into powder. Swirl gently until powder dissolves completely.
• Know that reconstituted solution should be clear and colorless. Do not use if discolored.
• Administer within 3 hours of reconstitution.
Do not mix with infusion solutions.
• Discard unused solution.

Infusion considerations
Give only by slow I.V. bolus over 2 to 5 minutes, depending on dosage.

Monitoring
Monitor for signs and symptoms of coagulation activation or thrombosis.
• Be aware that laboratory coagulation parameters may be used in addition to clinical evaluation of hemostasis to monitor drug efficacy and treatment schedule. However, these parameters lack direct correlation with achieving hemostasis.

Storage
• Before reconstitution, refrigerate at 2° to 8°C (36° to 46°F). Protect from sunlight.

Contraindications and precautions

Contraindicated in hypersensitivity to drug or mouse, hamster, or bovine products.

Use cautiously in pregnant or breast-feeding patients and in ***children*** (dosages based on weight, not age).

Adverse reactions

CNS: headache
CV: hypertension, hypotension, bradycardia
GU: renal dysfunction
Hematologic: purpura, **hemorrhage, hemarthrosis, disseminated intravascular coagulation, coagulation disorders, decreased fibrinogen plasma, thrombosis**
Musculoskeletal: arthrosis
Skin: pruritus, rash
Other: fever, edema, pain, redness or reaction at injection site, hypersensitivity reaction

Interactions

Drug-drug. *Activated prothrombin complex concentrates, prothrombin complex concentrates:* risk of potential interaction

Toxicity and overdose

• Known overdoses have not caused significant complications. Expect extension of adverse reactions.
• Provide symptomatic and supportive therapy.

Patient teaching

• Instruct patient to report swelling, pain, burning, or itching at infusion site.
• Tell patient to inform prescriber if she is pregnant or intends to become pregnant.
• As appropriate, review all other significant and life-threatening adverse reactions and interactions, especially those related to the drugs mentioned above.

codeine phosphate

Pharmacologic class: Opioid agonist
Therapeutic class: Opioid analgesic
Controlled substance schedule II
Pregnancy risk category C

Action

Binds to opiate receptors in CNS, altering perception of painful stimuli. Causes generalized CNS depression, decreases cough reflex, and reduces GI motility.

Pharmacokinetics

Drug distributes widely throughout tissues, crosses placental barrier, and is secreted in breast milk. It is metabolized mainly in the liver, and is excreted mainly in urine as unchanged drug, norcodeine, and free and conjugated morphine.

Onset	Peak	Duration
Rapid	Unknown	Unknown

How supplied

Solution for injection: 30 mg/mL, 60 mg/mL

Indications and dosages

➢ Mild to moderate pain

Adults: 15 to 60 mg I.V. q 4 to 6 hours. Usual daily dosage is 30 mg; maximum daily dosage is 360 mg.

Dosage adjustment

- Reduce dosage as appropriate in elderly or debilitated patients; consider effect of initial dosage in determining subsequent dosages.
- When giving with other opioid analgesics, sedative-hypnotics, or other CNS depressants, reduce dosage of one or both drugs.
- Reduce dosage in renal disease. With creatinine clearance of 10 to 50 mL/minute, give 75% of dose; with clearance below 10 mL/minute, give 50% of dose.

Administration

Preparation

- When changing administration route, be aware that oral dose is two-thirds as effective as parenteral dose.

Do not give I.V. to children.

Dilution and compatibility

- Do not mix with other solutions; drug is not compatible with other drugs.

Infusion considerations

- Place patient in supine position during administration.
- Titrate dosage to appropriate analgesic effect.

Monitoring

- Monitor vital signs and CNS status.
- Assess pain level and efficacy of pain relief.
- Evaluate patient for adverse reactions.
- Assess other drugs in patient's regimen for those that could cause additive or adverse interactions.
- Monitor patient for signs and symptoms of drug dependence and tolerance.

Storage

- Store at room temperature, protected from light.

Contraindications and precautions

Contraindicated in hypersensitivity to opioids, respiratory disease, labor and delivery of preterm neonate, and ***preterm neonates.***

Use cautiously in severe renal, hepatic, or pulmonary disease; adrenal insufficiency; head trauma; hypothyroidism; increased intracranial pressure; prostatic hypertrophy; undiagnosed abdominal pain; alcoholism; ***elderly patients;*** and pregnant or breastfeeding patients.

Adverse reactions

CNS: confusion, sedation, malaise, agitation, euphoria, floating feeling, headache, hallucinations, unusual dreams, apathy, mood changes

CV: hypotension, bradycardia, peripheral vasodilation, reduced peripheral resistance

EENT: blurred or double vision, miosis, reddened sclera

GI: nausea, vomiting, constipation, decreased gastric motility

GU: urine retention, urinary tract spasms, urinary urgency

Respiratory: suppressed cough reflex, **respiratory depression**

Skin: flushing, sweating

Other: physical or psychological drug dependence, drug tolerance

Interactions

Drug-drug. *Antidepressants, antihistamines, sedative-hypnotics:* additive CNS depression
Nalbuphine, pentazocine: decreased analgesic effect
Opioid partial agonists (buprenorphine, butorphanol, nalbuphine, pentazocine): precipitation of opioid withdrawal in physically dependent patients
Drug-herb. *Chamomile, hops, kava, skullcap, valerian:* increased CNS depression
Drug-behaviors. *Alcohol use:* increased CNS depression

Toxicity and overdose

- In overdose, expect CNS and respiratory depression, GI cramping, constipation, hypotension, bradycardia, and clammy skin.
- Protect airway and support ventilation. Maintain vital signs, serum electrolytes, and blood gas values. Give naloxone I.V., as prescribed; repeat administration, as needed (up to manufacturer's recommended maximum dosage) to reverse toxic effects. Do not give antagonist in absence of clinically significant respiratory or cardiovascular depression.

Patient teaching

- Instruct patient to report shortness of breath, difficulty breathing, or pronounced nausea, vomiting, or constipation.
- Advise patient to increase fluid intake (unless prescriber orders fluid restriction) to relieve constipation and to take stool softener or mild laxative, as prescribed.
- Caution patient to avoid driving and other hazardous activities until drug's effects on concentration, alertness, vision, coordination, and physical dexterity are known.
- Instruct patient to move slowly when sitting up or standing to avoid dizziness or light-headedness from sudden blood pressure decrease.
- As appropriate, review all other significant and life-threatening adverse reactions and interactions, especially those related to the drugs, herbs, and behaviors mentioned above.

colchicine

Pharmacologic class: Colchicum alkaloid
Therapeutic class: Antigout drug
Pregnancy risk category C

Action

Unclear. Antigout action may occur through white blood cell (WBC) migration and reduced lactic acid production by WBCs. This action in turn decreases uric acid deposition, kinetin formation, and phagocytosis, leading to reduction in inflammatory response.

Pharmacokinetics

Drug concentrates in WBCs and distributes rapidly into many body tissues (except skeletal muscle, heart, and brain). It is partially metabolized in the liver and some other tissues. It is excreted primarily in urine, with some excretion in feces and breast milk.

Onset	Peak	Duration
12 hr	24-72 hr	Unknown

How supplied

Solution for injection: 1 mg/2-mL (0.5 mg/mL) vials

Indications and dosages

➤ Acute gouty arthritis

Adults: 2 mg I.V., followed by 0.5 mg I.V. q 6 hours as needed, not to exceed 4 mg daily

Dosage adjustment
- Reduce dosage in mild hepatic or renal impairment.

Off-label uses
- Chronic progressive multiple sclerosis
- Dermatitis herpetiformis
- Hepatic cirrhosis
- Psoriasis
- Pyoderma gangrenosum associated with Crohn's disease

Administration
Preparation
Follow hazardous drug guidelines on page S19 for handling, preparation, and administration.
- Initiate therapy at first sign of acute gout attack.

Dilution and compatibility
Do not dilute with D_5W. If dilution is required, use normal saline solution.

Infusion considerations
Do not administer I.M. or subcutaneously, as severe local irritation may occur.
- Give by slow I.V. push over 2 to 5 minutes.

Use extreme caution during I.V. injection to avoid extravasation. Know that fluid extravasation may lead to shock.

Monitoring
Stay alert for signs and symptoms of toxicity (nausea, vomiting, abdominal pain, bloody diarrhea, burning sensation, muscle weakness, oliguria, hematuria, ascending paralysis, delirium, and seizures).
- Monitor complete blood count and renal function test results regularly.
- Be aware that opioids may be needed to control drug-induced diarrhea, especially if patient is receiving maximum dosage.

Storage
- Store at controlled room temperature of 15° to 30°C (59° to 86°F).

Contraindications and precautions
Contraindicated in hypersensitivity to drug; blood dyscrasias; or serious GI, renal, hepatic, or cardiac disorders.

Use cautiously in renal impairment, debilitated or ***elderly patients,*** pregnant or breastfeeding patients, and ***children*** (safety not established).

Adverse reactions
CNS: peripheral neuritis, neuropathy
GI: nausea, vomiting, diarrhea, abdominal pain
GU: anuria, hematuria, reversible azoospermia, renal impairment
Hematologic: purpura, **agranulocytosis, aplastic anemia, thrombocytopenia**
Metabolic: vitamin B_{12} malabsorption
Musculoskeletal: myopathy
Skin: dermatosis, alopecia
Other: hypersensitivity reactions

Interactions
Drug-drug. *Vitamin B_{12}:* reversible vitamin malabsorption
Cyclosporine: colchicine-induced myopathy
Drug-diagnostic tests. *Alkaline phosphatase, aspartate aminotransferase:* increased
Hematocrit, hemoglobin, platelets: decreased
Urinary red blood cells, urine hemoglobin: false-positive results
Drug-herb. *Caffeine, herbal teas, St. John's wort:* decreased drug effect
Drug-behaviors. *Alcohol use:* increased uric acid level

Toxicity and overdose
- Early signs and symptoms of overdose are nausea, vomiting, abdominal pain, and diarrhea (which may become

bloody). Be aware that latent period of several hours may separate overdose and symptom onset. Myocardial injury may lead to profound shock. Muscle weakness or paralysis may cause respiratory failure. Hepatic damage, renal failure, lung parenchymal infiltrates, leukopenia, thrombocytopenia, and coagulopathy may occur. Eventually, patient suffers delirium and seizures. Lethal dose may be as low as 7 mg I.V. Cumulative doses above 4 mg may cause organ failure and death from respiratory failure.

- Provide respiratory assistance and measures to prevent shock, as needed. Give atropine or morphine to relieve abdominal pain, as prescribed. Hemodialysis or peritoneal dialysis may be beneficial. Otherwise, provide symptomatic and supportive therapy.

Patient teaching

- Instruct patient to report rash, sore throat, fever, unusual bleeding, bruising, tiredness, weakness, numbness, or tingling.

Tell patient to immediately report muscle tremors, weakness, fatigue, bruising, bleeding, yellowing of skin or eyes, pale stools, dark urine, severe vomiting, watery or bloody diarrhea, and abdominal pain.

- Advise patient to increase fluid intake to prevent renal calculi (unless prescriber orders fluid restrictions).
- Instruct patient to avoid alcohol, herbal teas, and caffeine during therapy.
- As appropriate, review all other significant and life-threatening adverse reactions and interactions, especially those related to the drugs, tests, herbs, and behaviors mentioned above.

cyclophosphamide

Cytoxan, Endoxana, Procytox

Pharmacologic class: Alkylating agent, nitrogen mustard
Therapeutic class: Antineoplastic
Pregnancy risk category D

Action

Unclear. Thought to prevent cell division by cross-linking DNA strands and interfering with growth of susceptible cancer cells.

Pharmacokinetics

Drug distributes throughout the body, but does not penetrate cerebrospinal fluid. It is metabolized to active (alkylating) forms and inactive (nonalkylating) forms in the liver. Unchanged drug has low plasma protein-binding, but some metabolites are approximately 60% protein-bound. Elimination half-life is 3 to 12 hours in urine. Drug is eliminated mainly as metabolites, with 5% to 10% eliminated unchanged; a small amount is secreted in breast milk.

Onset	Peak	Duration
Unknown	2-3 hr	Unknown

How supplied

Powder for reconstitution for injection (white, lyophilized cake): 500 mg, 1 g, and 2 g in single-use vials

Indications and dosages

➤ Hodgkin's disease, malignant lymphoma, multiple myeloma, leukemia, advanced mycosis fungoides, neuroblastoma, ovarian cancer, breast cancer, certain other tumors

Adults: Initially, 40 to 50 mg/kg I.V. in divided doses over 2 to 5 days; or 10 to

15 mg/kg I.V. q 10 days; or 3 to 5 mg/kg I.V. twice weekly
Children: Initially, 2 to 8 mg/kg or 60 to 250 mg/m^2 I.V. daily in divided doses for 6 or more days, followed by oral maintenance doses twice weekly

Dosage adjustment

• Know that dosage may need to be decreased when drug is given with other antineoplastics or to patients receiving radiation therapy.
• Adjust dosage based on antitumor activity and leukopenia.

Off-label uses

• Selected cases of severe progressive rheumatoid arthritis and systemic lupus erythematosus
• Severe rheumatologic conditions

Administration

Preparation

Follow hazardous drug guidelines on page S19 for handling, preparation, and administration.
• Verify that patient is not pregnant before administering.
• Prehydrate patient with 500 to 1,000 mL normal saline solution I.V., as prescribed.

Dilution and compatibility

• Dilute each 100 mg powder with 5 mL sterile water for injection, to yield 20 mg/mL. Shake well until completely dissolved.
• Further dilute with compatible fluid, such as D_5W, 5% dextrose and normal saline solution, 5% dextrose and lactated Ringer's solution, or 5% dextrose and half-normal saline solution.
• Use solution prepared with sterile water for injection within 24 hours if stored at room temperature or within 6 days if refrigerated.

Infusion considerations

• For direct I.V. injection, give each 100 mg over at least 1 minute.
• When giving doses above 500 mg diluted in 100 to 250 mL compatible solution, administer by intermittent I.V. infusion over 20 to 60 minutes.

Monitoring

• To minimize bladder toxicity, increase patient's fluid intake during therapy and for 1 to 2 days afterward. Most adults require fluid intake of at least 2 L/day.
Monitor for signs and symptoms of hypersensitivity reactions. Be aware that fatal reactions may occur.
• Monitor hematologic profile to gauge degree of hematopoietic suppression. Be aware that leukopenia is an expected drug effect that is used to help determine dosage.
• Monitor urine regularly for red blood cells (RBCs), which may precede hemorrhagic cystitis.
Be aware that serious and sometimes fatal infections may result from immunosuppression; be prepared to interrupt therapy.
Monitor for signs and symptoms of cardiotoxicity, especially congestive heart failure (which may occur at high dosages).

Storage

• Store at or below 25°C (77°F); protect from temperatures above 30°C (86°F).
• Know that reconstituted drug may be refrigerated for 6 days at 2° to 8°C (36° to 46°F).

Contraindications and precautions

Contraindicated in hypersensitivity to drug or severe bone marrow depression.

Use cautiously in renal or hepatic impairment, adrenalectomy, mild to moderate bone marrow depression, other chronic debilitating illnesses, females of childbearing potential, and pregnant or breastfeeding patients.

Adverse reactions

CV: cardiotoxicity

GI: nausea, vomiting, diarrhea, abdominal pain or discomfort, stomatitis, oral mucosal ulcers, anorexia, **hemorrhagic colitis**
GU: urinary bladder fibrosis, hematuria, amenorrhea, decreased sperm count, sterility, **acute hemorrhagic cystitis, renal tubular necrosis, hemorrhagic ureteral inflammation**
Hematologic: anemia, **leukopenia, thrombocytopenia, bone marrow depression, neutropenia**
Hepatic: jaundice
Metabolic: hyperuricemia
Respiratory: interstitial pulmonary fibrosis
Skin: nail and pigmentation changes, alopecia
Other: poor wound healing, infections, allergic reactions including **anaphylaxis, secondary cancers**

Interactions

Drug-drug. *Allopurinol, thiazide diuretics:* increased risk of leukopenia
Cardiotoxic drugs (such as cytarabine, daunorubicin, doxorubicin): additive cardiotoxicity
Chloramphenicol: prolonged cyclophosphamide half-life
Digoxin: decreased digoxin blood level
Phenobarbital: increased risk of cyclophosphamide toxicity
Quinolones: decreased antimicrobial effect
Succinylcholine: prolonged neuromuscular blockade
Warfarin: increased anticoagulant effect
Drug-diagnostic tests. *Hemoglobin, platelets, pseudocholinesterase, RBCs, white blood cells:* decreased
Uric acid: increased

Toxicity and overdose

- In overdose, expect myelosuppression, nausea, vomiting, and extension of other adverse reactions.
- No known antidote exists. Provide supportive interventions, which may include blood transfusions. Dialysis may provide limited benefit.

Patient teaching

- Advise patient to promptly report unusual bleeding or bruising, fever, chills, sore throat, cough, shortness of breath, seizures, lack of menstrual flow, unusual lumps or masses, flank or stomach pain, joint pain, mouth or lip sores, and yellowing of skin or eyes.
- Instruct patient to drink 2 to 3 L of fluids daily (unless prescriber orders fluid restriction) and to urinate frequently to help prevent cystitis.
- Tell patient drug may cause hair loss, but hair usually grows back after treatment ends.
- Advise female patient to use barrier contraception during therapy and for 1 month afterward.
- As appropriate, review all other significant and life-threatening adverse reactions and interactions, especially those related to the drugs and tests mentioned above.

cyclosporine

Sandimmun, Sandimmune

Pharmacologic class: Polypeptide antibiotic
Therapeutic class: Immunosuppressant
Pregnancy risk category C

FDA BOXED WARNING

- Drug should be prescribed only by physicians experienced in managing systemic immunosuppressive therapy for indicated disease. At doses used for solid-organ transplantation, it should

be prescribed only by physicians experienced in immunosuppressive therapy and management of organ transplant recipients. Patient should be managed in facility with adequate laboratory and medical resources. Physician responsible for maintenance therapy should have complete information needed for patient follow-up.
• Drug should be given with adrenal corticosteroids but not other immunosuppressants. In transplant patients, increased susceptibility to infection and development of lymphoma and other neoplasms may result from increased immunosuppression.
• Sandimmune and Neoral are not bioequivalent. Do not use interchangeably without physician supervision.

Action
Exact action unknown. May cause specific and reversible inhibition of immunocompetent lymphocytes in G_0 or G_1 cell-cycle phases. Preferentially inhibits T lymphocytes; T-helper cell is main target, although T-suppressor cell also may be suppressed. Also inhibits lymphokine production and release, including interleukin-2 or T-cell growth factor.

Pharmacokinetics
Drug distributes widely into body tissues and crosses placental barrier. It is metabolized by P4503A enzyme system in the liver and forms at least 24 metabolites; it is not protein-bound. Plasma elimination half-life is 10 hours. Excretion is primarily biliary, with small amounts excreted in urine, feces, and breast milk.

Onset	Peak	Duration
Rapid	1-2 hr	Unknown

How supplied
Solution for injection: 50 mg/mL in 5-mL vials

Indications and dosages
➤ To prevent organ rejection in kidney, liver, or heart transplantation
Adults and children: 5 to 6 mg/kg I.V. 4 to 12 hours before transplantation as a continuous infusion

Off-label uses
• Aplastic anemia
• Atopic dermatitis

Administration
Preparation
Follow hazardous drug guidelines on page S19 for handling, preparation, and administration.
Dilution and compatibility
• Dilute each 1 mL (50 mg) of drug concentrate in 20 to 100 mL of D_5W for injection or normal saline solution.
Infusion considerations
• Administer I.V. infusion over 2 to 6 hours, as prescribed.
Monitoring
• Observe patient for first 30 to 60 minutes of infusion; monitor frequently thereafter.
• Monitor cyclosporine blood level, electrolyte levels, CBC with differential, and liver and kidney function test results.
• Assess for signs and symptoms of hyperkalemia in patient receiving concurrent potassium-sparing diuretic.
• Monitor for signs and symptoms of infection.
Storage
• Store at controlled room temperature of 15° to 30°C (59° to 86°F). Do not freeze; protect from light.

Contraindications and precautions
Contraindicated in hypersensitivity to drug, rheumatoid arthritis, psoriasis in

patients with abnormal renal function, and uncontrolled hypertension.

Use cautiously in hepatic impairment, renal dysfunction, active infection, hypertension, pregnant or breastfeeding patients, and ***children.***

Adverse reactions

CNS: tremor, headache, confusion, paresthesia, insomnia, anxiety, depression, lethargy, weakness
CV: hypertension, chest pain, **myocardial infarction**
EENT: visual disturbances, hearing loss, tinnitus, rhinitis
GI: nausea, vomiting, diarrhea, constipation, abdominal discomfort, gastritis, peptic ulcer, mouth sores, difficulty swallowing, anorexia, **upper GI bleeding, pancreatitis**
GU: gynecomastia, hematuria, **nephrotoxicity, renal dysfunction, glomerular capillary thrombosis**
Hematologic: anemia, **leukopenia, thrombocytopenia**
Metabolic: hyperglycemia, hypomagnesemia, hyperuricemia, **hyperkalemia, metabolic acidosis**
Musculoskeletal: muscle and joint pain
Respiratory: cough, dyspnea, ***Pneumocystis jiroveci*** **pneumonia, bronchospasm**
Skin: acne, hirsutism, brittle fingernails, hair breakage, night sweats
Other: gum hyperplasia, flulike symptoms, edema, fever, weight loss, hiccups, infection, **neoplasia, anaphylaxis**

Interactions

Drug-drug. *Acyclovir, aminoglycosides, amphotericin B, cimetidine, diclofenac, gentamicin, ketoconazole, melphalan, naproxen, ranitidine, sulfamethoxazole, sulindac, tacrolimus, tobramycin, trimethoprim, vancomycin:* increased risk of nephrotoxicity
Allopurinol, amiodarone, bromocriptine, clarithromycin, colchicine, danazol, diltiazem, erythromycin, fluconazole, imipenem and cilastatin, itraconazole, ketoconazole, methylprednisolone, nicardipine, prednisolone, quinupristin and dalfopristin, verapamil: increased cyclosporine blood level
Azathioprine, corticosteroids, cyclophosphamide: increased immunosuppression
Carbamazepine, isoniazid, nafcillin, ocreotide, orlistat, phenobarbital, phenytoin, rifabutin, rifampin, ticlopidine: decreased cyclosporine blood level
Digoxin: decreased digoxin clearance
Live-virus vaccines: decreased antibody response to vaccine
Lovastatin: decreased lovastatin clearance, increased risk of myopathy and rhabdomyolysis
Potassium-sparing diuretics: increased risk of hyperkalemia
Drug-diagnostic tests. *Alanine aminotransferase, aspartate aminotransferase, bilirubin, blood urea nitrogen, creatinine, glucose, low-density lipoproteins:* increased
Hemoglobin, platelets, white blood cells: decreased
Drug-herb. *Alfalfa sprouts, astragalus, echinacea, licorice:* interference with immunosuppressant action
St. John's wort: reduced cyclosporine blood level, possibly leading to organ rejection

Toxicity and overdose

- Overdose signs and symptoms include dizziness, confusion, and possibly seizures.
- Provide symptomatic and supportive therapy. Monitor vital signs and electrolytes closely. Dialysis has little benefit.

Patient teaching

- Inform patient that drug increases risk of infection. Caution patient to avoid crowds and exposure to illness.
- Tell patient about the need for repeated laboratory testing during therapy.

• As appropriate, review all other significant and life-threatening adverse reactions and interactions, especially those related to the drugs, tests, and herbs mentioned above.

cytarabine

Cytosar✦, Cytosar-U

cytarabine liposome

DepoCyt

Pharmacologic class: Antimetabolite, pyrimidine analogue
Therapeutic class: Antineoplastic
Pregnancy risk category D

FDA BOXED WARNING

• Drug should be given only by physicians experienced in cancer chemotherapy. For induction therapy, patients should be in facility with adequate resources to monitor drug tolerance and treat drug toxicity. Main toxic effect is bone marrow suppression with leukopenia, thrombocytopenia, and anemia. Less serious toxicities include nausea, vomiting, diarrhea, abdominal pain, oral ulcers, and hepatic dysfunction.
• Prescriber must weigh possible benefit against known toxic effects and should be familiar with complete package insert information.
• Give DepoCyt (liposomal injection) only under supervision of physician experienced with intrathecal cancer chemotherapy, in facility with adequate diagnostic and treatment resources. In all clinical studies, chemical arachnoiditis (manifested mainly by nausea, vomiting, headache, and fever) was a common adverse event; unless treated, it may be fatal. Patients receiving DepoCyt should receive dexamethasone concurrently to mitigate arachnoiditis symptoms.

Action

Unclear. Cytotoxic effect may stem from inhibition of DNA polymerase by drug's active metabolite.

Pharmacokinetics

Drug's distribution half-life is approximately 10 minutes; elimination half-life, approximately 1 to 3 hours. Drug penetrates cerebrospinal fluid well when given by continuous I.V. infusion. It is metabolized primarily in the liver and has biphasic elimination, with initial half-life of 8 minutes and terminal half-life of 1 to 3 hours. Excretion occurs primarily through urine as metabolites.

Onset	Peak	Duration
Unknown	Unknown	Unknown

How supplied

Powder for reconstitution for injection (white to off-white): 100-mg, 500-mg, 1-g, and 2-g vials

Indications and dosages

➤ To induce remission of acute nonlymphocytic leukemia
Adults: 100 mg/m^2/day by continuous I.V. infusion on days 1 through 7, or 100 mg/m^2 I.V. q 12 hours on days 1 through 7, given with other antineoplastics
➤ Postremission therapy in acute nonlymphocytic leukemia
Adults and children: 1 to 3 g/m^2 by I.V. infusion over 1 to 3 hours q 12 hours for 3 to 6 days; or 3 g/m^2 infused I.V. over 3 hours q 12 hours on days 1, 3, and 5 for six doses in patients younger than age 60; given with other antineoplastics
➤ Acute lymphocytic leukemia

Adults and children: A common high-dose regimen is 1 to 3 g/m^2 I.V. piggyback over 1 to 3 hours for two to four doses. For induction phase, 75 to 150 mg/m^2/day I.V. on designated days.

Dosage adjustment

- As needed, adjust dosage if given with blood dyscrasia–causing drugs or two or more bone-marrow depressant therapies (including radiation).
- Know that dosage modification or drug withdrawal may be needed if drug-induced bone marrow depression results in platelet count below 50,000/mm^3 or polymorphonuclear granulocyte count below 1,000/mm^3.

Administration

Preparation

Follow hazardous drug guidelines on page S19 for handling, preparation, and administration.

Do not confuse conventional form (powder) with liposomal form (solution) intended for intrathecal route.

- Be aware that patients can tolerate higher total dosages when drug is given by rapid I.V. injection rather than slow infusion.
- Give dexamethasone eyedrops before administering high doses.

Dilution and compatibility

- Reconstitute each 100 mg with 5 mL bacteriostatic water for injection with benzyl alcohol. Resulting solution will contain cytarabine 20 mg/mL.
- For I.V. infusion, dilute further with 50 to 100 mL D_5W or normal saline solution.
- Discard solution if slight haze develops.

Infusion considerations

- For I.V. injection, give each 100-mg dose over 1 to 3 minutes.
- For I.V. infusion, give over 30 minutes to 24 hours (depending on dosage and concentration).

Monitoring

Observe for signs and symptoms of cytarabine syndrome (malaise, fever, muscle ache, bone pain, occasional chest pain, maculopapular rash, and conjunctivitis), which may arise 6 to 12 hours after administration. Be prepared to give corticosteroids, if indicated.

- Monitor liver function test results, CBC with differential, platelet count, blood urea nitrogen, and serum creatinine and uric acid levels.

Monitor for signs and symptoms of infection, which may occur anywhere in body. Infection may be mild but sometimes is severe and fatal.

- Be aware that nausea and vomiting are most likely to follow rapid I.V. injection.
- Continue dexamethasone eyedrops for at least 24 hours after high-dose therapy.

Storage

- Store at controlled room temperature of 20° to 25°C (68° to 77°F). Reconstituted solution may be stored at controlled room temperature of 15° to 30°C (59° to 86°F) for 48 hours.

Contraindications and precautions

Contraindicated in hypersensitivity to drug.

Use cautiously in renal or hepatic disease, active infection, decreased bone marrow reserve, other chronic illnesses, females of childbearing potential, pregnant or breastfeeding patients, and ***children.***

Adverse reactions

CNS: malaise, dizziness, headache, neuritis, **neurotoxicity**
CV: chest pain, **thrombophlebitis**
EENT: conjunctivitis
GI: nausea, vomiting, diarrhea, anorexia, abdominal pain, anal ulcers, esophagitis, esophageal ulcers, oral ulcers (in 5 to 10 days), **bowel necrosis**
GU: urine retention, **renal dysfunction**

Hematologic: bleeding, anemia, **megaloblastosis, reticulocytopenia, leukopenia, thrombocytopenia**
Hepatic: hepatic dysfunction
Metabolic: hyperuricemia
Musculoskeletal: muscle ache, bone pain
Respiratory: pneumonia, shortness of breath
Skin: rash, pruritus, freckling, skin ulcers, urticaria, alopecia
Other: cytarabine syndrome, flulike symptoms, edema, infection, fever, sepsis, cellulitis at injection site, **anaphylaxis**

Interactions

Drug-drug. *Digoxin, fluorocytosine:* decreased blood levels of these drugs
Gentamicin: decreased gentamicin effects
Drug-diagnostic tests. *Hemoglobin, platelets, red blood cells, reticulocytes, white blood cells:* decreased
Megaloblasts, uric acid: increased

Toxicity and overdose

- Overdose may cause nausea, vomiting, pulmonary toxicity, myelosuppression, irreversible CNS toxicity, and death.
- No antidote exists. Provide symptomatic and supportive therapy, possibly including blood transfusions.

Patient teaching

Tell patient to immediately report signs and symptoms of cytarabine syndrome (malaise, fever, muscle ache, bone pain, chest pain, rash, and eye infection).

Inform patient that drug may reduce body's ability to fight infection. Instruct patient to promptly report fever, chills, unusual cough, and persistent sore throat.

- Advise patient to increase fluid intake to promote uric acid excretion.
- As appropriate, review all other significant and life-threatening adverse reactions and interactions, especially those related to the drugs and tests mentioned above.

cytomegalovirus immune globulin intravenous (human) (CMV-IG-IV)

CytoGam

Pharmacologic class: Immune globulin
Therapeutic class: Immune serum
Pregnancy risk category C

Action

Contains Ig G antibodies from pooled adult human plasma chosen for high levels of antibodies against CMV. May raise antibody levels sufficiently to decrease incidence of serious CMV disease in persons exposed to CMV.

Pharmacokinetics

Drug has mean half-life of 21 days (shorter in transplant recipients). It is eliminated primarily by catabolism.

Onset	Peak	Duration
Rapid	Unknown	Unknown

How supplied

Powder for reconstitution for injection (colorless, translucent): 1,000 mg in 20-mL single-dose vial; 2,500 mg in 50-mL single-dose vial

Indications and dosages

➤ Prophylaxis of CMV disease associated with kidney, lung, liver, pancreas, or heart transplantation
Adults: Maximum recommended total dosage per infusion is 150 mg/kg, given according to table below. (For transplants other than kidney from CMV-seropositive donors to seronegative recipients, drug may be given in combination with ganciclovir.)

Lung, liver, pancreas, heart transplants (mg/kg)	Kidney transplant (mg/kg)	Administer within
150	150	72 hours of transplant
150	100	2 weeks after transplant
150	100	4 weeks after transplant
150	100	6 weeks after transplant
150	100	8 weeks after transplant
100	50	12 weeks after transplant
100	50	16 weeks after transplant

Off-label uses

- Immunocompromised patients with CMV pneumonia or prevention of CMV disease
- Prevention or attenuation of primary CMV disease in immunosuppressed organ-transplant recipients

Administration

Preparation

- Assess vital signs before starting infusion.
- Ensure that patient is not volume-depleted; before administering, assess renal function, including blood urea nitrogen (BUN) and serum creatinine levels.
- Because of potentially increased risk of thrombosis, assess baseline blood viscosity in patients at risk for hyperviscosity, including those with cryoglobulins, fasting chylomicronemia, markedly high tricylglyceride levels, or monoclonal gammopathies.
- Ensure that emergency drugs, equipment, and oxygen are available before administering.

Dilution and compatibility

- Know that drug dilution before infusion is not recommended; but if necessary do not dilute drug more than a ratio of 1:2 (drug volume vs. solution volume) with compatible solution.
- Drug is compatible with either sodium chloride injection or one of the following: 2.5% dextrose in water, 5% dextrose in water, 10% dextrose in water, or 20% dextrose in water (with or without sodium chloride added).
- Do not shake vial, to avoid foaming.
- Be aware that drug does not contain preservative; therefore, enter vial only once and use within 6 hours.
- Use only if drug is clear and colorless, not turbid.
- Do not mix with other drugs.

Infusion considerations

- Give through I.V. line using administration set containing inline filter (pore size 15 microns) and constant infusion pump. Smaller inline filter (0.2 micron) also is acceptable.
- Administer through separate I.V. line. If this is not possible, piggyback into preexisting line if that line contains a compatible solution.
- Give initial dose I.V. at 15 mg Ig/kg/hour. If no adverse reactions occur after 30 minutes, increase rate to 30 mg Ig/kg/hour. If no adverse reactions occur after subsequent 30 minutes, increase rate to 60 mg Ig/kg/hour (with volume not exceeding 75 mL/hour).
- Give subsequent doses at 15 mg Ig/kg/hour for 15 minutes. If no adverse reactions occur, increase to 30 mg Ig/kg/hour for 15 minutes and then to a maximum rate of 60 mg Ig/kg/hour (with volume not exceeding 75 mL/hour).

Do not exceed recommended dosage or administration rate.

• Be aware that infusion must be completed within 12 hours.

Monitoring

• Assess vital signs midway through infusion, after infusion, and before any rate increase.

Be aware that minor adverse reactions, such as nausea, back pain, and flushing, may relate to infusion rate. If patient develops these, slow rate or temporarily interrupt infusion. If anaphylaxis occurs or blood pressure drops, immediately discontinue infusion and give diphenhydramine and epinephrine, as indicated and ordered.

Know that drug is linked to thrombotic events, especially in high-risk patients (including those with history of atherosclerosis, multiple cardiovascular risk factors, advanced age, impaired cardiac output, or known or suspected hyperviscosity).

Be aware that drug may cause noncardiogenic pulmonary edema or transfusion-related acute lung injury (TRALI). In TRALI, expect severe respiratory distress, pulmonary edema, hypoxemia, and fever. Typically, it arises within 1 to 6 hours after transfusion. In suspected TRALI, tests will be done for presence of antineutrophil antibodies in both product and patient serum. Be prepared to provide oxygen with adequate ventilatory support, if indicated.

Aseptic meningitis syndrome (AMS) occasionally occurs within several hours to 2 days after IGIV therapy. Monitor for signs and symptoms, including severe headache, nuchal rigidity, drowsiness, fever, photophobia, painful eye movements, nausea, and vomiting. If these occur, patient should receive thorough neurologic examination (including cerebrospinal fluid studies) to rule out other meningitis causes. AMS may be more likely with high-dose (2 g/kg) therapy. After drug discontinuation, AMS may remit within several days with no sequelae.

Monitor hydration status and renal function tests closely. If renal function deteriorates, know that drug discontinuation may be warranted.

If signs or symptoms of hemolysis occur after infusion, be prepared to perform appropriate laboratory testing.

Storage

• Store between 2° and 8°C (36° and 46°F).

Contraindications and precautions

Contraindicated in hypersensitivity to human immune globulins and patients with selective IgA deficiency.

Use cautiously in patients with renal insufficiency (including those with diabetes mellitus, age older than 65, volume depletion, paraproteinemia, or sepsis, and those receiving known nephrotoxic drugs), pregnant or breastfeeding patients, and ***children*** (safety and efficacy not established).

Adverse reactions

CNS: dizziness, **AMS**
CV: hypotension, **thrombosis**
GI: nausea, vomiting
GU: oliguria, anuria, acute renal failure, acute tubular necrosis, proximal tubular nephropathy and osmotic nephrosis
Hematologic: hemolysis
Musculoskeletal: muscle cramps, back pain, arthralgia
Respiratory: wheezing, **noncardiogenic pulmonary edema**
Other: fever, flushing, chills, reactions related to infusion rate, hypersensitivity reactions including **angioneurotic edema** and **anaphylaxis,** possible transmission of blood-borne viruses including **Creutzfeldt-Jakob disease** (rare)

Interactions

Drug-drug. *Live-virus vaccines (such as mumps, measles, rubella):* decreased antibody response to vaccine
Drug-diagnostic tests. *BUN, serum creatinine:* increased

Toxicity and overdose

- In overdose, expect major signs and symptoms to reflect volume overload.
- In suspected overdose, immediately discontinue drug, provide symptomatic and supportive therapy, and resuscitate, as indicated.

Patient teaching

Instruct patient to immediately report decreased urine output, sudden weight gain, and shortness of breath (which may suggest kidney damage).
Advise patient to promptly report severe headache, stiff neck, drowsiness, fever, light sensitivity, painful eye movements, nausea, and vomiting.
- Advise patient to defer live-virus vaccinations until about 3 months after receiving drug.
- As appropriate, review all other significant and life-threatening adverse reactions and interactions, especially those related to the drugs and tests mentioned above.

dacarbazine

DTIC✱, DTIC-Dome

Pharmacologic class: Alkylating drug, triazene
Therapeutic class: Antineoplastic
Pregnancy risk category C

FDA BOXED WARNING

- Give under supervision of physician experienced in cancer chemotherapy.
- Hematopoietic depression is most common toxicity; hepatic necrosis also has occurred.
- Drug is carcinogenic and teratogenic in animals.
- Prescriber must weigh potential benefit against toxicity risk.

Action

Unclear. Thought to inhibit DNA synthesis by acting as purine analogue. Also causes alkylation and may interact with sulfhydryl groups.

Pharmacokinetics

Volume of distribution exceeds total body water content, suggesting tissue localization (most likely in the liver). Drug distributes minimally into cerebrospinal fluid. Protein binding is slight. Plasma disappearance is biphasic, with initial half-life of 19 minutes and terminal half-life of 5 hours. Half-lives decrease in renal and hepatic dysfunction. Approximately 40% of dose is excreted unchanged in urine.

Onset	Peak	Duration
Unknown	Unknown	Unknown

How supplied

Powder for reconstitution for injection (colorless to ivory): 100-mg and 200-mg vials

Indications and dosages

➤ Hodgkin's disease
Adults: 150 mg/m² I.V. daily for 5 days in combination with other drugs, repeated q 4 weeks. Or 375 mg/m² I.V. on day 1 of combination therapy, repeated q 15 days.
➤ Metastatic malignant melanoma
Adults: 2 to 4.5 mg/kg I.V. daily for 10 days, repeated q 4 weeks. Or

250 mg/m^2 I.V. daily for 5 days, repeated q 3 weeks.

Off-label uses

- Malignant pheochromocytoma

Administration

Preparation

Follow hazardous drug guidelines on page S19 for handling, preparation, and administration.

Dilution and compatibility

- Reconstitute 100-mg and 200-mg vials with sterile water for injection (9.9 mL and 19.7 mL, respectively). Resulting solution contains dacarbazine 10 mg/mL.
- Further dilute reconstituted drug in 50 to 250 mL D_5W or normal saline solution.

Infusion considerations

Administer over 30 to 60 minutes by I.V. infusion only.

Take steps to prevent extravasation, which may cause tissue damage and severe pain.

Monitoring

Monitor for hypersensitivity reactions; be prepared to intervene appropriately.

Frequently monitor CBC with white cell differential and platelet count. Know that hematopoietic depression is most common toxicity.

Continue to assess infusion site closely for extravasation.

- Monitor hepatic and renal function regularly.

Storage

- Refrigerate powder at 2° to 8°C (36° to 46°F).
- After reconstitution, store solution in vial at 4°C (39°F) for up to 72 hours or at normal room temperature and light for up to 8 hours.
- If reconstituted solution is further diluted, store solution at 4°C (39°F) for up to 24 hours or at normal room temperature and light for up to 8 hours.

Contraindications and precautions

Contraindicated in hypersensitivity to drug.

Use cautiously in hepatic dysfunction, impaired bone marrow function, concurrent radiation therapy, ***elderly patients,*** pregnant or breastfeeding patients, and ***children*** (safety and efficacy not established).

Adverse reactions

CNS: malaise, paresthesia
GI: nausea, vomiting, dyspepsia, anorexia
Hematologic: anemia, **leukopenia, thrombocytopenia, bone marrow depression**
Hepatic: hepatic toxicity, hepatic vein thrombosis, hepatocellular necrosis (rare)
Musculoskeletal: myalgia
Skin: dermatitis, erythematous or urticarial rash, alopecia, flushing, photosensitivity
Others: flulike symptoms, fever, **hypersensitivity reactions** including **anaphylaxis**

Interactions

Drug-diagnostic tests. *Platelets, red blood cells, white blood cells:* decreased
Drug-behaviors. *Sun exposure:* photosensitivity reaction

Toxicity and overdose

- In overdose, expect extensions of adverse reactions, including nausea, vomiting, diarrhea, and myelosuppression.
- Provide supportive interventions and monitor blood cell counts.

Patient teaching

Instruct patient to immediately report pain, burning, or swelling at infusion site; numbness in arms or legs; gait changes; respiratory distress; difficulty breathing; rash; nausea; fatigue; malaise;

itching; black tarry stools; yellowing of skin or eyes; easy bruising; and bleeding.

- Advise patient to minimize adverse GI effects by eating small, frequent servings of healthy food and drinking plenty of fluids. Inform patient that symptoms usually subside after first 1 or 2 days.
- Teach patient about the need for regular blood testing during therapy.
- Inform patient that hair loss is a common adverse effect, but usually reverses after therapy ends.
- Caution females of childbearing potential to avoid becoming pregnant during therapy.
- As appropriate, review all other significant and life-threatening adverse reactions and interactions, especially those related to the tests and behaviors mentioned above.

dantrolene sodium

Dantrium Intravenous

Pharmacologic class: Hydantoin derivative
Therapeutic class: Skeletal muscle relaxant (direct-acting), malignant hyperthermia agent
Pregnancy risk category C

FDA BOXED WARNING

- Drug may be hepatotoxic and should be used only for recommended conditions. Daily doses of 400 mg are less likely to cause fatal and nonfatal hepatitis than daily doses above 800 mg. Overt hepatitis is most common during months 3 and 12, but may occur at any time; females, patients older than age 35, and those receiving concurrent therapy are at higher risk. Use only in conjunction with liver monitoring. Monitor liver function at baseline and regularly during therapy. Discontinue drug if values are abnormal.
- Use lowest possible effective dosage. If no benefit occurs after 45 days, discontinue.

Action

Relaxes skeletal muscle by affecting excitation-contraction coupling response at site beyond myoneural junction, probably by interfering with calcium release from sarcoplasmic reticulum

Pharmacokinetics

Drug appears in measurable amounts in blood and urine. Major metabolites in body fluids are 5-hydroxydantrolene and acetylamino metabolite. Significant amount of drug is bound to plasma proteins (mostly albumin); such binding is readily reversible. Mean biologic half-life varies from 4 to 8 hours. Slightly greater amounts of drug are associated with red blood cells than with plasma.

Onset	Peak	Duration
Rapid	Unknown	Unknown

How supplied

Powder for reconstitution for injection (lyophilized): 20 mg/vial

Indications and dosages

➢ Malignant hyperthermic crisis

Adults and children: Initially, 1 mg/kg by I.V. push, repeated as needed up to a cumulative dose of 10 mg/kg/day, followed by oral dantrolene for 1 to 3 days

➢ To prevent or minimize malignant hyperthermia in patients who require surgery

Adults and children: 2.5 mg/kg I.V. infused over 1 hour before anesthetics are given

Off-label uses

- Heat stroke
- Neuroleptic malignant syndrome

Administration

Dilution and compatibility

- Add 60 mL sterile water for injection to each vial; shake until solution is clear.
- Do not use bacteriostatic water for injection.
- Protect from direct light. Know that although solution is stable for 6 hours, drug should be prepared immediately before administration.

Infusion considerations

- Give therapeutic or emergency dose by rapid I.V. push. Administer follow-up dose over 2 to 3 minutes.

Prevent extravasation; drug causes tissue irritation.

Monitoring

- Monitor vital signs, ECG, serum electrolyte levels, and urine output regularly.

Watch for signs and symptoms of pulmonary edema (rare) during treatment of malignant hyperthermia crisis. (Diluent volume and mannitol needed to deliver I.V. drug may contribute to crisis.)

Storage

- Before reconstitution, store at controlled room temperature of 15° to 30°C (59° to 86°F). Avoid prolonged light exposure.

Contraindications and precautions

Use cautiously in cardiac, hepatic, renal, or respiratory dysfunction or impairment; women (especially pregnant or breastfeeding women); adults older than age 35; and ***children younger than age 5.***

Adverse reactions

CNS: dizziness, drowsiness, fatigue, malaise, weakness, confusion, depression, insomnia, nervousness, headache, light-headedness, speech disturbances,

CV: tachycardia, blood pressure fluctuations, phlebitis

EENT: double vision, excessive tearing

GI: nausea, vomiting, diarrhea, constipation, abdominal cramps, GI reflux and irritation, hematemesis, difficulty swallowing, anorexia

GU: urinary frequency, dysuria, urinary incontinence, nocturia, hematuria, crystalluria, prostatitis

Musculoskeletal: myalgia, backache

Respiratory: suffocating sensation, **respiratory depression, pulmonary edema** (rare)

Skin: rash, urticaria, pruritus, eczema-like eruptions, sweating, photosensitivity, abnormal hair growth

Other: altered taste, chills, fever, edema

Interactions

Drug-drug. *CNS depressants:* increased CNS depression

Estrogen: increased risk of hepatotoxicity

Verapamil (I.V.): cardiovascular collapse

Drug-diagnostic tests. *Alanine aminotransferase, alkaline phosphatase, aspartate aminotransferase, bilirubin, blood urea nitrogen:* increased

Drug-behaviors. *Alcohol use:* increased CNS depression

Sun exposure: phototoxicity

Toxicity and overdose

- In overdose, expect extensions of adverse reactions, including nausea and vomiting, renal problems, and CNS depression.
- No known antidote exists. Provide supportive interventions, such as giving large amounts of I.V. fluids to prevent crystalluria, maintaining patent airway, monitoring ECG, and providing other emergency measures, as indicated.

Patient teaching

- Inform patient drug may cause drowsiness, dizziness, or light-headedness.
- As appropriate, review all other significant and life-threatening adverse reactions and interactions, especially those related to the drugs, tests, and behaviors mentioned above.

daptomycin

Cubicin

Pharmacologic class: Cyclic lipopeptide
Therapeutic class: Anti-infective
Pregnancy risk category B

Action

Unlike other antibiotics, binds to bacterial membranes and causes rapid depolarization of membrane potential, which leads to disruption of cell membrane and bacterial cell death. Exhibits bactericidal activity against aerobic gram-positive bacteria.

Pharmacokinetics

Drug binds reversibly to plasma proteins (primarily serum albumin); overall mean binding is approximately 90%. Inactive metabolites have been detected in urine. Drug is excreted mainly by the kidneys (approximately 60% excreted in 24 hours), with a small amount excreted in feces.

Onset	Peak	Duration
Unknown	Unknown	Unknown

How supplied

Powder for reconstitution for injection (preservative-free, pale yellow to light brown, lyophilized cake): 500 mg in 10-mL single-use vials

Indications and dosages

➢ Complicated skin and skin-structure infections

Adults: 4 mg/kg by I.V. infusion over 30 minutes q 24 hours for 7 to 14 days

➢ Bacteremia caused by *Staphylococcus aureus* (including right-sided endocarditis) resulting from methicillin-susceptible and methicillin-resistant strains

Adults: 6 mg/kg over 30 minutes by I.V. infusion q 24 hours for at least 2 to 6 weeks

Dosage adjustment

- Adjust dosage in severe renal insufficiency as follows: For creatinine clearance below 30 mL/minute (including patients on dialysis), recommended dosage is 4 mg/kg for complicated skin and skin-structure infections and 6 mg/kg for *S. aureus* bacteremia q 48 hours.

Administration

Preparation

- Be aware that dosages above 6 mg/kg have not been approved.
- Administer on hemodialysis days, after hemodialysis session ends.

Dilution and compatibility

Know that drug is not compatible with dextrose-containing diluents.

- Be aware that drug is compatible only with normal saline injection and lactated Ringer's injection.
- Reconstitute 500-mg vial with 10 mL normal saline injection.
- Further dilute with appropriate amount of normal saline solution for I.V. infusion.
- Be aware that freshly reconstituted solutions range from pale yellow to light brown.
- Discard unused solution.

Do not mix with other drugs.

Infusion considerations
• Give by I.V. infusion over 30 minutes.
Do not infuse simultaneously through same I.V. line with other drugs or solutions. If same line is used for sequential infusion of several different drugs, flush with compatible solution before and after each daptomycin infusion.
Monitoring
• Perform repeated blood cultures in patients with persisting or relapsing *S. aureus* infection or poor clinical response.
• In patients with renal insufficiency, monitor both renal function and serum creatine kinase (CK) frequently.
Stay alert for complaints of muscle pain or weakness, particularly of distal extremities.
Discontinue drug in patients with unexplained signs or symptoms of myopathy in conjunction with CK above 1,000 U/L , or in asymptomatic patients with CK levels above 2,000 U/L. Consider temporarily suspending drugs linked to rhabdomyolysis (such as HMG-CoA reductase inhibitors) in patients receiving daptomycin.
Monitor for signs and symptoms of pseudomembranous colitis, which may range from mild to life-threatening. Be prepared to discontinue drug and provide appropriate therapy.
Storage
• Refrigerate original packages at 2° to 8°C (36° to 46°F); avoid excessive heat.
• Store reconstituted solution in vial for 12 hours at room temperature or up to 48 hours when refrigerated at 2° to 8°C (36° to 46°F).
• Store diluted solution in infusion bag for 12 hours at room temperature or 48 hours in refrigerator.
• Know that combined time (vial and infusion bag) at room temperature should not exceed 12 hours at room temperature or 48 hours when refrigerated.

Contraindications and precautions

Contraindicated in hypersensitivity to drug.

Use cautiously in renal insufficiency, ***elderly patients,*** pregnant or breastfeeding patients, and ***children younger than age 18*** (safety and efficacy not established).

Adverse reactions

CNS: dizziness, headache, insomnia, fatigue, anxiety, asthenia
CV: hypotension, hypertension, **heart failure**
EENT: sore throat, laryngopharyngeal pain
GI: nausea, vomiting, diarrhea, constipation, abdominal pain, dyspepsia, pseudomembranous colitis, GI hemorrhage
GU: urinary tract infections, **renal failure**
Hematologic: anemia
Metabolic: hypoglycemia, hyperglycemia, hypokalemia
Musculoskeletal: muscle pain or weakness, back pain, limb pain, sternal osteomyelitis, mediastinitis
Respiratory: dyspnea, cough, pneumonia, **pleural effusion**
Skin: rash, pruritus, erythema
Other: sweating, decreased appetite, fever, bacteremia, fungal infections, superinfection, sepsis, edema, cellulitis, peripheral edema, injection site reactions, hypersensitivity reaction

Interactions

Drug-drug. *HMG-CoA reductase inhibitors:* increased CK level
Tobramycin: increased daptomycin level, decreased tobramycin level
Drug-diagnostic tests. *Alkaline phosphatase, CK:* increased

Blood glucose: decreased or increased
Liver function tests: abnormal results
Potassium: decreased

Toxicity and overdose

- In overdose, expect extensions of adverse reactions, including electrolyte imbalances and CNS, cardiovascular, GI, renal, musculoskeletal, and respiratory adverse reactions.
- Provide supportive care, including maintaining glomerular filtration. Drug clears slowly from body with hemodialysis (approximately 15% recovered over 4 hours) or peritoneal dialysis (11% recovered over 48 hours). Observe for increase in CK level and muscle pain.

Patient teaching

Instruct patient to immediately report swelling, bloody diarrhea, change in urine output, respiratory problems, or rash.
- Advise patient to report muscle pain in arms or legs.
- As appropriate, review all other significant and life-threatening adverse reactions and interactions, especially those related to the drugs and tests mentioned above.

darbepoetin alfa

Aranesp

Pharmacologic class: Recombinant human erythropoietin
Therapeutic class: Hematopoietic
Pregnancy risk category C

FDA BOXED WARNING

- Use lowest dosage that will increase hemoglobin gradually to lowest level sufficient to avoid the need for red blood cell (RBC) transfusion.
- Drug increases risk of death and serious cardiovascular events when given to target hemoglobin level above 12 g/dL.
- In patients receiving radiation therapy for advanced head and neck cancer, drug shortens time to tumor progression when given to target hemoglobin level above 12 g/dL.
- In patients receiving chemotherapy for metastatic breast cancer, drug shortens overall survival and increases deaths from disease progression at 4 months when given to target hemoglobin level above 12 g/dL.
- In patients with active cancer who are receiving neither chemotherapy nor radiation therapy, drug increases risk of death when given to target hemoglobin level of 12 g/dL. Drug is not indicated for these patients.
- Patients who received epoetin alfa preoperatively to reduce the need for allogeneic RBC transfusion but were not receiving prophylactic anticoagulation had a higher incidence of deep vein thrombosis. Darbepoetin alfa is not approved to reduce the need for RBC transfusion.

Action

Stimulates erythropoiesis in bone marrow, increasing RBC production

Pharmacokinetics

Distribution is confined to vascular space. Serum concentration is biphasic, with distribution half-life of about 1.4 hours and mean terminal half-life of about 21 hours. With once-weekly dosing, steady-state serum level occurs within 4 weeks. Accumulation is negligible.

Onset	Peak	Duration
2-6 wk	Unknown	Unknown

How supplied

Albumin solution for injection: 25 mcg/0.42 mL, 40 mcg/0.4 mL, 60 mcg/0.3 mL, 100 mcg/0.5 mL, and 150 mcg/0.3 mL in single-dose prefilled syringe (SingleJect)
Polysorbate solution for injection: 25 mcg/0.42 mL, 40 mcg/0.4 mL, 60 mcg/0.3 mL, 100 mcg/0.5 mL, 150 mcg/0.3 mL, 200 mcg/0.4 mL, 300 mcg/0.6 mL, and 500 mcg/mL in single-dose prefilled syringe (SingleJect)

Indications and dosages

➢ Anemia caused by chronic renal failure
Adults: Initially, 0.45 mcg/kg I.V. as a single dose once weekly. Titrate dosage to maintain target hemoglobin level no higher than 12 g/dL.

➢ Chemotherapy-induced anemia in patients with nonmyeloid malignancies
Adults: 2.25 mcg/kg I.V. once weekly. Titrate dosage to maintain target hemoglobin level no higher than 12 g/dL.

Dosage adjustment

- Use lowest dosage that will increase hemoglobin gradually to lowest level sufficient to avoid the need for RBC transfusion.
- If hemoglobin is rising and approaching 12 g/dL, reduce dosage by approximately 25%. If hemoglobin continues to rise, withhold doses until hemoglobin begins to decrease; then reinitiate at dosage approximately 25% below previous dosage. If hemoglobin increases more than 1 g/dL in 2-week period, decrease dosage by approximately 25%. If hemoglobin increases less than 1 g/dL over 4 weeks and iron stores are adequate, increase dosage by approximately 25%. Further increases may be made at 4-week intervals until specified hemoglobin level is reached.
- Do not adjust dosage more often than once a month.

Administration

Preparation

🔊 Know that drug supplied in prefilled SureClick Autoinjector is indicated for subcutaneous, not I.V., use.

🔊 Ask patient about latex allergy before administering. Needle cover of prefilled syringe contains dry natural rubber (latex derivative).

- Assess hemoglobin, serum iron status, serum transferrin, and serum transferrin saturation before starting therapy.
- Be aware that when formulated with albumin, drug carries extremely remote risk of transmitting viral diseases and a theoretical risk of transmitting Creutzfeldt-Jakob disease.
- Know that supplemental iron is recommended for patients with serum ferritin levels below 100 mcg/mL or serum transferrin saturation less than 20%.

Dilution and compatibility

🔊 Do not dilute or give with other drug solutions.

🔊 Do not shake. Vigorous shaking may denature drug, making it biologically inactive.

- Do not use if solution is discolored.
- Do not use vial or prefilled syringe more than once. Discard unused solution.

Infusion considerations

- After removing prefilled syringe from carton, keep it covered to protect from room light until administration.
- After administration using prefilled syringe, activate UltraSafe needle guard until you hear an audible click, to prevent accidental needlestick.

Monitoring

- Monitor hemoglobin and hematocrit weekly during therapy.

🔊 Observe closely for serious CNS and cardiovascular adverse reactions.

Storage

- Store at 2° to 8°C (36° to 46°F); do not freeze. Protect from light.

Contraindications and precautions

Contraindicated in hypersensitivity to drug or its components and in uncontrolled hypertension.

Use cautiously in anemia, thalassemia, porphyria, seizures, underlying hematologic disease (including hemolytic and sickle cell anemia), pregnant or breastfeeding patients, and ***children*** (safety and efficacy not established).

Adverse reactions

CNS: dizziness, headache, fatigue, weakness, **seizures, transient ischemic attack, cerebrovascular accident**
CV: hypertension, hypotension, chest pain, peripheral edema, **arrhythmias, heart failure, cardiac arrest, myocardial infarction, vascular access thrombosis**
GI: nausea, vomiting, diarrhea, constipation, abdominal pain
Metabolic: fluid overload
Musculoskeletal: myalgia; joint, back, and limb pain
Respiratory: cough, upper respiratory tract infection, dyspnea, bronchitis
Skin: pruritus
Other: fever, flulike symptoms, infection, pain at injection site

Interactions

Drug-diagnostic tests. *Serum transferrin saturation:* decreased

Toxicity and overdose

- In overdose, expect cardiovascular and neurologic adverse events with excessive or rapid hemoglobin rise.
- No known antidote exists. Monitor closely for cardiovascular and hematologic abnormalities. If polycythemia occurs, temporarily withhold drug; physician may consider phlebotomy. After overdose effects resolve, drug may be reintroduced, with close monitoring for rapid hemoglobin rise (above 1 g/dL in 2-week period).

Patient teaching

- Instruct patient to report chest pain or other pain, muscle tremors, weakness, and cough or other respiratory symptoms.
- Teach patient to avoid driving and other hazardous activities until drug's effects on concentration and alertness are known.
- Advise patient to minimize GI upset by eating small, frequent servings of healthy food and drinking plenty of fluids.
- Tell patient about the need for frequent blood testing during therapy to help determine correct dosage.
- As appropriate, review all other significant and life-threatening adverse reactions and interactions, especially those related to the tests mentioned above.

daunorubicin citrate liposome

DaunoXome

Pharmacologic class: Anthracycline glycoside
Therapeutic class: Antibiotic antineoplastic
Pregnancy risk category D

FDA BOXED WARNING

- Monitor cardiac function regularly during therapy, because of potential cardiotoxicity and congestive heart failure (CHF). Also monitor cardiac function in patients who have cardiac disease or have previously received anthracyclines.
- Severe myelosuppression may occur.
- Give under supervision of experienced physician.
- Reduce dosage in patients with hepatic impairment.
- Drug may cause triad of back pain, flushing, and chest tightness. Triad usually

occurs within first 5 minutes of infusion, subsides with infusion interruption, and does not recur when infusion resumes at slower rate.

Action

Specific action is not known, but liposome formulation protects entrapped daunorubicin from chemical and enzymatic degradation, minimizes protein binding, and decreases uptake by normal tissues. Direct binding to DNA (intercalation) and inhibition of DNA repair (topoisomerase II inhibition) apparently cause blockade of DNA and RNA synthesis and fragmentation.

Pharmacokinetics

Drug has small volume of distribution compared to nonencapsulated form. Parent drug distributes slowly from peripheral tissues to the liver for metabolism, resulting in its major metabolite, daunorubicinol. Elimination half-life is about 4 hours. It is excreted mainly in feces, and to a lesser extent in urine.

Onset	Peak	Duration
Unknown	Unknown	Unknown

How supplied

Solution for injection (red, translucent dispersion): 2 mg/mL in single-use vial

Indications and dosages

➢ First-line cytotoxic therapy for advanced Kaposi's sarcoma associated with HIV

Adults: 40 mg/m^2 I.V. over 1 hour. Repeat q 2 weeks until evidence of disease progression or other complications occur.

Dosage adjustment

• Limited clinical experience exists regarding use of drug in patients with hepatic or renal impairment. Based on experience with daunorubicin hydrochloride, reduce recommended dosage if serum bilirubin or creatinine level is elevated, as follows: With bilirubin level of 1.2 to 3 mg/dL, give 75% of normal dosage; with bilirubin or creatinine level above 3 mg/dL, give 50% of normal dosage.

• Be aware that dosage adjustment may be required in patients receiving blood dyscrasia–causing drugs or when two or more bone marrow depressants (including radiation) are used concurrently or consecutively with this drug.

Administration

Preparation

Follow hazardous drug guidelines on page S19 for handling, preparation, and administration.

• Although no reliable means exist for predicting CHF, anthracycline-induced cardiomyopathy usually is associated with decreased left ventricular ejection fraction (LVEF). Determine LVEF before therapy starts.

• Assess cardiac, renal, and hepatic function before each course of therapy.

• Evaluate CBC with white cell differential before each dose.

• Control systemic infection before starting therapy.

• If prescribed, premedicate with allopurinol to help prevent hyperuricemia.

Dilution and compatibility

• Dilute each single dose 1:1 with D_5W. Recommended concentration after dilution is 1 mg/mL of solution.

Do not mix with other drugs or solutions.

• Know that drug is a translucent, red liposomal dispersion. Do not use if opaque.

Infusion considerations

Do not use inline filter for I.V. infusion.

• Administer by I.V. infusion slowly over 1 hour.
• Check for free-flowing I.V. line. Monitor site for patency throughout administration. Although no local tissue necrosis has been seen with liposomal form, daunorubicin hydrochloride may cause local tissue necrosis at extravasation site.

Monitoring

Continue to monitor cardiac function, including LVEF, in patients with preexisting cardiac disease or who previously received anthracyclines.

Continue to monitor CBC with differential. Withhold dose if granulocyte count drops below 750 cells/mm^3.

• Continue to monitor renal and hepatic function.
• Monitor serum uric acid level.
• Monitor patient for back pain, flushing, and chest tightness, which generally occur during first 5 minutes of infusion, subside with interruption of infusion, and do not recur if infusion resumes at slower rate.

Storage

• Refrigerate undiluted drug at 2° to 8°C (36° to 46°F). Do not freeze; protect from light. Refrigerate reconstituted solution for maximum of 6 hours.

Contraindications

Contraindicated in hypersensitivity to drug or its components.

Use cautiously in renal or hepatic impairment, bone marrow depression, cardiac disease, gout, infections, ***elderly patients*** (safety and efficacy not established), pregnant or breastfeeding patients, and ***children*** (safety and efficacy not established).

Adverse reactions

CNS: headache, fatigue, malaise, confusion, depression, dizziness, drowsiness, emotional lability, anxiety, hallucinations, syncope, tremors, rigors, insomnia, neuropathy, amnesia, hyperactivity, abnormal thinking, abnormal gait, **meningitis, seizures**
CV: hypertension, chest pain, palpitations, **myocardial infarction, cardiac arrest**
EENT: abnormal vision, conjunctivitis, eye pain, hearing loss, earache, tinnitus, rhinitis, sinusitis
GI: nausea, vomiting, diarrhea, constipation, abdominal pain, dyspepsia, gastritis, enlarged spleen, fecal incontinence, hemorrhoids, tenesmus, melena, difficulty swallowing, dry mouth, oral inflammation, **GI hemorrhage**
GU: dysuria, nocturia, polyuria
Hematologic: thrombocytopenia, neutropenia
Hepatic: hepatomegaly
Metabolic: hyperuricemia, dehydration
Musculoskeletal: joint pain, myalgia, muscle rigidity, back pain
Respiratory: dyspnea, cough, hemoptysis, increased sputum, **pulmonary infiltrations, pulmonary hypertension**
Skin: pruritus, dry skin, seborrhea, folliculitis, alopecia, sweating
Other: bleeding gums, dental caries, altered taste, lymphadenopathy, opportunistic infections, fever, hot flashes, hiccups, thirst, infusion site inflammation, edema, allergic reactions

Interactions

Drug-diagnostic tests. *Granulocytes:* decreased
Uric acid: increased

Toxicity and overdose

• Be aware that primary toxicity is myelosuppression, especially of granulocytes. Other signs and symptoms may include fatigue, nausea, and vomiting.
• No known antidote exists. Provide supportive and symptomatic therapy. Know that whole blood products and blood modifiers may have some benefit in treating bone marrow toxicity.

Patient teaching

Instruct patient to immediately report swelling, pain, burning, or redness at infusion site, as well as persistent nausea, vomiting, diarrhea, chest pain, arm or leg swelling, difficulty breathing, palpitations, rapid heartbeat, yellowing of skin or eyes, abdominal pain, or bloody stools.
- Inform patient that drug increases susceptibility to infection. Urge patient to avoid crowds and exposure to illness.
- Advise patient to minimize GI upset by eating small, frequent servings of healthy food, drinking plenty of fluids, and chewing gum.
- Tell patient about the need for regular blood testing during therapy.
- Inform patient that hair loss is a common adverse reaction and usually reverses once therapy ends.
- Caution females of childbearing potential to avoid becoming pregnant during therapy.
- Advise HIV-infected women not to breastfeed infants, to avoid HIV transmission.
- As appropriate, review all other significant and life-threatening adverse reactions and interactions, especially those related to the tests mentioned above.

daunorubicin hydrochloride

Cerubidine

Pharmacologic class: Anthracycline glycoside
Therapeutic class: Antibiotic antineoplastic
Pregnancy risk category D

FDA BOXED WARNING

- Administer into rapidly flowing I.V. infusion; never give I.M. or subcutaneously. Severe local tissue necrosis results if extravasation occurs.
- Myocardial toxicity (manifested most severely as potentially fatal congestive heart failure [CHF]) may occur during therapy or months to years afterward. Incidence increases with total cumulative dose above 550 mg/m^2 in adults, 300 mg/m^2 in children older than age 2, or 10 mg/kg in children younger than age 2.
- Therapeutic doses cause severe myelosuppression. Drug should be given only by physician experienced in leukemia chemotherapy, in facility with adequate diagnostic and treatment resources for monitoring drug tolerance and treating toxicity. Physician and facility must be capable of responding rapidly and completely to severe hemorrhagic conditions and overwhelming infection.
- Reduce dosage in patients with hepatic or renal impairment.

Action

Antimitotic and cytotoxic (although exact action is not clear). Forms complexes with DNA by intercalation between base pairs. Inhibits topoisomerase II activity by stabilizing topoisomerase II complex; causes breaks in single- and double-stranded DNA. May also inhibit polymerase activity, influence regulation of gene expression, and cause free-radical damage to DNA.

Pharmacokinetics

Drug undergoes rapid tissue uptake and distributes extensively, with highest concentration in the heart, liver, lungs, spleen, and kidneys. It does not cross blood-brain barrier. Drug is 63% bound to albumin. It is metabolized in the liver to active and inactive metabolites. Terminal half-life of parent drug is 18.5 hours; active metabolite (daunorubicinol), about 28 hours. About 40% of dose is excreted in bile and about 25% in urine.

Onset	Peak	Duration
Unknown	Unknown	Unknown

How supplied

Powder for reconstitution for injection (reddish color, lyophilized): 21.4-mg and 53.5-mg vials
Solution for injection: 5 mg/mL in single-dose vials

Indications and dosages

➤ Acute nonlymphocytic leukemia
Adults older than age 60: 30 mg/m^2/day I.V. on days 1, 2, and 3 of first course and on days 1 and 2 of subsequent courses; given with cytarabine I.V. infusion for 7 days during first course and for 5 days during subsequent courses
Adults younger than age 60: 45 mg/m^2/day I.V. on days 1, 2, and 3 of first course and on days 1 and 2 of subsequent courses; given with cytarabine I.V. infusion for 7 days during first course and for 5 days during subsequent courses
➤ Acute lymphocytic leukemia
Adults: 45 mg/m^2/day I.V. on days 1, 2, and 3 and vincristine I.V. on days 1, 8, and 15 and prednisone P.O. on days 1 through 22, then tapered between days 22 and 29; then asparaginase is given I.V. on days 22 to 32.
Children age 2 and older: 25 mg/m^2/day I.V. on day 1 every week; may be given in combination with vincristine I.V. on first day of every week and prednisone P.O. daily

Dosage adjustment

- Reduce dosage 25% in patients with serum bilirubin level of 1.2 to 3 mg/100 mL; reduce dosage 50% in patients with serum bilirubin or creatinine level above 3 mg/100 mL.
- For children younger than age 2 or less than 0.5 m^2 body surface area (BSA), base dosage on weight (1 mg/kg) instead of BSA.
- Know that dosage reduction may be required when two or more bone marrow depressants (including radiation) are used concurrently or consecutively.

Off-label uses

- Chronic myelogenous leukemia in blastic phase

Administration

Preparation

Follow hazardous drug guidelines on page S19 for handling, preparation, and administration.
- Although no reliable means exists for predicting CHF, ECG change showing decrease of 30% or more in limb-lead QRS voltage or decrease in systolic ejection fraction from pretreatment baseline is linked to significant risk of drug-induced cardiomyopathy. Obtain ECG and left ventricular ejection fraction (LVEF) results before therapy starts.
- Monitor cardiac, renal, and hepatic function before each course of therapy.
- Evaluate CBC with white cell differential before each dose.
- Control systemic infection, as ordered, before starting therapy.
- If prescribed, premedicate with allopurinol to help prevent hyperuricemia.

Dilution and compatibility

- Reconstitute powder with 4 mL sterile water for injection to yield 5 mg/mL solution. Agitate gently until powder dissolves completely. For intermittent I.V.

infusion, mix with 100 mL normal saline solution for injection.
- Prepare solution by withdrawing desired dosage into syringe containing 10 to 15 mL normal saline solution.
- Do not mix with other drugs or heparin.
- Discard unused portion of drug.

Infusion considerations
- For intermittent I.V. infusion, infuse over 30 to 45 minutes.
- For single-dose I.V. injection, inject into tubing or sidearm of rapidly flowing I.V. infusion of D_5W or normal saline solution over 3 to 5 minutes.

Check I.V. site for patency frequently throughout administration; drug causes severe local tissue necrosis. If extravasation occurs, stop infusion immediately; according to facility policy, intervene to avoid severe tissue necrolysis, severe cellulitis, thrombophlebitis, and painful induration.

Monitoring

Continue to monitor cardiac function, including ECG and LVEF, in patients with preexisting cardiac disease.

Continue to monitor CBC with differential. Withhold dose if granulocyte count is below 750 cells/mm^3.

Watch for hypersensitivity reaction; be prepared to intervene appropriately.
- Continue to monitor renal and hepatic function.
- Monitor serum uric acid level.

Storage
- Store powder at controlled room temperature of 15° to 30°C (59° to 86°F). Reconstituted solution is stable for 24 hours at room temperature and 48 hours when refrigerated. Protect from light. Keep in carton until use.
- Refrigerate unopened vials at 2° to 8°C (36° to 46°F).
- Reconstituted solution may be stored at room temperature of 15° to 30°C (59° to 86° F) for approximately 24 hours. Protect from light.

Contraindications
Contraindicated in hypersensitivity to drug.

Use cautiously in renal or hepatic impairment, bone marrow depression, cardiac disease, gout, infections, ***elderly patients,*** and pregnant or breastfeeding patients.

Adverse reactions
CV: cardiotoxicity
GI: acute nausea, vomiting, GI mucosal inflammation
GU: urine discoloration
Hematologic: bone marrow depression
Metabolic: hyperuricemia
Skin: rash, contact dermatitis, urticaria, reversible alopecia
Other: hypersensitivity reactions including **anaphylactoid reactions** (rare)

Interactions
Drug-drug. *Other antineoplastic, hepatotoxic, and myelosuppressive drugs:* increased risk of toxicity
Drug-diagnostic tests. *Granulocytes:* decreased
Uric acid: increased

Toxicity and overdose
- Be aware that primary toxicity is myelosuppression, especially of granulocytes. Other signs and symptoms may include fatigue, nausea, and vomiting.
- No known antidote exists. Provide supportive and symptomatic treatment. Know that whole blood products and blood modifiers may have some benefit in treating bone marrow toxicity.

Patient teaching

Instruct patient to immediately report swelling, pain, burning, or redness at infusion site, as well as persistent nausea, vomiting, diarrhea, bloody stools, abdominal or chest pain, swollen arm or leg, difficulty breathing, palpitations, rapid heartbeat, or yellowing of skin or eyes.

- Inform patient that drug increases susceptibility to infection. Urge patient to avoid crowds and exposure to illness.
- Advise patient to minimize GI upset by eating small, frequent servings of healthy food, drinking plenty of fluids, and chewing gum.
- Tell patient drug may temporarily redden urine.
- Teach patient about the need for regular blood testing during therapy.
- Inform patient that hair loss is a common adverse reaction but usually reverses once therapy ends.
- Caution females of childbearing potential to avoid becoming pregnant during therapy.
- Advise breastfeeding females to discontinue breastfeeding during therapy.
- As appropriate, review all other significant and life-threatening adverse reactions and interactions, especially those related to the drugs and tests mentioned above.

deferoxamine mesylate

Desferal, PMS-Deferoxamine

Pharmacologic class: Heavy-metal antagonist

Therapeutic class: Chelating agent, antidote

Pregnancy risk category C

Action

Complexes with iron (free serum iron and iron from ferritin and hemosiderin, but minimally with transferrin) to slow hepatic accumulation and prevent iron from reacting chemically

Pharmacokinetics

Drug is metabolized rapidly by plasma enzymes. Chelate is readily soluble in water and easily passes through the kidneys. It is excreted in urine, with some excretion by bile in feces.

Onset	Peak	Duration
Unknown	Unknown	Unknown

How supplied

Powder for reconstitution for injection (white to off-white): 500-mg vials

Indications and dosages

➤ Adjunctive therapy in acute iron intoxication with cardiovascular collapse

Adults and children older than age 3: Usual initial dosage—1 g by slow I.V. infusion (not exceeding 15 mg/kg/hour), followed by 500 mg over 4 hours for two doses, at rate not exceeding 125 mg/hour. If necessary, give subsequent doses of 500 mg over 4 to 12 hours at rate not exceeding 125 mg/hour. Maximum recommended dosage is 6 g/24 hour.

Off-label uses

- Aluminum accumulation in bone in patients with renal failure
- Aluminum-induced dialysis encephalopathy

Administration

Preparation

Know that I.V. route should be used only in patients with cardiovascular collapse—and then drug should be given only by slow infusion.

As soon as patient's condition permits, discontinue I.V. administration and administer drug I.M., if more therapy is indicated.

Know that in children younger than age 3 who have relatively little iron overload, iron mobilization with drug is relatively poor. Withhold drug in these patients unless significant iron mobilization occurs.

• Be aware that patients with iron overload usually become vitamin C–deficient (probably because iron oxidizes vitamin C). As adjuvant to iron chelation therapy, vitamin C may be given in divided doses (up to 200 mg for adults), starting after first month of regular deferoxamine therapy.

Dilution and compatibility

• Reconstitute each vial with 2 mL sterile water for injection.

• Know that reconstituted solution should be clear and colorless to slightly yellow.

• Further dilute with normal saline solution, D_5W, or lactated Ringer's solution.

• Discard unused solution.

Infusion considerations

Be aware that drug must be given by slow I.V. infusion at a rate not exceeding 15 mg/kg/hour for first infusion. Subsequent doses, if needed, must be given at a slower rate (not exceeding 125 mg/hour).

Be aware that rapid infusion may cause flushing, urticaria, hypotension, and shock.

Monitoring

• Closely monitor serum iron concentration, renal function, arterial blood gas values, central venous pressure, and cardiac output.

Be aware that patient may need larger-than-normal amounts of I.V. fluids to maintain intravascular volume and avoid kidney damage.

Monitor for mucormycosis, a rare but severe fungal infection. Discontinue drug until mycologic tests are performed and immediate treatment has begun.

• Be aware that drug causes iron excretion in urine, making urine appear reddish.

Storage

• Do not store solutions reconstituted with sterile water for injection for more than 1 week at 25°C (77°F). Protect from light.

Contraindications and precautions

Contraindicated in severe renal disease or anuria.

Use cautiously in ***elderly patients,*** pregnant patients, and ***children younger than age 3*** (safety and efficacy not established).

Adverse reactions

CNS: dizziness; peripheral sensory, motor, or mixed neuropathy; paresthesia; **exacerbation or precipitation of aluminum-related dialysis encephalopathy** (with high doses)

CV: tachycardia; **hypotension and shock** (with rapid I.V. administration)

EENT: visual disturbances, high-frequency sensorineural hearing loss, tinnitus (with excessive doses or in patients with low ferritin levels)

GI: nausea, vomiting, diarrhea, abdominal discomfort

GU: reddish urine, dysuria, impaired renal function

Hematologic: blood dyscrasias (rare)

Metabolic: growth retardation (with excessive doses or in patients with low ferritin levels)

Musculoskeletal: leg cramps

Respiratory: acute respiratory distress syndrome (with excessive doses)

Skin: generalized erythema

Other: allergic reactions including generalized rash, urticaria, angioedema, and **anaphylaxis; *Yersinia* infection or mucormycosis** (rare)

Interactions

Drug-drug. *Ascorbic acid:* increased availability of iron to chelation
Prochlorperazine: possible transient impairment of consciousness
Drug-diagnostic tests. *Gallium-67:* distortion of imaging results due to rapid urinary excretion of drug-bound gallium-67

Toxicity and overdose

- Inadvertent overdose, I.V. bolus, or rapid I.V. infusion may lead to hypotension, tachycardia, and GI disturbances. Other effects may include acute but transient vision or hearing loss, aphasia, agitation, headache, nausea, bradycardia, and acute renal failure.
- No known antidote exists. Discontinue infusion and provide symptomatic and supportive therapy, including dialysis and resuscitation, as indicated. In most cases, vision and hearing disturbances reverse once therapy ends.

Patient teaching

- Tell patient that vision and hearing disturbances should reverse when therapy ends.
- As appropriate, review all other significant and life-threatening adverse reactions and interactions, especially those related to the drugs and tests mentioned above.

desmopressin acetate (1-deamino-8-D-arginine vasopressin)

DDAVP

Pharmacologic class: Posterior pituitary hormone
Therapeutic class: Antidiuretic hormone
Pregnancy risk category B

Action

Enhances water reabsorption by increasing permeability of renal collecting ducts to adenosine monophosphate and water, thereby reducing urine output and increasing urine osmolality. Also increases factor VIII (antihemophilic factor) activity.

Pharmacokinetics

Biphasic half-lives are 7.8 minutes for fast phase and 75.5 minutes for slow phase.

Onset	Peak	Duration
15-30 min	1.5-3 hr	4-12 hr

How supplied

Solution for injection (aqueous): 4 mcg/mL in single-dose 1-mL ampules and multidose 10-mL vials

Indications and dosages

➤ Diabetes insipidus
Adults and children older than age 12: 0.5 mL (2 mcg) to 1 mL (4 mcg) I.V. daily, usually in two divided doses
➤ Hemophilia A and mild to moderate von Willebrand's disease (VWD) type 1
Adults and children: 0.3 mcg/kg I.V.; may repeat dose if needed. If required to maintain hemostasis during surgery, give I.V. dose 30 minutes before surgery.

Administration

Preparation

- Be aware that drug is not indicated in severe VWD type 1.
- Do not give to patients with VWD type 2B, because platelet aggregation may occur.
- In patients with hemophilia A, determine factor VIII coagulant activity before starting drug. If level is lower than 5%, desmopressin may not be recommended.

Dilution and compatibility
• For adults and children weighing more than 10 kg (22 lb) who have hemophilia A or VWD type 1, dilute in 50 mL normal saline solution.
• For children weighing less than 10 kg (22 lb) who have hemophilia A or VWD type 1, dilute in 10 mL normal saline solution.
• Administer immediately after dilution.
Infusion consideration
• When giving to patient with diabetes insipidus, adjust morning and evening dosages as appropriate to minimize frequent urination and risk of water intoxication.
🔈 When giving to child with diabetes insipidus, carefully restrict fluid intake to prevent hyponatremia and water intoxication.
• For patients with diabetes insipidus, give by direct I.V. injection over 1 minute.
• For patients with hemophilia A or VWD type 1, give by slow I.V. infusion over 15 to 30 minutes.
Monitoring
• Monitor pulse rate and blood pressure throughout infusion.
• Monitor urine volume and specific gravity, plasma and urine osmolality, and electrolyte levels in patients with diabetes insipidus.
• Monitor factor VIII antigen levels, activated partial thromboplastin time, and bleeding time in patients with hemophilia.
Storage
• Refrigerate at 2° to 8°C (36° to 46°F).

Contraindications and precautions

Contraindicated in hypersensitivity to drug or its components and in moderate to severe renal impairment (creatinine clearance below 50 mL/minute).

Use cautiously in hemophilia A with factor VIII levels of 5% or lower, severe VWD type 1, VWD type 2B, coronary artery disease, hypertensive cardiovascular disease, fluid and electrolyte imbalances, and pregnant or breast-feeding patients.

Adverse reactions

CNS: transient headache
CV: slight blood pressure changes
GI: nausea, mild abdominal pain
GU: vulval pain
Other: burning after injection, edema, local erythema, facial flushing

Interactions

Drug-drug. *Carbamazepine, chlorpropamide, pressors:* potentiation of desmopressin effects

Toxicity and overdose

• Overdose signs and symptoms may include abdominal pain, dyspnea, facial flushing, fluid retention, and headache.
• No known antidote exists. Depending on overdose severity, reduce dosage or frequency or discontinue drug, as ordered. Provide symptomatic and supportive interventions.

Patient teaching

🔈 Instruct patient to immediately report headache, shortness of breath, nausea, abdominal pain, and vulval pain.
• Instruct patient with diabetes insipidus to avoid overhydration, obtain daily weights, and report weight gain or swelling of arms or legs.
• Caution elderly patient with diabetes insipidus not to increase fluid intake beyond that sufficient to satisfy thirst.
• As appropriate, review all significant adverse reactions and interactions, especially those related to the drugs mentioned above.

dexrazoxane

Zinecard

Pharmacologic class: Cytoprotective agent

Therapeutic class: Chelator, anthracycline antidote

Pregnancy risk category C

Action

Exact action unknown. Drug is a potent intracellular chelating agent and ethylenediamine tetra-acidic acid derivative that readily penetrates cell membranes. Appears to undergo intracellular conversion to ring-opened chelating agent that impedes iron-mediated free-radical generation (partly responsible for anthracycline-induced cardiomyopathy). Also inhibits topoisomerase II, diminishing tissue damage from anthracycline extravasation.

Pharmacokinetics

Drug is partially metabolized, mainly in the liver. It distributes widely and rapidly, with highest concentrations in the liver and kidneys. It is not bound to plasma protein. Elimination half-life is 2.1 to 2.5 hours. Parent drug and metabolite are excreted primarily in urine.

Onset	Peak	Duration
Unknown	Unknown	Unknown

How supplied

Powder for reconstitution for injection (white, lyophilized): 250-mg and 500-mg single-use vials

Indications and dosages

➤ To reduce cardiomyopathy incidence and severity associated with doxorubicin in women with metastatic breast cancer

Adults: 10:1 ratio of dexrazoxane: doxorubicin (for example, 500 mg/m^2 dexrazoxane to 50 mg/m^2 doxorubicin) by slow I.V. push or rapid I.V. infusion, followed by doxorubicin within 30 minutes of starting dexrazoxane

Dosage adjustment

- Know that because doxorubicin dosage should be reduced in hyperbilirubinemia, dexrazoxane dosage should be reduced proportionately to maintain 10:1 ratio in patients with hepatic impairment.
- Reduce dosage by 50% in renal impairment (creatinine clearance below 40 mL/minute).

Off-label uses

- Anthracycline extravasation during chemotherapy
- Prophylaxis for anthracycline-induced cardiotoxicity

Administration

Preparation

Use caution when handling and preparing reconstituted solution. Wear gloves; if powder contacts skin or mucous membranes, immediately wash area with soap and water.

Be aware that drug is indicated only to reduce incidence and severity of cardiomyopathy associated with doxorubicin in women with metastatic breast cancer who have received cumulative doxorubicin dosages of 300 mg/m^2 and will continue to receive that drug to maintain tumor control.

Know that drug is not recommended for use at doxorubicin initiation.

- Obtain baseline CBC, prothrombin time (PT), partial thromboplastin time (PTT), ECG, serum iron and zinc levels, and hepatic and renal function tests before starting therapy.

Dilution and compatibility
• Reconstitute with 0.167 molar sodium lactate injection to yield a concentration of 10 mg dexrazoxane/mL sodium lactate injection.
• Further dilute with normal saline solution or D_5W to a concentration of 1.3 to 5 mg/mL in infusion solution.
• Do not mix with other drugs.
• Discard unused solution.
Infusion considerations
• Give reconstituted solution by slow I.V. push or rapid I.V. infusion.
🔊 After completing dose by I.V. push or infusion and before total elapsed time of 30 minutes from beginning of dexrazoxane administration, give doxorubicin I.V. injection. Do not give doxorubicin before I.V. injection of dexrazoxane.
Monitoring
• Continue to monitor CBC, PT, PTT, ECG, serum iron and zinc levels, and hepatic and renal function tests results throughout therapy.
🔊 Frequently observe for bone marrow depression, as drug may exacerbate myelosuppression caused by antineoplastic agents.
🔊 Closely monitor cardiac function, because of possible anthracycline-induced cardiotoxicity.
Storage
• Store at controlled room temperature of 25°C (77°F); excursions permitted to 15° to 30°C (59° to 86°F).
• Be aware that reconstituted solutions remain stable for 6 hours at controlled room temperature or when refrigerated at 2° to 8°C (36° to 46°F).

Contraindications and precautions

Contraindicated with chemotherapy regimens not containing anthracyclines.

Use cautiously in combination with other cytotoxic drugs and in ***elderly patients,*** pregnant or breastfeeding patients, and ***children*** (long-term safety and efficacy not established).

Adverse reactions

CNS: fatigue, malaise, **neurotoxicity**
CV: phlebitis
EENT: esophagitis
GI: nausea, vomiting, diarrhea, anorexia, stomatitis, dysphagia
Hepatic: abnormal liver function
Skin: alopecia, streaking or erythema at injection site
Other: fever, infection, sepsis, pain at injection site

Interactions

Drug-drug. *FAC (fluorouracil, doxorubicin, and cyclophosphamide) regimen:* interference with FAC antitumor efficacy
Other cytotoxic drugs: increased myelosuppressive effects
Drug-diagnostic tests. *CBC:* bone marrow depression
Liver function tests: abnormal

Toxicity and overdose

• Primary toxic effect is bone marrow depression.
• No known antidote exists. Until bone marrow depression and related conditions resolve, provide symptomatic and supportive therapy, including treatment of infection, fluid regulation, and adequate nutrition. Dialysis may have some benefit in drug removal.

Patient teaching

🔊 Instruct patient to immediately report fever, signs and symptoms of local infection, and sore throat.
• Inform patient that alopecia usually reverses 2 to 3 months after last dose and that new hair growth may differ in texture or color.
• Tell patient about the need for repeated laboratory testing during therapy.

- Advise breastfeeding patient to stop breastfeeding during therapy.
- As appropriate, review all other significant and life-threatening adverse reactions and interactions, especially those related to the drugs and tests mentioned above.

dextran, high-molecular-weight (dextran 70, dextran 75)

Gentran 70, Macrodex

dextran, low-molecular-weight (dextran 40, 10% LMD)

Gentran 40

Pharmacologic class: Polysaccharide
Therapeutic class: Plasma volume expander
Pregnancy risk category C

Action

Expands plasma volume through colloidal osmotic effects during hypovolemic shock; pulls fluid from interstitial space, moving it into intravascular space

Pharmacokinetics

High-molecular-weight (HMW) dextran: Molecules below 50,000 molecular weight are excreted renally, with approximately 50% appearing in urine within 24 hours in normovolemic patients. Remaining drug is degraded by enzymes to glucose at a rate of about 70 to 90 mg/kg/day. Because of larger molecules and slower excretion rates, HMW dextran more efficiently expands plasma volume 2 to 3 hours after infusion than dextran of low molecular weight.
Low-molecular-weight (LMW) dextran: Molecules are distributed evenly in vascular system. Drug distributes according to molecular weight, shifting toward higher molecular weights as the kidneys excrete smaller molecules. Approximately 50% appears in urine within 3 hours, 60% within 6 hours, and 75% within 24 hours in normovolemic patients. Remaining 25% is partially hydrolyzed and excreted in urine, partially excreted in feces, and partially oxidized. It degrades slowly by enzymes to glucose.

Onset	Peak	Duration
Immediate	Immediate	Unknown

How supplied

Solution for injection (clear): HMW dextran—6% dextran 70 or dextran 75 in normal saline solution or D_5W; LMW dextran—10% dextran 40 in normal saline solution or D_5W

Indications and dosages

➤ Plasma volume expansion

Adults: *HMW dextran*—Usual initial dosage is 500 mL of 6% solution I.V., not to exceed 20 mL/kg during first 24 hours. *LMW dextran*—Usual initial dosage is 500 mL of 10% solution I.V., not to exceed 20 mL/kg during first 24 hours. Beyond 24 hours, usual total daily dosage should not exceed 10 mL/kg, and therapy should not exceed 5 days for either HMW or LMW dextran.
Children: Dosage based on weight or body surface area, not to exceed 20 mL/kg I.V. daily

Administration

Dilution and compatibility

- Know that solutions do not require dilution.
- Be aware that solution must be clear.

• If crystals form in solution, place in warm water and dissolve all crystals before administering.
• Discard unused portion.

Infusion considerations
• Be aware that infusion rate is based on amount of fluid lost and hemoconcentration.
• Give by I.V. infusion only.
• In normovolemic patients, infuse no faster than 4 mL/minute.
• Monitor central venous pressure, especially during initial infusion.
• Replace I.V. administration apparatus at least once every 24 hours.

Monitoring
Observe patient closely for signs and symptoms of anaphylaxis during first 30 minutes of infusion.
Assess vital signs frequently. Suspect circulatory overload if patient has increased heart and respiratory rates, shortness of breath, and wheezing.
• Evaluate for dehydration after infusion. Maintain hydration with additional I.V. fluids, but avoid overhydration.
• Know that bleeding time may be prolonged temporarily in patients receiving more than 1,000 mL.
Carefully monitor amount and pattern of fluid intake and output. If no increase in diuresis follows infusion of 500-mL dose, discontinue drug until adequate diuresis develops spontaneously or can be induced by other means.
If infusion reaction or extravasation occurs, discontinue drug and treat appropriately.

Storage
• Store HMW solution at constant temperature no higher than 25°C (77°F).
• Store LMW solution at constant temperature of 15° to 30°C (59° to 86°F), not exceeding 40°C (104°F).

Contraindications and precautions

Contraindicated in hypersensitivity to drug, pulmonary edema, cardiac decompensation, severe congestive heart failure, thrombocytopenia, renal disease with severe oliguria or anuria, hypovolemic conditions, or when sodium or chloride use could be detrimental (sodium chloride–containing preparations).

Use cautiously in active hemorrhage, diabetes mellitus, chronic hepatic disease, abdominal conditions, and pregnant or breastfeeding patients.

Adverse reactions

CV: hypotension, **thrombophlebitis, cardiac arrest**
GI: nausea, vomiting
GU: increased urine viscosity, **osmotic nephrosis, renal failure**
Hematologic: reduced platelet function, **prolonged bleeding time, decreased coagulation times**
Metabolic: hyponatremia
Respiratory: wheezing, dyspnea, **bronchospasm, pulmonary edema**
Skin: urticaria, rash, flushing, pruritus, angioedema
Other: chills, infection at injection site, infusion reaction (such as fever, thrombosis, or phlebitis), **anaphylaxis**

Interactions

Drug-drug. *Abciximab, aspirin, heparin, thrombolytics, warfarin:* increased bleeding
Drug-diagnostic tests. *Alanine aminotransferase, aspartate aminotransferase:* increased
Bilirubin, glucose, hematocrit, hemoglobin, total protein, urine protein: false increases
Bleeding time: prolonged
Blood typing and cross-matching, Rh typing: test interference
Hematocrit: decreased

Toxicity and overdose

- In overdose, expect extension of adverse reactions.
- Discontinue infusion. Provide symptomatic and supportive therapy. Know that factor VIII infusion may help reverse excessive bleeding.

Patient teaching

- As appropriate, review all other significant and life-threatening adverse reactions and interactions, especially those related to the drugs and tests mentioned above.

dextrose (d-glucose)

Pharmacologic class: Monosaccharide
Therapeutic class: Carbohydrate, caloric parenteral nutritional supplement
Pregnancy risk category C

Action

Decreases protein and nitrogen loss; promotes glycogen deposition and ketone accumulation (at sufficient dosages)

Pharmacokinetics

Drug is metabolized readily and excreted by the kidneys.

Onset	Peak	Duration
2-3 min	Unknown	Unknown

How supplied

Solution for injection (clear): 2.5% and 5% in water
Solution for injection (clear, hypertonic): 10%, 20%, 25%, 30%, 40%, 50%, and 70% concentrated in water in flexible plastic containers

Indications and dosages

➤ Insulin-induced hypoglycemia
Adults and children: Initially, 20 to 50 mL by I.V. infusion or injection of 50% solution given at a rate of 3 mL/minute. Maintenance dosage is 10% solution by continuous I.V. infusion until blood glucose reaches therapeutic level.
Infants and neonates: 2 mL/kg of 10% to 25% solution by slow I.V. infusion until blood glucose reaches therapeutic level
➤ Calorie replacement
Adults and children: 2.5%, 5%, or 10% solution given through peripheral I.V. line, with dosage tailored to patient's need for fluid or calories; or 10% to 70% solution given through large central vein if needed (typically mixed as total parenteral nutrition)

Off-label uses

- Insulin-secreting islet-cell adenoma
- Varicose veins

Administration

Preparation
- Perform blood glucose sample before administering; however, in emergency, give prescribed dose without waiting for results.

Dilution and compatibility
- Be aware that hypertonic dextrose at 20% concentration or higher is considered a high-alert drug.
- Use extremely cautious aseptic technique when preparing solution; bacteria thrive in glucose environment.
- Do not use unless solution is clear.
- Do not store after mixing any additive in dextrose solution.
- Discard unused portion of solution.

Infusion considerations
- Pay particular attention to concentration of solution to be given.

Infuse hypertonic solutions (above 5% concentration) slowly, preferably through small-bore needle into large vein, to minimize venous irritation and avoid hyperosmolar syndrome and significant hyperglycemia.
Infuse concentrations above 10% through central vein after appropriate dilution to avoid risk of thrombosis.
Do not infuse concentrated solution rapidly (unless indicated); doing so may cause hyperglycemia and fluid shifts.
After abrupt withdrawal of concentrated dextrose infusion, give 5% or 10% dextrose, as ordered, to avoid rebound hypoglycemia.
Do not administer simultaneously with blood through same infusion set, as pseudoagglutination of red blood cells may occur.
Do not use plastic containers in series connections. Such use could result in air embolism due to residual air being drawn from primary container before administration of fluid from secondary container ends.

Monitoring

Avoid fluid and solute overload, which may cause serum electrolyte dilution, overhydration, congestion, or pulmonary edema.
Monitor infusion site frequently to prevent irritation, tissue sloughing, necrosis, and phlebitis.

- Check blood glucose level regularly.
- Monitor fluid intake and output.
- Weigh patient regularly.
- Assess patient for confusion.

Storage

- Protect from freezing and extreme heat.

Contraindications and precautions

Contraindicated in hypersensitivity to drug, hyperglycemia, diabetic coma, hemorrhage, heart failure, intracranial or intraspinal hemorrhage, delirium tremens in dehydrated patients, severe dehydration (concentrated solutions), anuria, hepatic coma, and glucose-galactose malabsorption syndrome.

Use cautiously in renal, cardiac, or hepatic impairment and diabetes mellitus.

Adverse reactions

CNS: hyperosmolar syndrome (mental confusion and loss of consciousness)
CV: hypertension, phlebitis, **venous thrombosis, heart failure**
GU: glycosuria, osmotic diuresis
Metabolic: hyperglycemia, electrolyte imbalances, **hypervolemia, hypovolemia, hyperosmolar coma**
Respiratory: pulmonary edema
Skin: flushing, urticaria
Other: chills, fever, dehydration, injection site reaction, infection

Interactions

Drug-drug. *Corticosteroids, corticotropin:* increased risk of fluid and electrolyte imbalance
Drug-diagnostic tests. *Glucose:* increased

Toxicity and overdose

- If fluid or solute overload occurs, expect extension of adverse reactions.
- Reevaluate patient's condition and institute corrective treatment as indicated.

Patient teaching

- Teach patient how to recognize signs and symptoms of hypoglycemia and hyperglycemia.
- Provide instructions on glucose self-monitoring to patient with diabetes mellitus.
- As appropriate, review all other significant and life-threatening adverse reactions and interactions, especially those related to the drugs and tests mentioned above.

[redacted]

diazepam

Diazemuls🍁❉, Valium

Pharmacologic class: Benzodiazepine
Therapeutic class: Anxiolytic, anticonvulsant, sedative-hypnotic, skeletal muscle relaxant (centrally acting)
Controlled substance schedule IV
Pregnancy risk category D

Action

Produces anxiolytic effect and CNS depression by stimulating gamma-aminobutyric acid receptors. Relaxes skeletal muscles of spine by inhibiting polysynaptic afferent pathways. Controls seizures by enhancing presynaptic inhibition.

Pharmacokinetics

Drug distributes widely throughout body tissues (including brain) and crosses placental barrier. Highly protein-bound, it undergoes hepatic biotransformation to active metabolite with long half-life. It is excreted mainly in urine, with some secretion in breast milk.

Onset	Peak	Duration
1-5 min	15-30 min	15-60 min

How supplied

Solution for injection (colorless): 5 mg/mL

Indications and dosages

➢ Anxiety

Adults: For moderate anxiety, 2 to 5 mg I.V., repeated in 3 to 4 hours if needed. For severe anxiety, 5 to 10 mg I.V., repeated in 3 to 4 hours if needed.

➢ Before cardioversion

Adults: 5 to 15 mg I.V. 5 to 10 minutes before cardioversion

➢ Before endoscopy

Adults: Dosage individualized; usually, 10 mg I.V. is sufficient. If response is inadequate, repeat dose, to a maximum total dosage of 20 mg I.V.

➢ Status epilepticus and severe recurrent seizures

Adults: 5 to 10 mg I.V. slowly, repeated as needed q 10 to 15 minutes to a maximum of 30 mg; repeat regimen in 2 to 4 hours if needed.

Children age 5 and older: 1 mg I.V. slowly q 2 to 5 minutes, to a maximum of 10 mg; repeat in 2 to 4 hours if needed.

Children ages 31 days to 5 years: 0.2 to 0.5 mg I.V. slowly q 2 to 5 minutes, to a maximum of 5 mg I.V.

➢ Muscle spasm associated with local pathology, cerebral palsy, athetosis, "stiff-man" syndrome, or tetanus

Adults: 5 to 10 mg I.V., repeated in 3 to 4 hours if needed. Tetanus may necessitate higher dosages.

Children age 5 and older: 5 to 10 mg I.V., repeated q 3 to 4 hours as needed to control tetanus spasm

Children ages 31 days to 5 years: 1 to 2 mg I.V. slowly; repeated q 3 to 4 hours as needed to control tetanus spasm

➢ Acute alcohol withdrawal

Adults: Initially, 10 mg I.V.; then 5 to 10 mg I.V. in 3 to 4 hours p.r.n.

Dosage adjustment

- Give lower dosage and increase dosage slowly in children, elderly or debilitated patients, and patients receiving other sedatives concurrently.

Off-label uses

- Adjunct to general anesthesia
- Panic attack

Administration

Preparation

- Assess blood pressure and liver function test results before administering.

Dilution and compatibility
Do not dilute or mix with other drugs or solutions in syringe or container.
Do not use if solution is darker than slightly yellow or contains precipitate.
Infusion considerations
• Know that I.V. route is preferred over I.M. route because of slow or erratic I.M. absorption.
Give slowly by direct I.V. injection into large vein over at least 1 minute for each 5 mg in adults or at least 3 minutes for each 0.25 mg/kg in children.
Be aware that I.V. infusion is not recommended because of possible precipitate formation in I.V. fluids and drug instability in plastic bags and I.V. tubing.
If direct I.V. injection is not feasible, give slowly through I.V. infusion tubing as close as possible to vein insertion site, taking at least 1 minute for each 5 mg in adults or at least 3 minutes for each 0.25 mg/kg in children.
Avoid sudden withdrawal. Taper dosage gradually to termination.
Monitoring
• Monitor vital signs and respiratory and neurologic status.
• Enforce bed rest for at least 3 hours after I.V. injection.
• Supervise ambulation, especially in elderly patients.
• Monitor kidney and liver function test results.
Storage
• Store at room temperature of 15° to 30°C (59° to 86°F); protect from light.

Contraindications and precautions

Contraindicated in hypersensitivity to drug, other benzodiazepines, alcohol, or tartrazine; coma or CNS depression; and narrow-angle glaucoma.

Use cautiously in lung disease or unstable cardiovascular disease, hepatic dysfunction, severe renal impairment, ***elderly patients,*** pregnant or breastfeeding patients (use not recommended), and ***children younger than 1 month*** (safety and efficacy not established).

Adverse reactions

CNS: dizziness, drowsiness, stupor, lethargy, depression, light-headedness, disorientation, anger, manic or hypomanic episodes, restlessness, paresthesia, headache, slurred speech, dysarthria, tremor, dystonia, vivid dreams, extrapyramidal reactions, mild paradoxical excitation
CV: bradycardia, tachycardia, hypertension, hypotension, palpitations, **cardiovascular collapse**
EENT: blurred vision, diplopia, nystagmus, nasal congestion
GI: nausea, vomiting, diarrhea, constipation, gastric disorders, difficulty swallowing, increased salivation
GU: urine retention or incontinence, menstrual irregularities, gynecomastia, libido changes
Hematologic: blood dyscrasias (including eosinophilia)
Hepatic: hepatic dysfunction
Musculoskeletal: muscle rigidity, muscular disturbances
Respiratory: respiratory depression
Skin: dermatitis, rash, pruritus, urticaria, diaphoresis
Other: weight gain or loss, decreased appetite, edema, hiccups, fever, physical or psychological drug dependence or tolerance

Interactions

Drug-drug. *Antidepressants, antihistamines, barbiturates, opioids:* additive CNS depression
Cimetidine, disulfiram, fluoxetine, hormonal contraceptives, isoniazid, ketoconazole, metoprolol, propoxyphene, propranolol, valproic acid: decreased metabolism and enhanced action of diazepam

Levodopa: decreased levodopa efficacy
Rifampin: increased metabolism and decreased efficacy of diazepam
Theophylline: decreased sedative effect of diazepam
Drug-diagnostic tests. *Alanine aminotransferase, alkaline phosphatase, aspartate aminotransferase, lactate dehydrogenase:* increased
Drug-herb. *Chamomile, hops, kava, skullcap, valerian:* increased CNS depression
Drug-behaviors. *Alcohol use:* increased CNS depression

Toxicity and overdose

- Overdose signs and symptoms may include confusion, drowsiness, somnolence, lethargy, impaired coordination, and diminished reflexes. Life-threatening reactions (including hypotension and respiration or circulatory depression) also may occur.
- Discontinue drug. Monitor vital signs closely and provide I.V. fluids, if indicated and ordered. In severe overdose, maintain patent airway, provide artificial ventilation and oxygen, provide symptomatic therapy, and resuscitate, as indicated and ordered. Know that flumazenil (specific benzodiazepine-receptor antagonist) may be indicated for complete or partial reversal of sedative effects. Dialysis has limited benefit.

Patient teaching

- Caution patient to avoid driving and other hazardous activities until drug's effects on concentration and alertness are known.
- Teach patient to move slowly when sitting up or standing, to avoid dizziness or light-headedness from blood pressure decrease. Advise patient to dangle legs briefly before getting out of bed.
- As appropriate, review all other significant and life-threatening adverse reactions and interactions, especially those related to the drugs, tests, herbs, and behaviors mentioned above.

D

digoxin

Lanoxin, Lanoxin Injection Pediatric

Pharmacologic class: Cardiac glycoside
Therapeutic class: Inotrope, antiarrhythmic
Pregnancy risk category C

Action

Increases force and velocity of myocardial contraction and prolongs refractory period of atrioventricular (AV) node by increasing calcium entry into myocardial cells. Slows conduction through sinoatrial and AV nodes and produces antiarrhythmic effect.

Pharmacokinetics

Drug concentrates in tissues, has a wide volume of distribution, and crosses blood-brain and placental barriers. It is partially protein-bound; only a small percentage is metabolized. Drug is excreted primarily in the kidneys by glomerular filtration, with approximately 50% to 70% excreted in urine unchanged. Renal excretion is proportional to glomerular filtration rate and largely independent of urine flow.

Onset	Peak	Duration
5-30 min	1-5 hr	2-4 days

How supplied

Solution for injection (clear): 0.05 mg/mL, 0.1 mg/mL, and 0.25 mg/mL

Solution for injection, pediatric (clear): 0.1 mg/mL

Indications and dosages

➤ Heart failure; tachyarrhythmias; atrial fibrillation and flutter; paroxysmal atrial tachycardia

Adults: For rapid digitalizing, 0.6 to 1 mg I.V. over 24 hours, with 50% of total dosage given initially and additional fractions given at 4- to 8-hour intervals; or oral digitalizing dose given over 24 hours, followed by oral maintenance dosages based on lean body weight, renal function, and drug blood level

Children older than age 10: For rapid digitalizing, 8 to 12 mcg/kg I.V. over 24 hours, with 50% of total dosage given initially and additional fractions given at 4- to 8-hour intervals, followed by oral maintenance dosages as determined by renal function

Children ages 5 to 10: For rapid digitalizing, 15 to 30 mcg/kg I.V. over 24 hours, with 50% of total dosage given initially and additional fractions given at 4- to 8-hour intervals, followed by oral maintenance dosages as determined by renal function

Children ages 2 to 5: For rapid digitalizing, 25 to 35 mcg/kg I.V. over 24 hours, with 50% of total dosage given initially and additional fractions given at 4- to 8-hour intervals, followed by oral maintenance dosages as determined by renal function

Children ages 1 to 2: For rapid digitalizing, 30 to 50 mcg/kg I.V. over 24 hours, with 50% of total dosage given initially and additional fractions given at 4- to 8-hour intervals, followed by oral maintenance dosages as determined by renal function

Infants (full-term): For rapid digitalizing, 20 to 30 mcg/kg I.V. over 24 hours, with 50% of total dosage given initially and additional fractions given at 4- to 8-hour intervals, followed by oral maintenance dosages as determined by renal function

Infants (premature): For rapid digitalizing, 15 to 25 mcg/kg I.V. over 24 hours, with 50% of total dosage given initially and additional fractions given at 4- to 8-hour intervals, followed by oral maintenance dosages as determined by renal function

Dosage adjustment

- Be aware that patients with renal impairment or thyroid disorders may require smaller-than-usual maintenance dosages or prolonged dosing intervals.

Off-label uses

- Intrauterine tachyarrhythmias
- Supraventricular tachyarrhythmias

Administration

Preparation

Because of drug's narrow therapeutic index, monitor dosage regularly and monitor patient for signs and symptoms of toxicity.

Be aware that preterm and immature infants are particularly sensitive to drug and require smaller dosages individualized based on degree of maturity.

Double-check vial to ensure that Lanoxin Injection Pediatric is being used for infants and children.

Be aware that drug affects cardiac contraction and excitability in same way calcium does; therefore, hypercalcemia may predispose patient to digoxin toxicity.

- Know that for rapid effect, initial digitalizing dosage generally is given in several divided doses over 12 to 24 hours.

• Be aware that dosages used for atrial arrhythmias generally are higher than those used for inotropic effect.
Assess baseline electrolyte levels; be aware that potassium or magnesium depletion sensitizes myocardium to digoxin and may cause digoxin-induced arrhythmias despite therapeutic digoxin serum levels.
Dilution and compatibility
• Give drug undiluted, or dilute with more than fourfold volume of sterile water for injection, normal saline solution for injection, or D_5W for injection, as directed.
Be aware that less than fourfold volume of diluent may lead to drug precipitation.
• Do not mix with other drugs or administer simultaneously through same line.
• Use diluted solution immediately.
Infusion considerations
Be aware that slow I.V. infusion (over at least 5 minutes) is preferable to bolus administration; too rapid infusion may cause systemic and coronary arteriolar constriction.
Monitoring
Monitor for signs and symptoms of drug toxicity (such as nausea, vomiting, visual disturbances, arrhythmias, and altered mental status). Be aware that therapeutic digoxin levels range from 0.5 to 2 ng/mL.
Continue to closely monitor ECG and blood digoxin, potassium, magnesium, calcium, and creatinine levels.
Storage
• Store at 25°C (77°F); excursions permitted to 15° to 30°C (59° to 86°F). Protect from light.

Contraindications and precautions

Contraindicated in hypersensitivity to drug, uncontrolled ventricular arrhythmias, AV block, idiopathic hypertrophic subaortic stenosis, and constrictive pericarditis.

Use cautiously in renal or hepatic impairment, electrolyte imbalance, myocardial infarction, thyroid disorders, obesity, ***elderly patients,*** and pregnant or breastfeeding patients.

Adverse reactions

CNS: fatigue, headache, asthenia, confusion
CV: bradycardia, ECG changes, **arrhythmias**
EENT: blurred or yellow vision
GI: nausea, vomiting, diarrhea
GU: gynecomastia
Hematologic: thrombocytopenia
Other: decreased appetite

Interactions

Drug-drug. *Amiodarone, cyclosporine, diclofenac, diltiazem, propafenone, quinidine, quinine, verapamil:* increased digoxin blood level, possibly leading to toxicity
Amphotericin B, corticosteroids, mezlocillin, piperacillin, thiazide and loop diuretics, ticarcillin: hypokalemia, increased risk of digoxin toxicity
Beta-adrenergic blockers, other antiarrhythmics (including disopyramide, quinidine): additive bradycardia
Laxatives (excessive use): hypokalemia, increased risk of digoxin toxicity
Spironolactone: reduced digoxin clearance, increased risk of digoxin toxicity
Thyroid hormones: decreased digoxin efficacy
Drug-diagnostic tests. *Creatine kinase:* increased
Drug-herb. *Coca seed, coffee seed, cola seed, guarana seed, horsetail, licorice, natural stimulants (such as aloe), yerba maté:* increased risk of digoxin toxicity and hypokalemia
Ephedra (ma huang): arrhythmias

Hawthorn: increased risk of adverse cardiovascular effects
Indian snakeroot: bradycardia
St. John's wort: decreased blood level and effects of digoxin

Toxicity and overdose

- Overdose may cause anorexia, nausea, vomiting, diarrhea, and CNS disturbances. Life-threatening toxicity may induce ventricular tachycardia or ventricular fibrillation, progressive bradyarrhythmias, heart block, or cardiac arrest. Life-threatening hyperkalemia may result from massive potassium shift from inside to outside of cells. Although digoxin may cause anorexia, nausea, vomiting, diarrhea, and CNS disturbances in young patients, these are rarely initial overdose manifestations. In infants and children, arrhythmias (including sinus bradycardia) are earliest and most common manifestation.
- Temporarily discontinue drug until adverse reactions resolve. Closely monitor cardiac function. Correct electrolyte imbalances as indicated. Know that digoxin immune FAB (ovine), atropine, or temporary pacemaker may be used to treat rhythm disturbances. Avoid potassium use in massive overdose. Dialysis or exchange transfusion does not effectively remove drug.

Patient teaching

- Stress importance of follow-up testing as directed by prescriber.
- As appropriate, review all other significant and life-threatening adverse reactions and interactions, especially those related to the drugs, tests, and herbs mentioned above.

digoxin immune FAB (ovine)

Digibind, DigiFab

Pharmacologic class: Digoxin-specific antigen-binding fragment
Therapeutic class: Cardiac glycoside antidote
Pregnancy risk category C

Action

Binds with free digoxin intravascularly and in extracellular fluid; resulting complex is excreted by the kidneys. As digoxin blood level falls, digoxin from tissues enters serum and is bound and excreted.

Pharmacokinetics

Drug distributes freely to extracellular space, has half-life of 15 to 20 hours, and is excreted in urine.

Onset	Peak	Duration
15-30 min	Unknown	8-12 hr

How supplied

Powder for reconstitution for injection (lyophilized): 40 mg/vial (binds 0.5 mg digoxin)
Solution for injection: 38 mg/vial (binds 0.5 mg digoxin)

Indications and dosages

➤ Digoxin toxicity when amount of drug ingested is known

Adults and children: I.V. dosage individualized based on amount of digoxin to be eliminated, calculated as follows: Amount of drug ingested (mg) times 0.8, divided by 0.5 and rounded to next whole vial. Average adult dosage is six vials (228 mg).

➤ Digoxin toxicity when amount of drug ingested is unknown

Adults and children: Twenty vials (760 mg) usually are adequate to treat life-threatening digoxin ingestion; alternatively, may give 10 vials followed by additional 10 vials if needed.

Administration

Preparation

- Perform allergy skin test before administering drug, if time permits.
- Assess baseline vital signs.
- Monitor digoxin and potassium blood levels before therapy.

Keep resuscitation equipment at hand during administration.

Dilution and compatibility

- Reconstitute each vial with 4 mL sterile water for injection.
- Mix gently. Resulting solution should be clear and colorless.
- Further dilute with normal saline solution to desired volume.
- Use reconstituted drug immediately.

Infusion considerations

- Give I.V. infusion over 30 minutes.
- Do not give by I.V. bolus injection unless cardiac arrest is imminent.

Monitoring

- Monitor vital signs, ECG, and cardiac status frequently during administration.
- Continue to monitor digoxin and potassium blood levels during and after therapy. Expect complete reversal of cardiovascular effects to take 3 to 4 hours.

Storage

- Store unreconstituted vials at 30°C (86°F) for up to 30 days, if needed.
- Refrigerate reconstituted drug at 2° to 8°C (36° to 46°F).

Contraindications and precautions

Contraindicated in hypersensitivity to drug, papain, or sheep products and in mild digoxin toxicity.

Use cautiously in cardiovascular disease, renal impairment, ***elderly patients,*** pregnant or breastfeeding patients, and ***children.***

Adverse reactions

CV: increased ventricular rate, **low cardiac output, atrial fibrillation, heart failure**
Metabolic: hypokalemia
Respiratory: impaired respiratory function, tachypnea
Skin: erythema
Other: facial swelling, hypersensitivity reactions including **anaphylaxis**

Interactions

Drug-diagnostic tests. *Immune digoxin assay:* test interference
Potassium: decreased

Toxicity and overdose

Unknown

Patient teaching

- Explain to patient (if alert) or caregiver the purpose of therapy and what to expect.
- As appropriate, review all other significant and life-threatening adverse reactions and interactions, especially those related to the tests mentioned above.

diltiazem hydrochloride

Cardizem

Pharmacologic class: Calcium channel blocker
Therapeutic class: Antianginal, antiarrhythmic (class IV), antihypertensive
Pregnancy risk category C

Action

Inhibits calcium from entering myocardial and vascular smooth-muscle cells, thereby depressing myocardial and smooth-muscle contraction and decreasing impulse formation, conduction velocity, and vasodilation. As a result, systolic and diastolic pressures decrease.

Pharmacokinetics

Drug is metabolized rapidly and almost completely in the liver, and is 70% to 85% protein-bound. It is excreted in urine and bile as active and inactive metabolites; some excretion occurs in breast milk.

Onset	Peak	Duration
2-5 min	2-4 hr	Unknown

How supplied

Powder for reconstitution for injection (white): 25-mg ready-to-use Lyo-Ject dual-chamber syringes; 25 mg in 5-mL vial, 50 mg in 10-mL vial
Solution for injection: 100-mg Monovial and Add-Vantage flexible containers

Indications and dosages

➤ Angina pectoris and vasospastic (Prinzmetal's) angina, hypertension, supraventricular tachyarrhythmias, atrial flutter, or atrial fibrillation
Adults: 0.25 mg/kg by I.V. bolus over 2 minutes; if response is inadequate, may give 0.35 mg/kg over 15 minutes; may follow with continuous I.V. infusion at initial rate of 10 mg/hour for up to 24 hours. May increase by 5 mg/hour to a maximum of 15 mg/hour for 24 hours.

Off-label uses

- Hyperthyroidism
- Migraine
- Raynaud's phenomenon
- Tardive dyskinesia
- Unstable angina, coronary artery bypass graft, myocardial infarction (MI)

Administration

Preparation
- Check blood pressure and ECG before starting therapy. Withhold dose if systolic pressure is below 90 mm Hg.

Dilution and compatibility
- Dilute in D_5W or normal saline solution.
- Mix thoroughly.
- Know that solution should be clear and colorless.
- Use within 24 hours of dilution.
- Discard unused portion of single-use container.

Infusion considerations
- Be aware that after reconstitution, Lyo-Ject syringe is intended for direct I.V. bolus injection and continuous I.V. infusion.
- Give I.V. bolus dose over 2 minutes; may give a second bolus after 15 minutes.
- Be aware that Monovial and Add-Vantage flexible containers are intended for continuous I.V. infusion.
- Administer continuous I.V. infusion at a rate of 5 to 15 mg/hour, based on patient's response.

Do not use plastic containers in series connections. Such use could result in air embolism due to residual air being drawn from primary container before administration of fluid from secondary container ends.

Monitoring
- Withhold dose if systolic blood pressure falls below 90 mm Hg, diastolic pressure falls below 60 mm Hg, or apical pulse is slower than 60 beats/minute.
- Continue to monitor blood pressure and ECG closely during dosage adjustment period.

Monitor for signs and symptoms of heart failure.
- Supervise patient during ambulation.

Storage
- Know that drug may be stored at room temperature for 1 month.

• Diluted drug is stable for up to 24 hours when stored at 15° to 30°C (59° to 86°F) or refrigerated at 2° to 8°C (36° to 46°F). Do not freeze.
• Store flexible containers at controlled room temperature of 20° to 25°C (68° to 77°F). Do not freeze.

Contraindications and precautions

Contraindicated in hypersensitivity to drug, atrial flutter or fibrillation associated with shortened refractory period (Wolff-Parkinson-White syndrome), or recent MI or pulmonary congestion.

Use cautiously in severe hepatic or renal impairment, heart failure, history of serious ventricular arrhythmias, ***elderly patients,*** or concurrent use with I.V. beta-adrenergic blockers (should not be given together or within a few hours), pregnant or breastfeeding patients, and ***children*** (safety not established).

Adverse reactions

CNS: headache, abnormal dreams, anxiety, confusion, dizziness, drowsiness, nervousness, psychiatric disturbances, asthenia, paresthesia, syncope, tremor
CV: peripheral edema, bradycardia, chest pain, hypotension, palpitations, tachycardia, **arrhythmias, heart failure**
EENT: blurred vision, tinnitus, epistaxis
GI: nausea, vomiting, diarrhea, constipation, dyspepsia, dry mouth
GU: urinary frequency, dysuria, nocturia, polyuria, gynecomastia, sexual dysfunction
Hematologic: anemia, **leukopenia, thrombocytopenia**
Metabolic: hyperglycemia
Musculoskeletal: joint stiffness, muscle cramps
Respiratory: cough, dyspnea
Skin: rash, dermatitis, flushing, diaphoresis, photosensitivity, pruritus, urticaria, **erythema multiforme**
Other: unpleasant taste, gingival hyperplasia, weight gain, decreased appetite, **Stevens-Johnson syndrome**

Interactions

Drug-drug. *Beta-adrenergic blockers, digoxin, disopyramide, phenytoin:* bradycardia, conduction defects, heart failure
Carbamazepine, cyclosporine, quinidine: decreased diltiazem metabolism, increased risk of toxicity
Cimetidine, ranitidine: increased blood level and effects of diltiazem
Fentanyl, nitrates, other antihypertensives, quinidine: additive hypotension
HMG-CoA reductase inhibitors, imipramine, sirolimus, tacrolimus: increased blood levels of these drugs
Lithium: decreased lithium blood level, reduced antimanic control
Nonsteroidal anti-inflammatory drugs: decreased antihypertensive effects of diltiazem
Theophylline: increased theophylline effects
Drug-diagnostic tests. *Hepatic enzymes:* increased
Drug-behaviors. *Acute alcohol ingestion:* additive hypotension

Toxicity and overdose

• Overdose signs and symptoms may include hypotension, heart failure, and serious arrhythmias.
• Provide symptomatic and supportive therapy, including vasopressors for hypotension, inotropic drugs and diuretics for heart failure, cardiac pacing, and resuscitation, as indicated and ordered. Dialysis does not remove drug.

Patient teaching

• Advise patient to change position slowly to minimize light-headedness and dizziness.

• As appropriate, review all other significant and life-threatening adverse reactions and interactions, especially those related to the drugs, tests, and behaviors mentioned above.

diphenhydramine hydrochloride
Benadryl

Pharmacologic class: Nonselective histamine$_1$-receptor antagonist
Therapeutic class: Antihistamine, antiemetic, antivertigo agent, sedative
Pregnancy risk category B

Action
Interferes with histamine effects at histamine$_1$-receptor sites; prevents but does not reverse histamine-mediated response. Also possesses CNS depressant and anticholinergic properties.

Pharmacokinetics
Drug distributes widely throughout body, including CNS. Drug is metabolized in the liver and excreted in urine with some evidence of secretion in breast milk.

Onset	Peak	Duration
Rapid	Unknown	4-8 hr

How supplied
Solution for injection: 10 mg/mL, 50 mg/mL

Indications and dosages
➢ Allergy symptoms caused by histamine release (including anaphylaxis, seasonal and perennial allergic rhinitis, and allergic dermatoses); nausea; vertigo
Adults and children older than age 12: 10 to 50 mg I.V. q 2 to 3 hours p.r.n. (Some patients may need up to 100 mg.) Do not exceed 400 mg/day.
Children ages 6 to 12: 1.25 mg/kg (37.5 mg/m^2) I.V. q.i.d. Do not exceed 150 mg/day.

Off-label uses
• Drug-induced extrapyramidal reactions

Administration
Preparation
Do not give within 14 days of monoamine oxidase (MAO) inhibitors.
• Know that injectable form should only be used when oral forms are impractical or contraindicated.
Dilution and compatibility
• Check compatibility carefully before mixing with other drugs.
• Drug is usually given undiluted.
Infusion considerations
• Inject slowly at a rate not exceeding 25 mg/minute.
Monitoring
• Monitor cardiovascular status, especially in patients with cardiovascular disease.
• Supervise patient during ambulation. Use side rails as necessary.
• Discontinue drug 4 days before allergy skin testing to avoid misleading results.
Storage
• Store at controlled room temperature of 15° to 30°C (59° to 86°F). Protect from freezing and light.

Contraindications and precautions
Contraindicated in hypersensitivity to drug, alcohol intolerance, acute asthma attacks, concurrent MAO inhibitor use, and breastfeeding.

Use cautiously in severe hepatic disease, angle-closure glaucoma, seizure disorders, prostatic hypertrophy, lower respiratory disease including asthma, ***elderly patients,*** and pregnant patients (safety not established).

Adverse reactions

CNS: drowsiness, dizziness, headache, paradoxical stimulation (especially in children)
CV: hypotension, palpitations
EENT: blurred vision, tinnitus
GI: diarrhea, constipation, dry mouth
GU: dysuria, urinary frequency, urine retention
Skin: photosensitivity
Other: decreased appetite

Interactions

Drug-drug. *Antihistamines, opioids, sedative-hypnotics:* additive CNS depression
Disopyramide, quinidine, tricyclic antidepressants: increased anticholinergic effects
MAO inhibitors: intensified and prolonged anticholinergic effects
Drug-diagnostic tests. *Hemoglobin, platelets:* decreased
Skin allergy tests: false-negative results
Drug-herb. *Angel's trumpet, jimsonweed, scopolia:* increased anticholinergic effects
Chamomile, hops, kava, skullcap, valerian: increased CNS depression
Drug-behaviors. *Alcohol use:* increased CNS depression

Toxicity and overdose

- In overdose, expect drowsiness and anticholinergic symptoms such as dry mouth. In severe overdose, hypotension, seizures, and possible ventricular arrhythmias may occur.
- Expect to give vasopressors (such as dopamine) for hypotension and diazepam or phenytoin for seizures. Do not give epinephrine for hypotension, as it may exacerbate hypotension. Do not give other stimulants (such as caffeine), as these may induce seizures. For arrhythmias, intervene as appropriate.

Patient teaching

- Caution patient to avoid driving and other hazardous activities until drug's effects on concentration and alertness are known.
- Caution patient to avoid alcohol and other CNS depressants (such as sedatives, tranquilizers) while taking drug.
- As appropriate, review all other significant adverse reactions and interactions, especially those related to the drugs, tests, herbs, and behaviors mentioned above.

dobutamine hydrochloride

Pharmacologic class: Sympathomimetic, adrenergic
Therapeutic class: Inotrope
Pregnancy risk category B

Action

Stimulates beta$_1$-adrenergic receptors of heart, causing a positive inotropic effect that increases myocardial contractility and stroke volume. Also reduces peripheral vascular resistance and decreases ventricular filling pressure.

Pharmacokinetics

Major metabolism routes are methylation of catechol and conjugation. Plasma half-life is 2 minutes. Drug is excreted in urine as dobutamine conjugates and inactive metabolite.

Onset	Peak	Duration
1-2 min	10 min	Brief

How supplied

Solution for injection: 12.5 mg/mL in 20-mL vial

Indications and dosages

➢ Short-term treatment of cardiac decompensation caused by depressed contractility (as during heart failure, cardiomyopathy, or cardiogenic shock); adjunct in cardiac surgery

Adults: 2.5 to 10 mcg/kg/minute I.V. as a continuous infusion, adjusted to hemodynamic response. Dosages above 10 mcg/kg/minute have minimal additional benefit.

Off-label uses

- Adjunct in myocardial infarction (MI) and septic shock
- Diagnostic aid in coronary artery disease (echocardiography stress test, ventriculography, computed tomography)

Administration

Preparation

- As needed, correct hypovolemia by giving volume expanders, as prescribed, before starting drug.

Make sure resuscitative equipment is available.

Dilution and compatibility

- Know that drug is not compatible with alkaline solutions such as sodium bicarbonate injection.
- Dilute to at least 50 mL of solution, using D_5W, normal saline solution, dextrose 5% in half-normal saline solution, dextrose 5% in normal saline solution, dextrose 10% in water, lactated Ringer's solution, D_5W in lactated Ringer's solution, Normosol-M in D_5W, or 20% Osmitrol in water.
- Be aware that solution containing drug may appear pink, from slight oxidation that increases over time but does not affect potency.
- Determine final volume based on patient's fluid requirements.
- Do not mix with other drugs or alkaline solutions such as sodium bicarbonate.

Infusion considerations

- Use infusion pump.
- Administer at 2.5 to 10 mcg/kg/minute I.V. as a continuous infusion. Be aware that rates up to 40 mcg/kg/minute occasionally are required.
- Adjust infusion rate according to response—heart rate, blood pressure, presence of ectopic activity, urine flow, and (when possible) central venous pressure, pulmonary wedge pressure, and cardiac output.

Monitoring

- Monitor ECG and blood pressure continuously during administration.
- Monitor fluid intake and output.

Closely monitor electrolyte levels. Stay especially alert for hypokalemia.

Storage

- Store vials at room temperature of 15° to 30°C (59° to 86°F).
- After dilution, solution is stable for 24 hours at room temperature. Avoid freezing, as crystallization may occur.

Contraindications and precautions

Contraindicated in hypersensitivity to drug and in idiopathic hypertrophic subaortic stenosis.

Use cautiously in hypertension, MI, atrial fibrillation, hypovolemia, ***elderly patients,*** pregnant or breastfeeding patients, and ***children*** (safety and efficacy not established).

Adverse reactions

CNS: headache
CV: hypertension, hypotension, tachycardia, premature ventricular contractions, angina, palpitations, nonspecific chest pain, phlebitis
GI: nausea, vomiting
Metabolic: hypokalemia

Respiratory: dyspnea
Skin: local inflammatory reactions (with extravasation)
Other: hypersensitivity reactions including **anaphylaxis**

Interactions

Drug-drug. *Beta-adrenergic blockers:* increased alpha-adrenergic effects
Bretylium: potentiation of vasopressor activity
Cyclopropane, halothane: serious arrhythmias
Guanethidine: decreased hypotensive effects
Thyroid hormone: increased cardiovascular effects
Tricyclic antidepressants: potentiation of cardiovascular and vasopressor effects
Drug-herb. *Rue:* increased inotropic potential

Toxicity and overdose

- Overdose signs and symptoms may include nausea, vomiting, anorexia, tremors, anxiety, palpitations, headache, shortness of breath, anginal or nonspecific chest pain, excessive blood pressure changes, myocardial ischemia, ventricular tachycardia, and ventricular fibrillation.
- Reduce infusion rate or temporarily discontinue infusion. Establish airway; administer propranolol or lidocaine as ordered for ventricular arrhythmias, and resuscitate as indicated.

Patient teaching

- Instruct patient to report angina, headache, leg cramps, and shortness of breath.
- Explain the need for close observation and monitoring.
- As appropriate, review all other significant and life-threatening adverse reactions and interactions, especially those related to the drugs and herbs mentioned above.

docetaxel

Taxotere

Pharmacologic class: Miotic inhibitor
Therapeutic class: Antineoplastic
Pregnancy risk category D

D

FDA BOXED WARNING

- Give under supervision of physician experienced in cancer chemotherapy, in facility with adequate diagnostic and treatment resources.
- Treatment-related death is more likely if patient has abnormal hepatic function, is receiving higher doses, or has non-small-cell lung cancer and history of platinum-based chemotherapy and is receiving drug as a single agent at a dosage of 100 mg/m^2.
- Generally, drug should not be given to patients with bilirubin level above upper limit of normal (ULN) or those with aspartate aminotransferase (AST) or alanine aminotransferase (ALT) level above 1.5 time ULN concomitant with alkaline phosphatase (ALP) level above 2.5 times ULN. Bilirubin elevations or transaminase abnormalities concurrent with ALP abnormalities increases risk of grade 4 neutropenia, febrile neutropenia, infections, severe thrombocytopenia, severe stomatitis, severe skin toxicity, and toxic death. Patients with isolated transaminase elevations above 1.5 times ULN have higher rate of grade 4 febrile neutropenia, but without increased incidence of toxic death. Before each cycle, obtain bilirubin, ALT or AST, and ALP values and have physician review them.
- Do not give drug to patients with neutrophil count below 1,500 cells/mm^3. Obtain frequent blood cell counts to

monitor for neutropenia (which may be severe and cause infection).
• Severe hypersensitivity reactions and fatal anaphylaxis (rare) have occurred in patients who received recommended 3-day dexamethasone premedication. If hypersensitivity reaction occurs, discontinue docetaxel immediately and give appropriate therapy. Do not give drug to patients with history of severe hypersensitivity reactions to it or other drugs containing polysorbate 80. Severe fluid retention may occur despite dexamethasone premedication regimen.

Action

Promotes assembly and blocks disassembly of microtubular network, preventing cancer cells from dividing and ultimately leading to cell death

Pharmacokinetics

Drug distributes widely throughout body. It is metabolized in the liver, primarily through cytochrome P4503A4 isoenzymes; protein binding is 94% to 97%. Pharmacokinetic profile is consistent with a three-compartment pharmacokinetic model, with half-lives of 4 minutes, 36 minutes, and 11.1 hours. Drug is eliminated in both urine and feces, but fecal excretion is main elimination route.

Onset	Peak	Duration
Rapid	Unknown	7 days

How supplied

Injection concentrate (nonaqueous, viscous): 20 mg and 80 mg in single-dose vials containing polysorbate 80

Indications and dosages

➢ Metastatic breast cancer unresponsive to previous regimens

Adults: 60 to 100 mg/m^2 I.V. over 1 hour q 3 weeks

➢ Non-small-cell lung cancer (NSCLC), metastatic NSCLC, androgen-independent (hormone-refractory) metastatic prostate cancer

Adults: 75 mg/m^2 I.V. over 1 hour q 3 weeks

➢ Gastric adenocarcinoma, head and neck cancer

Adults: 75 mg/m^2 I.V. as a 1-hour infusion, followed by cisplatin as a 1- to 3-hour infusion (both on day 1 only), followed by fluorouracil given as a 24-hour continuous I.V. infusion for 5 days starting at end of cisplatin infusion. Treatment is repeated q 3 weeks.

Dosage adjustment

• Adjust dosage to 75 mg/m^2 in breast cancer patients who received initial dose of 100 mg/m^2 and experience febrile neutropenia, neutrophil count below 500 cells/mm^3 for more than 1 week, or severe or cumulative cutaneous reactions during therapy. If patient continues to experience these reactions, decrease dosage further from 75 mg/m^2 to 55 mg/m^2 or discontinue drug, as ordered. Conversely, patients who received initial dose of 60 mg/m^2 and do not experience these reactions may tolerate higher doses. Discontinue drug entirely, as ordered, in patients who develop grade 3 or higher peripheral neuropathy.
• For patients receiving docetaxel monotherapy for NSCLC after failure of prior platinum-based chemotherapy who received initial dose of 75 mg/m^2 and experience febrile neutropenia, neutrophil count below 500 cells/mm^3 for more than 1 week, severe or cumulative cutaneous reactions, or other grade 3 or 4 nonhematologic toxicities during therapy, withhold dose until toxicity resolves; then resume at 55 mg/m^2.

Discontinue drug entirely, as ordered, in patients who develop grade 3 or higher peripheral neuropathy.
• For patients receiving combination therapy for hormone-refractory metastatic prostate cancer, administer drug when neutrophil count is 1,500 cells/mm^3 or higher. In patients who experience febrile neutropenia, neutrophil count below 500 cells/mm^3 for more than 1 week, severe or cumulative cutaneous reactions, or moderate neurosensory signs or symptoms during therapy, reduce dosage from 75 to 60 mg/m^2. If patient continues to experience these reactions at 60 mg/m^2, discontinue drug, as ordered.
• For patients with gastric or head and neck cancer who are receiving drug in combination with cisplatin and fluorouracil, granulocyte-colony stimulating factor (G-CSF) is recommended during second or subsequent cycles to support potential febrile neutropenia, documented infection with neutropenia, or neutropenia of more than 7 days. If episode of febrile neutropenia, prolonged neutropenia, or neutropenic infection occurs despite G-CSF use, reduce dosage from 75 to 60 mg/m^2. If subsequent episodes of complicated neutropenia occur, reduce dosage from 60 to 45 mg/m^2. For grade 4 thrombocytopenia, reduce dosage from 75 to 60 mg/m^2. Do not retreat with subsequent cycles until neutrophil count rises above 1,500 cells/mm^3 and platelet count rises above 100,000 cells/mm^3. As ordered, discontinue therapy if these toxicities persist. See table below for recommended dosage adjustments for diarrhea, stomatitis, and mucositis toxicities.

Toxicity	Dosage adjustment
Diarrhea grade 3	Episode 1: Reduce fluorouracil dosage 20%. Episode 2: Reduce docetaxel dosage 20%.
Diarrhea grade 4	Episode 1: Reduce docetaxel and fluorouracil dosages 20%. Episode 2: Discontinue therapy.
Stomatitis or mucositis grade 3	Episode 1: Reduce fluorouracil dosage 20%. Episode 2: Stop fluorouracil only in all subsequent cycles.
Stomatitis or mucositis grade 4	Episode 1: Stop fluorouracil only in all subsequent cycles. Episode 2: Reduce docetaxel dosage 20%.

Off-label uses

• Advanced or metastatic esophageal, gastric, or gastroesophageal junction carcinomas, including adenocarcinomas and squamous-cell carcinomas
• Bladder carcinoma
• Ovarian cancer after failure of platinum-based therapy
• Small-cell lung cancer after failure of first-line chemotherapy

Administration

Preparation

Follow hazardous drug guidelines on page S19 for handling, preparation, and administration.

Be aware that medication errors have occurred between docetaxel (Taxotere) and paclitaxel (Taxol) due to similarity in name.

• Assess baseline CBC with differential and liver function tests before starting therapy.

• Premedicate with antiemetic, as prescribed.
• Administer 3-day dexamethasone premedication regimen, as prescribed, to prevent or decrease fluid retention and hypersensitivity reactions.
• Be aware that patients with gastric cancer or head and neck cancer who will receive docetaxel in combination with cisplatin and fluorouracil must receive antiemetics and appropriate hydration, according to facility guidelines.
Dilution and compatibility
Do not let drug concentrate come in contact with plasticized polyvinyl chloride equipment or devices. Use bottles (glass, polypropylene) or plastic bags (polypropylene, polyolefin) and polyethylene-lined administration sets.
Be aware that drug concentrate requires two dilutions before administration.
• Dilute with accompanying diluent solution; rotate vial gently for at least 45 seconds to mix. Do not shake.
• Know that initial diluted solution should be clear; however, foam may appear on top of solution due to polysorbate 80.
• Once foam largely dissipates, withdraw prescribed amount of drug and mix in glass or polypropylene bottle or in plastic bag with 250 mL normal saline solution or D_5W.
• Use fully prepared infusion solution within 4 hours.
Infusion considerations
• Infuse over 1 hour in ambient room temperature and lighting conditions, using polyethylene-lined infusion set.
Monitoring
In patients with preexisting pleural or cardiac effusions, monitor closely for possible exacerbation.
Watch for signs and symptoms of anaphylaxis and other hypersensitivity reactions, especially with first two doses.
Monitor vital signs and fluid intake and output. Watch for signs and symptoms of fluid overload and bronchospasm.
Continue to closely monitor CBC with differential and platelet counts, and assess for signs and symptoms of blood dyscrasias.
• Observe I.V. site frequently for extravasation.
• Monitor neurologic status to detect neurosensory deficits and peripheral neuropathy.
Storage
• Keep in original package to protect from bright light.
• Know that infusion solution may be stored for 4 hours at 2° to 25°C (36° to 77°F).

Contraindications and precautions

Contraindicated in hypersensitivity to drug or polysorbate 80, hepatic impairment, neutrophil count below 1,500 cells/mm^3, bilirubin level above ULN, or AST or ALT level above 1.5 times ULN concomitant with ALP level above 2.5 times ULN.

Use cautiously in females of childbearing potential, pregnant or breastfeeding patients, and ***children younger than age 16*** (safety and efficacy not established).

Adverse reactions

CNS: fatigue, asthenia, neurosensory deficits, peripheral neuropathy
CV: peripheral edema, **cardiac tamponade, pericardial effusion**
GI: nausea, vomiting, diarrhea, stomatitis, ascites
Hematologic: anemia, **thrombocytopenia, leukopenia**
Musculoskeletal: myalgia, joint pain
Respiratory: bronchospasm, pulmonary edema
Skin: alopecia, rash, dermatitis, desquamation, erythema, nail disorders

Other: edema, infusion site reactions, hypersensitivity reactions including **anaphylaxis**

Interactions

Drug-drug. *Antineoplastics:* additive bone marrow depression
Cyclosporine, erythromycin, ketoconazole, troleandomycin: significant change in docetaxel effects
Live vaccines: increased risk of infection

Toxicity and overdose

- Expect overdose complications to include fluid retention, bone marrow suppression, peripheral neurotoxicity, and mucositis.
- No known antidote exists. Provide prompt symptomatic and supportive therapy.

Patient teaching

Instruct patient to obtain daily weights and immediately report sudden weight gain.
Advise patient to immediately report difficulty breathing or rash.
Teach patient which signs and symptoms of blood dyscrasias to report; reinforce the need for frequent blood testing to monitor for these effects.
- Tell patient that drug commonly causes hair loss, but hair will grow back after therapy ends.
- Advise female of childbearing potential to use effective contraception during therapy and to notify prescriber if she suspects she is pregnant.
- As appropriate, review all other significant and life-threatening adverse reactions and interactions, especially those related to the drugs mentioned above.

dolasetron mesylate

Anzemet

Pharmacologic class: Selective serotonin subtype 3 ($5\text{-}HT_3$) receptor antagonist
Therapeutic class: Antiemetic
Pregnancy risk category B

Action

Blocks serotonin activation at receptor sites in vagal nerve terminals and in CNS chemoreceptor trigger zone, suppressing the vomiting reflex

Pharmacokinetics

Drug is metabolized rapidly to active metabolite, hydrodolasetron, which is 50 times more potent than parent compound. Half-life is about 10 minutes for parent drug and 8 hours for hydrodolasetron. Metabolite is excreted unchanged in urine.

Onset	Peak	Duration
Unknown	15-30 min	Up to 24 hr

How supplied

Solution for injection (clear, colorless): 12.5 mg/0.625-mL single-use vials, 12.5 mg/0.625-mL single-use 2-mL Carpuject syringe, 100 mg/5 mL in 5-mL single-use vials, 500 mg/25 mL in 25-mL multidose vials

Indications and dosages

➤ Chemotherapy-induced nausea and vomiting
Adults: 1.8 mg/kg I.V. 30 minutes before chemotherapy
Children ages 2 to 16: 1.8 mg/kg I.V. (not to exceed 100 mg) 30 minutes before chemotherapy

➤ Prevention or treatment of postoperative nausea and vomiting
Adults: 12.5 mg I.V. 15 minutes before anesthesia cessation (for prevention) or as soon as nausea or vomiting begins (for treatment)
Children ages 2 to 16: 0.35 mg/kg I.V. (up to 12.5 mg) 15 minutes before anesthesia cessation (for prevention) or as soon as nausea or vomiting begins (for treatment)

Administration

Preparation

Before administering, check for changes in ECG intervals and use of concurrent drugs that may prolong ECG intervals.

Dilution and compatibility

- Do not dilute drug if giving by direct I.V. injection.
- For I.V. infusion, dilute in normal saline solution, D_5W, or lactated Ringer's solution.
- Do not mix with other drugs.

Infusion considerations

- For direct I.V. injection, administer over 30 seconds.
- For I.V. infusion, give single dose over at least 15 minutes.
- Flush I.V. line before and after infusion.

Monitoring

- Monitor closely for excessive diuresis.

Continue to watch for ECG changes, including prolonged PR interval and widened QRS complex, especially in patients receiving concurrent antiarrhythmics.

Storage

- Store at controlled room temperature of 20° to 25°C (68° to 77°F); protect from light.
- After dilution, drug may be stored under normal lighting conditions at room temperature for 24 hours or refrigerated for 48 hours.

Contraindications and precautions

Contraindicated in hypersensitivity to drug and in arrhythmias.

Use cautiously in risk factors for prolonged cardiac conduction intervals (including hypokalemia or hypomagnesemia), congenital QT syndrome, concurrent use of antiarrhythmics or other drugs that could prolong QT interval, concurrent use of diuretics that could induce electrolyte abnormalities, cumulative high-dose anthracycline therapy, pregnant or breastfeeding patients (safety not established), and ***children younger than age 2*** (safety and efficacy not established).

Adverse reactions

CNS: headache (increased in cancer patients), dizziness, fatigue, syncope
CV: bradycardia, tachycardia, ECG changes, hypertension, hypotension
GI: diarrhea, constipation, dyspepsia, abdominal pain
GU: urine retention, **oliguria**
Skin: pruritus, rash
Other: chills, fever, decreased appetite

Interactions

Drug-drug. *Antiarrhythmics, anthracyclines (high cumulative doses), diuretics, drugs that can prolong ECG intervals:* increased risk of conduction abnormalities
Drugs that affect hepatic microsomal enzymes: altered dolasetron blood level
Drug-diagnostic tests. *Alanine aminotransferase, aspartate aminotransferase:* increased

Toxicity and overdose

- In acute toxicity, signs and symptoms include severe hypotension, dizziness, tremors, depression, and seizures. Cardiac rhythm disturbances also may occur.

• No known antidote exists. Provide supportive care. If patient has second-degree or higher atrioventricular conduction block, institute cardiac telemetry monitoring. If ordered, give plasma expander, dopamine, and atropine. Value of dialysis in removing drug is not known.

Patient teaching

• Inform patient that drug commonly causes headache.
• As appropriate, review all other significant and life-threatening adverse reactions and interactions, especially those related to the drugs and tests mentioned above.

dopamine hydrochloride

Intropin, Revimine

Pharmacologic class: Catecholamine, adrenergic
Therapeutic class: Inotropic, vasopressor
Pregnancy risk category C

FDA BOXED WARNING

• Dilute full-strength injection before administering.
• If extravasation occurs, infiltrate area promptly with 10 to 15 mL saline solution containing 5 to 10 mg phentolamine to prevent sloughing and necrosis. Use syringe with fine hypodermic needle, and infiltrate solution liberally throughout area. Give phentolamine as soon as possible; its sympathetic blockade causes immediate local hyperemic changes if area is infiltrated within 12 hours.

Action

Causes norepinephrine release, leading to dose-dependent vasoconstriction. Also exerts inotropic effects on heart, which may increase heart rate, blood flow, myocardial contractility, and stroke volume.

Pharmacokinetics

Drug distributes widely throughout body, but does not cross blood-brain barrier. Metabolism to inactive metabolites takes place in the liver, kidneys, and plasma. Half-life is about 2 minutes. Approximately 80% of dose is excreted in urine within 24 hours as metabolites; a small portion is excreted unchanged.

Onset	Peak	Duration
1-2 min	Unknown	<10 min

How supplied

Premixed injection: 0.8 mg/mL, 1.6 mg/mL, and 3.2 mg/mL in 250 mL and 500 mL D_5W in plastic containers
Solution for injection (clear, practically colorless): 40 mg/mL, 80 mg/mL, and 160 mg/mL in ampules and vials

Indications and dosages

➤ Shock and hemodynamic imbalance unresponsive to fluid replacement; hypotension
Adults and children: Initially, 2 to 5 mcg/kg/minute by I.V. infusion. Titrate dosage to desired hemodynamic or renal response; may increase infusion by 1 to 4 mcg/kg/minute at 10- to 30-minute intervals. Generally, dosage should not exceed 20 mcg/kg/minute.

Off-label uses

• Chronic obstructive pulmonary disease
• Heart failure

Administration

Preparation

Do not give concurrently with monoamine oxidase (MAO) inhibitors. Reduce dosage if patient has received MAO inhibitor recently.

Dilution and compatibility

• Be aware that drug comes as premixed solution in plastic bags, which requires no dilution. Do not add other drugs to premixed solution. Do not use if solution is darker than slightly yellow or discolored in any other way.

Know that full-strength drug in ampules and vials must be diluted before administration.

• Dilute 200 to 400 mg dopamine in 250 to 500 mL of one of the following compatible solutions: normal saline solution, D5W, 5% dextrose and half-normal saline solution, 5% dextrose and normal saline solution, 5% dextrose and lactated Ringer's solution, lactated Ringer's solution, and sodium lactate solution (1/6 molar).

Do not add to sodium bicarbonate solution or other alkaline solutions, because this inactivates drug.

Infusion considerations

Do not give by direct I.V. injection.

Make sure I.V. line is free flowing.

• Give by I.V. infusion using metered pump or other device to control flow.

• Infuse into large (preferably central) vein to avoid extravasation.

Inspect I.V. site regularly for irritation and extravasation.

Do not use plastic containers in series connections. Such use could result in air embolism due to residual air being drawn from primary container before administration of fluid from secondary container ends.

Monitoring

• Monitor blood pressure, pulse, urine output, and pulmonary artery wedge pressure during infusion.

Monitor color and temperature of extremities, especially in patients with occlusive vascular disease. If skin color or temperature changes occur from suspected compromise of circulation to extremities, weigh benefits of continued dopamine infusion against risk of possible necrosis. To reverse these changes, decrease infusion rate or discontinue infusion, as ordered.

Never stop infusion abruptly, as this may cause severe hypotension. Taper gradually.

Storage

• Store vials and ampules at room temperature of 15° to 30°C (59° to 86°F); protect from light.

• Store plastic containers at room temperature of 25°C (77°F); brief exposure up to 40°C (104°F) is permitted.

Contraindications and precautions

Contraindicated in hypersensitivity to drug or bisulfites, tachyarrhythmias, ventricular fibrillation, and pheochromocytoma.

Use cautiously in myocardial infarction, hypovolemia, occlusive vascular disease, diabetic endarteritis, atrial embolism, concurrent MAO inhibitor use, pregnant or breastfeeding patients, and ***children.***

Adverse reactions

CNS: headache
CV: hypotension, angina, ECG changes, palpitations, tachycardia, vasoconstriction, **arrhythmias**
EENT: mydriasis
GI: nausea, vomiting
Metabolic: azotemia, hyperglycemia
Respiratory: dyspnea, asthma attacks
Skin: piloerection
Other: irritation at injection site, necrosis of fingers and toes (with prolonged high doses or in occlusive vascular disease)

Interactions

Drug-drug. *Alpha- or beta-adrenergic blockers:* antagonism of dopamine effects
Ergot alkaloids: extreme blood pressure rise
Guanethidine: decreased cardiostimulatory effects
Inhalation anesthetics: increased risk of hypertension, arrhythmias
MAO inhibitors: hypertensive crisis
Oxytocics: severe, persistent hypotension
Phenytoin: seizures, severe hypotension, bradycardia
Tricyclic antidepressants: decreased pressor response
Drug-diagnostic tests. *Glucose, nitrogenous compounds, urine catecholamines:* increased

Toxicity and overdose

- In overdose, expect severe blood pressure increase.
- Reduce infusion rate, which should resolve symptoms (because of drug's short duration). If patient does not stabilize after rate reduction, be prepared to give phentolamine.

Patient teaching

- Explain the need for close observation during infusion.
- Instruct patient to report adverse reactions and I.V. site discomfort.
- As appropriate, review all other significant and life-threatening adverse reactions and interactions, especially those related to the drugs and tests mentioned above.

doxapram hydrochloride

Dopram

Pharmacologic class: CNS and respiratory stimulant
Therapeutic class: Analeptic
Pregnancy risk category B

Action

Activates peripheral carotid, aortic, and other chemoreceptors to stimulate respiration. Increases tidal volume and respiratory rate by directly stimulating respiratory center in medulla oblongata.

Pharmacokinetics

Drug is extensively metabolized. Plasma half-life is 2.4 to 4.1 hours. It is excreted in urine mostly as metabolites, with a small amount excreted unchanged.

Onset	Peak	Duration
20-40 sec	1-2 min	5-12 min

How supplied

Solution for injection (clear, colorless): 20 mg/mL in multidose vials

Indications and dosages

➢ Respiratory depression after anesthesia
Adults and adolescents: 5 mg/minute by I.V. infusion until desired response occurs; then reduced to 1 to 3 mg/minute, to a maximum cumulative dosage of 4 mg/kg (or 300 mg). Or 0.5 to 1 mg/kg I.V. injection repeated q 5 minutes, if needed, to a maximum total dosage of 1.5 mg/kg.
➢ Chronic pulmonary disease related to acute hypercapnia
Adults: 1 to 2 mg/minute by I.V. infusion, using a concentration of 2 mg/mL, to a maximum of 3 mg/minute

➤ Drug-induced CNS depression
Adults: Initially, 2 mg/kg I.V., repeated in 5 minutes and then q 1 to 2 hours until patient awakens, to a maximum daily dosage of 3 g. For infusion, give priming dose of 2 mg/kg I.V.; if no response occurs, continue for 1 to 2 hours as needed; if some response occurs, give I.V. infusion of 250 mg in 250 mL saline solution or D_5W injection at 1 to 3 mg/minute until patient awakens. Do not exceed 3 g/day.

Off-label uses

- Laryngospasm secondary to postoperative tracheal extubation

Administration

Preparation

Do not use in conjunction with mechanical ventilation.

Ensure adequate airway and oxygenation before administering.

- Assess blood pressure, pulse rate, deep tendon reflexes, airway, and arterial blood gas (ABG) values before starting therapy.

Dilution and compatibility

- Know that drug is compatible with 5% and 10% dextrose in water and with normal saline solution.

Do not mix with thiopental sodium, bicarbonate, or aminophylline, because precipitates or gas may form.

Infusion considerations

Give I.V. slowly to avoid hemolysis.

- When administering for post-anesthesia respiratory depression, start I.V. infusion at 5 mg/minute until desired response occurs; then reduce to 1 to 3 mg/minute. Use infusion pump or microdrip for accuracy.
- When administering for chronic pulmonary disease related to acute hypercapnia, give at 1 to 2 mg/minute by I.V. infusion, using a concentration of 2 mg/mL, to a maximum of 3 mg/minute. Discontinue infusion after 2 hours.
- When administering for drug-induced CNS depression, give at 1 to 3 mg/minute until patient awakens. Do not infuse longer than 2 hours.
- Avoid vascular extravasation or use of a single injection site over extended period, as thrombophlebitis or local skin irritation may result.

Monitoring

- Monitor blood pressure, pulse rate, deep tendon reflexes, airway, and ABG values frequently during infusion.
- Monitor I.V. site frequently for irritation and thrombophlebitis.

Discontinue infusion immediately if severe hypotension or dyspnea suddenly develops.

Storage

- Store at controlled room temperature of 15° to 30°C (59° to 86°F).

Contraindications and precautions

Contraindicated in hypersensitivity to drug, cardiovascular disorders, cerebrovascular accident, head injury, seizures, respiratory failure, restrictive respiratory disease, and ***neonates.***

Use cautiously in bronchial asthma, arrhythmias, increased intracranial pressure, hyperthyroidism, pheochromocytoma, metabolic disorders, concurrent use of sympathomimetics or monoamine oxidase (MAO) inhibitors, pregnant or breastfeeding patients, and ***children younger than age 12*** (safety and efficacy not established).

Adverse reactions

CNS: weakness, dizziness, drowsiness, headache, dysarthria, disorientation, hyperactivity, paresthesia, **loss of consciousness, seizures**

CV: hypotension, bradycardia, chest pain or tightness, heart rate changes, **thrombophlebitis, atrioventricular block, arrhythmias, cardiac arrest**

EENT: lacrimation, diplopia, miosis, conjunctival hyperemia, sneezing, **laryngospasm**
GI: nausea, vomiting, diarrhea, abdominal cramps, increased salivation, dysphagia
GU: urinary frequency or incontinence, albuminuria
Musculoskeletal: muscle cramps, fasciculations
Respiratory: dyspnea, increased secretions, **respiratory muscle paralysis, central respiratory paralysis, bronchospasm, respiratory depression, respiratory arrest**
Skin: rash, diaphoresis, flushing, local irritation with extravasation
Other: burning or hot sensation in genitalia and perineal area

Interactions

Drug-drug. *General anesthetics:* increased risk of self-limiting arrhythmias
MAO inhibitors, sympathomimetics: potentiation of adverse cardiovascular effects
Skeletal muscle relaxants: masking of residual effects of these drugs
Drug-diagnostic tests. *Blood urea nitrogen:* increased
Erythrocytes, hematocrit, hemoglobin, red blood cells, white blood cells: decreased

Toxicity and overdose

- In overdose, expect excessive pressor effects, tachycardia, skeletal muscle hyperactivity, and enhanced deep tendon reflexes as early signs.
- No known antidote exists. Evaluate blood pressure, pulse rate, and deep tendon reflexes; adjust dosage or infusion rate as indicated. Provide symptomatic and supportive therapy as indicated and ordered, including short-acting barbiturates for seizures, oxygen, and resuscitation. Dialysis has no benefit.

Patient teaching

- Instruct patient to report adverse reactions promptly.
- As appropriate, review all other significant and life-threatening adverse reactions and interactions, especially those related to the drugs and tests mentioned above.

[redacted]

doxercalciferol

Hectorol

Pharmacologic class: Vitamin D analogue
Therapeutic class: Parathyroid stimulant
Pregnancy risk category B

Action

Undergoes transformation in the liver to active form of vitamin D_2 that helps regulate blood calcium. Biologically active vitamin D metabolites control intestinal absorption of dietary calcium, tubular reabsorption of calcium by the kidneys and, in conjunction with parathyroid hormone (PTH), calcium mobilization from skeleton.

Pharmacokinetics

Drug is metabolized in the liver by CYP27 to major (active) metabolite and minor (inactive) metabolite; activation does not require kidney involvement. Mean half-life is 32 to 96 hours. Drug is excreted in bile, with small amount excreted in urine.

Onset	Peak	Duration
Unknown	11-12 hr	Unknown

How supplied

Powder for reconstitution for injection: 4 mcg/2-mL (2-mcg/mL) ampules

Indications and dosages

➢ Hyperparathyroidism in dialysis patients with chronic kidney disease

Adults: Dosage individualized. Recommended initial dosage is 4 mcg I.V. bolus three times weekly (approximately every other day). Adjust initial dosage, as needed, to lower blood intact PTH (iPTH) level to target range of 150 to 300 pg/mL. May increase dosage by 1 to 2 mcg at 8-week intervals if iPTH does not decrease 50% and fails to reach target range.

Dosage adjustment

- Reduce dosage in impaired hepatic function.
- Suspend therapy if iPTH falls below 100 pg/mL; restart 1 week later at dosage at least 1 mcg lower than last administered dosage.
- If hypercalcemia or hyperphosphatemia occurs or if serum calcium times phosphorus product exceeds 70, immediately suspend therapy until these parameters decrease appropriately. Then restart drug at dosage at least 1 mcg lower.

Administration

Preparation

- Be aware that dosage must be individualized based on iPTH level.
- Monitor baseline serum calcium and phosphorus levels.
- Because drug is precursor of potent vitamin D_2 metabolite, withhold pharmacologic dosages of vitamin D and its derivatives during therapy to avoid possible additive effects and hypercalcemia.
- Know that dialysis patients should use oral calcium-based or other nonaluminum-containing phosphate binders and low-phosphate diet to control serum phosphorus levels. Uncontrolled serum phosphorus levels exacerbate secondary hyperparathyroidism and can reduce doxercalciferol efficacy in reducing blood PTH levels. After initiating doxercalciferol, decrease dosage of phosphate binders to correct persistent mild hypercalcemia (10.6 to 11.2 mg/dL for three consecutive tests) or increase dosage to correct persistent mild hyperphosphatemia (7 to 8 mg/dL for three consecutive tests).
- Be aware that patients on chronic renal dialysis should not take magnesium-containing antacids during doxercalciferol therapy; such use may lead to hypermagnesemia.

Dilution and compatibility

- Be aware that drug may be given undiluted.
- Discard unused portion of drug.

Infusion considerations

- Administer as a bolus I.V. dose at end of dialysis.

Monitoring

- During titration, monitor iPTH, serum calcium, and serum phosphorus levels at least weekly.
- Be aware that adverse reactions generally resemble those of excessive vitamin D intake.

Monitor patient closely for early signs and symptoms of vitamin D intoxication associated with hypercalcemia, including weakness, headache, somnolence, nausea, vomiting, dry mouth, constipation, muscle pain, bone pain, metallic taste, and anorexia.

Watch for late signs and symptoms of vitamin D intoxication associated with hypercalcemia, such as polyuria; polydipsia; anorexia; weight loss; nocturia; conjunctivitis; pancreatitis; photophobia; rhinorrhea; pruritus; hyperthermia; decreased libido; ectopic calcification; hypertension; arrhythmias; sensory disturbances; dehydration; apathy; arrested growth; urinary tract infections; overt psychosis (rare); albuminuria;

hypercholesterolemia; and elevated blood urea nitrogen, aspartate transaminase, and alanine transaminase levels.

Storage

• Store unopened vials at 25°C (77°F); excursions permitted to 15° to 30°C (58° to 86°F). Protect from light.

Contraindications and precautions

Contraindicated in hypersensitivity to drug or its components, vitamin D toxicity, hypercalcemia, and hyperphosphatemia.

Use cautiously in ***elderly patients,*** pregnant or breastfeeding patients, and ***children*** (safety and efficacy not established).

Adverse reactions

CNS: dizziness, headache, malaise, sleep disorder
CV: bradycardia
GI: nausea, vomiting, constipation, anorexia, dyspepsia
Metabolic: hypercalcemia, hyperphosphatemia, iPTH oversuppression, hypercholesterolemia, vitamin D intoxication
Musculoskeletal: arthralgia
Respiratory: dyspnea
Skin: pruritus
Other: edema, weight increase

Interactions

Drug-drug. *Digoxin:* increased risk of arrhythmias (secondary to hypercalcemia)
Magnesium-containing antacids: increased risk of hypermagnesemia

Toxicity and overdose

• In overdose, expect hypercalcemia, hypercalciuria, hyperphosphatemia, and increased PTH secretion
• If serum calcium level is more than 1 mg/dL above upper limit of normal, interrupt therapy immediately and withdraw any calcium supplements. Closely monitor serum calcium level, ECG, and fluid and electrolyte status. Persistent or marked serum calcium elevation may be corrected by dialysis using reduced-calcium or calcium-free dialysate.

Patient teaching

Instruct patient to report early signs and symptoms of hypercalcemia (weakness, headache, somnolence, nausea, vomiting, dry mouth, muscle or bone pain, and metallic taste).
• Urge patient to strictly adhere to dietary calcium and phosphorus supplement restrictions.
• Advise patient not to use over-the-counter products, especially those containing calcium, phosphorus, or magnesium, unless prescriber approves.
• As appropriate, review all other significant and life-threatening adverse reactions and interactions, especially those related to the drugs mentioned above.

doxorubicin hydrochloride

Adriamycin PFS, Adriamycin RDF

Pharmacologic class: Anthracycline
Therapeutic class: Antibiotic antineoplastic
Pregnancy risk category D

FDA BOXED WARNING

• Administer I.V. only—never I.M. or subcutaneously. Extravasation causes severe local tissue necrosis.
• Myocardial toxicity may occur during therapy or months to years afterward. Risk factors (cardiovascular disease, previous or concurrent radiotherapy to mediastinal or pericardial area, previous

therapy with doxorubicin or other anthracyclines, and concomitant use of other cardiotoxic drugs) may increase myocardial toxicity risk. Toxicity may occur at higher or lower cumulative doses even in patients without cardiac risk factors. Pediatric patients have increased risk of delayed cardiotoxicity.
• Secondary acute myelogenous leukemia (AML) may occur. Refractory secondary leukemia is more common when drug is given in combination with DNA-damaging antineoplastics, when patients have been heavily pretreated with cytotoxic drugs, and with dosage escalation. Pediatric patients are also at risk for secondary AML.
• Reduce dosage in hepatic impairment.
• Drug may cause severe myelosuppression.
• Give under supervision of physician experienced in cancer chemotherapy.

Action

Unclear. Thought to inhibit DNA and RNA synthesis by forming complex with DNA. Also exerts immunosuppressive activity. Cell-cycle–S-phase specific.

Pharmacokinetics

Drug distributes widely to body tissues, but does not cross blood-brain barrier. Highest concentrations occur in the lymph nodes, liver, bone marrow, fat, and skin. It is metabolized to several metabolites (some active, others inactive); major active metabolite is daunorubicinol. Drug is about 75% protein-bound (primarily to albumin). Terminal half-life is about 40 hours. Excretion occurs mainly via bile and feces, with small amount excreted in urine.

Onset	Peak	Duration
Rapid	2 hr	Unknown

How supplied

Powder for reconstitution for injection (red-orange, lyophilized) (Adriamycin RDF): 10-mg, 20-mg, and 50-mg single-dose vials; 150-mg multidose vial
Solution for injection (Adriamycin PFS): 10-mg, 20-mg, 50-mg, and 200-mg single-dose Cytosafe vials; 150-mg multidose vial

Indications and dosages

➣ Solid tumors, including bladder, breast, lung, stomach, and thyroid cancers; malignant lymphomas, including Hodgkin's disease; acute leukemia; Wilms' tumor; neuroblastoma
Adults: 60 to 75 mg/m^2 I.V. as a single dose in 21-day cycles; or 30 mg/m^2 I.V. as a single daily dose on first to third days of 4-week cycle; or 20 mg/m^2 I.V. once weekly. Maximum cumulative dosage is 550 mg/m^2.
➣ Ewing's sarcoma
Adults: In combination with vincristine and cyclophosphamide, alternating with ifosfamide, mesna, and etoposide, 40 to 60 mg/m^2 I.V. by slow I.V. infusion q 21 to 28 days.

Dosage adjustment

• Reduce dosage in inadequate marrow reserves.
• Reduce dosage in hepatic impairment if hyperbilirubinemia occurs. For serum bilirubin level of 1.2 to 3 mg/dL, reduce dosage 50%; for bilirubin level of 3.1 to 5 mg/dL, reduce dosage 75%.

Off-label uses

• Bladder carcinoma
• Carcinoid tumors
• Cervical, endometrial, head, neck, pancreatic, prostatic, or testicular carcinoma
• Chronic lymphocytic leukemia
• Germ-cell tumors
• Islet-cell carcinoma

- Multiple myeloma
- Primary hepatocellular carcinoma
- Retinoblastoma

Administration

Preparation

Follow hazardous drug guidelines on page S19 for handling, preparation, and administration.
- Assess baseline cardiac, hepatic, and renal function before starting therapy.
- Administer allopurinol to decrease risk of hyperuricemia, as prescribed.

Use caution to prevent inadvertent overdose when using multidose vials for administration.

Do not interchange doxorubicin hydrochloride with doxorubicin liposomal.

Do not give I.M. or subcutaneously.

Dilution and compatibility
- Dilute as directed with normal saline solution for injection to a final concentration of 2 mg/mL.

Do not dilute solution with bacteriostatic diluent.

Do not mix with other drugs or solutions.
- Discard unused portion from single-dose vials.

Infusion considerations

Confirm that I.V. line is free flowing to avoid extravasation.
- Administer slowly over 3 to 5 minutes into tubing of free-flowing I.V. infusion of normal saline solution or D_5W.
- Deliver into large vein using butterfly needle. Avoid veins over joints or extremities with compromised venous or lymphatic drainage.

Avoid rapid infusion, as this may increase risk of acute infusion-related reactions (back pain, chest tightness, and flushing).

Monitor I.V. site frequently. If extravasation occurs, stop infusion immediately, apply ice, and notify prescriber.

Monitoring

Watch for acute life-threatening arrhythmias, which may occur during or within a few hours after administration.

Monitor for cardiomyopathy and subsequent heart failure with chronic overdose (more common in children).
- Stay alert for erythematous streaking along vein next to injection site, which may indicate too-rapid infusion.
- Watch for nausea and vomiting. Administer antiemetics as needed and ordered.

Check for superinfection or hemorrhage caused by persistent bone marrow depression. However, expect white blood cell (WBC) counts as low as 1,000/mm^3 during therapy.

Monitor closely for infusion-related reactions and anaphylaxis; be prepared to intervene appropriately.
- Monitor CBC, hepatic profile, coagulation tests, ejection fraction, and glucose, uric acid, and calcium blood levels before each course of therapy.

Storage
- Store single-dose and multidose vials in cartons at controlled temperature of 15° to 30°C (59° to 86°F); protect from light.
- Refrigerate single-dose and multidose glass and Cytosafe vials in cartons at 2° to 8°C (36° to 46°F); protect from light. Reconstituted solution is stable for 7 days at room temperature under normal room light. It is stable for 15 days when refrigerated at 2° to 8°C. Protect from sunlight.

Contraindications and precautions

Contraindicated in hypersensitivity to drug, severe bone marrow depression, or previous treatment with maximum cumulative doses of doxorubicin, other anthracyclines

Use cautiously in cardiac disease, hepatic impairment, depressed bone marrow reserve, CNS metastases, brain tumor, malignant melanoma, renal carcinoma, ***elderly patients,*** females of childbearing potential, pregnant or breastfeeding patients, and ***children.***

Adverse reactions

CNS: drowsiness, dizziness, asthenia, fatigue, malaise, paresthesia, headache, depression, insomnia, anxiety, emotional lability
CV: chest pain, hypotension, tachycardia, peripheral edema, **cardiomyopathy, heart failure, arrhythmias, pericardial effusion**
GI: nausea, vomiting, diarrhea, constipation, enlarged abdomen, abdominal pain, dyspepsia, oral candidiasis, candidiasis, stomatitis, glossitis, esophagitis, dysphagia
GU: albuminuria, hyperuricosuria, red urine
Hematologic: anemia, **leukopenia, thrombocytopenia, neutropenia, bone marrow depression**
Metabolic: hyperglycemia, hypocalcemia
Musculoskeletal: myalgia, back pain
Respiratory: dyspnea, increased cough, pneumonia
Skin: rash, dry skin, pruritus, skin discoloration, alopecia, diaphoresis, exfoliative dermatitis, palmar-plantar erythrodysesthesia
Other: abnormal taste, infection, chills, fever, herpes zoster, injection site reactions including severe necrosis (with extravasation), hypersensitivity reactions including **anaphylaxis, acute infusion-associated reactions**

Interactions

Drug-drug. *Antineoplastics:* additive bone marrow depression
Cyclophosphamide: increased risk of hemorrhagic cystitis, increased cardiotoxicity
Cyclosporine: profound and prolonged hematologic toxicity, increased risk of coma and seizures
Dactinomycin (in children): increased risk of pneumonitis
Live-virus vaccines: decreased antibody response to vaccine, increased risk of adverse reactions
Mercaptopurine: hepatitis
Paclitaxel (if given first): reduced doxorubicin clearance, increased incidence and severity of neutropenia and stomatitis
Phenobarbital: increased clearance and decreased effects of doxorubicin
Phenytoin: decreased phenytoin blood level
Progesterone: increased incidence and severity of neutropenia and thrombocytopenia
Streptozocin: increased doxorubicin half-life
Verapamil: increased doxorubicin blood level
Drug-diagnostic tests. *Alkaline phosphatase, bilirubin, glucose, prothrombin time, serum and urine uric acid:* increased
Calcium, hemoglobin, neutrophils, platelets, WBCs: decreased

Toxicity and overdose

• In overdose, expect mucositis, leukopenia, thrombocytopenia, and possible increased risk of acute cardiomyopathy with resultant heart failure, even when cumulative dosage is below 300 mg/m^2.
• In acute overdose, expect to give anti-infectives, blood transfusions, and possibly hematopoietic growth factor (G-CSF, GM-CSF). For mucositis, provide symptomatic therapy. For cardiomyopathy, provide vigorous heart failure management with digitalis preparations, diuretics, beta-adrenergic blockers, and afterload reducers (such as angiotensin-converting enzyme inhibitors), as ordered.

Patient teaching

Instruct patient to promptly report irregular heartbeat, easy bruising or bleeding, and signs or symptoms of hypersensitivity reaction (such as rash).
- Advise home caregivers to take precautions (such as wearing gloves) to prevent contact with patient's urine and other body fluids for at least 5 days after course of therapy.
- Caution patient to avoid people with colds, flu, or other contagious illnesses.
- Explain that drug may cause complete but reversible hair loss.
- Inform patient that drug may turn urine red for 1 or 2 days.
- Instruct patient about the need for frequent laboratory tests.
- Caution females of childbearing potential to avoid becoming pregnant during therapy.
- Advise breastfeeding women to discontinue breastfeeding during therapy.
- As appropriate, review all other significant and life-threatening adverse reactions and interactions, especially those related to the drugs and tests mentioned above.

doxorubicin hydrochloride liposomal (liposomal encapsulated doxorubicin, LED)

Caelyx, Doxil, Myocet

Pharmacologic class: Anthracycline
Therapeutic class: Antibiotic antineoplastic
Pregnancy risk category D

FDA BOXED WARNING

- Drug may cause cardiotoxicity. Myocardial damage may lead to heart failure and may occur as total cumulative dose (including previous use of other anthracyclines or anthracenediones) approaches 550 mg/m^2. Toxicity may arise at lower cumulative doses in patients who have had previous mediastinal irradiation or are receiving concurrent cyclophosphamides.
- Acute infusion-related reactions occur in up to 10% of patients. These usually resolve over several hours to 1 day after infusion ends; in some patients, they resolve with slower infusion rate. Serious and sometimes life-threatening allergic or anaphylactoid-like infusion reactions may develop. Keep emergency equipment and drugs to treat reaction available for immediate use.
- Drug may cause severe myelosuppression.
- Reduce dosage in hepatic impairment.
- Accidental substitution of liposomal form for doxorubicin hydrochloride may cause severe adverse effects. Do not substitute on mg-per-mg basis.

Action

Unclear. Thought to inhibit DNA and RNA synthesis by forming complex with DNA. Also has immunosuppressive activity. Liposomal encapsulation increases uptake by tumor, prolongs drug action, and may decrease toxicity. Cell-cycle–S-phase specific.

Pharmacokinetics

Drug distributes primarily to intravascular space; half-life is approximately 55 hours. It is excreted primarily in bile.

Onset	Peak	Duration
10 days	14 days	Unknown

How supplied

Liposomal dispersion for injection (red): 20 mg/10 mL in 10-mL single-use vials

Indications and dosages

➢ First-line therapy for AIDS-related Kaposi's sarcoma
Adults: 20 mg/m^2 I.V. over 30 minutes once q 3 weeks

➢ Metastatic ovarian carcinoma in patients with disease that resists paclitaxel- and platinum-based chemotherapy
Adults: Initially, 50 mg/m^2 I.V. at a rate of 1 mg/minute q 4 weeks for at least four courses. If no adverse reactions occur, increase infusion rate to complete infusion over 1 hour.

Dosage adjustment

- Reduce dosage in hepatic impairment if hyperbilirubinemia occurs. For serum bilirubin level of 1.2 to 3 mg/dL, reduce dosage 50%; for level of 3.1 to 5 mg/dL, reduce dosage 75%.
- Reduce dosage or delay dose after first appearance of grade 2 or higher adverse event. Once dosage has been reduced, do not increase it later.

Administration

Preparation

🔊 Follow hazardous drug guidelines on page S19 for handling, preparation, and administration.

- Assess baseline cardiac, hepatic, and renal function before starting therapy.

🔊 Do not interchange doxorubicin hydrochloride and doxorubicin liposomal.

🔊 Do not give I.M. or subcutaneously.

Dilution and compatibility

- Know that drug is a translucent red dispersion, not a clear solution.
- Dilute dose (up to 90 mg) in 250 mL D_5W.

🔊 Do not dilute solution with bacteriostatic diluent. Do not mix with other diluents or drugs.

Infusion considerations

🔊 Avoid rapid infusion or bolus injection, as this may increase risk of acute infusion-related reactions (back pain, chest tightness, flushing).

- Administer slowly into tubing of free-flowing I.V. infusion line with good blood return.
- Deliver into large vein using butterfly needle. Avoid veins over joints or extremities with compromised venous or lymphatic drainage.

🔊 Do not use inline filter.

🔊 Avoid rapid flushing of infusion line.

- Administer within 24 hours of dilution.

Monitoring

🔊 Do not administer undiluted.

🔊 If extravasation occurs, stop infusion immediately, apply ice, and notify prescriber.

🔊 Observe patient closely for anaphylaxis and bleeding problems.

🔊 Stay alert for acute life-threatening arrhythmias, which may occur during or within a few hours after administration.

🔊 Assess for cardiomyopathy and subsequent heart failure with chronic overdose (more common in children).

🔊 Monitor closely for acute infusion reaction.

🔊 Assess for and report liver engorgement and yellowing of skin or eyes.

- Before each course of therapy, monitor CBC, coagulation tests, hepatic profile, and bilirubin, glucose, calcium and uric acid levels.
- Watch for nausea and vomiting. Give antiemetics as needed and prescribed.
- Assess for constipation; give fluids and stool softeners, as needed and prescribed.

Storage

- Refrigerate diluted drug at 2° to 8°C (36° to 46°F).

Contraindications and precautions

Contraindicated in hypersensitivity to drug and marked bone marrow depression.

Use cautiously in cardiac disease, hepatic impairment, depressed bone marrow reserve, CNS metastases, brain tumor, malignant melanoma, renal carcinoma, ***elderly patients,*** females of childbearing potential, pregnant patients, and ***children*** (safety and efficacy not established).

Adverse reactions

CNS: drowsiness, dizziness, asthenia, fatigue, malaise, paresthesia, headache, depression, insomnia, anxiety, emotional lability
CV: chest pain, hypotension, tachycardia, peripheral edema, **cardiomyopathy, heart failure, arrhythmias, pericardial effusion**
GI: nausea, vomiting, diarrhea, constipation, abdominal pain, enlarged abdomen, dyspepsia, candidiasis, esophagitis, stomatitis, glossitis, oral candidiasis, dysphagia
GU: albuminuria, red urine
Hematologic: anemia, **leukopenia, thrombocytopenia, neutropenia, bone marrow depression**
Hepatic: jaundice
Metabolic: hypocalcemia, hyperglycemia
Musculoskeletal: myalgia, back pain
Respiratory: dyspnea, increased cough, pneumonia
Skin: rash, dry skin, pruritus, skin discoloration, alopecia, diaphoresis, exfoliative dermatitis, palmar-plantar erythrodysesthesia
Other: altered taste, fever, chills, infection, herpes zoster, injection site reactions, hypersensitivity reactions including **anaphylaxis, acute infusion reaction**

Interactions

Drug-drug. *Antineoplastics:* additive bone marrow depression
Cyclophosphamide: increased risk of hemorrhagic cystitis
Cyclosporine: profound and prolonged hematologic toxicity, increased risk of coma and seizures, increased cardiotoxicity
Dactinomycin (in children): increased risk of pneumonitis
Live-virus vaccines: decreased antibody response to vaccine, increased risk of adverse reactions
Mercaptopurine: hepatitis
Paclitaxel (if given first): reduced doxorubicin clearance, increased incidence and severity of neutropenia and stomatitis
Phenobarbital: increased clearance and decreased effects of doxorubicin
Phenytoin: decreased phenytoin blood level
Progesterone: increased risk and severity of neutropenia and thrombocytopenia
Streptozocin: prolonged doxorubicin half-life
Verapamil: increased doxorubicin blood level
Drug-diagnostic tests. *Alkaline phosphatase, bilirubin, glucose, prothrombin time, serum and urine uric acid:* increased
Calcium, hemoglobin, neutrophils, platelets, white blood cells: decreased

Toxicity and overdose

- Acute overdose causes increased mucositis, leukopenia, and thrombocytopenia.
- In severely myelosuppressed patient, expect to give anti-infectives and blood transfusions. Provide symptomatic therapy for mucositis.

Patient teaching

Instruct patient to immediately report shortness of breath, peripheral edema, rash, chest pain, and palpitations
- Advise patient to avoid people with colds, flu, and other contagious illnesses.

• Inform patient that drug may turn urine red for 1 or 2 days.
• Explain that drug may cause complete but reversible hair loss.
• Instruct patient about the need for frequent laboratory tests.
• Caution females of childbearing potential to avoid becoming pregnant during therapy.
• Advise breastfeeding women to discontinue breastfeeding during therapy.
• As appropriate, review all other significant and life-threatening adverse reactions and interactions, especially those related to the drugs and tests mentioned above.

doxycycline hyclate

Doxylar (UK), Vibramycin Hyclate

Pharmacologic class: Tetracycline
Therapeutic class: Anti-infective
Pregnancy risk category D

Action

Unclear. Thought to inhibit bacterial protein synthesis at 30S and 50S ribosomal subunit and to alter cytoplasmic membrane of susceptible organisms; bacteriostatic.

Pharmacokinetics

Drug is highly lipid-soluble and readily penetrates cerebrospinal fluid, brain, eye, and prostate. Half-life is independent of renal or hepatic function. Drug is excreted in inactive form into intestinal lumen and eliminated in feces.

Onset	Peak	Duration
Rapid	End of infusion	Unknown

How supplied

Powder for reconstitution for injection: 100 mg, 200 mg

Indications and dosages

➢ Infections caused by unusual organisms, including *Mycoplasma, Chlamydia,* and *Rickettsia* organisms

Adults and children weighing more than 45 kg (99 lb): 200 mg I.V. once daily; or 100 mg I.V. q 12 hours on first day, followed by 100 to 200 mg I.V. once daily; or 50 to 100 mg I.V. q 12 hours

Children weighing 45 kg or less: 4.4 mg/kg I.V. once daily; or 2.2 mg/kg I.V. q 12 hours on first day, followed by 2.2 to 4.4 mg/kg I.V. once daily; or 1.1 to 2.2 mg/kg I.V. q 12 hours

➢ Anthrax

Adults and children weighing more than 45 kg: 100 mg I.V. q 12 hours for 60 days; change to oral route when appropriate.

Children weighing 45 kg or less: 100 mg I.V. q 12 hours for 60 days; change to oral route when appropriate.

Administration

Preparation

Be aware that outdated product may cause nephrotoxicity.
• Know that parenteral therapy is indicated only when oral therapy is not indicated. Switch to oral therapy as soon as possible.
• Before giving first dose, obtain specimens for culture and sensitivity testing and hepatic and renal function tests.
Do not give in conjunction with methoxyflurane anesthetic or other potentially nephrotoxic drugs. Severe or fatal kidney damage may result.
Do not give with other potentially hepatotoxic drugs.
Do not give during last half of pregnancy or to children younger than age 8

unless other anti-infectives are contraindicated or likely to be ineffective. Drug may retard bone growth and cause tooth discoloration and malformation.

Do not inject I.M. or subcutaneously.

Dilution and compatibility

- Reconstitute powder for injection with compatible solution in 10-mL (100-mg) or 20-mL (200-mg) vial.
- Know that compatible solutions include sterile water for injection, D_5W, normal saline solution, lactated Ringer's solution, dextrose 5% in lactated Ringer's solution, 10% invert sugar in water, Normosol-M in D_5W, and Plasma-Lyte 56 in D_5W.
- Be aware that reconstituted solution will be a pale yellow to yellow viscous liquid.
- Dilute further with compatible solution in 100- to 1,000-mL (100-mg) vial or 200- to 2,000-mL (200-mg) vial, to yield final concentration of 0.1 mg/mL to 1 mg/mL, respectively.

Do not infuse solution with concentrations of more than 1 mg/mL.

Avoid rapid administration. Infuse 100-mg dose over at least 1 hour.

- Complete infusion within 12 hours of dilution, unless diluted with lactated Ringer's solution or dextrose 5% in lactated Ringer's solution; in this case, complete infusion within 6 hours.
- Evaluate I.V. site regularly. Apply cool compresses as needed.

Monitoring

Monitor for hypersensitivity reactions, including anaphylaxis. Be prepared to intervene appropriately.

- Monitor hepatic profile, CBC, and blood urea nitrogen (BUN) and creatinine levels.
- Assess for hypercoagulability in patients receiving warfarin concurrently
- Monitor for digoxin toxicity in patients receiving digoxin concurrently.

Storage

- When diluted with solution other than lactated Ringer's solution or dextrose 5% in lactated Ringer's solution, drug may be stored up to 72 hours before infusion.

Contraindications and precautions

Contraindicated in hypersensitivity to drug, other tetracyclines, or bisulfites (with some products).

Use cautiously in renal disease, hepatic impairment, nephrogenic diabetes insipidus, cachexia, pregnant or breastfeeding patients, and ***children younger than age 8.***

Adverse reactions

CNS: paresthesia, **pseudotumor cerebri**
CV: phlebitis, **thrombophlebitis, pericarditis**
EENT: vestibular reactions, hoarseness, pharyngitis
GI: nausea, vomiting, diarrhea, esophagitis, epigastric distress, enterocolitis, anogenital lesions or inflammation, glossitis, oral candidiasis, black hairy tongue, **pancreatitis**
GU: dark yellow or brown urine, vaginal candidiasis
Hematologic: hemolytic anemia, neutropenia, thrombocytopenia
Hepatic: hepatotoxicity
Musculoskeletal: bone growth retardation (in children younger than age 8)
Skin: photosensitivity, maculopapular or erythematous rash, hyperpigmentation, urticaria
Other: tooth discoloration (yellow-brown-gray) in children who are younger than age 8 or whose mothers received tetracyclines during last half of pregnancy, increased appetite, phlebitis at I.V. site, superinfection, hypersensitivity reactions including **anaphylaxis**

Interactions

Drug-drug. *Barbiturates, carbamazepine, hormonal contraceptives containing estrogen, phenytoin, rifamycin:* decreased doxycycline efficacy
Methoxyflurane: increased nephrotoxicity
Penicillin: decreased penicillin activity
Warfarin: enhanced warfarin effects
Drug-diagnostic tests. *Alkaline phosphatase, alanine aminotransferase, amylase, aspartate aminotransferase, bilirubin, BUN, eosinophils:* increased
Hemoglobin, neutrophils, platelets, white blood cells: decreased
Urine catecholamines: false elevations
Drug-behaviors. *Alcohol use:* decreased anti-infective effect
Sun exposure: increased risk of photosensitivity

Toxicity and overdose

- In overdose, expect extension of pharmacologic effects and adverse reactions.
- Discontinue drug; provide symptomatic and supportive therapy. Dialysis has no benefit.

Patient teaching

Tell patient to immediately report painful swallowing, abdominal pain, easy bruising or bleeding, and signs and symptoms of hypersensitivity (such as rash).
- Instruct patient to avoid alcohol use.
- Stress importance of good oral hygiene.
- Tell patient drug may discolor urine.
- Advise female patient to tell prescriber if she is pregnant.
- As appropriate, review all other significant and life-threatening adverse reactions and interactions, especially those related to the drugs, tests, and behaviors mentioned above.

droperidol

Inapsine

Pharmacologic class: Butyrophenone
Therapeutic class: Anesthesia adjunct, antiemetic
Pregnancy risk category C

FDA BOXED WARNING

- QT prolongation and torsades de pointes may occur at or below recommended dosages, even in patients with no known risk factors. (Risk factors for prolonged QT syndrome include heart failure, bradycardia, cardiac hypertrophy, hypokalemia, hypomagnesemia, age older than 65, alcohol abuse, and use of diuretics, drugs that prolong the QT interval, benzodiazepines, volatile anesthetics, or I.V. opioids.) Some cases have been fatal. Reserve drug for patients with refractory disease. Use with extreme caution in patients at risk for prolonged QT interval.
- Drug is contraindicated in patients with known or suspected QT prolongation.

Action

Blocks action of dopamine by binding to dopamine receptors. Produces marked sedation by directly blocking subcortical receptors. Produces antiemetic effect by blocking CNS receptors in chemoreceptor trigger zone.

Pharmacokinetics

Drug is metabolized in the liver and excreted in urine and feces.

Onset	Peak	Duration
3-10 min	30 min	2-4 hr

How supplied

Solution for injection: 2.5 mg/mL in 1-mL, 2-mL, and 5-mL ampules and in 2-mL, 5-mL, and 10-mL vials

Indications and dosages

➤ Nausea and vomiting associated with surgical and diagnostic procedures

Adults: Initially, 2.5 mg slow I.V. infusion with additional doses of 1.25 mg given as needed to achieve desired effect. Dosages are highly individualized based on patient's age, weight, physical status, and underlying clinical condition.

Children ages 2 to 12: Maximum recommended initial dosage is 0.1 mg/kg I.V., highly individualized based on patient's age, weight, physical status, and underlying clinical condition. Additional doses may be given with caution.

Dosage adjustment

- Adjust dosage as appropriate in high-risk patients (such as those who are older than age 65, have heart failure, abuse alcohol, or have other factors that predispose to prolonged QT interval).
- Adjust dosage as appropriate in patients who have received other CNS depressants (such as analgesics or anesthesia).

Off-label uses

- Breakthrough chemotherapy-induced nausea and vomiting

Administration

Preparation

- Know that drug is indicated to relieve perioperative nausea and vomiting only in patients who do not respond adequately to other treatment.

🔊 Before starting drug, assess ECG status for risk of potentially serious arrhythmias.

🔊 Be aware that all patients should undergo 12-lead ECG before drug administration to detect prolonged QT interval (QTc interval greater than 440 msec in males or 450 msec in females).

🔊 Use with extreme caution in patients with risk factors for prolonged QT syndrome, such as congestive heart failure, bradycardia, cardiac hypertrophy, hypokalemia, hypomagnesemia, diuretic therapy, monoamine oxidase (MAO) inhibitor use, or use with other drugs known to increase QT interval (such as Class I and II antiarrhythmics).

🔊 Know that drug may cause sudden death at high dosages (above 25 mg) in patients at risk for arrhythmias.

- Be aware that drug action lasts 2 to 4 hours, although altered alertness may persist up to 12 hours.

Dilution and compatibility

- Be aware that drug does not require dilution for I.V. use.

Infusion considerations

- Give by slow I.V. injection.

Monitoring

🔊 For patient at risk for potentially serious arrhythmias, continue ECG monitoring for 2 to 3 hours after drug administration ends.

🔊 Monitor for signs and symptoms of neuroleptic malignant syndrome (rare), such as hyperthermia, severe extrapyramidal symptoms, altered mental status, stupor, coma, hypertension, tachycardia, pallor, and diaphoresis.

🔊 Monitor vital signs frequently. Stay alert for orthostatic hypotension and tachycardia. Keep I.V. fluids and vasopressors on hand in case of pronounced hypotension.

🔊 Do not place hypotensive patient in Trendelenburg position, as this may deepen anesthesia, precipitating respiratory arrest.

- Assess respiratory status frequently if drug is used with opioids or depressants.
- Avoid abrupt position changes.

• Monitor for and report extrapyramidal symptoms, such as restlessness, tremor, and facial tics.

Storage

• Store at room temperature of 15° to 25°C (59° to 77°F); protect from light.

Contraindications and precautions

Contraindicated in hypersensitivity to drug and known or suspected QT prolongation (QTc interval greater than 440 msec in males or 450 msec in females), including congenital long-QT syndrome.

Use cautiously in severe cardiac or renal disease, diabetes mellitus, respiratory insufficiency, prostatic hypertrophy, angle-closure glaucoma, CNS depression, CNS tumors, intestinal obstruction, bone marrow depression, Parkinson's disease, electrolyte imbalance, pheochromocytoma, ***elderly patients,*** pregnant or breastfeeding patients, and ***children younger than age 2*** (safety and efficacy not established).

Adverse reactions

CNS: drowsiness, weakness, dysarthria, dysphonia, dizziness, extrapyramidal reactions, headache, postoperative hallucinatory episodes with transient depression, tremor, irritability, paresthesia, aggression, vertigo, ataxia, **loss of consciousness, seizures, neuroleptic malignant syndrome** (rare)

CV: chest pain, hypertension, vasodilation, **hypotension, QT prolongation, torsades de pointes, cardiac arrest** (with high doses in high-risk patients), **ventricular tachycardia, atrial fibrillation**

EENT: cataracts, blurred vision, eye irritation, sore throat, **laryngospasm** (rare)

GI: nausea, vomiting, diarrhea, abdominal cramps, bloating, epigastric pain, fecal incontinence, increased salivation, dysphagia

GU: urinary frequency, increased libido

Hepatic: cholestatic jaundice

Metabolic: dehydration

Musculoskeletal: muscle cramps, arthritis, bone fractures

Respiratory: bronchitis, dyspnea, decreased pulmonary artery pressure, **bronchospasm** (rare)

Skin: bruising, rash, urticaria, diaphoresis, pruritus, flushing

Other: toothache, weight loss, hot flashes, influenza, chills, hypersensitivity reactions including **anaphylaxis** (rare)

Interactions

Drug-drug. *Antihypertensives, nitrates:* additive hypertension

Class I or II antiarrhythmics, MAO inhibitors, other drugs that may prolong QT interval: QT prolongation

CNS depressants (including antidepressants, antihistamines, and opioids): additive CNS depression

Drug-herb. *Chamomile, hops, kava, skullcap, valerian:* increased CNS depression

Drug-behaviors. *Alcohol use:* additive CNS depression

Toxicity and overdose

• Overdose signs and symptoms are extensions of pharmacologic and adverse reactions, including exaggerated sedation, QT prolongation, respiratory distress, hypotension, and serious arrhythmias.

• If respiratory distress occurs, maintain patent airway and provide oxygen and assisted ventilation, as indicated and ordered. Closely monitor patient for at least 24 hours. Maintain body warmth and hydration. For severe or persistent hypotension, consider hypovolemia and administer I.V. fluids, as ordered. For extrapyramidal symptoms, give anticholinergic, as ordered.

Patient education

- Advise patient not to drink alcohol or take CNS depressants for 24 hours after receiving drug.
- Tell patient drug may cause extreme drowsiness for several hours after administration.
- Caution patient not to drive or perform other activities requiring mental alertness until drug's effects dissipate completely.
- Instruct patient to change positions slowly.
- As appropriate, review all other significant and life-threatening adverse reactions and interactions, especially those related to the drugs, herbs, and behaviors mentioned above.

drotrecogin alfa (activated)

Xigris

Pharmacologic class: Activated protein C (recombinant)

Therapeutic class: Antisepsis drug

Pregnancy risk category C

Action

Antisepsis action unknown. May produce indirect profibrinolytic activity by hindering plasminogen activator inhibitor-1 and limiting generation of activated thrombin-activatable fibrinolysis inhibitor. Produces anti-inflammatory effect by inhibiting human tumor necrosis factor production and suppressing thrombin-induced inflammatory responses.

Pharmacokinetics

Drug rapidly achieves steady-state concentrations proportional to infusion rates. In most patients, plasma concentrations drop below quantitation limits of 10 mg/mL within 2 hours after infusion ends.

Onset	Peak	Duration
Rapid	Unknown	Unknown

D

How supplied

Powder for reconstitution for injection (white to off-white, lyophilized): 5 mg, 20 mg

Indications and dosages

➤ Prevention of death in adults with severe sepsis who are at high risk for death

Adults: 24 mcg/kg/hour I.V. for total duration of 96 hours (based on actual body weight)

Administration

Preparation

Be aware that drug efficacy has not been established in adults with severe sepsis who are at lower risk for death.

Discontinue drug 2 hours before invasive procedures. Once adequate hemostasis is restored, drug initiation may be reconsidered 12 hours after major invasive procedures or surgery, or drug may be restarted immediately after uncomplicated, less-invasive procedures.

- Before starting drug, assess International Normalized Ratio (INR), prothrombin time (PT), platelet count, and bleeding risk.

Dilution and compatibility

- Reconstitute 5-mg vial with 2.5 mL sterile water for injection or reconstitute 20-mg vial with 10 mL sterile water for injection by slowly adding diluent to vial. Gently swirl until powder dissolves completely; avoid inverting or shaking vial.

• Further dilute with normal saline solution by directing drug stream at side of infusion bag to minimize agitation. Gently invert infusion bag to mix thoroughly.
• Do not mix with other drugs
• Prepare immediately before use. Hang infusion bag within 3 hours of reconstitution.

Infusion considerations
• Administer only with infusion pump through dedicated infusion line. Be aware that only the following solutions can be given through same I.V. line: normal saline solution, lactated Ringer's solution, D_5W, and dextrose and saline mixture solutions.
• Infuse I.V. at 24 mcg/kg/hour for total duration of 96 hours.
Know that dosage escalation and bolus doses are not recommended.

Monitoring
Monitor closely for signs and symptoms of hemorrhage. Stop infusion if clinically significant bleeding occurs.
• Continue to monitor INR, PT, and CBC (especially platelet count).
• Be aware that drug may variably prolong activated partial thromboplastin time (APTT) and thus does not reliably indicate coagulopathy.

Storage
• Store vials at 2° to 8°C (36° to 46°F). Protect unreconstituted vials from heat and light.
• Know that reconstituted solution not used immediately can be stored at controlled room temperature of 15° to 30° C (59° to 86° F) for 3 hours.

Contraindications and precautions

Contraindicated in hypersensitivity to drug or its components, intracranial neoplasm or lesion, evidence of cerebral herniation, intracranial or intraspinal surgery within last 2 months, hemorrhagic stroke within last 3 months, severe head trauma or trauma with increased risk of life-threatening bleeding, active bleeding, severe thrombocytopenia, high risk of bleeding, current use of epidural catheter, and bone marrow therapy.

Use cautiously in intracranial arteriovenous malformation; chronic severe hepatic disease; recent GI bleeding; concurrent use of heparin, thrombolytics, oral anticoagulants, or aspirin; pregnant or breastfeeding patients; and ***children*** (safety and efficacy not established).

Adverse reactions

CNS: intracranial hemorrhage
GI: intra-abdominal, retroperitoneal, or other GI bleeding
GU: GU tract bleeding
Hematologic: bleeding
Skin: bruising
Other: skin and soft-tissue bleeding

Interactions

Drug-drug. *Anticoagulants, aspirin (dosages above 650 mg), glycoprotein IIb/IIIa inhibitors, heparin (therapeutic dosages) indomethacin, phenylbutazone, thrombolytics:* increased risk of bleeding
Drug-diagnostic tests. *APTT, PT:* prolonged
Hematocrit: decreased

Toxicity and overdose

• In overdose, expect minor to severe bleeding.
• No known antidote exists. Immediately stop infusion and monitor patient closely for hemorrhage.

Patient teaching

• As appropriate, review all other significant and life-threatening adverse reactions and interactions, especially those related to the drugs and tests mentioned above.

edrophonium chloride

Enlon, Tensilon

Pharmacologic class: Anticholinesterase

Therapeutic class: Diagnostic drug, muscle stimulant, antidote

Pregnancy risk category C

Action

Reversibly inhibits cholinesterase. Binds to acetylcholinesterase, which in turn prevents this enzyme from binding to acetylcholine and leads to acetylcholine accumulation at cholinergic synapses.

Pharmacokinetics

Distribution and metabolism are not clearly understood. Drug is primarily excreted in urine.

Onset	Peak	Duration
<1 min	Unknown	5-20 min

How supplied

Solution for injection (clear): 10 mg/mL in 1-mL ampules and 15-mL vials

Indications and dosages

➢ Diagnostic aid in myasthenia gravis

Adults: 1 to 2 mg I.V. over 15 to 30 seconds; if no response occurs within 45 seconds, give 8 mg.

Children weighing more than 34 kg (75 lb): 2 mg I.V.; if no response occurs within 45 seconds, give 1 mg q 45 seconds, to a maximum of 10 mg.

Children weighing 34 kg or less: 1 mg I.V.; if no response occurs within 45 seconds, give 1 mg q 45 seconds, to a maximum of 5 mg.

➢ To differentiate myasthenic crisis from cholinergic crisis

Adults: 1 mg I.V.; if no response occurs in 1 minute, repeat dose once. Increased muscle strength confirms myasthenic crisis; weakness or no increase in muscle strength confirms cholinergic crisis.

➢ Antidote to reverse nondepolarizing neuromuscular blockade

Adults: 10 mg I.V. given over 30 to 45 seconds; repeat dose q 5 to 10 minutes p.r.n. to a maximum of 40 mg.

Administration

Preparation

- Withdraw anticholinesterase drugs (cholinergics) at least 8 hours before diagnostic use of this agent.

Keep atropine (edrophonium antidote) readily available.

Keep advanced life-saving equipment on hand during administration, as drug may cause respiratory distress.

Administer only where continuous ECG monitoring is available.

Dilution and compatibility

- Know that drug may be given undiluted.
- Be aware that maximum concentration is 10 mg/mL.

Infusion considerations

- Give at rate prescribed for specific indication.
- Monitor I.V. site closely.

Monitoring

When giving drug to diagnose myasthenia gravis, monitor closely for cholinergic crisis (skeletal muscle fasciculations and increased muscle weakness, especially in respiratory muscles) after 2-mg dose. If cholinergic crisis occurs, discontinue drug and give atropine I.V. as prescribed.

Assess for bradycardia, hypotension, and cardiac arrest.

• Frequently assess muscle strength when giving drug for diagnostic or differentiating indications.

Storage

• Store at controlled room temperature of 15° to 30°C (59° to 86°F).

Contraindications and precautions

Contraindicated in hypersensitivity to drug or sulfites and in mechanical GI or urinary tract obstruction.

Use cautiously in bronchial asthma, peptic ulcer, peritonitis, bradycardia, arrhythmias, vagotonia, hyperthyroidism, epilepsy, recent coronary occlusion, and pregnant or breastfeeding patients.

Adverse reactions

CNS: asthenia, dysarthria, dysphonia, dizziness, drowsiness, headache, syncope, loss of consciousness, **seizures**

CV: hypotension, **thrombophlebitis, atrioventricular block, cardiac arrest, bradycardia**

EENT: lacrimation, diplopia, miosis, conjunctival hyperemia

GI: nausea, vomiting, diarrhea, abdominal cramps, increased salivation, dysphagia

GU: urinary frequency or incontinence

Musculoskeletal: muscle cramps, fasciculations

Respiratory: increased secretions, dyspnea, **respiratory muscle paralysis, respiratory depression, central respiratory paralysis, respiratory arrest, bronchospasm, laryngospasm**

Skin: rash, diaphoresis, flushing

Other: anaphylaxis

Interactions

Drug-drug. *Aminoglycosides:* prolonged or increased muscle weakness

Anesthetics (local and general): antagonism of cholinergic effects

Cholinergics: increased cholinergic effects that mimic myasthenia weakness

Corticosteroids, magnesium, procainamide, quinidine: antagonism of cholinergic effects

Depolarizing neuromuscular blockers: increased neuromuscular blockade, prolonged respiratory depression

Drug-diagnostic tests. *Urine cannabinoid test:* false-positive result

Drug-herb. *Jaborandi, pill-bearing spurge:* additive effects

Toxicity and overdose

• In overdose, expect muscarinic-like signs and symptoms (such as nausea, vomiting, diarrhea, sweating, increased bronchial and salivary secretions, and bradycardia) and possible airway obstruction caused by bronchial secretions.

• Discontinue drug and provide symptomatic and supportive therapy, including suctioning of bronchial secretions, I.V. atropine sulfate to counteract most adverse reactions, I.V. pralidoxime chloride (with caution), assisted ventilation, oxygen, cardiac monitoring, and appropriate measures to treat seizures or shock, as ordered.

Patient teaching

• Tell patient increased muscle strength is a positive response to drug.

• As appropriate, review all other significant and life-threatening adverse reactions and interactions, especially those related to the drugs, tests, and herbs mentioned above.

enalaprilat

Vasotec IV

Pharmacologic class: Angiotensin-converting enzyme (ACE) inhibitor
Therapeutic class: Antihypertensive
Pregnancy risk category C (first trimester), *D* (second and third trimesters)

FDA BOXED WARNING

• When used during second or third trimester of pregnancy, drug can cause fetal injury and even death. Discontinue as soon as pregnancy is detected.

Action

Inhibits conversion of angiotensin I to angiotensin II, a potent vasoconstrictor; inactivates bradykinin and prostaglandins. Also increases plasma renin and potassium levels and reduces aldosterone levels, resulting in systemic vasodilation.

Pharmacokinetics

Approximately 90% of dose is excreted unchanged in urine.

Onset	Peak	Duration
15 min	3-4 hr	6 hr

How supplied

Solution for injection (clear, colorless): 1.25 mg/mL

Indications and dosages

➤ Hypertension

Adults: For patients not taking concomitant diuretics, initially 1.25 mg I.V. q 6 hours. For patients who are receiving diuretics or have signs or symptoms of hypovolemia, initially 0.625 mg I.V.

Dosage adjustment

• Reduce dosage in impaired renal function. If creatinine clearance is 30 mL/minute or lower, give initial dose of 0.625 mg I.V. If response is inadequate after 1 hour, repeat 0.625-mg dose. Additional 1.25 mg may be given I.V. at 6-hour intervals. For patients on dialysis, give initial dose of 0.625 mg or lower over 5 minutes or longer but less than 1 hour.

Off-label uses

• Diabetic nephropathy
• Hypertensive emergency

Administration

Preparation

Find out if patient has history of angioedema (swelling of face, extremities, lips, tongue, glottis, or larynx) before starting drug.
• Know that I.V. administration usually is reserved for patients who cannot take oral form.
• Be aware that I.V. use is not recommended for pediatric patients.
• Discontinue diuretics for 2 to 3 days before starting drug, if possible.
• Evaluate serum potassium level before administering drug.

Dilution and compatibility

• Be aware that drug may be given either undiluted or diluted in 50 mL D_5W, normal saline solution, dextrose 5% in normal saline solution, or dextrose 5% in lactated Ringer's solution.

Infusion considerations

• Give I.V. slowly over 5 minutes.
• If patient is at risk for hypotension, give by slow I.V. infusion over 1 hour.

Monitoring

• After initial dose, observe patient closely for at least 2 hours until blood pressure stabilizes. Thereafter, continue to observe patient for an additional hour.

Assess for rapid blood pressure decline leading to cardiovascular collapse, especially when giving drug with diuretics.
In patient with renal insufficiency or renal artery stenosis, monitor for worsening renal function.
Watch for angioedema (rare reaction).
- Monitor vital signs, fluid intake and output, and daily weight.
- Supervise patient during ambulation until drug's effects are known.
- Monitor liver function tests and blood urea nitrogen (BUN), creatinine, and electrolyte levels.

Storage
- Store below 30°C (86°F). After dilution, drug may be stored up to 24 hours.

Contraindications and precautions
Contraindicated in hypersensitivity to drug or other ACE inhibitors, angioedema related to previous ACE inhibitor therapy or hereditary angioedema, and pregnancy.

Use cautiously in renal or hepatic impairment, hypovolemia, hyponatremia, aortic stenosis, hypertrophic cardiomyopathy, cerebrovascular or cardiac insufficiency, black patients with hypertension, concurrent diuretic use, ***elderly patients,*** breastfeeding patients, and ***children.***

Adverse reactions
CNS: dizziness, fatigue, headache, insomnia, drowsiness, vertigo, asthenia, paresthesia, ataxia, confusion, depression, nervousness, **cerebrovascular accident**
CV: palpitations, angina pectoris, tachycardia, peripheral edema, **hypotension, arrhythmias, cardiac arrest**
EENT: sinusitis
GI: nausea, vomiting, constipation, dyspepsia, abdominal pain, dry mouth, **pancreatitis**
GU: proteinuria, urinary tract infection, erectile dysfunction, decreased libido, **oliguria**
Hematologic: agranulocytosis, bone marrow depression
Hepatic: hepatitis
Metabolic: hyponatremia, **hyperkalemia**
Respiratory: cough, upper respiratory tract infection, asthma, bronchitis, dyspnea, **eosinophilic pneumonitis**
Skin: rash, alopecia, photosensitivity, diaphoresis, exfoliative dermatitis, **angioedema, erythema multiforme**
Other: altered taste, fever, increased appetite, anaphylactoid reactions

Interactions
Drug-drug. *Allopurinol:* increased risk of hypersensitivity reaction
Cyclosporine, indomethacin, potassium-sparing diuretics, potassium supplements: hyperkalemia
Digoxin, lithium: increased blood levels of these drugs and possible toxicity
Diuretics, nitrates, other antihypertensives, phenothiazines: additive hypotension
Nonsteroidal anti-inflammatory drugs: decreased antihypertensive response
Drug-diagnostic tests. *Alanine aminotransferase, alkaline phosphatase, aspartate aminotransferase, bilirubin, BUN, creatinine, potassium:* increased
Antinuclear antibodies: positive titer
Sodium: decreased
Drug-food. *Salt substitutes containing potassium:* hyperkalemia
Drug-herb. *Capsaicin:* increased incidence of cough
Drug-behaviors. *Acute alcohol ingestion:* additive hypotension
Sun exposure: photosensitivity reaction

Toxicity and overdose

- In overdose, expect severe hypotension.
- Discontinue drug. Provide symptomatic and supportive therapy, including volume expansion with I.V. normal saline solution to treat hypotension, as ordered. Hemodialysis may be beneficial.

Patient teaching

Tell patient to immediately report swelling of face, eye area, tongue, lips, hands, or feet; irregular heartbeat; rash, hives, or severe itching; unexplained fever; unusual tiredness; yellowing of skin or eyes; abdominal pain; and easy bruising.

- Instruct patient to move slowly when sitting up or standing, to avoid dizziness or light-headedness from sudden blood pressure decrease.
- As appropriate, review all other significant and life-threatening adverse reactions and interactions, especially those related to the drugs, tests, foods, herbs, and behaviors mentioned above.

epinephrine hydrochloride

Pharmacologic class: Sympathomimetic (direct-acting)

Therapeutic class: Bronchodilator, sympathomimetic, vasopressor, anaphylaxis agent

Pregnancy risk category C

Action

Stimulates alpha- and beta-adrenergic receptors, causing vasoconstriction and relaxing bronchial smooth muscle, which leads to bronchodilation. Directly stimulates beta-1 receptors in heart, resulting in tachycardia and increased cardiac output.

Pharmacokinetics

I.V. dose causes immediate intense response, with rapid drug disappearance from bloodstream. Drug becomes fixed in tissues and is rapidly inactivated, primarily by enzymatic transformation. It undergoes rapid and systematic degradation in the liver and other tissues by monoamine oxidase (MAO) and catechol-O-methyltransferase. Circulating drug unaccounted for by such mechanisms is deactivated by reuptake at synaptic receptor sites. Inactivated drug compounds are excreted in urine.

Onset	Peak	Duration
Immediate	5 min	4-8 hr

How supplied

Solution for injection: 1:1,000 (1 mg/mL) in 1-mL ampules, 1:2,000 (0.5 mg/mL) in prefilled syringes, 1:10,000 (0.1 mg/mL) in prefilled syringes, 1:100,000 (0.01 mg/mL) in prefilled syringes

Indications and dosages

➢ Bronchodilation, anaphylaxis, hypersensitivity reaction

Adults: 0.1 to 0.25 mL of 1:10,000 solution I.V. slowly over 5 to 10 minutes; may repeat q 5 to 15 minutes p.r.n. or follow with continuous I.V. infusion of 1 mcg/minute, increased to 4 mcg/minute p.r.n.

➢ To restore cardiac rhythm in cardiac arrest

Adults: 0.5 to 1 mg (5 to 10 mL of 1:10,000 solution) I.V., repeated q 3 to 5 minutes, if needed. If no response occurs, give 3 to 5 mg I.V. q 3 to 5 minutes.

Administration

Preparation

Do not give within 2 weeks of MAO inhibitors.

Be aware that not all epinephrine solutions can be given IV. Know that EpiPen and EpiPen Jr. are for I.M. use only. Always check manufacturer's label.

Dilution and compatibility

- Be aware that drug is available as prediluted solution in 10-mL syringes.

When administering in cardiac arrest, dilute 0.5 to 1 mg of 1:10,000 solution in 10 mL normal saline solution.

Know that epinephrine is incompatible with alkaline solutions (such as sodium bicarbonate). Administer separately.

- Do not use if solution is pinkish or darker than slightly yellow.
- Discard unused portion of drug.

Infusion considerations

- Give each 1-mg dose over at least 1 minute.

When giving as continuous I.V. infusion, use rate-control device set at 1 to 10 mcg/minute, adjusting to desired response.

Monitoring

- Assess drug's effect on underlying problem (such as anaphylaxis or asthma attack), and repeat dose as needed.

Monitor vital signs, ECG, and cardiovascular and respiratory status. Watch for ventricular fibrillation, tachycardia, arrhythmias, and signs and symptoms of shock. Ask patient about anginal pain.

Monitor neurologic status, particularly for decreased level of consciousness and other signs and symptoms of cerebral hemorrhage or cerebrovascular accident.

- Monitor fluid intake and output; watch for urine retention or decreased urine output.

Storage

- Store at 15° to 30°C (59° to 86°F). Protect from light, extreme heat, and freezing.

Contraindications and precautions

Contraindicated in hypersensitivity to drug, its components, or sulfites; angle-closure glaucoma; cardiac disease; cerebral arteriosclerosis; within 2 weeks of MAO inhibitors; labor; and breastfeeding.

Use cautiously in hypertension, hyperthyroidism, diabetes, prostatic hypertrophy, ***elderly patients,*** pregnant patients, and ***children.***

Adverse reactions

CNS: nervousness, anxiety, tremors, vertigo, headache, disorientation, agitation, drowsiness, fear, dizziness, asthenia, **cerebral hemorrhage, cerebrovascular accident**

CV: palpitations, widened pulse pressure, hypertension, tachycardia, angina, ECG changes, **ventricular fibrillation, shock**

GI: nausea, vomiting

GU: decreased urine output, urine retention, dysuria

Respiratory: dyspnea, **pulmonary edema**

Skin: urticaria, pallor, diaphoresis

Interactions

Drug-drug. *Alpha-adrenergic blockers:* hypotension

Antihistamines, thyroid hormone, tricyclic antidepressants: severe sympathomimetic effects

Beta-adrenergic blockers (such as propranolol): vasodilation and reflex tachycardia

Cardiac glycosides, general anesthetics: increased risk of ventricular arrhythmias

Diuretics: decreased vascular response

Doxapram, mazindol, methylphenidate: enhanced CNS stimulation or pressor effects

Ergot alkaloids: decreased vasoconstriction

Guanadrel, guanethidine: enhanced pressor effects of epinephrine

Levodopa: increased risk of arrhythmias
Levothyroxine: potentiation of epinephrine effects
MAO inhibitors: increased risk of hypertensive crisis
Drug-diagnostic tests. *Glucose:* transient increase

Toxicity and overdose

- Signs and symptoms of overdose may include sudden and severe blood pressure increase, unusually pale and cold skin, severe anxiety, severe nausea and vomiting, severe respiratory distress, pulmonary edema, renal failure, metabolic acidosis, and irregular heart rhythm.
- Provide symptomatic and supportive therapy, which may be sufficient because drug is rapidly inactivated. Monitor vital signs closely.

Patient teaching

- As appropriate, review all other significant and life-threatening adverse reactions and interactions, especially those related to the drugs and tests mentioned above.

epirubicin hydrochloride

Ellence

Pharmacologic class: Anthracycline
Therapeutic class: Antibiotic antineoplastic
Pregnancy risk category D

FDA BOXED WARNING

- Extravasation during administration causes severe local tissue necrosis.
- Myocardial toxicity, manifested most severely by potentially fatal heart failure, may occur during therapy or months to years afterward. Risk rises rapidly with increasing total cumulative doses above 900 mg/m^2; exceed this cumulative dose only with extreme caution. Active or dormant cardiovascular disease, previous or concurrent radiotherapy to mediastinal or pericardial area, previous anthracycline or anthracenedione therapy, or concurrent use of other cardiotoxic drugs may increase myocardial toxicity risk. Toxicity may occur at lower cumulative doses even if patient has no cardiac risk factors.
- Secondary acute myelogenous leukemia (AML) has occurred in breast cancer patients who have received this drug. Refractory AML is more common when drug is given in combination with DNA-damaging antineoplastics, when patients have been heavily pretreated with cytotoxic drugs, or when epirubicin dosage has been escalated.
- Reduce dosage in patients with hepatic impairment.
- Drug may cause severe myelosuppression.
- Give under supervision of physician experienced in cancer chemotherapy.

Action

Forms complex with DNA by intercalation with nucleotide base pairs, causing inhibition of DNA, RNA, and protein synthesis. This inhibition, in turn, leads to cytocidal activity (cell-cycle nonspecific).

Pharmacokinetics

Drug distributes rapidly and widely. It is metabolized extensively by the liver; epirubicinol is principal active metabolite. Drug is strongly protein-bound and concentrated in red blood cells; whole-blood concentrations are approximately twice those of plasma. Half-life is approximately 30 to 35 hours. Parent drug and metabolites are glucuronidated and excreted primarily in bile, with some renal excretion.

Onset	Peak	Duration
Unknown	Unknown	Unknown

How supplied

Solution for injection (clear, red): 2 mg/mL, 50 mg/25 mL, and 200 mg/dL in single-use vials

Indications and dosages

➤ Adjunct in patients with axillary-node tumor involvement after resection of primary breast cancer
Adults: 100 to 120 mg/m² by I.V. infusion over 3 to 5 minutes on first day of each cycle or divided equally in two doses on days 1 and 8 of each cycle; repeat cycle q 3 to 4 weeks for six cycles in conjunction with cyclophosphamide and fluorouracil.

Dosage adjustment

- After first cycle, base dosage adjustment on toxicity. For patients with platelet counts below 50,000/mm³, absolute neutrophil count (ANC) below 250/mm³, neutropenic fever, or grade 3 or 4 nonhematologic toxicity, reduce first day's dosage in subsequent cycles to 75% and delay subsequent cycles until platelet count is at least 100,000/mm³, ANC is at least 1,500/mm³, and nonhematologic toxicity recovers to grade 1 or better.
- Reduce dosage in impaired hepatic function or severe renal impairment.

Off-label uses

- Bladder cancer
- Esophageal carcinoma, esophagogastric junction carcinomas, and adenocarcinomas in combination with other agents
- Hodgkin's and non-Hodgkin's lymphoma
- Locally unresectable and metastatic gastric carcinoma
- Non-small-cell lung carcinoma
- Primary hepatocellular carcinoma
- Prostate cancer
- Small-cell lung carcinoma
- Soft-tissue sarcoma
- Stage III and IV (FIGO) ovarian carcinoma

Administration

Preparation

- Follow hazardous drug guidelines on page S19 for handling, preparation, and administration.
- Know that previous anthracycline use must be considered when determining dosage because of increased risk of heart failure.

Dilution and compatibility

- Be aware that drug solution provided is preservative-free and ready to use.
- Do not mix with alkaline solutions, because drug hydrolysis may occur.
- Do not mix with heparin or fluorouracil, because precipitation may occur.
- Discard unused portion of drug.

Infusion considerations

- Never give I.M. or subcutaneously.
- Know that direct I.V. push is not recommended because of extravasation risk.
- Make sure I.V. line is free flowing before administering.
- Administer premixed solution by slow I.V. infusion over 3 to 5 minutes into tubing of free-flowing I.V. line containing D_5W or normal saline solution for injection.
- Check I.V. patency frequently throughout infusion to avoid extravasation. If patient complains of burning or stinging, switch infusion to different vein.

Clinical alert: If patient develops facial flushing or red streak in infused vein, slow infusion rate.

Clinical alert: Do not exceed cumulative dosage of 900 mg/m^2 due to risk of cardiomyopathy.

Monitoring

Clinical alert: Monitor vital signs, left ventricular ejection fraction, and cardiovascular status carefully. Watch for signs and symptoms of cardiomyopathy and heart failure.

Clinical alert: Monitor CBC with white cell differential; watch for signs and symptoms of blood dyscrasias.

- Check temperature regularly. Stay alert for fever and other signs and symptoms of infection.
- Assess nutritional status and hydration regularly.

Storage

- Refrigerate between 2° and 8°C (36° and 46°F). Do not freeze; protect from light.

Contraindications and precautions

Contraindicated in hypersensitivity to drug, myocardial insufficiency, severe hepatic dysfunction, baseline neutrophil count below 1,500/mm^3, or cumulative doses above 900 mg/m^2.

Use cautiously in heart disease, hepatic disease, previous or recent radiation therapy, ***elderly patients (particularly females older than age 70),*** pregnant or breastfeeding patients, and ***children*** (safety and efficacy not established).

Adverse reactions

CNS: lethargy
CV: cardiomyopathy, heart failure
EENT: conjunctivitis, keratitis
GI: nausea, vomiting, diarrhea, mucositis
GU: reddish urine, amenorrhea
Hematologic: anemia, **leukopenia, neutropenia, thrombocytopenia**
Skin: alopecia; rash; pruritus; darkening of soles, palms, or nails
Other: increased appetite, infection, fever, hot flashes, tissue necrosis

Interactions

Drug-drug. *Calcium channel blockers:* increased risk of heart failure
Cimetidine: increased epirubicin blood level
Cytotoxic drugs: additive toxicity
Live-virus vaccines: increased risk of infection
Trastuzumab: increased risk of cardiac dysfunction
Drug-diagnostic tests. *Hemoglobin, neutrophils, platelets, white blood cells:* decreased

Toxicity and overdose

- In overdose, expect signs and symptoms similar to adverse reactions, which may progress to multisystemic failure and death.
- Provide supportive therapy, including antibiotics, blood and platelet transfusions, colony-stimulating factors, and intensive care, as needed and ordered, until recovery. Delayed heart failure may occur months after drug administration; patient must be observed carefully over time for signs and symptoms of heart failure and given appropriate supportive therapy.

Patient teaching

Clinical alert: Instruct patient to immediately report pain, burning, or swelling at I.V site.

Clinical alert: Advise patient to immediately report sudden weight gain, swelling, or shortness of breath.

Clinical alert: Tell patient to promptly report unusual bruising or bleeding, fever, and signs and symptoms of infection.

• Explain that drug will probably cause hair loss but that hair should grow back within a few months after therapy.
• Advise female patient that drug may cause premature menopause or permanent menses cessation.
• Instruct female patient to tell prescriber if she is pregnant or breastfeeding.
• As appropriate, review all other significant and life-threatening adverse reactions and interactions, especially those related to the drugs and tests mentioned above.

epoetin alfa

Epogen, Eprex♣❉, Procrit

Pharmacologic class: Recombinant human erythropoietin
Therapeutic class: Biological response modifier
Pregnancy risk category C

FDA BOXED WARNING

• Use lowest dosage that will gradually increase hemoglobin to lowest level sufficient to avoid the need for red blood cell (RBC) transfusion.
• Drug may increase risk of death and serious cardiovascular events when given to target hemoglobin above 12 g/dL.
• Drug may shorten time to tumor progression in patients with advanced head and neck cancer receiving radiation therapy when given to target hemoglobin above 12 g/dL. It may shorten overall survival and increase deaths from disease progression at 4 months in patients with metastatic breast cancer receiving chemotherapy when given to target hemoglobin above 12 g/dL, and may increase risk of death when given to target hemoglobin of 12 g/dL in patients with active cancer who are receiving neither chemotherapy nor radiation therapy. Drug is not indicated for these patients.
• When drug was given preoperatively to reduce allogeneic RBC transfusions, higher incidence of deep vein thrombosis occurred in patients not receiving prophylactic anticoagulation.

Action

Binds to erythropoietin, stimulating mitotic activity of erythroid progenitor cells in bone marrow and causing release of reticulocytes from bone marrow into bloodstream, where they become mature RBCs

Pharmacokinetics

In patients with chronic renal failure, circulating half-life is 4 to 13 hours. Drug is eliminated by first-order kinetics.

Onset	Peak	Duration
Unknown	Immediate	Unknown

How supplied

Solution for injection (colorless): 2,000 units/mL, 3,000 units/mL, and 4,000 units/mL in 1-mL single-use vials; 10,000 units/mL and 20,000 units/mL in multidose vials

Indications and dosages

➤ Anemia associated with chronic renal failure
Adults: Initially, 50 to 100 units/kg I.V. three times weekly. May be increased after 8 weeks if hematocrit is still below target range.
➤ Anemia caused by zidovudine therapy in patients with HIV infection
Adults: 100 units/kg I.V. three times weekly for 8 weeks or until hematocrit level is adequate. If desired response does not occur after 8 weeks, dosage

may be increased by 50 to 100 units/kg I.V. three times weekly; after 4 to 8 weeks, dosage may be further increased, as prescribed, to a maximum of 300 units/kg I.V. three times weekly.

➢ Anemia in children with chronic renal failure who are on dialysis

Children ages 1 month to 16 years: 50 units/kg I.V. three times weekly. Individualize maintenance dosage to maintain hematocrit within target range.

Administration

Preparation

Follow hazardous drug guidelines on page S19 for handling, preparation, and administration.

Avoid use of multidose vials in premature infants because of benzyl alcohol content.

- Be aware that because of time required for erythropoiesis (several days for erythroid progenitors to mature and be released into circulation), clinically significant increase in hematocrit usually takes at least 2 weeks, and may take up to 6 weeks in some patients.
- Know that supplemental iron may be needed to support erythropoiesis and avoid iron depletion.
- Assess transferrin and transferrin saturation before giving serum iron. Transferrin should be at least 100 mg/mL and transferrin saturation should be at least 20%.

Dilution and compatibility

Do not shake solution, as this may cause biological inactivation.

- Know that drug may be given undiluted.
- Be aware that single-dose vials contain no preservatives and must be entered only once. Discard unused portion.
- Do not mix with other drugs.

Infusion considerations

- For I.V. use, give single dose by direct I.V. injection over at least 1 minute, and follow with saline flush.
- If patient is on hemodialysis, administer drug into venous return line of dialysis tubing after dialysis session ends.

Monitoring

- Monitor vital signs and cardiovascular status, especially for hypertension and edema.
- Assess arteriovenous graft for patency, as drug may increase clotting at graft.
- Monitor electrolyte and uric acid levels. Watch closely for hyperuricemia, hyperkalemia, and hyperphosphatemia.
- Check temperature for fever.
- Monitor neurologic status for signs and symptoms of impending seizures.
- Evaluate nutritional status and hydration.

Storage

- Store between 2° and 8°C (36° and 46°F). Do not freeze.

Contraindications and precautions

Contraindicated in hypersensitivity to drug, human albumin, or products derived from mammal cells and in uncontrolled hypertension.

Use cautiously in pregnant or breastfeeding patients and ***children.***

Adverse reactions

CNS: headache, paresthesia, fatigue, dizziness, asthenia, **tonic-clonic seizures**

CV: increased clotting of arteriovenous grafts, hypertension

GI: nausea, vomiting, diarrhea

Metabolic: hyperuricemia, hyperphosphatemia, **hyperkalemia**

Musculoskeletal: joint pain

Respiratory: cough, dyspnea

Skin: rash, urticaria

Other: fever, edema

Interactions

Drug-diagnostic tests. *Blood urea nitrogen, creatinine, phosphate, potassium, uric acid:* increased

Toxicity and overdose

- Although maximum dosage has not been established, large dosages have been given without toxicity. If overdose occurs, expect polycythemia.
- Temporarily withhold dose until hematocrit returns to normal level. If polycythemia persists, phlebotomy may be needed.

Patient teaching

Instruct patient to monitor weight and blood pressure regularly and to immediately report hypertension, sudden weight gain, or swelling.

- Advise female patient to discuss pregnancy or breastfeeding with prescriber before starting drug.
- As appropriate, review all other significant and life-threatening adverse reactions and interactions, especially those related to the tests mentioned above.

epoprostenol sodium

Flolan

Pharmacologic class: Peripheral vasodilator

Therapeutic class: Antihypertensive

Pregnancy risk category B

Action

Causes direct vasodilation of pulmonary and systemic arterial vascular beds and inhibition of platelet aggregation

Pharmacokinetics

Drug is hydrolyzed rapidly at neutral blood pH and is degraded by enzymes. Half-life is approximately 6 minutes. It is metabolized into two active metabolites and excreted primarily in urine, with a small amount in feces.

Onset	Peak	Duration
Unknown	Unknown	Unknown

How supplied

Powder for reconstitution for injection (white to off-white): 0.5 mg in 17-mL vial, 1.5 mg in 17-mL vial

Indications and dosages

➤ Long-term treatment of primary pulmonary hypertension (PPH) and pulmonary hypertension associated with scleroderma spectrum of disease (PH/SSD) in New York Heart Association Class III and Class IV patients who have responded inadequately to conventional therapy

Adults: Initially, 2 ng/kg/minute by I.V. infusion

Dosage adjustment

- Consider dosage increases in increments of 2 ng/kg/minute every 15 minutes or longer until drug tolerance or dose-limiting pharmacologic effects occur and further infusion rate increases are not warranted.
- Decrease dosage gradually in 2-ng/kg/minute decrements every 15 minutes or longer until dose-limiting effects resolve. Avoid abrupt withdrawal and sudden large reductions in infusion rates.

Administration

Preparation

Drug is a potent pulmonary and systemic vasodilator and should be used only by clinicians experienced in diagnosing and treating pulmonary hypertension when diagnosis of PPH or PH/SSD has been established. Initiate doses in setting with adequate personnel and equipment for physiologic monitoring and emergency care.

Unless contraindicated, administer anticoagulant to patients with PPH and PH/SSD, as prescribed, to reduce risk of pulmonary thromboembolism or systemic embolism.

Dilution and compatibility

- Reconstitute only with sterile diluent that comes with drug.
- Do not mix with any other parenteral drugs or solutions.
- Use a concentration of a compatible solution that is also compatible with infusion pump to be used, in terms of minimum and maximum flow rates, reservoir capacity, and infusion pump criteria.
- When administering for long-term therapy, prepare in drug-delivery reservoir with total reservoir volume of at least 100 mL.
- Prepare drug with two vials of sterile diluent for use during 24-hour period.
- Know that 3,000 ng/mL and 10,000 ng/mL generally are satisfactory concentrations for delivering between 2 and 16 ng/kg/minute in adults. Patients receiving long-term therapy may require concentrations above 15,000 ng/mL.
- To prepare 3,000-ng/mL concentration, dissolve contents of one 0.5-mg vial with 5 mL sterile diluent. Withdraw 3 mL and add to sufficient diluent to yield a total of 100 mL.
- To prepare 5,000-ng/mL concentration, dissolve contents of one 0.5-mg vial with 5 mL sterile diluent. Withdraw entire vial contents and add sufficient sterile diluent to make a total of 100 mL.
- To prepare 10,000-ng/mL concentration, dissolve contents of two 0.5-mg vials with 5 mL sterile diluent. Withdraw entire vial contents and add sufficient sterile diluent to make a total of 100 mL.
- To prepare 15,000-ng/mL concentration, dissolve contents of one 1.5-mg vial with 5 mL sterile diluent. Withdraw entire vial contents and add sufficient sterile diluent to make a total of 100 mL.
- Do not use reconstituted solutions for more than 8 hours when administering at room temperature.

Infusion considerations

Except in life-threatening situations (such as unconsciousness or collapse), adjust infusion rate only under physician's direction.

Know that for initiation, drug may be given temporarily through peripheral I.V. infusion line until central line can be established.

For continuous long-term I.V. infusion, give only through central venous catheter using ambulatory infusion pump.

Monitoring

After new long-term infusion rate is established, observe patient and monitor standing and supine blood pressure and heart rate for several hours to ensure that new dosage is tolerated.

Avoid abrupt drug withdrawal (even for brief periods) or sudden large dosage reductions, as these may cause signs and symptoms associated with rebound pulmonary hypertension (including dyspnea, dizziness, and asthenia).

Be aware that sepsis may occur, particularly in patients on long-term therapy. Take steps to reduce infection risk during reconstitution, administration, and catheter care.

Storage

- Before reconstitution, store at room temperature of 15° to 25°C (59° to 77°F); protect from light.
- Refrigerate reconstituted solutions at 2° to 8°C (36° to 46°F) for no more than 40 hours; protect from light.

E

Contraindications and precautions

Contraindicated in hypersensitivity to drug or structurally related compounds; congestive heart failure caused by severe left ventricular systolic dysfunction (with long-term therapy); and patients who develop pulmonary edema during drug initiation.

Use cautiously in ***elderly patients,*** pregnant or breastfeeding patients, and ***children*** (safety and efficacy not established).

Adverse reactions

CNS: dizziness, headache, anxiety, nervousness, agitation, hyperesthesia, paresthesia, tremor
CV: tachycardia, syncope, **hypotension, bradycardia, heart failure**
GI: nausea, vomiting, diarrhea, abdominal pain, dyspepsia, anorexia
Musculoskeletal: back pain, jaw pain, neck pain, myalgia, arthralgia
Respiratory: dyspnea, **hypoxia**
Skin: flushing, ulcer, eczema, rash, urticaria
Other: nonspecific pain, chest pain, sweating, fever, chills, flulike symptoms, **sepsis**

Interactions

Drug-drug. *Antiplatelet agents, anticoagulants:* increased risk of bleeding
Diuretics, other antihypertensives and vasodilators: additive hypotension

Toxicity and overdose

- In overdose, expect dose-limiting pharmacologic effects, including flushing, headache, hypotension, tachycardia, nausea, vomiting, and diarrhea.
- Because drug metabolizes rapidly, dosage reduction may relieve symptoms.

Patient teaching

Teach patient receiving long-term therapy on continuous ambulatory basis through permanent indwelling central venous catheter to use only diluent supplied with drug. Stress importance of not interrupting drug delivery and of performing infusion pump care and meticulous sterile catheter care.

- Inform patient that drug may be needed for prolonged periods—possibly years.
- As appropriate, review all other significant and life-threatening adverse reactions and interactions, especially those related to the drugs mentioned above.

eptifibatide

Integrilin

Pharmacologic class: Platelet aggregation inhibitor
Therapeutic class: Antiplatelet agent
Pregnancy risk category B

Action

Inhibits platelet aggregation by binding to platelet-receptor glycoprotein (GP) IIb/IIIa, preventing binding of fibrinogen to platelets and subsequent thrombus formation

Pharmacokinetics

Drug has limited metabolism and is approximately 25% protein-bound. About 50% of dose clears from plasma by renal excretion.

Onset	Peak	Duration
Immediate	Immediate	4-6 hr

How supplied

Solution for injection (clear, colorless): 10-mL and 100-mL vials (2 mg/mL), 100-mL vials (0.75 mg/mL)

Indications and dosages

➢ Acute coronary syndrome (unstable angina or non-Q-wave myocardial infarction)
Adults: 180 mcg/kg I.V. (to a maximum of 22.6 mg) given over 1 to 2 minutes, followed by continuous infusion of 2 mcg/kg/minute (to a maximum of 15 mg/hour) for up to 72 hours
➢ To prevent thrombosis related to percutaneous coronary intervention (PCI)
Adults: 180 mcg/kg (to a maximum of 22.6 mg) I.V. bolus immediately before PCI, then continuous infusion of 2 mcg/kg/minute (to a maximum of 15 mg/hour), followed by second 180-mcg/kg bolus 10 minutes after first. Continue infusion until discharge or for up to 24 hours.

Dosage adjustment

- In acute coronary syndrome patients with estimated creatinine clearance below 50 mL/minute, give I.V. bolus of 180 mcg/kg as soon as possible after diagnosis, followed immediately with continuous infusion of 1 mcg/kg/minute.
- When giving drug for PCI in patients with estimated creatinine clearance below 50 mL/minute, administer I.V. bolus of 180 mcg/kg immediately before procedure begins; follow immediately with continuous infusion of 1 mcg/kg/minute and a second bolus of 180 mcg/kg given 10 minutes after first.

Administration

Preparation
- Before starting drug, obtain hematocrit or hemoglobin, platelet count, serum creatinine, and prothrombin time or activated partial thromboplastin time (APTT). In patients undergoing PCI, also measure activated clotting time.

Dilution and compatibility
- Know that drug does not require dilution.
- Withdraw single bolus dose from 10-mL vial into syringe.
- Discard unused portion left in vial.

Infusion considerations
- Give single bolus dose by I.V. push over 1 to 2 minutes.
- Follow I.V. push with continuous I.V. infusion given undiluted from 100-mL vial spiked with infusion set connected to infusion control device.
- Do not administer through same I.V. line as furosemide.

Monitoring
- Monitor vital signs and assess cardiovascular status, especially for syncope and hypotension.
- Monitor coagulation studies, CBC, and platelet count. Watch for signs and symptoms of abnormal bleeding, bruising, and hematuria.
- Maintain APTT between 50 and 70 seconds, unless PCI will be done.
- Check carefully for bleeding at all invasive procedure sites, particularly femoral access site.

Before femoral artery sheath removal in patients undergoing PCI, ensure that heparin is discontinued for 3 to 4 hours and APTT is less than 45 seconds. At least 4 hours before hospital discharge, both heparin and eptifibatide should be withdrawn and sheath hemostasis should be achieved by standard compressive techniques.

Storage
- Refrigerate vials at 2° to 8°C (36° to 46°F) or store at room temperature for 2 months; protect from light.

Contraindications and precautions

Contraindicated in hypersensitivity to drug or its components, severe hypertension (systolic pressure above 200 mm Hg or diastolic pressure above 110 mm Hg) inadequately controlled on antihypertensive therapy, history of bleeding diathesis, evidence of active abnormal bleeding within previous 30 days, history of hemorrhagic cerebrovascular accident (CVA) or CVA within past 30 days, major surgery within past 6 weeks, renal dialysis, or current or planned administration of another parenteral GP IIb/IIIa inhibitor.

Use cautiously in platelet count below 100,000/mm^3, renal insufficiency, ***elderly patients,*** pregnant or breastfeeding patients, and ***children*** (safety and efficacy not established).

Adverse reactions

CNS: headache, dizziness, asthenia, syncope, **intracranial hemorrhage** (rare)
CV: hypotension
GI: nausea, diarrhea, constipation
GU: hematuria
Hematologic: bleeding tendency, thrombocytopenia
Skin: flushing
Other: bleeding at femoral access site

Interactions

Drug-drug. *Clopidogrel, dipyridamole, nonsteroidal anti-inflammatory drugs, oral anticoagulants, thrombolytics, ticlopidine:* increased risk of bleeding
Other platelet aggregation inhibitors: serious bleeding
Drug-diagnostic tests. *Platelets:* decreased
Drug-herb. *Most commonly used herbs:* increased anticoagulant effect

Toxicity and overdose

- In overdose, expect extension of pharmacologic and adverse effects, including bleeding.
- Provide symptomatic and supportive therapy. Dialysis may clear drug because it is not extensively bound to plasma proteins.

Patient teaching

- Tell patient that drug causes serious adverse effects but can help prevent more chest pain or a heart attack. Provide reassurance that patient will be monitored closely during therapy.

Instruct patient to immediately report fainting or abnormal bruising or bleeding.

- Teach patient safety measures to avoid bruising and bleeding.
- As appropriate, review all other significant and life-threatening adverse reactions and interactions, especially those related to the drugs, tests, and herbs mentioned above.

ertapenem sodium

Invanz

Pharmacologic class: Carbapenem
Therapeutic class: Anti-infective
Pregnancy risk category B

Action

Inhibits bacterial cell-wall synthesis, causing cell death

Pharmacokinetics

Drug is highly bound to plasma proteins (mainly albumin). In healthy young adults, mean plasma half-life is approximately 4 hours and plasma clearance is approximately 1.8 L/hour. It is eliminated primarily by the kidneys; small amounts appear in breast milk.

Onset	Peak	Duration
Rapid	30 min	Unknown

How supplied

*Powder for reconstitution for infusion (white to off-white, lyophilized):*1 g/vial

Indications and dosages

➢ Community-acquired pneumonia, skin and skin-structure infections, complicated genitourinary (GU) infections, complicated intra-abdominal infections, acute pelvic infections
Adults and children older than age 13: 1 g I.V. daily. Duration of therapy varies with type of infection: community-acquired pneumonia, 10 to 14 days; skin and skin structures, 7 to 14 days; GU, 10 to 14 days; intra-abdominal, 5 to 14 days; acute pelvic, 3 to 10 days.
Children ages 3 months to 12 years: 15 mg/kg I.V. twice daily, not to exceed 1 g/day. May be given by I.V. infusion for up to 14 days.

➢ Prophylaxis of surgical-site infection after elective colorectal surgery
Adults: 1 g I.V. as a single dose given 1 hour before surgical incision

Dosage adjustment

- Reduce dosage to 500 mg daily in patients with advanced or end-stage renal insufficiency.

Administration

Dilution and compatibility
- Reconstitute by adding 10 mL sterile or bacteriostatic water or normal saline solution to vial. Shake well to dissolve; then immediately transfer contents of reconstituted vial for further dilution.
- Further dilute reconstituted drug in 50 mL normal saline solution.

🔊 Do not use diluents containing dextrose.
- Do not mix or infuse with other drugs.

Infusion considerations
- Give by I.V. infusion over 30 minutes.

Monitoring

🔊 Monitor vital signs, ECG, and cardiovascular status closely. Stay alert for arrhythmias, edema, blood pressure changes, and signs and symptoms of heart failure.

🔊 Assess neurologic status; watch for signs and symptoms of impending seizures.

🔊 Monitor bowel pattern; stay alert for indications of pseudomembranous colitis.

🔊 Watch for indications of erythema multiforme (sore throat, rash, cough, iris lesions, mouth sores, fever). Report early signs and symptoms before condition progresses to Stevens-Johnson syndrome. Also stay alert for other hypersensitivity reactions, including anaphylaxis.

🔊 Stay alert for respiratory distress, abnormal breath sounds, and dyspnea.
- Inspect injection site for evidence of thrombophlebitis and induration.
- Monitor for signs and symptoms of new infections.

Storage
- Do not store lyophilized powder above 25°C (77°F).
- Store reconstituted solution at room temperature of 25°C (77°F) and use within 6 hours. Or refrigerate it for 24 hours at 5°C (41°F) and use within 4 hours after removing from refrigerator.

Contraindications and precautions

Contraindicated in hypersensitivity to drug or its components, other carbapenems, or beta-lactams.

Use cautiously in penicillin hypersensitivity, seizure disorder, pregnant or breastfeeding patients, and ***children*** (not recommended in infants younger than 3 months).

Adverse reactions

CNS: headache, dizziness, asthenia, fatigue, insomnia, altered mental status, anxiety, **seizures**
CV: hypotension, hypertension, chest pain, phlebitis, **thrombophlebitis, arrhythmias, heart failure**

EENT: pharyngitis
GI: nausea, vomiting, diarrhea, constipation, abdominal pain, dyspepsia, gastroesophageal reflux disease, **pseudomembranous colitis**
GU: vaginitis
Hepatic: hepatotoxicity
Respiratory: crackles, cough, dyspnea, wheezing, **respiratory distress**
Skin: rash, **erythema multiforme, Stevens-Johnson syndrome, toxic epidermal necrolysis**
Other: fever, pain, induration, and inflammation at I.V. site; edema; overgrowth of susceptible organisms; hypersensitivity reactions including **anaphylaxis**

Interactions

Drug-drug. *Probenecid:* increased blood level and half-life of ertapenem

Toxicity and overdose

• Overdose may cause increased nausea, diarrhea, and transient dizziness.
• Discontinue drug and provide general supportive therapy until drug is eliminated renally. Although hemodialysis can remove drug, no information is available on its use in treating overdose.

Patient teaching

• Tell patient to notify nurse right away if drug causes pain or swelling at injection site.
• Inform patient that drug can be toxic to many organ systems. Tell patient to report significant adverse reactions right away.
• Advise female patient to inform prescriber of pregnancy or breastfeeding before taking drug.
• Provide reassurance that patient will be closely monitored.
• As appropriate, review all other significant and life-threatening adverse reactions and interactions, especially those related to the drug mentioned above.

erythromycin lactobionate

Erythrocin

Pharmacologic class: Macrolide
Therapeutic class: Anti-infective
Pregnancy risk category B

Action

Binds with 50S subunit of susceptible bacterial ribosomes, suppressing protein synthesis in bacterial cells and causing cell death

Pharmacokinetics

Drug diffuses readily into most body fluids, with tissue levels exceeding serum levels. It crosses placental barrier, but fetal plasma levels are low. In absence of meningeal inflammation, cerebrospinal concentrations are low; in meningitis, drug passage across blood-brain barrier increases. In normal hepatic function, drug concentrates in the liver and is excreted in bile; effect of hepatic dysfunction on excretion by the liver into bile is unknown. Up to 15% of dose is excreted unchanged in urine, with a significant amount excreted in bile and some in breast milk.

Onset	Peak	Duration
Rapid	End of infusion	6-12 hr

How supplied

Powder for reconstitution for injection (lyophilized): 500-mg and 1-g vials

Indication and dosages

➢ Mild to moderate upper and lower respiratory tract infections, skin and skin-structure infections, diphtheria, and erythrasma; prevention of initial and recurrent attacks of rheumatic fever in penicillin-allergic patients

Adults and children: 15 to 20 mg/kg/day I.V. divided into equal doses every 6 hours. Higher dosages (up to 4 g/day) may be given for severe infections.

➢ Acute pelvic inflammatory disease caused by *Neisseria gonorrhoeae* in adult females with penicillin hypersensitivity

Adults (females): 500 mg I.V. q 6 hours for 3 days, followed by oral therapy with erythromycin stearate or base

➢ Legionnaires' disease

Adults: 1 to 4 g I.V. daily in divided doses

Dosage adjustment

• Dosage may need to be reduced in hepatic impairment.

Administration

Preparation

• Know that I.V. therapy should be replaced with oral therapy as soon as possible.

🔊 Be aware that drug has been reported to significantly alter metabolism of terfenadine, astemizole, and cisapride (not available in the United States) when taken concomitantly. Rare cases of serious cardiovascular adverse events (including QT/QTc interval prolongation, cardiac arrest, torsades de pointes, and other ventricular arrhythmias) have occurred. Several deaths have been reported with coadministration of terfenadine and erythromycin.

Dilution and compatibility

• Dilute 500-mg or 1-g vial with 10 mL or 20 mL, respectively, of sterile water for injection only to yield a concentration of 50 mg/mL.

• Before administration, add initial dilution to normal saline solution, lactated Ringer's solution, or Normosol-R solution to yield a concentration of 1 g/L (1 mg/mL) for continuous I.V. infusion or 1 to 5 mg/mL for intermittent infusion.

• Alternatively, dilute with D_5W, D_5W and lactated Ringer's solution, or dextrose 5% in normal saline solution only, after first buffering with 4% sodium bicarbonate to yield alkaline solution.

🔊 Do not use other diluents.

🔊 Do not add other drugs or chemicals.

Infusion considerations

• Administer final diluted solution within 8 hours.

🔊 Do not administer by direct I.V. injection.

• Know that slow, continuous I.V. infusion is preferred. Administer over 6 to 24 hours, as directed.

• For intermittent I.V. infusion, infuse 25% of daily dose in no less than 100 mL diluent slowly over 20 to 60 minutes to minimize pain along vein.

Monitoring

🔊 Assess for hypersensitivity reaction; be prepared to intervene appropriately.

🔊 Monitor liver function test results. Watch for signs and symptoms of hepatotoxicity.

🔊 Monitor for serious arrhythmias, especially in elderly patients.

• Assess patient's hearing for signs and symptoms of ototoxicity. Know that risk of drug-induced hearing loss is higher in reduced renal or hepatic function, high-dose therapy, and elderly patients.

• Check temperature, and watch for signs and symptoms of superinfection.

Storage

• Store vials at controlled room temperature of 15° to 30°C (59° to 86°F).

• If necessary, reconstituted solutions may be stored for 14 days if refrigerated or for 24 hours at room temperature.

Contraindications and precautions

Contraindicated in hypersensitivity to drug and concurrent use of terfenadine or astemizole.

E

Use cautiously in myasthenia gravis, hepatic disease, ***elderly patients,*** and pregnant patients.

Adverse reactions

CV: torsades de pointes, arrhythmias
EENT: ototoxicity
GI: nausea, vomiting, diarrhea, abdominal pain or cramps
Hepatic: hepatic dysfunction, hepatitis
Skin: rash; **erythema multiforme, toxic epidermal necrolysis, Stevens-Johnson syndrome** (rare)
Other: increased appetite, aggravated weakness in myasthenia gravis, superinfection, phlebitis at I.V. site, allergic reactions ranging from urticaria to **anaphylaxis**

Interactions

Drug-drug. *Benzodiazepines (alprazolam, diazepam, midazolam, triazolam):* decreased clearance and increased effects of these drugs
Cyclosporine, tacrolimus: elevated concentrations with increased risk of nephrotoxicity and neurotoxicity
Digoxin: increased digoxin blood level
Drugs metabolized by CYP3A4 system (such as felodipine): several-fold increase in plasma felodipine level, increased felodipine effects
Drugs metabolized by P450 system (alfentanil, astemizole, bromocriptine, buspirone, carbamazepine, disopyramide, hexobarbital, lovastatin, phenytoin, pimozide, terfenadine, valproate): elevated blood levels of these drugs
Ergot alkaloids: increased risk of acute ergot toxicity
Fluoroquinolones such as sparfloxacin: increased risk of life-threatening arrhythmias (including torsades de pointes)
HMG-CoA reductase inhibitors: increased risk of myopathy and rhabdomyolysis
Hormonal contraceptives: decreased contraceptive efficacy
Lincosamides (clindamycin, lincomycin): antagonism of erythromycin's effects
Methylprednisolone: greatly reduced clearance of this drug
Nonsedating antihistamines (astemizole, terfenadine): significantly altered metabolism of these drugs, leading to serious cardiac disorders
Oral anticoagulants: increased anticoagulant effect
Penicillins: antagonism and synergism of erythromycin
Rifabutin, rifampin: decreased erythromycin effects, increased risk of adverse GI reactions
Theophylline: increased theophylline blood level, decreased erythromycin blood level
Vinblastine: increased risk of vinblastine toxicity
Warfarin: increased blood levels of erythromycin and risk of toxicity
Drug-diagnostic tests. *Alanine aminotransferase, alkaline phosphatase, aspartate aminotransferase, bilirubin:* increased
Urine catecholamines: false elevations

Toxicity and overdose

- In overdose, expect extension of pharmacologic actions and adverse reactions.
- Discontinue drug and provide symptomatic and supportive therapy. Dialysis does not remove drug.

Patient teaching

Advise patient to immediately report irregular heartbeats, unusual tiredness, yellowing of skin or eyes, and signs or symptoms of new infection.
- Tell patient about the need for repeated laboratory testing during therapy.
- As appropriate, review all other significant and life-threatening adverse reactions and interactions, especially those related to the drugs and tests mentioned above.

esmolol hydrochloride

Brevibloc

Pharmacologic class: Beta-adrenergic blocker (cardioselective)
Therapeutic class: Antiarrhythmic, antihypertensive
Pregnancy risk category C

Action

Blocks stimulation of beta-adrenergic receptors (primarily $beta_1$ receptors), thereby reducing atrioventricular conduction and cardiac output and decreasing blood pressure

Pharmacokinetics

Drug is metabolized rapidly by hydrolysis of ester linkage primarily in red blood cells. Metabolism is not limited by rate of blood flow to metabolizing tissues or affected by renal or hepatic blood flow. Drug is about 55% bound to plasma proteins. Distribution half-life is rapid (about 2 minutes); elimination half-life is about 9 minutes. One metabolite is excreted in urine, with clearance approximately equivalent to glomerular filtration rate.

Onset	Peak	Duration
Immediate	30 min	30 min after infusion

How supplied

Concentrate for dilution for injection (clear, colorless to slightly yellow): 2,500 mg (250 mg/mL) in 10-mL ampules
Solution for injection (clear, colorless to slightly yellow): 100 mg (10 mg/mL) ready-to-use 10 mL vials
Solution for injection (clear, colorless to slightly yellow): 100 mg (20 mg/mL) double-strength ready-to-use 5 mL-vials
Solution for injection (clear, colorless to slightly yellow): 2,000 mg (20 mg/mL) double-strength in 100 mL ready-to-use bags
Solution for injection (clear, colorless to slightly yellow): 2,500 mg (10 mg/mL) in 250-mL ready-to-use bags

Indications and dosages

➤ Supraventricular tachycardia

Adults: Initially, loading dose of 500 mcg/kg/minute by I.V. infusion over 1 minute, followed by maintenance infusion of 50 mcg/kg/minute over 4 minutes. If desired response does not occur after 5 minutes, repeat loading dose and increase maintenance infusion to 100 mcg/kg/minute for 4 minutes. Repeat sequence as needed, with maintenance dosage increased in increments of 50 mcg/kg/minute, to a maximum maintenance infusion of 200 mcg/kg/minute for 48 hours.

➤ Sinus tachycardia or hypertension

Adults: Initially, 80 mg (1 mg/kg) by I.V. bolus over 30 seconds; then, if needed, 150 mcg/kg/minute by I.V. infusion, to a maximum of 300 mcg/kg/minute

Off-label uses

- Acute myocardial ischemia

Administration

Preparation

Be aware that concentrate (250 mg/mL in 10-mL ampule) has been discontinued due to concerns involving improper dilution and dosage and resultant risk of potentially serious medication errors. Do not confuse or substitute 10-mg/mL strength with 250-mg/mL strength that may still be available in your pharmacy.

Dilution and compatibility

Know that 10-mg/mL and 20 mg/mL strengths are prediluted to provide ready-to-use concentration that may be used for I.V. bolus dose while maintenance infusion is being prepared.

Do not add other drugs or solutions to vials or bags.

• Be aware that loading dose may be withdrawn from medication port of premixed bag. Use remainder of bag within 24 hours.

• Discard unused portion of drug.

• Do not remove overwrap from bag until ready to use.

• Do not use if solution is discolored.

Infusion considerations

• Give at rate prescribed for indicated condition.

• Because large fluid volumes may be needed to infuse drug, use caution when excessive fluids could be harmful.

Be aware that safety of dosages above 300 mcg/kg/minute has not been established.

Do not use plastic containers in series connections. Such use could result in air embolism due to residual air being drawn from primary container before administration of fluid from secondary container ends.

Monitoring

Watch for signs and symptoms of heart failure; withdraw drug at first sign or symptom.

• Monitor vital signs and ECG, particularly for hypotension. Decreasing dosage or terminating infusion usually reverses hypotension within 30 minutes.

• Assess neurologic status; institute safety measures as needed.

• Monitor fluid intake and output, watching for urine retention.

Storage

• Store at controlled room temperature of 15° to 30°C (59° to 86°F). Do not freeze.

Contraindications and precautions

Contraindicated in sinus bradycardia, heart block greater than first degree, cardiogenic shock, and overt heart failure.

Use cautiously in hypotension, renal impairment, hypertension caused mainly by vasoconstriction associated with hypothermia (use not recommended), bronchospastic disease, diabetes mellitus and hypoglycemia, pregnant or breastfeeding patients, and ***children*** (safety and efficacy not established).

Adverse reactions

CNS: anxiety, depression, dizziness, drowsiness, headache, agitation, fatigue, confusion, asthenia
CV: peripheral ischemia, chest pain, bradycardia, hypotension
GI: nausea, vomiting, heartburn
GU: urine retention
Respiratory: wheezing, dyspnea
Skin: flushing, pallor, erythema
Other: altered taste, chills, edema, inflammation or induration at infusion site

Interactions

Drug-drug. *Catecholamine-depleting agents (such as reserpine):* increased bradycardia and hypotension
Digoxin: increased digoxin blood level
Morphine: increased esmolol blood level
Succinylcholine: prolonged neuromuscular blockade
Verapamil: increased risk of cardiac arrest in patients with depressed myocardial function
Drug-herb. *Ephedra (ma huang), St. John's wort, yohimbe:* decreased antihypertensive effect

Toxicity and overdose

• Overdose can cause cardiac arrest, bradycardia, hypotension, electromechanical dissociation, and loss of consciousness. Be aware that dilution errors have led to massive accidental overdoses—some fatal and others causing permanent disability. Bolus doses in range of 625 mg to 2.5 g (12.5 to 50 mg/kg) have been fatal. Patients who survived overdose were those whose circulation could be supported until drug effects resolved.

• Discontinue infusion. Based on clinical effects, expect to give I.V. atropine or another anticholinergic for bradycardia; beta$_2$-stimulating agent and theophylline derivative for bronchospasm; diuretic and cardiac glycoside for cardiac failure; dopamine, dobutamine, isoproterenol, or amrinone for shock; and fluids and pressors for symptomatic hypotension.

Patient teaching

• Inform patient that drug is an emergency measure to control blood pressure, arrhythmias, or heart rate.
• Assure patient he will be monitored closely throughout therapy.
• Tell patient to report pain or redness at I.V. site.
• As appropriate, review all other significant adverse reactions and interactions, especially those related to the drugs and herbs mentioned above.

esomeprazole sodium

Nexium I.V.

Pharmacologic class: Proton pump inhibitor
Therapeutic class: Antiulcer agent
Pregnancy risk category B

Action

Reduces gastric acid production by inhibiting enzyme activity in gastric parietal cells; through its action specifically on proton pump, drug blocks final step in acid production, thereby reducing gastric acidity.

Pharmacokinetics

Drug is extensively metabolized in the liver by P450 (CYP) enzyme system; it is 97% protein-bound. Drug is excreted primarily as metabolites in urine, with some excretion in feces. Less than 1% is excreted as unchanged drug. Plasma elimination half-life is 1.1 to 1.4 hours.

Onset	Peak	Duration
Unknown	Unknown	Unknown

How supplied

Powder for reconstitution for injection: 20 mg and 40 mg in 5-mL single-use vials

Indications and dosages

➢ Short-term treatment of gastroesophageal reflux disease (GERD) in patients with history of erosive esophagitis

Adults: 20 to 40 mg daily by I.V. injection or infusion for up to 10 days

Dosage adjustments

• Do not exceed daily dosage in patients with severe hepatic insufficiency.

Administration

Preparation

• Know that I.V. route is indicated only for short-term treatment of GERD (up to 10 days) in patients with history of erosive esophagitis as alternative to oral therapy when use of delayed-release capsules is not possible or appropriate.
• When oral therapy is possible or appropriate, discontinue I.V. therapy.

Dilution and compatibility

• For direct I.V. injection, reconstitute with 5 mL normal saline solution.

Withdraw 5 mL of reconstituted solution for injection.
- For I.V. infusion, reconstitute one vial with 5 mL normal saline solution, lactated Ringer's solution, or D_5W. Further dilute resulting solution to a final volume of 50 mL before infusing.

Infusion considerations
- Give by direct I.V. injection over no less than 3 minutes.
- Administer by I.V. infusion over 10 to 30 minutes.
- Do not give with other drugs through same I.V. site or tubing.
- Before and after administration, flush I.V. line with normal saline solution, lactated Ringer's solution, or D_5W.

Monitoring
- Monitor neurologic status, especially for dizziness and headache.
- Watch for signs and symptoms of eye, ear, nose, throat, and respiratory infections.
- Assess nutritional and hydration status.

Storage
- Store vials at controlled room temperature of 15° to 30°C (59° to 86°F); protect from light.
- Store solution reconstituted for direct I.V. injection at room temperature up to 30°C (86°F), and administer within 12 hours of reconstitution.
- Store solution reconstituted for I.V. infusion at room temperature up to 30°C (86°F); administer within 12 hours if reconstituted with normal saline solution or lactated Ringer's solution, or within 6 hours if reconstituted with D_5W.

Contraindications and precautions
Contraindicated in hypersensitivity to drug, its components, or substituted benzimidazoles.

Use cautiously in severe hepatic impairment, pregnant or breastfeeding patients, and ***children younger than age 18*** (safety not established).

Adverse reactions
CNS: headache, dizziness
EENT: sinusitis
GI: nausea, abdominal pain, diarrhea, constipation, dyspepsia, flatulence, dry mouth
Respiratory: respiratory tract infection
Skin: pruritus
Other: injection site reaction

Interactions
Drug-drug. *Atazanavir:* reduced atazanavir plasma level
Digoxin, iron salts, ketoconazole: altered absorption and effects of these drugs
Drug-diagnostic tests. *Hemoglobin, platelets, potassium, sodium, thyroxine, white blood cells:* decreased

Toxicity and overdose
- Overdose signs and symptoms (which may be transient and variable) may include confusion, drowsiness, blurred vision, tachycardia, nausea, diaphoresis, flushing, headache, and dry mouth.
- No specific antidote is known. Provide symptomatic and supportive therapy. Dialysis does not remove drug.

Patient teaching
- Caution patient to avoid driving and other hazardous activities until drug's effects on concentration and alertness are known.
- Advise patient to minimize GI upset by eating small, frequent servings of healthy food and drinking plenty of fluids.
- Instruct female patient to inform prescriber if she is pregnant or breastfeeding.
- As appropriate, review all other significant adverse reactions and interactions, especially those related to the drugs and tests mentioned above.

estrogens, conjugated

Premarin Intravenous

Pharmacologic class: Estrogen
Therapeutic class: Replacement hormone, antineoplastic, antiosteoporotic
Pregnancy risk category X

FDA BOXED WARNING

- Drug increases endometrial cancer risk in postmenopausal women.
- Drug may increase risk of cardiovascular disease, breast cancer, and dementia.
- Drug should not be used during pregnancy.
- Warnings may vary somewhat among specific brands. See package insert for complete warning information.

Action

Bind to nuclear receptors in estrogen-responsive tissues (such as female genital organs, breasts, and pituitary gland), enhancing DNA, RNA, and protein synthesis. In androgen-dependent prostate cancer, estrogens compete for androgen receptor sites, inhibiting androgen activity. Also decrease pituitary release of follicle-stimulating hormone and luteinizing hormone.

Pharmacokinetics

Drug distributes widely throughout body, largely bound to sex hormone-binding globulin and albumin. Generally, concentrations are higher in sex-hormone target organs. Estradiol converts reversibly to estrone; both can be converted to estriol (major urinary metabolite). Estrogens also undergo enterohepatic recirculation in the liver, biliary secretion of conjugates into the intestine, and hydrolysis in the gut, followed by reabsorption. Estradiol, estrone, and estriol are excreted in urine along with glucuronide and sulfate conjugates.

Onset	Peak	Duration
Rapid	Unknown	6-12 hr

E

How supplied

Powder for reconstitution for injection (lyophilized cake): 25-mg ampules

Indications and dosages

➢ Uterine bleeding caused by hormonal imbalance in absence of organic disease
Adults: 25 mg I.V., repeated in 6 to 12 hours if necessary

Off-label uses

- Bleeding diathesis in platelet-refractory patients

Administration

Preparation

Follow hazardous drug guidelines on page S19 for handling, preparation, and administration.

- Be aware that drug is indicated for short-term use only, to produce rapid and temporary rise in estrogen levels.

Dilution and compatibility

- Know that drug is supplied with one 5-mL ampule of sterile diluent with 2% benzyl alcohol in sterile water.
- To reconstitute, flow sterile diluent slowly against side of vial, and agitate gently. Do not shake violently.
- Know that drug is compatible with D_5W, normal saline solution, and invert sugar solution, but not with acid solutions.
- Use reconstituted solution within a few hours or refrigerate for 60 days. Do not use stored solution if darkening or precipitation occurs.

Infusion considerations
- Inject slowly to prevent flushing.
- Do not give with other drugs or solutions. However, for expediency in emergencies, if infusion has already begun, drug may be injected into tubing just distal to infusion needle. (Be sure to consider solution compatibility.)

Monitoring

Know that drug increases risk of thromboembolism, cerebrovascular accident (CVA), and myocardial infarction (MI).

Closely monitor diagnostic tests, including endometrial sampling when indicated, to rule out cancer in all cases of undiagnosed persistent or recurring abnormal vaginal bleeding.

- Evaluate patient for breast tenderness and swelling. As needed, give analgesics and apply cool compresses.
- Monitor fluid intake and output, and weigh patient daily.
- Closely monitor liver function tests and serum calcium and glucose levels.

Storage
- Before reconstitution, refrigerate at 2° to 8°C (36° to 46°F).
- Refrigerate reconstituted solution at 2° to 8°C (36° to 46°F) for 60 days.

Contraindications and precautions

Contraindicated in hypersensitivity to drug or its components, thromboembolic disease (current or previous), undiagnosed vaginal bleeding, breast cancer, estrogen-dependent neoplasms, hepatic dysfunction or disease, and pregnancy.

Use cautiously in cardiovascular disease, severe hepatic or renal disease, asthma, bone disease, migraine, seizures, breast disease, family history of breast or genital tract cancer, and breastfeeding patients.

Adverse reactions

CNS: headache, migraine, dizziness, depression, chorea, nervousness, dementia, **exacerbation of epilepsy, CVA**

CV: hypertension, chest pain, thrombophlebitis, **MI, thromboembolism**

EENT: contact lens intolerance, worsening of myopia or astigmatism, retinal vascular thrombosis, otitis media, sinusitis, rhinitis, pharyngitis

GI: nausea, vomiting, diarrhea, abdominal cramps, bloating, enlarged abdomen, dyspepsia, flatulence, gastritis, gastroenteritis, hemorrhoids, colitis, gallbladder disease, cholestatic jaundice, anorexia, **pancreatitis**

GU: urinary incontinence; dysuria; urinary tract infection; amenorrhea; dysmenorrhea; breakthrough bleeding; endometrial hyperplasia; vaginal candidiasis; change in degree of cervical secretion; genital eruptions; breast pain, tenderness, or enlargement; libido changes; **increased risk of breast cancer, ovarian cancer, and endometrial cancer; hemolytic uremic syndrome**

Hepatic: hepatic adenoma

Metabolic: hyperglycemia, hypercalcemia, sodium and fluid retention, reduced carbohydrate tolerance

Musculoskeletal: leg cramps, back pain, skeletal pain

Respiratory: upper respiratory tract infection, bronchitis, **asthma exacerbation, pulmonary embolism**

Skin: acne, oily skin, pigmentation changes (chloasma, melasma), rash, urticaria, pruritus, erythema nodosum, hemorrhagic eruption, skin hypertrophy, hirsutism, scalp hair loss, **erythema multiforme**

Other: edema; weight changes; increased appetite; porphyria exacerbation; injection site pain, edema, and phlebitis; hypersensitivity reactions including anaphylactoid reactions, **angioedema,** and **anaphylaxis**

Interactions

Drug-drug. *Corticosteroids:* enhanced corticosteroid effects
CYP450 inducers (such as barbiturates, carbamazepine, rifampin): possible decreased estrogen efficacy
CYP450 inhibitors (clarithromycin, erythromycin, itraconazole, ketoconazole, ritonavir): possible increased estrogen levels
Hypoglycemics, warfarin: altered requirements for these drugs
Phenytoin: loss of seizure control
Tamoxifen: interference with tamoxifen effects
Tricyclic antidepressants: reduced antidepressant effects
Drug-diagnostic tests. *Antithrombin III, folate, low-density lipoproteins, pyridoxine, total cholesterol, urine pregnanediol:* decreased
Cortisol; factors VII, VIII, IX, and X; glucose; high-density lipoproteins; phospholipids; prolactin; prothrombin; sodium; triglycerides: increased
Metyrapone test: false decrease
Thyroid function tests: false interpretation
Drug-food. *Caffeine:* increased blood caffeine level
Grapefruit juice: possible increased plasma estrogen levels
Drug-herb. *Black cohosh:* increased risk of adverse reactions
Red clover: interference with estrogen effects
Saw palmetto: antiestrogenic effects
St. John's wort: possible decreased drug blood level and effects
Drug-behaviors. *Smoking:* increased risk of adverse cardiovascular reactions

Toxicity and overdose

- Overdose may cause nausea and vomiting.
- Provide symptomatic and supportive therapy.

Patient teaching

Teach patient to recognize and immediately report signs and symptoms of thromboembolism.

Caution patient not to take drug if she is pregnant or plans to become pregnant.

- Advise patient to inform prescriber if she is breastfeeding, because estrogen passes into breast milk.
- As appropriate, review all other significant and life-threatening adverse reactions and interactions, especially those related to the drugs, tests, foods, herbs, and behaviors mentioned above.

etomidate

Amidate

Pharmacologic class: Nonbarbiturate hypnotic
Therapeutic class: General anesthetic
Pregnancy risk category C

Action

Reduces subcortical inhibition at hypnosis onset while inducing neocortical sleep; causes minimal cardiovascular effects. Reduces cerebral blood flow and cerebral oxygen consumption while maintaining perfusion pressure; slightly lowers intracranial and intraocular pressure.

Pharmacokinetics

Drug is metabolized rapidly in the liver; protein binding (primarily to albumin) is approximately 76%. Half-life is about 75 minutes. Approximately 75% of dose is excreted in urine, primarily as metabolite; small amounts are secreted in breast milk.

Onset	Peak	Duration
Rapid	1 min	3-5 min

How supplied

Solution for injection (clear): 20 mg (2 mg/mL) in 10-mL single-dose vials

Indications and dosages

➤ Induction of general anesthesia

Adults and children older than age 10: Dosage individualized; 0.2 to 0.6 mg/kg I.V. over 30 to 60 seconds

Dosage adjustment

- During short operative procedures, smaller increments may be given to adults to supplement subpotent anesthetics.
- Elderly patients may require lower dosages.

Off-label uses

- Sedation for diagnosis of seizure foci

Administration

Preparation

Do not confuse drug with etidronate.

Give drug under direct supervision of personnel trained in administering general anesthetics and managing complications, in facility with adequate emergency equipment.

- Know that lidocaine preadministration may be considered to reduce vein irritation.
- Be aware that patient may require I.V. opioid or benzodiazepine to reduce involuntary muscle movements.
- Know that exogenous corticosteroid replacement may be considered for patients undergoing severe stress, because etomidate can reduce plasma cortisol and aldosterone levels.

Dilution and compatibility

- Know that drug is compatible with alfentanil, atracurium, atropine, doxacurium, ephedrine, fentanyl, lidocaine, lorazepam, midazolam, mivacurium, morphine, pancuronium, phenylephrine, succinylcholine, and sufentanil.
- Be aware that drug is incompatible with ascorbic acid and vecuronium.
- Drug may be given undiluted. Discard unused portion.
- Do not use unless solution is clear.

Infusion considerations

- Be aware that drug is highly irritating. Avoid administration into small veins.
- Administer I.V. push over 30 to 60 seconds.

Be aware that too-rapid administration may cause hypotension.

Monitoring

Perform close cardiac monitoring and measure blood pressure frequently.

Assess laboratory test results, therapeutic effect, and adverse effects—particularly for signs of adrenal insufficiency (including hypotension, hyperkalemia).

Monitor respiratory status, including pulse oximetry.

- Monitor infusion site closely for potential vein irritation.

Storage

- Store at controlled room temperature of 15° to 30°C (59° to 86°F).

Contraindications and precautions

Contraindicated in hypersensitivity to drug or its components.

Use cautiously in ***elderly patients,*** during labor and delivery, pregnant or breastfeeding patients, and ***children younger than age 10*** (safety and efficacy not established).

Adverse reactions

CV: transient venous pain, tachycardia, hypertension, **hypotension, bradycardia, arrhythmias**
EENT: uncontrolled eye movements, **laryngospasm**
GI: nausea, vomiting
Metabolic: adrenal suppression
Musculoskeletal: transient skeletal muscle movements (myoclonic), tonic movements
Respiratory: hyperventilation, hypoventilation, **apnea** (transient)
Other: hiccups, injection site pain

Interactions

Drug-drug. *Fentanyl:* decreased etomidate elimination
Verapamil: increased etomidate effects, leading to prolonged respiratory depression and apnea

Toxicity and overdose

- Overdose may result from too-rapid or repeated injections (which may cause hypotension). No other cardiovascular or respiratory effects have been reported.
- Discontinue drug. Provide supportive therapy, including oxygen, ventilation, and resuscitation, as indicated and ordered.

Patient teaching

- Instruct patient to avoid alcohol and other CNS depressants for at least 24 hours before anesthesia induction.
- Advise patient not to drive or engage in other hazardous activities for 24 hours after anesthesia.
- As appropriate, review all other significant and life-threatening adverse reactions and interactions, especially those related to the drugs mentioned above.

etoposide (VP-16-213)

Eposin, VePesid

etoposide phosphate

Etopophos

Pharmacologic class: Podophyllotoxin derivative
Therapeutic class: Antineoplastic
Pregnancy risk category D

E

FDA BOXED WARNING

- Give under supervision of physician experienced in cancer chemotherapy. Severe myelosuppression may occur, resulting in infection or bleeding.

Action

Damages DNA before mitosis by inhibiting topoisomerase II enzyme. This action impairs DNA synthesis and inhibits selected cancer cell growth. Cell-cycle-phase specific.

Pharmacokinetics

Drug does not accumulate in plasma with daily administration. Distribution half-life is about 1.5 hours; terminal elimination half-life ranges from 4 to 11 hours. Cerebrospinal fluid penetration is poor. Drug is metabolized in the liver and is extensively protein-bound. It is excreted unchanged in urine (less than 50% of dose) and bile (about 6% of parent drug).

Onset	Peak	Duration
7-14 days	9-16 days	20 days

How supplied

Solution for injection (clear, nearly colorless to yellow): 20 mg/mL in 5-, 10-, 12.5-, and 25-mL vials

Solution for injection (phosphate): 100 mg in single-dose vials

Indications and dosages

➤ Refractory testicular tumors (in combination with other approved chemotherapeutic agents) in patients who have received appropriate surgical, chemotherapeutic, and radiotherapeutic therapy
Adults: Dosage ranges from 50 to 100 mg/m^2 I.V. daily (etoposide or equivalent doses of etoposide phosphate) on days 1 through 5, to 100 mg/m^2 I.V. daily on days 1, 3, and 5. Repeat course at 2- to 4-week intervals after recovery from toxicity.

➤ Small-cell lung cancer as first-line treatment (in combination with other approved chemotherapeutic agents)
Adults: Dosage ranges from 35 mg/m^2 I.V. daily for 4 days (etoposide or equivalent dose of etoposide phosphate) to a maximum of 50 mg/m^2 I.V. daily for 5 days q 3 to 4 weeks.

Dosage adjustment

- Modify dosage if patient is receiving other myelosuppressive drugs or has received previous radiation therapy or chemotherapy.
- Withhold therapy if platelet count drops below 50,000/mm^3 or absolute neutrophil count drops below 500/mm^3.
- In renal impairment, base initial dosage adjustment on creatinine clearance. For creatinine clearance of 15 to 50 mL/minute, give 75% of recommended dosage. Base subsequent dosages on tolerance and clinical effect. Consider further dosage reduction in creatinine clearance below 15 mL/minute.
- Administer 50% of normal dosage if bilirubin level is one to two times upper limit of normal (ULN); if level is two to four times ULN, reduce dosage to 25%; if level is above four times ULN, discontinue drug.

Off-label uses

- Acute myelocytic leukemia
- Advanced neuroblastoma
- AIDS-related Kaposi's sarcoma
- Carcinoma of unknown primary site
- Ewing's sarcoma
- Hodgkin's lymphoma
- Non-small-cell lung carcinoma
- Osteosarcoma and soft-tissue sarcoma (in combination with ifosfamide and platinum)

Administration

Preparation

Follow hazardous drug guidelines on page S19 for handling, preparation, and administration.

- Administer with antiemetics, as prescribed.

Dilution and compatibility

- For etoposide, dilute each 100-mg (5-mL) dose in 250 to 500 mL D_5W or normal saline solution to yield a final concentration of 0.2 to 0.4 mg/mL, respectively.
- For etoposide phosphate, dilute 100-mg vial with 5 to 10 mL D_5W, normal saline solution, sterile bacteriostatic water for injection with benzyl alcohol, or bacteriostatic sodium chloride with benzyl alcohol, to yield 20 mg/mL or 10 mg/mL, respectively. May give without further dilution; or further dilute with D_5W or normal saline solution to a concentration of 0.1 mg/mL.

Be aware that precipitation may occur in solutions with concentrations above 0.4 mg/mL.

Infusion considerations

- Administer etoposide by slow I.V. infusion over 30 to 60 minutes.
- Give etoposide phosphate by I.V. infusion over 5 to 210 minutes.
- Do not use inline filter.

Avoid rapid infusion, which may cause severe hypotension and bronchospasm.
During infusion, monitor closely for precipitates in solution.

Monitoring

Monitor blood pressure during and after infusion. Stop infusion if severe hypotension occurs.
- Monitor infusion rate closely to prevent infusion reactions.
- Throughout infusion, check I.V. site for extravasation, which may cause thrombophlebitis.

Keep diphenhydramine, hydrocortisone, epinephrine, and artificial airway at hand in case anaphylaxis occurs.
- Assess for CNS adverse effects. Assist patient during ambulation as needed.

Monitor for signs and symptoms of bone marrow depression.
- Monitor CBC, liver function test results, and blood urea nitrogen and creatinine levels. Report platelet count below 50,000/mm^3 or neutrophil count below 500/mm^3.

Storage
- Know that unopened etoposide vials can be stored for up to 2 years at room temperature of 25°C (77°F). Solutions diluted to 0.2 to 0.4 mg/mL are stable for 96 and 48 hours, respectively, at room temperature under normal room fluorescent light, in both glass and plastic containers.
- Refrigerate unopened etoposide phosphate vials at 2° to 8°C (36° to 46°F) in original package. When reconstituted as directed, solutions can be refrigerated in glass or plastic containers at 2° to 8°C for 7 days. Store at controlled room temperature of 20° to 25°C (68° to 77°F) for 24 hours after reconstitution with D_5W, normal saline solution injection, or sterile water for injection. Store at controlled room temperature of 20° to 25°C for 48 hours after reconstitution with bacteriostatic water for injection with benzyl alcohol or bacteriostatic sodium chloride for injection with benzyl alcohol. When further diluted as directed, solutions can be refrigerated at 2° to 8°C for 24 hours.

Contraindications and precautions

Contraindicated in hypersensitivity to drug or its components.

Use cautiously in active infections, low serum albumin level, decreased bone marrow reserve, renal or hepatic impairment, pregnant patients and patients with childbearing potential, breastfeeding patients, and ***children*** (safety and efficacy not established).

Adverse reactions

CNS: drowsiness, fatigue, headache, vertigo, peripheral neuropathy
CV: hypotension, heart failure, myocardial infarction
GI: nausea, vomiting, anorexia, diarrhea, stomatitis
GU: sterility
Hematologic: anemia, **leukopenia, thrombocytopenia, bone marrow depression**
Hepatic: hepatotoxicity
Metabolic: hyperuricemia
Musculoskeletal: muscle cramps
Respiratory: pulmonary edema, bronchospasm
Skin: alopecia
Other: fever, phlebitis at I.V. site, allergic reactions including **anaphylaxis**

Interactions

Drug-drug. *Live-virus vaccines:* increased risk of adverse reactions
Other antineoplastics: additive bone marrow depression
Drug-diagnostic tests. *Hemoglobin, neutrophils, platelets, red blood cells, while blood cells:* decreased
Uric acid: increased

Toxicity and overdose

- In overdose, expect extension of pharmacologic and adverse effects, including neurotoxicity, hepatotoxicity, and hematologic and respiratory changes.
- No proven antidote is known. Provide symptomatic and supportive therapy.

Patient teaching

- Instruct patient to inspect mouth daily for ulcers and bleeding gums.
- Tell patient to immediately report difficulty breathing or signs and symptoms of allergic reaction.
- Instruct patient to move slowly when sitting up or standing, to avoid lightheadedness or dizziness from sudden blood pressure decrease.
- Inform patient that drug may cause hair loss.
- Caution female of childbearing age to avoid pregnancy and breastfeeding during drug therapy.
- As appropriate, review all other significant and life-threatening adverse reactions and interactions, especially those related to the drugs and tests mentioned above.

[redacted]

factor IX (human)

AlphaNine SD, Mononine

factor IX (recombinant)

BeneFix

factor IX complex (human)

Bebulin VH, Defix, Hipfix, Profilnine SD, Proplex T (heat-treated), Replenine

Pharmacologic class: Blood modifier
Therapeutic class: Antihemophilic
Pregnancy risk category C

Action

Converts fibrinogen to fibrin, increasing levels of clotting factors; increases factor IX plasma levels, reducing the risk of hemorrhage in patients with factor IX deficiency

Pharmacokinetics

In factor IX-deficient patients, mean half-life is approximately 22 hours (range, 11 to 36 hours). After I.V. infusion, mean increase in circulating factor IX activity is 0.67 to 1.15 units/dL per units/kg body weight.

Onset	Peak	Duration
Immediate	Unknown	Unknown

How supplied

Powder for reconstitution for injection: Various strengths; units specified on label

Indications and dosages

Note: Dosage and duration of therapy for all factor IX products depend on severity of factor IX deficiency, location and extent of bleeding, and patient's clinical condition, age, and recovery of factor IX. Titrate dosage using factor IX activity and pharmacokinetic parameters, such as half-life and recovery; also consider clinical situation when adjusting dosage, as appropriate.

➤ Factor IX deficiency (hemophilia B or Christmas disease), anticoagulant overdose

Adults and children: Dosage individualized according to patient's condition and desired blood level percentage. The dosage range is 10 to 75 IU/kg of body weight. Use the following equations to calculate approximate number of units needed: *Human product:* unit/kg × body weight (in kg) × desired increase in factor IX level, expressed as a percentage of normal

Recombinant product: 1.2 units/kg × body weight (in kg) × desired increase in factor IX level, expressed as percentage of normal
Proplex T: 0.5 unit/kg × body weight (in kg) × desired increase in factor IX level, expressed as a percentage of normal

Off-label uses

- Hepatic dysfunction
- Unspecified GI hemorrhage (human product)

Administration

Preparation

- Know that dosage is highly individualized based on degree of factor IX deficiency, patient weight, and bleeding severity.
- Administer hepatitis B vaccine before giving factor IX, if prescribed.

Dilution and compatibility

- Warm drug to room temperature before reconstitution.
- Do not use glass syringe; use plastic syringe, to avoid binding to glass surfaces.
- Use diluent provided with drug; direct stream to side of vial to gently moisten all contents.
- Do not shake reconstituted solution. Swirl gently for a few minutes to mix; avoid foaming.
- Be aware that resulting solution should be clear and colorless.
- Do not mix with other I.V. solutions.
- Use within 3 hours of reconstitution.

Infusion considerations

- Base infusion rate on patient's condition.
- Administer by slow I.V. infusion. Average infusion rate is 2 to 3 mL/minute; do not exceed 10 mL/minute.
- Reduce infusion rate if patient develops adverse effects, such as transient fever, chills, urticaria, flushing, headache, blood pressure or pulse rate changes, nausea and vomiting, tingling, or burning or pain at injection site.

Monitoring

- Be aware that factor IX complex may transmit hepatitis.
- Closely monitor vital signs during infusion.

Observe for hemolytic reaction. If it occurs, stop infusion, flush I.V. line with saline solution, and notify prescriber immediately.

- Monitor I.V. injection site closely.

Monitor coagulation studies closely. Be aware that drug may cause thromboembolic disorders, including myocardial infarction (MI) and disseminated intravascular coagulation (DIC).

- Monitor factor IX assays to ensure that desired factor IX activity level has been achieved.

Storage

- Refrigerate at 2° to 8°C (36° to 46°F). Do not freeze diluent.

Contraindications and precautions

Contraindicated in hypersensitivity to mouse protein (human product) or hamster protein (recombinant product) and in fibrinolysis.

Use cautiously in hepatic disease, recent surgery, patients at risk for thromboembolic phenomena or DIC, pregnant patients, and ***children younger than age 6*** (safety and efficacy not established).

Adverse reactions

CNS: light-headedness, paresthesia, headache
CV: blood pressure changes, **thromboembolic reactions, MI**
EENT: allergic rhinitis
GI: nausea, vomiting
GU: nephrotic syndrome
Hematologic: DIC
Respiratory: dry cough, **pulmonary embolism**

F

Skin: rash, flushing, diaphoresis, pruritus, urticaria
Other: sneezing, altered taste, fever, chills, burning sensation in jaw and skull, pain at I.V. injection site, hypersensitivity reactions including **anaphylaxis**

Interactions

Drug-drug. *Aminocaproic acid:* increased risk of thrombosis

Toxicity and overdose

- In overdose, expect extension of adverse reactions, including DIC.
- Discontinue drug. Provide prompt supportive therapy, as appropriate.

Patient teaching

- Inform patient that drug may transmit diseases.
- Instruct patient to immediately report signs and symptoms of hypersensitivity reaction, including rash, hives, tightness in chest, wheezing, shortness of breath, and swelling of throat or lips.
- Advise patient to immediately report unusual bleeding or bruising.
- Caution patient to avoid activities that can cause injury.
- Tell patient to wear medical identification that lists blood-clotting disorder.
- Instruct patient to notify surgeon or dentist of blood-clotting disorder before surgery or invasive dental procedure.
- As appropriate, review all other significant and life-threatening adverse reactions and interactions, especially those related to the drug mentioned above.

famotidine

Pepcid injection

Pharmacologic class: Histamine$_2$-receptor antagonist
Therapeutic class: Antiulcer drug
Pregnancy risk category B

Action

Blocks action of histamine at histamine$_2$-receptor sites in gastric parietal cells, inhibiting concentration and volume of gastric acid secretion and stabilizing pepsin

Pharmacokinetics

Drug distributes widely to body tissues and is partially metabolized in the liver. In severe renal insufficiency, elimination half-life may exceed 20 hours. Drug is excreted in urine mostly unchanged, with remainder excreted as metabolites.

Onset	Peak	Duration
Rapid	0.5 hr	10-12 hr

How supplied

Solution for injection (clear, colorless): 10 mg/mL in 1-mL and 2-mL single-dose vials; 10 mg/mL in 4-mL, 20-mL, and 50-mL multidose vials; 20 mg/50 mL premixed in single-dose containers

Indications and dosages

➣ Hospitalized patients with pathologic hypersecretory conditions or intractable ulcers; patients unable to take oral drugs
Adults: 20 mg I.V. q 12 hours
➣ Gastroesophageal reflux disease (GERD)
Children ages 1 to 16: 0.25 mg/kg I.V. q 12 hours, up to 40 mg/day

Dosage adjustment
- In moderate or severe renal insufficiency, reduce dosage 50% or increase dosing interval to 36 to 48 hours, as indicated.

Administration

Preparation
- Be aware that drug may be given I.V. until oral therapy can begin.

Dilution and compatibility
- Be aware that multidose-vial solution contains benzyl alcohol 0.9%.
- Know that commonly used I.V. solutions for dilution are D_5W, dextrose 10% in water, normal saline solution, sterile water for injection, lactated Ringer's solution, and 5% sodium bicarbonate. However, precipitate may form if mixed with sodium bicarbonate in famotidine concentrations above 0.2 mg/mL.
- For direct injection, dilute 2-mL vial (solution containing 10 mg/mL) with 10 mL D_5W, normal saline solution, or other compatible solution to a total volume of either 5 mL or 10 mL.
- For I.V. piggyback administration, dilute 2-mL vial with 100 mL D_5W or other compatible solution.
- Know that drug also comes as isomotic solution (20 mg in 50 mL diluent) premixed with normal saline solution for I.V. piggyback administration.
- Do not add other drugs to premixed solution.
- Do not use unless solution is clear.
- Use immediately after dilution.

Infusion considerations
- Give I.V. push dose over 2 minutes.
- Administer intermittent dose by I.V. piggyback infusion over 30 minutes.
- In children receiving drug for GERD, give by I.V. push over not less than 2 minutes, or as 15-minute I.V. infusion.

Do not use plastic containers in series connections. Such use could result in air embolism due to residual air being drawn from primary container before administration of fluid from the secondary container ends.

Monitoring
- Monitor for transient irritation at I.V. site.
- Assess patient for GI signs and symptoms.
- Monitor blood urea nitrogen and creatinine levels in patients with renal impairment.

Storage
- If drug is not used immediately after dilution, refrigerate and use within 48 hours.
- Store nonpremixed vials at 2° to 8°C (36° to 46°F).
- Store premixed containers at controlled room temperature of 25°C (77°F).

Contraindications and precautions

Contraindicated in hypersensitivity to drug or other histamine$_2$-receptor antagonists.

Use cautiously in renal impairment, ***elderly patients,*** pregnant or breast-feeding patients, and ***children younger than age 1*** (safety and efficacy not established).

Adverse reactions

CNS: dizziness, headache, paresthesia, asthenia
CV: palpitations
GI: nausea, diarrhea, constipation, dry mouth, anorexia
EENT: orbital edema, conjunctival redness, tinnitus
Musculoskeletal: musculoskeletal pain
Skin: flushing, acne, dry skin
Other: altered taste, fever, pain at injection site, **hypersensitivity reactions**

F

Interactions

Drug-herb. *Yerba maté:* decreased famotidine clearance

Toxicity and overdose

- In overdose, expect extension of adverse reactions.
- Discontinue drug and provide supportive therapy. Hemodialysis does not remove drug.

Patient teaching

- Tell female patient to inform prescriber if she is pregnant or breastfeeding.
- As appropriate, review all other significant and life-threatening adverse reactions and interactions, especially those related to the herb mentioned above.

fat emulsions

Pharmacologic class: Parenteral lipids
Therapeutic class: Nutritional caloric agents, fatty acids
Pregnancy risk category C

Action

Increase plasma triglyceride levels and convert triglycerides to free fatty acids; increase oxygen consumption and heat production and serve as caloric source

Pharmacokinetics

Drug distributes through plasma compartments and is metabolized to energy source. Free fatty acids enter tissues or circulate in plasma bound to albumin. Fat particles may clear from plasma in manner similar to that of chylomicrons.

Onset	Peak	Duration
Rapid	Immediate	Unknown

How supplied

Solution for injection (white to slightly off-white): 50 mL (10%, 20%), 100 mL (10%, 20%), 200 mL (10%, 20%), 250 mL (10%, 20%), 500 mL (10%, 20%, 30%)

Indications and dosages

➤ Prevention of fatty acid deficiency

Adults: 500 mL (10% of total caloric intake) I.V. twice weekly, initially infused at 1 mL/minute for 30 minutes, not to exceed 500 mL over 4 to 6 hours

➤ Treatment of fatty acid deficiency

Adults and children: 8% to 10% of total caloric intake I.V.

➤ Adjunct to total parenteral nutrition (TPN)

Adults: 1 mL/minute I.V. for 15 to 30 minutes (10% emulsion), or 0.5 mL/minute I.V. for 15 to 30 minutes (20% emulsion), or equivalent of 0.1 g fat/minute for 15 to 30 minutes (30% emulsion). If no adverse effects occur, increase rate to 2 mL/minute, not to exceed 2.5 g/kg/day (10% emulsion) or 3 g/kg/day (20% emulsion); or increase infusion rate to equivalent of 0.2 g fat/minute with daily dosage not to exceed 2.5 g/kg/day (30% emulsion).
Children: 0.1 mL/minute I.V. for 10 to 15 minutes (10% emulsion), or 0.05 mL/minute I.V. for 10 to 15 minutes (20% emulsion), or 0.01 g fat/minute for 15 to 30 minutes (30% emulsion). If no adverse effects occur, increase rate to 1 g/kg over 4 hours (10% and 20% emulsion) or to 0.1 g/kg/hour (30% emulsion), not to exceed 3 g/kg/day. Fat emulsion provides up to 60% of daily caloric intake; protein-carbohydrate TPN should supply remaining 40%.

Administration

Preparation

Ask patient about allergy to eggs before starting therapy. If patient is allergic, withhold dose.

• Before giving emulsion, add 1 to 2 mL heparin to activate lipoprotein lipase.

Dilution and compatibility

• Know that drug is usually given as prepared by manufacturer.

• Do not mix other drugs or additives directly into fat emulsion solution or I.V. tubing (except low-dose heparin, if prescribed).

Do not use if "oiling out" (yellow droplets or streaking) of emulsion occurs.

Infusion considerations

• Be aware that lipid-containing fluids may extract phthalates from phthalate-plasticized polyvinyl chloride product. Use nonphthalate infusion set provided with drug, when available.

• Infuse at prescribed rate using administration pump.

• Do not use inline filter (drug particles are bigger than filter).

• Drug may be piggybacked into TPN infusion proximal to infusion site but past filter.

• Hang drug higher than TPN bag to prevent backup into bag.

• Change I.V. tubing with each new bottle to prevent bacterial growth.

• Discard remainder of partial doses.

Monitoring

Observe closely for serious adverse reactions, including hypersensitivity reaction and respiratory distress, during first few hours of infusion.

Assess for hepatomegaly and splenomegaly. Report positive findings.

• Monitor CBC, lipid and hepatic profile, coagulation studies, and electrolyte and glucose levels.

• Monitor fluid intake and output; assess for fluid overload (caused by osmotic pull of fat emulsion).

• Monitor I.V. site closely for infiltration.

• Change site as needed.

Storage

• Store at room temperature no higher than 25°C (77°F), or refrigerate.

Contraindications and precautions

Contraindicated in hypersensitivity to drug, allergy to eggs, acute pancreatitis accompanied by hyperlipidemia, pathologic hyperlipidemia, and lipid nephrosis.

Use cautiously in renal impairment, severe hepatic impairment, pulmonary disease, anemia, blood coagulation disorders, pregnant patients, and ***premature infants.***

F

Adverse reactions

GI: splenomegaly (with prolonged use)
Hematologic: hypercoagulability, leukocytosis, thrombocytopenia, leukopenia (with prolonged use)
Hepatic: jaundice, **hepatomegaly** (with prolonged use)
Metabolic: metabolic acidosis
Respiratory: reduced pulmonary diffusion capacity, **pulmonary edema**
Other: flushing, injection site reactions, overloading syndrome with prolonged use (causing **focal seizures, fever, leukocytosis, splenomegaly, shock), sepsis, hypersensitivity reaction**

Interactions

Drug-diagnostic tests. *Bilirubin, hepatic enzymes, lipids:* increased
Liver function tests: abnormal results
Platelets, white blood cells: decreased

Toxicity and overdose

• Signs and symptoms of overloading syndrome include focal seizures, fever, leukocytosis, splenomegaly, and shock.

• Discontinue infusion. Obtain blood for analysis of triglyceride levels, and measurement of light-scattering activity that confirms lipid clearance. Provide supportive therapy, as appropriate.

Patient teaching

• Instruct patient to report shortness of breath or injection site reaction.

• Tell female patient to inform prescriber if she is pregnant.
• As appropriate, review all other significant and life-threatening adverse reactions and interactions, especially those related to the tests mentioned above.

fentanyl citrate
Sublimaze

Pharmacologic class: Opioid agonist
Therapeutic class: Opioid analgesic, anesthesia adjunct
Controlled substance schedule II
Pregnancy risk category C

Action
Binds to specific opioid receptors in CNS, inhibiting pain pathways, altering pain perception, and increasing the pain threshold

Pharmacokinetics
Redistribution may be main reason for drug's brief effect. Drug is metabolized in the liver and excreted in urine unchanged and as metabolites. Elimination half-life is about 3.5 hours.

Onset	Peak	Duration
Immediate	3-5 min	0.5-1 hr

How supplied
Solution for injection (clear, colorless): 0.05 mg/mL in 2-, 5-, 10- and 20-mL ampules and 30- and 50-mL single-dose vials

Indications and dosages
➢ General anesthesia for open-heart surgery and other major surgical procedures (to protect myocardium from excess oxygen demand) and for complicated neurologic and orthopedic procedures
Adults: Dosage individualized; 50 to 100 mcg/kg with oxygen and muscle relaxant when reducing response to surgical stress is crucial. Some patients may require up to 150 mcg/kg.
➢ Adjunct to general anesthesia
Adults: Individualized *total low dosage,* 2 mcg/kg I.V. in small doses for minor, painful surgical procedures and postoperative pain relief. Maintenance dosage—2 mcg/kg I.V. Additional doses occasionally are needed in minor procedures.
Adults: Individualized *total moderate dosage,* 2 to 20 mcg/kg I.V. Maintenance dosage—2 to 20 mcg/kg I.V. Give 25 to 100 mcg I.V. when movement, vital sign changes, or both indicate surgical stress or lightening of analgesia.
Adults: Individualized *total high dosage,* 20 to 50 mcg/kg I.V. for "stress-free" anesthesia. Used during open-heart surgery and complicated neurosurgical and orthopedic procedures where surgery is prolonged and stress response is detrimental (in conjunction with nitrous oxide/oxygen to reduce stress response), and when postoperative ventilation and observation are ensured. Maintenance dosage—20 to 50 mcg/kg I.V., ranging from 25 mcg to 50% of initial loading dosage, administered when vital signs indicate surgical stress and lightening of analgesia.
➢ Short-term analgesia during anesthesia and immediate preoperative and postoperative periods
Adults: Individualized; maintenance dosage during surgery is 0.025 to 0.1 mg I.V.
Children ages 2 to 12: 2 to 3 mcg/kg I.V., depending on vital signs

➢ Adjunct to regional anesthesia
Adults: Individualized dosage; 0.05 to 0.1 mg (50 to 100 mcg) slow I.V. over 1 to 2 minutes

Dosage adjustment
• Be aware that elderly and debilitated patients may need lower initial dosages.

Administration
Preparation
Have opioid antagonist (naloxone) and emergency equipment available before giving drug; know that drug should be administered only by personnel specially trained in use of I.V. anesthetics and managing complications.
• To determine dosage, consider such factors as patient age, weight, physical status, underlying pathologic conditions, use of other drugs, type of anesthesia, and surgical procedure involved.
• Be aware that drug is not recommended to control mild or intermittent pain.
• Know that when drug is used for general anesthesia, oxygen and a muscle relaxant must be given.
Dilution and compatibility
• Be aware that small volumes may be given undiluted by anesthesiologist.
• Know that drug may be diluted in 5 mL of a commonly used solution for injection, such as normal saline solution or sterile water for injection.
• Use immediately after dilution.
Infusion considerations
• Inject I.V. dose slowly over 3 to 5 minutes; titrate dosage to patient's response.
Be aware that rapid administration may cause severe respiratory distress, including apnea.
• Monitor vital signs continuously.
Monitoring
Assess for muscle rigidity in patients receiving high doses; discuss need for neuromuscular blockers with prescriber. Patient will need ventilator if blocker is given.
• Monitor respiratory and cardiovascular function and urine output.
• If patient develops fever, assess for signs and symptoms of opioid toxicity (more drug is absorbed at higher body temperatures).
• Carefully monitor hematologic studies and hepatic enzyme levels.
Storage
• Store at room temperature, protected from light.

F

Contraindications and precautions
Contraindicated in hypersensitivity to drug or other opioids.

Use cautiously in hepatic or renal disease, susceptibility to respiratory depression (as in comatose patient with head injury or brain tumor), chronic obstructive pulmonary disease, decreased respiratory reserve, potentially compromised respiration, bradycardia, monoamine oxidase (MAO) inhibitor use within 14 days, ***elderly*** and debilitated patients, labor and delivery (use not recommended), pregnant or breastfeeding patients, and ***children younger than age 2*** (safety not established).

Adverse reactions
CNS: dizziness, headache, vertigo, floating feeling, lethargy, confusion, lightheadedness, nervousness, hallucinations, delirium, insomnia, anxiety, fear, mood changes, tremor, sedation, **coma, seizures**
CV: palpitations, hypertension, tachycardia, **hypotension, bradycardia, arrhythmias, circulatory depression, cardiac arrest, shock**
EENT: blurred vision, diplopia, **laryngospasm**
GI: nausea, vomiting, constipation, biliary tract spasm, dry mouth, anorexia
GU: urine retention or urinary hesitancy, ureteral or vesical sphincter spasm,

decreased libido, erectile dysfunction, **oliguria**
Musculoskeletal: skeletal and thoracic muscle rigidity
Respiratory: slow and shallow respirations, suppressed cough reflex, **bronchospasm, respiratory depression, apnea**
Skin: pruritus, urticaria, rash, diaphoresis, flushing, erythema, cold sensitivity
Other: phlebitis at injection site, hypersensitivity reactions including **anaphylaxis**

Interactions

Drug-drug. *Barbiturate anesthetics:* decreased effects of both drugs
Buprenorphine, dezocine, nalbuphine: decreased analgesic effect
CNS depressants (including antidepressants, other opioid analgesics, sedating antihistamines, sedative-hypnotics, skeletal muscle relaxants): profound sedation, hypoventilation, and hypotension
Erythromycin, ketoconazole, some protease inhibitors: decreased metabolism and increased effects of fentanyl, possibly leading to profound sedation, hypoventilation, and hypotension
MAO inhibitors: severe, unpredictable reactions
Opioid antagonists, partial-antagonist opioid analgesics: withdrawal in physically dependent patients
Drug-diagnostic tests. *Amylase, lipase:* increased
Granulocytes, hemoglobin, neutrophils, platelets, white blood cells: decreased
Drug-herb. *Chamomile, hops, kava, skullcap, valerian:* increased CNS depression
Drug-behaviors. *Alcohol use:* profound sedation, hypoventilation, and hypotension

Toxicity and overdose

- In overdose, expect extension of pharmacologic and adverse effects, including CNS and respiratory depression, hypotension, bradycardia, and shock.
- Discontinue drug, monitor vital signs closely, and ensure patent airway. As needed and ordered, give I.V. fluids for shock and opioid antagonist (such as naloxone) to counteract drug's effects; repeat dose as needed. Do not give antagonist in absence of significant respiratory or cardiovascular depression. Resuscitate, if indicated.

Patient teaching

- Caution patient to avoid driving and other hazardous activities until drug's effects on concentration and alertness are known.
- As appropriate, review all significant and life-threatening adverse reactions and interactions, especially those related to the drugs, tests, herbs, and behaviors mentioned above.

filgrastim

Neupogen

Pharmacologic class: Granulocyte colony–stimulating factor
Therapeutic class: Hematopoietic stimulator, antineutropenic
Pregnancy risk category C

Action

Induces formation of neutrophil progenitor cells by binding directly to receptor on surface of granulocyte, stimulating cell proliferation and differentiation. Also potentiates effects of mature neutrophils, and reduces fever and risk of infection associated with severe neutropenia.

Pharmacokinetics

Drug is metabolized in the liver and kidneys. Elimination half-life is about 3.5 hours.

Onset	Peak	Duration
5-60 min	24 hr	1-7 days

How supplied

SingleJect prefilled syringes: 300 mcg, 480 mcg
Solution for injection: 300 mcg/mL in single-dose, preservative-free vials containing 300 mcg (1 mL) of filgrastim (300 mcg/mL) or 480 mL (1.6 mL) of filgrastim (300 mcg/mL)

Indications and dosages

➣ Febrile neutropenia in nonmyeloid cancer patients receiving myelosuppressive chemotherapy; acute myeloid leukemia after chemotherapy
Adults and children: 5 mcg/kg/day by I.V. infusion over 15 to 30 minutes or by continuous I.V. infusion, increased by 5 mcg/kg with each chemotherapy cycle if needed

➣ Febrile neutropenia in patients with nonmyeloid cancer who are undergoing myeloablative chemotherapy followed by bone marrow transplantation
Adults and children: 10 mcg/kg/day I.V. infusion over 4 or 24 hours, starting no sooner than 24 hours after chemotherapy and bone marrow infusion

➣ Harvesting of peripheral blood stem cells
Adults and children: 10 mcg/kg/day continuous I.V. infusion, given at least 4 days before first leukapheresis and continued until last leukapheresis session

Dosage adjustment

• When giving drug to prevent infection after myelosuppressive chemotherapy, increase dosage in increments of 5 mcg/kg for each chemotherapy cycle, according to duration and severity of absolute neutrophil count (ANC) nadir. Discontinue if ANC exceeds 10,000/mm^3 after expected chemotherapy-induced ANC nadir.
• When administering for neutrophil recovery after bone marrow transplantation, titrate daily dosage to neutrophil response. If ANC exceeds 1,000/mm^3 for 3 consecutive days, reduce to 5 mcg/kg/day. Discontinue drug if ANC remains above 1,000/mm^3 for 3 more days.

F

Off-label uses

• Agranulocytosis
• AIDS- or zidovudine-associated neutropenia
• Aplastic anemia
• Hairy-cell leukemia
• Myelodysplasia
• Radiation-induced neutropenia

Administration

Preparation

• Do not give within 24 hours of chemotherapy, bone marrow transplantation, or radiation therapy.
• Obtain CBC and platelet count before starting therapy.

Dilution and compatibility

🔈 Dilute with D_5W. Never use saline solution, which can cause precipitation.
🔈 Dilute to a final concentration no less than 5 mcg/mL.
• Do not shake; do not mix with other drugs.

Infusion considerations

• Administer single dose intermittently over 15 to 30 minutes or by continuous infusion over 4 to 24 hours.
• Know that drug may be injected into venous return line of dialysis tubing after dialysis ends.

Monitoring

🔈 Be aware that allergic reactions may occur with initial or subsequent treatment (usually within first 30 minutes of infusion). These reactions typically include systemic symptoms involving at least two body systems—most often skin (rash, urticaria, facial edema), respiratory (wheezing, dyspnea), and cardiovascular (hypotension, tachycardia). Be prepared to give antihistamines, steroids, bronchodilators, and epinephrine.

- Continue to monitor CBC and platelet count.
- Monitor cardiovascular status carefully.

Assess for signs and symptoms of sickle cell crisis or splenic rupture.

Storage

- Refrigerate at 2° to 8°C (36° to 46°F).

Contraindications and precautions

Contraindicated in hypersensitivity to drug, its components, or *Escherichia coli*–derived proteins.

Use cautiously in patients receiving lithium or other drugs that can potentiate neutrophil release, pregnant or breastfeeding patients, and ***children.***

Adverse reactions

CNS: headache, fever, weakness
CV: chest pain, hypotension, transient supraventricular tachycardia, **myocardial infarction, arrhythmias**
EENT: sore throat
GI: nausea, vomiting, diarrhea, constipation, abdominal pain, splenomegaly, stomatitis
GU: bleeding
Hematologic: leukocytosis, sickle cell crisis, thrombocytopenia, splenic rupture
Metabolic: hyperuricemia
Musculoskeletal: bone, joint, muscle, arm, or leg pain
Respiratory: dyspnea, cough
Skin: pruritus, rash, erythema, alopecia, cutaneous necrotic vasculitis
Other: fever, mucositis, pain at injection site, edema, hypersensitivity reactions

Interactions

Drug-drug. *Lithium:* increased neutrophil production
Topotecan: prolonged neutropenia
Vincristine: increased risk of severe atypical peripheral neuropathy
Drug-diagnostic tests. *Alkaline phosphatase, creatinine, lactate dehydrogenase, uric acid:* increased
Platelets: decreased

Toxicity and overdose

- In overdose, expect excessive leukocytosis and extension of other adverse reactions.
- Discontinue drug and provide symptomatic and supportive therapy.

Patient teaching

Teach patient to recognize and promptly report signs and symptoms of allergic response.

- Caution patient to avoid driving and other hazardous activities until drug's effects on concentration and alertness are known.
- Advise patient to discuss possible need for iron supplements, vitamin B_{12}, and folic acid with prescriber.
- Teach patient how to monitor blood pressure at home.
- Advise patient to minimize GI upset by eating small, frequent servings of healthy food and drinking adequate fluids.
- Inform patient of the need for repeated laboratory testing during therapy.
- Advise female patient to inform prescriber if she is breastfeeding.
- As appropriate, review all other significant and life-threatening adverse reactions and interactions, especially those related to the drugs and tests mentioned above.

[redacted]

fluconazole

Diflucan, Fluconazole Omega ✦

Pharmacologic class: Synthetic azole
Therapeutic class: Systemic antifungal
Pregnancy risk category C

Action

Inhibits fungal sterol synthesis, causing aggregation of 14 alpha-methyl sterols in fungi; loss of normal sterols may explain fungistatic activity.

Pharmacokinetics

Drug distributes widely into all body fluids, including CNS, sputum, saliva, blister fluid, skin, and urine. It is partially metabolized and clears primarily by renal excretion, with about 11% excreted as metabolite.

Onset	Peak	Duration
Rapid	1 hr	2-4 days

How supplied

Solution for injection (clear): 2 mg/mL in 100- or 200-mL bottles or plastic containers

Indications and dosages

➢ Oropharyngeal candidiasis
Adults: 200 mg I.V. on first day, followed by 100 mg daily for at least 2 weeks
Children: 6 mg/kg I.V. on first day, followed by 3 mg/kg/day for at least 2 weeks

➢ Esophageal candidiasis
Adults: 200 mg I.V. on first day, followed by 100 mg/day for 3 weeks and for 2 weeks after symptoms resolve. Up to 400 mg/day may be given in severe cases.
Children: 6 mg/kg I.V. on first day, followed by 3 mg/kg/day for 3 weeks and for at least 2 weeks after symptoms resolve

➢ Systemic candidiasis
Adults: 400 mg I.V. on first day, followed by 200 mg/day for 4 weeks and for at least 2 weeks after symptoms resolve
Children: 6 to 12 mg/kg/day I.V.

➢ Cryptococcal meningitis
Adults: 400 mg I.V. on first day, followed by 200 or 400 mg/day for 10 to 12 weeks after cerebrospinal fluid (CSF) is negative
Children: 12 mg/kg I.V. on first day, followed by 6 mg/kg/day for 10 to 12 weeks after CSF is negative

➢ To suppress cryptococcal meningitis in patients with AIDS
Adults: 200 mg daily I.V.

➢ To prevent candidiasis after bone marrow transplantation
Adults: 400 mg I.V. daily for several days before and 7 days after neutrophil count rises above 1,000/mm^3

Dosage adjustment

- Reduce dosage in renal impairment based on creatinine clearance.

Administration

Dilution and compatibility

- Be aware that drug is supplied prediluted in glass bottles and plastic containers.
- Do not use if solution is cloudy.
- Do not mix with other drugs.

Infusion considerations

- Keep overwrap on I.V. bag until just before use.

🔊 Do not use plastic containers in series connections. Such use could result in air embolism due to residual air being drawn from primary container before administration of fluid from secondary container ends.

🔊 Limit single I.V. infusion to 200 mg/hour or less, using infusion pump.

- Do not piggyback with other I.V. infusions.

• Know that plastic container may be opaque; this does not affect drug and decreases over time.

Monitoring

Stay alert for signs and symptoms of anaphylaxis. Stop drug immediately if these occur.

• Monitor liver function tests and hematologic studies.

Assess for rash; if lesions develop, monitor patient. Stop drug and notify prescriber if lesions progress (may signal Stevens-Johnson syndrome).

• Be aware that patients with HIV infection have greater risk of adverse reactions.

Storage

• Store plastic containers between 5° and 25°C (41° and 77°F).

• Store glass bottles between 5° and 30°C (41° and 86°F).

Contraindications and precautions

Contraindicated in hypersensitivity to drug or its components.

Use cautiously in hypersensitivity to other azole antifungals, renal impairment, hepatic disease, pregnant or breastfeeding patients, and ***children younger than age 6 months*** (safety and efficacy not established).

Adverse reactions

CNS: headache, dizziness
GI: nausea, vomiting, diarrhea, dyspepsia, abdominal discomfort
Hematologic: leukopenia, thrombocytopenia
Hepatic: hepatotoxicity
Skin: rash, pruritus, exfoliative skin disorders (including **Stevens-Johnson syndrome**)
Other: altered taste, **anaphylaxis**

Interactions

Drug-drug. *Alfentanil, cyclosporine, phenytoin, rifabutin, tacrolimus, theophylline, zidovudine:* increased blood levels of these drugs, greater risk of toxicity
Benzodiazepines, buspirone, losartan, nisoldipine, tricyclic antidepressants, zolpidem: increased blood levels and effects of these drugs
CYP3A4 inducers: inhibited CYP3A4 enzyme system, altered actions of CYP3A4 inducers (with fluconazole dosages above 200 mg/day)
Rifampin: increased rifampin and decreased fluconazole blood levels
Sulfonylureas (glipizide, glyburide, tolbutamide): increased hypoglycemic effect of these drugs
Thiazide diuretics: increased fluconazole blood level
Warfarin: increased warfarin activity
Drug-diagnostic tests. *Alanine aminotransferase, alkaline phosphatase, bilirubin, gamma-glutamyltransferase, hepatic enzymes:* increased
Platelets, white blood cells: decreased

Toxicity and overdose

• In overdose, expect extension of adverse reactions.

• Provide symptomatic and supportive therapy.

Patient teaching

Teach patient to recognize and immediately report signs and symptoms of allergic response.

Urge patient to contact prescriber if rash occurs to determine if Stevens-Johnson syndrome is developing.

• Caution patient to avoid driving and other hazardous activities until drug's effects on concentration and alertness are known.

• Advise patient to minimize GI upset by eating frequent, small servings of healthy food and drinking adequate fluids.

• Instruct female patient to inform prescriber if she is pregnant or breastfeeding.

• As appropriate, review all other significant and life-threatening adverse reactions and interactions, especially those related to the drugs and tests mentioned above.

fludarabine phosphate

Fludara

Pharmacologic class: Antimetabolite
Therapeutic class: Antineoplastic
Pregnancy risk category D

FDA BOXED WARNING

• Give under supervision of physician experienced in cancer chemotherapy. Severe bone marrow suppression may occur. When given in high doses to patients with acute leukemia, drug has caused severe neurologic effects, including blindness, coma, and death. This severe CNS toxicity occurred in 36% of patients receiving dosages approximately four times greater than recommended dosage. Similar severe CNS toxicity has been reported in rare cases in patients who received dosages in range of that recommended for chronic lymphocytic leukemia (CLL).
• Life-threatening and sometimes fatal autoimmune hemolytic anemia has occurred after one or more treatment cycles. Evaluate patient closely and monitor for hemolysis.
• In study using drug in combination with pentostatin to treat refractory CLL, unacceptably high incidence of fatal pulmonary toxicity occurred. Use of fludarabine with pentostatin is not recommended.

Action

Not completely understood. Converts to active metabolite 2-fluoro-ara-ATP, which appears to inhibit DNA polymerase alpha, ribonucleotide reductase, and DNA primase. These effects lead to inhibition of DNA synthesis.

Pharmacokinetics

Drug converts to 2-fluoro-ara-A (active metabolite) within minutes of I.V. infusion. It distributes widely. Plasma protein binding ranges between 19% and 29%. Metabolite has terminal half-life of approximately 20 hours. Drug is eliminated primarily by the kidneys.

Onset	Peak	Duration
Unknown	1 hr	Unknown

How supplied

Powder for reconstitution for injection (lyophilized; white, solid cake): 50-mg vial

Indications and dosages

➤ Chronic B-cell lymphocytic leukemia after treatment with at least one standard alkylating-agent regimen
Adults: 25 mg/m^2 I.V. over 30 minutes daily for 5 consecutive days, with each 5-day course of therapy starting every 28 days

Dosage adjustment

• Decrease dosage or delay dose if hematologic or nonhematologic toxicity (other than neurotoxicity) occurs. Delay dose or discontinue drug if neurotoxicity occurs.
• Modify dosage in patients with advanced age or bone marrow impairment, as indicated.
• Decrease dosage by 20% in moderate renal impairment. Do not administer to patients with severe renal impairment.

Off-label uses

- Acute lymphocytic leukemia in children
- Hairy-cell leukemia
- Hodgkin's lymphoma
- Mycosis fungoides
- Prolymphocytic leukemia or prolymphocytoid CLL variant
- Relapsed non-Hodgkin's lymphoma
- Solid tumors in children
- Waldenstrom's macroglobulinemia

Administration

Preparation

Follow hazardous drug guidelines on page S19 for handling, preparation, and administration.

- Be prepared to give irradiated blood products to patients requiring transfusions while receiving drug. (Non-irradiated blood transfusions carry slight risk of graft vs. host disease.)

Dilution and compatibility

- Reconstitute powder with 2 mL sterile water for injection, to yield a concentration of 25 mg/mL. Solid powder cake should dissolve in about 15 seconds. Further dilute in 100 mL normal saline solution or D_5W.

Infusion considerations

- Give drug within 8 hours of reconstitution.
- Administer each dose by I.V. infusion over 30 minutes.

Monitoring

- Closely monitor CBC and platelet count during therapy to gauge degree of hematopoietic suppression. Be aware that clinically significant cytopenia may last 2 months to 1 year.

Monitor for tumor lysis syndrome, marked by flank pain, hematuria, hyperuricemia, hyperphosphatemia, hypocalcemia, metabolic acidosis, hyperkalemia, urate crystalluria, and renal failure.

Storage

- Refrigerate at 2° to 8°C (36° to 46°F).

Contraindications and precautions

Contraindicated in hypersensitivity to drug and in pregnancy or breastfeeding.

Use cautiously in renal impairment, patients at risk for tumor lysis syndrome, ***elderly patients,*** and ***children*** (safety and efficacy not established).

Adverse reactions

CNS: fatigue, malaise, weakness, paresthesia, headache, sleep disorder
EENT: visual disturbances, hearing loss, sinusitis
GI: nausea, vomiting, diarrhea
Hematologic: anemia, **neutropenia, thrombocytopenia**
Respiratory: cough, pneumonia
Other: fever, chills, infection, pain, diaphoresis

Interactions

Drug-drug. *Antigout agents:* decreased effects of these drugs
Bone marrow depressants: increased risk of bone marrow depression
Live-virus vaccines: possible potentiation of virus replication, increased vaccine side effects, decreased response to vaccine
Pentostatin: severe pulmonary toxicity
Drug-diagnostic tests. *Alkaline phosphatase, aspartate aminotransferase, uric acid:* possible increases
Calcium: decreased

Toxicity and overdose

- In overdose, expect lethargy, coma, blindness, and bone marrow depression. When used at high doses, drug may cause severe neurologic adverse effects, including blindness, coma, and death. Similar toxicity rarely occurs at recommended doses.

• No specific antidote exists. Discontinue drug and provide symptomatic and supportive therapy.

Patient teaching

Instruct patient to immediately report indications of bone marrow suppression, such as unusual bleeding or bruising and signs and symptoms of infection.
• Advise patient to avoid crowds, exposure to infection, and individuals who have recently received live-virus vaccines.
• Advise females of childbearing potential to avoid pregnancy.
• Instruct breastfeeding patient not to breastfeed during therapy.
• As appropriate, review all other significant and life-threatening adverse reactions and interactions, especially those related to the drugs and tests mentioned above.

flumazenil

Anexate, Romazicon

Pharmacologic class: Benzodiazepine receptor antagonist
Therapeutic class: Antidote
Pregnancy risk category C

FDA BOXED WARNING

• Drug has been linked to seizures—most commonly in patients who have received benzodiazepines for long-term sedation, or in overdose where patients show signs and symptoms of serious cyclic antidepressant overdose. Individualize dosage, and be prepared to manage seizures.

Action

Antagonizes CNS-depressant effects of benzodiazepines and inhibits activity at gamma-aminobutyric acid–benzodiazepine receptor sites

Pharmacokinetics

Drug distributes extensively in extravascular space. Initial distribution half-life is 7 to 15 minutes. Drug is 99% metabolized, with about 50% protein binding. Clearance occurs primarily via hepatic metabolism. Elimination is complete within 72 hours, with 90% to 95% of dose appearing in urine and 5% to 10% in feces as metabolites. Less than 1% of unchanged drug appears in urine. Terminal half-life is 41 to 79 minutes.

Onset	Peak	Duration
1-2 min	6-10 min	Unknown

How supplied

Solution for injection: 0.1 mg/mL in 5- and 10-mL vials

Indications and dosages

➢ To completely or partially reverse sedative effects of benzodiazepines after general anesthesia or diagnostic or therapeutic procedures
Adults: 0.2 mg I.V. given over 15 seconds. Additional doses may be given at 1-minute intervals until desired results occur, up to a total dosage of 1 mg. If resedation occurs, may repeat regimen at 20-minute intervals, not to exceed 3 mg/hour.
Children: 0.01 mg/kg I.V. (up to 0.2 mg) given over 15 seconds. If desired results do not occur after 45 seconds, may give further injections of 0.01 mg/kg (up to 0.2 mg) at 1-minute intervals (up to four additional doses), to a maximum total dosage of 0.05 mg/kg or 1 mg, whichever is lower.

➤ Suspected benzodiazepine overdose
Adults: 0.2 mg I.V. given over 30 seconds. If desired results do not occur after 30 seconds, may give 0.3 mg over 30 seconds. If necessary, may give further doses of 0.5 mg over 30 seconds at 1-minute intervals, to a total dosage of 3 mg. Usual required dosage is 1 to 3 mg. If resedation occurs, may give additional doses of 0.5 mg/minute over 2 minutes at 20-minute intervals (no more than 1 mg at a time or 3 mg/hour).

Administration
Preparation
Confirm that airway is stable before giving drug.
Dilution and compatibility
• Dilute with D_5W, lactated Ringer's, or normal saline solutions.
Infusion considerations
• Inject into large vein through free-flowing I.V. solution over 15 to 30 seconds.
Monitoring
• Be aware that drug has short duration. Monitor patient for sedation, and give additional doses as needed.
Assess neurologic status frequently. Stay alert for seizures.
Monitor cardiovascular status, watching closely for arrhythmias.
• Watch for extravasation into surrounding tissue.
Storage
• Store in vial until ready for use. Drug remains stable in syringe for 24 hours.

Contraindications and precautions
Contraindicated in hypersensitivity to drug or benzodiazepines.

Use cautiously in head injury, history of seizures, pregnant or breastfeeding patients, and ***children*** (safety not established).

Adverse reactions
CNS: dizziness, drowsiness, vertigo, ataxia, agitation, confusion, fatigue, headache, sleep disorders, paresthesia, rigors, **seizures**
CV: chest pain, hypertension, palpitations, **arrhythmias**
EENT: blurred or abnormal vision, abnormal hearing
GI: nausea, vomiting
Respiratory: hyperventilation
Skin: flushing, sweating
Other: shivering, pain at injection site

Interactions
Drug-drug. *Tricyclic antidepressants:* reversal of benzodiazepine effects, leading to arrhythmias or seizures (when given for mixed overdose)

Toxicity and overdose
• In overdose, expect extension of pharmacologic action in reversing benzodiazepine effect. Excessively high doses may cause anxiety, agitation, increased muscle tone, hyperesthesia, and seizures.
• Provide symptomatic and supportive therapy, including barbiturates, phenytoin, and benzodiazepines, as ordered.

Patient teaching
• Before giving drug and on discharge, inform patient that resedation may occur despite a feeling of alertness.
• Inform patient that drug may impair memory and judgment.
• Caution patient not to drive or engage in other hazardous activities requiring complete alertness for at least 24 hours after discharge.
• Tell patient to avoid alcohol and over-the-counter drugs for at least 24 hours after receiving drug.
• Advise female patient to inform prescriber if she is pregnant or breastfeeding.

• As appropriate, review all other significant and life-threatening adverse reactions and interactions, especially those related to the drugs mentioned above.

fluorouracil (5-fluorouracil, 5-FU)

Adrucil

Pharmacologic class: Antimetabolite
Therapeutic class: Antineoplastic
Pregnancy risk category D

FDA BOXED WARNING

• Patient should be hospitalized during first course of therapy, as drug may cause severe toxic reactions.

Action

Inhibits DNA and RNA synthesis, leading to death of rapid-growing neoplastic cells. Cell-cycle–S-phase specific.

Pharmacokinetics

About 7% to 20% of drug is excreted in urine in 6 hours, with more than 90% excreted in first hour. Remainder is metabolized in the liver, with inactive metabolites excreted by the kidneys. No intact drug is detected in plasma 3 hours after administration. Elimination half-life is 20 minutes. Drug distributes into tumors, intestinal mucosa, bone marrow, liver, and other tissues throughout the body and diffuses readily across the blood-brain barrier and distributes into cerebrospinal fluid and brain tissue.

Onset	Peak	Duration
1-9 days	9-21 days	30 days

How supplied

Solution for injection (clear, colorless to faint yellow): 50 mg/mL in 10-mL ampules and 10-, 20-, 50-, and 100-mL vials

Indications and dosages

➤ Advanced colorectal cancer

Adults: 370 mg/m^2 I.V. for 5 days, preceded by leucovorin 200 mg/m^2 daily for 5 days; may be repeated q 4 to 5 weeks. No single daily dose should exceed 800 mg.

➤ Palliative management of carcinoma of colon, rectum, breast, stomach, or pancreas

Adults: Various dosing regimens, including 12 mg/kg I.V. daily for 4 days, then 6 mg/kg I.V. daily on days 6, 8, 10, 12 (maximum dosage 800 mg/day). Maintenance therapy may be considered in patients who tolerate drug toxicity by repeating first course every 30 days, after last day of previous treatment cycle. Alternatively, a single maintenance dose of 10 to 15 mg/kg/week I.V. may be given after toxic signs resulting from initial course subside; maximum dosage is 1 g/week.

Poor-risk patients: 6 mg/kg/day I.V. for 3 days, then 3 mg/kg/day I.V. on days 5, 7, and 9 (not to exceed 400 mg/dose)

Administration

Preparation

Clinical alert: Follow hazardous drug guidelines on page S19 for handling, preparation, and administration.

Clinical alert: Consult facility's cancer protocols to ensure that drug is given appropriately. Protocols vary in dosage, administration technique, and cycle length.

Clinical alert: Be aware that drug is highly toxic and has narrow margin of safety.

• Know that all dosages are based on patient's actual weight. However, use estimated lean body mass (dry weight)

if patient is obese or has had spurious weight gain from edema, ascites, or other abnormal fluid retention.
- Give antiemetic before drug, as prescribed, to reduce GI upset.
- Obtain white blood count (WBC) before each dose.

Be aware of importance of leucovorin rescue, when prescribed.
- Know that pyridoxine may be given with fluorouracil to reduce risk of palmar-plantar erythrodysesthesia (hand-foot syndrome).

Dilution and compatibility
- Be aware that drug may be given without dilution by direct I.V. injection.
- For I.V. infusion, dilute with D_5W, sterile water, or normal saline solution in plastic bag (not glass bottle). Infusion may be given for up to 24 hours or more.
- If precipitate forms from exposure to low temperatures, resolubilize by heating to 77°C (171°F) and shaking vigorously. Cool to body temperature before using.

Infusion considerations
- Give by direct I.V. injection over 1 to 3 minutes.
- Give by I.V. infusion over 24 hours or as prescribed.
- Check infusion site frequently to detect extravasation.

Monitoring

Watch for signs and symptoms of toxicity, especially stomatitis, diarrhea, esophagopharyngitis, neutropenia (WBC below 3,500/mm^3 or rapidly falling), thrombocytopenia (platelet count below 100,000/mm^3), severe nausea and vomiting, or bleeding. If these occur, stop drug and notify prescriber. Note that toxicity may take 1 to 3 weeks to develop.
- Monitor CBC, WBC, platelet count, and kidney and liver function test results.
- Assess fluid intake and output.
- With long-term use, watch for serious rash on hands and feet. If it occurs, consult prescriber regarding possible need for pyridoxine.
- Assess for bleeding tendency.
- Monitor blood glucose level in patients at risk for hyperglycemia.

Storage
- Store at room temperature of 15° to 30°C (59° to 86°F); protect from light.

Contraindications and precautions

Contraindicated in hypersensitivity to drug or its components, bone marrow depression, poor nutritional status, serious infection, and pregnancy or breastfeeding.

Use cautiously in renal or hepatic impairment, poor-risk patients with history of high-dose pelvic irradiation or previous use of alkylating agents, widespread involvement of bone marrow by metastatic tumors, dihydropyrimidine dehydrogenase enzyme deficiency, serious infection, edema, ascites, obesity, and ***children*** (safety and efficacy not established).

Adverse reactions

CNS: confusion, disorientation, euphoria, ataxia, headache, weakness, malaise, acute cerebellar syndrome or dysfunction
CV: angina, **myocardial ischemia, thrombophlebitis**
EENT: vision changes, photophobia, lacrimation, lacrimal duct stenosis, nystagmus, epistaxis
GI: nausea, vomiting, diarrhea, stomatitis, anorexia, GI ulcer, **GI bleeding**
Hematologic: anemia, **leukopenia, thrombocytopenia**
Skin: alopecia, maculopapular rash, melanosis of nails, nail loss, palmar-plantar erythrodysesthesia, photosensitivity, dermatitis
Other: fever, **anaphylaxis**

Interactions

Drug-drug. *Bone marrow depressants (including other antineoplastics):* additive bone marrow depression
Irinotecan: dehydration, neutropenia, sepsis
Leucovorin calcium: increased risk of fluorouracil toxicity
Live-virus vaccines: decreased antibody response to vaccine, increased risk of adverse reactions
Drug-diagnostic tests. *Alanine aminotransferase, alkaline phosphatase, aspartate aminotransferase, bilirubin, lactate dehydrogenase, urinary 5-hydroxyindoleacetic acid:* increased
Albumin, granulocytes, platelets, red blood cells, WBCs: decreased
Drug-behaviors. *Sun exposure:* increased risk of phototoxicity

Toxicity and overdose

- In overdose (unlikely), expect nausea, vomiting, diarrhea, GI ulcers and bleeding, and bone marrow depression.
- No specific antidote exists. Provide symptomatic and supportive therapy. Monitor hematologic status for at least 4 weeks, and intervene as needed.

Patient teaching

Emphasize importance of taking leucovorin as prescribed with high-dose fluorouracil therapy.

Instruct patient to report signs and symptoms of toxicity, particularly stomatitis and diarrhea. Tell patient these may not occur for 1 to 3 weeks.

- Caution patient to avoid driving and other hazardous activities until drug's effects on concentration and alertness are known.
- Advise patient to avoid activities that can cause injury and to use soft toothbrush and electric razor to avoid gum and skin injury.
- Teach patient to minimize GI upset by eating frequent, small servings of healthy food and drinking adequate fluids.
- Inform patient that drug may cause reversible hair loss.
- Emphasize the need for repeated laboratory testing during therapy.

Advise female to inform prescriber immediately if she is pregnant. Caution her not to breastfeed.

- As appropriate, review all other significant and life-threatening adverse reactions and interactions, especially those related to the drugs, tests, and behaviors mentioned above.

[redacted]

folic acid

Folvite

Pharmacologic class: Vitamin
Therapeutic class: Nutritional supplement
Pregnancy risk category A

Action

Stimulates production of red blood cells, white blood cells, and platelets in certain megaloblastic anemias

Pharmacokinetics

Drug clears rapidly from plasma and distributes to all body tissues, crossing placental barrier. Cerebrospinal fluid levels are several times more than serum levels. Drug is metabolized in the liver, stored primarily in the liver, and excreted in urine and breast milk.

Onset	Peak	Duration
Unknown	Unknown	Unknown

How supplied

Solution for injection: 5 mg/mL in 10-mL vials

Indications and dosages

➢ Megaloblastic anemia; anemias of nutritional origin

Adults and children older than age 4: Up to 1 mg I.V. daily; resistant cases may require higher dosages. Maintenance dosage varies with age and clinical condition.

Administration

Preparation

- Be aware that parenteral administration is not recommended but may be necessary for some patients with severe megaloblastic anemia or severely impaired GI absorption.
- Obtain CBC with white cell differential before giving drug.

Dilution and compatibility

- Dilute each dose in at least 50 mL normal saline solution, D_5W, or sterile water for injection.
- May further dilute by adding to a compatible I.V. solution.

Infusion considerations

- Administer at prescribed rate.

Monitoring

- Monitor CBC with differential throughout therapy.
- Supervise patient closely; adjust maintenance dosage if relapse appears imminent.
- Know that maintenance dosage may need to be increased in alcoholism, hemolytic anemia, anticonvulsant therapy, or chronic infection.

Storage

- Store at controlled room temperature of 15° to 30°C (59° to 86°F). Do not freeze; protect from light.

Contraindications and precautions

Contraindicated in hypersensitivity to drug, pernicious anemia, and other megaloblastic anemias marked by vitamin B_{12} deficiency.

Use cautiously in undiagnosed anemia, ***elderly patients,*** pregnant or breastfeeding patients, and ***children.***

Adverse reactions

CNS: altered sleep pattern, poor concentration, irritability, overactivity, excitement, depression, confusion, impaired judgment

GI: nausea, abdominal distention, anorexia, flatulence

Metabolic: decreased vitamin B_{12} level (with prolonged therapy)

Other: rare hypersensitivity reactions including **anaphylaxis**

Interactions

Drug-drug. *Aminosalicylic acid:* decreased folate level

Dihydrofolate reductase inhibitors (such as methotrexate, trimethoprim): interference with folic acid utilization

Phenytoin: decreased efficacy of both drugs

Sulfasalazine: possible folate deficiency

Toxicity and overdose

- In overdose (unlikely), expect mostly GI adverse effects.
- Provide symptomatic and supportive therapy.

Patient teaching

- Teach patient about food sources of folic acid (whole grain, yeast, leafy vegetables, nuts, beans, and fruit). Instruct patient to avoid overcooked or canned food, as folic acid may have been destroyed.
- Stress importance of taking folic acid only as prescribed.

• As appropriate, review all other significant and life-threatening adverse reactions and interactions, especially those related to the drugs mentioned above.

[redacted]

fomepizole injection

Antizol

Pharmacologic class: Synthetic competitive alcohol dehydrogenase inhibitor
Therapeutic class: Antidote
Pregnancy risk category C

Action

Competitively inhibits alcohol dehydrogenase, blocking formation of ethylene glycol (main component of most antifreeze and coolant products) and methanol (main component of windshield-wiper fluid) toxic metabolites, including glycolic and oxalic acids (ethylene glycol intoxication) and formic acid (methanol intoxication).

Pharmacokinetics

Drug distributes rapidly to total body water. Plasma half-life varies with dose. Drug is primarily excreted in urine as metabolites with a small percentage excreted unchanged.

Onset	Peak	Duration
Unknown	Unknown	Unknown

How supplied

Concentrate for injection (clear to yellow): 1 g/mL in 1.5-mL vials

Indications and dosages

➤ Ethylene glycol or methanol poisoning, used alone or in combination with hemodialysis

Adults: Loading dose of 15 mg/kg I.V., followed by 10 mg/kg q 12 hours for four doses; then 15 mg/kg q 12 hours thereafter until ethylene glycol or methanol concentration is undetectable or drops below 20 mg/dL and patient is asymptomatic with normal pH

Dosage adjustment

• Be aware that patients on hemodialysis may need doses every 4 hours.

F

Administration

Preparation

Obtain baseline ethylene glycol or methanol (as appropriate) blood and urine concentrations, arterial blood gas (ABG) values, liver enzyme tests, and white blood cell count.

• Be aware that patients with anuria may need hemodialysis.

Dilution and compatibility

Be aware that drug is a concentrate and must be diluted before use.

• If drug has solidified in vial (as when stored at temperatures below 25°C (77°F), liquefy by running warm water over vial. Solidification does not affect drug efficacy, safety, or stability.

Dilute with at least 100 mL normal saline solution or D_5W; mix well.

• Do not use if solution is hazy or discolored.

Infusion considerations

• Use within 24 hours of dilution.

Do not give undiluted or by I.V. bolus, as serious vein damage may occur.

• Administer by slow I.V. infusion over 30 minutes.

Monitoring

Watch for and be prepared to manage hypocalcemia and toxic effects of ethylene glycol poisoning (acute renal failure, metabolic acidosis) or methanol poisoning (adult respiratory distress syndrome, visual disturbances).

Maintain patent airway and provide ventilation, as indicated.
Watch for sudden CNS or respiratory depression.
Provide continuous ECG monitoring.
Continue to monitor ABGs to determine drug's effect on toxins, pH, creatinine, blood urea nitrogen, electrolytes, hepatic enzymes, white blood cell (WBC) count, and urinalysis.
Meticulously monitor urine output.
Frequently monitor ethylene glycol or methanol blood and urine levels.
Monitor for signs and symptom of allergic reactions and be prepared to intervene appropriately.

Storage

- Store at controlled room temperature of 20° to 25°C (68° to 77°F).

Contraindications and precautions

Contraindicated in serious hypersensitivity to drug or other pyrazoles.

Use cautiously in ***elderly patients,*** pregnant or breastfeeding patients, and ***children*** (safety and efficacy not established).

Adverse reactions

CNS: dizziness, headache, increased drowsiness, vertigo, light-headedness, agitation, anxiety, feeling of drunkenness, strange feeling, decreased environmental awareness, **seizures**
CV: bradycardia, sinus bradycardia, tachycardia, phlebitis, phlebosclerosis, shock, hypotension
EENT: visual disturbances, nystagmus, "roaring" in ears, pharyngitis, abnormal smell
GI: nausea, diarrhea, abdominal pain, dyspepsia, heartburn
GU: anuria
Hematologic: anemia, **disseminated intravascular coagulation**
Musculoskeletal: backache
Skin: rash
Other: unpleasant or metallic taste, facial flushing, lymphangitis, hiccups, decreased appetite, speech disturbance, fever, hangover, injection site inflammation, pain on injection, **multisystemic failure**

Interactions

Drug-diagnostic tests. *Eosinophils, transaminases:* increased

Toxicity and overdose

- Short-term nausea, dizziness, and vertigo have occurred in patients who received six times the recommended dosage.
- Monitor patient closely and provide symptomatic and supportive therapy. Hemodialysis is beneficial.

Patient teaching

- Inform patient about the need for repeated laboratory testing during therapy.
- As appropriate, review all other significant and life-threatening adverse reactions and interactions, especially those related to the tests mentioned above.

furosemide

Furoside✦, Lasix

Pharmacologic class: Sulfonamide loop diuretic
Therapeutic class: Diuretic
Pregnancy risk category C

Action

Unclear. Thought to inhibit sodium and chloride reabsorption from ascending loop of Henle and proximal and distal renal tubules. Increases potassium excretion and plasma volume, promoting renal excretion of water, sodium, chloride, magnesium, and calcium.

Pharmacokinetics

Drug is approximately 30% to 40% metabolized, largely protein-bound, and excreted primarily in urine.

Onset	Peak	Duration
5 min	20-60 min	2 hr

How supplied

Solution for injection: 10 mg/mL in 2-, 4-, and 10-mL vials

Indications and dosages

➢ Acute pulmonary edema

Adults: 40 mg I.V. given over 1 to 2 minutes. If adequate response does not occur within 1 hour, give 80 mg. I.V. over 1 to 2 minutes.

➢ Edema secondary to heart failure, cirrhosis of the liver, or renal disease

Adults: Usual initial I.V. dosage is 20 to 40 mg as a single injection; if response is inadequate, may increase second dose and each succeeding dose in 20-mg increments, given no more often than q 2 hours until desired diuretic response occurs. Then single dose may be given once or twice daily.

Off-label uses

- Hypercalcemia associated with cancer

Administration

Preparation

- Know that parenteral injection is given when patient requires rapid onset of diuresis or cannot receive oral doses.

Dilution and compatibility

- Know that drug may be given undiluted by direct I.V. injection.
- Although not usually given by I.V. infusion, drug may be diluted in D_5W, normal saline solution, or lactated Ringer's solution for high dose administration.
- Do not mix with highly acidic solutions (pH below 5.5).
- Do not use discolored solutions.

Infusion considerations

- Be aware that I.V. dose may be given slowly by direct injection over 1 to 2 minutes.

🔈 For controlled I.V. infusion, do not infuse faster than 4 mg/minute.

Monitoring

🔈 Assess for evidence of drug toxicity (ototoxicity, arrhythmias, renal dysfunction, abdominal pain, sore throat, fever).

- Monitor CBC and blood urea nitrogen (BUN), electrolyte, uric acid, and CO_2 levels.
- Monitor blood pressure, pulse, fluid intake and output, and weight.
- Monitor blood glucose levels in patients with diabetes mellitus.
- Monitor dietary potassium intake. Watch for signs and symptoms of hypokalemia.

Storage

- Store at room temperature of 15° to 30°C (59° to 86°F); protect from light.

Contraindications and precautions

Contraindicated in hypersensitivity to drug or other sulfonamides and in anuria.

Use cautiously in diabetes mellitus, severe renal or hepatic disease, gout, systemic lupus erythematosus, ***elderly patients,*** pregnant or breastfeeding patients, and ***neonates.***

Adverse reactions

CNS: dizziness, light-headedness, headache, vertigo, weakness, lethargy, paresthesia, drowsiness, restlessness

CV: hypotension, orthostatic hypotension, tachycardia, volume depletion, **necrotizing angiitis, thrombophlebitis, arrhythmias**

EENT: blurred vision, xanthopsia, hearing loss, tinnitus

GI: nausea, vomiting, diarrhea, constipation, dyspepsia, cramping, oral and gastric irritation, anorexia, dry mouth, **acute pancreatitis**

GU: excessive and frequent urination, nocturia, glycosuria, bladder spasm, **oliguria, interstitial nephritis**
Hematologic: anemia, purpura, **leukopenia, thrombocytopenia, hemolytic anemia**
Hepatic: jaundice
Metabolic: hyperglycemia, hyperuricemia, dehydration, hypokalemia, hypomagnesemia, hypocalcemia, **hypochloremic alkalosis**
Musculoskeletal: muscle pain or cramps
Skin: photosensitivity, rash, diaphoresis, urticaria, pruritus, exfoliative dermatitis, **erythema multiforme**
Other: fever

Interactions

Drug-drug. *Aminoglycosides, ethacrynic acid, other ototoxic drugs:* increased risk of ototoxicity
Amphotericin B, corticosteroids, corticotropin, potassium-wasting diuretics, stimulant laxatives: additive hypokalemia
Antihypertensives, diuretics, nitrates: additive hypotension
Cardiac glycosides: increased risk of glycoside toxicity and fatal arrhythmias
Clofibrate: exaggerated diuretic response, muscle pain and stiffness
Hydantoins, nonsteroidal anti-inflammatory drugs, probenecid: diuresis inhibition
Insulin, oral hypoglycemics: decreased hypoglycemic effect
Lithium: decreased excretion and possible toxicity of lithium
Norepinephrine: decreased arterial response to norepinephrine
Propranolol: increased propranolol blood level
Salicylates: increased risk of salicylate toxicity at lower-than-usual dosages
Succinylcholine: potentiation of succinylcholine effect
Sucralfate: decreased naturietic and antihypertensive effects of furosemide
Sulfonylureas: decreased glucose tolerance, resulting in hyperglycemia
Theophyllines: altered, enhanced, or inhibited theophylline effects
Tubocurarine: antagonism of tubocurarine effects
Drug-diagnostic tests. *BUN:* transient increase
Calcium, magnesium, platelets, potassium, sodium: decreased
Cholesterol, creatinine, glucose, nitrogenous compounds, uric acid: increased
Drug-herb. *Dandelion:* interference with diuretic effect
Ephedra (ma huang), ginseng: decreased furosemide efficacy
Licorice: rapid potassium loss
Drug-behaviors. *Acute alcohol ingestion:* additive hypotension
Sun exposure: increased risk of photosensitivity

Toxicity and overdose

- Overdose causes profound water loss with dehydration, volume and electrolyte depletion (leading to weakness, dizziness, mental confusion, lethargy, anorexia, vomiting, and muscle cramps), circulatory collapse, and possibly vascular thrombosis and embolism.
- Replace fluids and electrolytes with careful monitoring of urine output and serum and urine electrolyte levels. Provide supportive measures (including oxygen) and resuscitate as indicated and ordered.

Patient teaching

- Instruct patient to move slowly when rising, to avoid light-headedness or dizziness from sudden blood pressure decrease.
- Tell patient about the need for repeated laboratory testing during therapy.

• As appropriate, review all other significant and life-threatening adverse reactions and interactions, especially those related to the drugs, tests, herbs, and behaviors mentioned above.

gallium nitrate

Ganite

Pharmacologic class: Heavy metal
Therapeutic class: Calcium regulator
Pregnancy risk category C

FDA BOXED WARNING

• Concurrent use with other potentially nephrotoxic drugs (such as aminoglycosides or amphotericin B) may increase risk of severe renal insufficiency in patients with cancer-related hypercalcemia. If use of potentially nephrotoxic drug is indicated during gallium nitrate therapy, discontinue this drug and continue hydration for several days after administration of potentially nephrotoxic drug. Monitor serum creatinine level and urine output closely during and after this period. Discontinue gallium nitrate if serum creatinine level exceeds 2.5 mg/dL.

Action

Accumulates in metabolically active areas of high bone turnover and reversibly inhibits osteoclast-mediated bone resorption; reduces flow of calcium from resorbing bone into blood, effectively decreasing total and ionized serum calcium

Pharmacokinetics

Drug is significantly excreted by the kidneys. Plasma half-life depends on dosage.

Onset	Peak	Duration
Unknown	Unknown	Unknown

How supplied

Solution for injection (clear, colorless): 500 mg in 20-mL single-dose vial (25 mg/mL)

Indications and dosages

➤ Symptomatic cancer-related hypercalcemia
Adults: 200 mg/m^2 by I.V. infusion daily for 5 consecutive days

Dosage adjustment

• Reduce dosage in mild to moderate renal impairment based on serum creatinine clearance.
• Reduce dosage in patients with few symptoms and mild hypercalcemia.
• Discontinue drug when serum calcium level falls into normal range.

Off-label uses

• Bone metastasis
• Malignant lymphoma

Administration

Preparation

• Know that drug is intended for patients with symptomatic cancer-related hypercalcemia (nausea, vomiting, anorexia, constipation, dehydration, fatigue, muscle weakness, cardiac arrest, and coma) who have not responded adequately to hydration.
• Obtain baseline plasma pH and serum calcium (corrected for serum albumin), serum phosphorus, electrolyte, serum creatinine, and blood urea nitrogen (BUN) levels.

• Know that pretreatment urine output of 2 L/day is recommended.
• Ensure that patient is adequately hydrated before starting therapy—preferably using normal saline solution to promote renal excretion of calcium and correct dehydration.
• If underlying cancer is corticosteroid-sensitive, administer corticosteroid, as prescribed.

Dilution and compatibility
• Dilute single daily dose, preferably in normal saline solution or D_5W.
• Use less diluent if absolutely necessary in patients with compromised cardiovascular status.
• Administer single daily dose evenly distributed over 24 hours using microdrip or infusion pump.
Be aware that too-rapid infusion may lead to overdose.

Monitoring
• Continue to closely monitor plasma pH and serum calcium (corrected for serum albumin), serum phosphorus, electrolyte, serum creatinine, and BUN levels.
If hypocalcemia occurs, stop gallium nitrate and initiate short-term calcium therapy, as prescribed.
Observe frequently for signs and symptoms of fluid overload, especially in patients with cardiovascular compromise.

Storage
• Store at controlled room temperature of 20° to 25°C (68° to 77°F). When added to normal saline solution or D_5W, drug is stable for 48 hours at room temperature of 15° to 30°C (59° to 86°F), or for 7 days if refrigerated at 2° to 8°C (36° to 46°F).

Contraindications and precautions

Contraindicated in hypersensitivity to drug or severe renal impairment.

Use cautiously in renal impairment, mild to moderate hypocalcemia, concurrent use of other nephrotoxic drugs, ***elderly patients,*** pregnant or breastfeeding patients, and ***children*** (safety and efficacy not established).

Adverse reactions

CNS: confusion, dreams and hallucinations, lethargy, paresthesia
CV: asymptomatic blood pressure decrease
EENT: acute optic neuritis, hearing loss, tinnitus
GI: nausea, vomiting, diarrhea, constipation
GU: acute renal failure
Hematologic: anemia, leukopenia
Metabolic: hypocalcemia, hypophosphatemia, decreased serum bicarbonate
Respiratory: dyspnea, wheezing, rhonchi, **pleural effusion, pulmonary infiltrates, respiratory alkalosis**
Skin: rash
Other: edema of legs, fever, fluid overload, hypothermia

Interactions

Drug-drug. *Aminoglycosides, amphotericin B, other nephrotoxic drugs:* increased risk of renal insufficiency
Drug-diagnostic tests. *BUN, creatinine:* increased
Calcium, phosphate, serum bicarbonate: decreased

Toxicity and overdose

• Overdose may cause nausea, vomiting, anemia, hypocalcemia, hypophosphatemia, and acute renal failure.
• Discontinue drug, monitor serum calcium level, institute vigorous I.V. hydration, and monitor fluid intake and output for at least 2 days, as ordered. Know that patient may require oral phosphorus therapy for hypophosphatemia and red blood cell transfusion for anemia.

Patient teaching

Instruct patient to immediately report abdominal cramps, chills, confusion, fever, muscle spasms, sore throat, and any new symptoms.
- Inform patient that dietary calcium and vitamin D restrictions may be required.
- Teach patient about the need for strict measurements of fluid intake and output.
- Inform patient about the need for repeated laboratory testing during therapy.
- Advise patient to take prescribed medications only during drug therapy.
- Tell female to tell prescriber if she is pregnant.
- Advise breastfeeding patient to stop breastfeeding during therapy.
- As appropriate, review all other significant and life-threatening adverse reactions and interactions, especially those related to the drugs and tests mentioned above.

ganciclovir (DHPG)

Cymevene❄, Cytovene

Pharmacologic class: Acyclic purine nucleoside analogue of 2′-deoxyguanosine
Therapeutic class: Antiviral
Pregnancy risk category C

FDA BOXED WARNING

- Drug may lead to granulocytopenia, anemia, and thrombocytopenia. In animal studies, it was carcinogenic and teratogenic and caused aspermatogenesis.
- Drug is indicated only to treat cytomegalovirus (CMV) retinitis in immunocompromised patients and to prevent CMV disease in at-risk transplant patients.

Action

Inhibits binding of deoxyguanosine triphosphate to DNA polymerase by terminating DNA synthesis, thereby inhibiting viral replication

Pharmacokinetics

Drug distributes into cerebrospinal fluid in low concentrations. Plasma-protein binding is low. Half-life is approximately 4 hours. Approximately 91% of dose is eliminated renally, with no evidence of metabolites.

Onset	Peak	Duration
Unknown	Unknown	Unknown

How supplied

Powder for reconstitution for injection (lyophilized): 500 mg in 10-mL vials

Indications and dosages

➢ To prevent CMV disease in at-risk transplant recipients

Adults: 5 mg/kg I.V. q 12 hours for 7 to 14 days; then 5 mg/kg daily for 7 days per week or 6 mg/kg daily for 5 days per week

➢ CMV retinitis in immunocompromised patients

Adults: Initially, 5 mg/kg I.V. q 12 hours for 14 to 21 days, followed by maintenance dosage of 5 mg/kg/day for 7 days per week or 6 mg/kg for 5 days per week, followed by oral maintenance therapy

Dosage adjustment

- In renal impairment, reduce dosage as shown in table on the next page:

CrCl (mL/min)	Induction dosage	Maintenance dosage
70 or higher	5 mg/kg q 12 hr	5 mg/kg q 24 hr
50 to 69	2.5 mg/kg q 12 hr	2.5 mg/kg q 24 hr
25 to 49	2.5 mg/kg q 24 hr	1.25 mg/kg q 24 hr
10 to 24	1.25 mg/kg q 24 hr	0.625 mg/kg q 24 hr
Below 10	1.25 mg/kg three times weekly after hemodialysis	0.625 mg/kg three times weekly after hemodialysis

• In neutropenia, anemia, or thrombocytopenia, reduce dosage even more than shown in table. Do not give drug in severe neutropenia (absolute neutrophil count below 500/mm^3) or severe thrombocytopenia (platelets below 25,000/mm^3).

Off-label uses

• CMV gastroenteritis, CMV pneumonia, CMV colitis, or CMV hepatitis
• Epstein-Barr virus
• Hepatitis B

Administration

Preparation

Follow hazardous drug guidelines on page S19 for handling, preparation, and administration.
• Obtain CBC with white cell differential, platelet count, serum creatinine level, and creatinine clearance before starting therapy.
• Ensure adequate hydration before starting therapy.

Dilution and compatibility

• Reconstitute 500-mg vial with 10 mL sterile water for injection; shake vial to dissolve drug.
• Dilute further in one of the following I.V. solutions: normal saline, D_5W, lactated Ringer's, or Ringer's.
Do not use bacteriostatic water for injection; parabens in solution are incompatible with drug and may cause precipitation.
• If patient is on fluid restriction, dilute to a concentration of 10 mg/mL or less.
• Give I.V. solution within 24 hours of dilution to reduce risk of bacterial contamination.
• Do not use if solution is discolored.

Infusion considerations

Do not give by I.V. bolus or by I.M. or subcutaneous route.
• Administer into large vein with adequate blood flow to permit rapid dilution and distribution, which helps prevent phlebitis and pain at I.V. site.
Administer single dose by I.V. infusion slowly (over at least 1 hour) using infusion pump or microdrip (60 drops/mL).

Monitoring

• Continue to monitor CBC and platelet counts frequently.
• Monitor serum creatinine level and creatinine clearance carefully in patients with renal impairment.
• Assess fluid intake and output regularly to ensure adequate hydration.
• Make sure patient has regular ophthalmic examinations during both induction and maintenance therapy.
Monitor neurologic status closely; watch for seizures and coma.
Check for signs and symptoms of infection, particularly sepsis.

Storage

• Store vials below 40°C (104°F).
• Store reconstituted solution at room temperature for 12 hours. Do not refrigerate.

Contraindications and precautions

Contraindicated in hypersensitivity to drug or acyclovir.

Use cautiously in renal impairment, history of cytopenia or cytopenic reactions, neutropenia, thrombocytopenia, ***elderly patients***, pregnant or breastfeeding patients, and ***children*** (safety and efficacy not established).

Adverse reactions

CNS: ataxia, confusion, dizziness, headache, drowsiness, tremor, abnormal thinking, agitation, amnesia, neuropathy, paresthesia, **seizures, coma**
CV: hypertension, hypotension, phlebitis, **arrhythmias**
GI: nausea, vomiting, diarrhea, abdominal pain, dyspepsia, flatulence, anorexia, dry mouth
Hematologic: anemia, **agranulocytosis, thrombocytopenia, leukopenia**
Respiratory: pneumonia
Skin: rash, diaphoresis, pruritus, dry skin, alopecia
Other: fever; infection; chills; inflammation, pain, and phlebitis at injection site; **sepsis**

Interactions

Drug-drug. *Amphotericin B, cyclosporine, other nephrotoxic drugs:* increased risk of renal impairment and ganciclovir toxicity
Cilastatin, imipenem: increased seizure activity
Cytotoxic drugs: increased toxic effects
Immunosuppressants: increased immunosuppression and bone marrow depression
Probenecid: increased ganciclovir blood level
Zidovudine: increased risk of agranulocytosis
Drug-diagnostic tests. *Alanine aminotransferase, alkaline phosphatase, aspartate aminotransferase, creatinine, gamma-glutamyltransferase:* increased
Creatinine clearance, granulocytes, hemoglobin, neutrophils, platelets, white blood cells: decreased
Liver function tests: abnormal results

Toxicity and overdose

- Overdose may lead to GI symptoms, irreversible pancytopenia, acute renal failure, persistent bone marrow suppression, reversible neutropenia or granulocytopenia, hepatitis, renal toxicity, and seizures.
- Maintain adequate hydration. Hematopoietic factors and hemodialysis may be needed to reduce serum drug level.

Patient teaching

[Clinical alert] Advise patient to report signs and symptoms of infection, including those at infusion site.
- Instruct patient to avoid driving and other hazardous activities until drug's effects on concentration and alertness are known.
- Inform patient that drug may cause birth defects. Advise females to use effective birth control during therapy; advise males to use barrier contraception during therapy and for 90 days afterward.
- Advise patient to minimize GI upset by eating frequent, small servings of healthy food.
- Inform patient about the need for repeated laboratory testing during therapy.
- Explain that drug does not cure CMV retinitis and that patient should have eye exams every 4 to 6 weeks during therapy.
- As appropriate, review all other significant and life-threatening adverse reactions and interactions, especially those related to the drugs and tests mentioned above.

gemcitabine hydrochloride

Gemzar

Pharmacologic class: Antimetabolite, pyrimidine nucleoside analogue
Therapeutic class: Antineoplastic
Pregnancy risk category D

Action

Kills malignant cells undergoing DNA synthesis; arrests progression of cells at S phase and G1/S phase border

Pharmacokinetics

Drug does not extensively distribute into tissues after short I.V. infusion. It is largely metabolized, with negligible protein binding. Half-life ranges from 42 to 94 minutes for short infusion and 245 to 638 minutes for long infusion (depending on age and gender). Clearance is lower in females and elderly patients, leading to increased concentrations. Small amount is excreted unchanged in urine.

Onset	Peak	Duration
Unknown	Unknown	Unknown

How supplied

Powder for reconstitution for injection (white, lyophilized): 200 mg (10-mL single-use vial) or 1 g (50-mL single-use vial)

Indications and dosages

➢ Monotherapy for locally advanced (nonresectable stage II or III) or metastatic (stage IV) adenocarcinoma of pancreas in patients previously treated with fluorouracil
Adults: 1,000 mg/m^2 I.V. q week for 7 weeks, followed by 1 week of rest. May continue with cycles of once-weekly administration for 3 weeks, followed by 1 week of rest.

➢ Inoperable, locally advanced (stage IIIA or IIIB) or metastatic (stage IV) non-small-cell lung cancer (in combination with cisplatin)
Adults: 1,000 mg/m^2 I.V. on days 1, 8, and 15 of each 28-day cycle, with cisplatin given on day 1 after gemcitabine; or 1,250 mg/m^2 on days 1 and 8 of each 21-day cycle, with cisplatin given on day 1 after gemcitabine

➢ Breast cancer (in combination with paclitaxel after failure of anthracycline-containing adjuvant chemotherapy, unless anthracyclines were contraindicated)
Adults: 1,250 mg/m^2 I.V. on days 1 and 8 of each 21-day cycle, with paclitaxel given on day 1 before gemcitabine

➢ Advanced ovarian cancer in combination with carboplatin for patients who relapsed at least 6 months after platinum-based therapy
Adults: 1,000 mg/m^2 I.V. on days 1 and 8 of each 21-day cycle, plus carboplatin I.V. on day 1 after gemcitabine

Dosage adjustment

- Increase dosage by 25% in patients who complete entire cycle of therapy, provided absolute granulocyte count (AGC) and platelet nadirs exceed 1,500 × 10^6/L and 100,000 × 10^6/L, respectively, and nonhematologic toxicity does not exceed World Health Organization (WHO) Grade 1. If patient tolerates subsequent course at increased dosage, dosage for next cycle can be further increased by 20%, provided AGC and platelet nadirs exceed 1,500 × 10^6/L and 100,000 × 10^6/L, respectively, and nonhematologic toxicity does not exceed WHO Grade 1.
- In pancreatic cancer therapy, if bone marrow suppression occurs, modify

dosage or withhold dose based on degree of hematologic toxicity, according to guidelines below:

Pancreatic cancer therapy

AGC ($\times 10^6$/L)	and/ or	Platelet count ($\times 10^6$/L)	% of full dosage to give
1,000 or higher	and	100,000 or higher	100%
500 to 999	or	50,000 to 99,000	75%
Below 500	or	Below 50,000	Withhold dose

• In non-small-cell lung cancer therapy, adjust gemcitabine and cisplatin dosages for hematologic toxicity. Base gemcitabine adjustment on AGC and platelet counts taken on day of therapy. If marrow suppression is detected, modify or suspend therapy according to guidelines given in breast cancer table (below). For Grade 3 or 4 nonhematologic toxicity (except alopecia, nausea, or vomiting), withhold dose or decrease gemcitabine and cisplatin dosages by 50%.

• In breast cancer therapy, adjust gemcitabine dosage for hematologic toxicity based on AGC and platelet counts taken on day 8 of therapy. For Grade 3 or 4 nonhematologic toxicity (except alopecia, nausea, or vomiting), withhold dose or decrease gemcitabine dosage by 50% and follow manufacturer's guidelines for paclitaxel adjustment. If bone marrow suppression occurs, modify dosage or withhold dose based on degree of hematologic toxicity, according to guidelines below.

Breast cancer therapy

AGC ($\times 10^6$/L)	and/ or	Platelet count ($\times 10^6$/L)	% of full dosage to give
1,200 or higher	and	Above 75,000	100%
1,000 to 1,199	or	50,000 to 75,000	75%
700 to 999	and	50,000 or more	50%
Below 700	or	Above 50,000	Withhold dose

G

• In ovarian cancer therapy, AGC should be 1,500 × 10^6/L or higher and platelet count should be 100,000 × 10^6/L before each cycle. Adjust dosage for hematologic toxicity within treatment cycle based on AGC and platelet counts taken on day 8 of therapy. For Grade 3 or 4 nonhematologic toxicity (except alopecia, nausea, or vomiting), withhold gemcitabine dose or decrease dosage 50% and follow manufacturer's guidelines for carboplatin adjustment. If marrow suppression occurs, modify gemcitabine dosage on day 8 according to guidelines shown below.

Ovarian cancer therapy

AGC ($\times 10^6$/L)	and/ or	Platelet count ($\times 10^6$/L)	% of full dosage to give
1,500 or higher	and	100,000 or higher	100%
1,000 to 1,499	and/ or	75,000 to 99,999	50%
Below 1,000	and/ or	Below 75,000	Withhold dose

• For gemcitabine given in combination with carboplatin for subsequent cycles, base dosage adjustment on observed toxicity. In subsequent cycles, reduce gemcitabine dosage to 800 mg/m² on days 1 and 8 if any of the following hematologic toxicities occurs: AGC below 500 × 10^6/L for more than 5 days; AGC below 100 × 10^6/L for more than 3 days; febrile neutropenia; platelet count below 25,000 × 10^6/L; cycle delay of more than 1 week due to toxicity. If any of these toxicities recurs after initial dosage reduction, give gemcitabine on day 1 only at 800 mg/m² for subsequent cycle.

Off-label uses

- Advanced or relapsed epithelial ovarian carcinoma
- Cervical cancer
- Head and neck cancer
- Hodgkin's or non-Hodgkin's lymphoma
- Kaposi's sarcoma (classic)
- Locally advanced, unresectable, or metastatic biliary tract or gallbladder carcinoma
- Metastatic bladder carcinoma
- Relapsed, refractory, progressive, metastatic, or nonseminomatous gonadal and extragonadal germ-cell tumors

Administration

Preparation

Follow hazardous drug guidelines on page S19 for handling, preparation, and administration.

- Obtain CBC with differential (particularly neutrophil and platelet counts) and renal and hepatic function tests before each dose.

Dilution and compatibility

- Reconstitute by adding 5 mL normal saline solution to 200-mg vial or adding 25 mL normal saline solution to 1-g vial. Shake to dissolve.
- Know that these dilutions each yield drug concentration of 38 mg/mL. Do not reconstitute at concentrations greater than 40 mg/mL.
- Be aware that complete withdrawal of vial contents provides 200 mg or 1 g of gemcitabine, respectively.
- Administer as prepared, or further dilute with normal saline solution to concentration as low as 0.1 mg/mL.
- Know that reconstituted drug is a clear, colorless to light straw-colored solution.
- Discard unused portion of drug.

Infusion considerations

- Give by I.V. infusion over 30 minutes.
- Know that infusion time beyond 60 minutes and dosing more often than weekly increase toxicity.

Monitoring

Stop infusion and notify prescriber immediately if patient develops signs or symptoms of allergic reaction.

Continue to monitor CBC with white cell differential and platelet count. Suspend or modify therapy according to dosage adjustment guidelines given above when bone marrow suppression is detected.

Watch for signs and symptoms of infection and bleeding tendencies, even after therapy ends.

- Monitor temperature, especially during first 12 hours of therapy.
- Evaluate respiratory status regularly.
- Monitor renal and hepatic function periodically.

Storage

- Store powder at room temperature of 20° to 25°C (68° to 77°F).
- Know that solution is stable for 24 hours at controlled room temperature of 20° to 25°C (68° to 77°F). Do not refrigerate reconstituted solutions, as crystallization may occur.

Contraindications and precautions

Contraindicated in hypersensitivity to drug.

Use cautiously in significant renal or hepatic impairment, concurrent radiation therapy, females of childbearing potential, pregnant or breastfeeding patients, and ***children*** (safety and efficacy not established).

Adverse reactions

CNS: paresthesia
GI: nausea, vomiting, diarrhea, stomatitis
GU: hematuria, proteinuria, **hemolytic uremic syndrome, renal failure**
Hematologic: anemia, **leukopenia, thrombocytopenia**
Respiratory: dyspnea, **bronchospasm**
Skin: alopecia, rash, cellulitis
Other: flulike symptoms, fever, edema, injection site reactions, **anaphylactoid reactions**

Interactions

Drug-drug. *Live-virus vaccines:* decreased antibody response to vaccine, increased risk of adverse reactions
Other antineoplastics: additive bone marrow depression
Drug-diagnostic tests. *Alanine aminotransferase, alkaline phosphatase, aspartate aminotransferase, bilirubin:* transient increases
Blood urea nitrogen, serum creatinine: increased

Toxicity and overdose

- In overdose, main toxicities are myelosuppression, paresthesia, and severe rash.
- No known antidote exists. Monitor CBC with differential and platelet counts, and provide symptomatic and supportive therapy.

Patient education

Instruct patient to immediately report signs or symptoms of allergic reaction.
Advise patient to watch for and immediately report signs or symptoms of infection (especially flulike symptoms).
Instruct patient to report unusual bleeding or bruising, change in urination pattern, or difficulty breathing.
- Advise patient to avoid crowds and exposure to infection.
- Caution patient to avoid driving and other hazardous activities until drug's effects on concentration and alertness are known.
- Advise patient to avoid activities that can cause injury and to use soft toothbrush and electric razor to avoid gum and skin injury.
- Tell patient to minimize GI upset by eating frequent, small servings of healthy food.
- Inform patient about the need for repeated laboratory testing during therapy.
- Advise women of childbearing potential to use adequate birth control.
- Advise breastfeeding patient not to breastfeed during therapy.
- As appropriate, review all other significant and life-threatening adverse reactions and interactions, especially those related to the drugs and tests mentioned above.

gemtuzumab ozogamicin

Mylotarg

Pharmacologic class: Monoclonal antibody
Therapeutic class: Antineoplastic
Pregnancy risk category D

FDA BOXED WARNING

- Give under supervision of physician experienced in cancer chemotherapy, in facility equipped to monitor and treat leukemia patients.

• No controlled trials have shown that drug is safe and effective when used in combination with other chemotherapeutic agents. Use only as single-agent chemotherapy and not in combination chemotherapy regimens (outside clinical trials).
• Severe myelosuppression occurs when drug is used at recommended dosages.
• Drug can cause severe hypersensitivity reactions (including anaphylaxis) and other infusion-related reactions, which may include severe pulmonary events. In rare cases, hypersensitivity reactions and pulmonary events have been fatal. Usually, infusion-related symptoms arise during or within 24 hours after infusion, and subsequently resolve. Interrupt infusion if patient experiences dyspnea or clinically significant hypotension. Monitor patient until signs and symptoms resolve completely. Strongly consider withdrawing drug if patient develops anaphylaxis, pulmonary edema, or acute respiratory distress syndrome. Patients with high peripheral blast counts may be at greater risk for pulmonary events and tumor lysis syndrome; therefore, physicians should consider leukoreduction with hydroxyurea or leukapheresis to reduce peripheral white blood cell (WBC) count below 30,000/mm^3 before gemtuzumab administration.
• Hepatotoxicity, including severe hepatic veno-occlusive disease (VOD), has occurred when drug was used as a single agent or as part of combination chemotherapy and in patients without history of hepatic disease or hematopoietic stem-cell transplant (HSCT). Patients who receive drug before or after HSCT, those with underlying hepatic disease or abnormal hepatic function, and those receiving drug in combination with other chemotherapeutic agents are at increased risk for developing VOD. Death from hepatic failure or VOD has occurred in patients who received drug. Monitor patient carefully for signs and symptoms of hepatotoxicity, particularly VOD (including rapid weight gain, right upper quadrant pain, hepatomegaly, ascites, and bilirubin and/or liver enzyme elevations). However, know that careful monitoring may not identify all at-risk patients or prevent complications of hepatotoxicity.

Action

Binds to CD33 antigen on surface of leukemic blasts, leading to formation of complex that is internalized by cell. Derivative is released inside myeloid cell lysosomes and binds to DNA, causing DNA double-strand breakage and cell death.

Pharmacokinetics

Drug is metabolized in the liver and crosses placental barrier.

Onset	Peak	Duration
Unknown	Unknown	Unknown

How supplied

Powder for reconstitution for injection (lyophilized): 5 mg in 20-mL single-use vial

Indications and dosages

➤ CD33-positive acute myeloid leukemia in first relapse in patients age 60 or older who are not eligible for cytotoxic chemotherapy
Adults: 9 mg/m^2 I.V. infusion over 2 hours given q 14 days for two doses

Administration

Preparation

Follow hazardous drug guidelines on page S19 for handling, preparation, and administration.

• Know that second dose can be given even if patient has not recovered fully from hematologic toxicities.
• To reduce risk of infusion reactions (fever, chills, and possibly hypotension and dyspnea), give diphenhydramine and acetaminophen 1 hour before gemtuzumab, as prescribed.

Dilution and compatibility
• Protect drug from direct and indirect sunlight and unshielded fluorescent light when preparing and administering infusion.
• Allow drug to come to room temperature before reconstituting.
• Reconstitute vial contents with 5 mL sterile water for injection; swirl vial gently. Final concentration is 1 mg/mL.
• Further dilute by injecting drug into 100-mL bag of normal saline solution. Place 100-mL bag into ultraviolet protectant bag; use resulting solution immediately.

Infusion considerations
Do not administer by I.V. push or bolus.
• Give by I.V. infusion over 2 hours through separate peripheral or central I.V. line using low-protein-binding 1.2-micron terminal filter.
• Monitor vital signs during infusion and for 4 hours afterward.

Monitoring
• Closely monitor CBC and platelet count daily for 14 days or until neutrophil and platelets recover.
Monitor patient carefully for signs and symptoms of hepatotoxicity—particularly those of VOD, such as rapid weight gain, right upper quadrant pain, hepatomegaly, ascites, and bilirubin and liver enzyme elevations.
Watch for postinfusion reaction for up to 24 hours after infusion; interrupt infusion if dyspnea or significant hypotension occurs. To reduce these reactions, give additional acetaminophen every 4 hours as needed and ordered.
• Monitor electrolyte levels and liver function tests results.

Storage
• Refrigerate at 2° to 8°C (36° to 46°F); protect from light.
• Refrigerate reconstituted drug in vial at 2° to 8°C (36° to 46°F) for up to 8 hours; protect from light.

G

Contraindications and precautions

Contraindicated in hypersensitivity to drug or its components.

Use cautiously in hepatic impairment, pregnant or breastfeeding patients, and ***children*** (safety and efficacy not established).

Adverse reactions

CNS: headache, asthenia, **cerebral hemorrhage**
CV: hypotension, hypertension
EENT: epistaxis
GI: diarrhea, nausea, vomiting, abdominal pain, stomatitis
Hematologic: severe myelosuppression (neutropenia, anemia, thrombocytopenia), disseminated intravascular coagulation
Hepatic: hepatotoxicity (including **severe VOD**)
Skin: rash, pruritus, cutaneous herpes simplex
Other: tumor lysis syndrome, postinfusion reactions (fever, chills, nausea, vomiting, headache, dyspnea, hypoxia, hypotension, hypertension, hyperglycemia), **sepsis**

Interactions

Drug/diagnostic tests. *Alanine aminotransferase, aspartate aminotransferase, bilirubin:* increased
Hematocrit, hemoglobin, platelets, potassium, magnesium, WBCs: decreased

Toxicity and overdose

- No cases of overdose have been reported.
- Provide supportive measures and carefully monitor blood pressure and blood counts. Dialysis does not remove drug.

Patient teaching

🔊 Instruct patient to promptly report unusual bruising or bleeding and signs and symptoms of infection.

- Advise patient to avoid crowds, exposure to infection, and persons who have recently received live-virus vaccines.
- Teach patient to minimize GI upset by eating frequent, small servings of healthy food.
- Inform patient about the need for repeated laboratory testing during therapy.
- Advise women of childbearing potential to use adequate birth control.
- Tell breastfeeding patient not to breastfeed during therapy.
- As appropriate, review all other significant and life-threatening adverse reactions and interactions, especially those related to the tests mentioned above.

gentamicin sulfate

Cidomycin🍁❉, Genticin❉

Pharmacologic class: Aminoglycoside
Therapeutic class: Anti-infective
Pregnancy risk category D

FDA BOXED WARNING

- Observe patient closely for potential ototoxicity and nephrotoxicity. Safety in therapy exceeding 14 days has not been established.
- Neuromuscular blockade and respiratory paralysis have occurred after administration.
- Monitor renal function and eighth-nerve function closely, especially in patients with known or suspected renal impairment at onset of therapy, as well as those with initially normal renal function who develop signs of renal dysfunction during therapy.
- Avoid concurrent use with potent diuretics (such as furosemide or ethacrynic acid), as diuretics may cause ototoxicity. Also, I.V. diuretics may increase gentamicin toxicity by altering antibiotic serum and tissue levels.
- Avoid concurrent and sequential systemic, oral, or topical use of other neurotoxic or nephrotoxic agents and other aminoglycosides. Advanced age and dehydration also may increase toxicity risk.
- Drug may harm fetus when given to pregnant women.

Action

Kills gram-negative bacteria by irreversibly binding to 30S subunit of bacterial ribosomes and blocking protein synthesis, leading to misreading of genetic code and separation of ribosomes from messenger RNA

Pharmacokinetics

Drug distributes well throughout all body fluids, accumulates in serum and tissues, and crosses placental barrier.

Metabolic transformation is minimal; protein binding is low. Half-life varies with patient age and renal function. Drug is excreted renally, principally by glomerular filtration; clearance is slower in patients with impaired renal function.

Onset	Peak	Duration
Immediate	30-90 min	6 to 8 hr

How supplied

Solution for infusion (clear): 40 mg, 60 mg, 70 mg, 80 mg, 90 mg, 100 mg, and 120 mg premixed in flexible containers
Solution for injection (clear): 40 mg/mL (adult) in 2-mL and 20-mL vials and 1.5-mL and 2-mL cartridge needle units; 10 mg/mL (pediatric) in ADD-Vantage 60-mg, 80-mg, 100-mg, and 2-mL vials

Indications and dosages

➢ Serious infections caused by *Pseudomonas aeruginosa, Escherichia coli,* and *Proteus, Klebsiella, Serratia, Enterobacter, Citrobacter,* and *Staphylococcus* species and susceptible gram-negative organisms
Adults: 3 mg/kg daily in three divided doses by I.V. infusion q 8 hours. For life-threatening infections, up to 5 mg/kg/day in three to four divided doses; reduce dosage to 3 mg/kg/day as indicated.
Children: 2 to 2.5 mg/kg q 8 hours by I.V. infusion
Infants older than 1 week: 2.5 mg/kg q 8 hours by I.V. infusion
Neonates younger than 1 week, preterm infants: 2.5 mg/kg q 12 hours by I.V. infusion. In preterm infants of less than 32 weeks' gestational age, 2.5 mg/kg q 18 hours or 3 mg/kg q 24 hours may produce satisfactory peak and trough blood levels.
➢ Endocarditis prophylaxis before surgery
Adults: 1.5 mg/kg I.V. 30 minutes before surgery, to a maximum dosage of 80 mg. Give with ampicillin or vancomycin, as prescribed.
Children: 2 mg/kg I.V. 30 minutes before surgery, to a maximum dosage of 80 mg

Dosage adjustment

- In renal impairment, adjust dosage or dosing intervals.

Off-label uses

- Pelvic inflammatory disease

Administration

Preparation
- Before starting therapy, obtain specimens as needed for culture and sensitivity testing.
- Give cephalosporin or parenteral penicillin 1 hour before or after gentamicin, as prescribed.
- Ensure that patient is well hydrated during treatment.

Dilution and compatibility
- For I.V. infusion, dilute vial with 50 to 200 mL D_5W or normal saline solution.
- Be aware that drug is available premixed in several concentrations.
- Do not mix with other drugs.

Infusion considerations
- Administer I.V. over 30 minutes to 2 hours.
- After infusion, flush line with normal saline or D_5W.

Do not use plastic containers in series connections. Such use could result in air embolism due to residual air being drawn from primary container before administration of fluid from secondary container ends.

Monitoring
- Obtain peak drug blood level 30 minutes after 30-minute infusion; obtain trough level within 30 minutes of next scheduled dose.
- Watch for signs and symptoms of hypersensitivity reactions.

Know that blood drug level monitoring is especially important in therapy lasting more than 5 days, acute or chronic renal impairment, extracellular fluid volume changes, obesity, infants younger than 3 months, concomitant use of nephrotoxic drugs, patients requiring higher dosages or dosage-interval adjustments (such as those with cystic fibrosis, endocarditis, or critical illness), and

patients with signs or symptoms of nephrotoxicity or ototoxicity.
• Assess fluid intake and output, urine specific gravity, and urinalysis for signs of nephrotoxicity.
• Monitor CBC, blood urea nitrogen (BUN), creatinine level, and creatinine clearance.
• Weigh patient regularly.
• Assess for signs and symptoms of ototoxicity (hearing loss, tinnitus, ataxia, vertigo).

Storage

• Store at controlled room temperature of 15° to 30°C (59° to 86°F).

Contraindications and precautions

Contraindicated in hypersensitivity to drug or other aminoglycosides.

Use cautiously in neuromuscular disease, renal impairment, hearing impairment, sulfite sensitivity, obesity, ***elderly patients,*** pregnant or breastfeeding patients, ***infants, neonates, and premature infants.***

Adverse reactions

CNS: dizziness, vertigo, tremors, numbness, depression, confusion, lethargy, headache, paresthesia, ataxia, peripheral neuropathy, **encephalopathy, neuromuscular blockade, seizures, neurotoxicity**
CV: hypotension, hypertension, palpitations
EENT: visual disturbances, dry eyes, nystagmus, photophobia, ototoxicity, hearing loss, tinnitus
GI: nausea, vomiting, stomatitis, increased salivation, splenomegaly, anorexia
GU: increased urinary casts, polyuria, dysuria, oliguria, azotemia, erectile dysfunction, **nephrotoxicity**
Hematologic: eosinophilia, **leukemoid reaction, hemolytic anemia, aplastic anemia, neutropenia, agranulocytosis, leukopenia, thrombocytopenia, pancytopenia**
Hepatic: hepatomegaly, hepatotoxicity, hepatic necrosis
Musculoskeletal: joint pain, muscle twitching
Respiratory: apnea
Skin: exfoliative dermatitis, rash, pruritus, urticaria, purpura, alopecia
Other: weight loss, superinfection, injection site pain

Interactions

Drug-drug. *Acyclovir, amphotericin B, carboplatin, cephalosporins, cisplatin, loop diuretics, other ototoxic or nephrotoxic drugs, vancomycin:* increased risk of ototoxicity and nephrotoxicity
Dimenhydrinate, other antiemetics: masking of ototoxicity symptoms
General anesthetics, neuromuscular blockers: increased activity of these drugs
Indomethacin: increased gentamicin peak and trough levels
Penicillins (such as ampicillin, ticarcillin): synergistic effect
Tacrolimus: nephrotoxicity
Drug-diagnostic tests. *Alanine aminotransferase, aspartate aminotransferase, bilirubin, BUN, creatinine, lactate dehydrogenase:* increased
Granulocytes, hemoglobin, platelets, white blood cells: decreased
Reticulocytes: increased or decreased

Toxicity and overdose

• In overdose, nephrotoxicity, ototoxicity, neuromuscular blockade, or respiratory paralysis may occur.
• Establish airway and ensure oxygenation and ventilation. Provide adequate hydration, as ordered, and carefully monitor fluid balance. Hemodialysis may reduce drug blood levels. In newborns, exchange transfusions may be considered. Resuscitate as indicated.

Patient teaching

Teach patient to recognize and immediately report signs and symptoms of hypersensitivity reaction, infection, unusual tiredness, yellowing of skin or eyes, or muscle twitching.
- Advise patient to report signs and symptoms of ototoxicity (hearing loss, ringing in ears, vertigo).
- Instruct patient to drink plenty of fluids to ensure adequate urine output.
- Teach patient to monitor urine output and report significant changes.
- Caution patient to avoid driving and other hazardous activities until drug's effects on concentration and alertness are known.
- As appropriate, review all other significant and life-threatening adverse reactions and interactions, especially those related to the drugs and tests mentioned above.

[redacted]

glucagon

GlucaGen, GlucaGen Diagnostic Kit, Glucagon Emergency Kit

Pharmacologic class: Antihypoglycemic
Therapeutic class: Insulin antagonist
Pregnancy risk category B

Action

Increases blood glucose concentration by converting glycogen in the liver to glucose. Also relaxes GI smooth muscle.

Pharmacokinetics

Drug is extensively degraded in the liver and kidneys. Plasma half-life is up to 18 minutes.

Onset	Peak	Duration
10 min	30 min	60-90 min

How supplied

Powder for reconstitution for injection: 1-mg vials in disposable syringes with 1 mL of diluent
Solution for injection: 1-mg syringes

Indications and dosages

➤ Hypoglycemia
Adults and children weighing more than 20 kg (44 lb): 1 mg I.V.
Children weighing 20 kg or less: 20 to 30 mcg/kg or 0.5-mg dose I.V.
➤ Diagnostic aid for radiologic examination
Adults: 0.25 to 2 mg I.V. before radiologic procedure

Administration

Preparation

Except when used as diagnostic aid, give drug only in hypoglycemic emergencies to patients with diabetes mellitus.

Dilution and compatibility
- Mix drug in 1-mg vial with 1 mL diluent supplied by manufacturer.
- For diagnostic use, dilute doses above 2 mg with sterile water for injection.
- Do not use in concentrations greater than 1 mg/mL (1 unit/mL).
- Use drug immediately; discard unused portion.
- Use reconstituted solution only if clear, with waterlike consistency.

Infusion considerations
- For I.V. injection, give 1 mg over 1 minute.

Monitoring

If patient does not respond within 15 minutes, give I.V. glucose, as ordered.
- When patient is alert and able to swallow, provide carbohydrate-rich food.
- Closely monitor blood glucose level.
- Monitor patient for aspiration.

• Assess blood pressure, electrolyte levels, and respiratory status.

Storage

• Store vials or syringes at room temperature of 15° to 30°C (59° to 86°F).

Contraindications and precautions

Contraindicated in hypersensitivity to drug, pheochromocytoma, or insulinoma.

Use cautiously in cardiac disease, adrenal insufficiency, chronic hypoglycemia, prolonged fasting, history suggesting insulinoma or pheochromocytoma, ***elderly patients,*** and pregnant or breastfeeding patients.

Adverse reactions

CV: hypotension
GI: nausea, vomiting
Metabolic: hypokalemia (with overdose)
Respiratory: bronchospasm, respiratory distress
Skin: urticaria, rash

Interactions

Drug-drug. *Anticoagulants:* enhanced anticoagulant effect
Drug-diagnostic tests. *Potassium:* decreased

Toxicity and overdose

• Overdose signs and symptoms include nausea, vomiting, diarrhea, gastric hypotonicity, and possibly hypokalemia and transient rise in blood pressure and pulse.
• Because of drug's short half-life, symptomatic treatment is adequate.

Patient teaching

• Teach patient and family members proper technique and timing for using this emergency drug.
Emphasize importance of contacting prescriber right away if hypoglycemic emergency occurs.
Instruct caregiver or family member to arouse patient immediately and give additional carbohydrate by mouth as soon as patient can tolerate it.
• As appropriate, review all other significant and life-threatening adverse reactions and interactions, especially those related to the drugs and tests mentioned above.

[redacted]

glycopyrrolate, glycopyrronium

Robinul

Pharmacologic class: Anticholinergic
Therapeutic class: Antispasmodic, antimuscarinic, parasympatholytic
Pregnancy risk category B

Action

Inhibits action of acetylcholine on structures innervated by postganglionic cholinergic nerves and on smooth muscles that respond to acetylcholine but lack cholinergic innervation. This inhibition diminishes volume and free acidity of gastric secretions and controls excessive pharyngeal, tracheal, and bronchial secretions.

Pharmacokinetics

After I.V. administration of 0.2-mg drug, 85% of dose was recovered in urine 48 hours later; some radioactivity also was recovered in bile. Renal failure severely impairs elimination.

Onset	Peak	Duration
1 min	Unknown	3-7 hr

How supplied

Solution for injection: 0.2 mg/mL in 1-mL single-dose vials, 2-mL single-dose vials,

5-mL multidose vials, and 20-mL multidose vials

Indications and dosages

➢ Adjunct therapy in peptic ulcer disorders

Adults: 0.1 mg I.V. q 4 hours up to three or four times daily; for more profound effect, may give 0.2 mg. Patient response should guide dosing frequency, to a maximum of four times daily; some patients may need only one dose.

➢ To diminish or block cholinergic effects caused by anticholinesterase agents

Adults and children: Recommended dosage is 0.2 mg for each 1 mg of neostigmine or 5 mg of pyridostigmine.

Administration

Preparation

Keep resuscitation equipment on hand to treat curare-like effects (neuromuscular blockade leading to muscle weakness and possible paralysis).

Be aware that drug is not intended for neonates because it contains benzyl alcohol.

Dilution and compatibility

- Be aware that drug may be given undiluted.
- Know that drug is compatible with dextrose 5% and 10% in water, dextrose 5% and 10% in normal saline solution, dextrose 5% in half-normal saline solution, and Ringer's solution.
- Be aware that drug is not compatible with lactated Ringer's solution.
- Do not use if discolored.

Infusion considerations

- Give each 0.2 mg over 1 to 2 minutes.
- When administering to diminish or block cholinergic effects of anticholinesterase, glycopyrrolate and anticholinesterase may be given simultaneously by I.V. injection and may be mixed in same syringe.

Monitoring

Check for signs and symptoms of anaphylaxis and malignant hyperthermia.

Monitor closely for curare-like effects (muscle weakness and possible paralysis) caused by overdose.

- Monitor neurologic and cardiovascular status.
- Assess fluid intake and output. Have patient void before each dose to avoid urine retention.

Storage

- Store at controlled room temperature of 20° to 25°C (68° to 77°F).

Contraindications and precautions

Contraindicated in hypersensitivity to drug or its components, glaucoma, obstructive uropathy, GI obstructive disease, paralytic ileus, unstable cardiovascular status in acute hemorrhage, severe ulcerative colitis, toxic megacolon complicating ulcerative colitis, intestinal atony in elderly or debilitated patients, and myasthenia gravis (when used to manage peptic ulcer patients).

Use cautiously in cardiovascular disease, heart failure, arrhythmias, hypertension, asthma, renal or hepatic disease, Down syndrome, hyperthyroidism, hiatal hernia, ulcerative colitis, mild to moderate prostatic hypertrophy, autonomic neuropathy, spasticity, suspected brain damage, cyclopropane anesthesia, high environmental temperatures, ***elderly patients,*** pregnant or breastfeeding patients, and ***children younger than age 12*** (safety and efficacy not established in peptic ulcer management).

Adverse reactions

CNS: weakness, nervousness, insomnia, drowsiness, dizziness, headache, confusion, excitement

CV: palpitations, tachycardia

G

EENT: blurred vision, photophobia, mydriasis, increased intraocular pressure, cycloplegia
GI: nausea, vomiting, constipation, abdominal distention, epigastric distress, heartburn, gastroesophageal reflux, dry mouth, **paralytic ileus**
GU: urinary hesitancy, urine retention, lactation suppression, erectile dysfunction
Skin: urticaria, decreased sweating or anhidrosis
Other: taste loss, fever, allergic reaction, **anaphylaxis, malignant hyperthermia**

Interactions

Drug-drug. *Amantadine, antihistamines, antiparkinsonian drugs, disopyramide, glutethimide, meperidine, phenothiazines, procainamide, quinidine, tricyclic antidepressants:* additive anticholinergic effects
Cyclopropane anesthesia: ventricular arrhythmias

Toxicity and overdose

- In overdose, expect curare-like effects and CNS signs and symptoms, including excitement, restlessness, seizures, and psychotic behavior. Hypotension and fever also may occur.
- If patient experiences curare-like effect on respiratory muscles, institute artificial respiration as ordered, and maintain it until effective respiratory action returns. With close monitoring for decreased heart rate and return of bowel sounds, neostigmine 0.25 mg I.V. may be given to adults to counteract anticholinergic effects, with doses repeated every 5 to 10 minutes until anticholinergic overactivity reverses (or up to a maximum of 2.5 mg is given). For adults, administer physostigmine 0.5 to 2 mg I.V. slowly, and repeat as needed to a total of 5 mg to counteract CNS effects. Use smaller neostigmine and physostigmine dosages in children. For hypotension, expect to provide I.V. fluids, pressor agents, and supportive care. For fever, provide symptomatic therapy.

Patient teaching

- Instruct patient to immediately report signs and symptoms of serious adverse effects, especially anaphylaxis.
- Caution patient to avoid driving and other hazardous activities until drug's effects on concentration, vision, and alertness are known.
- Advise patient to report urinary hesitancy or urine retention.
- As appropriate, review all other significant and life-threatening adverse reactions and interactions, especially those related to the drugs mentioned above.

granisetron hydrochloride

Kytril

Pharmacologic class: 5-hydroxytryptamine$_3$ antagonist
Therapeutic class: Antiemetic
Pregnancy risk category B

Action

Binds to serotonin receptors in chemoreceptor trigger zone and vagal nerve terminals, thereby blocking serotonin release and controlling nausea and vomiting

Pharmacokinetics

Drug is metabolized in the liver. Plasma-protein binding is 65%; half-life is 3 to 14 hours. It is excreted in urine and feces.

Onset	Peak	Duration
Rapid	30 min	Up to 24 hr

How supplied

Solution for injection (clear, colorless): 1 mg/mL in 1-mL single-dose and 4-mL multi-use vials with benzyl alcohol, 0.1 mg/mL in single-use vials (no preservative)

Indications and dosages

➤ To prevent nausea and vomiting caused by emetogenic chemotherapy

Adults and children ages 2 to 16: 10 mcg/kg I.V. 30 minutes before chemotherapy

➤ Acute postoperative nausea and vomiting

Adults: 1 mg I.V. given undiluted over 30 seconds

Administration

Dilution and compatibility

- Know that drug may be give undiluted or diluted with normal saline solution or 5% dextrose for infusion.
- Do not mix with other drugs.
- Prepare I.V. infusion just before administration.
- Once multidose vial is penetrated, use contents within 30 days.

Infusion considerations

- For direct I.V. injection, give undiluted over 30 seconds.
- For I.V. infusion, give over 5 minutes.

Monitoring

- Know that drug may mask progressive ileus or gastric distention in patients who have undergone abdominal surgery or have chemotherapy-induced nausea and vomiting.
- Monitor hepatic enzyme levels and CBC with white cell differential.
- Monitor temperature and blood pressure. Have patient ambulate cautiously to avoid orthostatic hypotension.

Storage

- Store vials at 25°C (77°F); excursions permitted to 15° to 30°C (59° to 86°F). Do not freeze; protect from light.

Contraindications and precautions

Contraindicated in hypersensitivity to granisetron or its components.

Use cautiously in pregnant or breast-feeding patients and ***children younger than age 2*** (safety not established).

Adverse reactions

CNS: headache, anxiety, stimulation, weakness, drowsiness, dizziness, asthenia, somnolence
CV: hypertension
GI: nausea, vomiting, diarrhea, constipation, abdominal pain
Hematologic: anemia, **leukopenia, thrombocytopenia**
Skin: alopecia
Other: altered taste, decreased appetite, fever, chills, shivering

Interactions

Drug-diagnostic tests. *Alanine aminotransferase, aspartate aminotransferase:* increased
Electrolytes: altered
Hemoglobin, platelets, white blood cells: decreased
Drug-herb. *Horehound:* enhanced serotonergic effects

Toxicity and overdose

- Overdoses of up to 38.5 mg have occurred without symptoms or with only slight headache.
- No specific antidote exists. Provide symptomatic therapy.

Patient teaching

- Caution patient to avoid driving and other hazardous activities until drug's effects on concentration and alertness are known.
- As appropriate, review all other significant and life-threatening adverse reactions and interactions, especially those related to the tests and herbs mentioned above.

heparin sodium

Hepalean🍁, Hepalean Lok🍁, Heparin Leo🍁, HepFlush 10, Hep-Lock🍁, Hep-Lock U/P

Pharmacologic class: Antithrombotic
Therapeutic class: Anticoagulant
Pregnancy risk category C

Action

Inhibits thrombus by preventing conversion of prothrombin to thrombin and fibrinogen to fibrin, thereby preventing clot formation. Does not lyse existing clot, but prevents clot enlargement and extension.

Pharmacokinetics

Drug distributes extensively in plasma. Primary biotransformation sites are the liver and reticuloendothelial system; secondary metabolism site may be the kidneys. Drug is nonspecifically and extensively protein-bound. Half-life (which is dose-dependent) ranges from about 30 to 180 minutes; it may be prolonged in hepatic disease. Drug is excreted in urine unchanged and as degradation products.

Onset	Peak	Duration
Immediate	5-10 min	2-6 hr

How supplied

I.V. solution (clear, colorless): 12,500/250 mL, 25,000/250 mL, 25,000/500 mL (premixed)
Heparin Lock Flush I.V. solution (clear, colorless): 1 unit/mL, 2 units/mL, 10 units/mL, 100 units/mL
HepFlush 10 I.V. solution (clear, colorless): 10 units/mL
Hep-Lock I.V. *solution (clear, colorless):* 10 units/mL, 100 units/mL
Monoject Prefill Advanced Heparin Lock Flush I.V. solution (clear, colorless): 100 units/mL
Monoject Prefill Heparin Lock Flush I.V. solution (clear, colorless): 10 units/mL, 100 units/mL
Solution for injection (clear, colorless): 1,000 units/mL, 5,000 units/mL, 10,000 units/mL, 20,000 units/mL, 5,000 units/0.5 mL
Vasceze Heparin Lock Flush I.V. *solution (clear, colorless):* 10 units/mL, 100 units/mL

Indications and dosages

➢ Therapeutic anticoagulation in prophylaxis and treatment of venous thrombosis and its extension, pulmonary embolism, peripheral arterial embolism, atrial fibrillation with embolization

Adults: 10,000 units I.V. by intermittent bolus, then 5,000 to 10,000 units I.V. q 4 to 6 hours. Or 5,000 units I.V. by continuous infusion, then 20,000 to 40,000 units I.V. over 24 hours (about 1,000 units/hour or 15 to 18 units/kg/hour).
Children: 50 units/kg I.V. by intermittent bolus, then 50 to 100 units/kg I.V. q 4 hours. Or 50 units/kg I.V. by continuous infusion, followed by 100 units/ kg/4 hours or 20,000 units/ m^2/24 hours.

➢ To prevent blood clotting during cardiovascular surgery

Adults: At least 150 units/kg I.V. (300 units/kg if procedure is less than 60 minutes; 400 units/kg if more than 60 minutes)

➢ I.V. flush

Adults and children: 10 to 100 units/mL I.V. heparin sodium solution to fill heparin lock set

Off-label uses

- Adjunct in treatment of coronary occlusion with acute myocardial infarction (MI)
- Prevention of cerebral thrombosis in evolving cerebrovascular accident (CVA)
- Prophylaxis of CVA after MI
- Prophylaxis of left ventricular thrombi
- Treatment of myocardial ischemia in unstable angina refractory to conventional treatment (as a continuous infusion)

Administration

Preparation

- Draw baseline blood sample for clotting studies before starting drug.
- With intermittent I.V. infusion, withdraw blood 30 minutes before dose, using arm without I.V. infusion.

Do not give heparin products containing benzyl alcohol to premature infants.

- Place note at bedside to remind personnel to apply pressure dressing after withdrawing blood.
- Have protamine available as heparin antagonist.

Dilution and compatibility

- Be aware that drug may be given diluted or undiluted.
- Know that compatible solutions include normal saline solution, D_5W, and Ringer's solution.
- When mixing with compatible solution for I.V. infusion, invert container at least six times to ensure adequate mixing and prevent pooling of heparin.
- Be aware that unit-dose heparin flush syringes are not intended for multiple use. Discard remaining drug after each use.
- Know that slight discoloration does not affect potency.

Infusion considerations

Do not give heparin I.M.

Use infusion pump to administer I.V. dose. Check regularly to ensure infusion rate is correct.

- Give continuous infusion over 4 to 24 hours, depending on dosage and volume of infusion solution.
- For direct I.V. injection, give single-dose injection over at least 1 minute.
- When using for I.V. flush to prevent clot formation in heparin lock, inject diluted heparin solution by injection hub to fill entire set to needle tip.

Monitoring

- Draw blood for partial thromboplastin time (PTT) from opposite arm 4 hours after continuous I.V. infusion begins.
- Monitor infusion rate closely, even when using infusion pump.
- Evaluate vital signs frequently.

Watch for signs and symptoms of anaphylactoid reaction.

Assess for white clot syndrome (new thrombus formation in association with thrombocytopenia caused by irreversible platelet aggregation). If it occurs, discontinue drug.

Stay alert for signs and symptoms of bleeding tendency.

- Check PTT and platelet count frequently.
- Monitor liver function test results.
- In long-term therapy, periodically assess stool for occult blood.
- Monitor potassium level in patients with diabetes or renal disease. (Drug may cause hyperkalemia.)

Storage

- Store drug at controlled room temperature of 20° to 25°C (68° to 77°F).

Contraindications and precautions

Contraindicated in hypersensitivity to drug, active bleeding disorders (except when caused by disseminated intravascular coagulation), severe thrombocytopenia, and patients who cannot have regular blood coagulation tests.

Use cautiously in severe hepatic or renal disease, bacterial endocarditis, hypertension, brain injury, retinopathy, ulcer disease, recent CNS or ophthalmologic surgery, immediate postpartum period, women older than age 60, and pregnant patients.

Adverse reactions

EENT: rhinitis
Hematologic: anemia, **bleeding, thrombocytopenia, white clot syndrome, severely prolonged clotting time**
Hepatic: hepatitis
Metabolic: hyperkalemia
Musculoskeletal: osteoporosis (with long-term use)
Skin: irritation, rash, urticaria, hematoma, ulceration, cutaneous or subcutaneous necrosis, pruritus, alopecia (with long-term use)
Other: fever, pain at injection site, hypersensitivity reactions including **anaphylactoid reactions**

Interactions

Drug-drug. *Antihistamines, digoxin, nicotine, tetracyclines:* decreased anticoagulant effect
Plicamycin, quinidine, valproic acid, and other drugs that cause hypoprothrombinemia; drugs that affect platelet function (including abciximab, aspirin, clopidogrel, dextran, dipyridamole, eptifibitide, nonsteroidal anti-inflammatory drugs, some penicillins, thrombolytics, ticlopidine, tirofiban): increased bleeding risk
Drug-diagnostic tests. *Alanine aminotransferase, aspartate aminotransferase, free fatty acids, thyroxine, triiodothyronine resin:* increased
Cholesterol, triglycerides: decreased
^{125}I fibrinogen uptake: false-negative results
Prothrombin time: prolonged
Drug-herb. *Anise, arnica, chamomile, clove, dong quai, feverfew, garlic, ginger, ginseng:* increased bleeding risk
Drug-behaviors. *Smoking:* increased bleeding risk

Toxicity and overdose

- Bleeding is major sign of overdose; hemoptysis, hematuria, or tarry stools may be first sign of bleeding. Easy bruising or petechiae may precede frank bleeding.
- When bleeding requires heparinization reversal, give 1% protamine sulfate solution by very slow I.V. infusion, as ordered, to neutralize heparin. Give no more than 50 mg protamine in any 10-minute period; each mg neutralizes approximately 100 USP heparin units. Amount of protamine required decreases over time as heparin is metabolized. To determine protamine dosage, assume heparin has half-life of about 30 minutes after I.V. injection. Be aware that protamine can cause severe hypotensive and anaphylactoid reactions (possibly fatal); give only if resuscitation techniques and treatment of anaphylactoid shock are readily available.

Patient teaching

Tell patient to immediately report nosebleed, blood in urine, or black stools, as these may be first sign of overdose.

Instruct patient to promptly report other unusual bleeding or bruising.

- Urge patient to avoid activities that can cause injury, and to use soft toothbrush and electric razor to avoid gum and skin injury.
- Inform patient about the need for repeated laboratory testing during therapy.
- As appropriate, review all other significant and life-threatening adverse reactions and interactions, especially those related to the drugs, tests, herbs, and behaviors mentioned above.

hetastarch

Hespan, Hextend, Voluven

Pharmacologic class: Nonprotein colloid

Therapeutic class: Plasma volume expander

Pregnancy risk category C

Action

Expands plasma volume through osmotic effect; increases erythrocyte sedimentation rate when added to whole blood

Pharmacokinetics

Molecules below molecular weight of 50,000 are eliminated rapidly by renal excretion, with a small amount of biliary excretion.

Onset	Peak	Duration
Immediate	Immediate	24-36 hr

How supplied

Solution for injection (clear, pale yellow to amber): 500 mL (6 g/100 mL in normal saline) in 500-mL containers

Indications and dosages

➤ Adjunctive therapy for plasma volume expansion in shock caused by hemorrhage, burns, surgery, sepsis, or other trauma

Adults: 500 to 1,000 mL I.V., depending on blood loss and hemoconcentration. Do not exceed total daily dosage of 1,500 mL.

➤ Continuous-flow centrifugation leukapheresis

Adults: 250 to 700 mL I.V. infused at a constant fixed ratio to venous whole blood (usually 1:8 to 1:13) up to twice weekly for a total of seven to ten treatments

Administration

Preparation

Ask patient about sensitivity to corn, which is associated with hetastarch sensitivity.

Dilution and compatibility

- Do not add solutions or other drugs to premixed container.

Infusion considerations

- Do not remove plastic container from overwrap until immediately before use.
- Give by I.V. infusion only.
- Know that infusion rate depends on indication and response. For acute hemorrhagic shock, drug can be given at a rate of up to 20 mL/kg/hour.
- Use only if solution is clear.

Do not use plastic containers in series connections. Such use could result in air embolism due to residual air being drawn from primary container before administration of fluid from secondary container ends.

Monitoring

Stay alert for signs and symptoms of hypersensitivity reaction; discontinue infusion immediately if these occur.

Assess for signs and symptoms of fluid overload, including peripheral edema of legs and periorbital edema.

Check closely for bleeding tendency.

- Monitor vital signs and temperature frequently.
- Closely monitor CBC, white blood cell count, platelet count, hematocrit, prothrombin time (PT), and partial thromboplastin time (PTT).

Storage

- Store at room temperature of 25°C (77°F); brief excursion up to 40°C (104°F) permitted.

Contraindications and precautions

Contraindicated in hypersensitivity to drug, severe bleeding disorders, severe heart failure, and renal failure.

Use cautiously in corn allergy, increased risk of congestive heart failure (CHF) or pulmonary edema, renal or hepatic disorders, pregnant or breastfeeding patients, and ***children*** (safety and efficacy not established).

Adverse reactions

CNS: headache, restlessness, **intracranial bleeding**
CV: peripheral edema of legs, bradycardia, tachycardia, **severe hypotension, cardiac arrest, ventricular fibrillation, circulatory overload, CHF**
EENT: periorbital edema, **laryngeal edema**
GI: nausea, vomiting, submaxillary and parotid glandular enlargement
Hematologic: anemia and dilution of clotting factors, **increased bleeding and clotting times, factor VIII deficiency, acquired von Willebrand–like disease, disseminated intravascular coagulation and hemolysis** (rare)
Musculoskeletal: muscle pain
Metabolic: fluid overload, metabolic acidosis
Respiratory: wheezing, tachypnea, stridor, shortness of breath, coughing, sneezing, **pulmonary edema, bronchospasm**
Skin: rash, urticaria, pruritus, erythema multiforme
Other: chills, fever, flulike symptoms, chest pain, facial and periorbital edema, flushing, hypersensitivity reactions including **anaphylaxis, angioedema, death**

Interactions

Drug-diagnostic tests. *PT, PTT:* prolonged
Serum amylase: transient increase
Urine specific gravity: increased

Toxicity and overdose

- In overdose, expect extension of adverse reactions, including bleeding, fluid overload, and other cardiovascular effects.
- Discontinue drug and provide supportive therapy. Hemodialysis does not remove drug.

Patient teaching

Teach patient to recognize and promptly report signs and symptoms of allergic response and other adverse reactions, including swelling and unusual bleeding or bruising.
- Advise patient to minimize GI upset by eating frequent, small servings of healthy food.
- Tell patient to avoid activities that can cause injury, and to use soft toothbrush and electric razor to avoid gum and skin injury.
- Inform patient about the need for repeated laboratory testing during therapy.
- As appropriate, review all other significant and life-threatening adverse reactions and interactions, especially those related to the tests mentioned above.

[redacted]

hydrocortisone sodium succinate

Solu-Cortef

Pharmacologic class: Short-acting corticosteroid
Therapeutic class: Anti-inflammatory (steroidal)
Pregnancy risk category C

Action

Suppresses inflammatory and immune responses, mainly by inhibiting migration of leukocytes and phagocytes and by decreasing inflammatory mediators

Pharmacokinetics

Drug is reversibly bound to corticosteroid-binding globulin and albumin. It is metabolized by the liver. Excretion is nearly complete within 12 hours.

Onset	Peak	Duration
Immediate	Unknown	1-1.5 days

How supplied

Powder for reconstitution for injection: 100 mg, 250 mg, 500 mg, and 1,000 mg in single-dose ACT-O-VIAL system with benzyl alcohol

Indications and dosages

➤ Replacement therapy in adrenocortical insufficiency; hypercalcemia caused by cancer; arthritis; collagen diseases; dermatologic diseases; autoimmune and hematologic disorders; trichinosis; ulcerative colitis; multiple sclerosis; proctitis; nephrotic syndrome; aspiration pneumonia

Adults and children: 100 to 500 mg I.V.; may repeat at 2-, 4-, or 6-hour intervals, depending on patient response and clinical condition

Off-label uses

- Phlebitis

Administration

Preparation

Do not give powder for injection to premature infants, because 100-mg, 250-mg, 500-mg, and 1,000-mg ACT-O-VIAL systems contain benzyl alcohol (associated with fatal gasping syndrome in premature infants).

Dilution and compatibility

- For direct I.V. injection, prepare 100-mg vial solution by adding no more than 2 mL bacteriostatic water for injection or bacteriostatic sodium chloride injection to contents of one vial.
- For I.V. infusion, prepare 100-mg vial solution by adding no more than 2 mL bacteriostatic water for injection to contents of one vial. Then add this diluted dose to 100 to 1,000 mL D_5W, normal saline solution, or dextrose 5% in normal saline solution if patient is not on sodium restriction.
- When reconstituting ACT-O-VIAL powder for direct I.V. injection, press down on plastic activator to force diluent into lower compartment; gently agitate to effect solution, insert needle squarely through center of stopper until tip is just visible, and then invert vial and withdraw dose. Further dilution is not necessary.
- When reconstituting ACT-O-VIAL powder for I.V. infusion, first prepare solution as described above. Add 100-mg solution to 100 to 1,000 mL D_5W (or normal saline solution or dextrose 5% in normal saline solution if patient is not on sodium restriction). Or add 250-mg solution to 250 to 1,000 mL, 500-mg solution to 500 to 1,000 mL, and 1,000-mg solution to 1,000 mL of same diluents. If administration of small fluid volume is desirable, 100 to 3,000 mg of drug may be added to 50 mL of above diluents.
- Know that when prepared as described above, resulting solutions are stable for at least 4 hours.
- Use solution only if clear.

Infusion considerations

- Give direct I.V. injection over 30 seconds to 10 minutes.
- Know that drug may be given as intermittent or continuous I.V. infusion.

Never abruptly discontinue high-dose or long-term systemic therapy.

Monitoring

In high-dose therapy (which should not exceed 48 hours), watch closely for signs and symptoms of depression or psychotic episodes.

- Monitor blood pressure, weight, and electrolyte levels regularly.
- Assess blood glucose level in diabetic patients. Expect to increase insulin or oral hypoglycemic dosage.

Monitor patient's response during weaning. Watch for adrenal crisis (fever, myalgia, arthralgia, malaise, anorexia, nausea, orthostatic hypotension, fainting, and dyspnea), which may occur if drug is withdrawn too quickly.

Storage

- Store unreconstituted product at controlled room temperature of 20° to 25°C (68° to 77°F).
- Store solution at controlled room temperature of 20° to 25°C (68° to 77°F); protect from light.

Contraindications and precautions

Contraindicated in hypersensitivity to drug, alcohol, bisulfites, or tartrazine (with some products); systemic fungal infections; concurrent use of other immunosuppressive corticosteroids; concurrent administration of live-virus vaccines; and ***premature infants*** (powder with benzyl alcohol).

Use cautiously in hypertension, osteoporosis, glaucoma, renal or GI disease, hypothyroidism, cirrhosis, thromboembolic disorders, myasthenia gravis, heart failure, pregnant or breastfeeding patients, and ***children age 6 and younger*** (safety not established).

Adverse reactions

CNS: headache, nervousness, depression, euphoria, personality changes, psychoses, vertigo, paresthesia, insomnia, restlessness, conus medullaris syndrome, **meningitis, increased intracranial pressure, seizures**

CV: hypotension, hypertension, **thrombophlebitis, heart failure, shock, fat embolism, thromboembolism, arrhythmias**

EENT: cataracts, glaucoma, increased intraocular pressure, epistaxis, nasal congestion, perforated nasal septum, dysphonia, hoarseness, nasopharyngeal or oropharyngeal fungal infections

GI: nausea, vomiting, abdominal distention, esophageal candidiasis or ulcer, dry mouth, **rectal bleeding, peptic ulcer, pancreatitis**

Hematologic: purpura

Metabolic: sodium and fluid retention, hypokalemia, hypocalcemia, hyperglycemia, hypercholesterolemia, amenorrhea, growth retardation, diabetes mellitus, cushingoid appearance, **hypothalamic-pituitary-adrenal suppression with secondary adrenal insufficiency** (with abrupt withdrawal or prolonged high-dose use)

Musculoskeletal: osteoporosis, aseptic joint necrosis, muscle pain or weakness, steroid myopathy, loss of muscle mass, tendon rupture, spontaneous fractures

Respiratory: cough, wheezing, rebound congestion, **bronchospasm**

Skin: rash, pruritus, urticaria, contact dermatitis, acne, bruising, hirsutism, petechiae, striae, acneiform lesions, skin fragility and thinness, angioedema

Other: altered taste; anosmia; appetite changes; weight gain; facial edema; increased susceptibility to infection; masking or aggravation of infection; adhesive arachnoiditis; injection site pain, burning, or atrophy; immunosuppression; hypersensitivity reactions including **anaphylaxis**

Interactions

Drug-drug. *Amphotericin B, loop and thiazide diuretics, mezlocillin, piperacillin, ticarcillin:* additive hypokalemia

Fluoroquinolones: increased risk of tendon rupture

Hormonal contraceptives: prolonged half-life and increased effects of hydrocortisone

Insulin, oral hypoglycemics: increased requirements for these drugs
Live-virus vaccines: decreased antibody response to vaccine, increased risk of adverse reactions
Nonsteroidal anti-inflammatory drugs: increased risk of adverse GI reactions
Phenobarbital, phenytoin, rifampin: decreased hydrocortisone efficacy
Somatrem: inhibition of growth-promoting effect
Drug-diagnostic tests. *Calcium, potassium, thyroxine, triiodothyronine:* decreased
Cholesterol, glucose: increased
Digoxin assays: false elevation (with some methods)
Nitroblue tetrazolium test: false-negative result
Drug-herb. *Echinacea:* increased immunostimulation
Ginseng: potentiation of immunomodulation
Drug-behaviors. *Alcohol use:* increased risk of gastric irritation and GI ulcer

Toxicity and overdose

- Acute toxicity and overdose are rare. In overdose, expect extension of adverse reactions.
- Provide supportive therapy.

Patient teaching

Urge patient to immediately report unusual weight gain, facial or leg swelling, epigastric burning, vomiting of blood, black tarry stools, irregular menstrual cycles, fever, prolonged sore throat, cold or other infection, or worsening of symptoms.
- Instruct patient to eat small, frequent meals and to take antacids as needed to minimize GI upset.
- Advise patient receiving immunosuppressive hydrocortisone doses to avoid exposure to chickenpox or measles and, if exposed, to seek medical advice without delay.
- Tell patient that response to drug will be monitored regularly.
- In long-term use, instruct patient to have regular eye examinations.
- Instruct patient to wear medical identification listing this drug.

Caution patient not to stop drug abruptly because serious adverse reactions may occur.
- As appropriate, review all other significant and life-threatening adverse reactions and interactions, especially those related to the drugs, tests, herbs, and behaviors mentioned above.

hydromorphone hydrochloride

Dilaudid, Dilaudid-HP

Pharmacologic class: Opioid agonist
Therapeutic class: Opioid analgesic
Controlled substance schedule II
Pregnancy risk category C (*D* with long-term use or at term with high doses)

FDA BOXED WARNING

- Dilaudid-HP and generic high-potency hydromorphone (10 mg/mL) are highly concentrated solutions intended for use in opioid-tolerant patients. Do not confuse them with standard parenteral formulations of hydromorphone or other opioids, as overdose and death could result.

Action

Binds to opiate receptors in spinal cord and CNS, altering perception of and response to painful stimuli while producing generalized CNS depression

Pharmacokinetics

Drug is extensively metabolized in the liver by glucuronidation, with more than 95% of dose metabolized to hydromorphone-3-glucuronide, along with minor amounts of 6-hydroxy reduction metabolites. At therapeutic plasma levels, drug is approximately 8% to 19% protein-bound. It crosses placental barrier and appears in low levels in breast milk. Only a small amount is excreted unchanged in urine; most is excreted as hydromorphone-3-glucuronide. Terminal elimination half-life is about 2.3 hours.

Onset	Peak	Duration
10-15 min	15-30 min	2-3 hr

How supplied

Powder for reconstitution for injection (lyophilized): 250-mg vial
Solution for injection: 1-mg/mL, 2-mg/mL, and 4-mg/mL ampules and prefilled syringes; 2-mg ampules, prefilled syringes, and multidose vials
Solution for injection: 10-mg/mL (high-potency) ampules and vials

Indications and dosages

➢ Moderate to severe pain (for opioid-naïve patients or those not receiving high-potency formulations)
Adults weighing more than 50 kg (110 lb): Initially, 0.2 to 0.6 mg I.V. q 2 to 3 hours p.r.n.; individual dosage based on patient's pain, underlying disease, age, and size.

➢ Moderate to severe pain in opioid-tolerant patients who require higher-than-usual opioid dosages to obtain adequate pain relief (high-potency formulations)
Adults weighing more than 50 kg: Experience with I.V. dosing is limited; individualize dosage based on patient's pain level, underlying disease, age, and size.

Dosage adjustment

• For elderly patients and those with moderate hepatic or renal impairment, start with lower dosage. For patients with severe renal impairment, start with even lower dosage.

Administration

Preparation

Be aware that drug is a potent Schedule II opioid agonist with highest abuse potential and risk of causing respiratory depression. Alcohol, other opioids, and CNS depressants potentiate respiratory depressant effect, increasing risk of potentially fatal respiratory depression.
• For maximal analgesic effect, give before pain becomes severe.

Dilution and compatibility

Know that high-potency 10-mg/mL solution in amber ampules and vials is meant only for preparation of large-volume parenteral solutions.
• Reconstitute 250-mg powder for reconstitution immediately before use with 25 mL sterile water for injection to yield 10 mg/mL.
• For I.V. direct injection, drug may be given undiluted, or diluted with 5 mL normal saline solution or sterile water for injection.
• For I.V. infusion, further dilute in larger amounts of normal saline solution, D_5W, dextrose 5% in normal saline solution, or dextrose 5% in half-normal saline solution to a concentration of 0.1 mg (1 mg/mL).
• Be aware that slightly yellowish discoloration may develop in ampules, but does not affect potency.

Infusion considerations

• Give single-dose by slow I.V. injection, over 2 to 3 minutes depending on dosage. Titrate frequently based on symptom relief and respiratory rate.

• Give by I.V. infusion using infusion pump with extremely close titration to adhere to prescribed rate, symptom relief, and respiratory rate.

Monitoring

Monitor for respiratory depression. Keep resuscitation equipment and naloxone readily available.

• Assess for signs and symptoms of physical or psychological drug dependence.

• Closely monitor patient with renal impairment during titration.

• Monitor for constipation.

Storage

• Store at 25°C (77°F); excursions permitted to 15° to 30°C (59° to 86°F). Protect from light. Do not refrigerate, as precipitation or crystallization may occur.

Contraindications and precautions

Contraindicated in hypersensitivity to opioids or bisulfites, patients not already receiving large amounts of parenteral opioids (high-potency formulation), respiratory depression in absence of resuscitative equipment, acute or severe bronchial asthma, status asthmaticus, upper respiratory tract obstruction, obstetric analgesia, and ***premature neonates.***

Use cautiously in increased intracranial pressure; severe renal, hepatic, or pulmonary disease; hypothyroidism; adrenal insufficiency; prostatic hypertrophy; alcoholism; concurrent use of monoamine oxidase (MAO) inhibitors; ***elderly patients;*** pregnant or breastfeeding patients; and ***children*** (safety and efficacy not established).

Adverse reactions

CNS: confusion, sedation, dysphoria, euphoria, floating feeling, hallucinations, headache, unusual dreams, anxiety, dizziness, drowsiness

CV: hypotension, hypertension, palpitations, bradycardia, tachycardia

EENT: blurred vision, diplopia, miosis, nystagmus, tinnitus, laryngeal edema, **laryngospasm**

GI: nausea, vomiting, constipation, abdominal cramps, biliary tract spasm, anorexia

GU: urine retention, dysuria

Hepatic: hepatotoxicity

Respiratory: dyspnea, wheezing, **bronchospasm, respiratory depression**

Skin: flushing, diaphoresis

Other: physical or psychological drug dependence; drug tolerance; injection site pain, redness, or swelling

Interactions

Drug-drug. *Antidepressants, antihistamines, MAO inhibitors, sedative-hypnotics:* additive CNS depression

Antihypertensives, diuretics, guanadrel, guanethidine, mecamylamine: increased risk of hypotension

Atropine, belladonna alkaloids, difenoxin, diphenoxylate, kaolin and pectin, loperamide, paregoric: increased risk of CNS depression, severe constipation

Barbiturates: increased sedation

Buprenorphine, butorphanol, nalbuphine, pentazocine: precipitation of opioid withdrawal in physically dependent patients

Nalbuphine, pentazocine: decreased analgesia

Drug-diagnostic tests. *Amylase, lipase:* increased

Drug-herb. *Chamomile, hops, kava, skullcap, valerian:* increased CNS depression

Drug-behaviors. *Alcohol use:* increased CNS depression

Toxicity and overdose

• Serious overdose causes respiratory depression, somnolence progressing to stupor or coma, skeletal muscle flaccidity, cold and clammy skin, constricted pupils, and sometimes bradycardia and hypotension. Apnea, circulatory collapse, cardiac arrest, and death may occur.

• Reestablish adequate respiratory exchange by ensuring patent airway and instituting assisted or controlled ventilation, as ordered. Provide supportive measures (including oxygen and vasopressors) to manage circulatory shock and pulmonary edema accompanying overdose, as indicated and ordered. Cardiac arrest or arrhythmias may require cardiac massage or defibrillation. Naloxone (opioid antagonist) may be given—but only if patient has significant respiratory or circulatory depression. If ordered, give naloxone cautiously if patient has known or suspected physical dependence on drug; in this case, abrupt or complete reversal of opioid effects may trigger acute withdrawal syndrome. Because drug may have longer duration than naloxone, keep patient under continued surveillance. Be aware that repeated naloxone doses may be needed to maintain adequate respiration. Provide other supportive measures as indicated.

Patient teaching

• Advise patient to report difficulty breathing, nausea, vomiting, or dizziness.

• Caution patient to avoid driving and other hazardous activities until drug's effects on concentration and alertness are known.

• Instruct patient to avoid alcohol while taking drug.

• As appropriate, review all other significant and life-threatening adverse reactions and interactions, especially those related to the drugs, tests, herbs, and behaviors mentioned above.

ibandronate

Boniva IV

Pharmacologic class: Bisphosphonate
Therapeutic class: Calcium regulator
Pregnancy risk category C

Action

Inhibits osteoclast activity and reduces bone resorption and turnover. In postmenopausal women, reduces elevated rate of bone turnover, leading to (on average) a net gain in bone mass.

Pharmacokinetics

Drug either rapidly binds to bone or is excreted into urine; no evidence indicates it is metabolized. Portion not removed from circulation by bone absorption is eliminated unchanged by the kidneys (approximately 50% to 60% of dose). Plasma elimination is multiphasic. Renal clearance and distribution into bone account for rapid and early decline in plasma levels; this is followed by slower clearance phase as drug redistributes back into blood from bone. Observed apparent terminal half-life of 2- and 4-mg I.V. doses after 2-hour infusion ranges from 4.6 to 15.3 hours and 5 to 25.5 hours, respectively. Difference between apparent total and renal clearance probably reflects bone uptake.

Onset	Peak	Duration
Rapid	Unknown	Unknown

How supplied

Solution for injection (clear, colorless): 3 mg/3 mL in single-use prefilled glass syringe

Indications and dosages

➢ Treatment of osteoporosis in postmenopausal women
Adults: 3 mg I.V. injection every 3 months

Off-label uses

- Prevention and treatment of complications of metastatic bone disease in breast cancer patients

Administration

Preparation

- Evaluate for hypocalcemia and other disorders of bone and mineral metabolism; ensure effective treatment of these disorders before starting drug.
- Ensure that patient has adequate supplemental calcium and vitamin D intake, as appropriate.

Dilution and compatibility

- Be aware that drug is available as ready-to-use solution in prefilled syringe, and requires no dilution.
- Do not mix with calcium-containing solutions or other I.V. drugs.
- Know that prefilled syringes are for single use only. Discard unused portion.
- Do not use if discolored.

Infusion considerations

Clinical alert: Be aware that drug is intended for I.V. use only. Do not give by any other route, as tissue damage may occur.

- Give by I.V. injection only over 15 to 30 seconds.

Monitoring

Clinical alert: If I.V. dose is missed, give it as soon as it can be rescheduled; thereafter, give dose every 3 months from date of last injection. Do not administer more often than once every 3 months.

- Monitor creatinine clearance in patients with mild or moderate renal impairment.
- Be aware that drug is not recommended in severe renal impairment.
- Monitor serum calcium and phosphate levels.

Storage

- Store at 25°C (77°F); excursions from 15° to 30°C (59° to 86°F) permitted.

Contraindications and precautions

Contraindicated in hypersensitivity to drug or its components and in uncorrected hypocalcemia.

Use cautiously in patients (especially cancer patients) who will undergo major dental procedure (because of risk of jaw osteonecrosis); severe renal impairment; concurrent use of aspirin, nonsteroidal anti-inflammatory drugs (NSAIDs), or other bisphosphonates; pregnant or breastfeeding patients; and ***children younger than age 18*** (safety and efficacy not established).

Adverse reactions

CNS: insomnia, asthenia, headache, fatigue, dizziness, vertigo, nerve-root lesion
CV: hypertension
EENT: pharyngitis
GI: constipation, diarrhea, vomiting, abdominal pain, dysphagia, esophagitis, gastric ulcer, dyspepsia, gastritis, **esophageal ulcer**
GU: urinary tract infection
Metabolic: hypercholesterolemia
Musculoskeletal: osteonecrosis (primarily of jaw), localized osteoarthritis and muscle cramp, joint disorder, joint pain, muscle pain, back pain, extremity pain, arthritis
Respiratory: upper respiratory tract infection, bronchitis, pneumonia
Skin: rash
Other: tooth disorder, influenza, infection, injection site reactions, allergic reaction

Interactions

Drug-diagnostic tests. *Alkaline phosphatase, calcium:* decreased

Bone-imaging agents: possible interference with test results

Toxicity and overdose

- No overdoses have been reported. However, I.V. overdose may lead to hypocalcemia, hypophosphatemia, and hypomagnesemia.
- As ordered, give calcium gluconate, potassium or sodium phosphate, and magnesium sulfate I.V. to correct significant reductions in serum calcium, phosphorus, and magnesium levels, respectively. Dialysis is beneficial only if performed within 2 hours of overdose.

Patient teaching

Instruct patient to immediately report heartburn, serious vomiting, severe chest or abdominal pain, difficulty swallowing, or abdominal swelling.

- Inform patient that drug will be given every 3 months.
- Advise patient to take supplemental calcium and vitamin D as prescribed if dietary intake is inadequate.
- Teach patient to take only those pain relievers suggested by prescriber. Inform patient that some over-the-counter pain medicines (such as aspirin and NSAIDs) may worsen adverse effects.
- As appropriate, review all other significant and life-threatening adverse reactions and interactions, especially those related to the tests mentioned above.

ibritumomab tiuxetan

Zevalin

Pharmacologic class: Monoclonal antibody
Therapeutic class: Antineoplastic
Pregnancy risk category D

FDA BOXED WARNING

- Deaths from infusion reactions have occurred within 24 hours of infusion of rituximab (essential component of ibritumomab tiuxetan regimen), with roughly 80% occurring after first infusion. Signs and symptoms include hypoxia, pulmonary infiltrate, acute respiratory distress syndrome, myocardial infarction (MI), ventricular fibrillation, and cardiogenic shock. If infusion reaction occurs, discontinue rituximab, indium-111 (In-111) Zevalin, and yttrium-90 (Y-90) Zevalin infusions and provide supportive treatment.
- Y-90 Zevalin regimen causes severe, prolonged cytopenias in most patients. Do not give to patients with 25% or greater lymphoma bone marrow involvement or impaired marrow reserve (such as those who have had previous myeloablative therapy or those with platelet counts below 100,000/mm^3, neutrophil counts below 1,500/mm^3, or hypocellular bone marrow) or marked reduction in bone marrow precursors.
- Ibritumomab tiuxetan regimen has caused severe cutaneous and mucocutaneous reactions, with some deaths. Patients experiencing such reactions should not receive further regimen components and should obtain prompt medical evaluation.
- Do not exceed maximum Y-90 Zevalin dosage of 32 mCi (1,184 MBq).
- Y-90 Zevalin should not be given to patients with altered biodistribution, as determined by In-111 Zevalin imaging.
- In-111 Zevalin and Y-90 Zevalin are radiopharmaceuticals and should be used only by healthcare professionals qualified in safe radionuclide use and handling.

Action

Ibritumomab binds to CD20 antigen on malignant B lymphocytes and induces apoptosis. Tiuxetin binds radionuclides In-111 or Y-90 and is covalently linked to amino groups of lysines and argines in antibody. Beta emission from Y-90 damages cells by stimulating free radical formation in target and neighboring cells.

Pharmacokinetics

Mean effective half-life of Y-90 is 30 hours. Over 7 days, median of 7.2% of injected activity is excreted in urine.

Onset	Peak	Duration
Unknown	Unknown	Unknown

How supplied

Solution for injection (clear, colorless): Two separate and distinctly labeled kits, each containing four vials used to produce a single dose of either In-111 Zevalin or Y-90 Zevalin, as indicated on outer container label:

• One Zevalin vial containing 3.2 mg ibritumomab tiuxetan in 2 mL normal saline solution (1.6 mg/mL)

• One 50-mM sodium acetate vial containing 13.6 mg sodium acetate trihydrate in 2 mL water for injection

• One formulation buffer vial containing 750 mg albumin (human), 76 mg sodium chloride, 28 mg sodium phosphate dibasic dodecahydrate, 4 mg pentetic acid, 2 mg potassium phosphate monobasic, and 2 mg potassium chloride in 10 mL water for injection (adjusted to pH of 7.1 with sodium hydroxide or hydrochloric acid)

• One empty reaction vial (sterile, pyrogen-free).

Indications and dosages

➢ Non-Hodgkin's lymphoma

Adults: Use two-step regimen that includes predose of rituximab (not included in Zevalin kit)

Step 1: Single I.V. infusion of 250 mg/m^2 rituximab at 50 mg/hour. Increase rate by 50 mg/hour q 30 minutes, to a maximum of 400 mg/hour. If hypersensitivity or infusion-related reaction occurs, temporarily slow or interrupt infusion. If symptoms improve, may continue infusion at 50% of previous rate. Within 4 hours of rituximab dose, give 5 mCi of In-111 Zevalin I.V. over 10 minutes.

Step 2: In 7 to 9 days after step 1, I.V. infusion of 250 mg/m^2 rituximab at 100 mg/hour (50 mg/hour if infusion-related reaction occurred during first rituximab dose). Increase by 100 mg/hour q 30 minutes, to a maximum of 400 mg/hour, as tolerated. Within 4 hours of rituximab dose, 0.3 to 0.4 mCi/kg (depending on platelet count) of Y-90 Zevalin I.V. over 10 minutes, not to exceed absolute maximum allowable dose of 32 mCi, regardless of patient's weight.

Dosage adjustment

• Reduce Y-90 Zevalin dosage for baseline platelet count between 100,000 and 149,000/mm^3.

Administration

Preparation

🔊 Follow hazardous drug guidelines on page S19 for handling, preparation, and administration.

🔊 Assess for human antimurine antibody before treatment starts. If result is positive, patient may experience hypersensitivity reaction; keep epinephrine, antihistamines, and corticosteroids on hand to treat reaction.

• Obtain baseline CBC with platelet count.

• Be aware that the two Zevalin kits contain four vials used to produce a single dose of either In-111 Zevalin or Y-90 Zevalin, as indicated on outer container label.

• Be aware that In-111 and Y-90 must be ordered separately from Zevalin kit.

Do not give Y-90 Zevalin if platelet count is below 100,000/mm^3.

Know that ibritumomab should be used only as part of regimen that consists of ibritumomab-rituximab combination.

Know that each dose must be measured by radioactivity calibration in accordance with manufacturer's guidelines immediately before administration.

• Premedicate patient with acetaminophen and diphenhydramine, as prescribed, before each rituximab infusion.

Dilution and compatibility

• Be aware that significant differences exist in preparation of In-111 and Y-90; follow manufacturer's directions explicitly.

• Do not mix any component of regimens with other drugs.

• Administer Y-90 within 8 hours of radiolabeling.

• Administer In-111 ibritumomab tiuxetan within 12 hours of radiolabeling.

Infusion considerations

Give by slow I.V. infusion over 10 minutes; monitor closely.

Do not give by I.V. push or bolus.

Take steps to prevent extravasation of Y-90 Zevalin. If extravasation occurs, stop infusion immediately and restart in another vein.

Monitoring

Follow facility policy on radiation precautions to protect patients, visitors, and medical personnel from radiation exposure.

Monitor patient for severe infusion hypersensitivity reactions, which can be fatal. Know that these reactions usually occur within 30 minutes to 2 hours of administration. Signs and symptoms include hypotension, angioedema, hypoxia, and bronchospasm. The most severe reactions include pulmonary infiltrates, acute respiratory distress syndrome, MI, ventricular fibrillation, and cardiogenic shock. Be prepared to intervene appropriately.

Watch for unusual bleeding or bruising.

Institute infection control protocols. Protect patient from potential infection sources.

Monitor CBC and platelet count regularly during and after therapy; continue to monitor until these levels recover.

Continue to monitor for cytopenias for up to 3 months after therapy ends.

Storage

• Refrigerate at 2° to 8°C (36° to 46°F) until use. Do not freeze.

Contraindications and precautions

Contraindicated in hypersensitivity to any drug in therapeutic regimen, their components, or murine products.

Use cautiously in ***elderly patients,*** pregnant or breastfeeding patients, and ***children*** (safety and efficacy not established).

Adverse reactions

CNS: dizziness, anxiety, headache, insomnia, asthenia
CV: hypotension, peripheral edema
EENT: rhinitis, epistaxis, throat irritation
GI: nausea, vomiting, diarrhea, constipation, dyspepsia, abdominal pain or enlargement, melena, anorexia
Hematologic: anemia, **thrombocytopenia, neutropenia, pancytopenia, hemorrhage**
Musculoskeletal: joint pain, myalgia, back pain
Respiratory: increased cough, dyspnea, **apnea, bronchospasm**

Skin: flushing, bruising, diaphoresis, petechiae, pruritus, rash, urticaria, angioedema
Other: bacterial infection, I.V. site irritation, fever, chills, generalized pain, tumor pain, remote risk of transmission of viral disease (such as **Creutzfeldt-Jakob disease**), hypersensitivity reactions including **severe infusion reactions and anaphylaxis, myeloid cancers, dysplasias**

Interactions

Drug-drug. *Agents that interfere with platelet function or anticoagulants:* increased potential for prolonged, severe thrombocytopenia
Bone marrow depressants: increased risk of bone marrow depression
Live-virus vaccines: possible potentiation of virus replication, increased vaccine side effects, decreased response to vaccine
Drug-diagnostic tests. *Hematocrit, hemoglobin, platelets, white blood cells:* severely decreased

Toxicity and overdose

• In overdose, expect severe hematologic toxicities.
• Provide supportive care as appropriate; know that patient may require autologous stem-cell support to manage hematologic toxicity.

Patient teaching

Instruct patient to promptly report unusual bleeding or bruising.
Teach patient about signs and symptoms of bone marrow depression (unusual bleeding or bruising) and infection, which can occur up to 3 months after therapy ends.
• Tell patient to avoid crowds and potential or known sources of infection.
• Advise patient to eat small, frequent meals and take antiemetic drugs, as needed and prescribed, to control nausea and vomiting.
• Inform patient about the need for repeated laboratory testing during and after therapy to monitor drug effects.
• Caution women of childbearing potential not to become pregnant during therapy.
• Instruct breastfeeding patient not to breastfeed during therapy (whether drug is excreted in breast milk is unknown; however, human immunoglobulin G is excreted in breast milk).
• As appropriate, review all other significant and life-threatening adverse reactions and interactions, especially those related to the drugs and tests mentioned above.

[redacted]

ibutilide fumarate

Corvert

Pharmacologic class: Ibutilide derivative
Therapeutic class: Antiarrhythmic (Class III)
Pregnancy risk category C

FDA BOXED WARNING

• Drug can cause potentially fatal arrhythmias—particularly sustained polymorphic ventricular tachycardia, usually in association with QT prolongation (torsades de pointes). In studies, these arrhythmias arose within several hours of administration. They can be reversed if treated promptly. Drug must be given in setting of continuous ECG monitoring by personnel trained to identify and treat acute ventricular arrhythmias. Patients with atrial fibrillation of more than 2 to 3 days' duration must be adequately anticoagulated, generally for at least 2 weeks.

• Patients with chronic atrial fibrillation tend to revert after conversion to sinus rhythm, and treatments to maintain sinus rhythm carry risks. Therefore, candidates for this drug must be selected carefully, with expected benefits of maintaining sinus rhythm outweighing drug's immediate risks and the risks of maintenance therapy, and with drug offering benefits over alternative management.

Action

Prolongs myocardial action potential by slowing repolarization and atrioventricular (AV) conduction

Pharmacokinetics

After I.V. administration, plasma level decreases rapidly. Pharmacokinetics vary greatly among individuals. Drug has a high systemic plasma clearance that approximates liver blood flow, large steady-state volume of distribution (about 11 L/kg) in healthy patients, and minimal (about 40%) protein binding. It clears rapidly and is highly distributed; elimination half-life averages about 6 hours (range, 2 to 12 hours). Drug is excreted in urine, with remainder in feces.

Onset	Peak	Duration
Immediate	10 min	Unknown

How supplied

Solution for injection (clear, colorless): 0.1 mg/mL in 10-mL vials

Indications and dosages

➢ To convert atrial fibrillation or flutter to sinus rhythm

Adults weighing more than 60 kg (132 lb): 1 vial (1 mg) by I.V. infusion over 10 minutes; may repeat after 10 minutes if arrhythmia persists

Adults weighing less than 60 kg: 0.1 mL/kg (0.01 mg/kg) by I.V. infusion over 10 minutes; may repeat after 10 minutes if arrhythmia persists

Administration

Preparation

Do not give with amiodarone, disopyramide, procainamide, quinidine, or sotalol because of increased risk of dangerous arrhythmias.

Assess electrolyte levels before giving drug. Expect to correct electrolyte abnormalities (especially involving potassium and magnesium), as hypokalemia and hypomagnesemia can lead to arrhythmias.

Dilution and compatibility

• As appropriate, administer diluted or undiluted. To dilute, add 10-mL vial to 50 mL normal saline solution or D_5W to yield a concentration of 0.017 mg/mL.
• Do not use if solution is discolored.

Infusion considerations

• Administer by I.V. infusion only.
• Infuse over 10 minutes.

Monitor ECG continuously during and after infusion. Stop infusion as soon as presenting arrhythmia ends.

• Stop infusion immediately if sustained or nonsustained ventricular tachycardia develops or if marked QT or QTc prolongation occurs.

Monitoring

Keep emergency equipment (defibrillator, emergency cart and drug box, oxygen, suction, and intubation equipment) on hand during administration and for at least 4 hours afterward.

Stay alert for premature ventricular contractions, sinus tachycardia, sinus bradycardia, and heart block.

• Observe with continuous ECG monitoring for at least 4 hours after administration, or until QTc returns to baseline.

• Monitor prothrombin time, International Normalized Ratio, and activated partial thromboplastin time if patient is receiving anticoagulant therapy.
• Continue to monitor electrolyte levels frequently.

Storage
• Store at controlled room temperature of 20° to 25°C (68° to 77°F).
• Know that admixtures with approved diluents are chemically and physically stable for 24 hours at room temperature of 15° to 30°C (59° to 86°F) and for 48 hours when refrigerated at 2° to 8°C (36° to 46°F).

Contraindications and precautions

Contraindicated in hypersensitivity to drug or its components.

Use cautiously in ventricular and AV arrhythmias, concurrent use of Class I or other Class III antiarrhythmics (withhold these drugs for at least 5 half-lives before ibutilide infusion and for 4 hours afterward), elevated digoxin level (supraventricular arrhythmias may mask cardiotoxicity associated with excessive digoxin levels), and pregnant or breastfeeding patients.

Adverse reactions

CNS: headache, light-headedness, dizziness, numbness or tingling in arms
CV: hypotension, hypertension, bradycardia, **sustained ventricular tachycardia** (usually in association with QT prolongation), **bundle-branch block, ventricular extrasystoles, ventricular arrhythmias, ventricular tachycardia, AV heart block, heart failure**
GI: nausea
GU: renal failure

Interactions

Drug-drug. *Amiodarone, disopyramide, procainamide, quinidine, sotalol:* increased risk of dangerous arrhythmias
Antihistamines, phenothiazines, tricyclic antidepressants: increased proarrhythmic effect (causing prolonged QT interval)

Toxicity and overdose

• In overdose, expect prolongation of repolarization seen at usual clinical doses.
• For events that follow overdose, such as proarrhythmia or AV block, use appropriate measures as ordered.

Patient teaching

• Instruct patient to immediately report chest pain, dizziness, numbness, palpitations, headache, or difficulty breathing.
• Tell patient he will be monitored closely for at least 4 hours after drug administration.
• As appropriate, review all other significant and life-threatening adverse reactions and interactions, especially those related to the drugs mentioned above.

idarubicin hydrochloride

Idamycin PFS, Zavedos

Pharmacologic class: Anthracycline antibiotic
Therapeutic class: Antineoplastic
Pregnancy risk category D

FDA BOXED WARNING

• Administer slowly I.V.–never I.M. or subcutaneously. Extravasation may cause severe local tissue necrosis.
• Drug may cause myocardial toxicity leading to heart failure, especially in patients who previously received anthracyclines or have preexisting cardiac disease.

• Severe bone marrow depression may occur when drug is used at effective therapeutic dosages.
• Reduce dosage in hepatic or renal impairment.
• Give under supervision of physician experienced in using leukemia chemotherapeutic drugs, in facility with adequate diagnostic and treatment resources.

Action
Inhibits nucleic acid synthesis by disrupting DNA and RNA polymerase, thereby causing cell death

Pharmacokinetics
Drug has rapid distributive phase with high volume of distribution, presumably reflecting extensive tissue binding. It undergoes extensive extrahepatic metabolism; primary active metabolite is idarubicinol. On average, idarubicin is 97% bound to plasma proteins; idarubicinol, 94%. Estimated mean terminal half-life is 22 hours (range, 4 to 48 hours) when used as single agent and 20 hours (range, 7 to 38 hours) when given with cytarabine. Idarubicinol is eliminated much more slowly than parent drug, with estimated mean terminal half-life exceeding 45 hours; hence, its plasma levels are sustained for more than 8 days. Drug is eliminated mainly by biliary and to a lesser extent renal excretion, mostly as idarubicinol.

Onset	Peak	Duration
Immediate	Several min	Unknown

How supplied
Powder for reconstitution and infusion (lyophilized, red-orange): 20-mg single-use vial
Solution for injection (red-orange): 1 mg/mL in 5-mL (5-mg), 10-mL (10-mg) and 20-mL (20-mg) single-use vials

Indications and dosages
➢ Acute myeloid leukemia
Adults: 12 mg/m²/day by slow I.V. injection over 10 to 15 minutes for 3 days in combination with cytarabine, as prescribed

Dosage adjustment
• Consider reducing dosage in renal or hepatic impairment. Do not administer if bilirubin level exceeds 5 mg%.
• In severe mucositis, delay second course if necessary until full recovery; then reduce dosage by 25%.

Off-label uses
• Acute nonlymphocytic and chronic myelogenous leukemias
• Breast cancer
• Non-Hodgkin's lymphoma

Administration
Preparation
Follow hazardous drug guidelines on page S19 for handling, preparation, and administration.
When preparing drug, wear goggles and gloves, as exposure may cause severe skin reaction. If exposure occurs, wash affected area immediately with soap and water. If drug gets in eyes, follow standard eye irrigation procedure.
Dilution and compatibility
• Do not mix with other drugs.
• Know that precipitation occurs with heparin and that prolonged contact with alkaline solution causes drug degradation.
• Reconstitute 5-, 10-, or 20-mg vial with 5, 10, or 20 mL normal saline solution, respectively, to yield a concentration of 1 mg/mL.
• Do not use if discolored.
• Discard unused solution.

Infusion considerations

- Attach tubing to butterfly needle or other suitable device, and insert into large vein.
- Administer slowly over 10 to 15 minutes into free-flowing I.V. infusion of normal saline solution or D_5W.

Monitoring

Evaluate injection site for burning, stinging, and extravasation. Be aware that extravasation may occur with or without accompanying stinging or burning sensation, even if blood returns well on aspiration of infusion needle. If extravasation occurs, stop infusion and restart in another vein. Then rinse area with normal saline solution and apply cold compresses. (Local infiltration with corticosteroids may be indicated.)

- Monitor patient's response to therapy regularly.
- Assess serum uric acid level and CBC.
- Monitor hemodynamic status and cardiac output. Assess for S_3 heart sound (which signals heart failure).
- Assess fluid intake and output. Make sure patient is adequately hydrated, to prevent hyperuricemia.

Storage

- Keep in carton protected from light until ready to use.
- Be aware that reconstituted solutions are physically and chemically stable for 72 hours when refrigerated at 2° to 8°C (36° to 46°F) or when stored at controlled room temperature of 15° to 30°C (59° to 86°F).

Contraindications and precautions

Contraindicated in hypersensitivity to drug, cardiac disease, or pregnant or breastfeeding patients.

Use cautiously in renal or hepatic impairment, bone marrow depression, previous treatment with anthracyclines or cardiotoxic drugs, and ***children*** (safety and efficacy not established).

Adverse reactions

CNS: headache, mental status changes, peripheral neuropathy, **seizures**
CV: chest pain, **heart failure, atrial fibrillation, myocardial infarction, arrhythmias**
GI: nausea, vomiting, diarrhea, cramps, mucositis, **GI hemorrhage**
GU: red urine, **renal failure**
Hematologic: bone marrow depression
Hepatic: hepatic function changes
Metabolic: hyperuricemia
Skin: alopecia, urticaria, bullous erythematous rash on palms and soles, erythema at previously irradiated site, tissue necrosis or urticaria at injection site
Other: fever, infection, hypersensitivity reaction

Interactions

None known

Toxicity and overdose

- In overdose, expect severe, prolonged myelosuppression and possible increased severity of GI toxicity. With very high doses, cardiotoxicity (including severe arrhythmias and delayed cardiac failure) may occur.
- No known antidote exists. Provide supportive care, including platelet transfusions, antibiotics, and symptomatic care for mucositis, as ordered. Peritoneal dialysis or hemodialysis is not likely to yield benefits.

Patient teaching

Instruct patient to immediately report unusual bleeding or bruising, difficulty breathing, or sudden weight gain.

- Advise patient to eat small, frequent meals.
- If patient becomes pregnant while receiving drug, discuss potential hazards to fetus and risk of pregnancy loss.
- Advise breastfeeding patient to stop breastfeeding before therapy starts.

- Urge patient to keep follow-up appointments for assessment, regular blood testing, and monitoring of drug effects.
- As appropriate, review all other significant and life-threatening adverse reactions.

ifosfamide

Ifex, Ifex/Mesnex, Mitoxana

Pharmacologic class: Alkylating agent, nitrogen mustard
Therapeutic class: Antineoplastic
Pregnancy risk category D

FDA BOXED WARNING

- Give under supervision of physician experienced in using cancer chemotherapy, in facility with adequate diagnostic and treatment resources. Adverse urotoxic effects (especially hemorrhagic cystitis) and CNS toxicities (such as confusion and coma) have occurred; these effects may warrant drug discontinuation.
- Severe myelosuppression may occur.

Action

Alkylates DNA, thereby interfering with replication and synthesis of susceptible cells and ultimately causing cell death

Pharmacokinetics

Drug is metabolized in the liver, producing two major metabolites. Parent drug and metabolites are excreted in urine. Elimination half-life is 7 to 15 hours.

Onset	Peak	Duration
Immediate	Unknown	Unknown

How supplied

Powder for reconstitution for injection: 1 g and 3 g in single-dose vials; 1-g (ifosfamide) single-dose vial plus 1-g (mesna) multidose vials, 3-g (ifosfamide) single-dose vial plus 1-g (mesna) multidose vials, 1-g (ifosfamide) single-dose vial plus 3-g (mesna) multidose vials

Indications and dosages

➤ Germ-cell testicular cancer

Adults: 1.2 g/m^2/day by I.V. infusion over 30 minutes for 5 days. May repeat q 3 weeks or after recovery from hematologic toxicity (platelet level of 100,000/mm^3 or higher and white blood cell count of 4,000/mm^3 or higher).

Off-label uses

- Acute leukemia
- Breast, lung, ovarian, and pancreatic cancer
- Malignant lymphomas
- Sarcomas

Administration

Preparation

Follow hazardous drug guidelines on page S19 for handling, preparation, and administration.

- Be aware that drug is usually given with other antineoplastics as well as mesna.
- Before therapy begins, assess hematopoietic function tests, such as CBC with white cell differential.

To prevent bladder toxicity, give drug with extensive hydration consisting of at least 2 L/day of oral or I.V. fluids. Know that protective drug such as mesna should be given to prevent hemorrhagic cystitis.

Dilution and compatibility

- To reconstitute and dilute, add sterile water or bacteriostatic water for injection to vial, and shake gently.

• Mix 20 mL diluent with 1-g vial or 60 mL diluent with 3-g vial to yield a concentration of 50 mg/mL. For smaller concentrations, dilute solution further with normal saline solution, D_5W, lactated Ringer's solution, or sterile water for injection.
• Refrigerate reconstituted admixtures and use within 24 hours.
Infusion considerations
• Administer I.V. slowly over at least 30 minutes.
Monitoring
• Assess fluid intake; ensure intake of at least 2 L of fluids daily to prevent bladder toxicity.
Monitor urine output for hematuria and hemorrhagic cystitis.
• Monitor hematopoietic function test results (such as CBC with white cell differential) weekly during therapy.
Be aware that drug is associated with urotoxicity, especially hemorrhagic cystitis, as well as CNS toxicities (such as confusion and coma); these effects require cessation of therapy.
Storage
• Store at controlled room temperature of 20° to 25°C (68° to 77°F). Protect from temperatures above 30°C (86°F).

Contraindications and precautions

Contraindicated in hypersensitivity to drug or severe bone marrow depression.

Use cautiously in impaired renal or hepatic function, mild to moderate bone marrow depression, extensive bone marrow metastases, prior radiation therapy, prior therapy with other cytotoxic agents, pregnant or breast-feeding patients, and ***children*** (safety and efficacy not established).

Adverse reactions

CNS: drowsiness, dizziness, confusion, disorientation, ataxia, hallucinations, depressive psychosis, cranial nerve dysfunction, **coma, seizures**
CV: phlebitis
GI: nausea, vomiting, diarrhea, anorexia, stomatitis
GU: hematuria, bladder fibrosis, gonadal suppression, **nephrotoxicity, hemorrhagic cystitis**
Hematologic: anemia, **leukopenia, thrombocytopenia, bone marrow depression**
Metabolic: metabolic acidosis
Skin: alopecia
Other: infection, **secondary neoplasms**

Interactions

Drug-drug. *Anticoagulants, aspirin, nonsteroidal anti-inflammatory drugs:* increased risk of bleeding
Barbiturates, chloral hydrate, fosphenytoin, phenytoin: increased risk of toxicity
Corticosteroids: decreased ifosfamide effects
Cyclophosphamide: increased risk of cardiac tamponade
Myelosuppressants: increased hematologic toxicity
Drug-diagnostic tests. *Hepatic enzymes, uric acid:* increased
Platelets, white blood cells: decreased

Toxicity and overdose

• In overdose, expect nausea, vomiting, hemorrhagic cystitis, and bone marrow depression.
• No known specific antidote exists. Provide general supportive measures as needed.

Patient teaching

Instruct patient to immediately report jaundice, unusual bleeding or bruising, bloody urine, pain on urination, fever, chills, sore throat, cough, difficulty breathing, unusual lumps or masses, mouth sores, or pain in flank, stomach, or joints.

- Advise patient to maintain adequate nutrition and hydration (10 to 12 glasses of fluid daily).
- Inform patient that drug may cause hair loss.
- Advise both male and female patients to use reliable contraception during and immediately after therapy, because drug may cause severe birth defects.
- Urge patient to keep regular follow-up appointments for blood testing and monitoring of drug effects.
- As appropriate, review all other significant and life-threatening adverse reactions and interactions, especially those related to the drugs and tests mentioned above.

[redacted]

imipenem and cilastatin sodium

Primaxin

Pharmacologic class: Carbapenem
Therapeutic class: Anti-infective
Pregnancy risk category C

Action

Acts against various gram-positive and gram-negative organisms by binding to bacterial cell wall, leading to cell death. Addition of cilastatin prevents renal inactivation of imipenem, resulting in increased urinary concentration. Imipenem resists actions of many enzymes that degrade most other penicillins and penicillin-like agents.

Pharmacokinetics

Drug distributes to many body fluids and tissues. Plasma half-life of both components is approximately 1 hour. Imipenem is approximately 20% protein-bound; cilastatin, 40%. When given alone, imipenem is metabolized by the kidneys by dehydropeptidase; however, cilastatin inhibits this enzyme and prevents renal metabolism of drug. About 70% of both components is recovered in urine within 10 hours.

Onset	Peak	Duration
Rapid	End of infusion	6-8 hr

How supplied

Powder for reconstitution for I.V. injection: 250 mg imipenem/250 mg cilastatin, 500 mg imipenem/500 mg cilastatin in single-dose infusion bottles and vials

Indications and dosages

➢ Infections caused by susceptible microorganisms, including lower respiratory tract infections, urinary tract infections, intra-abdominal infections, gynecologic infections, bacterial septicemia, bone and joint infections, skin infections, endocarditis, and polymicrobial infections

Adults: For mild infections, 250 to 500 mg I.V. q 6 hours to a maximum of 2 g/day, depending on infection severity. For moderate infections, 500 mg I.V. q 6 to 8 hours or 1 g I.V. q 8 hours to a maximum of 3 g/day, depending on infection severity. For severe, life-threatening infections, 500 mg I.V. q 6 hours to 1 g q 6 to 8 hours to a maximum of 4 g/day, depending on infection severity.

Children age 3 months and older: 15 to 25 mg/kg I.V. q 6 hours

Infants ages 4 weeks to 3 months: 25 mg/kg I.V. q 6 hours

Infants ages 1 to 4 weeks: 25 mg/kg I.V. q 8 hours

Infants age 1 week or younger: 25 mg/kg I.V. q 12 hours

Dosage adjustment

• Reduce dosage in creatinine clearance of 70 mL/minute/1.73 m^2 or lower, and in patents weighing less than 70 kg (154 lb), according to manufacturer's guidelines.

Administration

Preparation

Ask patient about previous hypersensitivity to penicillins, cephalosporins, or other beta-lactams before starting therapy.

• Know that patients with creatinine clearance of 5 mL/minute/1.73 m^2 or lower should not receive drug I.V. unless hemodialysis begins within 48 hours.

Do not use diluent containing benzyl alcohol for preterm infants, because of link with fatal gasping syndrome.

• Be aware that based on studies in adults only, maximum daily dosage for adults and children should not exceed 50 mg/kg or 4 g, whichever is lower.

Dilution and compatibility

• Know that drug is compatible with normal saline solution, D_5W, dextrose 10% in water, dextrose 5% in normal saline solution, dextrose 5% in 0.225% or 0.45% sodium chloride, dextrose 5% in 0.15% potassium chloride solution, and mannitol 5% and 10%.

• For I.V. use, reconstitute each 250- or 500-mg vial with 10 mL diluent; shake well.

• For piggyback infusion, add 250- or 500-mg I.V. dose to 100 mL diluent; shake solution until it is clear and drug has dissolved completely.

• Know that resulting suspension should be colorless to yellow; however, variations within this range do not affect potency.

• Do not mix in same container with other anti-infectives.

Infusion considerations

Do not give by direct I.V. injection.

• Infuse doses of 500 mg or less over 20 to 30 minutes; infuse doses of 750 to 1,000 mg over 40 to 60 minutes.

• Slow infusion rate if patient experiences nausea, vomiting, dizziness, or sweating.

Monitoring

Stay alert for seizures in patients with brain lesions, head trauma, or other CNS disorders and in those receiving more than 2 g daily.

Watch closely for severe diarrhea and hypersensitivity reaction.

• Assess tissue or fluid culture results obtained before and during therapy.

• Monitor for signs and symptoms of infection, such as fever and elevated white blood cell count. Also evaluate for bacterial and fungal superinfection.

• Monitor electrolyte levels, especially sodium.

• Monitor renal function (particularly creatinine clearance) to determine need for dosage adjustment.

Storage

• Store dry powder at temperature below 25°C (77°F).

• When reconstituted with compatible solution, drug may be stored for up to 4 hours at room temperature or for 24 hours if refrigerated at 5°C (41°F). Do not freeze.

Contraindications and precautions

Contraindicated in hypersensitivity to drug or its components.

Use cautiously in hypersensitivity to penicillins, cephalosporins, or other beta-lactams; history of multiple hypersensitivity reactions; seizure disorder; renal impairment; ***elderly patients,*** and pregnant or breastfeeding patients.

Adverse reactions

CNS: dizziness, drowsiness, **seizures**

CV: hypotension

GI: nausea, vomiting, diarrhea, **pseudomembranous colitis**
Hematologic: eosinophilia
Skin: rash, pruritus, diaphoresis, urticaria
Other: phlebitis at I.V. site, fever, superinfection, allergic reactions including **anaphylaxis**

Interactions

Drug-drug. *Aminoglycosides:* interference with imipenem effects
Cyclosporine, ganciclovir: increased risk of seizures
Probenecid: decreased renal excretion of imipenem
Drug-diagnostic tests. *Alanine aminotransferase, alkaline phosphatase, aspartate aminotransferase, bilirubin, blood urea nitrogen, creatinine, lactate dehydrogenase:* increased
Direct Coombs' test: positive result
Hematocrit, hemoglobin: decreased

Toxicity and overdose

- In overdose, expect extension of adverse reactions, including seizures.
- Discontinue drug and provide supportive therapy. Although drug is hemodialyzable, usefulness in overdose is questionable.

Patient teaching

- Instruct patient to immediately report rash, hives, difficulty breathing, and signs or symptoms of superinfection (such as diarrhea, mouth sores, and vaginal itching or discharge).
- Instruct patient to report I.V. site discomfort.
- As appropriate, review all other significant and life-threatening adverse reactions and interactions, especially those related to the drugs and tests mentioned above.

immune globulin for I.V. use, human (IGIV)

Carimune NF, Flebogamma, Gamimune N, Gammagard Liquid, Gammagard S/D, Gamunex✤, Iveegam EN, Iveegam Immuno✤, Octagam, Polygam S/D

Pharmacologic class: Immune serum
Therapeutic class: Antibody production stimulator
Pregnancy risk category C

FDA BOXED WARNING

- IGIV products have been linked to renal dysfunction, acute renal failure, osmotic nephrosis, and death. Patients predisposed to acute renal failure include those with preexisting renal insufficiency, diabetes mellitus, age greater than 65, volume depletion, sepsis, or paraproteinemia and those receiving known nephrotoxic drugs. In such patients, give drug at minimum infusion rate possible. IGIV products containing sucrose as stabilizer account for disproportionate share of renal dysfunction and acute renal failure cases.

Action

Improves immunity by binding to and neutralizing pathogens, thereby increasing antibodies against bacterial, viral, parasitic, and mycoplasmic antigens. Acts through antimicrobial and antitoxin neutralization.

Pharmacokinetics

Drug reaches peak level immediately after infusion. It distributes relatively rapidly between plasma and extravascular fluid until approximately half is partitioned in extravascular space;

therefore, rapid initial drop in serum levels is expected. Half-life is approximately 23 to 53 days. Drug is eliminated mainly by catabolism.

Onset	Peak	Duration
Unknown	2 days	21-28 days

How supplied

Dried concentrate for reconstitution for injection: 2.5 g, 5 g, and 10 g in single-use bottles (Gammagard S/D)
Powder for reconstitution for injection: 2.5 g, 5 g, and 10 g in single-use bottles (Polygam S/D)
Powder for reconstitution for injection: 500-mg, 1,000-mg, 2,500-mg, and 5,000-mg vials (Iveegam EN)
Powder for reconstitution for injection (white): 1-, 3-, 6-, and 12-g vials (Carimune NF)
Solution for injection: 1 g in 20-mL, 2.5 g in 50-mL, 5 g in 100-mL, and 10 g in 200-mL single-use bottles (Octagam)
Solution for injection (clear): 0.5 g in 10-mL vial, 2.5 g in 50-mL vial, 5 g in 100-mL vial, 10 g in 200-mL vial (Flebogamma)
Solution for injection (clear, slightly opalescent or pale yellow): 1 g in 10 mL-bottle, 2.5 g in 25-mL bottle, 5 g n 50 mL-bottle, 10 g in 100-mL bottle, 20 g in 200-mL bottle (Gammagard Liquid)
Solution for injection (10%): 1-g, 2.5-g, 5-g, 10-g, and 20-g vials (Gamunex)

Indications and dosages

➤ Immunodeficiency
Carimune NF—
Adults and children: 0.2 g/kg I.V. monthly. If response is inadequate, may increase to 0.3 g/kg or increase infusion frequency.
Flebogamma 5%, Gamunex, Gammagard Liquid, Octagam—
Adults and children: 300 to 600 mg/kg I.V. q 3 to 4 weeks
Gammagard Liquid—
Adults and children: 300 to 600 mg/kg I.V. at 3- to 4-week intervals, adjusted to response
Gammagard S/D—
Adults and children: 200 to 400 mg/kg I.V., then in monthly doses based on response
Iveegam EN—
Adults and children: 200 mg/kg I.V. monthly; may be increased up to 800 mg/kg/month based on response
Polygam S/D—
Adults and children: 100 to 400 mg/kg I.V. monthly

➤ Idiopathic thrombocytopenic purpura
Gammagard S/D—
Adults and children: 1,000 mg/kg I.V.; may give up to three doses on alternating days, depending on platelet count
Polygam S/D—
Adults and children: 1 g/kg I.V.; may give additional doses depending on response

➤ Kawasaki disease
Gammagard S/D—
Adults and adolescents: 1 g/kg I.V. as a single dose; alternatively, 400 mg/kg/day for 4 consecutive days with aspirin
Iveegam EN—
Adults and children: 400 mg/kg/day I.V. with aspirin
Polygam S/D—
Adults and children: 1 g/kg I.V. as a single dose, or 400 mg/kg I.V. for 4 consecutive days starting within 7 days of fever onset. Give with aspirin, as prescribed.

➤ To prevent bacterial infection in patients with hypogammaglobulinemia or recurrent bacterial infection associated with B-cell chronic lymphocytic leukemia
Adults and adolescents: 400 mg/kg I.V. (Gammagard S/D or Polygam S/D) q 3 to 4 weeks

Off-label uses

- Chronic inflammatory demyelinating polyneuropathy
- Guillain-Barré syndrome

Administration

Preparation

Before starting therapy, determine if patient has risk factors for acute renal failure (such as use of nephrotoxic drugs; history of diabetes mellitus, renal insufficiency, sepsis, volume depletion, or paraproteinemia; or age 65 or older). Also perform baseline assessment of blood viscosity in patient with hyperviscosity risk factors (such as markedly high fasting triglycerides or monoclonal gammopathies).

Ensure that epinephrine is available to treat acute anaphylactoid reactions.

Do not mix products of different formulations or from different manufacturers.

Do not confuse IGIV with IGIM (intended for I.M. use).

Dilution and compatibility

General—

- Do not shake vigorously, as foaming may occur.
- Know that cold drug or cold diluent may take up to 20 minutes to dissolve.
- Be aware that reconstituted drug should be a clear to slightly opalescent and colorless to pale yellow solution. Do not use if discolored or turbid.
- If sterile laminar airflow conditions are not available for drug reconstitution, administer immediately; discard unused portion.
- Do not mix with other drugs or with IGIV products of different formulations or from different manufacturers.

Carimune NF, Gammagard S/D, Iveegam EN, Polygam S/D—

- Know that Carimune NF and Iveegam EN powder for reconstitution and Gammagard S/D dried concentrate are supplied with diluent (sterile water for injection), transfer device, and administration set with 1.5-micron filter.
- To reconstitute, remove plastic caps from drug and diluent bottles. After disinfecting both rubber stoppers, remove protective cover from one end of transfer set, and insert exposed needle through center of rubber stopper into bottle containing diluent. Remove protective cover from other end of transfer set, grasp both bottles, and quickly plunge diluent bottle into drug bottle and bring bottles to upright position so diluent can flow into drug bottle. Once appropriate amount of diluent is transferred, lift diluent bottle off transfer spike and remove spike. Swirl drug bottle vigorously, but do not shake (to prevent foaming).
- When reconstituting with diluent other than that supplied with drug, use normal saline solution, D_5W, or sterile water for injection only.
- Know that dilution of Gammagard S/D with I.V. fluids is not recommended. If dilution is required, use only D_5W for injection.
- To prepare 5% Polygam S/D solution, use 50 mL, 96 mL, or 192 mL diluent for 2.5 g, 5 g, or 10 g of drug, respectively. To prepare 10% Polygam S/D solution, use 25 mL, 48 mL, or 96 mL diluent for 2.5 g, 5 g, or 10 g of drug, respectively.

Flebogamma—

- Know that dilution with I.V. fluids is not recommended.

Gammagard Liquid, Octagam—

- Be aware that drug is supplied as ready-to-use solution and requires no dilution.
- Promptly use any vial or bottle that has been entered. Discard unused portion.

Infusion considerations

General—

Give I.V. only.

- Use antecubital vein for administration, if possible, to decrease infusion site discomfort.

• Reduce infusion rate 50% to 25% for patients at risk for renal dysfunction.
• Be prepared to reduce infusion rate or discontinue infusion if severe adverse reactions occur.
• Monitor vital signs continuously during I.V. infusion. Stay alert for hypotension.
Carimune NF—
• In previously untreated patients with hypogammaglobulinemia, give first infusion as 3% solution by using total volume of diluent provided.
• Start with flow rate of 10 to 20 gtt (0.5 to 1 mL)/minute. After 15 to 30 minutes, increase to 30 to 50 gtt (1.5 to 2.5 mL)/minute.
• After first bottle of 3% solution is infused and patient shows tolerance, give subsequent infusions at higher rate or concentration. Make increases gradually, allowing 15 to 30 minutes before each increment.
Flebogamma—
• Initially, give 5% solution by I.V. infusion through separate infusion line at a rate of 0.01 mL/kg/minute (0.5 mg/kg/minute). If patient shows tolerance during first 30 minutes, may increase rate gradually to a maximum of 0.1 mL/kg/minute (5 mg/kg/minute).
• In elderly patients, give at a rate less than 2 mg/kg/minute.
Gamimune N—
• Administer by I.V. infusion through separate line at 0.01 to 0.02 mL/kg/minute for 30 minutes. If patient shows tolerance, may increase to a maximum rate of 0.08 mL/kg/minute.
• If adverse reactions occur, reduce or interrupt infusion until symptoms subside; then resume at a rate patient tolerates.
Gammagard Liquid—
• Give at initial I.V. infusion rate of 0.5 mL/kg/hour (0.8 mg/kg/minute); may increase gradually every 30 minutes to 5 mL/kg/hour (8.9 mg/kg/minute).
• For patients at risk for renal dysfunction or thrombotic complications, gradually titrate up to a maximum rate of less than 2 mL/kg/hour (3.3 mg/kg/minute).
Iveegam EN—
• Initially, give by I.V. infusion through separate infusion line at a rate of 0.01 mL/kg/minute (0.5 mg/kg/minute). If well tolerated, may increase rate gradually to a maximum of 0.08 mL/kg/minute (4 mg/kg/minute).
• If other drugs are given, flush line with normal saline solution for injection before Iveegam EN infusion.
Octagam—
• Initially, give 5% solution by I.V. infusion through separate line at a rate of 0.01 mL/kg/minute (30 mg/kg/hour) for 30 minutes. If well tolerated, advance to 0.02 mL/kg/minute (60 mg/kg/hour) for second 30 minutes. If further tolerated, advance to 0.04 mL/kg/minute (120 mg/kg/hour) for third 30 minutes. Thereafter, maintain infusion at a rate up to but not exceeding 0.07 mL/kg/minute (200 mg/kg/hour).
Polygam S/D—
• Initially, give 5% solution by I.V. infusion at 0.5 mL/kg/hour. If well tolerated, may increase rate gradually to 4 mL/kg/hour.
• Know that too-rapid infusion rate may cause flushing and pulse and blood pressure changes. Slow or stop infusion until symptoms subside.

Monitoring

Closely monitor patient for anaphylaxis; be prepared to intervene appropriately.

Watch for acute inflammatory reaction in patients receiving drug for first time (reaction usually arises within 30 to 60 minutes after infusion begins), in those whose last treatment was more than 8 weeks earlier, and when initial infusion rate exceeds 1 mL/minute.

I

Monitor for transfusion-related acute lung injury, characterized by acute respiratory depression, noncardiac pulmonary edema, hypoxemia, and fever that may occur within 1 to 6 hours after infusion. If suspected, perform appropriate tests for antineutrophil antibodies in product and patient serum.
• Monitor CBC, platelet count, and clotting factors for signs of hemolysis.
Assess fluid volume status and blood urea nitrogen and creatinine levels. If renal function deteriorates, consider discontinuing drug.
• After infusion is complete, monitor patient closely for nausea, vomiting, drowsiness, and severe headache.

Storage

• Store Carimune NF at room temperature not exceeding 30°C (86°F).
• Store Flebogamma at 2° to 25°C (36° to 77°F). Do not freeze.
• Refrigerate Gammagard Liquid at 2° to 8°C (36° to 46°F) for 36 months and at room temperature of 25°C (77°F) for 9 months. Do not freeze.
• Refrigerate Iveegam EN at 2° to 8°C (36° to 46°F).
• Store Octagam at a temperature not exceeding 25°C (77°F) for up to 18 months, or refrigerate at 2° to 8°C (36° to 46°F) for 24 months.
• Store Gammagard S/D and Polygam S/D at a temperature not exceeding 25°C (77°F); do not freeze (to prevent diluent bottle from breaking).

Contraindications and precautions

Contraindicated in hypersensitivity to drug or its components, selective immunoglobulin A (IgA) deficiency, and isolated IgA deficiency.

Use cautiously in bleeding disorders, renal impairment, acute renal failure, risk factors for renal insufficiency, ***elderly patients,*** and pregnant patients.

Adverse reactions

CNS: headache, malaise
CV: chest pain, tachycardia, **thromboembolism**
GI: nausea, vomiting, abdominal pain
Hematologic: hemolysis
Musculoskeletal: joint pain, back pain, myalgia
Respiratory: dyspnea, **transfusion-related acute lung injury**
Skin: pruritus
Other: chills, lymphadenopathy, pain at injection site, possible **viral transmission (including hepatitis C and Creutzfeldt-Jakob disease), anaphylaxis**

Interactions

Drug-drug. *Live-virus vaccines:* decreased antibody response to vaccine
Drug-diagnostic tests. *Blood and urine glucose:* test interference (with products containing maltose)

Toxicity and overdose

• In overdose, expect extension of pharmacologic effects and adverse reactions.
• Provide symptomatic and supportive therapy.

Patient teaching

• Instruct patient to report symptoms occurring during or after drug administration.
• Advise patient to avoid live-virus vaccines for 3 months after therapy; drug may delay or inhibit response to vaccine.
• As appropriate, review all other significant and life-threatening adverse reactions and interactions, especially those related to the drugs and tests mentioned above.

inamrinone lactate

Amrinone

Pharmacologic class: Bipyridine derivative
Therapeutic class: Inotropic, vasodilator
Pregnancy risk category C

Action

Inhibits cyclic adenosine monophosphate (cAMP) phosphodiesterase activity in myocardium, thereby increasing cellular levels of cAMP (which regulates intracellular and extracellular calcium levels). These actions increase myocardial contraction force. Also relaxes and dilates vascular smooth muscle, decreasing preload and afterload.

Pharmacokinetics

Drug is partially protein-bound and partially metabolized to several metabolites. It is excreted primarily in urine as both parent drug and metabolites, with some excretion in feces.

Onset	Peak	Duration
2-5 min	10 min	30-120 min

How supplied

Solution for injection (clear to yellow): 5 mg/mL in 20-mL ampules and vials

Indications and dosages

➢ Short-term management of heart failure

Adults: Initially, 0.75 mg/kg I.V. bolus given over 2 to 3 minutes; may give additional bolus of 0.75 mg/kg over 30 minutes. Then start maintenance infusion of 5 to 10 mcg/kg/minute. Maximum daily dosage is 10 mg/kg.

Off-label uses

- Open-heart surgery

Administration

Preparation

Do not confuse inamrinone with amiodarone, an adrenergic blocker.

- Assess electrolyte levels, especially potassium, before starting drug; be prepared to provide potassium supplements to correct hypokalemia, if indicated.

Dilution and compatibility

- Administer either undiluted or diluted in normal or half-normal saline solution to yield a concentration of 1 to 3 mg/mL, as prescribed.

Do not mix with solutions containing dextrose, because slow chemical reaction may occur.

Do not mix with furosemide. Do not inject furosemide into same I.V. line as inamrinone infusion, as immediate precipitation will occur.

- Do not use if discolored.

Infusion considerations

- Give I.V. bolus over 2 to 3 minutes, followed by maintenance infusion using infusion pump or microdrip (60 gtt/mL) at recommended dosage.

Monitoring

Monitor vital signs frequently. Expect to slow or stop infusion if significant hypotension occurs.

- Monitor hemodynamic indicators (including cardiac output, cardiac index, central venous pressure, and pulmonary artery wedge pressure) to assess drug efficacy.
- Assess daily weight and fluid intake and output.

Watch closely for ventricular arrhythmias, especially if patient has atrial fibrillation or flutter.

Assess for signs and symptoms of thrombocytopenia, such as bleeding or bruising.

I

• Monitor platelet count and electrolyte levels before and during therapy.

Storage

• Store at controlled room temperature of 15° to 30°C (59° to 86°F); protect from light.

Contraindications and precautions

Contraindicated in hypersensitivity to drug or bisulfites.

Use cautiously in renal or hepatic disease, atrial fibrillation or flutter, severe aortic or pulmonic valvular disease, acute phase of myocardial infarction, ***elderly patients,*** pregnant or breastfeeding patients, and ***children.***

Adverse reactions

CV: hypotension, **arrhythmias**

GI: nausea, vomiting

Hematologic: thrombocytopenia

Hepatic: hepatotoxicity

Other: hypersensitivity reaction

Interactions

Drug-drug. *Cardiac glycosides:* increased inotropic effects

Disopyramide: excessive hypotension

Drug-herb. *Aloe, buckthorn bark, cascara sagrada, ephedra (ma huang), senna leaf:* increased drug action

Toxicity and overdose

• Overdose may cause hypotension.

• No specific antidote is known. Reduce dosage or discontinue drug. Provide general supportive measures and circulatory support.

Patient teaching

• Instruct patient to report dizziness or light-headedness.

• As appropriate, review all other significant and life-threatening adverse reactions and interactions, especially those related to the drugs and herbs mentioned above.

infliximab

Remicade

Pharmacologic class: Monoclonal antibody

Therapeutic class: Antirheumatic, GI anti-inflammatory

Pregnancy risk category B

FDA BOXED WARNING

• Drug increases risk of infection, including progression to serious infections leading to hospitalization or death. Infections have included bacterial sepsis, tuberculosis (TB), and invasive fungal and other opportunistic infections. Teach patient signs and symptoms of infection; monitor closely for these during and after treatment, and ensure that patient has access to appropriate medical care. If infection occurs, evaluate for appropriate antimicrobial therapy; for serious infection, discontinue drug.

• Evaluate patient for TB risk factors and test for latent TB infection before and during therapy. Start treatment of latent TB before infliximab therapy.

• Rare postmarketing cases of hepatosplenic T-cell lymphoma have occurred in adolescents and young adults with Crohn's disease. This lymphoma is highly aggressive and usually fatal. All cases have occurred in patients receiving concomitant azathioprine or 6-mercaptopurine.

Action

Neutralizes and prevents activity of tumor necrosis factor-alpha (TNF-alpha) by binding to soluble and transmembrane forms of TNF and inhibiting its receptors, resulting in anti-inflammatory and antiproliferative activity. Reduces rate of joint destruction in rheumatoid arthritis and eases symptoms of Crohn's disease.

Pharmacokinetics

Steady-state volume of distribution is dose-independent; drug distributes mainly within vascular compartment. Clearance or volume of distribution is not significantly affected by patient's age, weight, or gender. Terminal half-life is prolonged.

Onset	Peak	Duration
1-2 wk	Unknown	12-48 wk

How supplied

Powder for reconstitution for injection (white, lyophilized): 100 mg in 20-mL single-use vials

Indications and dosages

➢ Rheumatoid arthritis (given with methotrexate)
Adults: Initially, 3 mg/kg I.V., followed by 3 mg/kg 2 and 6 weeks after initial dose, then q 8 weeks. In partial responders, may adjust dosage up to 10 mg/kg or repeat treatment as often as q 4 weeks.
➢ Moderately to severely active Crohn's disease or fistulizing Crohn's disease
Adults: 5 mg/kg I.V. as a single infusion starting as induction regimen at 0, 2, and 6 weeks, followed by maintenance regimen of 5 mg/kg q 8 weeks thereafter. For patients who respond initially but stop responding later, dosage of 10 mg/kg may be warranted.
Children ages 6 and older: 5 mg/kg I.V. as a single infusion starting as induction regimen at 0, 2, and 6 weeks, followed by maintenance regimen of 5 mg/kg q 8 weeks thereafter
➢ Ankylosing spondylitis
Adults: 5 mg/kg I.V. infusion, followed by additional similar doses at 2 and 6 weeks after first infusion and q 6 weeks thereafter
➢ Psoriatic arthritis
Adults: 5 mg/kg I.V. infusion, followed by additional doses at 2 and 6 weeks after first infusion and q 8 weeks thereafter (with or without methotrexate)
➢ Chronic severe plaque psoriasis
Adults: 5 mg/kg I.V infusion, followed by additional doses at 2 and 6 weeks after first infusion and q 8 weeks thereafter
➢ Moderately to severely active ulcerative colitis
Adults: 5 mg/kg I.V. given as induction regimen at 0, 2, and 6 weeks, followed by maintenance regimen of 5 mg/kg q 8 weeks thereafter

Off-label uses

- Sarcoidosis

Administration

Preparation

- Premedicate with antihistamines, acetaminophen, and corticosteroids, as prescribed.

Dilution and compatibility

- To reconstitute, use 21G or smaller needle to add 10 mL sterile water to each vial.
- To mix, swirl—do not shake. Solution may foam and appear clear or light yellow; do not use if discolored.
- Withdraw volume equal to amount of reconstituted drug from 250-mL polypropylene or polyolefin infusion bag or glass bottle of normal saline solution. Slowly add reconstituted drug to infusion bag or bottle, and gently mix. Use within 3 hours.

I

• Know that concentration of infusion should be 0.4 to 4 mg/mL.
• Do not mix with other drugs.
• Discard unused portions of infusion solution.

Infusion considerations
• Give I.V. infusion over at least 2 hours.
• Use polyethylene-lined infusion set with inline filter, with pore size of 1.2 microns or less.
• Do not infuse in same I.V. line as other agents.

Monitoring
Stay alert for signs and symptoms of hypersensitivity reaction, including fever, chills, itching, rash, chest pain, dyspnea, facial flushing, and headache. Be prepared to intervene appropriately.
Watch for evidence of infection, especially in patients who have chronic infections or are receiving immunosuppressants. Drug increases risk of life-threatening opportunistic infections (histoplasmosis, listeriosis, pneumocystosis) and TB. Discontinue drug if patient develops serious infection.
Assess for heart failure in patients with history of cardiac disease.
Monitor liver function. If jaundice occurs or liver enzyme levels rise to five times upper limit of normal or higher, discontinue drug and help determine cause.
Stay alert for nonmelanoma skin cancers, particularly in patients who have had previous prolonged phototherapy.
• Monitor CBC with white cell differential and platelet count.
• Be aware that patients who do not respond by week 14 are unlikely to respond, and therapy should end.

Storage
• Refrigerate powder at 2° to 8°C (36° to 46°F). Do not freeze.

Contraindications and precautions

Contraindicated in hypersensitivity to drug, murine proteins, or other drug components and (at dosages above 5 mg) in heart failure (New York Heart Association Class III or IV).

Use cautiously in active infection (use not recommended), chronic infection or history of recurrent infection, history of TB, active TB, exposure to TB, active hepatitis B virus carrier status, preexisting or recent onset of CNS demyelinating or seizure disorders, ***elderly patients***, pregnant or breastfeeding patients, and ***children*** (safety not established, except in Crohn's disease in children age 6 and older, for no longer than 1 year).

Adverse reactions

CNS: fatigue, headache, anxiety, depression, dizziness, insomnia
CV: chest pain, hypertension, hypotension, tachycardia, peripheral edema, **worsening of heart failure**
EENT: conjunctivitis, rhinitis, sinusitis, laryngitis, pharyngitis
GI: nausea, vomiting, diarrhea, constipation, abdominal pain, dyspepsia, flatulence, ulcerative stomatitis, oral pain, **intestinal obstruction**
GU: dysuria, urinary frequency, urinary tract infection
Hematologic: hematoma, **pancytopenia**
Hepatic: hepatotoxicity, **hepatosplenic T-cell lymphoma**
Musculoskeletal: arthritis, joint pain, back pain, myalgia, involuntary muscle contractions
Respiratory: upper respiratory tract infection, bronchitis, cough, dyspnea
Skin: acne, diaphoresis, dry skin, bruising, eczema, erythema, flushing, pruritus, urticaria, rash, alopecia, **nonmelanoma skin cancer**

Other: tooth pain, candidiasis, chills, hot flashes, flulike symptoms, herpes simplex, herpes zoster, lupuslike syndrome, infections, hypersensitivity reaction, **anaphylaxis**

Interactions

Drug-drug. *Anakinra, etanercept:* increased risk of serious infections and neutropenia
Vaccines: decreased antibody response to vaccine
Drug-diagnostic tests. *Antinuclear antibodies:* positive titer
Hepatic enzymes: increased
Hemoglobin: decreased

Toxicity and overdose

- Single doses up to 20 mg/kg have been given without direct toxic effects.
- In overdose, monitor for signs or symptoms of adverse reactions; provide symptomatic therapy immediately.

Patient teaching

Instruct patient to report signs and symptoms of hypersensitivity reaction, such as fever, chills, itching, rash, chest pain, dyspnea, facial flushing, and headache (may occur up to 12 days after therapy).

Tell patient to report infection symptoms, such as fever, burning on urination, cough, and sore throat.

- Advise patient to avoid potential infection sources, such as crowds and people with known illness or infection.
- As appropriate, review all other significant and life-threatening adverse reactions and interactions, especially those related to the drugs and tests mentioned above.

insulin, regular (insulin injection)

Actrapid, Humulin R, Insulin-Toronto, Novolin ge Toronto, Novolin R, Novolin R PenFill

Pharmacologic class: Pancreatic hormone
Therapeutic class: Hypoglycemic
Pregnancy risk category B

Action

Promotes glucose transport, which stimulates carbohydrate metabolism in skeletal and cardiac muscle and adipose tissue. Also promotes phosphorylation of glucose in liver, where it is converted to glycogen. Directly affects fat and protein metabolism, stimulates protein synthesis, inhibits free fatty acid release, and indirectly decreases phosphate and potassium.

Pharmacokinetics

Drug distributes rapidly and widely and takes effect quickly. The onset of action may vary considerably among individuals or at different times in same individual. Duration depends on dosage, injection site, blood supply, temperature, and physical activity. Drug is eliminated to some extent in urine.

Onset	Peak	Duration
10-30 min	15-30 min	5-8 hr

How supplied

Regular insulin injection (clear): 100 units/mL in vials

Indications and dosages

➢ Diabetic ketoacidosis

Adults and children: Loading dose of 0.15 units/kg (nonconcentrated regular insulin) I.V. bolus, followed by continuous infusion of 0.1 unit/kg/hour until glucose level drops; followed by subcutaneous administration at dosage adjusted to glucose level

Administration

Preparation

Give nonconcentrated regular insulin I.V. only; otherwise, anaphylactic reaction may occur.

Dilution and compatibility

- For I.V. bolus, drug may be given undiluted.
- For I.V. infusion, mix 100 units regular insulin with normal or half-normal saline solution, as prescribed, to yield a concentration of 1 unit/mL.
- Do not use solution unless absolutely clear.

Infusion considerations

- Know that drug may be given by direct I.V. injection into vein, through three-way stopcock or Y-tube, or by I.V. infusion.
- For I.V. bolus, give every 50 units I.V. over at least 1 minute.
- For I.V. infusion, give 0.1 unit/kg/hour.

Monitoring

Monitor glucose level frequently to assess drug efficacy and appropriateness of dosage.

Monitor for signs and symptoms of hypoglycemia (such as CNS changes). Keep glucose source at hand in case hypoglycemia occurs.

Assess for signs and symptoms of hyperglycemia, such as polydipsia, polyphagia, polyuria, and diabetic ketoacidosis (as shown by blood and urine ketone, metabolic acidosis, extremely elevated blood glucose level, and hypovolemia).

Monitor for glycosuria.

- Closely evaluate kidney and liver function test results in patients with renal or hepatic impairment.

Storage

- Refrigerate unopened vials at 2° to 8°C (36° to 46°F).
- Store opened vials in cool, dark room for up to 1 month; protect from sunlight.

Contraindications and precautions

Contraindicated in hypersensitivity to drug or its components and in hypoglycemia.

Use cautiously in hepatic or renal impairment, hypothyroidism, hyperthyroidism, ***elderly patients,*** pregnant or breastfeeding patients, and ***children.***

Adverse reactions

Metabolic: hypokalemia, sodium retention, **hypoglycemia, rebound hyperglycemia (Somogyi effect)**

Interactions

Drug-drug. *Acetazolamide, albuterol, antiretrovirals, asparaginase, calcitonin, corticosteroids, cyclophosphamide, danazol, dextrothyroxine, diazoxide, diltiazem, diuretics, dobutamine, epinephrine, estrogens, hormonal contraceptives, isoniazid, morphine, niacin, phenothiazines, phenytoin, somatropin, terbutaline, thyroid hormones:* decreased hypoglycemic effect

Anabolic steroids, angiotensin-converting enzyme inhibitors, calcium, chloroquine, clofibrate, clonidine, disopyramide, fluoxetine, guanethidine, mebendazole, monoamine oxidase inhibitors, octreotide, oral hypoglycemics, phenylbutazone, propoxyphene, pyridoxine, salicylates, sulfinpyrazone, sulfonamides, tetracyclines: increased hypoglycemic effect

Beta-adrenergic blockers (nonselective): masking of some hypoglycemia symptoms, delayed recovery from hypoglycemia

Lithium carbonate: decreased or increased hypoglycemic effect

Pentamidine: increased hypoglycemic effect, possibly followed by hyperglycemia
Drug-diagnostic tests. *Glucose, inorganic phosphate, magnesium, potassium:* decreased
Liver and thyroid function tests: interference with test results
Urine vanillylmandelic acid: increased
Drug-herb. *Basil, burdock, glucosamine, sage:* altered glycemic control
Chromium, coenzyme Q10, dandelion, eucalyptus, fenugreek, marshmallow: increased hypoglycemic effect
Garlic, ginseng: decreased blood glucose level
Drug-behaviors. *Alcohol use:* increased hypoglycemic effect
Marijuana use: increased blood glucose level
Smoking: increased blood glucose level, decreased response to insulin

Toxicity and overdose

- Expect overdose to cause profound hypoglycemia.
- Immediately give I.V. glucagon, as ordered. Because of serious adverse reactions linked to prolonged cerebral hypoglycemia, administer I.V. glucose if patient does not respond to glucagon within 15 minutes. Give carbohydrate-rich foods as soon as patient is alert. Closely monitor blood glucose level. Monitor patient for aspiration and assess blood pressure, electrolyte levels, and respiratory status.

Patient teaching

Teach patient to recognize and report signs and symptoms of hypoglycemia and hyperglycemia. Advise patient to carry glucose source at all times.
- Instruct patient how to monitor and record blood glucose level and, if indicated, urine glucose and ketone levels.
- Inform patient that dietary changes, activity, and stress can alter blood glucose level and insulin requirements.
- Advise patient to wear medical identification stating that patient is diabetic and takes insulin.
- Urge patient to have regular medical examinations, including eye and dental checkups.
- As appropriate, review all other significant and life-threatening adverse reactions and interactions, especially those related to the drugs, tests, herbs, and behaviors mentioned above.

interferon alfa-2b, recombinant

Intron A, Viraferon

Pharmacologic class: Biological response modifier
Therapeutic class: Antineoplastic, antiviral
Pregnancy risk category C

Action

Unknown. Antitumor and antiviral activity may relate to drug's direct antiproliferative action against tumor or viral cells, inhibition of viral replication, and modulation of host immune response.

Pharmacokinetics

Drug level is undetectable 4 hours after administration. The kidneys may be primary metabolism site. Elimination half-life is 2 to 3 hours.

Onset	Peak	Duration
Unknown	15-60 min	4 hr

How supplied

Powder for reconstitution for injection: 10 million, 18 million, and 50 million international units/vial (with diluent)

Indications and dosages

➤ Malignant melanoma (as adjunct to surgery in patients at high risk for systemic recurrence for up to 8 weeks after surgery)
Adults: Induction dosage of 20 million international units/m^2 I.V. for 5 consecutive days per week for 4 weeks (followed by subcutaneous maintenance dose three times weekly for 48 weeks), followed by subcutaneous maintenance doses, as prescribed

Dosage adjustment

• Temporarily discontinue drug if granulocyte level falls below 500/mm^3 or alanine aminotransferase (ALT) or aspartate aminotransferase (AST) level rises above five to ten times upper limit of normal. Resume when adverse reactions abate at 50% of previous dosage. Discontinue drug if intolerance persists or severe adverse reactions recur after dosage decrease, granulocyte level falls below 250/mm^3, or ALT or AST level exceeds 10 times upper limit of normal.

Off-label uses

• Carcinoid tumor
• Chronic granulocytic or chronic myelogenous leukemia
• Non-Hodgkin's lymphoma (low-grade)
• Renal cell carcinoma

Administration

Preparation

Do not confuse drug with interferon alfa-2a (intended for I.M. or subcutaneous use only).

Know that interferon alfa-2b solution for injection in vials or multidose pens is not recommended for I.V. administration and should not be used for induction phase of malignant melanoma treatment. Only the sterile powder is used for I.V. administration.

Know that not all dosage forms and strengths are appropriate for certain indications and routes. Read labeling information carefully.

Before therapy, assess CBC with white cell differential, granulocyte count, bone-marrow hairy cells, glucose and electrolyte levels, thyroid stimulating hormone (TSH), and liver and kidney function test results.

• Be aware that patient should undergo baseline eye examination.
• Give antiemetic to prevent or reduce nausea and vomiting, as prescribed.
• Give antipyretic (acetaminophen) to reduce flulike symptoms, as prescribed.
• Ensure that patient is well hydrated, especially during initial treatment stages.

Dilution and compatibility

• Only use powder for reconstitution for injection for I.V. use.
• Reconstitute powder with diluent provided by manufacturer (bacteriostatic water for injection), according to chart provided with drug. Mix gently, draw drug up into sterile syringe, and inject into 100 mL normal saline solution. Be aware that final concentration should be no less than 10 million international units/100 mL.

Infusion considerations

• Administer by slow I.V. infusion over 20 minutes.

Monitoring

Monitor CBC with white cell differential, granulocyte count, bone-marrow hairy cells, glucose and electrolyte levels, TSH, and liver and kidney function test results monthly during therapy.

Withdraw drug if patient develops thyroid abnormalities and thyroid function cannot be normalized with treatment.

Withhold drug if patient has severe adverse reactions. When reactions ease, resume therapy at prescribed dosage; withdraw drug if reactions persist.
• Monitor fluid intake and output. Keep patient well hydrated.
• Assess for GI upset. Provide small, frequent meals and give antiemetics, as prescribed, to ease severe nausea and vomiting.
Monitor for mental status changes, depression, and suicidal ideation.
• Assess for bleeding and bruising.
• Institute infection-control measures. Monitor for signs and symptoms of infection.
• Be aware that patients with preexisting eye conditions should have periodic eye exams after therapy.

Storage
• Store powder for injection (before and after reconstitution) between 2° and 8°C (36° and 46°F).

Contraindications and precautions
Contraindicated in hypersensitivity to drug or its components, autoimmune hepatitis, pregnant women, and female partners of males receiving drug.

Use cautiously in cardiac or pulmonary disease; bone marrow, autoimmune, seizure, or psychiatric disorders; thyroid abnormalities (patients must not keep receiving drug unless thyroid function normalizes with treatment); ophthalmic conditions; diabetic patients prone to ketoacidosis; pregnant or breastfeeding patients, and ***children younger than age 18*** (safety and efficacy not established).

Adverse reactions
CNS: dizziness, confusion, paresthesia, rigors, lethargy, depression, difficulty thinking or concentrating, insomnia, anxiety, fatigue, asthenia, amnesia, malaise, nervousness, drowsiness, **suicidal ideation**
CV: chest pain, hypertension, palpitations, **arrhythmias**
EENT: visual disturbances, stye, hearing disorders, nasal congestion, sinusitis, rhinitis, pharyngitis
GI: nausea, vomiting, diarrhea, constipation, abdominal pain, dyspepsia, flatulence, eructation, stomatitis, dry mouth, **intestinal obstruction**
GU: gynecomastia, impaired fertility in women, transient erectile dysfunction
Hematologic: anemia, **leukopenia, thrombocytopenia, neutropenia**
Metabolic: hyperglycemia, hypocalcemia
Musculoskeletal: joint pain, back pain, myalgia
Respiratory: cough, dyspnea
Skin: flushing, rash, dry skin, pruritus, alopecia, dermatitis, diaphoresis
Other: gingivitis, flulike symptoms, candidiasis, edema, weight loss

Interactions
Drug-drug. *Aminophylline, theophylline:* reduced clearance of these drugs
CNS depressants: additive CNS effects
Live-virus vaccines: decreased antibody response to vaccine, increased risk of adverse reactions
Zidovudine: synergistic effects
Drug-diagnostic tests. *Alkaline phosphatase, ALT, AST, bilirubin, blood urea nitrogen, calcium, creatinine, fasting glucose, International Normalized Ratio, lactate dehydrogenase, neutralizing antibodies, partial thromboplastin time, phosphate, prothrombin time, uric acid, triglycerides:* increased
Hemoglobin, platelets, white blood cells: decreased
TSH: altered

Toxicity and overdose
• In overdose, expect extension of pharmacologic effects and adverse reactions,

including hepatic enzyme abnormalities, renal failure, hemorrhage, and myocardial infarction.
• No specific antidote exists. Provide symptomatic and supportive therapy. Dialysis does not remove drug.

Patient teaching

Instruct patient to immediately report depression, suicidal thoughts, mental status changes, signs or symptoms of infection (such as fever, chills, or sore throat), unusual bleeding or bruising, dizziness, palpitations, and chest pain.
• Caution patient to avoid driving and other hazardous activities until drug's effects on concentration, alertness, and vision are known.
• Inform female patient that drug has been linked to fetal abnormalities. Caution her not to become pregnant during therapy, and advise her to use barrier contraception.
• Advise patient to eat small, frequent meals to combat nausea, vomiting, and appetite loss.
• Urge female patient not to breastfeed while receiving drug.
• Advise patient to avoid potential infection sources, such as crowds and people with known infections.
• Inform male patient that drug may cause transient erectile dysfunction.
• Teach patient about the need for regular follow-up examinations and blood tests to gauge drug's effects.
• As appropriate, review all other significant and life-threatening adverse reactions and interactions, especially those related to the drugs and tests mentioned above.

irinotecan hydrochloride

Campto, Camptosar

Pharmacologic class: Topoisomerase I inhibitor
Therapeutic class: Antineoplastic
Pregnancy risk category D

FDA BOXED WARNING

• Give under supervision of physician experienced in using cancer chemotherapy, in facility with adequate diagnostic and treatment resources.
• Drug can cause both early and late forms of diarrhea that may be severe. Early diarrhea (arising during or shortly after drug infusion) may be accompanied by cholinergic symptoms; atropine may prevent or relieve it. Late diarrhea (generally arising more than 24 hours after administration) can be life-threatening and prolonged, and may lead to dehydration, electrolyte imbalance, or sepsis. For late diarrhea, give loperamide promptly.
• Drug may cause severe myelosuppression.

Action

Inhibits topoisomerase I (an enzyme that allows DNA replication) by binding to it. This action prevents religation of DNA strand, which leads to breakage of double-stranded DNA and cell death.

Pharmacokinetics

Drug is converted to active metabolite SN-38 primarily in the liver. SN-38 subsequently undergoes conjugation to form a glucuronide metabolite. Parent drug has moderate plasma protein–binding (30% to 68%); SN-38 is approximately 95% protein-bound. Urinary excretion of drug is 11% to 20%; SN-38 glucuronide, 3%; and SN-38, less than 1%.

Onset	Peak	Duration
Immediate	1-2 hr	Unknown

How supplied

Solution for injection (pale yellow, clear): 20 mg/mL in 2-mL and 5-mL single-dose vials

Indications and dosages

➢ Component of first-line therapy in combination with 5-fluorouracil (5-FU) and leucovorin for patients with metastatic carcinoma of colon or rectum

Adults: Administer as I.V. infusion over 90 minutes. For all regimens, give leucovorin immediately after irinotecan and give 5-FU immediately after leucovorin. Follow currently recommended irinotecan dosages and modifications for both combination and single-agent therapy.

➢ Recurrence or progression of metastatic colorectal carcinoma after 5-FU therapy

Adults: Single-dose regimen, follow currently recommended dosage and modifications. Give by I.V. infusion once weekly for 4 weeks, followed by 2-week rest period. After adequate recovery, repeat additional doses in similar 6-week cycle; continue indefinitely in patients who achieve response or whose disease remains stable.

Dosage adjustment

• Base all dosage adjustments on worst preceding toxicity. After first treatment, patients with active diarrhea should have resumed pretreatment bowel function without requiring antidiarrheals for at least 24 hours before next chemotherapy administration. Monitor patient carefully for toxicity, and evaluate before each treatment. Modify irinotecan and 5-FU dosages as needed according to tolerance. Based on current recommended dosage levels, adjust subsequent doses.

• Modify starting dosage in patients age 70 and older to 300 mg/m^2 in single-agent, once-every-3-week regimen.

Off-label uses

• Most cancers (including brain, gastric, cervical, ovarian, non-small-cell lung, and pancreatic cancer)

Administration

Preparation

Follow hazardous drug guidelines on page S19 for handling, preparation, and administration.

• Administer antiemetic for nausea and vomiting, as needed and prescribed.

• Consider prophylactic or therapeutic administration of atropine in patients experiencing early diarrhea and other cholinergic symptoms.

Dilution and compatibility

• Dilute in D_5W or normal saline solution, to a concentration of 0.12 to 2.8 mg/mL.

• Do not mix with other drugs.

• Do not use if discolored.

Infusion considerations

• Infuse within 6 hours if drug is stored at room temperature or within 24 hours if refrigerated.

• Give each dose by I.V. infusion over 90 minutes.

Monitoring

Assess CBC before each infusion. Withhold dose if neutrophil count is below 1,500/mm^3.

• Monitor infusion site for extravasation; if it occurs, flush with sterile water and apply ice.

• Assess fluid intake and output. Keep patient well hydrated.

• Monitor oral intake. Evaluate for nausea and vomiting.

Assess for diarrhea. In severe diarrhea, expect to decrease dosage or withhold dose.

• Institute infection-control protocols to help guard patient from infection sources.

• Monitor liver function test results.

Storage

• Store at controlled room temperature of 15° to 30°C (59° to 86°F); protect from light. Keep vial (with backing and plastic blister) in carton until use.

Contraindications and precautions

Contraindicated in hypersensitivity to drug.

Use cautiously in bone marrow depression, severe diarrhea, patients undergoing radiation therapy, ***elderly patients,*** pregnant or breastfeeding patients, and ***children.***

Adverse reactions

CNS: insomnia, dizziness, asthenia, headache, akathisia
CV: vasodilation, orthostatic hypotension
EENT: rhinitis
GI: nausea, vomiting, constipation, diarrhea, flatulence, dyspepsia, abdominal pain or enlargement, stomatitis, anorexia
Hematologic: anemia, **neutropenia, leukopenia, thrombocytopenia**
Hepatic: hepatotoxicity
Metabolic: dehydration
Musculoskeletal: back pain
Respiratory: dyspnea, increased cough
Skin: alopecia, diaphoresis, rash
Other: weight loss, edema, fever, pain, chills, minor infections

Interactions

Drug-drug. *Dexamethasone:* increased risk of lymphocytopenia
Diuretics: increased risk of dehydration
Laxatives: increased risk of diarrhea
Other antineoplastics: additive adverse effects
Drug-diagnostic tests. *Alkaline phosphatase:* increased
Hemoglobin, neutrophils, white blood cells: decreased

Toxicity and overdose

• In overdose, expect adverse events similar to those reported with recommended dosage and regimen.

• No known antidote exists. Monitor patient extremely closely and provide maximum supportive care to prevent dehydration caused by diarrhea. Intervene as appropriate for infectious complications.

Patient teaching

• Inform patient that blood tests will be done before each dose.

• Instruct patient to report pain at infusion site; severe nausea or vomiting; severe, increased, or bloody diarrhea; infection; or injury.

Advise patient to immediately report unusual tiredness or yellowing of skin or eyes.

• Tell patient drug increases risk of infection. Advise patient to avoid crowds and other potential infection sources.

• Caution female patient not to breastfeed or become pregnant during therapy. Recommend use of barrier contraception methods.

• As appropriate, review all other significant and life-threatening adverse reactions and interactions, especially those related to the drugs and tests mentioned above.

iron dextran

CosmoFer, DexFerrum, DexIron, InFeD, Infufer

Pharmacologic class: Trace element

Therapeutic class: Iron supplement, hematinic agent

Pregnancy risk category C

FDA BOXED WARNING

• Parenteral use has caused anaphylactic-type reactions, some resulting in death. Use only in patients with clearly established indications when laboratory tests confirm iron deficiency not amenable to oral iron therapy. Give drug only where resuscitation techniques and treatment of anaphylactic and anaphylactoid shock are readily available.

Action

Replenishes depleted stores of iron (a component of hemoglobin) in bone marrow

Pharmacokinetics

Half-life ranges from 5 hours to more than 20 hours; however, these values do not represent iron clearance from the body. Iron is not easily eliminated, and accumulation can be toxic.

Onset	Peak	Duration
4 days	1-2 wk	Wks-mos

How supplied

Injection (dark brown, slightly viscous liquid complex): 50 mg/mL in 2-mL single-dose vials

Indications and dosages

➤ Iron-deficiency anemia secondary to blood loss when oral administration is unsatisfactory or impossible

Adults and children weighing more than 15 kg (33 lb): Direct therapy toward replacing equivalent amount of iron represented in blood loss. (Formula below does *not* apply to simple iron replacement values.) Quantitative estimates of patient's periodic blood loss and hematocrit during bleeding episode provide a convenient way to calculate required iron dosage. Formula shown below is based on approximation that 1 mL of normocytic normochromic red cells contains 1 mg elemental iron:

Replacement iron (in mg) = blood loss (in mL) × hematocrit

Example: Blood loss of 500 mL with 20% hematocrit

Replacement iron = 500 × 0.20 = 100 mg

Iron dextran dosage = 100 mg = 2 mL

Administration

Preparation

Follow hazardous drug guidelines on page S19 for handling, preparation, and administration.

Ensure that vial label states "For I.V. use."

Discontinue oral iron preparations before starting I.V. therapy.

Dilution and compatibility

• Know that drug may be given undiluted for direct injection.

• For I.V. infusion, dilute desired dosage in 50 to 1,000 mL normal saline solution.

• Do not mix with other drugs or with D_5W.

• Do not add to parenteral nutrition solutions.

Infusion considerations

• For direct I.V. injection, administer undiluted at a rate no faster than 1 mL/minute.

- For I.V. infusion, administer over 1 to 8 hours, depending on dosage, diluent amount, and response.

Be aware that too-rapid infusion may cause flushing and hypotension.

Monitoring

Monitor for hypersensitivity reaction. Keep epinephrine and other emergency supplies on hand in case reaction occurs.

Watch for signs and symptoms of iron overload, such as decreased activity, sedation, and GI or respiratory tract bleeding.

- Regularly assess serum ferritin levels, which correlate with iron stores. However, know that correlation of iron stores and serum ferritin may not be valid in patients on chronic renal dialysis who are receiving iron dextran complex.
- Monitor hemoglobin, hematocrit, serum iron, total iron-binding capacity, and transferrin saturation.
- In patients with rheumatoid arthritis, monitor for acute exacerbation of joint pain and swelling. Provide appropriate comfort measures.
- Be aware that after administration, evidence of therapeutic response may appear in a few days as increased reticulocyte count.
- Know that in patients with high serum ferritin levels or after iron dextran infusion, bone scans with ^{99m}Tc-labeled bone-seeking agents may show reduction in bony uptake, marked renal activity, and excessive blood pool and soft-tissue accumulation.
- Be aware that doses of 5 mL or greater may give serum a brownish tinge when sample is drawn 4 hours after administration.

Storage

- Store at controlled room temperature of 15° to 30°C (59° to 86°F).

Contraindications and precautions

Contraindicated in hypersensitivity to drug, alcohol, tartrazine, or sulfites; anemias not associated with iron deficiency; or hemolytic anemia.

Use cautiously in autoimmune disorders, arthritis, severe hepatic impairment, acute phase of infectious renal disease (use not recommended), ***elderly patients,*** pregnant or breastfeeding patients, and ***children.***

Adverse reactions

CNS: dizziness, headache, syncope, **seizures**
CV: chest pain, tachycardia, hypotension
GI: nausea, vomiting
Hematologic: hemochromatosis, **hemolysis, hemosiderosis**
Musculoskeletal: joint pain, myalgia
Respiratory: dyspnea
Other: abnormal or metallic taste, fever, lymphadenopathy, hypersensitivity reactions including **anaphylaxis**

Interactions

Drug-drug. *Chloramphenicol:* increased serum iron level caused by decreased iron clearance and erythropoiesis
Drug-diagnostic tests. *Serum bilirubin:* falsely elevated
Serum calcium: falsely decreased

Toxicity and overdose

- Overdose rarely causes acute manifestations. Dosages in excess of requirements for restoring hemoglobin and iron stores may cause hemosiderosis. Signs and symptoms of iron overload include decreased activity, sedation, and GI or respiratory tract bleeding.
- Periodic serum ferritin monitoring may aid recognition of harmful progressive iron accumulation caused by impaired iron uptake from reticuloendothelial system in such concurrent medical conditions as chronic renal

failure, Hodgkin's disease, and rheumatoid arthritis. Dialysis provides negligible iron dextran removal.

Patient teaching

- Caution patient not to take oral iron preparations or vitamins containing iron during I.V. iron therapy.
- Instruct patient to report difficulty breathing, itching, or rash.
- Inform patient about the need for periodic blood testing to monitor response to therapy.
- As appropriate, review all other significant and life-threatening adverse reactions and interactions, especially those related to the drugs and tests mentioned above.

[redacted]

iron sucrose

Venofer

Pharmacologic class: Trace element
Therapeutic class: Iron supplement
Pregnancy risk category B

Action

Replenishes depleted stores of iron (a component of hemoglobin) in bone marrow

Pharmacokinetics

Drug distributes mainly in blood and to some extent in extravascular fluid; significant amount distributes in the liver, spleen, and bone marrow. Drug is dissociated into iron and sucrose by reticuloendothelial system. Sucrose component is eliminated mainly by urinary excretion; some iron also is eliminated in urine. Elimination half-life is 6 hours.

Onset	Peak	Duration
4 days	1-2 wk	Wks-mos

How supplied

Aqueous complex for injection (brown): 20 mg elemental iron/mL in 5-mL single-use vials (100 mg of elemental iron)

Indications and dosages

➤ Iron-deficiency anemia in patients undergoing chronic hemodialysis who are concurrently receiving erythropoietin
Adults: 100 mg elemental iron (5 mL) I.V. directly into dialysis line or by slow I.V. injection or infusion during dialysis session (up to three times weekly) for 10 doses (total of 1,000 mg).

➤ Iron-deficiency anemia in patients with non-dialysis-dependent chronic kidney disease (NDD-CKD), whether or not they are receiving erythropoietin
Adults: 200 mg by slow I.V. injection over 2 to 5 minutes on five different occasions, to a total cumulative dosage of 1,000 mg over 14-day period

➤ Iron-deficiency anemia in patients with hemodialysis-dependent chronic kidney disease (HDD-CKD) who are receiving erythropoietin
Adults: 100 mg by slow I.V. injection over 2 to 5 minutes or I.V. infusion of 100 mg diluted in maximum of 100 mL normal saline solution over at least 15 minutes per consecutive hemodialysis session, for a total cumulative dosage of 1,000 mg

➤ Iron-deficiency anemia in patients with peritoneal dialysis–dependent chronic kidney disease (PDD-CKD) who are receiving erythropoietin
Adults: Total cumulative dosage of 1,000 mg in three divided doses, diluted in a maximum of 250 mL normal saline solution given by slow I.V. infusion within 28-day period as follows: two 300-mg infusions given over 1.5 hours 14 days apart, followed 14 days later by one 400-mg infusion given over 2.5 hours

Off-label uses

- Autologous blood donation
- Bloodless surgery

Administration

Preparation

- Be aware that no test dose is required; however, 50 mg (2.5 mL) I.V. over 3 to 10 minutes may be prescribed.
- Do not give with oral iron preparations.
- Assess hemoglobin, hematocrit, serum ferritin, and transferrin saturation levels before therapy starts.

Dilution and compatibility

- Know that drug may be given undiluted for direct slow I.V. injection over 2 to 5 minutes.
- For I.V. infusion in HDD-CKD patients, dilute each 100-mg dose in no more than 100 mL normal saline solution, and give by I.V. infusion over at least 15 minutes.
- Know that for NDD-CKD patients, experience with I.V. infusion of 500 mg diluted in a maximum of 250 mL normal saline solution given over 3.5 to 4 hours (as alternative to direct slow I.V. injection) is limited.
- For I.V. infusion in PDD-CKD patients, dilute each dose in a maximum of 250 mL normal saline solution over 1.5 hours.
- Do not mix with other drugs or add to parenteral nutrition solutions.
- Use immediately after preparation.
- Discard unused portion.

Infusion considerations

- When administering by direct I.V. or by I.V. infusion into dialysis line, give at 20 mg/minute, not to exceed 100 mg/injection.
- For slow I.V. infusion, give over at least 15 minutes.

🔊 Be aware that too-rapid infusion may cause hypotension, dyspnea, headache, vomiting, nausea, dizziness, joint aches, paresthesia, abdominal and muscle pain, edema, and cardiovascular collapse.

Monitoring

🔊 Monitor for hypersensitivity reaction. Keep epinephrine and other emergency supplies available in case reaction occurs.

🔊 Monitor blood pressure. Stay alert for hypotension.

🔊 Watch for signs and symptoms of iron overload, such as decreased activity, sedation, and GI or respiratory tract bleeding.

- Assess hemoglobin, hematocrit, serum ferritin, and transferrin saturation levels during and after therapy.

Storage

- Store in original carton at 25°C (77°F); excursions permitted to 15° to 30°C (59° to 86°F). Do not freeze.

Contraindications and precautions

Contraindicated in hypersensitivity to drug or its components, hemolytic anemias and other anemias not caused by iron deficiency, primary hemochromatosis, and evidence of iron overload.

Use cautiously in autoimmune disorders, arthritis, severe hepatic impairment, ***elderly patients,*** pregnant or breastfeeding patients, and ***children.***

Adverse reactions

CNS: dizziness, headache, syncope, **seizures**
CV: chest pain, tachycardia, hypotension
GI: nausea, vomiting
Hematologic: hemochromatosis, **hemolysis, hemosiderosis**
Musculoskeletal: muscle cramps, aches, or weakness; joint pain
Respiratory: dyspnea
Other: abnormal or metallic taste, fever, lymphadenopathy, allergic reactions including **anaphylaxis**

Interactions

None significant

Toxicity and overdose

- Dosages in excess of iron needs may cause iron to accumulate in storage sites, leading to hemosiderosis. Signs and symptoms of overdose (or too-rapid infusion) include hypotension, dyspnea, headache, vomiting, nausea, dizziness, joint aches, paresthesia, abdominal and muscle pain, edema, and cardiovascular collapse.
- Discontinue drug until serum ferritin levels equal or exceed established guidelines. Be aware that most symptoms can be treated successfully with I.V. fluids, hydrocortisone, and antihistamines. Solution infused as recommended or at a slower rate also may relieve symptoms. Drug removal by dialysis is negligible.

Patient teaching

- Caution patient not to take oral iron preparations or vitamin supplements containing iron during I.V. iron therapy.
- Instruct patient to report dyspnea, itching, or rash.
- Inform patient about the need for periodic blood testing to monitor response to therapy.
- As appropriate, review all other significant and life-threatening adverse reactions mentioned above.

isoproterenol hydrochloride

Isuprel

Pharmacologic class: Sympathomimetic, $beta_1$-adrenergic and $beta_2$-adrenergic agonist
Therapeutic class: Vasopressor, bronchodilator, antiasthmatic
Pregnancy risk category C

Action

Acts on $beta_2$-adrenergic receptors to cause relaxation of bronchial smooth muscle; acts on $beta_1$-adrenergic receptors in heart to cause positive inotropic and chronotropic effects and increase cardiac output. Also lowers peripheral vascular resistance in skeletal muscle and inhibits antigen-induced histamine release.

Pharmacokinetics

Drug is readily absorbed when given parenterally and metabolized primarily in the liver and other tissues by catechol-O-methyltransferase (COMT) inhibitors. It is a relatively poor substrate for monoamine oxidase, and is not taken up by sympathetic neurons to same extent as are epinephrine and norepinephrine. Therefore, its duration may exceed that of epinephrine but is still brief.

Onset	Peak	Duration
Immediate	Unknown	<1 hr

How supplied

Solution for injection (clear): 0.2 mg/mL (1:5,000) in 1-mL ampule, 0.2 mg/mL in 5-mL ampule, 0.2 mg/mL (1:5,000) in 5-mL vials, 0.2 mg/mL in 10-mL vials, 0.02- or 200-mcg/mL (1:50,000) syringes

Indications and dosages

➢ Adjunctive treatment of hypovolemia, septic shock, cardiogenic shock, low cardiac output, or congestive heart failure

Adults and children: 0.5 to 5 mcg/minute by continuous I.V. infusion

➢ Serious episodes of heart block, Adams-Stokes attacks (except when caused by ventricular tachycardia or fibrillation), or cardiac arrest (until electric shock or pacemaker therapy is available)

Adults: Initially, 0.02 to 0.06 mg I.V. bolus, with subsequent doses of 0.01 to 0.2 mg by I.V. bolus or 5 mcg/minute by I.V. infusion

➤ Bronchospasm during anesthesia
Adults: 0.01 to 0.02 mg I.V., repeated when necessary
➤ Status asthmaticus
Children: 0.08 to 1.7 mcg/kg/minute by I.V. infusion

Administration

Dilution and compatibility

- Be aware that for direct I.V. injection, 1:50,000 solution may be given undiluted.
- For I.V. direct injection, dilute 1 mL of 0.2 mg/mL (1:5,000 solution) in 10 mL normal saline solution or D_5W to achieve a concentration of 1:50,000.
- For I.V. infusion, dilute 10 mL of 0.2 mg/mL (1:5,000 solution) in 500 mL D_5W, or dilute 5 mL of 0.2 mg/mL (1:5,000 solution) in 250 mL D_5W to achieve a concentration of 1:250,000.
- Do not use if pinkish or darker than slightly yellow.

Infusion considerations

- Give each I.V. infusion dose at rate prescribed for condition being treated.
- Be aware that American Heart Association recommends initial infusion rate of 0.1 mcg/kg/minute, with usual range of 0.1 to 1 mcg/kg/minute for children.

Always use continuous infusion pump when administering I.V. infusion.

Assess patient's response to drug, and adjust I.V. infusion rate accordingly.

Know that if patient's heart rate exceeds 110 beats/minute, infusion rate may need to be decreased or infusion discontinued temporarily.

Monitoring

- During administration, monitor ECG and vital signs carefully.
- Closely monitor arterial blood gas values, acid-base and electrolyte balance, urine output, and central venous pressure.

Stay alert for rebound bronchospasm.

Storage

- Store in a cool place between 8° and 15°C (46° and 59°F); protect from light. Keep in opaque container until use.

Contraindications and precautions

Contraindicated in angina pectoris, tachyarrhythmias, tachycardia or heart block caused by digitalis intoxication, and ventricular arrhythmias that warrant inotropic therapy.

Use cautiously in sensitivity to sympathomimetic amines or sulfites, renal impairment, unstable vasomotor disorders, hypertension, coronary insufficiency, coronary artery disease, chronic obstructive pulmonary disease, diabetes mellitus, hyperthyroidism, history of cerebrovascular accident or seizures, ***elderly patients,*** labor, delivery, and breastfeeding.

Adverse reactions

CNS: tremors, anxiety, insomnia, headache, dizziness, asthenia
CV: palpitations, tachycardia, angina, rapid blood pressure changes, **arrhythmias, cardiac arrest, Stokes-Adams attacks**
EENT: pharyngitis
GI: nausea, vomiting, heartburn
Metabolic: hyperglycemia
Respiratory: bronchitis, increased sputum, **pulmonary edema, bronchospasm**
Skin: diaphoresis
Other: parotid gland swelling (with prolonged use)

Interactions

Drug-drug. *Cyclopropane, epinephrine, halogenated general anesthetics:* increased risk of arrhythmias
Propranolol and other beta-adrenergic blockers: antagonism of bronchodilating effects
Drug-diagnostic tests. *Glucose:* increased

Toxicity and overdose

• Acute toxicity may manifest mainly as tachycardia or other arrhythmias, palpitations, angina, hypotension, or hypertension.
• Reduce administration rate or discontinue drug until patient's condition stabilizes. Monitor blood pressure, pulse rate, respirations, and ECG. Provide other supportive measures as indicated. Efficacy of dialysis on drug removal is unknown.

Patient teaching

• Assure patient that he will be monitored closely.
• As appropriate, review all other significant and life-threatening adverse reactions and interactions, especially those related to the drugs and tests mentioned above.

kanamycin sulfate

Pharmacologic class: Aminoglycoside
Therapeutic class: Anti-infective
Pregnancy risk category D

FDA BOXED WARNING

• Observe patient closely for signs and symptoms of toxicity. Drug's major toxic effects are actions on auditory and vestibular branches of eighth nerve and on renal tubules. Neurotoxicity manifests as bilateral auditory toxicity (which may be permanent) and vestibular ototoxicity. Loss of high-frequency perception usually precedes noticeable hearing loss and can be detected by audiometric testing. Patients may lack symptoms of developing cochlear damage. Vertigo may occur, signaling vestibular injury. Other neurotoxicity manifestations may include numbness, skin tingling, muscle twitching, and seizures. Risk of hearing loss increases with degree of exposure to high peak or high trough serum drug levels and continues to progress after drug withdrawal. Renal impairment may manifest as decreased creatinine clearance, urinary cells or casts, oliguria, proteinuria, decreased urine specific gravity, or evidence of increasing nitrogen retention, such as increasing blood urea nitrogen (BUN), nonprotein nitrogen, or serum creatinine levels.
• Risks of severe ototoxic and nephrotoxic reactions increase sharply in patients with impaired renal function and in those with normal renal function who receive high doses or prolonged therapy.
• Monitor renal and eighth nerve function closely, especially in patients with known or suspected reduced renal function at onset of therapy, and in those who initially have normal renal function but develop signs of renal dysfunction during therapy. Monitor serum drug level when feasible to ensure adequate levels and avoid potentially toxic levels. Examine urine for decreased specific gravity, increased protein excretion, and cells or casts.
• Measure BUN, serum creatinine, or creatinine clearance periodically. Obtain serial audiograms when feasible in patients old enough to be tested, particularly high-risk patients. Evidence of ototoxicity (dizziness, vertigo, tinnitus, roaring in ears, and hearing loss) or nephrotoxicity warrants dosage adjustment or drug withdrawal.
• Neuromuscular blockade with respiratory paralysis may develop when drug is instilled intraperitoneally, concomitantly with anesthesia and muscle-relaxing drugs. Neuromuscular blockade has occurred after parenteral injection and oral use of aminoglycosides. Consider possibility of neuromuscular blockade and respiratory paralysis when giving

K

drug by any route, especially in patients receiving anesthetics, neuromuscular blockers (such as tubocurarine, succinylcholine, or decamethonium), or massive transfusions of citrate-anticoagulated blood. If blockade occurs, calcium salts may reduce it, but patient may need mechanical respiratory assistance.
• Avoid concurrent or sequential systemic, oral, or topical use of kanamycin and other potentially nephrotoxic or neurotoxic drugs (particularly polymyxin B, bacitracin, colistin, amphotericin B, cisplatin, vancomycin, and all other aminoglycosides), as toxicity may be additive. Advanced age and dehydration also may increase toxicity risk.
• Do not give drug concurrently with potent diuretics (ethacrynic acid, furosemide, meralluride sodium, sodium mercaptomerin, or mannitol). Some diuretics cause ototoxicity, and I.V. diuretics may enhance aminoglycoside toxicity by altering antibiotic serum and tissue levels.

Action
Interferes with protein synthesis in bacterial cells by binding to 30S ribosomal subunit, causing misreading of genetic code. Formation of inaccurate peptide sequence in protein chain leads to bacterial death.

Pharmacokinetics
Drug diffuses rapidly into most body fluids, including synovial and peritoneal fluids and bile. In normal adults, only trace levels appear in spinal fluid. Little, if any, metabolism occurs. Drug is excreted almost entirely by glomerular filtration and is not reabsorbed by renal tubules. Thus, it attains high levels in nephron, leading to urine levels that may be 10 to 20 times higher than serum levels. Renal excretion is extremely rapid. In patients with normal renal function, approximately half of dose clears within 4 hours and excretion is complete within 24 to 48 hours. Excretion is slower in patients with impaired renal function or diminished glomerular filtration pressure.

Onset	Peak	Duration
Immediate	15-30 min	Unknown

How supplied
Solution for injection: 75 mg/2 mL, 500 mg/2 mL, 1,000 mg/3 mL

Indications and dosages
➢ Serious infections caused by susceptible strains of *Escherichia coli, Acinetobacter* species, *Proteus* species, *Klebsiella* species, *Serratia marcescens, Enterobacter aerogenes, Citrobacter* species, and *Staphylococcus* species
Adults and children: 7.5 mg/kg I.V. q 12 hours. To obtain continuously high drug blood level, may give daily dosage of 15 mg/kg in equally divided doses q 6 or 8 hours, not to exceed 1.5 g/day.

Dosage adjustment
• Reduce dosage or lengthen dosing interval in elderly patients and patients with renal impairment.

Administration
Preparation
• Collect specimens for culture and sensitivity testing as appropriate before therapy starts.
Dilution and compatibility
• Dilute I.V. dose by mixing 500 mg in 100 to 200 mL normal saline solution or D_5W, or by adding 1 g to 200 to 400 mL of either solution.
Do not mix with other anti-infectives (specifically penicillins, cephalosporins,

and beta-lactams) as inactivation of kanamycin may occur.
- Be aware that vials occasionally may darken during product shelf life, but this does not indicate potency loss.

Infusion considerations
- Infuse total single dose I.V. slowly over 30 to 60 minutes at a rate no faster than 3 to 4 mL/minute.

Monitoring

Monitor urine output, urinalysis, and BUN and creatinine levels. To avoid potential renal toxicity, watch for decreased specific gravity, increased protein excretion, and urinary cells or casts.
- Evaluate cardiovascular status carefully.
- Assess neurologic status. Institute safety measures as needed to prevent injury.
- Monitor peak and trough drug blood levels.
- Check for hearing loss based on audiogram recorded before first dose.
- Assess for bleeding tendency.
- Keep patient well hydrated; drug may cause nephrotoxicity.

Storage
- Protect from direct heat and light.

Contraindications and precautions

Contraindicated in hypersensitivity or toxic reaction to drug or other aminoglycosides and in intestinal obstruction.

Use cautiously in renal impairment, neuromuscular diseases (such as myasthenia gravis), hearing impairment, obesity, ***elderly patients,*** pregnant or breastfeeding patients, and ***infants and neonates*** (safety not established).

Adverse reactions

CNS: dizziness, vertigo, tremors, numbness, depression, confusion, lethargy, headache, paresthesia, **neuromuscular blockade, seizures, neurotoxicity**
CV: hypotension, hypertension, palpitations
EENT: visual disturbances, dry eyes, nystagmus, photophobia, hearing loss, tinnitus, ototoxicity
GI: nausea, vomiting, anorexia, splenomegaly, stomatitis, increased salivation
GU: polyuria, dysuria, azotemia, increased urinary casts, erectile dysfunction, **nephrotoxicity**
Hematologic: purpura, eosinophilia, **leukemoid reaction, hemolytic anemia, aplastic anemia, neutropenia, agranulocytosis, leukopenia, thrombocytopenia, pancytopenia**
Hepatic: hepatomegaly, hepatic necrosis, hepatotoxicity
Musculoskeletal: joint pain, muscle twitching
Respiratory: apnea
Skin: rash, urticaria, pruritus, exfoliative dermatitis, alopecia
Other: weight loss, superinfection

Interactions

Drug-drug. *Acyclovir, amphotericin B, cisplatin, potent diuretics, vancomycin:* increased risk of ototoxicity and nephrotoxicity
Dimenhydrinate: masking of ototoxicity symptoms
General anesthetics, neuromuscular junction blockers: increased neuromuscular blockade
Indomethacin: increased kanamycin peak and trough blood levels
Drug-diagnostic tests. *Alanine aminotransferase, aspartate aminotransferase, bilirubin, BUN, creatinine, low-density lipoproteins, nonprotein nitrogen:* increased
Granulocytes, hemoglobin, platelets, white blood cells: decreased
Reticulocytes: increased or decreased

Toxicity and overdose

• Overdose severity depends on dosage given; patient's renal function, state of hydration, and age; and whether patient is receiving concurrent drugs with similar toxicities. Nephrotoxicity, ototoxicity, and neuromuscular blockade with respiratory paralysis may occur.
• Establish airway and ensure oxygenation and ventilation. Provide adequate hydration and monitor fluid balance carefully. Hemodialysis or peritoneal dialysis can help remove drug. In neonates, exchange transfusion also may be considered. Resuscitate, if indicated.

Patient teaching

Teach patient to immediately report unusual bleeding or bruising, unusual tiredness, or yellowing of skin or eyes.
• Tell patient to promptly report tinnitus or difficulty hearing.
• Instruct patient to maintain adequate hydration and to report change in urination pattern.
• Advise patient to avoid activities that can cause injury and to use soft toothbrush and electric razor to avoid gum and skin injury.
• Caution patient to avoid driving and other hazardous activities until drug's effects on concentration and alertness are known.
• Advise female patient to inform prescriber if she is pregnant or breastfeeding.
• Inform patient about the need for repeated laboratory testing during therapy.
• As appropriate, review all other significant and life-threatening adverse reactions and interactions, especially those related to the drugs and tests mentioned above.

ketamine hydrochloride

Ketalar

Pharmacologic class: *N*-methyl-D-aspartate receptor antagonist
Therapeutic class: General anesthetic
Pregnancy risk category C

FDA BOXED WARNING

• About 12% of patients experience reactions when emerging from ketamine anesthesia (called emergence phenomena), ranging from pleasant dreamlike states and vivid imagery to hallucinations and delirium. In some cases, these states are accompanied by confusion, excitement, and irrational behavior. Duration usually is no more than a few hours, although recurrences have occurred up to 24 hours postoperatively. No known residual psychological effects have resulted. Incidence of emergence phenomena is lowest in patients age 15 or younger and those older than age 65, and when drug is given intramuscularly. Emergence phenomena may be reduced by giving lower recommended dosages in conjunction with I.V. diazepam during anesthesia induction and maintenance, or by minimizing verbal, tactile, and visual stimulation of patient during recovery. (However, this does not preclude vital sign monitoring.) To terminate severe emergence reaction, small hypnotic dose of short- or ultrashort-acting barbiturate may be required. When ketamine is used on outpatient basis, do not release patient until recovery from anesthesia is complete and ensure that responsible adult accompanies patient.

Action

Produces anesthetic state marked by profound analgesia, normal pharyngeal-laryngeal reflexes, normal or slightly enhanced skeletal muscle tone, cardiovascular and respiratory stimulation, and occasionally a transient and minimal respiratory depression. Produces dissociative anesthesia by selectively interrupting brain's association pathways before producing somesthetic sensory blockade. May selectively depress thalamoneocortical system before significantly dulling reticular activating and limbic systems.

Pharmacokinetics

Drug biotransformation includes cyclohexene derivative (metabolite II). Drug level has initial slope lasting about 45 minutes, with half-life of 10 to 15 minutes; this phase corresponds to its anesthetic effect. Anesthetic action ends by a combination of redistribution from CNS to slower equilibrating peripheral tissues and by hepatic biotransformation to metabolite I. Later drug half-life is 2.5 hours.

Onset	Peak	Duration
30 sec	Immediate	5 to 10 min

How supplied

Solution for injection (colorless to slightly yellowish): 50 mg/mL in 10-mL vial, 10 mg/mL in 20-mL vial, 100 mg/mL in 5-mL vial

Indications and dosages

➤ Sole anesthetic agent for diagnostic and surgical procedures not requiring skeletal muscle relaxation

Adults: Initially, 1 mg/kg to 4.5 mg/kg I.V. Average amount required to produce 5 to 10 minutes of surgical anesthesia is 2 mg/kg. Alternatively, dosage of 1 to 2 mg/kg I.V. at a rate of 0.5 mg/kg/minute may be given for anesthesia induction. Adjust maintenance dosage according to patient's anesthetic needs and whether additional anesthetic agent is used.

Administration

Preparation

🔊 Know that drug should be used by or under direction of physician experienced in administering general anesthetics and maintaining airway and controlling respiration.

- Know that drug is best suited for short procedures, but can be used with additional doses for longer procedures.
- Be aware that diazepam (given in separate syringe) may be used to reduce incidence of emergence phenomena.
- Because of rapid induction after initial I.V. injection, ensure that patient is in a supported position during administration.
- Know that atropine, scopolamine, or another drying agent should be given at appropriate interval before induction.

Dilution and compatibility

🔊 Do not use 100-mg/mL concentration without proper dilution. Dilute 5-mL vial by adding it to 500 mL D_5W or normal saline solution and mix well.

- To dilute solution containing 1 mg/mL, transfer 10 mL (50-mg/mL vial) to 500 mL D_5W or normal saline solution and mix well. Resulting solution contains 1 mg/mL.

🔊 Know that dilution is not recommended for 10-mg/mL vial.

- Consider patient's fluid requirements and anesthesia duration when choosing appropriate dilution. If fluid restriction is required, add drug to 250-mL infusion as described above to provide ketamine concentration of 2 mg/mL.

🔊 Know that ketamine and barbiturates are chemically incompatible and

K

may lead to precipitation if mixed in same syringe.
- Do not mix ketamine and diazepam in syringe or infusion flask.
- Know that solution may darken with prolonged exposure to light, but this does not affect potency.

Infusion considerations

Give I.V. slowly over 60 seconds. Be aware that more rapid administration may cause respiratory depression, apnea, and enhanced pressor response
- Titrate dosage based on patient's requirements.

Monitoring

In patients with hypertension or cardiac decompensation, monitor cardiac function continually during procedure.

Closely monitor cardiac function if ketamine and halothane are used together, as halothane blocks cardiovascular stimulatory effects of ketamine.

Storage
- Store at controlled room temperature of 15° to 30°C (59° to 86°F); protect from light.

Contraindications and precautions

Contraindicated in hypersensitivity to drug and when significant blood pressure increase would pose a serious hazard.

Use cautiously in chronic alcoholism, acute alcohol intoxication, preanesthesia elevation in cerebrospinal fluid pressure, ***elderly patients,*** pregnant patients (use not recommended), breastfeeding patients, and ***children.***

Adverse reactions

CNS: purposeless and tonic-clonic movements of extremities
CV: tachycardia, hypertension, **hypotension, bradycardia, arrhythmia**
EENT: diplopia, nystagmus, slight intraocular pressure increase
GI: mild anorexia, nausea and vomiting
Respiratory: laryngospasm and other forms of airway obstruction, severe respiratory depression or apnea (with too-rapid administration)
Skin: transient erythema, morbilliform rash
Other: local pain and exanthema at injection site

Interactions

Drug-drug. *Barbiturates, opioids:* prolonged recovery time
Halothane: decreased cardiac output, blood pressure, and pulse rate
Nondepolarizing muscle relaxants: prolonged respiratory depression
Theophylline: unpredictable extensor-type seizures
Thiopental: antagonism of thiopental's hypnotic effect
Thyroid hormones: possible hypertension and tachycardia

Toxicity and overdose

- Drug has wide margin of safety. Several cases of unintentional overdoses (up to 10 times the dose usually required) have been followed by prolonged but complete recovery. Respiratory depression or apnea may occur with overdose or too-rapid administration.
- Use supportive ventilation for respiratory depression or apnea; mechanical respiratory support is preferred to analeptic administration. Provide other supportive measures as indicated.

Patient teaching

- Caution patient not to drive, operate hazardous machinery, or engage in other hazardous activities for at least 24 hours after drug administration.
- As appropriate, review all other significant and life-threatening adverse reactions and interactions, especially those related to the drugs mentioned above.

ketorolac tromethamine

Toradol

Pharmacologic class: Nonsteroidal anti-inflammatory drug (NSAID)

Therapeutic class: Analgesic

Pregnancy risk category C (first and second trimesters), *D* (third trimester)

FDA BOXED WARNING

- Drug is indicated for short-term management (up to 5 days in adults) of moderately severe acute pain that requires opioid-level analgesia. It is not indicated for minor or chronic painful conditions. Drug carries many risks; adverse events from NSAIDs can be serious in certain patients, especially when used inappropriately. Raising dosage beyond recommendations increases risk of serious adverse events without increasing efficacy.
- Drug can cause peptic ulcers, GI bleeding, and perforation and is contraindicated in patients with active peptic ulcer disease, recent GI bleeding or perforation, or history of peptic ulcer disease or GI bleeding.
- Drug is contraindicated in advanced renal impairment and patients at risk for renal failure.
- Drug inhibits platelet function and is contraindicated in patients with suspected or confirmed cerebrovascular bleeding, hemorrhagic diathesis, incomplete hemostasis, or high risk of bleeding.
- Drug is contraindicated as prophylactic analgesic before major surgery, and intraoperatively when hemostasis is critical.
- Hypersensitivity reactions ranging from bronchospasm to anaphylactic shock have occurred. Keep appropriate counteractive measures at hand when giving first dose of injection form. Drug is contraindicated in known hypersensitivity to ketorolac or allergic reaction to aspirin or other NSAID.
- Drug is contraindicated for intrathecal or epidural administration (due to alcohol content), during labor and delivery (may impede fetal circulation and inhibit uterine contractions), in breastfeeding patients (due to potential adverse effects of prostaglandin-inhibiting drugs on neonates), and in patients currently receiving aspirin or other NSAIDs (due to cumulative risk of serious NSAID-related adverse effects).
- Tablet form is indicated only as continuation therapy to injection form; combined duration of use of both forms must not exceed 5 days.
- For tablets, recommended total daily dosage (maximum 40 mg) is significantly lower than for injection (maximum 120 mg).
- Adjust dosage in patients age 65 and older, those weighing less than 50 kg (110 lb), and those with moderately elevated serum creatinine level. With injection form, do not exceed 60 mg (total daily dosage) in these patients. Injection form is indicated as single-dose therapy in pediatric patients, not to exceed 30 mg for I.M. use or 15 mg for I.V. use.

Action

Interferes with prostaglandin biosynthesis by inhibiting cyclooxygenase pathway of arachidonic acid metabolism; also acts as potent inhibitor of platelet aggregation

Pharmacokinetics

Drug is metabolized largely in the liver. Although it is highly protein-bound (99%), even plasma levels as high as 10 mcg/mL occupy only about 5% of albumin binding sites; thus, unbound fraction for each metabolite is constant over therapeutic range. However, serum albumin decrease causes increased free concentrations. Principal elimination route of drug and metabolites is renal. About 92% of dose appears in urine (approximately 60% as unchanged drug and 40% as metabolites); drug also appears in breast milk.

Onset	Peak	Duration
10 min	1-2 hr	≥6 hr

How supplied

Solution for injection (clear and slightly yellow): 15 mg/mL in 1-mL preloaded syringes, 30 mg/mL in 1- and 2-mL preloaded syringes, 15 mg/mL and 30 mg/mL in 1-mL single-dose vials, 60 mg/2-mL single-dose vials, 300 mg/10-mL single-dose vials

Indications and dosages

➤ Short-term management of moderately severe pain

Adults younger than age 65: Initially, 30 mg I.V. as a single dose, or 30 mg I.V. q 6 hours, not to exceed 120 mg/day

Children ages 2 to 16: Single dose of 0.5 mg/kg, up to a maximum of 15 mg I.V.

Dosage adjustment

• Reduce dosage to 15 mg every 6 hours in mild to moderate renal impairment, elderly patients, and patients weighing less than 50 kg (110 lb); do not exceed maximum daily dosage of 60 mg.

Administration

Preparation

Know that adults should not receive more than 20 doses in 5 days, and patients should be switched to alternative analgesic as soon as possible.

Be aware that in children, drug is recommended only for single-dose use.

• Be aware that oral therapy may be used only as continuation of parenteral therapy.

Dilution and compatibility

• May be given undiluted.

• Drug is compatible with normal saline solution, D_5W, dextrose 5% in normal saline solution, or lactated Ringer's solution.

• Do not use if discolored.

Do not mix in small volume (such as in syringe) with morphine sulfate, meperidine hydrochloride, promethazine hydrochloride, or hydroxyzine hydrochloride, as this causes precipitation.

Infusion considerations

• Administer single I.V. bolus over 1 to 2 minutes.

Monitoring

Know that NSAIDs may increase risk of serious cardiovascular thrombotic events, myocardial infarction, and cerebrovascular accident, which can be fatal. Risk may increase with duration of use and in patients with risk factors.

• Monitor for adverse reactions, especially prolonged bleeding time and CNS reactions.

• Monitor fluid intake and output.

Storage

• Store at 20° to 25°C (68° to 77°F); protect from light. Keep in carton until use.

Contraindications and precautions

Contraindicated in hypersensitivity to drug, its components, aspirin, or other NSAIDs; concurrent use of aspirin, other NSAIDs, or probenecid; peptic ulcer disease (current or previous); GI bleeding or perforation (current or previous); advanced renal impairment or risk of renal failure due to volume depletion; increased risk of bleeding; suspected or confirmed cerebrovascular bleeding; hemorrhagic diathesis; incomplete hemostasis; prophylactic use before major surgery; intraoperative use when hemostasis is critical; neuraxial administration; labor and delivery; and breastfeeding.

Use cautiously in mild to moderate renal impairment, cardiovascular disease, ***elderly patients,*** pregnant patients, and ***children younger than age 2*** (safety and efficacy not established).

Adverse reactions

CNS: drowsiness, headache, dizziness
CV: hypertension
EENT: tinnitus
GI: nausea, vomiting, diarrhea, constipation, flatulence, dyspepsia, epigastric pain, stomatitis
Hematologic: thrombocytopenia
Skin: rash, pruritus, diaphoresis
Other: excessive thirst, edema

Interactions

Drug-drug. *Angiotensin-converting enzyme inhibitors, beta-adrenergic blockers:* decreased antihypertensive effect
Anticoagulants: prolonged prothrombin time
Aspirin: altered ketorolac distribution, metabolism, and excretion; increased risk of serious adverse reactions
Corticosteroids, other NSAIDs: additive adverse GI effects
Diuretics: decreased diuretic effect
Hydantoins, lithium: increased blood levels and greater risk of toxicity of these drugs
Methotrexate: increased risk of methotrexate toxicity
Probenecid: increased risk of ketorolac toxicity
Drug-diagnostic tests. *Bleeding time:* prolonged for 24 to 48 hours after therapy ends
Drug-herb. *Anise, arnica, chamomile, clove, dong quai, feverfew, garlic, ginger, ginkgo, ginseng:* increased risk of bleeding

Toxicity and overdose

- After acute overdose, symptoms usually are limited to lethargy, drowsiness, nausea, vomiting, and GI bleeding. Rarely, hypertension, acute renal failure, respiratory depression, and coma occur.
- No specific antidote exists. Provide symptomatic and supportive therapy. Dialysis does not significantly clear drug.

Patient teaching

- Inform patient that drug is meant only for short-term pain management.
- Tell patient to immediately report bleeding and adverse CNS reactions.
- Advise patient to minimize GI upset by eating small, frequent servings of healthy food.
- Instruct patient to avoid aspirin products and herbs during therapy.
- Caution female patient not to take drug if she is breastfeeding.
- Tell female patient to inform prescriber if she is pregnant.
- Caution patient to avoid driving and other hazardous activities until drug's effects on concentration and alertness are known.
- As appropriate, review all other significant and life-threatening adverse reactions and interactions, especially those related to the drugs, tests, and herbs mentioned above.

labetalol hydrochloride

Trandate

Pharmacologic class: Nonselective beta-adrenergic blocker, selective $alpha_1$-adrenergic blocker
Therapeutic class: Antihypertensive
Pregnancy risk category C

Action

Blocks stimulation of $beta_1$- and $beta_2$-adrenergic receptor sites and $alpha_1$-adrenergic receptors, decreasing myocardial contractile force and enhancing coronary artery blood flow and myocardial perfusion. Net effect is decreased heart rate and blood pressure.

Pharmacokinetics

Drug distributes widely throughout body and crosses placental barrier. It is metabolized in the liver and is approximately 50% protein-bound. About 55% to 60% of dose appears in urine as conjugates or unchanged drug, with some excretion in feces. Elimination half-life is 5.5 hours.

Onset	Peak	Duration
5-20 min	Unknown	Unknown

How supplied

Solution for injection: 5 mg/mL in 20-mL and 40-mL multidose vials

Indications and dosages

➢ Severe hypertension

Adults: Initially, 20 mg I.V. bolus over 2 minutes, followed by I.V. injection of 40 to 80 mg q 10 minutes until blood pressure falls to desired level; maximum dosage is 300 mg. Alternatively, 50 to 200 mg by continuous I.V. infusion at 2 mg/minute (some patients may require total dosage of 300 mg); continue infusion until desired blood pressure occurs. (Follow I.V. administration with P.O. dosing.)

Off-label uses

- Hypertension secondary to pheochromocytoma
- Hypertensive crisis

Administration

Preparation

- Know that injection form is intended for I.V. use in hospitalized patients. Individualize dosage based on severity of hypertension and response during dosing.
- Be aware that patient usually is switched from I.V. to oral dosing when desired blood pressure is reached.
- Ensure that patient is in supine position before giving drug.
- Measure blood pressure immediately before giving drug.

Dilution and compatibility

- Know that drug is compatible with normal saline solution, dextrose 5% in normal saline solution, dextrose 5% in 0.2% sodium chloride solution, dextrose 2.5% in 0.45% sodium chloride injection, dextrose 5% in 0.33% sodium chloride injection, dextrose 5% in water (D_5W), dextrose 5% in Ringer's solution, lactated Ringer's, Ringer's solution and sterile water for injection.
- Be aware that drug may be given undiluted for I.V. bolus injection.
- For continuous I.V. infusion, add 200 mg labetalol to 160 mL D_5W or normal saline solution to yield 1 mg/mL solution, to be given at 2 mL (2 mg)/minute.
- Alternatively, for continuous I.V. infusion, add 200 mg labetalol to 250 mL D_5W or normal saline solution yield 2 mg/3 mL solution, to be given at 3 mL (2 mg)/minute.
- Do not mix with 5% sodium bicarbonate injection.

Infusion considerations

- Give I.V. bolus injection over 2 minutes at 10-minute intervals.
- For continuous infusion, deliver with infusion control pump.
- Adjust infusion rate according to blood pressure response.

Monitoring

🔈 Measure blood pressure 5 and 10 minutes after giving drug.

🔈 Observe closely for first signs of cardiac failure; be prepared to treat with digitalis preparation and diuretics. If cardiac failure continues, discontinue drug.

🔈 Monitor closely for signs and symptoms of hepatic toxicity; discontinue drug if patient develops jaundice or liver function tests indicate hepatic injury.

- Closely monitor ECG and vital signs, especially blood pressure.
- Monitor CBC and blood glucose level.
- Assess respiratory and neurologic status closely to detect adverse reactions.

Storage

- Store between 2° and 8°C (36° and 46°F); protect from light.

Contraindications and precautions

Contraindicated in hypersensitivity to drug, bronchospastic disease, overt heart failure, cardiogenic shock, second- or third-degree atrioventricular block, severe bradycardia, and conditions associated with severe and prolonged hypotension.

Use cautiously in hepatic impairment, pulmonary disease, diabetes mellitus, hyperthyroidism, thyrotoxicosis, ***elderly patients,*** pregnant or breastfeeding patients, and ***children*** (safety and efficacy not established).

Adverse reactions

CNS: fatigue, asthenia, anxiety, depression, dizziness, paresthesia, drowsiness, insomnia, memory loss, nightmares, mental status changes

CV: orthostatic hypotension, peripheral vasoconstriction, bradycardia, **arrhythmias, heart failure**

EENT: blurred vision, dry eyes, nasal congestion

GI: nausea, diarrhea, constipation

GU: erectile dysfunction, decreased libido

Hematologic: purpura, **agranulocytosis, thrombocytopenia**

Hepatic: hepatotoxicity (rare)

Metabolic: hyperglycemia, **hypoglycemia**

Musculoskeletal: joint pain, back pain, muscle cramps

Respiratory: wheezing, **bronchospasm, pulmonary edema**

Skin: rash, pruritus

Interactions

Drug-drug. *Adrenergic bronchodilators, theophylline:* decreased efficacy of these drugs

Antihypertensives, nitrates: additive hypotension

Cimetidine, propranolol: increased labetalol effects

Digoxin: additive bradycardia

Dobutamine, dopamine: reduced cardiovascular benefits of these drugs

General anesthetics, verapamil: additive myocardial depression

Insulin, oral hypoglycemics: altered hypoglycemic efficacy

Monoamine oxidase inhibitors: hypertension

Nonsteroidal anti-inflammatory drugs: decreased antihypertensive action

Drug-diagnostic tests. *Alanine aminotransferase, alkaline phosphatase, antinuclear antibodies, aspartate aminotransferase, blood urea nitrogen, glucose, liver function tests, low-density lipoproteins, potassium, triglycerides, uric acid:* increased

Toxicity and overdose

- Overdose signs and symptoms include severe hypotension and bradycardia. Cardiac failure and bronchospasm also may occur.
- Place patient in supine position with legs elevated. As ordered, give vasopressors for hypotension, atropine or epinephrine for bradycardia, digitalis preparation and possibly dopamine or dobutamine for

L

cardiac failure, and epinephrine for bronchospasm. Dialysis does not remove drug.

Patient teaching

Instruct patient to immediately report adverse reactions, such as easy bruising or bleeding and respiratory problems.

- Tell patient dizziness may occur at start of therapy, especially if patient is receiving diuretic concurrently.
- Advise patient to move slowly when sitting up or standing, to avoid dizziness or light-headedness from sudden blood pressure decrease.
- Caution patient not to drive or perform other hazardous activities until drug's effects on concentration, vision, and alertness are known.
- Emphasize the need for follow-up care and regular blood pressure monitoring.

Caution patient to closely follow oral therapy protocol after I.V. therapy and not to stop taking drug abruptly, as this may cause heart attack or may worsen angina.

- Tell female patient to inform prescriber if she is pregnant or breastfeeding.
- As appropriate, review all other significant and life-threatening adverse reactions and interactions, especially those related to the drugs and tests mentioned above.

lepirudin

Refludan

Pharmacologic class: Thrombin inhibitor
Therapeutic class: Anticoagulant
Pregnancy risk category B

Action

Binds with thrombin, blocking its thrombogenic activity

Pharmacokinetics

Distribution is confined to extracellular fluids; initial half-life is approximately 10 minutes. Drug presumably is metabolized by release of amino acids via catabolic hydrolysis of parent drug. About 48% of dose is excreted in urine, 35% of this as unchanged drug and other fragments of parent drug. Elimination terminal half-life is about 1.3 hours. In hemodialysis patients with marked renal insufficiency, elimination half-live is prolonged up to 2 days.

Onset	Peak	Duration
Immediate	Unknown	Unknown

How supplied

Powder for reconstitution for injection (white): 50-mg vial

Indications and dosages

➤ Heparin-induced thrombocytopenia and associated thromboembolic disease

Adults: Initially, 0.4 mg/kg by I.V. bolus over 15 to 20 seconds (to a maximum of 44 mg), followed by 0.15 mg/kg continuous I.V. infusion for 2 to 10 days or longer if needed

Dosage adjustment

- Reduce bolus dosage and infusion rate in patients with renal impairment.
- In hemodialysis patients or acute renal failure, stop infusion; consider giving additional I.V. bolus doses of 0.1 mg/kg every other day only if activated partial thromboplastin time (APTT) falls below lower therapeutic limit of 1.5.
- If APTT is above target range, stop infusion for 2 hours. At restart, decrease infusion rate 50% (do not give additional I.V. bolus). Determine APTT again 4 hours later.
- If APTT is below target range, increase infusion rate in increments of 20%. Determine APTT again 4 hours later.

Administration

Preparation

- Check APTT before starting therapy.

Do not restart drug in patients with baseline APTT of 2.5 or more, to avoid initial overdosing.

- If patient will receive oral anticoagulant after lepirudin therapy, gradually reduce lepirudin dosage first, to reach APTT just above 1.5 before initiating oral anticoagulant. To avoid prothrombotic effects when starting oral anticoagulant, continue I.V. parenteral anticoagulation for 4 to 5 days; discontinue parenteral agent when International Normalized Ratio stabilizes within desired target range.

Dilution and compatibility

- For I.V. bolus injection, reconstitute 1 vial (50 mg) with 1 mL sterile water for injection or normal saline solution.
- Further dilute for I.V. bolus injection by transferring vial contents into single-use syringe of at least 10 mL, and dilute solution to total volume of 10 mL using sterile water for injection, normal saline solution, or D_5W to yield a final concentration of 5 mg/mL.
- For continuous I.V. infusion, reconstitute two vials (each containing 50 mg) with 1 mL each of sterile water for injection or normal saline solution for injection. Then further dilute by transferring contents of both vials into infusion bag containing 500 mL or 250 mL normal saline solution or D_5W to yield a final concentration of 0.2 mg/mL or 0.4 mg/mL, respectively.
- Do not mix with other solutions.
- Use immediately after reconstitution. Discard unused portion.

Infusion considerations

Administer I.V. bolus slowly over at least 15 to 20 seconds.

- Follow bolus with continuous I.V. infusion.
- For continuous I.V. infusion, set rate (mL/hour) according to body weight, as prescribed.

Reduce infusion rate in patients with renal impairment.

In general, do not exceed infusion rate of 0.21 mg/kg/hour without checking for coagulation abnormalities (which might prevent appropriate APTT response).

Monitoring

Obtain first APTT determination for monitoring treatment 4 hours after infusion starts; then monitor APTT at least daily. Target range is 1.5 to 2.5. More frequent APTT monitoring is highly recommended in patients with renal impairment or serious hepatic injury.

Watch closely for signs and symptoms of bleeding.

Check for adverse effects, particularly signs and symptoms of infection, multisystemic failure, and cardiorespiratory problems.

- Monitor CBC with white cell differential; assess liver function test results.
- Assess fluid intake and output and monitor creatinine clearance.
- Check vital signs frequently.

Storage

- Store unopened vials at 2° to 25°C (36° to 77°F).

Contraindications and precautions

Contraindicated in hypersensitivity to drug, its components, or hirudin.

Use cautiously in renal or hepatic disease, bleeding, bacterial endocarditis, recent cerebrovascular accident or neurosurgery, ***elderly patients,*** pregnant or breastfeeding patients, and ***children.***

Adverse reactions

CNS: depression

CV: heart failure, pericardial effusion, ventricular fibrillation

GI: GI bleeding

GU: hematuria, **abnormal renal function**
Hematologic: hemorrhage, thrombocytopenia
Respiratory: pneumonia, hemoptysis
Skin: rash, pruritus, urticaria
Other: chills, fever, bleeding at injection site, excessive wound bleeding, **multi-systemic failure, sepsis, anaphylaxis**

Interactions

Drug-drug. *Cefamandole, cefoperazone, cefotetan, clopidogrel, eptifibatide, nonsteroidal anti-inflammatory drugs, oral anticoagulants, platelet aggregation inhibitors, plicamycin, thrombolytics, ticlopidine, tirofiban, valproic acid:* increased risk of bleeding
Drug-diagnostic tests. *Liver function tests:* increased

Toxicity and overdose

- In overdose (indicated by excessively high APTT), risk of bleeding increases.
- No specific antidote exists. If life-threatening bleeding occurs and excessive plasma drug levels are suspected, immediately stop administration, determine APTT and other coagulation levels as appropriate, determine hemoglobin, and prepare for blood transfusion. Follow facility guidelines for treating patients with shock. Dialysis may be beneficial.

Patient teaching

- Teach patient to recognize and immediately report signs and symptoms of bleeding.
- Explain bleeding precautions which the patient should take.
- Inform patient of the need for repeated laboratory testing during therapy.
- Advise female patient to tell prescriber if she is pregnant or breastfeeding.
- As appropriate, review all other significant and life-threatening adverse reactions and interactions, especially those related to the drugs and tests mentioned above.

leucovorin calcium (calcium folinate ❋, citrovorum factor, folinic acid)

Pharmacologic class: Folic acid derivative
Therapeutic class: Antidote to folic acid antagonist, antianemic, antineoplastic adjunct
Pregnancy risk category C

Action

Counteracts therapeutic and toxic effects of folic acid antagonists; may enhance therapeutic and toxic effects of fluoropyrimidines used in cancer therapy. Also supplements folic acid in folic acid deficiency.

Pharmacokinetics

Drug is metabolized to active metabolite in the liver. Mean time to peak serum level is 10 minutes; terminal half-life is 6.2 hours. Sharp drop in parent compound coincides with appearance of active metabolite 5-methyl-THF, which is main circulating form of drug. Metabolites are excreted in urine, with a small amount in feces.

Onset	Peak	Duration
<5 min	Unknown	3-6 hr

How supplied

Powder for reconstitution for injection (expressed as base): 50 mg, 100 mg, and 350 mg in single-use vials
Solution for injection: 50 mg/5 mL (10 mg/mL) in single-dose ampules

Indications and dosages

➢ Leucovorin rescue after high-dose methotrexate therapy

Adults: Based on methotrexate dosage of 12 to 15 g/m^2 by I.V. infusion over 4 hours, give leucovorin 15 mg (approximately 10 mg/m^2) I.V. q 6 hours starting 24 hours after methotrexate infusion begins and continuing until serum methotrexate level drops below 10^{-8} M. If 24-hour serum creatinine level rises 50% over baseline or 24-hour methotrexate level exceeds 5×10^{-6} M or 48-hour level exceeds 9×10^{-7} M, increase leucovorin dosage to 100 mg/m^2 I.V. q 3 hours and continue hydration and urinary alkalization until methotrexate level drops below 10^{-8} M.

➢ To reduce toxicity and counteract effects of impaired methotrexate elimination or inadvertent overdose of folic acid antagonist

Adults: Within 24 hours of methotrexate administration if elimination is delayed, or starting promptly after inadvertent overdose, give leucovorin 15 mg (approximately 10 mg/m^2) I.V. q 6 hours until serum methotrexate level drops below 10^{-8} M. If 24-hour serum creatinine level rises 50% over baseline or if 24-hour methotrexate level exceeds 5×10^{-6} M or 48-hour level exceeds 9×10^{-7} M, increase leucovorin dosage to 100 mg/m^2 I.V. q 3 hours, and continue hydration and urinary alkalization until methotrexate level drops below 10^{-8} M.

➢ Advanced colorectal cancer

Adults: Usually given in one of the following regimens: 200 mg/m^2 slow I.V. injection over at least 3 minutes, followed by I.V. injection of 5-fluorouracil (5-FU); or 20 mg/m^2 I.V. injection followed by I.V. injection of 5-FU. Treatment may be repeated daily for 5 days, and may then be repeated at 28-day intervals for two courses and then at 4- to 5-week intervals (if patient has completely recovered from toxic effects of previous course).

Dosage adjustment

• Extend leucovorin rescue and adjust dosage based on the following guidelines:

Clinical situation	Laboratory findings	Leucovorin dosage and duration
Normal methotrexate elimination	Serum methotrexate level approximately 10 μmol at 24 hr after administration, 1 μmol at 48 hr and less than 0.2 μmol at 72 hr	15 mg I.V. q 6 hr for 60 hr (10 doses starting 24 hr after methotrexate infusion begins)
Delayed late methotrexate elimination	Serum methotrexate level remaining above 0.2 μmol at 72 hr and more than 0.05 μmol at 96 hr after administration	Continue 15 mg I.V. q 6 hr until methotrexate level is less than 0.05 μmol
Delayed early methotrexate elimination and/or evidence of acute renal injury	Serum methotrexate level of 50 μmol or more at 24 hr or 5 μmol or more at 48 hr after administration; or 100% or greater increase in serum creatinine level at 24 hr after methotrexate administration such as increase from 0.5 mg/dL to 1 mg/dL or more	150 mg I.V. q 3 hr until methotrexate level is less than 1 μmol; then 15 mg I.V. q 3 hr until methotrexate level is less than 0.05 μmol

L

Administration

Preparation

Recheck leucovorin dosage in current published protocols before giving drug for methotrexate rescue.

• Know that leucovorin must be given promptly when prescribed, to diminish methotrexate toxicity and counteract effects of impaired methotrexate elimination or folic acid antagonist overdose.

Dilution and compatibility

• Dilute 10 mg/mL solution in single-dose ampules with D_5W, normal saline solution, lactated Ringer's, or Ringer's solution, for a final concentration of 0.05 mg/mL.

• Reconstitute each 50-mg vial or 100-mg vial with 5 or 10 mL sterile or bacteriostatic water for injection containing benzyl alcohol, respectively, to yield a concentration of 10 mg/mL.

• Reconstitute each 350-mg vial with 17.5 mL sterile or bacteriostatic water for injection containing benzyl alcohol, to yield a concentration of 20 mg/mL.

• When giving with 5-FU for colorectal cancer in dosages above 10 mg/m^2, reconstitute only with sterile water for injection, because of benzyl alcohol in bacteriostatic water for injection.

Do not mix leucovorin injection with 5-FU, because precipitation will occur.

• Know that drug contains no preservative. When reconstituted with bacteriostatic water for injection, use resulting solution within 7 days. When reconstituted with sterile water for injection, use immediately and discard unused portion.

• Do not use if discolored.

• Discard diluted solution after 24 hours.

Infusion considerations

Give I.V. leucovorin slowly (no faster than 160 mg/minute) because of calcium content. Large doses may be infused over 1 to 6 hours as directed.

Do not give intrathecally; drug may be harmful or fatal by this route.

Know that 5-FU and leucovorin may be infused together through Y-site but should not be mixed together in same I.V. bag, to avoid precipitation.

Monitoring

Monitor serum creatinine and methotrexate levels carefully every 24 hours.

When giving as leucovorin rescue after high-dose methotrexate therapy or to diminish toxicity and counteract effects of impaired methotrexate elimination or inadvertent folic acid antagonist overdose, monitor patient closely for adverse reactions. Continue leucovorin therapy, hydration, and urinary alkalization, as ordered, until methotrexate level drops below 10^{-8} M.

Monitor CBC with white cell differential and platelet count before leucovorin–5-FU therapy starts. Repeat weekly during first two courses and then once each cycle at anticipated white blood cell nadir.

• Check electrolyte levels and liver function test results before each treatment for first three cycles. Thereafter, check before every other cycle.

• Watch for hypersensitivity reactions, especially anaphylactoid reactions.

Storage

• Store powder at controlled room temperature of 25°C (77°F). Keep in carton until use, protected from light.

• Know that diluted solution may be stored for 24 hours at room temperature.

Contraindications and precautions

Contraindicated in treatment of pernicious anemia and other megaloblastic anemias secondary to vitamin B_{12} deficiency.

Use cautiously in anemia (when vitamin B_{12} deficiency has been ruled out), patients receiving 5-FU concomitantly, pregnant or breastfeeding patients, and ***children.***

Adverse reactions

Skin: urticaria
Other: allergic sensitization reactions, **anaphylactoid reactions**

Interactions

Drug-drug. *5-FU:* increased fluorouracil toxicity
Methotrexate, other folic acid antagonists: negation of therapeutic and toxic effects of these drugs
Phenobarbital, phenytoin, primidone: negation of anticonvulsant effect, increased frequency of seizures in susceptible children

Toxicity and overdose

- Excessive leucovorin dosages may nullify chemotherapeutic effect of folic acid antagonists.
- Reduce dosage if indicated.

Patient teaching

- Teach patient about drug and treatment protocol. Emphasize that drug is not just a vitamin.

Tell patient to immediately report signs or symptoms of allergic reaction, such as hives.

- As appropriate, review all other significant and life-threatening adverse reactions and interactions, especially those related to the drugs mentioned above.

levofloxacin

Levaquin, Tavanic

Pharmacologic class: Fluoroquinolone
Therapeutic class: Anti-infective
Pregnancy risk category C

Action

Inhibits enzyme DNA gyrase in susceptible gram-negative and gram-positive aerobic and anaerobic bacteria, interfering with bacterial DNA synthesis

Pharmacokinetics

Drug distributes widely in body tissues, including lung tissues. It undergoes limited metabolism and is approximately 24% to 38% protein-bound. Stereochemically stable in plasma and urine, it does not invert metabolically to its enantiomer, *D*-ofloxacin. Less than 5% of dose is recovered in urine as desmethyl and *N*-oxide metabolites. Drug is primarily excreted unchanged in urine; about 4% of dose appears in feces. Mean terminal plasma elimination half-life ranges from approximately 6 to 8 hours after single or multiple doses.

Onset	Peak	Duration
Rapid	End of infusion	24 hr

How supplied

Premixed solution for injection: 5 mg/mL (250 mg/50 mL) in 100-mL flexible container, 5 mg/mL (500 mg/100 mL) in 100-mL flexible container, 5 mg/mL (750 mg/150 mL) in 150-mL flexible container
Solution for injection (concentrated, clear yellow to clear greenish yellow): 25 mg/mL (500 mg/20 mL)

Indications and dosages

➢ Acute bacterial exacerbation of chronic bronchitis caused by *Staphylococcus aureus, Streptococcus pneumoniae, Haemophilus influenzae, Haemophilus parainfluenzae,* or *Moraxella catarrhalis*
Adults: 500 mg I.V. q 24 hours for 7 days
➢ Community-acquired pneumonia caused by *S. aureus, S. pneumoniae* (including multi-drug-resistant strains),

H. influenzae, H. parainfluenzae, Klebsiella pneumoniae, M. catarrhalis, Chlamydia pneumoniae, Legionella pneumophila, or *Mycoplasma pneumoniae*
Adults: 500 mg I.V. q 24 hours for 7 to 14 days, or 750 mg I.V. q 24 hours for 5 days
➢ Nosocomial pneumonia caused by methicillin-susceptible strains of *S. aureus, Pseudomonas aeruginosa, Serratia marcescens, Escherichia coli, K. pneumoniae, H. influenzae,* or *S. pneumoniae;* complicated skin and skin-structure infections caused by *S. aureus, Enterococcus faecalis, Streptococcus pyogenes,* or *Proteus mirabilis*
Adults: 750 mg I.V. q 24 hours for 7 to 14 days
➢ Acute maxillary sinusitis caused by *S. pneumoniae, H. influenzae,* or *M. catarrhalis*
Adults: 500 mg I.V. q 24 hours for 10 to 14 days
➢ Uncomplicated skin and skin-structure infections caused by *S. aureus* or *S. pyogenes*
Adults: 500 mg I.V. q 24 hours for 7 to 10 days
➢ Complicated skin and skin-structure infections caused by methicillin-susceptible *S. aureus, Enterococcus faecalis, S. pyogenes,* or *P. mirabilis*
Adults: 750 mg I.V. q 24 hours for 7 to 14 days
➢ Complicated urinary tract infections caused by *E. coli, K. pneumoniae,* or *P. mirabilis* or acute pyelonephritis caused by *E. coli,* including cases with concurrent bacteremia
Adults: 750 mg I.V. q 24 hours for 5 days
➢ Complicated urinary tract infections (mild to moderate) caused by *E. faecalis, Enterobacter cloacae, E. coli, K. pneumoniae, P. mirabilis,* or *P. aeruginosa;* acute pyelonephritis (mild to moderate) caused by *E. coli*
Adults: 250 mg I.V. q 24 hours for 10 days
➢ Uncomplicated urinary tract infections (mild to moderate) caused by *E. coli, K. pneumoniae,* or *Staphylococcus saprophyticus*
Adults: 250 mg I.V. q 24 hours for 3 days
➢ Chronic bacterial prostatitis caused by *E. coli, E. faecalis,* or *Staphylococcus epidermidis*
Adults: 500 mg I.V. q 24 hours for 28 days

Dosage adjustment

• Adjust dosage in renal impairment to avoid drug accumulation caused by decreased clearance.

Administration

Dilution and compatibility

• Know that ready-to-use containers are premixed with D_5W for injection and require no dilution.
• To prepare concentrated contents of single-use vials for I.V. infusion, use compatible solution, such as normal saline solution, dextrose 5% in normal saline solution, D_5W, or dextrose 5% in lactated Ringer's solution. Dilute each 10 mL (250-mg dose) with at least 40 mL compatible solution to desired concentration of 5 mg/mL.
• When preparing two 250-mg doses from 20-mL concentrated vial containing 500 mg, withdraw full contents of vial at once using single-entry procedure, because product has no preservative or bacteriostatic agent. Prepare second dose and store for future use according to manufacturer's guidelines.
• Do not add other I.V. additives or drugs to premixed containers or vials.
• Do not use if cloudy.
• Discard unused drug from premixed containers and vials.

Infusion considerations

Give parenteral form by I.V. route only. Drug is not for I.M., subcutaneous, intrathecal, or intraperitoneal use.

- Infuse over 60 to 90 minutes, depending on dosage.
- Do not infuse through same line with solutions containing multivalent cations (such as magnesium).
- If same I.V. line is used for sequential infusion of several different drugs, flush line before and after infusion with solution compatible with levofloxacin injection and any other drug given through common line.

Avoid rapid or bolus I.V. administration, as this may cause severe hypotension.

Do not use plastic containers in series connections. Such use could result in air embolism due to residual air being drawn from primary container before administration of fluid from secondary container ends.

Monitoring

Assess for severe diarrhea, which may indicate pseudomembranous colitis.

Watch for hypersensitivity reaction. Discontinue drug immediately if rash or other signs or symptoms occur.

- Monitor vital signs, especially blood pressure.
- Closely monitor patient with renal insufficiency
- Monitor blood glucose level closely in diabetic patients.

Storage

- Store premixed containers at or below 25°C (77°F). Brief exposure up to 40°C (104°F) does not harm product. Avoid excessive heat and protect from freezing and light.
- Know that after dilution in compatible solution to a concentration of 5 mg/mL, drug is stable for 72 hours when stored at or below 25°C (77°F) and for 14 days when refrigerated at 5ϒC (41ϒF) in plastic I.V. container.

Contraindications and precautions

Contraindicated in hypersensitivity to drug, its components, or other quinolones.

Use cautiously in bradycardia, acute myocardial ischemia, prolonged QTc interval, cirrhosis, renal impairment, underlying CNS disease, uncorrected hypocalcemia, ***elderly patients,*** pregnant or breastfeeding patients, and ***children younger than age 18.***

Adverse reactions

CNS: dizziness, headache, insomnia, **seizures**

CV: chest pain, palpitations, hypotension

EENT: photophobia, sinusitis, pharyngitis

GI: nausea, vomiting, diarrhea, constipation, abdominal pain, dyspepsia, flatulence, **pseudomembranous colitis**

GU: vaginitis

Hematologic: lymphocytopenia

Metabolic: hyperglycemia, **hypoglycemia**

Musculoskeletal: back pain, tendon rupture, tendinitis

Skin: photosensitivity

Other: altered taste, reaction and pain at I.V. site, hypersensitivity reactions including **Stevens-Johnson syndrome**

Interactions

Drug-drug. *Cimetidine:* interference with levofloxacin elimination

Nonsteroidal anti-inflammatory drugs: increased risk of CNS stimulation and seizures

Drug-diagnostic tests. *EEG:* abnormal findings

Glucose: increased or decreased

Lymphocytes: decreased

Drug-herb. *Dong quai, St. John's wort:* phototoxicity

Drug-behaviors. *Sun exposure:* phototoxicity

Toxicity and overdose

- Drug has low potential for acute toxicity. In overdose, expect extension of adverse reactions.
- Observe patient and maintain adequate hydration. Dialysis does not remove drug.

Patient teaching

Tell patient to immediately report signs or symptoms of hypersensitivity reaction (rash, hives, or other skin reactions) or severe diarrhea (which may indicate pseudomembranous colitis).

- Caution patient to avoid driving and other activities requiring mental alertness until drug's CNS effects are known.
- As appropriate, review all other significant and life-threatening adverse reactions and interactions, especially those related to the drugs, tests, herbs, and behaviors mentioned above.

levorphanol tartrate

Levo-Dromoran

Pharmacologic class: Synthetic opioid agonist
Therapeutic class: Opioid analgesic
Controlled substance schedule II
Pregnancy risk category C

Action

Inhibits adenylate cyclase, which regulates release of pain neurotransmitters (acetylcholine, dopamine, substance P, and gamma-aminobutyric acid). Also stimulates mu and kappa opioid receptors, altering perception of and emotional response to pain.

Pharmacokinetics

After I.V. dose, drug distributes widely throughout body and crosses placental barrier. Terminal half-life is approximately 11 to 16 hours. Drug is extensively metabolized in the liver; only 40% is bound to plasma proteins. It is eliminated as inactive glucuronide metabolite in urine and is secreted in breast milk.

Onset	Peak	Duration
Unknown	20 min	6-8 hr

How supplied

Solution for injection: 2 mg/mL

Indications and dosages

➤ Pain management when opioid analgesics are appropriate

Adults: Up to 1 mg I.V. injection in divided doses; may repeat in 3 to 6 hours, as needed. Maximum daily dosage is 4 to 8 mg.

Dosage adjustment

- Reduce dosage in hepatic or renal insufficiency, conditions that affect respiratory reserve, concomitant use of drugs that may cause respiratory depression, and elderly patients, as appropriate.

Administration

Preparation

Make sure resuscitation equipment is available before starting therapy.

- Know that 2 mg is analgesically equivalent to 10 to 15 mg morphine and 100 mg meperidine.

Dilution and compatibility

- Be aware that drug may be given undiluted.
- If desired, dilute in 5 mL normal saline solution or sterile water for injection to aid titration.

Infusion considerations

- Give I.V. injection slowly, administering each 2 mg over at least 4 to 5 minutes. Monitor patient response.

Do not add to I.V. infusion solution or give by I.V. infusion.

Monitoring

- Check vital signs and respiratory status; monitor ECG carefully.
- Evaluate fluid intake and output.
- Assess neurologic status. Institute safety precautions as needed to prevent injury.
- Watch for signs and symptoms of depression.
- Monitor liver and kidney function test results.
- After administration, place patient in supine position with legs elevated to minimize adverse reactions.

Storage

- Store at 15° to 30°C (59° to 86°F).

Contraindications and precautions

Contraindicated in hypersensitivity to drug or other opioid agonists, bronchial asthma, increased intracranial pressure, respiratory depression, and acute alcoholism.

Use cautiously in renal or hepatic dysfunction, chronic obstructive pulmonary disease, acute abdominal conditions, cardiovascular disease, seizure disorders, cerebral arteriosclerosis, Addison's disease, prostatic hypertrophy, toxic psychosis, alcoholism, drug dependence, pregnant or breastfeeding patients, and ***children.***

Adverse reactions

CNS: personality disorders, nervousness, insomnia, hypokinesia, dyskinesia, drowsiness, light-headedness, dizziness, depression, delusions, confusion, amnesia, sedation, euphoria, delirium, mood changes, **coma, seizures**
CV: palpitations, hypotension, tachycardia, bradycardia, **shock, peripheral circulatory collapse, cardiac arrest**
EENT: diplopia, abnormal vision
GI: nausea, vomiting, constipation, abdominal pain, dyspepsia, increased colonic motility (in patients with chronic ulcerative colitis), dry mouth
GU: dysuria, urine retention, urinary hesitancy, ureteral or vesicle sphincter spasms, decreased libido, **oliguria**
Hepatic: biliary tract spasms, **hepatic failure**
Respiratory: suppressed cough reflex, hyperventilation, **periodic apnea**
Skin: urticaria, rash, pruritus, cyanosis
Other: facial flushing; injection site pain, redness, or swelling; physical or psychological drug dependence

Interactions

Drug-drug. *Alfentanil, fentanyl, sufentanil, other CNS depressants:* increased CNS and respiratory depression, increased risk of hypotension
Anticholinergics: increased risk of severe constipation
Antidiarrheals (such as atropine, difenoxin, kaolin, loperamide), antihypertensives: increased risk of hypotension
Buprenorphine, naloxone, naltrexone: decreased levorphanol efficacy
Metoclopramide: antagonism of metoclopramide effects
Neuromuscular blockers: increased risk of prolonged CNS and respiratory depression
Drug-diagnostic tests. *Amylase, lipase:* increased
Drug-behaviors. *Alcohol use:* increased CNS depression

Toxicity and overdose

- Overdose may result from intentional or accidental misuse of product (especially in infants and children). Overdose may cause signs and symptoms of respiratory depression, cardiovascular failure (especially in predisposed patients), and CNS depression. S erious overdose causes respiratory depression (reductions in respiratory rate and/or tidal volume, cyanosis), extreme somnolence progressing to

L

stupor or coma, skeletal muscle flaccidity, cold and clammy skin, constricted pupils, and sometimes bradycardia and hypotension. In severe overdose, apnea, circulatory collapse, cardiac arrest, and death may occur.

- In suspected overdose, immediately establish adequate airway and ventilation, followed (if necessary) by I.V. naloxone. Continuously monitor patient's respiratory and cardiac status and provide appropriate supportive measures, such as oxygen, I.V. fluids and/or vasopressors, if required and ordered. Be aware that levorphanol duration far exceeds naloxone duration, so repeated naloxone doses may be required. Give naloxone cautiously to patients with known or suspected physical dependence on levorphanol; in such patients, abrupt and complete reversal of opioid effects may trigger acute abstinence syndrome. If naloxone must be given to physically dependent patient, use extreme care, titrating with smaller-than-usual dosages. Do not give naloxone in absence of clinically significant respiratory or cardiovascular depression.

Patient teaching

- Explain need for continuous vital sign and ECG monitoring.
- To minimize adverse effects, instruct patient to lie supine after parenteral administration, if possible.
- Instruct patient or caregiver to report adverse reactions immediately.
- Tell patient or caregiver to use safety measures as needed to prevent injury, and to report significant problems.
- Caution patient to avoid driving and other hazardous activities until drug's effects on concentration and alertness are known.
- Advise female patient to inform prescriber if she is pregnant or breastfeeding.
- As appropriate, review all other significant and life-threatening adverse reactions and interactions, especially those related to the drugs, tests, and behaviors mentioned above.

lidocaine hydrochloride

Xylocaine, Xylocard

Pharmacologic class: Amide

Therapeutic class: Antiarrhythmic (class IB)

Pregnancy risk category B

Action

Suppresses automaticity of ventricular cells, decreasing diastolic depolarization and increasing ventricular fibrillation threshold. Produces local anesthesia by reducing sodium permeability of sensory nerves, which blocks impulse generation and conduction.

Pharmacokinetics

Drug is completely absorbed after I.V. administration and crosses blood-brain and placental barriers. Plasma binding depends on drug concentration; fraction bound decreases with increasing drug concentration. At level of 1 to 4 mcg of free base/mL, 60% to 80% is protein-bound. Binding also depends on plasma level of alpha-1-acid glycoprotein. Drug is rapidly metabolized by the liver; any condition affecting liver function may alter lidocaine kinetics. Typical elimination half-life after I.V. bolus is 1.5 to 2 hours. Half-life may lengthen twofold or more in patients with hepatic dysfunction. Renal dysfunction may increase metabolite accumulation. Metabolites and unchanged drug are excreted by the kidneys, approximately

90% as various metabolites and less than 10% as unchanged drug.

Onset	Peak	Duration
45-90 sec	Immediate	10-20 min

How supplied

Injection for direct I.V. use: 1% and 2% in syringes and vials; 0.5% in 50-mL single-dose and multidose vials; 1% and 2% in ampules, vials, multidose vials, and syringes; 1.5% in 10-mL and 20-mL ampules and 5-mL and 10-mL single-dose vials
Injection for I.V. infusion: 2 mg/mL, 4 mg/mL, 8 mg/mL
Injection for I.V injection admixtures: 40 mg/mL, 100 mg/mL, 200 mg/mL

Indications and dosages

➢ Life-threatening ventricular arrhythmias
Adults: Initially, 50 to 100 mg I.V. bolus given at a rate of 25 to 50 mg/minute. If desired response does not occur after 5 minutes, give second dose of 50 to 100 mg at a rate of 25 to 50 mg/minute; maximum dosage is 300 mg given over 1 hour. Maintenance dosage is 1 to 4 mg/minute by continuous I.V. infusion, usually for no more than 24 hours.
Children: Initially, 1 mg/kg I.V. bolus, repeated based on response; do not exceed 5 mg/kg. Maintenance dosage is 30 mcg/kg/minute by continuous I.V. infusion.
➢ I.V. regional infiltration (without epinephrine)
Adults: 50 to 300 mg I.V. as 0.5% solution. For I.V. regional anesthesia, maximum dosage is 4 mg/kg.
➢ I.V. local infiltration (without epinephrine)
Children: Up to 4.5 mg/kg I.V. as 0.25% to 1% solution

Off-label uses

- Cardiac arrest in pediatric patients who develop frequent premature ventricular contractions
- Status epilepticus

Administration

Preparation
Make sure resuscitation equipment and oxygen are available before giving drug.
Dilution and compatibility
- Know that I.V. bolus dose may be given undiluted.
- Before giving I.V. infusion, dilute injection in additive syringe and single-use vial according to manufacturer's instructions.
- Add 1 g lidocaine to 1 L D_5W to yield 1 mg/mL solution.

Infusion considerations
- For I.V. bolus injection, give doses of 25 to 50 mg over at least 1 minute.
- Deliver continuous I.V. infusion by infusion pump no faster than 4 mg/minute.

Know that too-rapid infusion may cause seizures.
Monitoring
Monitor vital signs and ECG continuously. Watch for cardiac depression.
Evaluate level of consciousness closely.
Watch for localized and systemic adverse reactions, particularly anaphylaxis.
Stay alert for seizures.
Monitor neurologic status for lower spinal segment deficits.
- Administer supportive oxygen therapy, as indicated and prescribed.
- Monitor electrolyte, blood urea nitrogen, and creatinine levels.

Storage
- Store at room temperature of approximately 25°C (77°F); protect from light.

L

Contraindications and precautions

Contraindicated in hypersensitivity to drug, its components, or other amide local anesthetics; heart failure; cardiogenic shock; second- or third-degree heart block; intraventricular block in absence of pacemaker; and Wolff-Parkinson-White or Adams-Stokes syndrome.

Use cautiously in renal or hepatic disorders, labor or delivery, and breast-feeding patients.

Adverse reactions

CNS: anxiety; confusion; difficulty speaking; dizziness; hallucinations; lethargy; paresthesia; light-headedness; fatigue; drowsiness; headache; persistent sensory, motor, or **autonomic deficit of lower spinal segment; septic meningitis; seizures**
CV: bradycardia, hypotension, new or worsening **arrhythmias, cardiac arrest**
EENT: diplopia, abnormal vision
GI: nausea, vomiting, dry mouth
GU: urine retention
Metabolic: methemoglobinemia
Respiratory: suppressed cough reflex, **respiratory depression, respiratory arrest**
Skin: rash; urticaria; pruritus; erythema; contact dermatitis; cutaneous lesions; tissue irritation, sloughing, and necrosis
Other: fever; edema; infection, burning, stinging, tenderness, and swelling at injection site; **anaphylaxis**

Interactions

Drug-drug. *Beta-adrenergic blockers, cimetidine:* increased lidocaine blood level
Mexiletine, tocainide: additive cardiac effects
Monoamine oxidase inhibitors, tricyclic antidepressants: prolonged hypertension
Phenytoin, procainamide: increased cardiac depression

Toxicity and overdose

- Drug blood levels may correlate with CNS toxicity, including seizures and cardiovascular depression resulting in hypoxia, acidosis, bradycardia, arrhythmias, and cardiac arrest unless treated immediately.
- At first sign of change in cardiovascular and respiratory vital signs and state of consciousness, maintain patent airway and give oxygen or controlled ventilation with oxygen, as indicated and ordered. Manage seizures with adequate respiratory support and (if circulatory status permits) small increments of ultra-short-acting barbiturate (such as thiopental or thiamylal) or benzodiazepine (such as diazepam) I.V. for persistent seizures. Evaluate circulation and provide supportive treatment of circulatory depression with I.V. fluids and, when appropriate, vasopressor. Resuscitate as indicated. Dialysis has little value in acute overdose.

Patient teaching

- Discuss reason for drug therapy with patient and family, when appropriate.
- Explain that patient will be monitored continuously during therapy.

🔊 Instruct patient to promptly report discomfort at I.V. site as well as adverse effects, especially cardiovascular, respiratory, or neurologic problems or allergic reaction.

- As appropriate, review all other significant and life-threatening adverse reactions and interactions, especially those related to the drugs mentioned above.

linezolid

Zyvox, Zyvoxam✤

Pharmacologic class: Oxazolidinone
Therapeutic class: Anti-infective
Pregnancy risk category C

Action

Selectively binds to bacterial 23S ribosomal RNA of 50S subunit, preventing formation of an essential component of bacterial protein synthesis. Bacteriostatic or bactericidal against gram-positive and some gram-negative bacteria.

Pharmacokinetics

Drug readily distributes into tissues. It is metabolized to two inactive metabolites, partially protein-bound, and excreted in urine as parent drug and metabolites, with a small amount excreted in feces.

Onset	Peak	Duration
Unknown	Unknown	Unknown

How supplied

Solution for injection: 2 mg/mL in 100-mL, 200-mL, and 300-mL ready-to-use infusion bags

Indications and dosages

➤ Vancomycin-resistant *Enterococcus faecium* infections

Adults and children age 12 and older: 600 mg I.V. infusion q 12 hours for 14 to 28 days

Children from birth to age 11: 10 mg/kg I.V. q 8 hours for 14 to 28 days

➤ Nosocomial pneumonia caused by *Staphylococcus aureus* (methicillin-susceptible and methicillin-resistant strains) or *Streptococcus pneumoniae* (multidrug-resistant strains); community-acquired pneumonia caused by *S. pneumoniae* (including multidrug-resistant strains) or *S. aureus*; complicated skin and skin-structure infections caused by *S. aureus* (methicillin-susceptible and methicillin-resistant strains), *Streptococcus pyogenes*, or *Streptococcus agalactiae*

Adults and children age 12 and older: 600 mg I.V. infusion q 12 hours for 10 to 14 days

Children from birth to age 11: 10 mg/kg I.V. q 8 hours for 10 to 14 days

Administration

Dilution and compatibility

- Keep bag in overwrap until ready to use.
- Know that single-use, ready-to-use infusion bag requires no dilution.
- Compatible I.V. solutions are D_5W, normal saline solution, and lactated Ringer's solution.
- Be aware that drug may have yellow color, which can intensify over time without affecting potency.

Infusion considerations

- Infuse over 30 minutes to 2 hours.

Clinical alert: Do not use plastic containers in series connections. Such use could result in air embolism due to residual air being drawn from primary container before administration of fluid from secondary container ends.

- Do not give concomitantly with other drugs.
- Flush I.V. line with compatible solution before and after administering drug, to avoid incompatibilities.

Monitoring

- Check I.V. site for infiltration.
- Monitor neurologic status. Institute safety measures as needed to prevent injury.
- Monitor CBC, coagulation studies, and culture and sensitivity tests.

Clinical alert: Watch for bleeding and signs and symptoms of other adverse reactions (especially pseudomembranous colitis).

Monitor for signs and symptoms of lactic acidosis, including repeated episodes of nausea and vomiting. Unexplained acidosis or low bicarbonate level warrants immediate medical evaluation.

Storage

- Store at room temperature. Do not freeze.

Contraindications and precautions

Contraindicated in hypersensitivity to drug or its components.

Use cautiously in hepatic dysfunction, hypertension, hyperthyroidism, pheochromocytoma, bone marrow depression, pseudomembranous colitis, and pregnant or breastfeeding patients.

Adverse reactions

CNS: dizziness, headache, insomnia, peripheral neuropathy, **seizures**
EENT: optic neuropathy
GI: nausea, vomiting, diarrhea, constipation, dyspepsia, abdominal pain, oral candidiasis, **pseudomembranous colitis**
GU: vaginal candidiasis
Hematologic: thrombocytopenia
Metabolic: lactic acidosis
Skin: rash, pruritus
Other: tongue discoloration, taste alteration, fever, fungal infection

Interactions

Drug-drug. *Monoamine oxidase inhibitors, pseudoephedrine:* increased risk of hypertension and associated adverse effects
Serotonergics: serotonin syndrome
Drug-diagnostic tests. *Bicarbonate, platelets:* decreased
Prothrombin time: altered
Drug-foods. *Tyramine-containing foods and beverages (such as beer; Chianti and certain other red wines; aged cheese; bananas; aged, cured, or spoiled meats; salted herring and other dried fish; avocado; bananas; bean curd; red plums; soy sauce; spinach; tofu; tomatoes; yeast):* hypertension

Toxicity and overdose

- In overdose, expect extension of adverse reactions.
- Provide symptomatic and supportive therapy. Hemodialysis may aid drug removal.

Patient teaching

Advise patient to promptly report bleeding or severe diarrhea.

- Instruct patient to minimize adverse GI effects by eating small, frequent servings of healthy food—but to avoid tyramine-containing foods.
- Tell patient to inform prescriber if taking medications containing pseudoephedrine, such as decongestants and cold remedies.
- Advise patient to report vision changes.
- Instruct female patient to inform prescriber if she is pregnant or breastfeeding.
- Caution patient to avoid driving and other hazardous activities until drug's effects on concentration and alertness are known.
- As appropriate, review all other significant and life-threatening adverse reactions and interactions, especially those related to the drugs, tests, and foods mentioned above.

lorazepam

Ativan

Pharmacologic class: Benzodiazepine
Therapeutic class: Anxiolytic
Controlled substance schedule IV
Pregnancy risk category D

Action
Unknown. Thought to depress CNS at limbic system and disrupt neurotransmission in reticular activating system by interacting with gamma-aminobutyric acid–benzodiazepine receptor complex in the brain.

Pharmacokinetics
Drug distributes widely in body tissues and crosses placental barrier. It is metabolized by the liver to inactive metabolites and is largely protein-bound. It undergoes slow excretion in urine as parent drug and metabolites, with some secretion in breast milk.

Onset	Peak	Duration
Rapid	15-20 min	6 to 8 hr

How supplied
Solution for injection (clear): 2 mg/mL in 1-mL and 10-mL vials, 4 mg/mL in 1-mL and 10-mL vials

Indications and dosages
➢ Premedication before surgery as anxiolytic, sedative hypnotic, or amnestic
Adults: 0.044 mg/kg (not to exceed 2 mg) I.V. 15 to 20 minutes before surgery. For greater amnestic effect, give up to 0.05 mg/kg (not to exceed 4 mg) I.V. 15 to 20 minutes before surgery.
➢ Status epilepticus
Adults: 4 mg I.V. given slowly (no faster than 2 mg/minute). If seizures continue or recur after 10 to 15 minutes, repeat dose. If second dose does not establish seizure control, other measures should be used. Do not give more than 8 mg in 12 hours.

Dosage adjustment
- Be aware that elderly or debilitated patients may require smaller initial dosages.

Off-label uses
- Acute alcohol withdrawal syndrome

Administration
Preparation
- Keep resuscitation equipment and oxygen at hand.
- Do not give parenteral form to children younger than age 18.

Dilution and compatibility
- Dilute with equal volume of compatible diluent, such as sterile water for injection, normal saline solution, or D_5W for injection. Invert gently to mix. Do not shake.
- Do not use if solution is discolored.

Infusion consideration
- Administer immediately after preparation.

🔊 Give I.V. at a rate not exceeding 2 mg/minute.

Monitoring

🔊 During administration, monitor ECG and cardiovascular and respiratory status.
- Monitor vital signs closely.
- Watch closely for CNS depression. Institute safety precautions as needed to prevent injury.
- Assess liver function test results and CBC.

Storage
- Refrigerate drug; protect from light.

Contraindications and precautions
Contraindicated in hypersensitivity to drug, other benzodiazepines, polyethylene or propylene glycol, or benzyl alcohol; acute angle-closure glaucoma; sleep-apnea syndrome; severe respiratory insufficiency (except in patients requiring relief of anxiety or diminished recall of events during mechanical ventilation).

Use cautiously in hepatic or renal impairment, history of suicide attempt, drug abuse, depressive disorder, psychosis, ***elderly patients,*** pregnant or breastfeeding patients, and ***children younger than age 18*** (use not recommended).

Adverse reactions

CNS: amnesia, ataxia, depression, dizziness, drowsiness, headache
CV: hypotension, bradycardia, tachycardia, apnea, **cardiac arrest, cardiovascular collapse** (with too-rapid I.V. administration)
EENT: blurred vision, diplopia
GI: nausea, vomiting

Interactions

Drug-drug. *CNS depressants (including antidepressants, antihistamines, benzodiazepines, sedative-hypnotics):* additive CNS depression
Hormonal contraceptives: increased lorazepam clearance
Valproate: decreased lorazepam clearance
Drug-herb. *Chamomile, hops, kava, skullcap, valerian:* increased CNS depression
Drug-behaviors. *Alcohol use:* increased CNS depression
Smoking: increased metabolism and decreased efficacy of lorazepam

Toxicity and overdose

• Overdose may cause confusion, hypotension, impaired coordination, diminished reflexes, coma, and labored breathing.
• Discontinue drug. Closely monitor vital signs and provide I.V. fluids, if indicated and ordered. In severe overdose, maintain patent airway, provide artificial ventilation and oxygen, implement symptomatic care, and resuscitate, as indicated. Flumazenil (specific benzodiazepine-receptor antagonist) may be indicated for complete or partial reversal of sedative effects. Dialysis provides limited benefit.

Patient teaching

• Tell patient and family about drug's possible CNS effects. Recommend appropriate safety precautions.
• Advise female patient to inform prescriber if she is pregnant or breastfeeding.
• As appropriate, review all other significant and life-threatening adverse reactions and interactions, especially those related to the drugs, herbs, and behaviors mentioned above.

magnesium sulfate

Pharmacologic class: Mineral
Therapeutic class: Electrolyte replacement, anticonvulsant
Pregnancy risk category A

Action

Precise action as nutritional adjunct is uncertain. Prevents or controls seizures by blocking neuromuscular transmission and decreasing amount of acetylcholine liberated at endplate by motor nerve impulse.

Pharmacokinetics

Effective anticonvulsant serum levels range from 2.5 to 7.5 mEq/L. Drug is excreted by the kidneys.

Onset	Peak	Duration
Immediate	Unknown	30 min

How supplied

Solution for injection: 10%, 12.5%, 25%, and 50% in single-dose vials

Indications and dosages

➤ Severe hypomagnesemia

Adults: 5 g (approximately 40 mEq) in 1 L D_5W or normal saline solution by I.V. infusion over 3 hours

➢ To prevent and control seizures in patients with preeclampsia or eclampsia

Adults: 4 to 5 g I.V. infusion in 250 mL D_5W or normal saline solution, not to exceed 3 mL/minute given simultaneously with I.M. injections. Alternatively, initial I.V. dose of 4 g may be given by diluting 50% solution to 10% or 20% concentration; diluted fluid (40 mL of 10% solution or 20 mL of 20% solution) may then be injected I.V. over 3 to 4 minutes. Subsequently, prescribed I.M. doses may be given, as needed, depending on continuing presence of patellar reflex and adequate respiratory function. Alternatively, after initial I.V. dose, some clinicians give 1 to 2 g/hour by constant I.V. infusion. Therapy should continue until paroxysms cease.

➢ Supplemental magnesium in total parenteral nutrition (TPN)

Adults: 8 to 24 mEq/day by I.V. infusion added to TPN solution

Infants: 2 to 10 mEq (0.25 to 1.25 g) daily added to TPN solution

Off-label uses

- Bronchodilation in some asthmatic patients
- Post–myocardial infarction hypomagnesemia

Administration

Preparation

🔈 Individualize dosage; discontinue drug as soon as desired effect occurs.

🔈 Know that I.V. use in eclampsia is reserved for life-threatening seizures.

🔈 Keep resuscitative equipment on hand.

Dilution and compatibility

🔈 Be aware that drug must be diluted to a concentration of 20% (200 mg/mL) or less in normal saline solution or D_5W.

Infusion considerations

🔈 Do not exceed concentration of 20% or infusion rate of 1.5 mL/minute of 10% solution. Too-rapid I.V. infusion may cause hypotension and asystole.

🔈 Give with caution if flushing or hypotension occurs.

Monitoring

🔈 Monitor blood magnesium level; desired level is 3 to 6 mg/dL or 2.5 to 5 mEq/L. Check for signs and symptoms of magnesium toxicity (hypotension, nausea, vomiting, ECG changes, muscle weakness, mental or respiratory depression, coma). Keep injectable calcium on hand to counteract magnesium toxicity.

🔈 When giving prolonged or repeated I.V. infusions, assess patellar reflex and monitor for respiratory rate of 16 breaths/minute or more.

🔈 If patient received I.V. magnesium before delivery, assess neonate for signs and symptoms of magnesium toxicity, such as neuromuscular or respiratory depression.

- Monitor urine output, which should measure at least 100 mL every 4 hours.
- Monitor electrolyte levels and liver function test results.

Storage

- Store at controlled room temperature of 15° to 30°C (59° to 86°F).

Contraindications and precautions

Contraindicated in heart block or myocardial damage.

Use cautiously in renal insufficiency, abdominal pain, nausea and vomiting, rectal bleeding, anuria, hypocalcemia, and pregnant patients.

Adverse reactions

CV: hypotension, **circulatory collapse, cardiac depression**

M

Metabolic: hypermagnesemia, hypocalcemia
Musculoskeletal: muscle weakness, flaccidity
Respiratory: respiratory paralysis
Skin: diaphoresis, flushing

Interactions

Drug-drug. *CNS depressants:* additive effects
Digoxin: heart block, conduction changes
Neuromuscular blockers: increased effects of these drugs
Drug-diagnostic tests. *Calcium, magnesium:* increased

Toxicity and overdose

• In toxicity, expect hypotension, nausea, vomiting, ECG changes, muscle weakness, mental or respiratory depression, and coma. As magnesium plasma levels begin to exceed 4 mEq/L, deep tendon reflexes decrease and may be absent at levels approaching 10 mEq/L.
• Administer 10 to 20 mL 5% calcium solution diluted with normal saline solution. Provide resuscitative measures as necessary. Physostigmine and dialysis may be beneficial.

Patient teaching

Teach patient about adverse reactions. Instruct patient to report symptoms that occur during administration.
• Tell pregnant female to make sure prescriber knows she is pregnant before taking drug (except when used to prevent or control seizures in preeclampsia or eclampsia).
• As appropriate, review all other significant and life-threatening adverse reactions and interactions, especially those related to the drugs and tests mentioned above.

mannitol

Osmitrol

Pharmacologic class: Osmotic diuretic
Therapeutic class: Diuretic
Pregnancy risk category B (25% fliptop vial), C (all other products)

Action

Increases plasma osmotic pressure in renal glomerular filtrate, inhibiting tubular reabsorption of water and electrolytes (including sodium and potassium). These actions enhance water flow from such tissues as brain tissue and ultimately decrease intracranial pressure (ICP) and intraocular pressure (IOP). Serum sodium level rises while potassium and blood urea levels fall. Also protects kidneys by preventing toxins from forming and blocking tubules.

Pharmacokinetics

Drug is confined to extracellular space. It is only slightly metabolized and is rapidly excreted by the kidneys. Approximately 80% of 100-g dose appears in urine in 3 hours.

Onset	Peak	Duration
Unknown (diuresis)	Unknown	Unknown
15 min (IOP)	30 to 60 min	Unknown
15 min (ICP)	Unknown	Unknown

How supplied

Solution for injection: 5%, 10%, 15%, and 20% in flexible containers; 25% in fliptop vials

Indications and dosages

➤ Test dose for marked oliguria or suspected inadequate renal function

Adults: 0.2 g/kg I.V. infusion (about 50 mL of 25% solution, 75 mL of 20% solution, or 100 mL of 15% solution) over 3 to 5 minutes. If urine flow does not increase, may give second dose; if response to second dose is inadequate, reevaluate patient.

➢ To prevent acute renal failure (oliguria) during cardiovascular and other surgeries

Adults: 50 to 100 g I.V. infusion as 5% to 25% solution

➢ Acute renal failure (oliguria)

Adults: 50 to 100 g I.V. infusion as 15% to 25% solution

➢ To reduce intracranial pressure and brain mass

Adults: 1.5 g/kg I.V. infusion as 25% solution given over 30 to 60 minutes or 0.25 g/kg given no more often than q 6 to 8 hours

➢ To reduce IOP

Adults: 1.5 to 2 g/kg I.V. infusion as 15% to 25% solution given over 30 to 60 minutes. For preoperative use, administer 60 to 90 minutes before surgery.

➢ To promote diuresis in drug toxicity

Adults: Generally, I.V. bolus dose followed by slower I.V. infusion of 5% to 25% solution given continuously to maintain high urine output, based on fluid requirement or urine output. If benefits do not occur after administration of 200 g mannitol, discontinue.

Administration

Preparation

Withhold drug until adequate renal function and urine output are established.

Dilution and compatibility

- Know that no dilution is required for drug in flexible containers.
- Dilute solution in fliptop vials in prescribed amount of I.V. fluid for infusion.
- Be aware that at low temperatures, solution may crystallize. To dissolve crystals in flexible container, warm unit to 70°C (158°F) with agitation. To dissolve crystals in fliptop vial, warm bottle in hot-water bath at 60° to 80°C (140° to 176°F) and shake periodically. Cool to body temperature or lower before administering.
- Discard unused portion of drug.

Infusion considerations

- When infusing 20% or 25% concentration, use administration set with filter.
- Do not give electrolyte-free mannitol solution with blood; when giving blood with mannitol, add 20 mEq or more of sodium chloride solution to each liter of mannitol solution to avoid pseudoagglutination.
- Give drug only as continuous or intermittent I.V. infusion.
- Infuse at prescribed rate using infusion device and inline filter. Give single I.V. dose over 30 to 90 minutes in adults.

Avoid too-rapid infusion of large amounts, because hyponatremia, congestive heart failure (CHF), and pulmonary edema may occur.

Do not use plastic containers in series connections. Such use could result in air embolism due to residual air being drawn from primary container before administration of fluid from secondary container ends.

Avoid extravasation, which may cause local edema and tissue necrosis.

Monitoring

Monitor I.V. site carefully to avoid extravasation and tissue necrosis.

- In comatose patient, insert indwelling urinary catheter as prescribed to monitor urine output.
- Monitor renal function tests, urine output, fluid balance, central venous pressure, and electrolyte levels (especially sodium and potassium).

Watch for excessive fluid loss and signs and symptoms of hypovolemia and dehydration.

M

Assess for evidence of circulatory overload, including pulmonary edema, water intoxication, and heart failure.

Storage

- Store flexible containers at room temperature of 25°C (77°F); brief excursions permitted up to 40°C (104°F).
- Store fliptop vials at controlled room temperature of 20° to 25°C (68° to 77°F). Avoid excessive heat; protect from freezing.

Contraindications and precautions

Contraindicated in active intracranial bleeding (except during craniotomy); anuria secondary to severe renal disease; progressive CHF, pulmonary congestion, renal damage, or renal dysfunction after mannitol therapy begins; severe pulmonary congestion or pulmonary edema; and severe dehydration.

Use cautiously in severe renal disease, CHF, mild to moderate dehydration, and pregnant or breastfeeding patients.

Adverse reactions

CV: chest pain, hypotension, hypertension, tachycardia, **thrombophlebitis, venous thrombosis**

EENT: blurred vision, rhinitis

GI: nausea, vomiting, diarrhea, dry mouth

GU: urine retention, **osmotic nephrosis**

Metabolic: dehydration, water intoxication, hypernatremia, hyponatremia, hypokalemia, hypervolemia, **hyperkalemia**

Respiratory: pulmonary edema

Skin: rash, urticaria, skin necrosis

Other: chills; fever; thirst; edema, tissue necrosis, edema, and arm pain with extravasation

Interactions

Drug-diagnostic tests. *Electrolytes:* increased or decreased

Toxicity and overdose

- Too-rapid infusion of large amounts causes intracellular water to shift into extracellular compartment, resulting in cellular dehydration and overexpansion of intravascular space with hyponatremia, CHF, and pulmonary edema. Dosages higher than recommended may increase excretion of electrolytes, particularly sodium, chloride, and potassium. Sodium depletion may lead to orthostatic tachycardia or hypotension and decreased central venous pressure. Potassium depletion may impair neuromuscular function and intestinal dilation and ileus. Other symptoms may include stupor and seizures. Always monitor dosage carefully, and adjust based on clinical situation to avoid overdose. Do not give repeated doses to patients with persistent oliguria, as this may cause hyperosmolar state and trigger CHF and pulmonary edema.
- In overdose, discontinue infusion immediately. Provide prompt supportive care to correct fluid and electrolyte imbalances. Hemodialysis may be beneficial.

Patient teaching

Advise patient to report pain at infusion site as well as adverse reactions, such as increased shortness of breath or pain in back, legs, or chest.

- Tell patient drug may cause thirst or dry mouth. Emphasize that fluid restrictions are necessary, but that frequent mouth care and comfort measures should ease these symptoms.
- As appropriate, review all other significant and life-threatening adverse reactions and interactions, especially those related to the tests mentioned above.

mechlorethamine hydrochloride (HN_2, mustine, nitrogen mustard)

Mustargen

Pharmacologic class: Alkylating agent, nitrogen mustard agent
Therapeutic class: Antineoplastic
Pregnancy risk category D

FDA BOXED WARNING

- Give only under supervision of physician experienced in using cancer chemotherapeutic agents.
- Drug is highly toxic. Handle and administer both powder and solution with care. Avoid inhaling dust or vapors or letting drug contact skin, mucous membranes, or eyes. Avoid exposure during pregnancy. Drug is corrosive, carcinogenic, mutagenic, and teratogenic. Review special handling procedures before handling, and follow these diligently.
- Drug extravasation into subcutaneous tissues causes painful inflammation, with induration and sloughing. If drug leakage is obvious, promptly infiltrate area with sterile isotonic sodium thiosulfate (1/6 M) and apply ice compress for 6 to 12 hours. For 1/6 M sodium thiosulfate solution, use 4.14 g sodium thiosulfate per 100 mL sterile water for injection or 2.64 g anhydrous sodium thiosulfate per 100 mL, or dilute 4 mL sodium thiosulfate injection (10%) with 6 mL sterile water for injection.

Action

Interferes with DNA and RNA synthesis by cross-linking strands of cellular DNA. Cell-cycle-phase nonspecific.

Pharmacokinetics

Drug undergoes rapid chemical transformation and combines with water or reactive compounds of cells; thus, it is no longer present in active form a few minutes after administration. A small amount of active drug and a significant amount of inactive metabolite are excreted in urine.

Onset	Peak	Duration
Unknown	Unknown	Unknown

How supplied

Powder for reconstitution for injection (light yellow brown, crystalline): 10 mg/vial

Indications and dosages

➤ Palliative combination therapy in chronic myelocytic or chronic lymphocytic leukemia, lymphosarcoma, polycythemia vera, mycosis fungoides, or bronchogenic carcinoma

Adults: 0.4 mg/kg I.V. given as a single dose or in divided doses of 0.1 to 0.2 mg/kg/day I.V., with subsequent doses given after hematologic recovery (usually 3 to 6 weeks)

➤ Palliative treatment of Hodgkin's disease (stages III and IV)

Adults: 6 mg/m^2 I.V. on days 1 and 8 of 28-day cycle as part of MOPP (mechlorethamine, vincristine, procarbazine, prednisone) regimen. During subsequent cycles, blood counts determine dosage.

Administration

Preparation

Follow hazardous drug guidelines on page S19 for handling, preparation, and administration.

Neutralize equipment or unused solution in equal volumes of 5% sodium thiosulfate and 5% sodium bicarbonate. Soak for 45 minutes; then discard unused solution according to facility policy.

M

Be aware that drug has narrow margin of safety. Use extreme caution with dosages.

- Know that severe nausea and vomiting may occur 1 to 3 hours after administration. Premedicate with antiemetics and sedatives, as prescribed.

Dilution and compatibility

- Reconstitute with 10 mL sterile water or sodium chloride for injection; shake vial several times to dissolve drug completely. Resulting solution yields a concentration of 1 mg/mL.
- Know that when reconstituted, drug is a clear, colorless solution. Do not use if solution is discolored or water droplets appear in vial before reconstitution.

Administer immediately after reconstitution; drug decomposes on standing.

Infusion considerations

- Withdraw calculated dosage and inject either directly into vein or into port of free-flowing I.V. line (preferred) over 3 to 5 minutes.

Check I.V. site carefully to avoid extravasation and tissue necrosis.

Monitoring

- If extravasation occurs, infiltrate area with sterile isotonic sodium thiosulfate, apply ice compresses for 6 to 12 hours, and notify prescriber.
- Monitor hematologic, kidney, and liver function studies.
- Watch for hyperuricemia. Maintain adequate hydration to prevent uric acid elevation.
- Monitor patient for infection. Lymphocytopenia occurs within 24 hours; significant granulocytopenia occurs in 6 to 8 days and lasts 10 to 21 days, with recovery within 2 weeks after nadir.

Storage

- Store at controlled room temperature of 15° to 30°C (59° to 86°F). Protect from light and humidity.

Contraindications and precautions

Contraindicated in hypersensitivity to drug and active infection.

Use cautiously in chronic lymphocytic leukemia, decreased bone marrow reserve, hematopoietic depression, amyloidosis, severe edema, obesity, previous radiation therapy or chemotherapy, ***elderly or debilitated patients,*** patients with childbearing potential, pregnant or breastfeeding patients, and ***children*** (safety and efficacy not established).

Adverse reactions

CNS: vertigo
GI: nausea, vomiting, diarrhea
EENT: tinnitus, diminished hearing
GU: infertility, delayed menses, oligomenorrhea, amenorrhea
Hematologic: anemia, **leukopenia, thrombocytopenia, lymphocytopenia, granulocytopenia, agranulocytosis, persistent pancytopenia**
Hepatic: jaundice
Metabolic: hyperuricemia
Skin: rash, alopecia, **erythema multiforme**
Other: herpes zoster reactivation, chromosomal abnormalities, tissue necrosis and phlebitis at I.V. site with extravasation, hypersensitivity reactions including **anaphylaxis, amyloidosis, secondary cancers**

Interactions

Drug-drug. *Other antineoplastics:* additive bone marrow depression
Live-virus vaccines: decreased antibody response to vaccine, increased risk of adverse reactions
Drug-diagnostic tests. *Granulocytes, lymphocytes, platelets, red blood cells:* decreased
Uric acid: increased

Toxicity and overdose

- Total single-course dosage exceeding 0.4 mg/kg may cause severe leukopenia, anemia, thrombocytopenia, and hemorrhagic complications with subsequent delayed bleeding. Death may result.
- Discontinue drug. Sole treatment is administration of repeated transfusions of blood products or blood modifiers, such as darbepoetin alfa, epoetin alfa, or filgrastim, to treat bone marrow toxicity; anti-infectives to treat complicating infections; and general supportive measures, such as hydration.

Patient teaching

Clinical alert: Instruct patient to immediately report pain or burning at injection site.

Clinical alert: Advise patient to immediately report signs or symptoms of infection, including fever, malaise, or sore throat.

Clinical alert: Tell patient to report bleeding gums, dark stools, or easy bruising or bleeding.

- Instruct patient to avoid crowds and practice good hand washing.
- Inform patient about the need for repeated laboratory testing during therapy.
- Advise patient to avoid pregnancy or breastfeeding.
- Inform patient that drug may cause sterility.
- As appropriate, review all other significant and life-threatening adverse reactions and interactions, especially those related to the drugs and tests mentioned above.

melphalan hydrochloride

Alkeran

Pharmacologic class: Alkylating agent, nitrogen mustard agent

Therapeutic class: Antineoplastic

Pregnancy risk category D

FDA BOXED WARNING

- Give under supervision of physician experienced in cancer chemotherapy, in facility with adequate diagnostic and treatment resources.
- Drug may cause severe bone marrow suppression leading to infection or bleeding. I.V. use causes greater myelosuppression than oral use, and also may lead to hypersensitivity reactions (including anaphylaxis).
- Drug may cause leukemia and is potentially mutagenic.

Action

Forms cross-links between strands of cellular DNA, disrupting DNA and RNA transcription and causing cell death

Pharmacokinetics

Plasma concentrations decline rapidly after administration, with distribution phase and terminal half-life of approximately 10 and 75 minutes, respectively. Drug is largely protein-bound. Only 10% is excreted unchanged in urine.

Onset	Peak	Duration
Unknown	Unknown	Unknown

How supplied

Powder for reconstitution for injection (lyophilized): 50 mg in single-use vial

Indications and dosages

➤ Palliative treatment of multiple myeloma in patients for whom oral therapy is not appropriate

Adults: 16 mg/m^2 by I.V. infusion over 15 to 20 minutes at 2-week intervals for four doses (usually with prednisone). I.V. dose can be repeated q 4 weeks after recovery from toxicity.

M

Dosage adjustment
- Reduce dosage up to 50% in patients with renal insufficiency.
- Adjust dosage based on blood counts at nadir and on treatment day.

Administration
Preparation
- Follow hazardous drug guidelines on page S19 for handling, preparation, and administration.
- Before starting therapy, obtain CBC with white cell differential and platelet count.

Dilution and compatibility
- For I.V. use, reconstitute by rapidly injecting 10 mL supplied diluent into vial with lyophilized powder, to yield a concentration of 5 mg/mL. Shake vigorously until solution is clear.
- After adding supplied diluent, immediately dilute desired dosage further in normal saline solution to a concentration no greater than 0.45 mg/mL.

Minimize time between reconstitution, dilution, and administration, because solution is unstable; product must be given within 60 minutes of reconstitution.

Infusion considerations
- Administer over 15 to 20 minutes. Be sure to give entire dose within 60 minutes of reconstitution.

Monitoring

Continue to monitor CBC with white cell differential and platelet count. Check for thrombocytopenia and leukopenia. If platelet count exceeds 100,000/mm^3 or white blood cell (WBC) count drops below 3,000/mm^3, discontinue drug until peripheral blood counts recover.

Watch closely for indications of bone marrow depression, including infection, anemia, and bleeding.

After multiple courses, watch for acute hypersensitivity reaction. If it occurs, discontinue drug and give volume expanders, corticosteroids, or antihistamines, as prescribed.
- Watch for signs and symptoms of GI or pulmonary toxicity.
- Evaluate renal and hepatic function closely.

Storage
- Store at 15° to 30°C (59° to 86°F); protect from light.
- Do not refrigerate reconstituted solution; precipitate will form if reconstituted solution is stored at 5°C (41°F) or below.

Contraindications and precautions
Contraindicated in hypersensitivity to drug and in patients whose disease has shown previous drug resistance.

Use cautiously in bone marrow depression, infection, renal disease, previous radiation therapy, patients with childbearing potential, pregnant or breastfeeding patients, and ***children*** (safety and efficacy not established).

Adverse reactions
CV: hypotension, tachycardia, vasculitis
GI: nausea, vomiting, diarrhea, oral ulcers, stomatitis
GU: amenorrhea, gonadal suppression, infertility
Hematologic: anemia, **bone marrow suppression, leukopenia, thrombocytopenia**
Hepatic: hepatotoxicity
Respiratory: dyspnea, **interstitial pneumonitis, bronchospasm, pulmonary fibrosis**
Skin: rash, urticaria, pruritus, alopecia
Other: edema, I.V. site reactions, allergic reactions including **anaphylaxis**

Interactions
Drug-drug. *Carmustine:* increased pulmonary toxicity
Cisplatin: increased risk of renal dysfunction, decreased melphalan clearance

Cyclosporine: increased risk of nephrotoxicity, severe renal failure
Live-virus vaccines: decreased antibody response to vaccine
Myelosuppressants: additive toxicity
Nalidixic acid: increased risk of severe hemorrhagic necrotic enterocolitis (in children)
Drug-diagnostic tests. *Hemoglobin, platelets, red blood cells, WBCs:* decreased
Nitrogenous compounds: increased

Toxicity and overdose

- Overdose may cause severe nausea and vomiting, decreased consciousness, seizures, muscle paralysis, veno-occlusive disease, increased liver function test results, hyponatremia, severe mucositis, stomatitis, colitis, diarrhea, GI hemorrhage, bone marrow depression, and death.
- Discontinue drug and provide general supportive measures. Give hematopoietic growth factors, such as sargramostim or filgrastim, as prescribed, to shorten pancytopenia. Administer blood transfusions and anti-infectives, as appropriate and prescribed. Hemodialysis and hemoperfusion are not helpful in drug removal. Closely follow hematologic parameters for 3 to 6 weeks.

Patient teaching

Advise patient to immediately report unusual bleeding or bruising, fever, chills, sore throat, shortness of breath, yellowing of skin or eyes, persistent cough, flank or stomach pain, joint pain, black tarry stools, rash, or unusual lumps or masses.

- Tell patient to consult prescriber before using over-the-counter medications.
- Instruct patient to use reliable contraception.
- Caution patient to avoid breastfeeding during therapy.
- Inform patient about the need for repeated laboratory testing during therapy.
- As appropriate, review all other significant and life-threatening adverse reactions and interactions, especially those related to the drugs and tests mentioned above.

meperidine hydrochloride (pethidine hydrochloride❋)

Demerol

Pharmacologic class: CNS agent, opioid agonist
Therapeutic class: Analgesic, adjunct to anesthesia
Controlled substance schedule II
Pregnancy risk category B; D (prolonged therapy, high dosages at term)

Action

Binds to and depresses opiate receptors in spinal cord and CNS, altering perception of and response to pain

Pharmacokinetics

Drug distributes widely throughout body and crosses placental barrier. It is metabolized by the liver to active or inactive metabolites. Half-life is 3 to 4 hours; half-life of normeperidine (active metabolite) is 15 to 30 minutes (which may lead to cumulative effects). Drug is excreted by the kidneys and secreted in breast milk.

Onset	Peak	Duration
Unknown	Unknown	Unknown

How supplied

Solution for injection (clear): 10 mg/mL, 25 mg/mL, 50 mg/mL, 75 mg/mL, 100 mg/mL

Indications and dosages

➤ For support of anesthesia

Adults: Initial dosage is usually 10 mg, with incremental dosages of 1 to 5 mg. For continuous I.V. infusion, usual dosage is 15 to 35 mg/hour.

Dosage adjustment

- Adjust dosage based on patient need, premedication, and type of anesthesia.
- Decrease dosage in renal impairment.
- Decrease dosage 25% to 50% when giving drug with phenothiazines or other tranquilizers.
- For elderly patients, use dosage at lower end of recommended range.

Administration

Preparation

Do not give drug I.V. unless opioid antagonist and facilities for assisted or controlled respiration are immediately available.

For I.V. administration, ensure that patient is lying down.

Dilution and compatibility

- Be aware that drug is compatible with dextrose 2.5%, 5% or 10% in water, lactated Ringer's solution, and dextrose–saline solution combinations.
- Know that drug is not compatible with soluble barbiturates, aminophylline, heparin, iodide, methicillin, morphine sulfate, phenytoin, sodium bicarbonate, sulfadiazine, or sulfisoxazole.
- Be aware that drug may be given undiluted or diluted.
- Do not use if discolored.

Infusion considerations

Administer by very slow I.V. injection undiluted, or preferably as diluted solution with 5 mL normal saline solution for injection, sterile water for injection, or other compatible I.V. solution. Closely observe respiratory rate and monitor symptom relief.

Be aware that rapid I.V. injection increases risk of serious adverse reactions (such as severe respiratory depression, apnea, hypotension, peripheral circulatory collapse, and cardiac arrest).

When giving as I.V. infusion, dilute each 10 mg in at least 1 mL normal saline solution, dextrose 5% in normal saline solution, D_5W, or other compatible infusion solution. Use controlled infusion device and adhere closely to prescribed dosage rate and interval.

Monitoring

- Reassess patient's pain level after administration.

Monitor vital signs and respiratory status. Discontinue drug if patient has significant respiratory or CNS depression.

Watch for seizures, agitation, irritability, nervousness, tremors, twitches, and myoclonus in patients at risk for normeperidine accumulation (such as those with renal or hepatic impairment and those with sickle cell anemia, burns, or cancer who are receiving high doses).

Use with extreme caution in head injury. Drug may increase intracranial pressure (ICP) and cause adverse reactions that obscure clinical course.

- Closely monitor patients with acute abdominal pain. Drug may obscure diagnosis and clinical course of GI condition.
- Evaluate bowel and bladder function.

Storage

- Store at controlled temperature of 20° to 25°C (68° to 77°F); protect from light.

Contraindications and precautions

Contraindicated in hypersensitivity to drug and monoamine oxidase (MAO) inhibitor use within 14 days.

Use cautiously in head trauma; increased ICP; severe renal, hepatic, or pulmonary disease; hypothyroidism; adrenal insufficiency; extensive burns; alcoholism; undiagnosed abdominal pain; prostatic hypertrophy; ***elderly or debilitated patients;*** pregnant patients (not recommended before labor); labor (drug may cause respiratory depression in neonate); breastfeeding patients; and ***children.***

Adverse reactions

CNS: light-headedness, dizziness, weakness, agitation, tremor, uncoordinated muscle movements, disorientation, confusion, sedation, dysphoria, euphoria, floating feeling, hallucinations, headache, unusual dreams, **seizures**
CV: hypotension, tachycardia, syncope, palpitations, **bradycardia, cardiac arrest, shock, circulatory depression**
EENT: blurred vision, diplopia, miosis
GI: constipation, biliary tract spasms, dry mouth
GU: urine retention
Respiratory: respiratory depression, respiratory arrest
Skin: flushing, sweating, pruritus, urticaria, rashes
Other: pain and phlebitis at injection site

Interactions

Drug-drug. *Anesthetics, antihistamines, barbiturates, opioid analgesics, phenothiazines, sedative-hypnotics, tricyclic antidepressants:* additive CNS and respiratory depression
MAO inhibitors, procarbazine: potentially fatal reaction
Opioid agonist-antagonists: precipitation of opioid withdrawal in physically dependent patients
Drug-diagnostic tests. *Amylase, lipase:* increased
Drug-herb. *Chamomile, hops, kava, skullcap, valerian:* increased CNS depression
Drug-behaviors. *Alcohol use:* increased CNS depression

Toxicity and overdose

- In overdose, expect respiratory depression, Cheyne-Stokes respiration, cyanosis, extreme somnolence progressing to stupor or coma, skeletal muscle flaccidity, cold and clammy skin, bradycardia, hypotension, and pulmonary edema. Severe I.V. overdose may cause apnea, circulatory collapse, cardiac arrest, and death.
- Maintain patent airway and provide assisted or controlled ventilation. As prescribed, give appropriate dosage of opioid antagonist (naloxone) and promptly provide respiratory resuscitation, as needed. In patients with physical dependence on drug, avoid naloxone, if possible; if it must be used to treat serious respiratory depression, administer with extreme care and titrate with smaller-than-usual dosages. Do not give naloxone or other antagonist in absence of significant respiratory or cardiovascular depression. Provide oxygen, I.V. fluids, vasopressors, and other supportive measures, as indicated and ordered. Atropine may be useful for treating bradycardia. Be aware that about 40% of patients experience noncardiac pulmonary edema.

Patient teaching

- Advise patient to report adverse reactions promptly.
- Instruct ambulatory patient to change positions slowly to avoid orthostatic hypotension.
- Caution patient to avoid alcohol during therapy.
- Tell female patient to inform prescriber if she is pregnant or breastfeeding.
- As appropriate, review all other significant and life-threatening adverse reactions and interactions, especially those related to the drugs, tests, herbs, and behaviors mentioned above.

M

[redacted]

meropenem

Merrem I.V., Merronem ⊕

Pharmacologic class: Carbapenem
Therapeutic class: Anti-infective
Pregnancy risk category B

Action

Inhibits bacterial cell-wall synthesis and penetrates gram-negative and gram-positive bacteria

Pharmacokinetics

Drug distributes widely into body tissues. It is metabolized into one inactive metabolite; a small amount is protein-bound. Half-life is 0.8 to 1.24 hours. Drug is excreted largely by the kidneys.

Onset	Peak	Duration
Unknown	1 hr	Unknown

How supplied

Powder for reconstitution for injection: 500 mg in 20-mL vial, 1 g in 30-mL vial

Indications and dosages

➤ Intra-abdominal infections caused by alpha-hemolytic streptococci, *Escherichia coli, Klebsiella pneumoniae, Pseudomonas aeruginosa, Bacteroides fragilis, Bacteroides thetaiotaomicron,* and *Peptostreptococcus* species

Adults: 1 g I.V. q 8 hours over 15 to 30 minutes by infusion or over 3 to 5 minutes as bolus injection

Children weighing 50 kg (110 lb) or more: 1 g I.V. q 8 hours over 15 to 30 minutes by infusion or over 3 to 5 minutes as bolus injection

Children age 3 months and older weighing less than 50 kg: 20 mg/kg q 8 hours over 15 to 30 minutes by infusion or over 3 to 5 minutes as bolus injection

➤ Bacterial meningitis caused by *Streptococcus pneumoniae, Haemophilus influenzae,* or *Neisseria meningitidis*

Children weighing 50 kg or more: 2 g I.V. q 8 hours over 15 to 30 minutes by infusion or over 3 to 5 minutes as bolus injection

Children age 3 months and older weighing less than 50 kg: 40 mg/kg I.V. q 8 hours over 15 to 30 minutes by infusion or over 3 to 5 minutes as bolus injection, to a maximum of 2 g q 8 hours

Dosage adjustment

- Reduce dosage in adults with renal impairment, as shown in the table below. (No information is available on children with renal impairment.)

CrCl (mL/min)	Dosage (infection-dependent)	Dosing interval
26 to 50	Recommended dosage	12 hours
10 to 25	Half of recommended dosage	12 hours
Below 10	Half of recommended dosage	24 hours

Off-label uses

- Acute pulmonary exacerbation caused by respiratory tract infection with susceptible organisms in patients with cystic fibrosis

Administration

Preparation

- Collect specimens for culture and sensitivity testing as needed. Be aware that drug therapy may begin pending results.

Dilution and compatibility

- For I.V. bolus, add 10 or 20 mL sterile water for injection to 500-mg or 1-g vial, respectively, to yield a concentration of 50 mg/mL. Shake until clear.
- For intermittent I.V. infusion, piggyback vials can be reconstituted with

compatible I.V. solution (normal saline solution or D_5W) to yield a concentration of 2.5 to 50 mg/mL. Or vials can be reconstituted as for I.V. bolus injection and added to compatible I.V. solution for further dilution. To reconstitute and administer ADD-Vantage system, follow manufacturer's instructions.
- Know that solution should be colorless to yellow.
- Do not mix with other drugs.
- Use diluted solution immediately, if possible.

Infusion considerations
- For I.V. bolus, give single dose over 3 to 5 minutes.
- For intermittent I.V. infusion, infuse drug over 15 to 30 minutes.

Monitoring

Monitor for hypersensitivity reaction or anaphylaxis. If either occurs, stop infusion immediately and initiate emergency measures.
- Monitor for CNS irritability and seizures.
- In prolonged therapy, evaluate hematopoietic, renal, and hepatic functions and watch for overgrowth of nonsusceptible organisms.
- If diarrhea occurs, check for pseudomembranous colitis and obtain stool cultures.
- Obtain hearing tests in child being treated for bacterial meningitis.

Storage
- Store dry powder at controlled room temperature of 20° to 25°C (68° to 77°F).

Contraindications and precautions
Contraindicated in hypersensitivity to drug, its components, or other beta-lactams.

Use cautiously in sulfite sensitivity, renal disease, seizure disorder, pregnant or breastfeeding patients, and ***children younger than 3 months*** (safety and efficacy not established).

Adverse reactions
CNS: headache, insomnia, dizziness, drowsiness, weakness, **seizures**
CV: hypotension, phlebitis, palpitations, **heart failure, cardiac arrest, myocardial infarction**
GI: nausea, vomiting, diarrhea, constipation, tongue discoloration, oral candidiasis, glossitis, **pseudomembranous colitis**
GU: vaginal candidiasis
Hematologic: anemia, eosinophilia, **leukopenia, bone marrow depression, thrombocytopenia, neutropenia**
Musculoskeletal: myoclonus
Respiratory: chest discomfort, dyspnea, hyperventilation
Skin: rash, urticaria, pruritus, erythema at injection site
Other: altered taste, fever, pain, fungal infection, **anaphylaxis**

Interactions
Drug-drug. *Probenecid:* increased meropenem blood level
Valproic acid: possible reduction of serum valproic acid to subtherapeutic level
Drug-diagnostic tests. *Alanine aminotransferase, alkaline phosphatase, amylase, aspartate aminotransferase, bilirubin, blood urea nitrogen, creatinine, eosinophils, gamma-glutamyl transpeptidase, lactate dehydrogenase, lipase:* increased
Hematocrit, hemoglobin, neutrophils, platelets, white blood cells: decreased
International Normalized Ratio, partial thromboplastin time, prothrombin time: increased or decreased

Toxicity and overdose
- In overdose, expect extension of adverse reactions.
- Discontinue drug and provide supportive measures. Know that hemodialysis effectively removes drug.

Patient teaching

Advise patient to promptly report such adverse reactions as diarrhea, rash, shortness of breath, and pain at infusion site.

- Instruct patient to notify prescriber if she is pregnant or breastfeeding.
- As appropriate, review all other significant and life-threatening adverse reactions and interactions, especially those related to the drugs and tests mentioned above.

mesna

Mesnex, Uromitexan♣ ❁

Pharmacologic class: Detoxifying agent
Therapeutic class: Hemorrhagic cystitis inhibitor
Pregnancy risk category B

Action

Reacts in kidney with urotoxic ifosfamide metabolites (acrolein and 4-hydroxy-ifosfamide), resulting in their detoxification. Also binds to double bonds of acrolein and to other urotoxic metabolites.

Pharmacokinetics

Drug is rapidly oxidized to its only major metabolite, mesna disulfide, which stays in intravascular compartment and does not distribute into tissues. It is reduced to free thiol compound, mesna, which the kidneys rapidly eliminate. Approximately 32% of dose is eliminated in urine in 24 hours as mesna and 33% as mesna disulfide. Half-life is 0.37 hours for mesna, 1.17 hours for mesna disulfide.

Onset	Peak	Duration
Unknown	Unknown	Unknown

How supplied

Solution for injection (clear, colorless): 100 mg/mL in 2-mL and 10-mL multidose vials

Indications and dosages

➤ To prevent hemorrhagic cystitis in patients receiving ifosfamide

Adults: I.V. bolus of mesna at 20% of ifosfamide dosage given at same time, repeated 4 and 8 hours after each ifosfamide dose

Administration

Preparation

- Be aware that drug commonly is prescribed in combination I.V. and oral regimen.
- Know that drug is available in combination with ifosfamide.

When adjusting ifosfamide dosage, maintain proper mesna-to-ifosfamide ratio.

Do not use multidose vials (contain benzyl alcohol) in neonates or infants. In older children, use with caution.

Dilution and compatibility

- Dilute with D_5W, 5% dextrose and 0.2% sodium chloride solution, 5% dextrose and 0.33% sodium chloride solution, 5% dextrose and half-normal saline solution, normal saline solution, or lactated Ringer's solution. Final concentration should be 20 mg mesna/mL.

Infusion considerations

- Give I.V. bolus over at least 1 minute with ifosfamide dose and at prescribed intervals after ifosfamide doses.
- Do not use if solution is discolored.

Monitoring

- Monitor nutritional and hydration status.

- Monitor vital signs and ECG. Watch closely for blood pressure changes and tachycardia.
- Assess body temperature. Stay alert for fever, flulike symptoms, and EENT infections.
- Monitor respiratory status carefully.

Storage

- Store vials at controlled room temperature of 20° to 25°C (68° to 77°F).
- Be aware that diluted solution is stable for 24 hours at 25°C (77°F).

Contraindications and precautions

Contraindicated in hypersensitivity to drug or other thiol compounds.

Use cautiously in autoimmune disorders, impaired renal or hepatic function, ***elderly patients,*** pregnant or breastfeeding patients, and ***children.***

Adverse reactions

CNS: fatigue, malaise, irritability, headache, dizziness, drowsiness, hyperesthesia
CV: hypertension, hypotension, ST-segment elevation, tachycardia
EENT: pharyngitis, rhinitis
GI: nausea, vomiting, diarrhea, constipation, anorexia, flatulence
Hematologic: hematuria
Respiratory: coughing, tachypnea
Skin: flushing, rash
Other: injection site reactions, fever, flulike symptoms, allergic reactions

Interactions

Drug-diagnostic tests. *Liver enzymes:* increased
Urinary erythrocytes: false-positive or false-negative results
Urine tests using Ames Multistix (during mesna/ifosfamide therapy): false-positive for ketonuria

Toxicity and overdose

- In overdose, expect extension of adverse reactions.
- No known antidote exists. Provide symptomatic and supportive therapy, as indicated.

Patient teaching

- Inform patient that drug may cause significant adverse effects. Reassure patient that he will be monitored closely.
- Encourage patient to request analgesics or other pain-relief measures for headache, back or joint pain, hyperesthesia, or muscle ache.

Advise patient to immediately report breathing difficulties and allergic symptoms.

- Inform patient about drug's adverse CNS effects. Explain safety measures used to prevent injury.
- As appropriate, review all other significant and life-threatening adverse reactions and interactions, especially those related to the tests mentioned above.

[redacted]

methocarbamol

Robaxin

Pharmacologic class: Autonomic nervous system agent
Therapeutic class: Skeletal muscle relaxant (centrally acting)
Pregnancy risk category C

Action

Unknown. Action presumably results from general CNS depression.

Pharmacokinetics

Drug distributes widely throughout body tissues and is metabolized to inactive metabolites that are excreted largely in urine, with small amount excreted in feces.

M

Onset	Peak	Duration
Unknown	Unknown	Unknown

How supplied

Solution for injection: 100 mg/mL in 10-mL vials

Indications and dosages

➢ Adjunct in muscle spasms associated with acute, painful musculoskeletal conditions

Adults: If oral dosing is not feasible or if condition is severe, 1 to 3 g/day I.V. given in 1-g doses q 8 hours for a maximum of 3 days

Off-label uses

• Tetanus

Administration

Preparation

• Know that drug may be given I.M. but not subcutaneously.

Do not give parenteral form to patients with renal impairment. Polyethylene glycol vehicle may irritate kidneys.

• Be aware that drug usually is given as part of regimen that includes rest and physical therapy.

Dilution and compatibility

• Know that for direct I.V. injection, drug may be given undiluted.

• For I.V. infusion, dilute 1 g with up to 250 mL D_5W or normal saline solution.

Infusion consideration

• For direct I.V. injection, give slowly at a maximum rate of 3 mL/minute.

• For I.V. infusion, adjust infusion rate based on patient comfort.

Avoid extravasation; drug is hypertonic.

Monitoring

• Assess for orthostatic hypotension, especially with parenteral use. Keep patient supine for 10 to 15 minutes after administration.

Stay alert for bradycardia and syncope after administration. As needed and prescribed, give epinephrine, corticosteroids, or antihistamines if syncope occurs.

Monitor I.V. site frequently to avoid extravasation, which may lead to sloughing and thrombophlebitis.

Storage

• Store at 20° to 25°C (68° to 77°F); excursions permitted to 15° to 30°C (59° to 86°F).

• Do not refrigerate infusion solution.

Contraindications and precautions

Contraindicated in hypersensitivity to drug, its components, or polyethylene glycol and in renal impairment.

Use cautiously in seizure disorders, pregnant or breastfeeding patients, and ***children younger than age 12*** (safety not established).

Adverse reactions

CNS: dizziness, light-headedness, drowsiness, syncope, insomnia, sedation, vertigo, headache, amnesia, confusion, **seizures**

CV: bradycardia, hypotension

EENT: blurred vision, conjunctivitis, nasal congestion

GI: nausea, GI upset, anorexia, vomiting, jaundice

Hematologic: leukopenia

Skin: flushing, pruritus, rash, urticaria

Other: fever, phlebitis at I.V. site

Interactions

Drug-drug. *Antihistamines, CNS depressants (such as opioids, sedative-hypnotics):* additive CNS depression

Drug-diagnostic tests. *Urinary 5-hydroxyindoleacetic acid, urine vanillylmandelic acid:* false elevations

Drug-herb. *Chamomile, hops, kava, skullcap, valerian:* increased CNS depression

Drug-behaviors. *Alcohol use:* increased CNS depression

Toxicity and overdose

- In overdose, signs and symptoms include drowsiness and light-headedness. Severe overdose may cause marked CNS depression, including coma.
- Discontinue drug and provide supportive therapy.

Patient teaching

- Advise patient to report adverse effects.
- Caution patient not to drive or perform other hazardous activities, as drug may cause drowsiness or dizziness.
- Instruct patient to move slowly when changing position, to avoid dizziness or light-headedness from sudden blood pressure decrease.
- As appropriate, review all other significant and life-threatening adverse reactions and interactions, especially those related to the drugs, tests, herbs, and behaviors mentioned above.

methotrexate sodium

Pharmacologic class: Antimetabolite, folic acid antagonist
Therapeutic class: Antineoplastic
Pregnancy risk category X

FDA BOXED WARNING

- Give drug under supervision of physician experienced in antimetabolite use.
- Use drug only for life-threatening neoplastic diseases or in patients with severe, recalcitrant, disabling psoriasis that responds inadequately to other therapies.
- Deaths have occurred when drug was used to treat cancer and psoriasis.
- Monitor patient closely for bone marrow, liver, lung, and kidney toxicities. Explain risks involved, and stress importance of adequate follow-up.
- Use caution when giving high-dose regimen for osteosarcoma. (High-dose regimens for other cancers are investigational.)
- Do not use preserved forms and diluents containing preservatives for intrathecal or high-dose therapy.
- Do not give to pregnant women or women with childbearing potential unless medical evidence suggests benefits may outweigh risks. Drug has caused fetal death and congenital anomalies.
- Drug elimination is reduced in patients with renal impairment, ascites, or pleural effusions. Monitor them carefully for toxicity; dosage may need to be reduced or drug may need to be stopped.
- Unexpectedly severe (sometimes fatal) bone marrow suppression and GI toxicity have occurred in patients receiving drug (usually in high doses) concurrently with nonsteroidal anti-inflammatory drugs (NSAIDs).
- Drug causes hepatotoxicity, fibrosis, and cirrhosis, but generally only after prolonged use. Acute liver enzyme elevations are common but usually transient and asymptomatic. Psoriasis patients receiving long-term therapy should have periodic liver biopsies.
- Potentially dangerous lung disease may arise acutely at any time during therapy. It has occurred at dosages as low as 7.5 mg/week and is not always fully reversible.
- Interrupt therapy for diarrhea and ulcerative stomatitis; otherwise, hemorrhagic enteritis and death from intestinal perforation may occur.
- Malignant lymphomas may occur at low dosages and may not require cytotoxic treatment. Discontinue drug first;

if lymphoma does not regress, begin appropriate treatment.

- Drug may induce tumor lysis syndrome in patients with rapidly growing tumors.
- Severe and occasionally fatal skin reactions have occurred within days of single or multiple I.V., P.O., I.M., or intrathecal doses. Drug withdrawal has led to recovery.
- Potentially fatal opportunistic infections may occur.
- When given concomitantly with radiation therapy, drug may increase risk of soft-tissue necrosis and osteonecrosis.

Action

Binds to dihydrofolate reductase, interfering with folic acid metabolism and inhibiting DNA synthesis and cellular replication

Pharmacokinetics

Drug distributes widely in body tissues, is metabolized primarily in the liver, and is about 50% protein-bound. Terminal half-life is about 3 to 10 hours (in high-dose therapy, 8 to 15 hours). It is excreted mainly by the kidneys.

Onset	Peak	Duration
Unknown	Unknown	Unknown

How supplied

Powder for reconstitution for injection (lyophilized, preservative-free): 20-mg and 1-g vials

Indications and dosages

➢ Acute lymphoblastic leukemia

Adults and children: As an alternative to oral and intramuscular use, may give 2.5 mg/kg I.V. q 14 days

➢ Osteosarcoma

Adults: As part of adjunctive regimen with other antineoplastics, initially 12 g/m^2 I.V. as 4-hour infusion, then 12 to 15 g/m^2 I.V. in subsequent 4-hour infusions given at weeks 4, 5, 6, 7, 11, 12, 15, 16, 29, 30, 44, and 45 until peak blood level reaches 1,000 micromoles. Leucovorin rescue must start 24 hours after methotrexate infusion begins; if patient cannot tolerate oral leucovorin, dose must be given I.V. on same schedule.

➢ Lymphosarcoma (stage III)

Adults: 0.625 to 2.5 mg/kg/day I.V.

➢ Psoriasis

Adults: After test dose, 10 to 25 mg I.V. as a single weekly dose, to a maximum dosage of 30 mg weekly; decrease dosage when adequate response occurs.

Dosage adjustment

- Reduce dosage or stop drug in renal impairment, ascites, or pleural effusions, as appropriate.
- Adjust or reduce dosage or discontinue therapy based on neurologic adverse effects (such as seizures).
- Reduce dosage or stop drug and take appropriate corrective measures to reverse common adverse reactions, such as vomiting, diarrhea, or stomatitis, or drug-induced lung disease, as appropriate.
- Be aware that elderly patients may require dosage reduction.

Off-label uses

- Relapsing-remitting multiple sclerosis
- Refractory Crohn's disease

Administration

Preparation

Follow hazardous drug guidelines on page S19 for handling, preparation, and administration.

For osteosarcoma, make sure leucovorin rescue is used appropriately in patients receiving high methotrexate doses. Rescue usually starts 24 hours after methotrexate infusion begins. Follow established safety guidelines meticulously.

Know that serum creatinine level must be normal and creatinine clearance must be above 60 mL/minute before giving drug. Obtain serum creatinine level before each course of therapy; if creatinine level increases at least 50% over previous value, obtain creatinine clearance to ensure it is still within normal range.

- Be aware that drug exits slowly from third-space compartments (ascites, pleural effusions). Before therapy starts, such fluids should be evacuated.

Know that patient must be adequately hydrated and treated with sodium bicarbonate for urinary alkalization before starting therapy.

Dilution and compatibility

- Reconstitute vial with 20-mg powder with preservative-free solution, such as D_5W or normal saline solution for injection to yield a concentration no greater than 25 mg/mL. Reconstitute 1-g vial with 19.4 mL to yield a concentration of 50 mg/mL.
- For high-dose I.V. infusion, dilute in D_5W.
- Reconstitute immediately before use.

Infusion considerations

- Administer by I.V. in infusion over 4 hours as directed.

Monitoring

- Watch for vomiting, diarrhea, or stomatitis, which may cause dehydration. Take appropriate measures to correct these problems.

Know that high-dose therapy may cause nephrotoxicity. Closely monitor renal function, hydration status, electrolytes, urine alkalization (for pH above 6.5), and methotrexate blood level.

Assess for fever, sore throat, bleeding, increased bruising, and other signs and symptoms of hematologic compromise or infection.

Monitor creatinine and methotrexate blood levels 24 hours after therapy starts and daily thereafter. Adjust leucovorin dosage as prescribed.

- Check hematologic studies at least monthly; blood or platelet transfusions may be necessary.
- Monitor liver and kidney function studies every 1 to 3 months. Evaluate uric acid levels.

Watch for signs and symptoms of pulmonary toxicity, such as fever, dry nonproductive cough, dyspnea, hypoxemia, and infiltrates on chest X-ray.

Storage

- Store at controlled temperature of 20° to 25°C (68° to 77°F); excursions permitted to 15° to 30°C (59° to 86°F). Protect from light.

Contraindications and precautions

Contraindicated in hypersensitivity to drug, psoriasis or rheumatoid arthritis in pregnant patients, and breastfeeding.

Use cautiously in severe myocardial, hepatic, or renal disease; decreased bone marrow reserve; active infection; hypotension; coma; ***elderly patients;*** patients with childbearing potential; and ***young children.***

Adverse reactions

CNS: malaise, fatigue, drowsiness, dizziness, headache, aphasia, hemiparesis, demyelination, **seizures, leukoencephalopathy**
EENT: blurred vision, pharyngitis
GI: nausea, vomiting, diarrhea, hematemesis, melena, GI ulcers, enteritis, pancreatitis, abdominal distress, gingivitis, stomatitis, anorexia, **GI bleeding**
GU: hematuria, cystitis, proteinuria, infertility, spontaneous abortion, menstrual dysfunction, defective spermatogenesis or oogenesis, **severe nephropathy, renal failure**
Hematologic: anemia, **leukopenia, thrombocytopenia, severe bone marrow depression**

M

Hepatic: hepatotoxicity
Metabolic: hyperuricemia, diabetes mellitus
Musculoskeletal: joint pain, myalgia, osteonecrosis, osteoporosis (with long-term use in children), stress fracture
Respiratory: dry nonproductive cough, **pneumonitis, pulmonary fibrosis, pulmonary interstitial infiltrates**
Skin: pruritus, rash, urticaria, alopecia, painful plaque erosions, photosensitivity
Other: chills, fever, increased susceptibility to infection, **septicemia, anaphylaxis, sudden death**

Interactions

Drug-drug. *Activated charcoal:* decreased methotrexate blood level
Azathioprine, retinoids, sulfasalazine: increased hepatotoxicity
Folic acid derivatives: antagonism of methotrexate effects
Fosphenytoin, phenytoin: decreased blood levels of these drugs
Hepatotoxic drugs: increased risk of hepatotoxicity
Mercaptopurine, theophylline: increased blood levels of these drugs
NSAIDs, phenylbutazone, phenytoin, probenecid, salicylates, sulfonamides: increased methotrexate toxicity
Penicillin, sulfonamide: increased methotrexate blood level
Procarbazine: increased nephrotoxicity
Vaccines: vaccine inefficacy
Drug-diagnostic tests. *Hemoglobin, platelets, red blood cells, white blood cells:* decreased
Pregnancy tests: false-positive results
Protein-bound iodine, transaminases, uric acid: increased
Drug-herb. *Astragalus, echinacea, melatonin:* interference with methotrexate-induced immunosuppression
Drug-behaviors. *Alcohol use:* increased hepatotoxicity
Sun exposure: photosensitivity

Toxicity and overdose

• In overdose, expect extension of pharmacologic effects and adverse reactions, including hematologic and GI reactions (such as anemia, leukopenia, thrombocytopenia, pancytopenia, bone marrow suppression, mucositis, stomatitis, oral ulcers, nausea, and vomiting). Aplastic anemia, sepsis or septic shock, and renal failure leading to death have been reported.
• Give leucovorin promptly, as prescribed, to reduce toxicity and counteract overdose effects. Be aware that as interval between overdose and leucovorin rescue increases, leucovorin's efficacy in counteracting hematologic toxicity decreases. Closely monitor serum methotrexate level to determine optimal dosage and duration of leucovorin therapy. In massive overdose, use hydration and urine alkalinization to prevent precipitation of drug or metabolites in renal tubules. Know that acute, intermittent hemodialysis using high-flux dialyzer may have some benefit in drug removal.

Patient teaching

Instruct patient to promptly report diarrhea, abdominal pain, clay-colored or black tarry stools, fever, chills, sore throat, unusual bleeding or bruising, sores in or around the mouth, cough or shortness of breath, yellowing of skin or eyes, dark or bloody urine, swelling of feet or legs, or joint pain.
• Teach patient to take temperature daily and to report fever or other signs or symptoms of infection.
• Instruct patient to drink 2 to 3 L of fluid daily.
• Advise male patient to use reliable contraception during therapy and for at least 3 months afterward. Advise female patient to use reliable contraception

during therapy and for one ovulatory cycle afterward.

- Caution breastfeeding patient not to breastfeed during therapy.
- Tell patient not to take over-the-counter medications or herbal supplements without consulting prescriber.
- Advise patients to avoid sun exposure and to use sunscreen and protective clothing (especially if they have psoriasis).
- Instruct patient to avoid alcohol.
- Inform patient about the need for repeated laboratory testing during therapy.
- As appropriate, review all other significant and life-threatening adverse reactions and interactions, especially those related to the drugs, tests, herbs, and behaviors mentioned above.

methyldopate hydrochloride

Aldomet

Pharmacologic class: Centrally acting antiadrenergic

Therapeutic class: Antihypertensive

Pregnancy risk category C

Action

Unclear. Drug is metabolized to alpha-methyl norepinephrine, which lowers arterial pressure by stimulation of central inhibitory alpha-adrenergic receptors, false neurotransmission, reduction in plasma renin activity, or a combination of these actions.

Pharmacokinetics

Drug is extensively metabolized; plasma half-life is 90 to 127 minutes. It crosses placental barrier and is secreted in breast milk. Approximately 49% is excreted in urine, with some excretion in feces.

Onset	Peak	Duration
Unknown	4-6 hr	10-16 hr

How supplied

Solution for injection (clear, colorless): 250 mg/5 mL (50 mg/mL) in single-dose vials

Indications and dosages

➤ Hypertension (when parenteral therapy is indicated), hypertensive crisis

Adults: 250 to 500 mg I.V. q 6 hours, as required. Maximum daily dosage is 1 g q 6 hours.

Children: 20 to 40 mg/kg I.V. in divided doses q 6 hours. Maximum daily dosage is 65 mg/kg or 3 g daily, whichever is lower.

Dosage adjustment

- Be aware that patients who are elderly or have renal impairment may require smaller dosages.

Administration

Preparation

Do not give within 14 days of monoamine oxidase (MAO) inhibitors.

- Obtain baseline CBC with white cell differential and direct Coombs' test before therapy starts.
- Be aware that patient should be switched to oral therapy once blood pressure is under control.

Dilution and compatibility

- Add desired dosage to 100 mL D_5W or add desired dosage to sufficient amount of D_5W to achieve a concentration of 100 mg/10 mL (10 mg/mL).
- Do not use if solution is discolored.

Infusion considerations

- Administer by slow I.V. infusion over 30 to 60 minutes.

Monitoring

Do not stop drug therapy abruptly.

Obtain direct Coombs' test 6 and 12 months after therapy to detect Coombs'-positive hemolytic anemia.

Check for edema or weight gain, which may be controlled with diuretic. Do not continue giving methyldopate if edema progresses or signs and symptoms of heart failure appear.

Be aware that rare involuntary choreoathetotic movements may develop in patients with severe bilateral cerebrovascular disease. Stop therapy in this case.

- Monitor CBC with white cell differential periodically to detect adverse hematologic reactions.
- Monitor hepatic function tests and check for signs and symptoms of hepatic dysfunction (particularly during first 6 to 12 weeks of therapy).
- Closely monitor blood pressure. Know that drug may cause paradoxical pressor response and that tolerance may occur during second and third months of therapy.

Storage

- Store at 15° to 30°C (59° to 86°F).

Contraindications and precautions

Contraindicated in hypersensitivity to drug or its components, including sulfites; active hepatic disease or history of methyldopa-associated hepatic disorders; and within 14 days of MAO inhibitors.

Use cautiously in history of previous hepatic disease or dysfunction, ***elderly patients,*** and pregnant or breastfeeding patients.

Adverse reactions

CNS: headache, asthenia, weakness, dizziness, sedation, decreased mental acuity, depression, paresthesia, parkinsonism, Bell's palsy, involuntary choreoathetotic movements (rare)
CV: angina aggravation, heart failure, prolonged carotid sinus sensitivity, paradoxical pressor response, bradycardia, orthostatic hypotension
EENT: nasal congestion
GI: nausea, vomiting, diarrhea, constipation, flatus, abdominal distention, colitis, dry mouth, sialadenitis, sore or black tongue, **pancreatitis**
GU: amenorrhea, breast enlargement, gynecomastia, lactation, hyperprolactinemia, erectile dysfunction, decreased libido
Hematologic: bone marrow depression, **hemolytic anemia**
Hepatic: hepatitis
Other: edema, hypersensitivity reaction

Interactions

Drug-drug. *Adrenergics, MAO inhibitors:* excessive sympathetic stimulation
Anesthetics, antihypertensives, nitrates: additive hypotension
Lithium: increased risk of lithium toxicity
Nonselective beta-adrenergic blockers: paradoxical hypertension
Drug-diagnostic tests. *Alanine aminotransferase, alkaline phosphatase, aspartate aminotransferase, bilirubin, blood urea nitrogen, creatinine, potassium, prolactin, sodium, uric acid:* increased
Direct Coombs' test: positive results
Liver function tests: abnormal results
Prothrombin time: prolonged
Drug-herb. *Capsicum:* reduced antihypertensive effect
Drug-behaviors. *Alcohol use:* increased hypotension

Toxicity and overdose

- Acute overdose may cause acute hypotension, excessive sedation, weakness, bradycardia, dizziness, light-headedness, constipation, abdominal distention, flatus, diarrhea, nausea, and vomiting.
- Provide symptomatic and supportive therapy, paying close attention to cardiac rate and output, blood volume, electrolyte balance, paralytic ileus,

urinary function, and cerebral activity. Sympathomimetic drugs (such as levarterenol, epinephrine, and metaraminol bitartrate) may be indicated. Dialysis may aid drug removal.

Patient teaching

- Inform patient that sedation usually occurs when therapy starts and during dosage titration.
- Caution patient not to stop taking drug abruptly.
- Instruct patient to report fever, yellowing of skin or eyes, fatigue, abdominal pain, flulike symptoms, swelling, or significant weight gain.
- Inform patient that urine may darken on exposure to air.
- Advise patient to move slowly when changing position, to avoid dizziness or light-headedness from sudden blood pressure decrease.
- Caution patient to avoid driving and other hazardous activities until drug's effects are known or dosage titration is completed.
- Tell female patient to inform prescriber if she is pregnant or breastfeeding.
- As appropriate, review all other significant and life-threatening adverse reactions and interactions, especially those related to the drugs, tests, herbs, and behaviors mentioned above.

methylprednisolone sodium succinate

Solu-Medrol

Pharmacologic class: Glucocorticoid
Therapeutic class: Antiasthmatic, anti-inflammatory (steroidal), immunosuppressant
Pregnancy risk category NR

Action

Reduces inflammation and prevents edema by stabilizing membranes and reducing permeability of leukocytic cells. Suppresses immune system by interfering with antigen-antibody interactions of macrophages and T cells.

Pharmacokinetics

Drug distributes rapidly in body tissues, crosses placental barrier, and is secreted in breast milk. It is metabolized in the liver to inactive metabolites. These metabolites and a small amount of parent drug are excreted in urine; an insignificant amount is excreted in feces.

Onset	Peak	Duration
Rapid	Unknown	Unknown

How supplied

Powder for reconstitution for injection (white, or nearly white): 40 mg, 125 mg, 500 mg, 1 g and 2 g in single-dose Act-O-Vial System

M

Indications and dosages

➤ Diseases and disorders of endocrine system, collagen, skin, eye, GI tract, respiratory system, or hematologic system; neoplastic diseases; allergies; edema; multiple sclerosis; tuberculous meningitis; trichinosis; rheumatic disorders; osteoarthritis; bursitis; localized inflammatory lesions

Adults: *When high doses are required*—30 mg/kg I.V. given over at least 30 minutes; may repeat q 4 to 6 hours for 48 hours
Other conditions—10 to 40 mg I.V., depending on clinical problem; subsequent dosages depend on both response and clinical condition
Infants and children: Dosages depend more on severity of condition and

patient response than on age and size. Dosage should not be less than 0.5 mg/kg I.V. every 24 hours; subsequent dosages depend on response and clinical condition.

Dosage adjustment

- Decrease dosage or discontinue drug gradually if it has been given for more than a few days. If spontaneous remission occurs during treatment of chronic condition, discontinue therapy.

Off-label uses

- Lupus nephritis
- *Pneumocystis jiroveci* (formerly *Pneumocystis carinii*) pneumonia in AIDS patients

Administration

Preparation

Do not use in premature infants because drug contains benzyl alcohol (associated with fatal gasping syndrome in premature infants).

- As needed and prescribed, give prophylactic antacids to prevent peptic ulcers in patients receiving high doses.

Dilution and compatibility

- Reconstitute with accompanying bacteriostatic water for injection containing 0.9% benzyl alcohol only, per manufacturer's instructions.
- For I.V. infusion, further dilute in compatible I.V. solution (such as D_5W, normal saline solution, or 5% dextrose in normal saline solution).
- Use solution within 48 hours after mixing.

Infusion considerations

- For direct I.V. injection, inject each 500-mg dose over 2 to 3 minutes or more.
- For I.V. infusion, give over 10 to 20 minutes.

Monitoring

- Monitor fluid and electrolyte balance, weight, and blood pressure.

Check for signs and symptoms of steroid-induced psychosis—delirium, euphoria, insomnia, mood swings, personality changes, and depression.

After dosage reduction or drug withdrawal, stay alert for signs and symptoms of adrenal insufficiency.

- Monitor routine laboratory studies (such as urinalysis), 2-hour postprandial blood glucose, blood pressure, and chest X-ray at regular intervals during prolonged therapy. Know that upper GI X-rays are desirable in patients with history of ulcers or significant dyspepsia.

Storage

- Store powder or reconstituted solution at controlled room temperature of 20° to 25°C (68° to 77°F).

Contraindications and precautions

Contraindicated in hypersensitivity to drug or its components, systemic fungal infections, and premature infants (due to benzyl alcohol in some products).

Use cautiously in cardiovascular, hepatic, renal, or GI disease; active untreated infections; thromboembolic tendency; idiopathic thrombocytopenic purpura; osteoporosis; myasthenia gravis; hypothyroidism; glaucoma; ocular herpes simplex; vaccinia or varicella; seizure disorders; metastatic cancer; pregnant or breastfeeding patients; and ***children.***

Adverse reactions

CNS: headache, restlessness, nervousness, depression, euphoria, personality changes, psychoses, vertigo, paresthesia, insomnia, adhesive arachnoiditis, conus medullaris syndrome, **increased intracranial pressure, seizures, meningitis**

CV: hypotension, hypertension, **arrhythmias, heart failure, shock, fat**

embolism, thrombophlebitis, thromboembolism
EENT: cataracts, glaucoma, exophthalmos, increased intraocular pressure, nasal irritation, nasal septum perforation, sneezing, epistaxis, nasopharyngeal or oropharyngeal fungal infection, dysphonia, hoarseness, throat irritation
GI: nausea, vomiting, abdominal distention, rectal bleeding, dry mouth, anorexia, esophageal candidiasis, **esophageal ulcer, peptic ulceration, pancreatitis**
GU: amenorrhea, irregular menses
Metabolic: decreased growth (in children), reduced carbohydrate tolerance, diabetes mellitus, hyperglycemia, sodium and fluid retention, hypokalemia, hypocalcemia, cushingoid state, **negative nitrogen balance, hypothalamic-pituitary-adrenal suppression** (with systemic use beyond 5 days), **adrenal suppression** (with long-term high-dose use), **acute adrenal insufficiency** (with abrupt withdrawal)
Musculoskeletal: muscle wasting, osteoporosis, osteonecrosis, tendon rupture, aseptic joint necrosis, muscle pain and weakness, steroid myopathy, arthralgia, vertebral compression fractures, long-bone fracture
Respiratory: cough, wheezing, **bronchospasm**
Skin: facial edema, rash, pruritus, urticaria, contact dermatitis, acne, decreased wound healing, bruising, hirsutism, thin and fragile skin, petechiae, purpura, striae, subcutaneous fat atrophy, skin atrophy, acneiform lesions, angioedema, hyperpigmentation, hypopigmentation
Other: anosmia, bad taste, increased appetite, Churg-Strauss syndrome, increased susceptibility to infection, aggravation or masking of infection, impaired wound healing, sterile abscess, hypersensitivity reaction including **anaphylactic reaction with or without circulatory collapse, cardiac arrest, or bronchospasm**

Interactions

Drug-drug. *Amphotericin B, mezlocillin, piperacillin, thiazide and loop diuretics, ticarcillin:* additive hypokalemia
Aspirin (high doses): increased aspirin clearance
Cyclosporine: inhibition of cyclosporine or methylprednisolone effects
Fluoroquinolones: increased risk of tendon rupture
Isoniazid, phenobarbital, phenytoin, rifampin: decreased methylprednisolone efficacy
Ketoconazole: decreased methylprednisolone clearance
Live-virus vaccines: decreased antibody response to vaccine, increased risk of adverse reactions
Nonsteroidal anti-inflammatory drugs: increased risk of adverse GI effects
Oral anticoagulants: altered anticoagulant requirement
Drug-diagnostic tests. *Calcium, potassium, thyroxine, triiodothyronine:* decreased
Cholesterol, glucose: increased
Nitroblue tetrazolium test for bacterial infection: false-negative result
Drug-herb. *Echinacea:* increased immune stimulation
Ginseng: immunomodulation
Drug-behaviors. *Alcohol use:* increased risk of gastric irritation and ulcers

Toxicity and overdose

- Toxicity signs and symptoms rarely occur with short-term use.
- In overdose, provide symptomatic and supportive therapy.

Patient teaching

- Inform patient that drug increases risk of infection. Urge patient to avoid exposure to people with such infections as measles and chickenpox and to contact prescriber if exposure occurs.

Advise patient to promptly report unusual weight gain, leg or foot swelling, facial swelling, muscle weakness, black and tarry stools, vomiting of blood, menstrual irregularities, sore throat, fever, or infection.

Tell patient to immediately report signs or symptoms of adrenal insufficiency (fatigue, appetite loss, nausea, vomiting, diarrhea, weight loss, weakness, and dizziness) after dosage reduction or drug withdrawal.

- Advise diabetic patient to monitor blood glucose level carefully.
- Tell female patient to inform prescriber if she is pregnant or breastfeeding.
- As appropriate, review all other significant and life-threatening adverse reactions and interactions, especially those related to the drugs, tests, herbs, and behaviors mentioned above.

[redacted]

metoclopramide hydrochloride

Metoclopramide Omega✤, Reglan

Pharmacologic class: Dopamine antagonist

Therapeutic class: Antiemetic, GI stimulant

Pregnancy risk category B

Action

Blocks dopamine receptors by disrupting CNS chemoreceptor trigger zone, increasing peristalsis and promoting gastric emptying

Pharmacokinetics

Drug distributes widely into body tissues and crosses placental barrier. It is not extensively metabolized, but a small amount is metabolized in the liver. It is excreted in urine, feces, and breast milk.

Onset	Peak	Duration
Unknown	Unknown	Unknown

How supplied

Solution for injection (clear, colorless): 5 mg/mL in 2-mL vials

Indications and dosages

➤ To prevent chemotherapy-induced vomiting

Adults: 1 to 2 mg/kg I.V. 30 minutes before chemotherapy, then q 2 hours for two doses, then q 3 hours for three additional doses

➤ To promote small-bowel intubation; radiologic examination when delayed gastric emptying interferes

Adults and children older than age 14: 10 mg I.V. as a single dose

Children ages 6 to 14: 2.5 to 5 mg I.V. as a single dose

Children younger than age 6: 0.1 mg/kg I.V. as a single dose

➤ Diabetic gastroparesis

Adults: 10 mg I.V. given slowly over 1 to 2 minutes. Up to 10 days of therapy may be required before symptoms subside, at which time patient may be switched to oral therapy.

Dosage adjustment

- Reduce dosage 50% in renal impairment.

Off-label uses

- Hiccups

Administration

Dilution and compatibility

- Know that drug does not require further dilution for direct I.V. injection.
- For dosages above 10 mg, dilute with 50 mL 5% dextrose in normal saline

solution, 5% dextrose in half-normal saline solution, or lactated Ringer's solution.

- Do not use solution if discolored.
- Discard unused portion.

Infusion considerations

- Administer low dosages (10 mg or less) by direct I.V. injection slowly over 2 minutes. Be aware that rapid injection may cause intense anxiety and restlessness followed by drowsiness.
- For I.V. infusion, administer over at least 15 minutes.

Monitoring

- Monitor blood pressure during I.V. administration.
- Stay alert for depression and other adverse CNS effects.

Clinical alert: Watch for extrapyramidal reactions, which usually occur within first 24 to 48 hours. To reverse symptoms, give diphenhydramine 50 mg I.M. or benztropine 1 to 2 mg I.M., as prescribed.

- Check for parkinsonian-like symptoms, which may develop within first 6 months of therapy and usually subside within 2 to 3 months after withdrawal.
- With long-term use, assess patient for tardive dyskinesia.
- In patients with diabetes mellitus, stay alert for gastric stasis. Insulin dosage may need to be adjusted.

Storage

- Store at 20° to 25°C (68° to 77°F).
- Know that diluted solution is stable for 24 hours in normal light and 48 hours when protected from light.

Contraindications and precautions

Contraindicated in hypersensitivity to drug; pheochromocytoma; Parkinson's disease; suspected GI obstruction, perforation, or hemorrhage; and history of seizure disorders.

Use cautiously in diabetes mellitus, history of depression, patients taking monoamine oxidase (MAO) inhibitors, ***elderly patients,*** pregnant or breastfeeding patients, and ***children.***

Adverse reactions

CNS: drowsiness, restlessness, anxiety, confusion, dizziness, depression with suicidal ideation, irritability, tardive dyskinesia, fatigue, lassitude, insomnia, headache, parkinsonian-like reactions, extrapyramidal reactions, akathisia, dystonia, hallucinations, **seizures**

CV: hypertension, hypotension, **acute congestive heart failure, atrioventricular block, arrhythmias**

EENT: visual disturbances

GI: nausea, diarrhea, bowel disturbances

GU: gynecomastia, galactorrhea, amenorrhea, erectile dysfunction secondary to hyperprolactinemia, urinary frequency, incontinence

Hematology: neutropenia, leukopenia, agranulocytosis

Hepatic: hepatotoxicity

Skin: rash, urticaria

Other: fluid retention, allergic reactions (including **angioneurotic edema and bronchospasm,** especially in patients with asthma)

Interactions

Drug-drug. *Anticholinergics, opioids:* antagonism of metoclopramide's GI motility effect

Antidepressants, antihistamines, other CNS depressants (such as opioids, sedative-hypnotics): additive CNS depression

Cimetidine, digoxin: decreased blood levels of these drugs

General anesthetics: exaggerated hypotension

Haloperidol, phenothiazines: increased risk of extrapyramidal reactions

Levodopa: decreased metoclopramide efficacy

MAO inhibitors: increased catecholamine release

M

Drug-diagnostic tests. *Aldosterone, prolactin:* increased
Drug-behaviors. *Alcohol use:* increased blood alcohol level, increased CNS depression

Toxicity and overdose

- In overdose (rare), expect extension of adverse reactions, including drowsiness, restlessness, anxiety, fatigue, lassitude, insomnia, and dystonia.
- Discontinue drug. As ordered and needed, give anticholinergic, antiparkinsonian drugs, and possibly antihistamines.

Patient teaching

- Instruct patient to report involuntary movements of face, eyes, or limbs.
- Caution patient to avoid driving and other hazardous activities until drug's effects are known.
- As appropriate, review all other significant and life-threatening adverse reactions and interactions, especially those related to the drugs, tests, and behaviors mentioned above.

metoprolol tartrate

Lopressor

Pharmacologic class: Beta-adrenergic blocker (selective)
Therapeutic class: Antihypertensive, antianginal
Pregnancy risk category C

FDA BOXED WARNING

- Exacerbations of angina pectoris and myocardial infarction (MI) may follow abrupt withdrawal of some beta blockers. When discontinuing long-term therapy, particularly in patients with ischemic heart disease, reduce dosage gradually over 1 to 2 weeks and monitor patient carefully. If angina worsens markedly or acute coronary insufficiency develops, reinstate drug promptly (at least temporarily) and take other appropriate measures to manage unstable angina. Caution patient not to interrupt or discontinue therapy without prescriber's advice. Because coronary artery disease is common and may be unrecognized, it may be prudent not to discontinue drug abruptly even in patients treated only for hypertension.

Action

Blocks stimulation of $beta_1$ (myocardial) adrenergic receptors, usually without affecting $beta_2$ (pulmonary, vascular, uterine) adrenergic receptor sites

Pharmacokinetics

Drug distributes widely in the body. It is metabolized primarily in the liver; a small amount is protein-bound. It is excreted as metabolites in urine.

Onset	Peak	Duration
Immediate	20 min	5-8 hr

How supplied

Solution for injection: 1 mg/mL in 5-mL vials

Indications and dosages

➤ Acute myocardial infarction (MI)
Adults: For early treatment, three bolus injections of 5 mg I.V. given at 2-minute intervals. If patient tolerates I.V. dose, give oral dose 15 minutes after last I.V. dose, as prescribed. Continue oral doses q 6 hours for 48 hours. Give maintenance dosages orally. If patient does not tolerate full I.V. dose, give oral dose (depending on degree of intolerance), starting 15 minutes after last I.V. dose

or when clinical condition allows. Discontinue drug if patient shows severe intolerance. For late treatment, administer oral doses when clinical condition allows; continue for at least 3 months.

Off-label uses

- Anxiety
- Tachycardia
- Tremors
- Ventricular arrhythmias

Administration

Preparation

- Measure blood pressure closely when starting therapy and titrating dosage.
- Monitor blood pressure and pulse before I.V. administration. If patient is hypotensive or has bradycardia, consult prescriber before giving dose.

Dilution and compatibility

- Know that drug requires no dilution.

Infusion considerations

- Give each dose by direct injection over at least 1 minute.

Monitoring

- Measure blood pressure closely. Once patient stabilizes, measure blood pressure every 3 to 6 hours.
- Watch for orthostatic hypotension in at-risk patients, particularly elderly patients.
- Assess glucose level in patient with diabetes mellitus. Be aware that drug may mask hypoglycemia signs and symptoms.
- Monitor for signs and symptoms of hyperthyroidism. Know that drug may mask these. Reduce dosage gradually in hyperthyroid patients.

When discontinuing drug, reduce dosage gradually over 1 to 2 weeks.

Storage

- Store at controlled room temperature of 20° to 25°C (68° to 77°F). Protect from light.

Contraindications and precautions

Contraindicated in heart rate below 45 beats/minute, second- or third-degree heart block, significant first-degree heart block, systolic blood pressure below 100 mm Hg, or moderate to severe cardiac failure.

Use cautiously in renal or hepatic impairment, pulmonary disease, diabetes mellitus, thyrotoxicosis, within 14 days of monoamine oxidase inhibitors, pregnant or breastfeeding patients, and ***children*** (safety not established).

Adverse reactions

CNS: depression, dizziness, sleep disturbances, memory loss, mental status changes, confusion
CV: bradycardia; hypotension; **first-, second-, or third-degree heart block; heart failure**
EENT: visual disturbances
GI: nausea, gastric pain
GU: decreased libido
Metabolic: hyperglycemia
Respiratory: dyspnea
Skin: rash

Interactions

Drug-drug. *Amphetamines, ephedrine, epinephrine, norepinephrine, phenylephrine, pseudoephedrine:* unopposed alpha-adrenergic stimulation (excessive hypertension, bradycardia)
Antihypertensives, catecholamine-depleting drugs (reserpine), nitrates: additive hypotension
Clonidine: increased rebound hypertension on clonidine withdrawal
Potent CYP2D6 inhibitors (such as cimetidine, diphenhydramine, fluoxetine, hydroxychloroquine, propafenone, quinidine, ritonavir, terbinafine, thioridazine): increased metoprolol blood level
Drug-diagnostic tests. *Aminotransferase, blood urea nitrogen, glucose, lactate*

dehydrogenase, lipoproteins, potassium, triglycerides, uric acid: increased
Drug-food. *Any food:* enhanced drug absorption
Drug-behaviors. *Acute alcohol ingestion:* additive hypotension
Cocaine use: unopposed alpha-adrenergic stimulation (excessive hypertension, bradycardia)

Toxicity and overdose

- In overdose, expect severe hypotension, bradycardia, heart failure, bronchospasm, and possibly hypoglycemia.
- Discontinue drug. Provide symptomatic and supportive therapy, including I.V. fluids and vasopressors, with extreme caution. For heart failure, expect to give digitalis preparation and diuretics.

Patient teaching

Advise patient with heart failure to report signs or symptoms of worsening condition, such as weight gain and shortness of breath.
- As appropriate, review all other significant and life-threatening adverse reactions and interactions, especially those related to the drugs, tests, food, and behaviors mentioned above.

metronidazole hydrochloride

Pharmacologic class: Nitroimidazole derivative
Therapeutic class: Anti-infective, antiprotozoal
Pregnancy risk category B

FDA BOXED WARNING

- Drug is carcinogenic in mice and rats. Avoid unnecessary use; reserve drug for indicated conditions.

Action

Disturbs DNA synthesis in susceptible bacterial organisms

Pharmacokinetics

Drug distributes into most body tissues and fluids and crosses blood-brain and placental barriers. Protein-binding is less than 20%. Metabolites are excreted in urine, with some excretion in feces and breast milk.

Onset	Peak	Duration
Unknown	Unknown	Unknown

How supplied

Solution for injection (premixed): 500 mg/100 mL in plastic containers

Indications and dosages

➤ Bacterial infections caused by susceptible anaerobic organisms
Adults: Initially, 15 mg/kg I.V. infused over 1 hour, followed by 7.5 mg/kg I.V. q 6 hours infused over 1 hour, not to exceed 4 g/day for 7 to 10 days
➤ Perioperative prophylaxis in colorectal surgery
Adults: Initially, 15 mg/kg I.V. infusion over 30 to 60 minutes, completed 1 hour before surgery; if necessary, 7.5 mg/kg I.V. infusion over 30 to 60 minutes at 6 and 12 hours after initial dose

Administration

Preparation

Follow hazardous drug guidelines on page S19 for handling, preparation, and administration.

Dilution and compatibility

- Be aware that drug is premixed and does not require dilution.
- Do not introduce additives into infusion.
- Do not use equipment containing aluminum, as solution may turn reddish brown.

Infusion considerations

- If used with primary I.V. fluid system, discontinue primary solution during metronidazole infusion.
- Administer only by slow-drip I.V. infusion, either by intermittent or continuous infusion over 1 hour for treatment of infection or over 30 to 60 minutes for prophylaxis of infection.

Do not use plastic containers in series connections. Such use could result in air embolism due to residual air being drawn from primary container before administration of fluid from secondary container ends.

Monitoring

- Monitor I.V. site. Avoid prolonged use of indwelling catheter.
- Evaluate hematologic studies, especially in patients with history of blood dyscrasias.

Storage

- Store at room temperature of 15° to 30°C (59° to 86°F); protect from light.

Contraindications and precautions

Contraindicated in hypersensitivity to drug or other nitroimidazole derivatives.

Use cautiously in severe hepatic impairment, history of blood dyscrasias, seizures, or other neurologic problems, pregnant or breastfeeding patients, and ***children.***

Adverse reactions

CNS: dizziness, headache, ataxia, syncope, confusion
GI: nausea, vomiting, diarrhea, abdominal pain
GU: dysuria, dark urine, incontinence
Hematologic: reversible **leukopenia**
Skin: rash, pruritus
Other: fever, unpleasant or metallic taste, superinfection, phlebitis at I.V. site

Interactions

Drug-drug. *Azathioprine, fluorouracil:* increased risk of leukopenia
Cimetidine: decreased metronidazole metabolism, increased risk of toxicity
Disulfiram: acute psychosis and confusion
Phenobarbital, phenytoin: increased metabolism and decreased efficacy of metronidazole
Warfarin: increased warfarin effects
Drug-diagnostic tests. *Alanine aminotransferase, aspartate aminotransferase, lactate dehydrogenase:* altered level
Drug-behaviors. *Alcohol use:* disulfiram-like reaction

Toxicity and overdose

- In overdose, expect extension of adverse reactions, including nausea, vomiting, and ataxia.
- No specific antidote exists. Provide symptomatic and supportive therapy.

Patient teaching

- Advise patient to report fever, sore throat, bleeding, or bruising.
- Inform patient that drug may cause metallic taste and may turn urine a deep brownish red.
- Tell female patient to consult prescriber if she is pregnant or plans to become pregnant.
- As appropriate, review all other significant and life-threatening adverse reactions and interactions, especially those related to the drugs, tests, and behaviors mentioned above.

midazolam hydrochloride

Pharmacologic class: Benzodiazepine
Therapeutic class: Anxiolytic, sedative-hypnotic, adjunct for general anesthesia induction
Controlled substance schedule IV
Pregnancy risk category D

M

FDA BOXED WARNING

- I.V. form is linked to respiratory depression and respiratory arrest, especially when used for sedation in noncritical care settings. In some cases in which this was not recognized promptly and treated effectively, hypoxic encephalopathy or death resulted. Use I.V. form only in hospital or ambulatory care setting that provides continuous monitoring of respiratory and cardiac function. Ensure immediate availability of resuscitative drugs and equipment, as well as personnel trained in their use and skilled in airway management. For deeply sedated pediatric patient, dedicated individual should monitor patient throughout procedure.
- Patients who are debilitated, older than age 60, or receiving concurrent opioids or other CNS depressants require lower dosages. Slowly titrate initial dose and all subsequent doses; give over at least 2 minutes and allow 2 or more additional minutes to fully evaluate sedative effect. In pediatric patients, calculate dosage on mg/kg basis, and titrate slowly.
- Do not give by rapid injection to neonates. Severe hypotension and seizures may result.

Action

Unknown. Thought to suppress CNS stimulation at limbic and subcortical levels by enhancing effects of gamma-aminobutyric acid, an inhibitory neurotransmitter.

Pharmacokinetics

Drug has large volume of distribution, accumulates in peripheral tissues, and crosses placental barrier. It is metabolized in the liver and is 98% protein-bound, primarily to albumin. Metabolites are excreted in urine. Elimination half-life is 1.8 to 6.4 hours.

Onset	Peak	Duration
1.5-5 min	Rapid	2-6 hr

How supplied

Concentrated solution for injection:
1 mg/mL in 2-, 5-, and 10-mL vials;
5 mg/mL in 1-, 2-, 5-, and 10-mL vials

Indications and dosages

➤ To induce general anesthesia

Adults younger than age 55: 0.3 to 0.35 mg/kg I.V. over 20 to 30 seconds if patient has not received premedication, or 0.15 to 0.35 mg/kg (usual dosage of 0.25 mg/kg) I.V. over 20 to 30 seconds if patient has received premedication. Wait 2 minutes to evaluate effect. Additional increments of 25% of initial dosage may be needed to complete induction.

➤ Continuous infusion to initiate sedation

Adults: When rapid sedation is required, give loading dose of 0.01 to 0.05 mg/kg I.V. slowly; repeat dose q 10 to 15 minutes until adequate sedation occurs. To maintain sedation, infuse at initial rate of 0.02 to 0.10 mg/kg/hour (1 to 7 mg/hour). Adjust infusion rate as needed.

➤ Preoperative sedation, anxiolysis, and amnesia

Adults younger than age 60: Give initial dose of 1 mg and titrate slowly to effect. Some patients may respond adequately to 1-mg dose. Do not give more than 2.5 mg over 2-minute period. Total dosage above 5 mg rarely is necessary. Wait at least 2 minutes after additional doses to assess effect. To maintain effect, may give additional doses, in increments of 25% of dosage used to achieve sedation, by slow titration.

Children ages 12 to 16: Patients in this age-group should receive adult dosages.

Children ages 6 to 12: 0.025 to 0.05 mg/kg I.V.; total dosage of 0.4 mg/kg may be needed to achieve desired endpoint. Total dosage should not exceed 10 mg.
Children ages 6 months to 5 years: 0.05 to 0.1 mg/kg I.V.; total dosage of up to 0.6 mg/kg may be needed to achieve desired endpoint. Total dosage should not exceed 6 mg.

Dosage adjustment

- Reduce dosage in chronic renal failure, congestive heart failure, and chronic obstructive pulmonary disease.
- Reduce dosage if patient is also receiving opioid premedication or other CNS depressant.
- Reduce dosage in elderly or debilitated patients.

Administration

Preparation

Keep oxygen and resuscitation equipment at hand in case severe respiratory depression occurs.

Dilution and compatibility

- Dilute concentrate for I.V. infusion to 0.5 mg/mL using D_5W or normal saline solution. Resulting solution is stable for 24 hours, or for 4 hours if diluted with lactated Ringer's solution for injection.
- Know that drug may be mixed in same syringe as meperidine, atropine, scopolamine, or morphine.

Infusion considerations

- Infuse over at least 2 minutes; wait at least 2 minutes before giving second dose. Be aware that excessive dosage or rapid I.V. delivery may cause severe respiratory depression.

Monitoring

- Monitor vital signs, ECG, respiratory status, and oxygen saturation.
- Assess neurologic status closely, especially in pediatric patients.
- Watch for nausea and vomiting.

Storage

- Store at 15° to 30°C (59° to 86°F).

Contraindications and precautions

Contraindicated in hypersensitivity to drug, its components, or other benzodiazepines and in acute angle-closure glaucoma.

Use cautiously in pulmonary disease, heart failure, renal impairment, severe hepatic impairment, ***elderly or debilitated patients,*** pregnant or breastfeeding patients, ***children, and neonates.***

Adverse reactions

CNS: headache, oversedation, drowsiness, agitation and excitement (in children), seizurelike activity
CV: hypotension, irregular pulse, bradycardia, tachycardia, bigeminy, vasovagal episode, nodal rhythm, premature ventricular contractions, **cardiac arrest**
GI: nausea, vomiting
Respiratory: decreased respiratory rate, hiccups, dyspnea, laryngospasm, bronchospasm, hyperventilation, tachypnea, **airway obstruction, apnea, respiratory arrest**
Other: injection site reaction (such as pain during injection or I.V. site redness, irritation, phlebitis, induration, or tenderness)

Interactions

Drug-drug. *Cimetidine, diltiazem, erythromycin, itraconazole, ketoconazole verapamil:* prolonged sedation (from decreased midazolam clearance)
CNS depressants (such as some antidepressants, antihistamines, barbiturates, opioids, and tranquilizers), respiratory depressants: potentiation of CNS effects of these drugs
Hormonal contraceptives: prolonged effect
Drug-herb. *Chamomile, kava, skullcap, valerian:* increased CNS depression

Drug-behaviors. *Alcohol use:* potentiation of midazolam effects

Toxicity and overdose

- Overdose signs and symptoms include sedation, somnolence, confusion, incoordination, and hypotension.
- Discontinue drug, monitor vital signs closely, and provide supportive therapy, including I.V. fluids and vasopressors for hypotension.

Patient teaching

- Inform patient that drug causes perioperative amnesia.
- Advise female patient to tell prescriber if she is pregnant or breastfeeding.
- As appropriate, review all other significant and life-threatening adverse reactions and interactions, especially those related to the drugs, herbs, and behaviors mentioned above.

milrinone lactate

Pharmacologic class: Bipyridine phosphodiesterase inhibitor
Therapeutic class: Inotropic
Pregnancy risk category C

Action

Increases cellular levels of cyclic adenosine monophosphate, causing inotropic action that relaxes vascular smooth muscle and increases myocardial contractility

Pharmacokinetics

Drug is partially metabolized, approximately 70% protein-bound, and excreted primarily in urine unchanged.

Onset	Peak	Duration
5-15 min	Unknown	Unknown

How supplied

Solution for injection (colorless to pale yellow): 1 mg/mL in 10-, 20-, and 50-mL single-dose vials
Solution for injection (premixed, colorless to pale yellow): 200 mcg/mL in 100-mL and 200-mL D_5W in plastic containers

Indications and dosages

➢ Acute decompensated heart failure
Adults: Initially, 50 mcg/kg I.V. bolus given slowly over 10 minutes, followed by continuous I.V. infusion of 0.375 to 0.75 mcg/kg/minute. Do not exceed total daily dosage of 1.13 mg/kg.

Dosage adjustment

- Reduce infusion rate in renal impairment.

Administration

Dilution and compatibility

- Know that loading dose may be given undiluted or diluted to a total volume of 10 or 20 mL.
- Dilute 1-mg/mL vial with half-normal saline solution, normal saline solution, or D_5W per manufacturer's instructions.
- Know that flexible containers provide ready-to-use solutions. Do not dilute or add supplementary medication.
- Do not use solution if discolored.

Infusion considerations

Do not administer through same I.V. line as furosemide or torsemide, as precipitate will form.
- Administer I.V. bolus loading dose slowly over 10 minutes.

• Use the following table below to determine infusion rate for maintenance dosage:

Infusion rate (mL/hr) using 200-mcg/mL concentration						
Maintenance dosage in mcg/kg/min	Patient weight (kg)					
	50	60	70	80	90	100
0.375	5.6	6.8	7.9	9	10.1	11.3
0.400	6	7.2	8.4	9.6	10.8	12
0.500	7.5	9	10.5	12	13.5	15
0.600	9	10.8	12.6	14.4	16.2	18
0.700	10.5	12.6	14.7	16.8	18.9	21
0.750	11.3	13.5	15.8	18	20.3	22.5

• In patients with renal impairment, reduce infusion rate based on creatinine clearance, as shown below:

Creatinine clearance (mL/min/1.73 m^2)	Infusion rate (mcg/kg/min)
50	0.43
40	0.38
30	0.33
20	0.28
10	0.23
5	0.20

Do not use plastic containers in series connections. Such use could result in air embolism due to residual air being drawn from primary container before administration of fluid from secondary container ends.

Monitoring

Monitor vital signs and ECG. Watch closely for ventricular arrhythmias and sustained tachycardia.

Stop drug and contact prescriber immediately if patient's systolic pressure drops 30 mm Hg or more.

• Assess cardiovascular status closely. Stay alert for complaints of chest pain.

• Monitor patient for headache. Provide analgesics as needed.

Storage

• Store at controlled room temperature of 15° to 30°C (59° to 86°F).

Contraindications and precautions

Contraindicated in hypersensitivity to drug.

Use cautiously in atrial flutter or fibrillation, supraventricular or ventricular arrhythmias, renal impairment, electrolyte abnormalities, decreased blood pressure, severe aortic or pulmonic valvular disease, acute phase of myocardial infarction (use not recommended), abnormal blood digoxin level, ***elderly patients,*** pregnant or breastfeeding patients, and ***children*** (safety and efficacy not established).

M

Adverse reactions

CNS: headache

CV: hypotension, chest pain, angina, **ventricular or supraventricular arrhythmias, ventricular ectopic activity, ventricular tachycardia or fibrillation**

Interactions

None significant

Toxicity and overdose

• In overdose, expect hypotension.

• No specific antidote exists. Temporarily discontinue drug or reduce dosage and provide supportive therapy, including I.V. fluids as ordered and appropriate.

Patient teaching

• Instruct patient to change position slowly, to avoid light-headedness or dizziness from hypotension.

• As appropriate, review all other significant and life-threatening adverse reactions.

mitomycin

Mutamycin

Pharmacologic class: Antitumor antibiotic
Therapeutic class: Antineoplastic
Pregnancy risk category NR

FDA BOXED WARNING

- Give under supervision of physician experienced in cancer chemotherapy, in facility with adequate diagnostic and treatment resources.
- Most common and severe toxic effect is bone marrow suppression.
- Some patients receiving drug systemically have experienced hemolytic uremic syndrome, a serious complication consisting primarily of microangiopathic hemolytic anemia, thrombocytopenia, and irreversible renal failure. Syndrome may arise at any time during systemic therapy, but most cases occur at doses of 60 mg or higher. Blood-product transfusion may exacerbate symptoms.

Action

Selectively inhibits DNA synthesis by causing cross-linking of DNA strands and suppressing RNA and protein synthesis, resulting in cell death

Pharmacokinetics

Drug clears rapidly from serum; clearance is affected primarily by hepatic metabolism to inactive form. Metabolism occurs in the spleen and kidneys. Drug and inactive metabolites are excreted in urine. Elimination half-life is about 1 hour.

Onset	Peak	Duration
Unknown	Unknown	Unknown

How supplied

Powder for reconstitution for injection: 5-mg, 20-mg, and 40-mg vials with mannitol

Indications and dosages

➤ Disseminated adenocarcinoma of stomach or pancreas (given with other chemotherapeutic agents); palliative treatment when other therapies fail
Adults: After full hematologic recovery from previous chemotherapy, 20 mg/m^2 I.V. as a single dose. Repeat cycle q 6 to 8 weeks, adjusting dosage if necessary.

Dosage adjustment

- Do not give drug to patients with renal impairment.
- Give 50% of previous dosage to patients with white blood cell (WBC) count below 2,000/mm^3 and platelet count below 25,000/mm^3.
- Give 70% of previous dosage to patients with WBC count between 2,000 and 2,999/mm^3 and platelet count between 25,000 and 74,999/mm^3.
- Give 100% of previous dosage to patients with WBC count of 3,000/mm^3 or higher and platelet count of 75,000/mm^3 or higher.
- Do not repeat dose until WBC count has risen to 4,000/mm^3 and platelet count to 100,000/mm^3.
- Expect to adjust dosage in patients receiving other myelosuppressants. If disease continues after two courses, stop drug, because chance of clinical response is minimal.

Off-label uses

- Bladder cancer
- Squamous-cell cancer of anus (combination therapy)

Administration

Preparation

🔈 Follow hazardous drug guidelines on page S19 for handling, preparation, and administration.

- Assess CBC with white cell differential and platelet count before starting therapy.

Dilution and compatibility

- For I.V. injection, reconstitute 5-, 20-, and 40-mg vials with 10, 40, or 80 mL sterile water for injection, respectively. Shake; let mixture stand until it dissolves completely.
- For I.V. infusion, further dilute with D_5W, normal saline solution, or sodium lactate solution.

Infusion considerations

- Administer direct I.V. injection through Y-tube or three-way stopcock over 5 to 10 minutes in I.V. line with running infusion of normal saline solution or D_5W solution.
- Administer I.V. infusion at prescribed rate depending on amount and type of solution.

🔈 Avoid extravasation; necrosis and tissue sloughing may occur with or without stinging or burning, even if blood return on aspiration is adequate.

Monitoring

🔈 Closely monitor CBC with white cell differential and platelet count. Stay alert for evidence of blood dyscrasias.

🔈 Watch for signs and symptoms of hemolytic uremic syndrome (irritability, fatigue, pallor, and decreased urine output).

🔈 Closely monitor I.V. site and skin integrity throughout infusion.

🔈 Assess respiratory status carefully to detect severe pulmonary problems.

- Assess kidney function tests. Measure fluid intake and output and evaluate fluid balance.

Storage

- Before reconstitution, store at room temperature. Avoid exposure to temperatures above 40°C (104°F).
- Know that when reconstituted with sterile water for injection to a concentration of 0.5 mg/mL, drug is stable for 7 days at room temperature or for 14 days when refrigerated.
- Know that when further diluted with D_5W, drug is stable for 3 hours; with normal saline solution, for 12 hours; and with sodium lactate, for 24 hours.

Contraindications and precautions

Contraindicated in hypersensitivity to drug, thrombocytopenia, coagulation disorders, and increased bleeding tendency.

Use cautiously in active infections, decreased bone marrow reserve, impaired hepatic function, history of pulmonary disorders, ***elderly patients,*** and pregnant or breastfeeding patients.

Adverse reactions

CNS: headache, confusion, drowsiness, syncope, fatigue

CV: congestive heart failure

EENT: blurred vision

GI: nausea, vomiting, diarrhea, stomatitis, mouth ulcers, anorexia

GU: renal failure, hemolytic uremic syndrome

Hematologic: anemia, hematemesis, **leukopenia, thrombocytopenia**

Respiratory: pulmonary toxicity, interstitial pneumonitis, respiratory distress syndrome

Skin: rash; reversible alopecia; pruritus; desquamation; phlebitis, necrosis, and sloughing with I.V. site extravasation; cellulitis at injection site

Other: fever, pain, edema

Interactions

Drug-drug. *Live-virus vaccines:* decreased antibody response to vaccine, increased risk of adverse reactions

Other antineoplastics: additive bone marrow depression

Vinca alkaloids: respiratory toxicity

M

Toxicity and overdose

- Overdose signs and symptoms include nausea, vomiting, and myelosuppression.
- No specific antidote exists. Provide supportive therapy, including antiemetics, anti-infectives, and blood components, as indicated and ordered.

Patient teaching

- Teach patient to recognize and immediately report signs and symptoms of hemolytic uremic syndrome, blood dyscrasias, and renal failure.
- Instruct patient to report cough or shortness of breath, even if it occurs several months after therapy ends.
- Advise patient to limit exposure to infections and to avoid live vaccines.
- Tell patient drug may cause hair loss, and discuss options for dealing with this problem.
- Advise female patient to inform prescriber if she is pregnant or breastfeeding.
- As appropriate, review all other significant and life-threatening adverse reactions and interactions, especially those related to the drugs mentioned above.

mitoxantrone hydrochloride

Mitoxana, Novantrone

Pharmacologic class: Anthracenedione
Therapeutic class: Antineoplastic, immune modifier
Pregnancy risk category D

FDA BOXED WARNING

- Give drug under supervision of physician experienced in use of cytotoxic chemotherapy agents.
- Administer slowly into free-flowing I.V. infusion. Never give I.M., subcutaneously, intra-arterially, or intrathecally; severe local tissue damage may occur with extravasation.
- Except in acute nonlymphocytic leukemia, drug generally should not be given to patients with baseline neutrophil count below 1,500/mm^3. Obtain frequent peripheral blood cell counts on all patients to monitor for bone marrow depression.
- Myocardial toxicity, whose severe form manifests as potentially fatal congestive heart failure (CHF), may occur during therapy or months to years afterward. Risk increases with cumulative dosage. In cancer patients, risk of symptomatic CHF is about 2.6% for those receiving cumulative dosages up to 140 mg/m^2. Monitor patients for evidence of cardiotoxicity and ask about CHF symptoms before starting therapy. In multiple sclerosis (MS) patients who reach cumulative dosage of 100 mg/m^2, monitor for evidence of cardiotoxicity before each subsequent dose; they should not receive cumulative dosage above 140 mg/m^2.
- Active or dormant cardiovascular disease, previous or concomitant radiation to mediastinal or pericardial area, previous anthracycline or anthracenedione therapy, and concurrent use of other cardiotoxic drugs may increase cardiotoxicity risk.
- Carefully assess all patients for cardiac signs and symptoms by history and physical examination before starting therapy. Baseline evaluation of left ventricular ejection fraction (LVEF) by echocardiography or multiple-gated radionuclide angiography should be done. MS patients with baseline LVEF below 50% should not receive drug; LVEF should be reevaluated before each dose for MS patients. Do not give additional doses to MS patients who experience LVEF decrease to below 50% or a clinically significant LVEF reduction during therapy. MS patients should not receive cumulative dosages above

140 mg/m². In cancer patients, estimated risk of symptomatic CHF is 2.6% for those receiving cumulative dosages of up to 140 mg/m². Current or previous cardiovascular disease, previous or concomitant radiotherapy to mediastinal or pericardial area, previous therapy with other anthracyclines or anthracenediones, or concomitant use of other cardiotoxic drugs may increase risk of cardiac toxicity. However, such toxicity may occur even with no cardiac risk factors present.
• Secondary acute myelogenous leukemia has occurred in MS and cancer patients. In cohort of mitoxantrone-treated MS patients followed for varying periods, elevated leukemia risk was 0.25%.

Action
Selectively inhibits DNA synthesis by causing cross-linking of DNA strands and suppressing RNA and protein synthesis, resulting in cell death

Pharmacokinetics
Drug distributes extensively in body tissues, but bioavailability is poor. It is metabolized in the liver, 78% protein-bound, and excreted in urine and feces as unchanged drug and metabolites.

Onset	Peak	Duration
Unknown	Unknown	Unknown

How supplied
Solution for injection, concentrate (dark blue, aqueous): 2 mg/mL in 10-, 12.5-, and 15-mL multidose vials

Indications and dosages
➢ Initial treatment of acute nonlymphocytic leukemia (given with other agents)
Adults: For induction—12 mg/m²/day I.V. on days 1 to 3, with 100 mg/m² of cytosine arabinoside given for 7 days as a continuous I.V. infusion (over 24 hours) on days 1 through 7. If remission does not occur, second course may follow, with mitoxantrone given for 2 days and cytosine arabinoside for 5 days at the same daily dosages. For consolidation therapy—12 mg/m²/day mitoxantrone I.V. on days 1 and 2 and 100 mg/m² cytosine arabinoside I.V. as a continuous infusion over 24 hours on days 1 through 5, given 6 weeks after induction therapy.
➢ Pain in patients with advanced hormone-refractory prostatic cancer (given with corticosteroids)
Adults: 12 to 14 mg/m² as a short I.V. infusion over 15 to 30 minutes q 21 days
➢ Multiple sclerosis
Adults: 12 mg/m² I.V. over 5 to 15 minutes q 3 months. Maximum cumulative lifetime dosage is 140 mg/m².

Off-label uses
• Breast cancer
• Chronic myelocytic leukemia in blast phase
• Non-Hodgkin's lymphoma

Administration
Preparation
Follow hazardous drug guidelines on page S19 for handling, preparation, and administration.
• Assess CBC, including platelet count, before each course and if signs or symptoms of infection develop. Monitor liver function tests before each course.
• Be aware that drug is not indicated for primary progressive multiple sclerosis.
Dilution and compatibility
Be aware that drug is a concentrate that must be diluted before injection.
• Dilute with 50 mL or more normal saline solution or D_5W. If desired, dilute further in normal saline solution, D_5W, or dextrose 5% in normal saline solution, and use immediately.
• Do not mix in same infusion with other drugs.

M

• Discard unused infusion solution promptly and appropriately.

Infusion considerations

• Infuse a single diluted dose I.V. slowly over at least 3 minutes or by intermittent infusion over 15 to 30 minutes.

• Infuse a single dose by continuous I.V. infusion over 24 hours.

If extravasation occurs, stop infusion immediately.

Monitoring

Monitor CBC with white cell differential. Watch for evidence of blood dyscrasias.

• Assess vital signs, ECG, and respiratory and cardiovascular status.

• Monitor kidney and liver function tests. Measure fluid intake and output and evaluate fluid balance.

• Monitor temperature. Stay alert for fever and signs and symptoms of urinary tract and other infections.

Storage

• Store at 15° to 25°C (59° to 77°F). Do not freeze.

Contraindications and precautions

Contraindicated in hypersensitivity to drug.

Use cautiously in bone marrow depression, CHF, chronic debilitating illness, hepatobiliary dysfunction, ***elderly patients,*** pregnant or breastfeeding patients, and ***children.***

Adverse reactions

CNS: headache, asthenia, fatigue, **seizures**
CV: heart failure, arrhythmias, cardiotoxicity
EENT: conjunctivitis, mucositis
GI: nausea, vomiting, diarrhea, constipation, abdominal pain, stomatitis, anorexia
GU: menstrual disorder, amenorrhea, menorrhagia, urinary tract infection, bluish green urine, **renal failure**
Hematologic: anemia, **bone marrow depression, leukopenia, thrombocytopenia, bleeding**
Hepatic: jaundice, **hepatotoxicity**
Metabolic: hyperuricemia
Musculoskeletal: back pain
Respiratory: cough, dyspnea, upper respiratory tract infection
Skin: rash, petechiae, bruising, alopecia, cutaneous mycosis
Other: fever, infection, hypersensitivity reaction

Interactions

Drug-drug. *Anthracycline antineoplastics (daunorubicin, doxorubicin, idarubicin):* increased risk of cardiomyopathy
Live-virus vaccines: decreased antibody response to vaccine
Other antineoplastics: additive bone marrow depression
Drug-diagnostic tests. *Alanine aminotransferase, aspartate aminotransferase, bilirubin, uric acid:* increased

Toxicity and overdose

• In overdose, expect extension of adverse reactions, including infection, severe leukopenia, and death.

• No specific antidote exists. Be prepared to provide hematologic support and anti-infectives during prolonged periods of severe myelosuppression. Dialysis is unlikely to aid drug removal.

Patient teaching

Advise patient to immediately report chest pain, seizure, easy bruising or bleeding, change in urination pattern, yellowing of skin or eyes, or difficulty breathing.

• Instruct patient to limit exposure to people with infections and to avoid live vaccines.

• Tell patient drug may turn urine bluish green.

• Advise patient to minimize GI upset by eating small, frequent servings of food and drinking plenty of fluids.

• Tell female patient to inform prescriber if she is pregnant or breastfeeding.
• As appropriate, review all other significant and life-threatening adverse reactions and interactions, especially those related to the drugs and tests mentioned above.

morphine sulfate

Astramorph PF, Duramorph

Pharmacologic class: Opioid agonist
Therapeutic class: Opioid analgesic
Controlled substance schedule II
Pregnancy risk category C

FDA BOXED WARNING

• Avinza (morphine sulfate) capsules are modified-release form indicated for once-daily P.O. administration to relieve moderate to severe pain requiring continuous, around-the-clock opioids for extended time. Instruct patients to swallow capsules whole or sprinkle contents on applesauce. Warn them never to chew, crush, or dissolve capsules or consume alcoholic beverages or use prescription or nonprescription drugs containing alcohol during therapy, as this may lead to rapid release and absorption of potentially fatal dose.
• Intrathecal dosage of morphine sulfate injection is usually one-tenth of epidural dosage.

Action

Interacts with opioid receptor sites, primarily in limbic system, thalamus, and spinal cord. This interaction modifies neurotransmitter release, ultimately altering perception of and tolerance for pain.

Pharmacokinetics

Drug crosses placental barrier and is metabolized in the liver; approximately 20% to 35% is protein-bound. It is excreted in urine and bile and secreted in breast milk.

Onset	Peak	Duration
Rapid	20 min	Unknown

How supplied

Solution for injection (clear): 1 mg/mL in 10-mL and 30-mL prefilled syringes and 10-mL vials
Solution for injection (clear): 2 mg/mL in 1-mL syringes
Solution for injection (clear): 4 mg/mL in 1-mL vials
Solution for injection (clear): 5 mg/mL in 1-mL ampules and vials and in 30-mL vials
Solution for injection (clear): 8 mg/mL in 1-mL syringes and vials
Solution for injection (clear): 10 mg/mL in 1-mL ampules, syringes, and vials and in 10-mL vials
Solution for injection (clear): 15 mg/mL in 1-mL ampules and vials and in 20-mL ampules
Solution for injection (for patient-controlled analgesia device, clear): 0.5 mg/mL, 1 mg/mL, 2 mg/mL, 3 mg/mL, 5 mg/mL
Solution for injection (preservative-free, clear): 0.5 mg/mL in 10-mL ampules and vials
*Solution for injection (preservative-free, clear):*1- and 2-mg/mL in prefilled syringes
Solution for injection (preservative-free, clear): 25 mg/mL in 4-mL, 10-mL, and 20-mL vials; 25 mg/mL in 4-mL, 10-mL, and 20-mL syringes
Solution for injection (preservative-free, clear): 50 mg/mL in 20-mL, 40-mL, and 50-mL vials

M

Indications and dosages

➤ Severe to moderate pain

Adults: 2 to 10 mg/70 kg I.V. p.r.n. given slowly over 4 to 5 minutes. As a continuous I.V. infusion, 0.1 to 1 mg/mL in D_5W delivered by controlled-infusion device. With patient-controlled anesthesia (PCA) device, 1-mg bolus with a range of 0.2 to 3 mg/incremental dose for 0.5 mg/mL and 1 mg/mL concentration and a range of 0.5 to 3 mg/incremental dose for 5 mg/mL concentration. Recommended lockout period for incremental doses is 6 minutes.

Dosage adjustment

- Adjust dosage based on pain severity, response, metabolism, and clinical condition. Maintain lowest dosage level that produces acceptable analgesia.
- Adjust dosage for adults weighing less than 50 kg (110 lb), elderly patients, and children.

Administration

Preparation

- For best response, administer at pain onset.
- To counteract opioid-induced respiratory depression, keep opioid antagonist (such as naloxone) readily available.

Dilution and compatibility

- For direct I.V. administration, give undiluted or dilute with at least 5 mL sterile water for injection or normal saline solution for injection.
- When giving by I.V. infusion, dilute each 0.1 to 1 mg in 1 mL normal saline solution or D_5W for use in PCA device, or dilute in larger amounts for selected situations.
- Do not use if solution is darker than pale yellow, is cloudy, or contains visible particulates.

Infusion considerations

- When giving by direct I.V., administer 2.5 to 10 mg over 4 to 5 minutes.
- For continuous I.V. infusion, use infusion pump or PCA pump. Titrate dosage to provide adequate pain relief.

Monitoring

Monitor vital signs. Contact prescriber if respiratory rate is 10 breaths/minutes or less.

- Assess pain character, location, and intensity; adjust dosage accordingly.
- Monitor fluid intake and output. Stay alert for urine retention.
- Monitor bowel elimination pattern. If constipation occurs, intervene as appropriate.
- Assess neurologic status. Implement safety measures as needed to prevent injury.
- Evaluate patient for signs and symptoms of physical or psychological dependence.

Storage

- Store at 20° to 25°C (68° to 77°F); protect from light and freezing. Keep in carton until use.

Contraindications and precautions

Contraindicated in hypersensitivity to morphine or other opioids, acute bronchial asthma, upper airway obstruction, and medical conditions that preclude I.V. opioid administration.

Use cautiously in head trauma; increased intracranial pressure; severe renal, hepatic, or pulmonary disease; hypothyroidism; adrenal insufficiency; prostatic hypertrophy; ***elderly or debilitated patients;*** pregnant or breastfeeding patients; and ***children.***

Adverse reactions

CNS: confusion, sedation, dizziness, dysphoria, euphoria, floating feeling,

hallucinations, headache, nightmares, anxiety, **seizures**
CV: hypotension, bradycardia
EENT: blurred vision, diplopia, miosis
GI: nausea, vomiting, constipation, dry mouth
GU: urine retention, decreased libido, menstrual irregularities, oliguria
Respiratory: apnea, respiratory depression, respiratory arrest
Skin: flushing, itching, sweating
Other: physical or psychological drug dependence, drug tolerance, interference with thermal regulation

Interactions

Drug-drug. *Antihistamines, barbiturates, clomipramine, sedative-hypnotics, tricyclic antidepressants:* additive CNS depression
Mixed opioid agonist-antagonists: withdrawal symptoms in physically dependent patients
Monoamine oxidase inhibitors: severe, unpredictable reactions
Nalbuphine, nalmefene, pentazocine: decreased analgesia
Drug-herb. *Chamomile, hops, kava, skullcap, valerian:* increased CNS depression
Drug-behaviors. *Alcohol use:* increased CNS depression

Toxicity and overdose

- In acute overdose, signs and symptoms include cold and clammy skin, respiratory depression, somnolence progressing to stupor or coma, skeletal muscle flaccidity, constricted pupils, and in some cases pulmonary edema, bradycardia, hypotension, and death.
- Establish secure airway and support ventilation and perfusion. Monitor heart filling pressures; be aware that noncardiac pulmonary edema may occur. Give opioid antagonist (such as naloxone), as ordered, to antagonize opioid effects; however, avoid antagonist in physically dependent patient if possible. If naloxone must be used to treat serious respiratory depression, administer with extreme care and titrate with smaller-than-usual dosages. Do not give antagonist in absence of clinically significant respiratory or cardiovascular depression. As indicated and ordered, give I.V. fluids and vasopressors for hypotension and atropine for bradycardia. Dialysis does not remove drug.

Patient teaching

- [Clinical alert] Tell patient and caregiver that drug may cause respiratory depression. Instruct them to immediately report respiratory rate of 10 breaths/minute or less.
- Advise patient using PCA pump to take drug at first sign of pain.
- Inform patient that drug may cause constipation or urine retention. Encourage high-fiber diet and high fluid intake.
- Advise female patient to tell prescriber if she is pregnant or breastfeeding.
- Caution patient to avoid driving and other hazardous activities until drug's effects on concentration, vision, and alertness are known.
- Teach patient and caregiver about appropriate home safety measures to prevent injury.
- Caution patient to avoid alcohol and other CNS depressants during and for 24 hours after therapy.
- Advise patient to avoid herbs, which may worsen adverse CNS effects.
- As appropriate, review all other significant and life-threatening adverse reactions and interactions, especially those related to the drugs, herbs, and behaviors mentioned above.

[redacted]

moxifloxacin hydrochloride

Avelox

Pharmacologic class: Fluoroquinolone
Therapeutic class: Anti-infective
Pregnancy risk category C

Action

Selectively inhibits DNA synthesis by disrupting DNA replication and transcription and suppressing protein synthesis, causing bacterial cell death

Pharmacokinetics

Drug distributes widely throughout body and is partially metabolized in the liver. Half-life is 5 to 17 hours. It is excreted as unchanged drug and metabolites in feces and urine, and secreted in breast milk.

Onset	Peak	Duration
Unknown	Unknown	24 hr

How supplied

Solution for injection (premixed): 400 mg/250 mL in single-use flexible bags

Indications and dosages

➢ Acute bacterial sinusitis caused by *Haemophilus influenzae, Moraxella catarrhalis,* or *Staphylococcus pneumoniae*
Adults: 400 mg I.V. q 24 hours for 10 days
➢ Acute bacterial exacerbation of chronic bronchitis
Adults: 400 mg I.V. q 24 hours for 5 days
➢ Community-acquired pneumonia
Adults: 400 mg I.V. q 24 hours for 7 to 14 days
➢ Uncomplicated skin and skin-structure infections
Adults: 400 mg I.V. q 24 hours for 7 days
➢ Complicated skin or skin-structure infections
Adults: 400 mg I.V. q 24 hours for 7 to 21 days
➢ Complicated intra-abdominal infections
Adults: 400 mg I.V. q 24 hours for 5 to 14 days

Administration

Dilution and compatibility

- Be aware that drug is available as ready-to-use solution and requires no dilution.
- Do not add additives or other solutions to premixed drug.

Infusion considerations

- Give premixed dose by I.V. infusion only over 60 minutes. Avoid bolus or rapid infusion.
- Do not mix with other drugs in same I.V. line.
- When using same I.V. line to administer other drugs, flush line before and after morphine infusion with compatible I.V. solution, such as normal saline solution, dextrose 5% in water, 10% dextrose in water, lactated Ringer's solution, or sterile water for injection.

Do not use plastic containers in series connections. Such use could result in air embolism due to residual air being drawn from primary container before administration of fluid from secondary container ends.

- Discard unused portion.

Monitoring

Watch for hypersensitivity reactions (such as anaphylaxis) and other allergic reactions after initial dose.

Assess GI status closely. Report signs or symptoms of pseudomembranous colitis.

- Monitor cardiovascular and neurologic status closely.
- Stay alert for tendinitis and Achilles tendon rupture.

- Monitor CNC and liver function tests.
- Watch closely for superinfection.

Storage

- Store at 25°C (77°F); excursions permitted to 15° to 30°C (59° to 86°F). Do not refrigerate.

Contraindications and precautions

Contraindicated in hypersensitivity to drug, its components, or other fluoroquinolones.

Use cautiously in underlying CNS diseases or disorders, renal impairment, cirrhosis, bradycardia, acute myocardial ischemia, prolonged QTc interval, uncorrected hypokalemia, dialysis, ***elderly patients,*** pregnant or breastfeeding patients (safety not established except in postexposure inhalation anthrax), and ***children younger than age 18*** (except in postexposure inhalation anthrax).

Adverse reactions

CNS: dizziness, drowsiness, headache, asthenia, confusion, light-headedness, insomnia, somnolence, anxiety, nervousness, vertigo, agitation, hallucinations, acute psychoses, tremor, **seizures**
CV: hypertension, vasodilation, tachycardia, palpitation, **prolonged QT interval, arrhythmias**
EENT: oral candidiasis, stomatitis, glossitis
GI: nausea, vomiting, diarrhea, constipation, abdominal pain, dyspepsia, flatulence, anorexia, dry mouth, **pseudomembranous colitis**
GU: vaginitis
Hematologic: eosinophilia, prothrombin decrease, **thrombocytopenia, leukopenia**
Musculoskeletal: joint pain, tendinitis, tendon rupture, myalgia
Skin: rash, pruritus, sweating, urticaria, photosensitivity, phototoxicity, **Stevens-Johnson syndrome**
Other: altered taste, pain, phlebitis at I.V. site, superinfection, malaise, hypersensitivity reactions including **anaphylaxis**

Interactions

Drug-drug. *Amiodarone, bepridil, disopyramide, erythromycin, pentamidine, phenothiazines, pimozide, procainamide, quinidine, sotalol, tricyclic antidepressants:* increased risk of serious adverse cardiovascular reactions
Antacids containing aluminum and/or magnesium, products containing iron: decreased moxifloxacin level
Drug-diagnostic tests. *Alanine aminotransferase, alkaline phosphatase, aspartate aminotransferase, bilirubin, lactate dehydrogenase, platelets:* increased
Drug-herb. *Dong quai, St. John's wort:* phototoxicity
Drug-behaviors. *Sun exposure:* phototoxicity

Toxicity and overdose

- Overdose may cause prolonged QT interval and other adverse reactions.
- No specific antidote exists. Monitor ECG closely and provide symptomatic and supportive therapy, including adequate hydration. Drug may not be dialyzable.

Patient teaching

Tell patient drug may cause serious allergic reactions even several days after therapy begins. Advise patient to report these immediately.

Urge patient to promptly report tendon pain, diarrhea with blood or pus, and signs or symptoms of superinfection.

- Caution patient to avoid driving and other hazardous activities until drug's effects on concentration and alertness are known.
- As appropriate, review all other significant and life-threatening adverse

reactions and interactions, especially those related to the drugs, tests, herbs, and behaviors mentioned above.

multivitamin infusion

Infuvite Adult, Infuvite Pediatric, M.V.I Adult, M.V.I. Pediatric

Pharmacologic class: Vitamin, parenteral multivitamin
Therapeutic class: Nutritional supplement
Pregnancy risk category C

Action

Provides a combination of important water-soluble and fat-soluble vitamins in system specially formulated for incorporation into I.V. infusions to contribute intake of vitamins needed to maintain normal resistance and repair processes

Pharmacokinetics

Fat-soluble vitamins (A, D, and E) may accumulate in body tissues. Water-soluble vitamins (B and C) are readily excreted in urine.

Onset	Peak	Duration
No information available		

How supplied

Solution for injection (Infuvite): 5-mL single-dose vial (adult); 1-mL and 4-mL single-dose vial (pediatric)
Solution for injection (M.V.I. Pediatric): 5 mL

Indications and dosages

➤ Treatment and prevention of vitamin deficiency
Adults and children: Preparations are not standardized and may vary substantially. See product prescribing information for components, indications, and dosages.

Administration

Preparation

Be aware that some products contain aluminum, which may be toxic, particularly in premature infants and patients with renal impairment.
- Know that low-birth-weight infants may need supplemental vitamin A.
- Do not exceed recommended daily dosage in infants.

Dilution and compatibility

Do not give undiluted.
- Know that certain multivitamin preparations are available in dual-vial and/or two-chambered vials. Use caution to ensure patient receives intended dose with these formulations.
- For adults, dilute daily dose in no less than 500 mL (preferably 1,000 mL) normal saline solution, D_5W, or similar compatible solution. Consult product prescribing information for dilution details.
- For children, dilute daily dose in no less than 100 mL normal saline solution, D_5W, or similar compatible infusion solution. Consult product prescribing information for dilution details.
- Use reconstituted or diluted drug immediately, or consult prescribing information to determine whether solution may be stored after dilution.
- Know that drug is physically incompatible with alkaline solutions or moderately alkaline drugs (such as acetazolamide, aminophylline, chlorothiazide, and sodium bicarbonate).
- Be aware that drug may not be compatible with tetracycline or ampicillin.
- Know that folic acid may be unstable in presence of calcium salts.

Do not add multivitamins directly to fat emulsions.

Infusion considerations

Do not give by direct I.V. injection, as dizziness, faintness, and vein irritation may occur.

- Administer by I.V. infusion at prescribed rate.

Monitoring

Monitor for signs and symptoms of allergic reaction, including anaphylaxis; be prepared to intervene appropriately.

- With long-term use (4 to 6 months), monitor blood levels of vitamins A, C, D, and folic acid; levels may decline if parenteral multivitamins remain sole source of these vitamins.
- When administering for more than a few weeks, monitor vitamin A and D levels occasionally to check for excess accumulation of these fat-soluble vitamins (especially in patients with renal impairment).
- Monitor prothrombin time and International Normalized Ratio in patients receiving warfarin.

Storage

- Refrigerate between 2° and 8°C (36° and 46°F). Protect from light and heat. Do not freeze.

Contraindications and precautions

Contraindicated in hypersensitivity to any vitamin in product, preexisting hypervitaminosis, and before blood tests to detect megaloblastic anemia.

Use cautiously in renal impairment, ***elderly patients,*** pregnant or breastfeeding patients, and ***children younger than age 11.***

Adverse reactions

CNS: dizziness, headache, agitation, anxiety

EENT: diplopia

Skin: rash, erythema, pruritus

Other: hypersensitivity reactions including urticaria, shortness of breath, periorbital and digital edema, angioedema, and **anaphylaxis** (rare)

Interactions

Drug-drug. *Anti-infectives (erythromycin, kanamycin, lincomycin, oxycycline, streptomycin):* decreased anti-infective action

Chloramphenicol: inhibited hematologic response to vitamin B_{12}

Hydralazine, isoniazid: reduced pyridoxine effect

Levodopa: reduced levodopa effect (caused by pyridoxine)

Methotrexate: decreased response to this drug (caused by folic acid)

Phenytoin: decreased phenytoin and folic acid serum levels, increased seizure risk

Warfarin: antagonism of hypothrombinemic response (caused by vitamin K)

Drug-diagnostic tests. *Alanine aminotransferase:* increased

Urine glucose: false-negative result

Toxicity and overdose

- Vitamins A, D, and E may accumulate to harmful levels. Vitamin A toxicity may cause alopecia, cracking at mouth corners, decreased appetite, and bulging fontanels in infants. Early signs and symptoms of vitamin D toxicity associated with hypercalcemia include weakness, headache, somnolence, nausea, vomiting, dry mouth, constipation, muscle and bone pain, and metallic taste; these may progress to more serious complications if vitamin D administration continues. Vitamin E may prolong prothrombin time by inhibiting vitamin K–dependent carboxylase; dosages of 1,600 international units/day also reduce platelet thromboxane production; may also impair hematologic response to iron in children with iron-deficiency anemia.
- In overdose, discontinue vitamins.

Patient teaching

- Explain to patient, parents, or home caregivers the reason for I.V. vitamin administration.

M

Instruct patient to immediately report rash, difficulty breathing, and other signs or symptoms of allergy.
- As appropriate, review all other significant and life-threatening adverse reactions and interactions, especially those related to the drugs and tests mentioned above.

muromonab-CD3

Orthoclone OKT3

Pharmacologic class: Murine monoclonal antibody
Therapeutic class: Immunosuppressant
Pregnancy risk category C

FDA BOXED WARNING

- Give under supervision of physician experienced in immunosuppressive therapy and management of solid-organ transplant patients, in facility equipped for cardiopulmonary resuscitation where patient can be monitored closely based on health status.
- Drug may cause anaphylactic and anaphylactoid reactions and occasionally life-threatening or lethal systemic, cardiovascular, or CNS reactions. Monitor patient's fluid status closely before and during therapy. Methylprednisolone pretreatment is recommended to minimize symptoms of cytokine release syndrome.

Action

Binds to and blocks function of T lymphocytes responsible for antigen recognition, thereby reversing graft rejection

Pharmacokinetics

A rapid decrease in the number of CD2, CD3, CD4, and CD8 positive T cells occurred within minutes after administration. Serum levels are measured with an enzyme-linked immunosorbent assay (ELISA). Mean serum levels rose over first 3 days and averaged 0.9 mcg/mL on days 3 to 14.

Onset	Peak	Duration
Immediate	Unknown	Unknown

How supplied

Solution for injection (clear, colorless): 1 mg/1 mL in 5-mL ampules

Indications and dosages

➢ Acute allograft rejection in kidney transplant patients; steroid-resistant acute allograft rejection in heart and liver transplant patients

Adults and children weighing more than 30 kg (66 lb): 5 mg/day as I.V. bolus for 10 to 14 days
Children weighing 30 kg or less: 2.5 mg/day as I.V. bolus for 10 to 14 days

Administration

Preparation

- In kidney transplant patients, start therapy as soon as acute renal rejection is diagnosed. In heart and liver transplant patients, start therapy when physician determines steroid therapy has not reversed allograft rejection.
- Give methylprednisolone 1 to 4 hours before first muromonab-CD3 dose, as prescribed.
- As prescribed, give antipyretics to decrease fever and corticosteroids to reduce allergic response.

Dilution and compatibility

- Give drug undiluted.
- For I.V. bolus injection, draw solution into syringe through low-protein-binding 0.2- or 0.22-micron filter. Do not shake.

Discard filter and attach needle-free adapter.
• Be aware that drug is a protein solution and may develop a few fine translucent particles, which do not affect potency.
• Use immediately after ampule has been opened. Discard unused portion.

Infusion considerations
• Administer by I.V. bolus over less than 1 minute.
• Do not mix with other drugs in same I.V. line.
• When administering other drugs through same line, flush line before and after muromonab infusion with normal saline solution.

Monitoring
• Evaluate vital signs and cardiovascular status. Monitor ECG closely.
Stay alert for signs and symptoms of cytokine release syndrome, including fever (temperature up to 41.6°C (107°F), chills, rigor, nausea, vomiting, abdominal pain, diarrhea, malaise, joint and muscle pain, headache, and tremors.
Be aware that most adverse reactions occur within 30 minutes to 6 hours of first dose.
Assess neurologic status and respiratory status closely. Evaluate for evidence of aseptic meningitis, encephalopathy, cerebral edema, pulmonary edema, and acute respiratory distress syndrome (ARDS).
• Monitor temperature closely. Stay alert for fever and other signs and symptoms of infection.

Storage
• Refrigerate at 2° to 8°C (36° to 46°F). Do not freeze.

Contraindications and precautions
Contraindicated in hypersensitivity to drug or other murine products, uncompensated heart failure, uncontrolled hypertension, predisposition to or history of seizures, anti-mouse antibody titer of 1:1,000 or higher, pregnancy, or breastfeeding.
Use cautiously in fever and ***children younger than age 2.***

Adverse reactions
CNS: fatigue, headache, lethargy, malaise weakness, tremors, hallucinations, **aseptic meningitis, cerebral edema, seizures, encephalopathy**
CV: chest pain, hypertension, hypotension, vasodilation, tachycardia, **heart failure, cardiac arrest, shock**
EENT: vision loss, blurred vision, conjunctivitis, photophobia, tinnitus, otitis media
GI: nausea, vomiting, diarrhea, abdominal pain, anorexia
GU: renal dysfunction, **oliguria, anuria**
Hematologic: leukopenia
Respiratory: dyspnea, wheezing, hyperventilation, respiratory congestion, abnormal chest sound, **severe pulmonary edema, ARDS**
Skin: flushing, sweating, pruritus, rash
Other: fever, chills, flulike symptoms, infection, pain, **anaphylaxis, cytokine release syndrome**

Interactions
Drug-drug. *Indomethacin:* increased muromonab blood level, encephalopathy and other adverse CNS effects
Live-virus vaccines: increased viral replication and effects
Other immunosuppressants: increased risk of infection
Drug-diagnostic tests. *Blood urea nitrogen, creatinine:* increased
Drug-herb. *Astragalus, echinacea, melatonin:* interference with immunosuppressant effect

Patient monitoring
• Overdose signs and symptoms include severe chills, hyperthermia, vomiting, diarrhea, myalgia, pulmonary edema,

M

hemolytic anemia, oliguria, and acute renal failure.
• Decrease dosage or discontinue drug and consider another immunosuppressant, if indicated and ordered. Carefully observe patient and provide symptomatic and supportive therapy.

Patient teaching

• Inform patient that drug can cause serious adverse reactions, but that he will be monitored closely and receive interventions to relieve these reactions. Teach patient which signs and symptoms to report immediately.
• Reassure patient that adverse reactions will subside as treatment progresses.
• Advise female patient to avoid becoming pregnant or breastfeeding during therapy.
• As appropriate, review all other significant and life-threatening adverse reactions and interactions, especially those related to the drugs, tests, and herbs mentioned above.

mycophenolate mofetil hydrochloride

CellCept Intravenous

Pharmacologic class: Mycophenolic acid derivative
Therapeutic class: Immunosuppressant
Pregnancy risk category D

FDA BOXED WARNING

• Give drug under supervision of physician experienced in immunosuppressive therapy and management of renal, cardiac, or hepatic transplant patients, in facility with adequate diagnostic and treatment resources. Physician responsible for maintenance therapy should have complete information needed for patient follow-up.
• Increased susceptibility to infection and possible lymphoma development may result from immunosuppression.
• Females with child-bearing potential must use contraception. Use of mycophenolate mofetil hydrochloride during pregnancy is associated with increased risk of pregnancy loss and congenital malformations.

Action

Drug's active metabolite, mycophenolic acid (MPA), inhibits guanosine nucleotide synthesis and has a cytostatic effect on T and B lymphocytes. MPA also suppresses antibody formation by B lymphocytes and may inhibit lymphocyte migration to inflammation and graft rejection sites.

Pharmacokinetics

Drug rapidly metabolizes to MPA. Mean apparent half-life is about 16.6 hours. Most of dose is excreted in urine unchanged, with a small amount excreted as metabolite.

Onset	Peak	Duration
Unknown	Unknown	Unknown

How supplied

Powder for reconstitution for injection (white to off-white, lyophilized): 500 mg/vial

Indications and dosages

➤ To prevent organ rejection in patients receiving allogeneic kidney or liver transplants
Adults: 1 g I.V. b.i.d. given over no less than 2 hours with corticosteroids and cyclosporine

Dosage adjustment

• In renal transplant patients with severe chronic renal impairment beyond immediate posttransplant period, avoid dosages above 1 g twice daily.
• If neutropenia (absolute neutrophil count below $1.3 \times 10^3/mm^3$) occurs, interrupt dosing or reduce dosage.

Administration

Preparation

Follow hazardous drug guidelines on page S19 for handling, preparation, and administration.
Be aware that drug is teratogenic. Avoid inhaling powder in capsules or letting powder contact skin, mucous membranes, or eyes. If contact occurs, wash skin thoroughly with soap and water or flush eyes with water.
• Know that safety and efficacy in children is not established except in renal transplant.

Dilution and compatibility

• Reconstitute with D_5W and dilute to 6 mg/mL.

Infusion considerations

Do not give by rapid I.V. push or bolus.
• Administer by I.V. infusion over no less than 2 hours

Monitoring

• Monitor CBC with white cell differential, electrolyte levels, lipid panel, blood chemistry, and liver function tests frequently.
• Evaluate vital signs. Assess cardiovascular and respiratory status carefully. Watch for signs and symptoms of bronchitis and pneumonia.
Assess all body systems carefully for signs and symptoms of infection.
Monitor patient closely for bleeding tendency.

Storage

• Store at 25°C (77°F); excursions permitted to 15° to 30°C (59° to 86°F).

Contraindications and precautions

Contraindicated in hypersensitivity to drug or its components, mycophenolic acid, or polysorbate 80.

Use cautiously in lymphoma, cancer, neutropenia, or GI disorders, ***elderly patients,*** pregnant or breastfeeding patients, and ***children.***

Adverse reactions

CNS: headache, dizziness, insomnia, asthenia, tremor, anxiety, paresthesia
CV: chest pain, hypertension, peripheral edema, tachycardia, cardiovascular disorder, hypotension
EENT: pharyngitis, oral candidiasis
GI: nausea, vomiting, diarrhea, constipation, abdominal pain, dyspepsia, **GI hemorrhage**
GU: urinary tract infection, hematuria, abnormal renal function, **renal tubular necrosis**
Hematologic: anemia, hypochromic anemia, **leukocytosis, leukopenia, thrombocytopenia**
Metabolic: hypophosphatemia, hyperglycemia, hypokalemia, hypercholesterolemia, **hyperkalemia**
Musculoskeletal: back pain
Respiratory: dyspnea, cough, bronchitis, pneumonia
Skin: acne, rash
Other: pain, fever, opportunistic infections, ascites, **fatal infections, lymphoma and other cancers** (especially of skin), **sepsis**

Interactions

Drug-drug. *Acyclovir, ganciclovir, other drugs that undergo renal tubular secretion:* increased risk of toxicity from either drug
Aluminum or magnesium-containing antacids, cholestyramine, norfloxacin and metronidazole (combined therapy), rifampin, sevelamer and other calcium-free

M

phosphate binders: decreased MPA concentration causing decreased effect
Cyclosporine: decreased mycophenolate level
Hormonal contraceptives: reduced contraceptive efficacy
Live-virus vaccines: vaccine inefficacy
Phenytoin, theophylline: increased blood levels of both drugs
Probenecid, salicylates: increased mycophenolate blood level
Drug-diagnostic tests. *Blood glucose, cholesterol:* increased
Potassium: increased or decreased
Phosphate: decreased
Drug-herb. *Astragalus, echinacea, melatonin:* interference with immunosuppressant effect

Toxicity and overdose

- In overdose, expect nausea, vomiting, diarrhea, and possibly hematologic abnormalities.
- Reduce dosage or discontinue drug if severe neutropenia occurs. Hemodialysis may remove small amount of drug.

Patient teaching

Instruct patient to promptly report fever and other signs or symptoms of infection.
Advise patient to immediately report unusual bleeding or bruising.
- Caution patient to avoid driving and other hazardous activities until drug's effects on concentration and alertness are known.
- Instruct patient to avoid crowds and people with known infections.
- Advise patient not to take herbs without consulting prescriber.
- Tell patient to avoid live-virus vaccines.

Teach patient to avoid excessive exposure to sunlight and ultraviolet light because of increased risk of skin cancer.
Tell female patient to use abstinence or two other contraceptive methods during therapy and for 6 weeks afterward (even if she has a history of infertility). Urge her to report suspected pregnancy immediately.
- Advise patient not to breastfeed during therapy.
- As appropriate, review all other significant and life-threatening adverse reactions and interactions, especially those related to the drugs, tests, and herbs mentioned above.

nafcillin sodium

Pharmacologic class: Penicillinase-resistant penicillin
Therapeutic class: Anti-infective
Pregnancy risk category B

Action

Inhibits cell-wall synthesis during microorganism multiplication; resists inactivation by staphylococcal penicillinase. Bactericidal.

Pharmacokinetics

Drug distributes extensively into most body tissues and fluids and crosses placental barrier; however, penetration into spinal fluid is poor. It is metabolized primarily in the liver, largely protein-bound, and excreted in bile, with a small amount excreted in urine. Drug is also secreted in breast milk.

Onset	Peak	Duration
Immediate	Unknown	Unknown

How supplied

I.V. infusion (piggyback): 1 g in 50-mL and 2-g in 100-mL premixed frozen solution in plastic containers

Indications and dosages

➤ Systemic infections caused by penicillinase-producing staphylococci
Adults: 500 mg I.V. q 4 hours; for more severe infections, 1 g I.V. q 4 hours. Duration depends on type and severity of infection.

Dosage adjustment

• In hepatic or renal impairment, measure drug blood levels and adjust dosage accordingly.

Administration

Preparation

Ask patient about penicillin allergy before giving.

Dilution and compatibility

• Know that drug is available as prediluted frozen solution.
• Thaw frozen container at room temperature of 25°C (77°F) or in refrigerator at temperature of 5°C (41°F).
Do not force-thaw by immersion in water bath or by microwave irradiation.
• Know that solution components may precipitate in frozen state and dissolve on reaching room temperature with little or no agitation; this does not affect potency. Agitate after solution reaches room temperature. If solution remains cloudy, insoluble precipitate appears, or seals or outlet ports are not intact, discard container.
• Know that thawed solution is stable for 21 days when refrigerated at 5°C (41°F) or for 72 hours at room temperature of 25°C (77°F).
Do not refreeze solution.
• Know that drug is inactivated if mixed with aminoglycosides. Do not mix with other drugs in same solution.
• Do not use if solution is cloudy or discolored.

Infusion considerations

• Administer slowly by I.V. over 30 to 60 minutes to minimize risk of vein irritation and extravasation.
Do not use plastic containers in series connections. Such use could result in air embolism due to residual air being drawn from primary container before administration of fluid from secondary container ends.

Monitoring

Assess for signs and symptoms of hypersensitivity reaction (including anaphylaxis, serum sickness, and angioedema), which may occur several days after therapy begins.
Monitor neurologic status. Stay alert for seizures, depression, and hallucinations.
• Evaluate CBC with white cell differential.
• In prolonged therapy, assess for superinfection.
• Be aware that therapy should continue until 48 hours after patient is afebrile and asymptomatic and has negative cultures.

Storage

• Store in freezer capable of maintaining temperature of –20°C (–4°F) or less.

Contraindications and precautions

Contraindicated in hypersensitivity to drug or other penicillins.

Use cautiously in cephalosporin hypersensitivity, renal disorders, GI distress, pregnant or breastfeeding patients, and ***children*** (safety and efficacy not established).

Adverse reactions

CNS: neurotoxic reactions
CV: thrombophlebitis
GI: pseudomembranous colitis
Hematologic: bone marrow depression, agranulocytosis

N

Skin: angioedema
Other: superinfection, vein irritation, injection site reaction, hypersensitivity reactions including **serum sickness** and **anaphylaxis**

Interactions

Drug-drug. *Cyclosporine:* subtherapeutic cyclosporine blood level
Probenecid: increased nafcillin blood level
Drug-diagnostic tests. *Granulocytes, neutrophils, platelets:* decreased

Toxicity and overdose

- Overdose signs and symptoms include neuromuscular irritability, such as twitching and seizures, and extension of other adverse reactions.
- Provide symptomatic and supportive therapy. Dialysis has little benefit in removing drug.

Patient teaching

- Instruct patient to complete entire course of therapy even if symptoms disappear.

Teach patient to recognize and immediately report signs and symptoms of hypersensitivity reaction (including serum sickness and angioedema).

- Instruct patient about signs and symptoms of superinfection. Advise patient to report these promptly.
- Caution patient to avoid driving and other hazardous activities until drug's effects on alertness and motor function are known.
- As appropriate, review all other significant and life-threatening adverse reactions and interactions, especially those related to the drugs and tests mentioned above.

nalbuphine hydrochloride

Nubain

Pharmacologic class: Opioid agonist-antagonist
Therapeutic class: Analgesic, adjunct to anesthesia
Pregnancy risk category B, D (prolonged use in high doses at term)

Action

Binds to opiate receptors in CNS, inhibiting ascending pain pathways. This inhibition alters perception of and response to painful stimuli.

Pharmacokinetics

Drug crosses placental barrier and is metabolized in the liver; it is minimally protein-bound. Plasma half-life is 5 hours. A small amount is excreted unchanged in urine, with some excretion in bile and breast milk.

Onset	Peak	Duration
2-3 min	Unknown	3-6 hr

How supplied

Solution for injection: 10 mg/mL and 20 mg/mL in 10-mL multidose vials; 10 mg/mL and 20 mg/mL in ampules

Indications and dosages

➤ Moderate to severe pain
Adults: 10 mg/70 kg I.V. q 3 to 6 hours p.r.n., up to 160 mg/day. Maximum for single dose is 20 mg.
➤ Adjunct to balanced anesthesia
Adults: 0.3 to 3 mg/kg I.V. over 10 to 15 minutes, followed by maintenance dosage of 0.25 to 0.5 mg/kg I.V. in single doses p.r.n.

Administration

Preparation

Make sure emergency resuscitation equipment and naloxone (antidote) are available before starting therapy.

Dilution and compatibility

- Know that drug requires no dilution.

Infusion considerations

- Infuse undiluted over 2 to 3 minutes into vein or I.V. line with compatible solution, such as D_5W, normal saline solution, or lactated Ringer's solution.
- For anesthesia induction, administer doses over 10 to 15 minutes.

Monitoring

- Monitor vital signs. Watch for respiratory depression and heart rate changes.
- Evaluate patient for CNS changes. Institute safety measures as needed to prevent injury.

Watch for hypersensitivity reactions, such as anaphylaxis.

Storage

- Store at controlled room temperature of 15° to 30°C (59° to 86°F); protect from light.

Contraindications and precautions

Contraindicated in hypersensitivity to drug.

Use cautiously in increased intracranial pressure, head trauma, myocardial infarction, severe heart disease, respiratory depression, renal or hepatic disease, impaired ventilation, hypothyroidism, adrenal insufficiency, prostatic hypertrophy, emotional instability, alcoholism, history of substance abuse or dependence, pregnant or breastfeeding patients, and ***children.***

Adverse reactions

CNS: dizziness, sedation, headache, vertigo
CV: hypertension, hypotension, tachycardia, bradycardia
GI: nausea, vomiting, dry mouth
Respiratory: dyspnea, **respiratory depression**
Skin: sweating, clammy skin
Other: hypersensitivity reactions including **anaphylaxis**

Interactions

Drug-drug. *CNS depressants (including general anesthetics, monoamine oxidase inhibitors, sedative-hypnotics, tranquilizers):* additive CNS effects
Drug-diagnostic tests. *Amylase, lipase:* increased
Drug-herb. *Chamomile, hops, kava, skullcap, valerian:* increased CNS depression
Drug-behaviors. *Alcohol use:* additive CNS and respiratory depression

Toxicity and overdose

- Overdose signs and symptoms include hypotension, bradycardia, pinpoint pupils, respiratory depression, pulmonary edema, CNS depression, shock, and seizures.
- Establish secure airway and support ventilation and perfusion. Monitor for pulmonary edema. Give nalmefene or naloxone promptly, as ordered to antagonize opioid effects; however, avoid giving antagonist to physically dependent patient, if possible. If antagonist must be used to treat serious respiratory depression, administer with extreme care and titrate with smaller-than-usual doses. Do not give antagonist in absence of clinically significant respiratory or cardiovascular depression. As indicated and ordered, give I.V. fluids and vasopressors for hypotension and atropine for bradycardia. Dialysis does not remove drug.

Patient teaching

- Instruct patient to change position slowly and carefully, to avoid dizziness or light-headedness from sudden blood pressure decrease.

N

• Caution patient to avoid CNS depressants (including alcohol, sedative-hypnotics, and some herbs) for at least 24 hours after taking nalbuphine.
• Advise patient to consult prescriber before taking herbs.
• Teach patient to avoid driving and other hazardous activities until drug's effects on concentration, vision, and alertness are known.
• As appropriate, review all other significant and life-threatening adverse reactions and interactions, especially those related to the drugs, tests, herbs, and behaviors mentioned above.

nalmefene hydrochloride

Revex

Pharmacologic class: Opioid antagonist
Therapeutic class: Antidote
Pregnancy risk category B

Action

Prevents or reverses opioid effects, including respiratory depression, sedation, and hypotension; has a longer duration of action than naloxone at fully reversing doses; lacks opioid agonist activity.

Pharmacokinetics

Drug distributes rapidly in body and is metabolized by the liver. Less than 5% of dose is excreted in urine unchanged; 17% is excreted in feces. Terminal elimination half-life is 7 to 75 and 5.6 to 16 hours.

Onset	Peak	Duration
Unknown	Unknown	Varies with drug being reversed

How supplied

Solution for injection: 100 mcg/mL in blue-labeled ampule containing 1 mL; 1 mg/mL in green-labeled ampule containing 2 mL

Indications and dosages

➢ Complete or partial reversal of postoperative opioid effects
Adults: Initially using 100-mcg/mL strength (blue-labeled ampule), 0.25 mcg/kg I.V. followed by 0.25-mcg/kg incremental doses at 2- to 5-minute intervals

➢ Known or suspected opioid overdose
Adults: Initially using 1-mg/mL strength (green-labeled ampule) for nonopioid-dependent patients, 0.5 mg/70 kg I.V. followed by second dose of 1 mg/70 kg 2 to 5 minutes later, if needed. If total dosage of 1.5 mg/70 kg has been given without clinical response, additional doses are unlikely to have an effect.

In reasonable suspicion of opioid dependency, give challenge dose of 0.1 mg/70 kg initially; if no evidence of withdrawal occurs in 2 minutes, give recommended dosage for nonopioid-dependent patients.

Dosage adjustment

• Give smaller initial and incremental dosages of 0.1 mcg/kg in postoperative setting in patients with known increased cardiovascular risk.

Administration

Preparation

Know that in most emergency settings, this drug should be given after, not before, establishment of patent airway and circulatory access, ventilatory assistance, and oxygen administration.

Be aware that drug comes in two concentrations that can be identified by color-coded container labels:

concentration for postoperative use (100 mcg/mL) in blue-labeled ampule containing 1 mL; and concentration for managing overdose supplied as 1 mg/mL (10 times as concentrated) in green-labeled ampule containing 2 mL. Take proper steps to prevent using incorrect concentration.
• Know that drug is longest-acting parenteral opioid antagonist. If respiratory depression recurs, titrate dosage again to clinical effect, using incremental doses to avoid overreversal.
• Be aware that in postoperative setting, goal is to reverse excessive opioid effects without inducing complete reversal and acute pain. Stop treatment as soon as desired degree of opioid reversal occurs; know that cumulative total dosage above 1 mcg/kg does not provide additional therapeutic effect.
• In managing known or suspected opioid overdose, drug has no effect when opioids do not cause sedation and hypoventilation. Therefore, patients should receive it only when likelihood of opioid overdose is high, based on history of opioid overdose or clinical presentation of respiratory depression with pupillary constriction. To minimize risk of cardiovascular stress and precipitating withdrawal syndrome, do not give more drug than needed to restore respiratory rate to normal. Using higher dosages or shorter intervals between incremental doses is likely to increase incidence and severity of acute withdrawal symptoms, such as nausea, vomiting, elevated blood pressure, and anxiety. If I.V. access is lost or not readily obtainable, a single 1-mg dose should be effective within 5 to 15 minutes after I.M. or subcutaneous injection.
Prevent dermal absorption of spilled drug by promptly removing contaminated clothing and rinsing skin thoroughly with cool water.

Dilution and compatibility
• Know that drug may usually be given undiluted.
• Dilute drug 1:1 with normal saline solution or sterile water for injection in postoperative setting when giving to patients at increased cardiovascular risk.

Infusion considerations
• Know that drug is given mainly as I.V. bolus over 15 to 60 seconds.
• To manage known or suspected opioid overdose, titrate dosage to reverse undesired opioid effects. Once adequate reversal is established, additional doses aren't required and may be harmful due to unwanted reversal of analgesia or precipitation of withdrawal.
In renal failure, deliver incremental doses slowly (over 60 seconds) to minimize hypertension and dizziness that may follow abrupt administration.

Monitoring
• Know that reversal of respiratory depression is primary efficacy criterion for complete or partial reversal of postoperative opioid effects. Positive reversal is defined as both an increase in respiratory rate of 5 breaths/minute and a minimum respiratory rate of 12 breaths/minute.
Know that drug may cause acute withdrawal symptoms in patients with some degree of opioid tolerance and dependence. Closely observe such patients for withdrawal symptoms after initial and subsequent injections.
Monitor for pulmonary edema, cardiovascular instability, hypotension or hypertension, ventricular tachycardia, and ventricular fibrillation in connection with opioid reversal in both postoperative and emergency department settings. In many cases, these effects appear to result from abrupt reversal of opioid effects.

N

Be aware that excessive opioid antagonist doses in postoperative setting have been linked to hypertension, tachycardia, and excessive deaths in patients at high risk for cardiovascular complications.
Know that drug may not completely reverse buprenorphine-induced respiratory depression.
Closely observe ECG, pupil dilation, and vital signs (especially respirations).

Storage
- Store at controlled room temperature.

Contraindications and precautions
Contraindicated in hypersensitivity to drug.

Use with extreme caution in known physical dependence on opioids or after surgery involving high opioid doses. Use cautiously in increased cardiovascular risk, patients who have received potentially cardiotoxic drugs, ***elderly patients,*** pregnant or breastfeeding patients, and ***children*** (safety and efficacy not established).

Adverse reactions
CNS: dizziness, dysphoria, headache
CV: tachycardia, hypertension, hypotension, vasodilation, **bradycardia** (rare), **arrhythmia** (rare)
GI: nausea, vomiting, diarrhea, abdominal cramps
Musculoskeletal: myalgia, joint pain
Other: fever, chills, postoperative pain

Interactions
Drug-drug. *Flumazenil:* potential risk of seizures

Toxicity and overdose
- I.V. doses up to 24 mg in absence of opioid agonists have produced no serious adverse reactions, severe signs or symptoms, or clinically significant laboratory abnormalities. As with all opioid antagonists, use in patients with physical opioid dependence may precipitate withdrawal reactions resulting in symptoms that require medical attention.
- Provide symptomatic and supportive therapy. Resuscitate as needed.

Patient teaching
- As appropriate, review all significant and life-threatening adverse reactions and interactions, especially those related to the drugs mentioned above.

[redacted]

naloxone hydrochloride
Narcan

Pharmacologic class: Opioid antagonist
Therapeutic class: Opioid antidote
Pregnancy risk category B

Action
Unclear. Thought to compete with opioids for same receptor sites in brain. Prevents or reverses opioid effects, including respiratory depression, sedation, and hypotension.

Pharmacokinetics
Drug distributes rapidly into body tissues and fluids, and is metabolized rapidly in the liver. Half-life is 30 to 81 minutes in adults. It is excreted in urine.

Onset	Peak	Duration
1-2 min	5-15 min	Variable

How supplied
Solution for injection: 0.4 mg/mL in 1-mL ampule, 1 mg/mL (with preservatives), 0.02 mg/mL, 0.4 mg/mL (paraben-free)

Indications and dosages

➤ Opioid overdose

Adults: 0.4 to 2 mg I.V. Repeat q 2 to 3 minutes p.r.n., up to 10 mg.

Children: Usual initial dosage is 0.01 mg/kg I.V.; if this does not produce desired improvement, may give subsequent dose of 0.1 mg/kg I.V.

➤ Partial reversal of postoperative narcotic depression

Adults: 0.1 to 0.2 mg I.V. at 2- to 3-minute intervals to desired degree of reversal (adequate ventilation and alertness without significant pain or discomfort). Repeat doses may be needed within 1- to 2-hour intervals, depending on amount, drug action (short- or long-acting), and interval since last administration.

Children: 0.005 to 0.01 mg/kg I.V. q 2 to 3 minutes p.r.n.

Neonates: Usual initial dosage is 0.01 mg/kg I.V. Repeat doses may be required within 1- or 2-hour intervals, depending on amount, drug action (short- or long-acting), and interval since last administration.

Off-label uses

- Dementia associated with Alzheimer's disease or schizophrenia
- Reversal of alcoholic coma

Administration

Preparation

Administer only if resuscitation equipment is available.

Use cautiously in patients with physical dependence on opioids. If drug must be used to treat serious respiratory depression, give with extreme care, titrating with smaller-than-usual dosages. Do not give in absence of significant respiratory or cardiovascular depression.

- If prescribed, give initial dose of 0.1 mg I.V. to assess response.
- If I.V. route is not readily available, give I.M. or subcutaneously.

Dilution and compatibility

- Know that drug may be given undiluted.
- For I.V. infusion, dilute in normal saline solution or D_5W.
- Know that dilution of 2 mg in 500 mL of compatible solution yields a concentration of 0.004 mg/mL.

Infusion considerations

- Give doses of 0.4 mg or less (undiluted) by direct injection over 15 seconds, or titrate based on response.
- As needed, give by continuous I.V. infusion, and titrate based on response.
- Use diluted solution within 24 hours.

Monitoring

- Monitor vital signs every 3 to 5 minutes until opioid effects are reversed.
- Assess arterial blood gas studies and oxygen saturation.
- Evaluate cardiac status with continuous ECG monitoring.
- If patient does not respond to 10-mg doses given for opioid overdose, reevaluate cause of underlying condition.

Assess neurologic status, including level of consciousness. Stay alert for seizures.

Once naloxone is effective (up to 2 hours after administration), watch for signs and symptoms of acute withdrawal syndrome in opioid-dependent patients.

Storage

- Store at controlled room temperature of 15° to 30°C (59° to 86°F); protect from light.

Contraindications and precautions

Contraindicated in hypersensitivity to drug or other opioid antagonists.

Use cautiously in cardiovascular disease, opioid dependency, pregnant or breastfeeding patients, and ***children.***

N

Adverse reactions

CNS: tremors, **seizures**
CV: tachycardia, hypotension, hypertension (with higher doses), **ventricular tachycardia, ventricular fibrillation, cardiac arrest**
GI: nausea, vomiting
Respiratory: hyperpnea, **pulmonary edema**
Skin: diaphoresis
Other: withdrawal syndrome

Interactions

None significant

Toxicity and overdose

- No clinical experience with overdose exists. As with all opioid antagonists, administration to patients with physical dependence on opioids can trigger withdrawal reactions that may result in symptoms requiring medical attention.
- Provide symptomatic and supportive therapy. Resuscitate as needed. Follow facility guidelines regarding follow-up treatment for drug overdose.

Patient teaching

- Reassure patient that environment is safe.

neostigmine methylsulfate

PMS-Neostigmine Methylsulfate ♣
Prostigmin, Robinul-Neostigmine ❉

Pharmacologic class: Anticholinesterase
Therapeutic class: Muscle stimulant
Pregnancy risk category C

Action

Inhibits the enzyme acetylcholinesterase, leading to increased acetylcholine concentration at synapse and prolonged acetylcholine effects. Exerts direct cholinomimetic effect on skeletal muscle.

Pharmacokinetics

Drug undergoes hydrolysis by cholinesterase, and is metabolized by microsomal enzymes in the liver. Protein binding ranges from 15% to 25%. Approximately 80% of dose is eliminated in urine within 24 hours, 50% as unchanged drug, and 30% as metabolites. Plasma half-life ranges from 47 to 60 minutes.

Onset	Peak	Duration
Unknown	Unknown	Unknown

How supplied

Solution for injection: 0.5 mg/mL and 1 mg/mL in flip-top multidose vials

Indications and dosages

➢ Antidote for nondepolarizing neuromuscular blockers

Adults: 0.5 to 2 mg I.V.; repeat p.r.n. up to a maximum of 5 mg. Precede initial dose with 0.6 to 1.2 mg atropine sulfate I.V., as prescribed.

Administration

Preparation

- Keep resuscitation equipment on hand.
- Before giving, ensure that atropine sulfate is available to treat cholinergic crisis.
- Be aware that only in exceptional cases should total dosage exceed 5 mg.
- Know that atropine may be combined with usual neostigmine dose to decrease risk of adverse reactions.

Dilution and compatibility

- Know that drug requires no dilution.

Infusion considerations

- Administer I.V. dose directly into vein or I.V. line.
- Give 0.5-mg dose slowly over 1 minute.
- Do not add drug to I.V. solutions.

Monitoring

Monitor vital signs. Assess patient for hypotension, bradycardia or tachycardia, atrioventricular (AV) block, and evidence of impending cardiac arrest.
- Evaluate respiratory and neurologic status.

Storage
- Store at controlled room temperature of 15° to 30°C (59° to 86°F). Keep in carton until use, protected from light.

Contraindications and precautions

Contraindicated in hypersensitivity to cholinergics, mechanical obstruction of GI or urinary tract, and peritonitis.

Use cautiously in asthma, peptic ulcer, bradycardia, arrhythmias, recent coronary occlusion, vagotonia, hyperthyroidism, seizure disorder, and pregnant or breast-feeding patients.

Adverse reactions

CNS: dizziness, headache, drowsiness, asthenia, **loss of consciousness**
CV: hypotension, tachycardia, bradycardia, **AV block, cardiac arrest**
EENT: vision changes, lacrimation, miosis
GI: nausea, vomiting, diarrhea, abdominal cramps, flatulence, increased peristalsis
GU: urinary frequency
Musculoskeletal: muscle cramps, spasms, and fasciculations; joint pain
Respiratory: dyspnea, **bronchospasm, respiratory depression, respiratory arrest, laryngospasm**
Skin: rash, urticaria, flushing
Other: anaphylaxis

Interactions

Drug-drug. *Aminoglycosides, anticholinergics, atropine, corticosteroids, local and general anesthetics:* reversal of anticholinergic effects
Cholinergics: additive toxicity
Kanamycin, neomycin, streptomycin: increased neuromuscular blockade
Succinylcholine: potentiation of neuromuscular blockade, prolonged respiratory depression

Toxicity and overdose

- Overdose signs and symptoms include cholinergic crisis marked by GI stimulation with epigastric distress, vomiting, diarrhea, abdominal cramps, excessive salivation, pallor, cold sweats, urinary urgency, blurred vision, and eventually fasciculation and paralysis of voluntary muscles.
- Because overdose has an abrupt onset, discontinue drug immediately at first sign or symptom. Give atropine 0.5 to 1 mg I.V. as prescribed, and provide other supportive therapy as indicated.

Patient teaching

Tell patient drug may alter respiratory and cardiac status. Teach patient to recognize and immediately report warning signs.
- Caution patient to avoid driving and other hazardous activities until drug's effects on concentration, vision, muscle function, and alertness are known.
- As appropriate, review all other significant and life-threatening adverse reactions and interactions, especially those related to the drugs mentioned above.

nesiritide

Natrecor

Pharmacologic class: Human B-type natriuretic peptide
Therapeutic class: Vasodilator
Pregnancy risk category C

Action

Binds to receptors on vascular smooth muscle and endothelial cells, causing smooth-muscle relaxation and vasodilation. As a result, systemic and pulmonary pressures decrease and diuresis occurs.

Pharmacokinetics

Drug has a mean elimination half-life of about 18 minutes. It clears from circulation by three mechanisms, including renal filtration.

Onset	Peak	Duration
Unknown	Unknown	Unknown

How supplied

Powder for reconstitution for injection (white to off-white, lyophilized): 1.5 mg in single-use vials

Indications and dosages

➢ Acutely decompensated heart failure in patients who have dyspnea at rest or with minimal activity

Adults: 2 mcg/kg I.V. bolus, followed by continuous infusion of 0.01 mcg/kg/minute

Administration

Preparation

Do not initiate at dosage above that recommended (2 mcg/kg).

Dilution and compatibility

- Know that recommended preservative-free diluents for reconstitution are 5% dextrose injection, normal saline solution, 5% dextrose and 0.45% sodium chloride, and 5% dextrose and 0.2% sodium chloride.
- Reconstitute 1.5-mg vial by adding 5 mL diluent removed from prefilled 250-mL plastic I.V. bag containing desired diluent, to yield 0.32 mg/mL.
- Do not shake vial. To ensure complete reconstitution, rock vial gently so all surfaces (including stopper) come in contact with diluent.
- Use solution only if clear and essentially colorless.
- Withdraw entire contents of reconstituted vial and add to 250-mL plastic I.V. bag to yield a concentration of approximately 6 mcg/mL. Invert I.V. bag several times to ensure complete mixing of solution.
- Use reconstituted solution within 24 hours.
- Draw bolus dose from reconstituted solution in infusion bag.

Do not mix with other drug solutions.

Infusion considerations

Be aware that drug is physically or chemically incompatible with heparin, insulin, ethacrynate sodium, bumetanide, enalaprilat, hydralazine, and furosemide. Do not administer through same I.V. line.

Know that drug is incompatible with sodium metabisulfite (a preservative). Do not administer injectable drugs containing sodium metabisulfite through same I.V. line.

- After withdrawing bolus from infusion bag, give bolus dose over approximately 60 seconds through I.V. port in tubing.
- Follow immediately with constant I.V. infusion. To calculate infusion flow rate to deliver 0.01 mcg/kg/minute, use the following formula: infusion flow rate (mL/hr) = patient weight (kg) × 0.1.

Do not titrate at frequent intervals.

Monitoring

- Be aware that therapy beyond 48 hours has not been studied.
- Monitor vital signs and pulmonary artery wedge pressure continuously during infusion and for several hours afterward.

Assess cardiovascular status closely, especially for hypotension. Nesiritide-induced hypotension may be prolonged, so observation period may be necessary before restarting drug.

Storage

- Keep in carton until use.
- Store at controlled room temperature of 20° to 25°C (68° to 77°F), with excursions permitted from 15° to 30°C (59° to 86°F); or refrigerate at 2° to 8°C (36° to 46°F).
- Store reconstituted vials at controlled room temperature or refrigerate for 24 hours.

Contraindications and precautions

Contraindicated in hypersensitivity to drug or its components, systolic blood pressure below 90 mm Hg, and primary therapy for cardiogenic shock.

Use cautiously in restrictive or obstructive cardiomyopathy, constrictive pericarditis, pericardial tamponade, renal dysfunction, hypotension, and pregnant or breastfeeding patients.

Adverse reactions

CNS: dizziness, headache, insomnia, anxiety
CV: hypotension, angina pectoris, bradycardia, ventricular extrasystole, **ventricular tachycardia**
GI: nausea, vomiting, abdominal pain
Musculoskeletal: leg cramps, back pain
Respiratory: cough, hemoptysis, **apnea**
Other: injection site reactions

Interactions

Drug-drug. *Angiotensin-converting enzyme inhibitors, nitrates:* increased hypotension
Bumetanide, enalaprilat, ethacrynate sodium, furosemide, heparin, hydralazine, insulin: physical and chemical incompatibility with nesiritide
Drug-diagnostic tests. *Hematocrit, hemoglobin:* decreased

Toxicity and overdose

- No data on overdose exist. In overdose, expect extreme hypotension and possibly other adverse reactions.
- Reduce dosage or discontinue drug. Provide symptomatic and supportive therapy as indicated.

Patient teaching

- Tell patient he will be monitored closely during infusion and for several hours afterward.
- Inform patient that drug may cause serious adverse effects, but that he will receive appropriate interventions to relieve symptoms.
- Instruct patient to report chest pain, dizziness, palpitations, and other uncomfortable symptoms.
- As appropriate, review all other significant and life-threatening adverse reactions and interactions, especially those related to the drugs and tests mentioned above.

nicardipine

Cardene IV

Pharmacologic class: Calcium channel blocker
Therapeutic class: Antihypertensive
Pregnancy risk category C

Action

Inhibits calcium transport into myocardial and vascular smooth-muscle cells, causing reductions in cardiac output and myocardial contractions

Pharmacokinetics

After administration, plasma concentrations decline, with a rapid early distribution phase (half-life of 2.7 minutes), an intermediate phase ((half-life of 44.8 minutes), and a slow terminal phase (half-life of 14.4 hours) that can be detected only after long-term infusion. Drug is metabolized rapidly and extensively by the liver, and is largely protein-bound.

Onset	Peak	Duration
Unknown	Unknown	Unknown

How supplied

Solution for injection (clear, yellow): 2.5 mg/mL in 10-mL ampules

Indications and dosages

➢ Short-term treatment of hypertension when oral therapy is not feasible or desirable

Adults: Continuous I.V. infusion of 0.5 mg/hour (equal to 20 mg P.O. q 8 hours), or 1.2 mg/hour (equal to 30 mg P.O. q 8 hours), or 2.2 mg/hour (equal to 40 mg P.O. q 8 hours)

Off-label uses

- Heart failure
- Migraine
- Raynaud's disease

Administration

Dilution and compatibility

- Dilute each 25-mg ampule with 240 mL compatible I.V. fluid to a concentration of 0.1 mg/mL. Compatible fluids include D_5W, normal saline solution, dextrose 5% with normal saline solution, and half-normal saline solution.

Know that drug is incompatible with sodium bicarbonate 5% and lactated Ringer's solution.

- Do not mix with furosemide, heparin, or thiopental.
- Do not use solution if discolored.

Infusion considerations

Give by slow I.V. infusion. Titrate dosage to blood pressure response.

Monitoring

- Assess vital signs and cardiovascular status.
- Monitor fluid intake and output. Assess for signs and symptoms of heart failure.

Storage

- Keep in carton until use.
- Store at controlled room temperature of 20° to 25°C (68° to 77°F); protect from light.
- Know that diluted solution may be stored at room temperature for 24 hours.

Contraindications and precautions

Contraindicated in hypersensitivity to drug and advanced aortic stenosis.

Use cautiously in hepatic or mild renal impairment, hypotension, heart failure, significant left ventricular dysfunction (especially when given with beta-adrenergic blockers), pheochromocytoma, pregnant or breastfeeding patients (safety not established), and ***children younger than age 18*** (safety not established).

Adverse reactions

CNS: dizziness, headache, asthenia, drowsiness, paresthesia
CV: hypotension, peripheral edema, chest pain, increased angina, palpitations, tachycardia
GI: nausea, dyspepsia, dry mouth
Musculoskeletal: myalgia
Skin: flushing

Interactions

Drug-drug. *Cimetidine:* increased nifedipine blood level
Cyclosporine: increased cyclosporine blood level
Fentanyl anesthesia: increased hypotension
Drug-herb. *Ephedra (ma huang), yohimbe:* antagonism of drug's antihypertensive effect
St. John's wort: decreased nifedipine blood level
Drug-behaviors. *Alcohol use:* additive hypotension, increased drowsiness or dizziness

Toxicity and overdose

- In overdose, expect severe hypotension, bradycardia, palpitations, flushing, drowsiness, confusion, and slurred speech.
- Reduce dosage or discontinue drug. Monitor cardiac and respiratory functions. Place patient in Trendelenburg position to avoid cerebral anoxia. Monitor blood pressure. As ordered and indicated, give vasopressors if patient has profound hypotension. Know that I.V. calcium gluconate may help reverse effects of calcium entry blockade, and that hemodialysis does not remove drug.

Patient teaching

- Teach patient how to monitor blood pressure and to report abnormal findings.

Advise patient to immediately report chest pain or blood pressure decrease.

- Instruct patient to consult prescriber before drinking alcohol or taking herbs or over-the-counter drugs (especially cold remedies).
- As appropriate, review all other significant adverse reactions and interactions, especially those related to the drugs, herbs, and behaviors mentioned above.

nitroglycerin

Pharmacologic class: Nitrate
Therapeutic class: Antianginal
Pregnancy risk category C

Action

Inhibits calcium transport into myocardial and vascular smooth-muscle cells, suppressing contractions. Dilates main coronary arteries and arterioles, inhibits coronary artery spasm, increases oxygen delivery to heart, and reduces frequency and severity of angina attacks.

Pharmacokinetics

Drug distributes widely in body tissues and is rapidly metabolized in the liver and serum; approximately 60% is protein-bound. It is excreted in urine.

Onset	Peak	Duration
Immediate	Unknown	Several min

How supplied

Injection: 0.5 mg/mL in 10-mL ampule, 5 mg/mL in 5-mL and 10-mL vials
Solution for injection: 25 mg/250 mL, 50 mg/250 mL, 50 mg/500 mL, 100 mg/250 mL, 200 mg/500 mL

Indications and dosages

➤ Perioperative hypertension
Adults: 5 mcg/minute I.V., increased by 5 mcg/minute q 3 to 5 minutes up to 20 mcg/minute, then increased by 10 to 20 mcg/minute q 3 to 5 minutes (dosage determined by hemodynamic parameters)

➤ Heart failure associated with acute myocardial infarction
Adults: 5 mcg/minute I.V. using nonabsorptive tubing. Initially, titrate in 5-mcg/minute increments at intervals of 3 to 5 minutes, guided by response; if no response occurs at 20 mcg/minute, may use incremental increases of 10 and 20 mcg/minute.

➤ Treatment of angina pectoris in patients who have not responded to sublingual nitroglycerin and beta blockers
Adults: Initially, 5 mcg/minute I.V using nonabsorptive tubing. Titrate by 5 mcg/minute q 3 to 5 minutes based on response; if no response occurs at 20 mcg/minute, may use incremental increases of 10 and 20 mcg/minute.

N

Administration

Dilution and compatibility

Know that solution for injection is a concentrate and must be diluted before use to a concentration not exceeding 400 mcg/mL for I.V. infusion.

- Dilute with D_5W or normal saline solution.
- Be aware that in fluid-restricted patients, concentration may be increased to approximately 400 mcg/mL (100 mg in 250 mL D_5W) if necessary.

Do not mix solution for injection with other drugs.

Be aware that solution for injection is affected by type of infusion set used. Dosages listed above are based on use of nonabsorbent tubing.

Infusion considerations

Do not give by direct I.V. injection.

- Administer with infusion pump. Increase dosage in increments of 5 mcg/minute every 3 to 5 minutes, as needed, to achieve desired blood pressure response. Once achieved, reduce dosage and lengthen dosage-adjustment intervals.

Do not give concurrently with sildenafil, as life-threatening hypotension may occur.

Monitoring

Frequently monitor blood pressure; titrate dosage to obtain desired blood pressure results.

- Monitor patient for angina relief.

Storage

- Store at room temperature, protected from freezing and light.

Contraindications and precautions

Contraindicated in hypersensitivity to drug, other organic nitrates, or nitrites; orthostatic hypotension; hypotension or uncorrected hypovolemia; increased intracranial pressure (as from head trauma or cerebral hemorrhage); severe anemia; pericardial tamponade or constrictive pericarditis; and concurrent sildenafil therapy.

Use cautiously in severe renal or hepatic impairment, glaucoma, hypertrophic cardiomyopathy, hypovolemia, normal or decreased pulmonary capillary wedge pressure, alcohol intolerance (with large doses), pregnant or breastfeeding patients, and ***children*** (safety not established).

Adverse reactions

CNS: dizziness, headache
CV: hypotension, syncope
Hematologic: methemoglobinemia
Skin: rash, exfoliative dermatitis, flushing

Interactions

Drug-drug. *Antihypertensives, beta-adrenergic blockers, calcium channel blockers, haloperidol, phenothiazines:* additive hypotension

Sildenafil: increased risk of potentially fatal hypotension

Drug-diagnostic tests. *Cholesterol:* false elevations

Methemoglobin: significant levels (with excessive doses)

Triglycerides: falsely elevated results in assays based on glycerol oxidase

Urine catecholamines, urine vanillylmandelic acid: increased

Drug-behaviors. *Acute alcohol ingestion, alcohol use:* increased risk of potentially fatal hypotension

Toxicity and overdose

- In overdose, expect reflex tachycardia and hypotension.
- Because I.V. nitroglycerin has short-lived hemodynamic effects, leg elevation and I.V. fluids may be sufficient to relieve symptoms. Know that epinephrine and related drugs are ineffective in treating hypotension and should not be used. If indicated and ordered, give I.V. alpha-adrenergic agonist such as phenylephrine. If methemoglobinemia

occurs, provide high-flow oxygen and administer methylene blue at 0.2 mL/kg I.V. slowly, as ordered.

Patient teaching

- As appropriate, review all significant and life-threatening adverse reactions and interactions, especially those related to the drugs, tests, and behaviors mentioned above.

nitroprusside sodium

Nipride, Nitropress

Pharmacologic class: Vasodilator
Therapeutic class: Antihypertensive
Pregnancy risk category C

FDA BOXED WARNING

- After reconstitution with appropriate diluent, drug is not suitable for direct injection. Dilute reconstituted solution further in sterile 5% dextrose injection before infusing.
- Drug may cause steep blood pressure decrease, which can lead to irreversible ischemic injury or death in patients not properly monitored. Give drug only when available equipment and personnel allow continuous blood pressure monitoring.
- Except when used briefly or at low infusion rates, drug gives rise to significant amount of cyanide ion, which can reach toxic and potentially lethal levels. Never infuse at maximum dosage rate for more than 10 minutes. If blood pressure is not adequately controlled after 10 minutes of maximum-rate infusion, end infusion immediately. Monitor acid-base balance and venous oxygen concentration, but be aware that although these tests may indicate cyanide toxicity, they provide imperfect guidance.
- Review these warnings thoroughly before giving drug.

Action

Interferes with calcium influx and intracellular activation of calcium, causing peripheral vasodilation and direct decrease in blood pressure

Pharmacokinetics

Drug distributes rapidly to extracellular space and is cleared from this volume by intra-erythrocytic reaction with hemoglobin; resulting circulatory half-life is about 2 minutes. Metabolism results in cyanide radical in the liver. Some cyanide leaves the body as expired hydrogen cyanide; otherwise, drug is excreted primarily by the kidneys, and has a half-life of about 20 minutes.

Onset	Peak	Duration
30-60 sec	1-2 min	1-10 min

N

How supplied

Powder for reconstitution for injection (reddish brown): 50 mg/vial in 2-mL and 5-mL vials

Indications and dosages

➤ Hypertensive emergencies; to produce controlled hypotension during anesthesia

Adults and children: 0.3 to 10 mcg/kg/minute I.V., titrated to patient's response

➤ Congestive heart failure

Adults: Initially, 0.3 mcg/kg/minute by I.V. infusion; titrate every few minutes to desired effect. Usual effective dosage is 3 mcg/kg/minute I.V.; maximum dosage, 10 mcg/kg/minute.

Administration

Preparation

Check on availability of antidote (cyanide) kit before starting drug. Kit usually contains amyl nitrite inhalant ampules and sodium nitrite to induce methemoglobinemia.

- Obtain baseline ECG.

Dilution and compatibility

Reconstitute 50 mg in 2 to 3 mL D_5W for injection. Do not use any other diluent.

- Further dilute in 250 to 1,000 mL D_5W solution.
- Know that solution is rapidly degraded by trace contaminants, often with resulting color changes. It also is sensitive to certain wavelengths of light, and must be shielded from light during preparation and administration.

Know that solution has a faint reddish brown tint. Discard immediately if highly colored, blue, green, or dark red.

- Use only freshly prepared solution; however, if properly shielded from light, reconstituted and diluted solution is stable for 24 hours.
- Immediately after dilution, wrap infusion solution in aluminum foil or other opaque material to shield from light.

Infusion considerations

Administer only with microdrip regulator, infusion pump, or other device that allows precise flow-rate measurement.

Be aware that if drug is given at a rate more than 500 mcg/kg faster than 2 mcg/kg/minute, cyanide is generated at a rate faster than patient can eliminate it.

Monitoring

Measure blood pressure frequently (preferably with continuous arterial line) to detect rapid decrease.

Monitor injection site closely to avoid extravasation. Ensure that infusion rate is precisely controlled to prevent too-rapid infusion.

Watch for signs and symptoms of cyanide toxicity (lactic acidosis, dyspnea, headache, vomiting, confusion, and loss of consciousness).

Monitor for signs and symptoms of methemoglobinemia. (Methemoglobin levels can be measured by most clinical laboratories.) Suspect this rare diagnosis in patients who have received more than 10 mg/kg and have signs of impaired oxygen delivery despite adequate cardiac output and arterial partial pressure of oxygen. Classically, methemoglobinemic blood appears chocolate brown, without color change on exposure to air. Treatment of choice is methylene blue I.V. In patients likely to have substantial amounts of cyanide bound to methemoglobin as cyanmethemoglobin, use extreme caution when giving methylene blue.

- Continue to monitor ECG.

Storage

- Store at controlled room temperature of 15° to 30°C (59° to 86°F).

Contraindications and precautions

Contraindicated in compensatory hypertension caused by aortic coarctation or atrioventricular shunting, to produce hypotension during surgery in patients with known inadequate cerebral circulation, acute heart failure caused by reduced peripheral vascular resistance, congenital (Leber's) optic atrophy, tobacco amblyopia, and moribund patients undergoing emergency surgery.

Use cautiously in hepatic or renal disease, fluid and electrolyte imbalances, hypothyroidism, ***elderly patients,*** pregnant or breastfeeding patients, and ***children.***

Adverse reactions

CNS: increased intracranial pressure
CV: ECG changes, bradycardia, tachycardia, **marked hypotension, too-rapid blood pressure decrease**
GI: ileus
Hematologic: decreased platelet aggregation, **methemoglobinemia**
Metabolic: hypothyroidism
Skin: rash, flushing
Other: pain, irritation, and venous streaking at injection site; **thiocyanate or cyanide toxicity** (initially, tinnitus, miosis, and hyperreflexia) at blood level of 60 mg/L; **life-threatening cyanide toxicity** (lactic acidosis, air hunger, confusion, death) at blood level of 200 mg/L

Interactions

Drug-drug. *Enflurane, ganglionic blockers, halothane, negative inotropic drugs, volatile liquid anesthetics:* severe hypotension
Sildenafil: potentiation of nitroprusside's hypotensive effects
Drug-diagnostic tests. *Creatinine:* increased
Methemoglobin: hemoglobin sequestration as methemoglobin

Toxicity and overdose

- Know that toxicity may occur at dosages well below recommended maximum of 10 mcg/kg/minute. Overdose signs and symptoms include excessive hypotension and cyanide or thiocyanide toxicity.
- Because acidosis may not arise for more than 1 hour after cyanide levels have become dangerous, do not wait for laboratory values. In reasonable suspicion of cyanide toxicity, use antidote kit, if available, and initiate treatment immediately, as ordered. Promptly discontinue drug; use I.V. sodium nitrite as buffer to convert as much hemoglobin to methemoglobin as patient can safely tolerate; then give sufficient sodium thiosulfate to convert cyanide into thiocyanate, as prescribed. Be aware that amyl nitrite inhalant ampules may be used when I.V. sodium nitrite administration may be delayed. In patient with preexisting patent I.V. line, amyl nitrite use has no benefit that is not provided by sodium nitrite infusion. Know that hemodialysis does not remove cyanide but may remove thiocyanate.

Patient teaching

- Tell patient he will be closely monitored during therapy.
- Instruct patient to immediately report headache, nausea, or pain at injection site.
- As appropriate, review all other significant and life-threatening adverse reactions and interactions, especially those related to the drugs and tests mentioned above.

norepinephrine bitartrate

Levophed

Pharmacologic class: Sympathomimetic
Therapeutic class: Alpha- and beta-adrenergic agonist, cardiac stimulant, vasopressor
Pregnancy risk category C

FDA BOXED WARNING

- If extravasation occurs, infiltrate area promptly with 10 to 15 mL of saline solution containing 5 to 10 mg phentolamine to prevent sloughing and necrosis. Use syringe with fine hypodermic needle, and infiltrate solution liberally throughout area. Give phentolamine as soon as possible; its sympathetic blockade causes immediate local hyperemic changes if area is infiltrated within 12 hours.

Action

Stimulates $beta_1$ and $alpha_1$ receptors in sympathetic nervous system, causing vasoconstriction, increased blood pressure, enhanced contractility, and decreased heart rate

Pharmacokinetics

Drug is rapidly inactivated in body by catechol-O-methyltransferase and monoamine oxidase. It is excreted in urine primarily as inactive form.

Onset	Peak	Duration
Immediate	Immediate	1-2 min after infusion ends

How supplied

Solution for injection (clear, colorless): 1 mg/mL

Indications and dosages

➢ Severe hypotension; adjunct in treatment of cardiac arrest and profound hypotension

Adults: 8 to 12 mcg/minute I.V.; then titrated based on blood pressure response. For maintenance, 2 to 4 mcg/minute.

Administration

Dilution and compatibility

Know that drug must be diluted before use.

• Mix with D_5W or dextrose 5% in normal saline solution.

• Inspect solution to make sure it is clear and colorless; do not infuse if brown or pink.

Infusion considerations

• Administer through infusion pump. Titrate infusion rate to achieve and maintain systolic blood pressure of 80 to 100 mm Hg.

To prevent delivery of large drug concentrations, avoid line stasis and flushing.

Never leave patient unattended during infusion.

• Continue infusion until blood pressure and tissue perfusion remain adequate without drug therapy.

• Gradually titrate dosage downward.

• To avoid extravasation, administer only into large vein (antecubital) or through central line. Do not use femoral vein in patients who are elderly or have occlusive vascular disorders.

Monitoring

• Monitor ECG and blood pressure continuously.

Check blood pressure every 2 minutes until desired pressure occurs. Recheck every 5 minutes for duration of infusion.

Be aware that headache may signal extreme hypertension and overdose.

Watch for signs and symptoms of peripheral vascular insufficiency (decreased capillary refill, pale to cyanotic to black skin color).

• Continue to monitor infusion site closely for extravasation; be prepared to intervene, as prescribed.

Storage

• Store at room temperature, protected from light.

Contraindications and precautions

Contraindicated in concurrent cyclopropane or halothane anesthesia, hypotension caused by blood volume deficit (except in emergencies until blood volume replacement therapy can be completed), profound hypoxia or hypercarbia, and mesenteric or peripheral vascular thrombosis.

Use cautiously in sulfite sensitivity (with some products), especially in asthmatic patients; arterial embolism; cardiac disease; peripheral vascular disease; hypertension; hyperthyroidism; concurrent use of monoamine oxidase (MAO) inhibitors or tricyclic antidepressants; ***elderly patients;*** pregnant or breastfeeding patients; and ***children*** (safety and efficacy not established).

Adverse reactions

CNS: headache, anxiety
CV: bradycardia, **severe hypertension, arrhythmias**
Respiratory: respiratory difficulty
Skin: irritation with extravasation, necrosis
Other: ischemic injury

Interactions

Drug-drug. *Alpha-adrenergic blockers:* antagonism of norepinephrine effects
Antihistamines, ergot alkaloids, guanethidine, MAO inhibitors, oxytocin, tricyclic antidepressants: severe hypertension
Bretylium, inhalation anesthetics: increased risk of arrhythmias

Toxicity and overdose

- Overdose signs and symptoms include headache, vomiting, diaphoresis, severe hypertension, photophobia, retrosternal or pharyngeal pain, cerebral hemorrhage, seizures, reflex bradycardia, marked increase in peripheral resistance, decreased cardiac output, and arrhythmias.
- Discontinue drug. Provide symptomatic and supportive therapy, including propranolol for arrhythmias, as ordered.

Patient teaching

- Once patient is alert, explain why drug was given.
- Reassure patient he will be monitored continuously until he is stable.

octreotide acetate

Sandostatin

Pharmacologic class: Somatostatin analogue
Therapeutic class: Antidiarrheal, growth hormone inhibitor
Pregnancy risk category B

Action

Suppresses secretion of serotonin, serotonin metabolites, and gastrohepatic peptides, resulting in increased fluid and electrolyte absorption from GI tract. Also suppresses growth hormone, insulin, and glucagon.

Pharmacokinetics

Drug distributes to plasma, where approximately 65% is protein-bound. Half-life is longer than that of natural hormone somatostatin. About 35% of unchanged drug is excreted in urine.

Onset	Peak	Duration
Unknown	0.4 hr	Up to 12 hr

O

How supplied

Solution for injection (clear): 0.05 mg/mL, 0.1 mg/mL, and 0.5 mg/mL in 1-mL ampules; 0.2 mg/mL and 1 mg/mL in 5-mL multidose vials

Indications and dosages

➤ Diarrhea and flushing associated with metastatic carcinoid tumors
Adults: 100 to 600 mcg I.V. daily in two to four divided doses for 2 weeks
➤ Diarrhea caused by vasoactive intestinal peptide tumors (VIPomas)
Adults: 200 to 300 mcg I.V. daily in two to four divided doses for 2 weeks
➤ To normalize growth hormone in patients with acromegaly

Adults: 50 to 100 mcg I.V. two or three times daily

Dosage adjustment
- Know that dosage may need to be reduced in severe renal impairment requiring dialysis.
- Be aware that elderly patients may require dosage adjustment due to significant increase in drug half-life and decrease in clearance.

Off-label uses
- Dumping syndrome (postprandial hypotension)
- GI and pancreatic fistulas
- Variceal bleeding

Administration
Preparation
- Know that octreotide suppression test and octreotide scintigraphy may be done to determine if drug will aid carcinoid tumor treatment.

Dilution and compatibility
- Dilute in 50 to 200 mL D_5W or normal saline solution.
- Diluted drug may be kept at room temperature for 24 hours.
- After initial use, discard multidose vials within 14 days. Open ampules just before administration. Discard unused portion.
- Do not use solution if discolored.

Infusion considerations
- Administer by direct I.V. injection over 3 minutes, or infuse over 15 to 30 minutes.
- Be aware that in emergencies (such as carcinoid crisis), drug may be given by rapid I.V. bolus.

Monitoring
- Assess bowel sounds and stool frequency and consistency.
- Monitor vital signs.
- Monitor fluid intake and output. Stay alert for dehydration or edema.
- Evaluate diabetic patient for hypoglycemia or hyperglycemia.
- To determine response, evaluate laboratory tests, such as urinary 5-hydroxyindole acetic acid and plasma serotonin in patients with carcinoid tumors, plasma vasoactive VIP in patients with VIPomas, and growth hormone levels in patients with acromegaly.

Storage
- For prolonged storage, refrigerate at 2° to 8°C (36° to 46°F) or at room temperature of 20° to 30°C (68° to 86°F) for 14 days if protected from light.

Contraindications and precautions
Contraindicated in hypersensitivity to drug or its components.

Use cautiously in renal impairment, gallbladder disease, hyperglycemia or hypoglycemia, fat malabsorption, pregnant or breastfeeding patients, and ***children.***

Adverse reactions
CNS: dizziness, drowsiness, fatigue, headache, weakness
CV: edema, bradycardia, conduction abnormalities, **arrhythmias**
EENT: vision disturbances
GI: nausea, vomiting, diarrhea, abdominal pain, cholelithiasis, fat malabsorption
Metabolic: hypothyroidism, hyperglycemia, **hypoglycemia**
Skin: flushing

Interactions
Drug-drug. *Cyclosporine:* reduced cyclosporine blood level
Beta blockers, calcium channel blockers, drugs used to control fluid and electrolyte balance, insulin, oral hypoglycemics: altered requirements for these drugs
Drug-diagnostic tests. *Glucose:* increased or decreased
Hepatic enzymes: slightly increased

Schilling's test: abnormal results
Thyroxine, vitamin B_{12}: decreased

Toxicity and overdose
- No cases of overdose have been reported. In healthy volunteers, no serious ill effects have occurred with bolus I.V. doses of 1,000 mcg and 30,000 mcg I.V. over 20 minutes, or 120,000 mcg I.V. over 8 hours. In overdose, expect extension of pharmacologic action and adverse reactions.
- Reduce dosage or discontinue drug, as indicated and ordered.

Patient teaching
- Instruct patient being treated for carcinoid tumor to keep track of number of daily stools or flushing episodes (which reflect drug efficacy in suppressing amine-induced symptoms).
- Teach patient to take daily weights and report significant changes.
- Caution patient to avoid driving and other hazardous activities until drug's effects on concentration, vision, and alertness are known.
- As appropriate, review all other significant and life-threatening adverse reactions and interactions, especially those related to the drugs and tests mentioned above.

ofloxacin
Floxin, Tarivid ❉

Pharmacologic class: Fluoroquinolone
Therapeutic class: Anti-infective
Pregnancy risk category C

Action
Inhibits bacterial DNA synthesis by inhibiting DNA gyrase in susceptible bacteria

Pharmacokinetics
Drug distributes widely to body tissues and fluids; liver metabolism is limited. Drug is excreted primarily in urine, with some excretion in feces.

Onset	Peak	Duration
Rapid	End of infusion	12 hr

How supplied
Premixed solution for injection: 200 mg/50 mL and 400 mg/100 mL in single-use flexible containers
Solution for injection: 400 mg (40 mg/mL) in 10-mL single-use vial

Indications and dosages
➢ Prostatitis caused by *Escherichia coli*
Adults: 300 mg I.V. q 12 hours for 6 weeks
➢ Complicated urinary tract infections caused by *E. coli, Klebsiella pneumoniae*, or *Proteus mirabilis*
Adults: 200 mg I.V. q 12 hours for 10 days
➢ Uncomplicated cystitis caused by *E. coli* or *K. pneumoniae*
Adults: 200 mg I.V. q 12 hours for 3 days
➢ Acute uncomplicated urethral and cervical gonorrhea
Adults: 400 mg I.V. as a single dose
➢ Nongonococcal cervicitis or urethritis caused by *Chlamydia trachomatis;* mixed infections of cervix or urethra caused by *C. trachomatis* or *Neisseria gonorrhoeae*
Adults: 300 mg I.V. q 12 hours for 7 days
➢ Acute bacterial exacerbation of chronic bronchitis, community-acquired pneumonia, or uncomplicated skin and skin-structure infections caused by susceptible organisms
Adults: 400 mg I.V. q 12 hours for 10 days
➢ Acute pelvic inflammatory disease
Adults: 400 mg I.V. q 12 hours for 10 to 14 days
➢ Community-acquired pneumonia caused by *Haemophilus influenzae* or

Streptococcus pneumoniae; uncomplicated skin and skin-structure infections caused by *Staphylococcus aureus, Streptococcus pyogenes,* or *Proteus mirabilis*
Adults: 400 mg I.V. q 12 hours for 10 days
➢ Mixed infections of urethra and cervix caused by *C. trachomatis* or *N. gonorrhoeae*
Adults: 300 mg I.V. q 12 hours for 7 days

Dosage adjustment

- In severe hepatic impairment, do not exceed maximum dosage of 400 mg daily, because drug excretion may be reduced.
- In renal impairment, adjust dosage based on creatinine clearance. With clearance of 20 to 50 mL/minute, give normal recommended dosage every 24 hours. With clearance below 20 mL/minute, give half of usual recommended dosage every 24 hours.

Administration

Dilution and compatibility

- For intermittent I.V. infusion, dilute single-use vials to a concentration of 4 mg/mL using normal saline solution, D_5W, dextrose 5% in normal saline solution, or dextrose 5% in lactated Ringer's solution.
- Do not add other solutions or drugs to premixed solution.
- Know that premixed solution is preservative-free. Discard unused portion.

Infusion considerations

- Administer by I.V. infusion slowly over at least 60 minutes.

Do not use plastic containers in series connections. Such use could result in air embolism due to residual air being drawn from primary container before administration of fluid from secondary container ends.

Monitoring

Monitor patient for fever with diarrhea, diarrhea containing pus, or severe persistent diarrhea.

- Inspect for rash. Check for signs and symptoms of other hypersensitivity reactions.
- Evaluate neurologic status closely.
- Assess for signs and symptoms of superinfection.

Storage

- Store single-use vials before reconstitution at controlled room temperature of 15° to 30°C (59° to 86°F); protect from light. When diluted in compatible solution to a concentration of 0.4 to 4 mg/mL, drug is stable for 72 hours when stored at or below 24°C (75°F) or for 14 days when refrigerated at 5°C (41°F).
- Store premixed flexible containers at or below 25°C (77°F); brief exposure at or below 40°C (104°F) does not affect stability. Avoid excessive heat, protect from light, and avoid freezing.

Contraindications and precautions

Contraindicated in hypersensitivity to drug or other fluoroquinolones.

Use cautiously in underlying CNS disease, renal impairment, cirrhosis, bradycardia, acute myocardial ischemia, history of tendinitis or tendon rupture with fluoroquinolone use, dialysis patients, ***elderly patients,*** pregnant or breastfeeding patients, and ***children younger than age 18***

Adverse reactions

CNS: dizziness, drowsiness, headache, light-headedness, insomnia, acute psychoses, agitation, confusion, tremors, hallucinations, **increased intracranial pressure, seizures**
CV: chest pain, vasodilation
GI: nausea, diarrhea, constipation, abdominal pain, **pseudomembranous colitis**
GU: interstitial cystitis, hematuria, pyuria, vaginitis
Hematologic: eosinophilia, leukocytosis, neutropenia, neutrophilia, increased

band forms, lymphocytopenia, lymphocytosis, **leukopenia**
Musculoskeletal: tendinitis, tendon rupture, joint pain, back pain
Skin: rash, photosensitivity, phototoxicity, **Stevens-Johnson syndrome**
Other: altered taste, superinfection, phlebitis at I.V. site, hypersensitivity reactions including **anaphylaxis**

Interactions

Drug-drug. *Amiodarone, bepridil, disopyramide, erythromycin, pentamidine, phenothiazines, pimozide, procainamide, quinidine, sotalol, tricyclic antidepressants:* increased risk of serious adverse cardiovascular reactions
Corticosteroids: increased risk of tendon rupture
Cyclosporine: elevated cyclosporine level
Nonsteroidal anti-inflammatory drugs: increased risk of CNS stimulation and seizures
Probenecid: decreased renal elimination of ofloxacin
Theophylline: increased theophylline blood level and possible toxicity
Warfarin: increased warfarin effects
Drug-diagnostic tests. *Alanine aminotransferase, alkaline phosphatase, aspartate aminotransferase, blood urea nitrogen, creatinine, erythrocyte sedimentation rate, platelets, urine glucose, urine protein:* increased
Blood glucose: increased or decreased
Hematocrit, hemoglobin: decreased
Drug-herb. *Dong quai, St. John's wort:* phototoxicity
Drug-behaviors. *Sun exposure:* phototoxicity

Toxicity and overdose

- In overdose, expect drowsiness, dizziness, nausea, and confusion.
- Expect to withdraw drug, which usually leads to symptom resolution. Observe patient closely and maintain appropriate hydration.

Patient teaching

- Instruct patient to drink at least 1,500 mL of fluids daily to prevent crystalluria.
- Advise patient being treated for gonorrhea that sexual partners must be treated.

Tell patient to promptly report fever and diarrhea, especially if stool contains blood, pus, or mucus. Caution patient not to treat diarrhea without consulting prescriber.

Instruct patient to immediately report rash or tendon pain or inflammation.

- Teach patient ways to counteract photosensitivity, such as wearing sunglasses and avoiding excessive exposure to bright light.
- Advise female patient to tell prescriber if she is pregnant before taking drug. Caution her not to breastfeed during therapy.
- As appropriate, review all other significant and life-threatening adverse reactions and interactions, especially those related to the drugs, tests, herbs, and behaviors mentioned above.

ondansetron hydrochloride

Zofran, Zofran Preservative Free

Pharmacologic class: Serotonin type 3 ($5\text{-}HT_3$) antagonist
Therapeutic class: Antiemetic
Pregnancy risk category B

Action

Blocks $5\text{-}HT_3$ receptors, which exist both peripherally on vagal nerve terminals and centrally in chemoreceptor trigger zone. It is not clear if antiemetic action in chemotherapy-induced nausea and vomiting is mediated centrally, peripherally, or both.

Pharmacokinetics

Drug is metabolized extensively in the liver by hydroxylation, and is 70% to 76% protein-bound. Patients older than age 75 have reduced clearance and increased elimination half-life. In mild to moderate hepatic impairment, clearance decreases twofold and mean half-life increases to 11.6 hours, compared to 5.7 hours in patients with normal hepatic function. In severe hepatic impairment, clearance decreases two- to threefold and apparent volume of distribution increases; as a result, half-life increases to 20 hours. Only 5% of dose is excreted in urine as parent drug.

Onset	Peak	Duration
Rapid	15-30 min	4-8 hr

How supplied

Solution for injection (clear, colorless): 2 mg/mL in 2- and 20-mL vials
Solution for injection (clear, premixed): 32 mg/50 mL in single-dose flexible containers
Solution for injection (clear, preservative-free): 2 mg/mL in 2-mL single-dose vials

Indications and dosages

➢ To prevent nausea and vomiting caused by highly emetogenic chemotherapy

Adults and children older than age 12: 32-mg I.V. infusion as a single dose infused over 15 minutes, starting 30 minutes before chemotherapy; or three 0.15-mg/kg doses I.V., with first dose infused over 15 minutes, starting 30 minutes before chemotherapy and repeated 4 hours and 8 hours later

➢ Prevention and treatment of postoperative nausea and vomiting

Adults and children older than age 12: 4 mg by I.V. injection before anesthesia or postoperatively
Children ages 2 to 12 weighing more than 40 kg (88 lb): 4 mg by I.V. injection before anesthesia or postoperatively
Children ages 2 to 12 weighing less than 40 kg: 0.1 mg/kg by I.V. injection before anesthesia or postoperatively

Dosage adjustment

- In severe hepatic impairment, single maximum dose of 8 mg I.V. infused over 15 minutes starting 30 minutes before emetogenic chemotherapy begins is recommended.

Administration

Preparation

- Give first dose at least 30 minutes before emetogenic event.

Dilution and compatibility

- When administering by direct I.V. injection to prevent or treat postoperative nausea and vomiting, give single dose undiluted.
- For I.V. infusion, dilute single dose from vial in 50 mL normal saline solution, D_5W, dextrose 5% in normal saline solution, dextrose 5% in 0.45% sodium chloride, or 3% sodium chloride solution.

Know that alkaline solutions may cause precipitation.

- Do not add other solutions or drugs to premixed solution in flexible containers.
- Know that premixed solution is preservative-free. Discard unused portion.
- Do not administer unless solution is clear.

Infusion considerations

- Give undiluted drug by direct I.V. immediately before anesthesia induction, or postoperatively if nausea and vomiting occur. Administer slowly, over at least 30 seconds (preferably over 2 to 5 minutes).

- For I.V. infusion, administer over 15 minutes.

Do not use plastic containers in series connections. Such use could result in air embolism due to residual air being drawn from primary container before administration of fluid from secondary container ends.

Monitoring

- Monitor GI status.
- Assess for extrapyramidal reactions.

Check vital signs frequently. Watch for hypotension and bronchospasm.

- Monitor fluid intake and output. Stay alert for urine retention.

Storage

- Store between 2° and 30° C (36° and 86° F); protect from light. With flexible containers, avoid excessive heat and protect from freezing.
- After dilution, do not use beyond 24 hours.

Contraindications and precautions

Contraindicated in hypersensitivity to drug.

Use cautiously in hepatic disease, pregnant or breastfeeding patients, and ***children younger than age 12.***

Adverse reactions

CNS: headache, dizziness, malaise, drowsiness, fatigue, weakness, extrapyramidal reactions
CV: chest pain, hypotension
GI: constipation, diarrhea, abdominal pain, dry mouth
GU: urine retention
Respiratory: bronchospasm
Skin: rash
Other: pain at injection site, shivering, **anaphylaxis**

Interactions

Drug-drug. *Drugs that alter hepatic enzyme activity:* altered ondansetron pharmacokinetics

Drug-diagnostic tests. *Alanine aminotransferase, aspartate aminotransferase, bilirubin:* transient increases

Toxicity and overdose

- No overdoses have been reported. Individual doses as large as 150 mg and total daily doses (three doses) as large as 252 mg have been given I.V. without significant adverse events. In overdose, expect extension of adverse reactions, including hypotension.
- No specific antidote exists. Provide symptomatic and supportive therapy.

Patient teaching

Instruct patient to immediately report extrapyramidal symptoms or allergic reaction.

- Caution patient to avoid driving and other hazardous activities until drug's effects on concentration and alertness are known.
- As appropriate, review all other significant and life-threatening adverse reactions and interactions, especially those related to the drugs and tests mentioned above.

[redacted]

orphenadrine citrate

Biorphen, Norflex

Pharmacologic class: Diphenhydramine derivative

Therapeutic class: Skeletal muscle relaxant (centrally acting)

Pregnancy risk category C

Action

Unclear. Action may be related to drug's analgesic properties. Acts centrally on brain stem; does not directly relax tense skeletal muscles. Also possesses anticholinergic actions.

Pharmacokinetics

Drug is metabolized extensively into several metabolites and excreted in urine and feces.

Onset	Peak	Duration
Unknown	Unknown	Unknown

How supplied

Solution for injection: 30 mg/mL in 2-mL ampules and 10-mL vials

Indications and dosages

➢ Adjunct in painful, acute musculoskeletal conditions

Adults: 60 mg I.V; may repeat q 12 hours

Administration

Preparation

• Be aware that drug is prescribed in conjunction with rest, physical therapy, and other measures to relieve discomfort associated with painful musculoskeletal conditions.

Dilution and compatibility

• Know that drug may be given undiluted or diluted as a single dose in 5 to 10 mL sterile water for injection.

Infusion considerations

• Administer 60 mg (2 mL) or fraction thereof I.V. over 5 minutes.

Monitoring

• Monitor for adverse effects. such as rash, urinary difficulties, and especially mental confusion (in elderly patients).

• Be aware that safety of continuous long-term therapy has not been established. In patients receiving drug for prolonged use, monitor blood, urine and liver function values periodically.

Storage

• Store at controlled room temperature of 15° to 30°C (59° to 86°F).

Contraindications and precautions

Contraindicated in hypersensitivity to drug, glaucoma, pyloric or duodenal obstruction, stenosing peptic ulcers, prostatic hypertrophy, bladder neck obstruction, cardiospasm, and myasthenia gravis.

Use cautiously in sulfite sensitivity, cardiac decompensation, coronary insufficiency, arrhythmias, tachycardia, long-term orphenadrine therapy, pregnant or breastfeeding patients, and ***children*** (safety and efficacy not established).

Adverse reactions

CNS: dizziness, headache, drowsiness, weakness, light-headedness, confusion (in elderly patients), hallucinations, agitation, tremor
CV: tachycardia, palpitations, transient syncope
EENT: blurred vision, pupil dilation, increased ocular pressure
GI: nausea, vomiting, constipation, gastric irritation, dry mouth
GU: urinary hesitancy, urine retention
Other: hypersensitivity reaction (including urticaria, pruritus, and other dermatoses)

Interactions

Drug-drug. *Amantadine:* increased anticholinergic effects
Haloperidol: decreased haloperidol blood level, tardive dyskinesia, worsening of schizophrenic symptoms
Phenothiazines: decreased phenothiazine effects
Propoxyphene: increased risk of confusion, anxiety, and tremors
Drug-behaviors. *Alcohol use:* increased CNS effects

Toxicity and overdose

• Overdose signs and symptoms include dry mouth, blurred vision, urine retention, tachycardia, confusion, paralytic ileus, coma, seizures, shock, respiratory arrest, arrhythmias, and death. In adults, lethal dosage is 2 to 3 g. Intoxication arises rapidly and death may occur in 3 to 5 hours, preceded by deep coma, seizures, and shock. Serious arrhythmias are common.

- In overdose, immediately discontinue drug, closely monitor vital signs and fluid and electrolyte balance, and provide supportive therapy, as indicated and ordered. Know that hemodialysis may not remove drug.

Patient teaching

- Instruct patient to notify prescriber if rash, itching, rapid heart rate, or mental confusion occurs.
- Tell patient about adverse effects, such as dry mouth, blurred vision, and GI upset. Instruct patient to notify prescriber if these effects persist.
- Instruct patient to move slowly when sitting up or standing, to avoid dizziness or light-headedness from blood pressure decrease. Advise patient to dangle legs briefly before getting out of bed.
- Caution patient to avoid driving and other hazardous activities until drug's effects on concentration and alertness are known.
- Advise patient to avoid alcohol use during therapy.
- As appropriate, review all other significant adverse reactions and interactions, especially those related to the drugs and behaviors mentioned above.

[redacted]

oxacillin sodium

Bactocill

Pharmacologic class: Penicillinase-resistant penicillin

Therapeutic class: Broad-spectrum anti-infective

Pregnancy risk category B

Action

Interferes with bacterial cell-wall synthesis during multiplication of susceptible organisms; overall, shows minimal immunosuppressant activity

Pharmacokinetics

Drug distributes widely throughout the body and crosses placental barrier. Although cerebrospinal fluid penetration is poor, drug appears in therapeutic concentrations in pleural, bile, and amniotic fluids. It is partially metabolized and approximately 90% protein-bound. It is rapidly excreted in urine, with some secretion in breast milk. Half-life is 20 to 30 minutes.

Onset	Peak	Duration
Immediate	Immediate	Unknown

How supplied

Solution: 250-mg, 500-mg, 1-g, 2-g, and 4-g vials

Solution: 1 g and 2 g in vials

Indications and dosages

➤ Systemic infections caused by penicillinase-producing staphylococci

Adults and children weighing more than 40 kg (88 lb): For mild to moderate infections, 250 to 500 mg I.V. q 4 to 6 hours, with follow-up oral therapy q 4 to 6 hours. For severe infections, 1 g I.V. q 4 to 6 hours, with follow-up oral therapy q 4 to 6 hours.

Children weighing less than 40 kg: For mild to moderate infections, 50 mg/kg I.V. q 6 hours, with follow-up oral therapy q 6 hours. For severe infections, 100 mg/kg I.V. q 4 to 6 hours, with follow-up oral therapy q 4 to 6 hours.

Premature infants and neonates: 25 mg/kg/day I.V.

Administration

Preparation

- Ask patient about penicillin allergy before giving drug.
- Obtain bacteriologic studies to determine causative organisms and their sensitivity to penicillinase-resistant penicillins.
- Know that duration of therapy varies with infection type and severity and patient's overall condition; in severe staphylococcal infections, therapy should last at least 14 days. Therapy should continue for at least 48 hours after patient becomes afebrile and asymptomatic and cultures are negative. Treatment of endocarditis and osteomyelitis may require longer duration.

Dilution and compatibility

- For direct I.V. injection dilute each 500 mg dose using 5 mL of normal saline solution or sterile water.
- For intermittent or continuous I.V. infusion, reconstitute as directed above before diluting in 50 to 1,000 mL of one of the following solutions only: D_5W; dextrose 5% in normal saline solution; normal saline solution; 10% D-fructose in water; 10% D-fructose in normal saline solution; lactated potassic saline; 10% invert sugar in normal saline solution; 10% invert sugar plus 0.3% potassium chloride in water; Travert 10% Electrolyte #1, #2, or #3; or lactated Ringer's solution. Dilute to a final concentration of 0.5 to 40 mg/mL.
- Know that drug is also available in ADD-Vantage vials with diluent and volume specified on label for use with ADD-Vantage infusion sets for piggyback administration. Discard solution after 24 hours at room temperature.
- Do not mix with other drugs.

Infusion considerations

- For direct I.V. injection, administer slowly over approximately 10 minutes.
- For intermittent I.V. infusion, administer slowly over 10 to 30 minutes.
- For continuous I.V. infusion, administer slowly for up to 6 hours.

Be aware that too-rapid infusion may cause vein irritation and seizures.

Monitoring

Stay alert for severe anaphylaxis; be prepared to intervene appropriately.

Monitor CBC with white cell differential. Watch for signs and symptoms of blood dyscrasias.

Assess neurologic status carefully. Stay alert for seizures and impending coma.

Observe bowel movements for severe persistent diarrhea (with or without fever) and pus in stool.

- Watch for signs and symptoms of infection. If therapeutic effects do not occur, obtain specimens for repeat culture tests.
- Monitor liver function tests.

Storage

- Know that when diluted with compatible solution for I.V. infusion, drug is stable at room temperature for 6 hours.

Contraindications and precautions

Contraindicated in hypersensitivity to drug or other penicillins.

Use cautiously in renal disorders, pregnant or breastfeeding patients, and ***neonates.***

Adverse reactions

CNS: depression, agitation, confusion, anxiety, hallucinations, lethargy, twitching, neuropathy, neuromuscular irritability, **seizures, coma**
CV: thrombophlebitis
GI: nausea, vomiting, diarrhea, abdominal pain, enterocolitis, oral lesions, **pseudomembranous colitis**
GU: proteinuria, hematuria, vaginitis, candidiasis, **oliguria, glomerulonephritis**

Hematologic: anemia, eosinophilia, **hemolytic anemia, thrombocytopenia, neutropenia, granulocytopenia, increased bleeding, bone marrow depression**
Hepatic: hepatotoxicity
Other: overgrowth of nonsusceptible organisms, hypersensitivity reactions including **anaphylaxis, serum sickness**

Interactions

Drug-drug. *Aminoglycosides:* aminoglycoside inactivation
Aspirin, disulfiram, probenecid: increased oxacillin blood level, increased bone marrow depression
Hormonal contraceptives: decreased contraceptive efficacy
Rifampin, tetracyclines: decreased antimicrobial activity
Drug-diagnostic tests. *Alanine aminotransferase, alkaline phosphatase, aspartate aminotransferase, eosinophils, low-density lipoproteins:* increased
Granulocytes, hemoglobin, neutrophils, platelets: decreased

Toxicity and overdose

- No information on overdose is available. Expect signs and symptoms to include neuromuscular sensitivity and seizures.
- Provide symptomatic and supportive therapy, as indicated. Know that dialysis may not remove drug.

Patient teaching

- Instruct patient to complete entire course of therapy even if he feels better.
- Advise patient to immediately report rash, easy bruising or bleeding, difficulty breathing, nausea, unusual fatigue, yellowing of skin or eyes, severe diarrhea, and black or furry tongue.
- Caution patient to avoid driving and other hazardous activities until drug's effects on concentration and alertness are known.
- As appropriate, review all other significant and life-threatening adverse reactions and interactions, especially those related to the drugs and tests mentioned above.

oxaliplatin

Eloxitan

Pharmacologic class: Alkylator
Therapeutic class: Antineoplastic
Pregnancy risk category D

FDA BOXED WARNING

- Give under supervision of physician experienced in cancer chemotherapy, in facility with adequate diagnostic and treatment resources.
- Anaphylaxis may occur within minutes of administration. Epinephrine, corticosteroids, and antihistamines have been used to relieve symptoms.

O

Action

Unclear. Thought to form reactive platinum complexes that inhibit DNA synthesis through formation of interstrand and intrastrand cross-linking of DNA molecules. Cell-cycle-phase nonspecific.

Pharmacokinetics

Drug distributes rapidly into body tissues after rapid, extensive biotransformation into active drug and metabolites. It is more than 90% protein-bound, and is eliminated in urine. Terminal half-life is long (about 390 hours).

Onset	Peak	Duration
Unknown	Unknown	Unknown

How supplied

Powder for reconstitution for injection (lyophilized): 50 mg and 100 mg in single-use vials

Indications and dosages

➢ Metastatic cancer of colon or rectum, given with 5-fluorouracil (5-FU) and leucovorin

Adults: On day 1, 85 mg/m^2 oxaliplatin I.V. infusion and 200 mg/m^2 leucovorin; give both drugs simultaneously over 2 hours, followed by 400 mg/m^2 I.V. bolus of 5-FU over 2 to 4 minutes, and then 600 mg/m^2 5-FU I.V. infusion as 22-hour continuous infusion. On day 2, 200 mg/m^2 leucovorin I.V. infusion over 2 hours, followed by 400 mg/m^2 5-FU I.V. bolus over 2 to 4 minutes, and then 600 mg/m^2 5-FU I.V. infusion as 22-hour continuous infusion.

➢ Adjuvant treatment of stage III colon cancer in patients who have undergone complete resection of primary tumor

Adults: In combination with infusional 5-FU/leucovorin as for first indication (metastatic cancer) above. Therapy is recommended for a total of 6 months (12 cycles), given every 2 weeks according to dosage schedule described for previously treated patients with advanced colorectal cancer.

Dosage adjustment

- Be aware that prolonging infusion time from 2 to 6 hours may help ease acute toxicities; 5-FU and leucovorin infusion times do not need to be changed.
- Reduce dosage in patients who experience persistent Grade 2 neurosensory toxicities that do not resolve. In those with persistent Grade 3 neurosensory toxicities, prescriber may decide to withdraw therapy. Be aware that 5-FU/leucovorin regimen dosages do not need to be altered.
- Know that dosage reductions for oxaliplatin and 5-FU are recommended after recovery from Grade 3 or 4 GI toxicity (despite prophylactic treatment) or Grade 4 neutropenia or Grade 3/4 thrombocytopenia. Delay next dose until neutrophil count is at least 1.5×10^9/L and platelet count is at least 75×10^9/L.

Off-label uses

- Esophageal cancer
- Head and neck cancer
- Non-small-cell lung cancer
- Ovarian cancer

Administration

Preparation

Follow guideline on page S19 for handling, preparation, and administering mutagenic, teratogenic, and carcinogenic drugs.

- Be aware that leucovorin is not used as a rescue agent when given as part of colon cancer regimen with oxaliplatin and 5-FU. Instead, it is used to enhance 5-FU cytotoxicity.
- Premedicate patient with antiemetics, as prescribed.

Dilution and compatibility

- Reconstitute 50-mg or 100-mg vial with 10 mL or 20 mL sterile water or D_5W for injection, respectively.

Know that reconstituted drug must be further diluted in 250 to 500 mL D_5W solution.

Do not reconstitute or dilute with normal saline solution for injection or other solutions containing chloride.

- Know that drug is incompatible with alkaline solution and drugs such as 5-FU, and must not be mixed with these.

Infusion considerations

Infuse over 2 hours simultaneously with leucovorin, but in a separate I.V. bag.

- Do not give simultaneously through same I.V. line with 5-FU or other alkaline solutions or drugs.

- Do not use administration sets or needles that contain aluminum.

Clinical alert: Avoid extravasation, which may cause necrosis and other severe reactions.

Monitoring

Clinical alert: Know that anaphylactic-like reactions may occur within minutes of administration. Be prepared to administer epinephrine, corticosteroids, and antihistamines.

Clinical alert: Continue to monitor I.V. site frequently to avoid extravasation.

Clinical alert: Watch closely for blood dyscrasias, hemolytic uremic syndrome, serious pulmonary problems, and anaphylaxis.

Clinical alert: Stay alert for unexplained respiratory symptoms, such as nonproductive cough, dyspnea, crackles, or radiologic pulmonary infiltrates. Know that drug should be discontinued until interstitial lung disease or pulmonary fibrosis is ruled out.

Clinical alert: Monitor patient closely for signs and symptoms of acute pharyngolaryngeal dysesthesia syndrome, such as dysphagia or dyspnea without laryngospasm or bronchospasm (stridor or wheezing).

- Monitor CBC, blood chemistry, and kidney and liver function tests before each treatment cycle.
- Perform complete neurologic examination before and after each dose; especially check for paresthesia, dysesthesia, hypoesthesia, and proprioceptive deficits.
- Monitor vital signs and ECG. Evaluate cardiovascular and respiratory status closely.
- Assess patient's comfort level. Keep patient warm during infusion to minimize neurologic effects.

Storage

- Store vials under normal lighting at 25°C (77°F); excursions permitted to 15° to 30°C (59° to 86°F).
- After reconstitution in original vial, refrigerate solution at 2° to 8°C (36° to 46°F) for up to 24 hours. After final dilution with D_5W, drug is stable for 6 hours at room temperature of 20° to 25°C (68° to 77°F) or for up to 24 hours when refrigerated at 2° to 8°C.

Contraindications and precautions

Contraindicated in hypersensitivity to drug or platinum products.

Use cautiously in renal impairment, ***elderly patients,*** pregnant or breastfeeding patients, and ***children.***

Adverse reactions

CNS: headache, dizziness, fatigue, insomnia, peripheral neuropathy
CV: cardiac abnormalities
EENT: decreased visual acuity, hearing loss, tinnitus, rhinitis, pharyngitis, acute pharyngolaryngeal dysesthesia syndrome
GI: severe nausea, vomiting, diarrhea, constipation, dyspepsia, gastroesophageal reflux, mucositis, flatulence, stomatitis, anorexia
GU: hematuria, dysuria
Hematologic: anemia, **thrombocytopenia, leukopenia, pancytopenia, neutropenia, hemolytic uremic syndrome**
Metabolic: hypokalemia, hyperglycemia, hyponatremia, hypocalcemia, hypoalbuminemia
Respiratory: dyspnea, cough, upper respiratory tract infection, **pulmonary fibrosis**
Skin: alopecia, rash, flushing, **Stevens Johnson syndrome**
Other: weight loss, fever, increased cold sensitivity, pain at injection site, extravasation, **angioedema, anaphylaxis**

Interactions

Drug-drug. *Aminoglycosides, loop diuretics:* increased risk of nephrotoxicity
Aspirin, nonsteroidal anti-inflammatory drugs: increased risk of bleeding
Live-virus vaccines: decreased antibody response to vaccine
Myelosuppressants: increased bone marrow depression

O

Drug-diagnostic tests. *Alanine aminotransferase, aspartate aminotransferase, bilirubin, blood glucose, creatinine:* increased
Albumin, calcium, hemoglobin, neutrophils, platelets, potassium, sodium, white blood cells: decreased
Drug-behaviors. *Alcohol use:* increased risk of bleeding

Toxicity and overdose

- Overdose may cause paresthesia, nausea, vomiting, diarrhea, thrombocytopenia, myelosuppression, and neurotoxicity.
- No known antidote exists. Monitor patient closely and provide symptomatic and supportive therapy.

Patient teaching

- Inform patient that chemotherapy drugs can cause many adverse effects.
- Tell patient to immediately report itching, hives, swelling of hands or face, chest tightness, difficulty breathing, unsteadiness, severe diarrhea or vomiting, and tingling sensation in hands, arms, legs, or feet.
- Instruct patient to promptly notify prescriber of unusual bleeding or bruising, black tarry stools, blood in urine or stools, or pinpoint red spots on skin.
- Advise patient of increased risk of infection. Instruct patient to avoid contact with persons who have infections and to notify prescriber at once if fever or other signs or symptoms of infection occur.
- Instruct patient to inform nurse immediately if pain or redness occurs at I.V. site.
- Tell patient that acute neurosensory toxicity may occur or worsen with exposure to cold. Instruct patient to avoid cold beverages and ice, cover exposed skin before exposure to cold temperatures or cold objects, avoid ice packs, avoid deep inhalations of cold air, and avoid running air conditioning at high levels in home or car.
- As appropriate, review all other significant and life-threatening adverse reactions and interactions, especially those related to the drugs, tests, and behaviors mentioned above.

oxymorphone hydrochloride

Opana

Pharmacologic class: Opioid agonist
Therapeutic class: Opioid analgesic
Controlled substance schedule II
Pregnancy risk category C

Action

Unclear. Thought to interact with opioid receptor sites primarily in limbic system, thalamus, and spinal cord, blocking pain impulse transmission.

Pharmacokinetics

Drug distributes widely in body tissues and crosses placental barrier. It is metabolized primarily in the liver. Less than 1% of dose is excreted in urine unchanged; remainder is excreted in urine and feces as metabolites.

Onset	Peak	Duration
5-10 min	30-60 min	3-6 hr

How supplied

Solution for injection: 1 mg/mL in 1-mL ampules, 1.5 mg/mL in 10-mL multidose vials

Indications and dosages

➤ Moderate to severe pain; preoperative medication for support of anesthesia; obstetric analgesia; anxiolysis in patients with dyspnea associated with pulmonary

edema secondary to acute left ventricular dysfunction
Adults: Initially, 0.5 mg I.V., increased cautiously until pain relief or desired response occurs

Dosage adjustment

- In mild hepatic impairment, start therapy at lowest dosage and titrate slowly while carefully monitoring for adverse effects.
- Titrate dosage to adequate pain relief (generally no pain or mild pain). Patients who experience breakthrough pain may require dosage adjustment or nonopioid pain-relief therapy, such as acetaminophen or nonsteroidal anti-inflammatory drugs.
- Adjust subsequent dosages to obtain appropriate balance between pain relief and opioid-related adverse reactions.

Administration

Preparation

Keep naloxone available to reverse respiratory depression, if necessary.

Dilution and compatibility

- Know that drug may be given undiluted, or may be diluted with 5 mL sterile water for injection or normal saline solution for injection.

Infusion considerations

- Give I.V. dose by direct injection over 2 to 3 minutes; titrate dosage based on symptom relief.

Monitoring

Closely monitor respiratory status. Stay alert for respiratory depression and allergic responses affecting bronchi and larynx.

- Monitor vital signs and ECG.
- Assess neurologic status carefully. Institute protective measures as needed.
- With prolonged use, watch for signs and symptoms of drug dependence.

Do not stop drug abruptly in physically dependent patient.

Storage

- Store at 25°C (77°F); excursions permitted from 15° to 30°C (59° to 86°F).

Contraindications and precautions

Contraindicated in hypersensitivity to drug, its components, or morphine analogues; respiratory depression (except in monitored setting); acute or severe bronchial asthma; upper airway obstruction; hypercarbia; suspicion of paralytic ileus; or moderate to severe hepatic impairment.

Use with extreme caution in conditions accompanied by hypoxia, hypercapnia, or decreased respiratory reserve (such as asthma, chronic obstructive pulmonary disease, severe obesity, myxedema, or sleep apnea). Use cautiously in mild hepatic impairment, renal impairment, pulmonary edema secondary to chemical irritant, circulatory shock, or head trauma; increased intracranial pressure; hypothyroidism; adrenal insufficiency; urethral stricture; undiagnosed abdominal pain or prostatic hypertrophy; extensive burns; alcoholism; biliary tract disease (including acute pancreatitis); history of substance abuse; prolonged or high-dose therapy; ***elderly or debilitated patients;*** labor and delivery; pregnant or breastfeeding patients; and ***children younger than age 1.***

Adverse reactions

CNS: headache, drowsiness, confusion, dysphoria, euphoria, dizziness, hallucinations, lethargy, impaired mental and physical performance, depression, restlessness, insomnia, paradoxical stimulation, **seizures**
CV: hypotension, orthostatic hypotension, palpitations, **bradycardia, tachycardia**
EENT: blurred vision, miosis, diplopia, visual disturbances, tinnitus

O

GI: nausea, vomiting, constipation, biliary tract spasm, cramps, dry mouth, anorexia, **paralytic ileus, toxic megacolon**
GU: urinary hesitancy, urine retention, urethral spasm, antidiuretic effect
Respiratory: suppressed cough reflex, **atelectasis, respiratory depression, allergic bronchospastic reaction, allergic laryngeal edema or laryngospasm, apnea**
Skin: rash, urticaria, pruritus, facial flushing, diaphoresis
Other: physical or psychological drug dependence, drug tolerance, allergic reaction, injection site reaction

Interactions

Drug-drug. *Antihistamines (first-generation), antipsychotics, barbiturates, general anesthetics, monoamine oxidase inhibitors, sedative-hypnotics, skeletal muscle relaxants, tricyclic antidepressants:* increased risk of respiratory depression
Drug-diagnostic tests. *Amylase, lipase:* increased
Drug-behaviors. *Alcohol use or abuse, opiate abuse:* increased risk of respiratory depression

Toxicity and overdose

- Overdose signs and symptoms include respiratory depression, skeletal muscle flaccidity, cold and clammy skin, constricted pupils, bradycardia, hypothermia, hypotension, circulatory collapse and shock, apnea, pulmonary edema, seizures, extreme somnolence leading to stupor or coma, and cardiopulmonary arrest. Death may occur.
- Establish patent airway and institute assisted or controlled ventilation, as ordered. Closely monitor vital signs, neurologic status, and electrolyte balance and other laboratory parameters. Use supportive measures (including oxygen and vasopressors), as ordered, to manage circulatory shock and pulmonary edema. Cardiac arrest or arrhythmias may warrant cardiac massage or defibrillation. Pure opioid antagonist (such as naloxone) is specific antidote for respiratory depression; nalmefene may be given as alternative. Do not give opioid antagonist unless patient has significant respiratory or circulatory depression secondary to oxymorphone overdose.

Patient teaching

- Instruct patient to immediately report seizures or difficulty breathing.
- Teach patient to rise slowly when changing position, to avoid dizziness from blood pressure decrease.
- Instruct patient to avoid alcohol.
- Caution patient not to drive or perform other hazardous activities during therapy.
- Advise patient not to stop taking drug suddenly after several weeks, because withdrawal symptoms may occur.
- As appropriate, review all other significant and life-threatening adverse reactions and interactions, especially those related to the drugs, tests, and behaviors mentioned above.

oxytocin

Pitocin, Syntocinon✤

Pharmacologic class: Posterior pituitary hormone
Therapeutic class: Uterine-active agent
Pregnancy risk category A

FDA BOXED WARNING

- Drug is not indicated for elective induction of labor (labor initiation in pregnant woman with no medical indications for induction). Available data are inadequate to evaluate benefits versus risk.

Action
Unclear. Thought to directly stimulate smooth-muscle contractions in uterus and cervix.

Pharmacokinetics
Drug distributes throughout extracellular fluid; small amounts may enter fetal circulation. It is metabolized rapidly in the liver and kidneys, and has a short half-life. Only small amounts are excreted in urine.

Onset	Peak	Duration
Immediate	40 min	1 hr

How supplied
Solution for injection (clear, colorless aqueous): 10-units/mL ampule or vial

Indications and dosages
➢ To induce or stimulate labor
Adults: Initially, 1-mL ampule (10 units) in compatible I.V. solution infused I.V. at 1 to 2 milliunits/minute (0.001 to 0.002 unit/minute). Increase rate in increments of 1 to 2 milliunits/minute q 15 to 30 minutes until acceptable contraction pattern is established.
➢ To control postpartum bleeding
Adults: 10 to 40 units in compatible I.V. solution infused I.V. at rate adequate to control bleeding
➢ Incomplete abortion
Adults: 10 units in compatible I.V. solution infused I.V. at 10 to 20 milliunits/minute (0.01 to 0.02 unit/minute)

Off-label uses
- Antepartal fetal heart rate testing

Administration
Preparation
Know that drug should be given only to inpatients at critical care facilities when prescriber is immediately available.
Dilution and compatibility
- Dilute by adding 1 mL (10 units) to 1,000 mL normal saline solution, lactated Ringer's solution, or D_5W.

Infusion considerations
Do not give by I.V. bolus injection.
- Infuse I.V. using controlled-infusion device.

Do not exceed 30 units in 12-hour period, because of risk of water intoxication.
Monitoring
Continuously monitor contractions, fetal and maternal heart rate, and maternal blood pressure and ECG. Discontinue infusion if uterine hyperactivity occurs.
Monitor patient extremely closely during first and second stages of labor, due to risk of cervical laceration, uterine rupture, and maternal and fetal death.
Assess fluid intake and output. Watch for signs and symptoms of water intoxication.
- When giving drug to control postpartum bleeding, monitor and record vaginal bleeding.

Storage
- Store at controlled room temperature.

Contraindications and precautions
Contraindicated in hypersensitivity to drug, cephalopelvic disproportion, fetal distress when delivery is not imminent, prolonged use in uterine inertia or severe toxemia, hypertonic or hyperactive uterine pattern, unfavorable fetal position or presentation that is undeliverable without conversion, and labor induction or augmentation when vaginal delivery is contraindicated (as in invasive cervical cancer, active genital herpes, or total placenta previa).

Use cautiously in patients with previous cervical or uterine surgery, history of uterine sepsis, and pregnant or breastfeeding patients.

Adverse reactions

CNS: seizures or coma (from water intoxication), **neonatal brain damage, subarachnoid hemorrhage**
CV: premature ventricular contractions, **arrhythmias, neonatal bradycardia**
GI: nausea, vomiting
GU: postpartum hemorrhage; pelvic hematoma; uterine hypertonicity, spasm, or tetanic contraction; abruptio placentae; uterine rupture (with excessive doses)
Hematologic: afibrinogenemia
Hepatic: neonatal jaundice
Other: hypersensitivity reactions including **anaphylaxis; low 5-minute Apgar score** (neonates)

Interactions

Drug-drug. *Sympathomimetics:* postpartum hypertension
Thiopental anesthetics: delayed anesthesia induction
Vasoconstrictors: severe hypertension (when given within 3 to 4 hours of oxytocin)
Drug-herb. *Ephedra (ma huang):* increased hypertension

Toxicity and overdose

- Uterine hyperstimulation with hypertonic or tetanic contractions and resting tone of 15 to 20 mm H_2O or higher between contractions can lead to such complications as tumultuous labor, uterine rupture, cervical and vaginal lacerations, postpartum hemorrhage, impaired uterine blood flow, and fetal hypoxia. Water intoxication with seizures may occur if large doses are infused for long periods.
- Because of drug's short half-life, withdrawal should relieve symptoms. As ordered and indicated, also restrict fluid intake, initiate diuresis, administer hypertonic saline solution, correct electrolyte imbalance, control seizures with barbiturate (using caution), and use other supportive measures.

Patient teaching

- Inform patient about risks and benefits of oxytocin-induced labor.
- Teach patient to recognize and immediately report adverse drug effects.
- As appropriate, review all other significant and life-threatening adverse reactions and interactions, especially those related to the drugs and herbs mentioned above.

paclitaxel

Onxol, Paxene ❉, Taxol

Pharmacologic class: Antimicrotubule agent
Therapeutic class: Antineoplastic
Pregnancy risk category D

FDA BOXED WARNING

- Give injection under supervision of physician experienced in use of cancer chemotherapy, in facility with adequate diagnostic and treatment resources.
- Anaphylaxis and severe hypersensitivity reactions may occur despite premedication. All patients should be pretreated with corticosteroids, diphenhydramine, and histamine$_2$ antagonists. Do not give drug to patients who have had previous severe reactions.
- Do not administer to patients with solid tumors whose baseline neutrophil counts are below 1,500/mm^3 or to patients with AIDS-related Kaposi's sarcoma whose baseline neutrophil counts are below 1,000/mm^3. To monitor for bone marrow suppression, obtain frequent peripheral blood cell counts on all patients.

• Albumin form of drug may substantially affect drug's functional properties. Do not substitute for or use with other paclitaxel forms.

Action

Stabilizes cellular microtubules to prevent depolymerization. This action inhibits microtubule network (essential for vital interphase and mitotic cellular functions) and induces abnormal microtubule arrays or bundles throughout cell cycle and during mitosis.

Pharmacokinetics

Drug is metabolized in the liver by several enzymes; it is largely protein-bound. Primary clearance route is not fully understood. A small amount of unchanged drug appears in urine.

Onset	Peak	Duration
Unknown	Unknown	Unknown

How supplied

Concentrate for injection: 30 mg/5-mL vial, 100 mg/16.7-mL vial, 300 mg/50-mL vial

Indications and dosages

➢ Advanced ovarian cancer

Adults: As first-line therapy, 175 mg/m² I.V. over 3 hours q 3 weeks, or 135 mg/m² I.V. over 24 hours q 3 weeks, followed by cisplatin. After failure of first-line therapy, 135 mg/m² I.V. or 175 mg/m² I.V. over 3 hours q 3 weeks.

➢ Breast cancer after failure of combination chemotherapy

Adults: As adjuvant treatment for node-positive breast cancer, 175 mg/m² I.V. over 3 hours q 3 weeks for four courses sequentially with doxorubicin combination chemotherapy. After chemotherapy failure for metastatic disease or relapse within 6 months of adjuvant therapy, 175 mg/m² I.V. over 3 hours q 3 weeks.

➢ Non-small-cell lung cancer

Adults: 135 mg/m² I.V. over 24 hours q 3 weeks, followed by cisplatin

➢ AIDS-related Kaposi's sarcoma

Adults: 135 mg/m² I.V. over 3 hours q 3 weeks, or 100 mg/m² I.V. over 3 hours q 2 weeks

Dosage adjustment

• For treatment of Kaposi's sarcoma, adjust dosages as follows for patients with advanced AIDS: Reduce dosage of dexamethasone (as one of three premedication drugs); initiate or repeat paclitaxel treatment only if neutrophil count is at least 1,000/mm³; reduce paclitaxel dosage in subsequent courses by 20% for patients with severe neutropenia (neutrophil count below 500/mm³ for 1 week or more); and initiate concomitant hematopoietic growth factor (G-CSF), as indicated. Do not repeat paclitaxel course until neutrophil count is 1,500/mm³ or higher and platelet count is 100,000/mm³ or higher. Reduce dosage by 20% for subsequent courses in patients who experience severe neutropenia or severe peripheral neuropathy during therapy.

• In patients with solid tumors (ovary, breast, or non-small-cell lung cancer), do not repeat paclitaxel course until neutrophil count is at least 1,500/mm³ and platelet count is at least 100,000/mm³.

• Be aware that patients with hepatic impairment may be at increased risk for toxicity (especially Grade 3-4 myelosuppression) and require dosage adjustment for first course.

Off-label uses

• Advanced gastric cancer
• Advanced head and neck cancer
• Metastatic esophageal cancer
• Prostate cancer

P

Administration

Preparation

Follow hazardous drug guidelines on page S19 for handling, preparation, and administration.

- To prevent severe hypersensitivity reaction, premedicate with dexamethasone 20 mg P.O., as prescribed, 12 and 6 hours before infusion. Also give diphenhydramine 50 mg I.V., plus either cimetidine 300 mg I.V. or ranitidine 50 mg I.V. 30 to 60 minutes before paclitaxel, as prescribed.

Dilution and compatibility

- Dilute in D_5W, normal saline solution, dextrose 5% in Ringer's solution, or dextrose 5% in normal saline solution to a final concentration of 0.3 mg/mL to 1.2 mg/mL.
- Do not use solution if discolored; however, haziness does not affect potency.

Infusion considerations

- Administer through polyethylene-lined administration set attached to 0.22-micron inline filter.
- Give at prescribed rate.

Monitoring

If severe hypersensitivity reaction occurs, stop infusion immediately and give epinephrine, I.V. fluids, and additional antihistamine and corticosteroid doses, as indicated and prescribed.

- Monitor heart rate and blood pressure.
- Continue to assess infusion site for local effects and extravasation, especially during prolonged infusions.

Monitor CBC with platelet count. If neutropenia develops, monitor patient for infection; if thrombocytopenia develops, watch for signs and symptoms of bleeding.

- If patient has preexisting cardiac conduction abnormality, maintain continuous cardiac monitoring.
- Monitor liver function tests results.

Storage

- Store unopened vials between 20° and 25°C (68° and 77°F) in original package.
- Know that diluted solutions can be stored at ambient lighting and ambient temperature of 25°C (77°F) for up to 27 hours.

Contraindications and precautions

Contraindicated in hypersensitivity to drug or castor oil, solid tumors in patients with baseline neutrophil count below 1,500/mm^3, and AIDS-related Kaposi's sarcoma in patients with baseline neutrophil count below 1,000/mm^3.

Use cautiously in increased serum bilirubin level, hepatic impairment, active infection, decreased bone marrow reserve, chronic debilitating illness, cardiovascular disease, CNS disorders, patients with childbearing potential, ***elderly patients,*** pregnant patients, breast-feeding patients (not recommended), and ***children*** (safety not established).

Adverse reactions

CNS: peripheral neuropathy
CV: hypotension, hypertension, syncope, abnormal ECG, bradycardia, **venous thrombosis**
GI: nausea, vomiting, diarrhea, stomatitis, mucositis
Hematologic: anemia, **bleeding, leukopenia, neutropenia, thrombocytopenia**
Musculoskeletal: joint pain, myalgia
Skin: alopecia, radiation reactions
Other: infection, injection site reaction, hypersensitivity reactions including **anaphylaxis**

Interactions

Drug-drug. *Cisplatin:* increased bone marrow depression (when paclitaxel dose follows cisplatin dose)
Cyclosporine, diazepam, doxorubicin, felodipine, ketoconazole, midazolam:

inhibited paclitaxel metabolism and greater risk of toxicity
CYP2C8 and 3A4 enzyme inducers (such as carbamazepine, efavirenz, nevirapine, phenytoin, rifampin): decreased paclitaxel blood level and efficacy
CYP2C8 and 3A4 inhibitors (such as erythromycin, fluoxetine, gemfibrozil): increased paclitaxel blood level and efficacy
Doxorubicin: increased doxorubicin blood level and toxicity
Live-virus vaccines: decreased antibody response to vaccine, increased risk of infection
Other antineoplastics: increased risk of bone marrow depression
Drug-diagnostic tests. *Hemoglobin, neutrophils, platelets:* decreased
Liver function tests: abnormal
Triglycerides: increased

Toxicity and overdose

- Overdose signs and symptoms may include bone marrow depression, peripheral neurotoxicity, mucositis, and other adverse reactions.
- No known antidote exists. Provide symptomatic and supportive therapy.

Patient teaching

- Instruct patient to promptly report pain or burning at injection site.
- Advise neutropenic patient to minimize infection risk by avoiding crowds.
- Tell thrombocytopenic patient to avoid activities that can cause injury and to use soft toothbrush and electric razor.

Clinical alert: Advise patient to promptly report signs and symptoms of infection, bleeding, or peripheral neuropathy (such as numbness and tingling of hands and feet).

- Explain that temporary hair loss is likely to occur.
- As appropriate, review all other significant and life-threatening adverse reactions and interactions, especially those related to the drugs and tests mentioned above.

paclitaxel protein-bound particles

Abraxane

Pharmacologic class: Antimicrotubule agent
Therapeutic class: Antineoplastic
Pregnancy risk category D

FDA BOXED WARNING

- Give injection under supervision of physician experienced in use of cancer chemotherapy, in facility with adequate diagnostic and treatment resources.
- Do not administer to patients with metastatic breast cancer who have baseline neutrophil counts below 1,500/mm^3. To detect bone marrow suppression (primarily neutropenia), which may be severe and result in infection, all patients should undergo frequent peripheral blood cell counts.
- Albumin form of drug may substantially affect functional properties relative to those of drug in solution. Do not substitute for or with other paclitaxel forms.

Action

Promotes assembly of microtubules from tubulin dimers and stabilizes microtubules by preventing depolymerization. This stability inhibits normal dynamic reorganization of microtubule network essential for vital interphase and mitotic cellular functions. Drug induces abnormal arrays or bundles of microtubules throughout cell cycle and multiple asters of microtubules during mitosis.

P

Pharmacokinetics

Protein-bound particle formulation enhances paclitaxel solubility. Large volume of distribution indicates extensive extravascular distribution, tissue binding, or both. Plasma levels fall in biphasic manner; initial rapid decline represents distribution to perpheral compartment, while slower second phase represents drug elimination. Terminal half-life is about 27 hours. Drug undergoes metabolism in the liver. It is excreted in feces, with a small amount excreted in urine.

Onset	Peak	Duration
Unknown	Unknown	Unknown

How supplied

Powder or cake for reconstitution for injection (white to yellow, lyophilized powder): 100-mg single-use vial

Indications and dosages

➤ Breast cancer treatment after failure of combination chemotherapy for metastatic disease or relapse within 6 months of adjuvant therapy. (Previous therapy should have included an anthracycline, unless contraindicated.)
Adults: 260 mg/m^2 I.V. over 30 minutes q 3 weeks

Dosage adjustment

- If severe sensory neuropathy or severe neutropenia (neutrophil count below 500/mm^3 for 1 week or longer) occurs during therapy, reduce dosage to 220 mg/m^2 for subsequent courses. If either condition recurs, make additional dosage decreases to 180 mg/m^2.
- For Grade 3 sensory neuropathy, withhold treatment until condition resolves to Grade 1 or 2, followed by dosage reduction for all subsequent courses.
- Be aware that appropriate dosage for patients with bilirubin levels above 1.5 mg/dL is unknown.

Administration

Preparation

Follow hazardous drug guidelines on page S19 for handling, preparation, and administration.

- Be aware that premedication to prevent hypersensitivity is not required.

Dilution and compatibility

- To reconstitute each vial, slowly inject 20 mL normal saline solution for injection over at least 1 minute by directing solution flow onto inside wall of vial.
- Do not inject solution directly onto lyophilized cake or powder, as this will cause foaming.
- Once injection into vial is complete, let vial sit for at least 5 minutes to ensure proper wetting of lyophilized cake or powder.
- Gently swirl or invert vial slowly for at least 2 minutes until cake or powder dissolves completely. Avoid foaming.
- If foaming or clumping occurs, let solution stand for at least 15 minutes until foam subsides. Do not filter.
- Know that each milliliter of reconstituted formulation contains 5 mg/mL paclitaxel. Use this formula to calculate exact total dosing volume of 5 mg/mL suspension required: dosing volume (mL) = total dose (mg)/5 (mg/mL).
- Ensure complete resuspension by agitating mildly before use. Discard reconstituted suspension if precipitation or discoloration appears.
- Use reconstituted suspension immediately.
- Discard unused portion.

Infusion considerations

- Administer by I.V. infusion over 30 minutes.

Monitoring
Be aware that patients should not be retreated in subsequent cycles until neutrophil count rises above 1,500/mm^3 and platelet count rises above 100,000/mm^3.
• Monitor ECG and liver function tests results.
• Because extravasation may occur, closely monitor infusion site for possible infiltration.
• Limit infusion to 30 minutes, as prescribed, to reduce likelihood of infusion-related reactions.
Storage
• Store vial in original carton at 20° to 25°C (68° to 77°F); protect from bright light.
• If reconstituted drug is not used immediately, store at 2° to 8°C (36° to 46°F) for a maximum of 8 hours if necessary.

Contraindications and precautions

Contraindicated in baseline neutrophil count below 1,500/mm^3.

Use cautiously in increased serum bilirubin level, hepatic impairment, cardiovascular disease, CNS disorder, ***elderly patients,*** pregnant or breast-feeding patients, and ***children*** (safety and efficacy not established).

Adverse reactions

CNS: sensory neuropathy, asthenia
CV: hypotension, severe cardiovascular events, abnormal ECG
EENT: vision disturbances
GI: nausea, vomiting, diarrhea, mucositis
Hematologic: anemia, **bleeding, leukopenia, neutropenia, febrile neutropenia, thrombocytopenia**
Musculoskeletal: myalgia, arthralgia
Respiratory: cough, dyspnea
Skin: alopecia
Other: fluid retention, edema, injection site reaction, hypersensitivity reaction

Interactions

Drug-diagnostic tests. *Alkaline phosphatase, aspartate aminotransferase, bilirubin:* increased
Hemoglobin, neutrophils, platelets: decreased

Toxicity and overdose

• In overdose, expect bone marrow suppression, sensory neurotoxicity, and mucositis.
• No known antidote exists. Provide symptomatic and supportive therapy.

Patient teaching

• Advise patient to promptly report pain or burning at injection site.
Inform patient that drug increases susceptibility to infection and fever. Instruct patient to promptly report fever or other signs or symptoms of infection.
• Teach neutropenic patient to minimize infection risk by avoiding crowds and persons with infections.
• Instruct thrombocytopenic patient to avoid activities that can cause injury and to use soft toothbrush and electric razor.
• Teach patient to report sensory neuropathy (numbness, tingling, or burning in hands and feet).
• Advise patient about potential side effects, such as blood pressure decrease, weakness, fatigue, muscle pains, and redness or sores of mouth or lips.
• Inform patient that drug may cause vision disturbances, particularly at higher doses.
• Tell patient drug usually causes complete hair loss (eyebrows, eyelashes, pubic hair, and scalp hair), but that hair generally grows back after treatment ends.
• Advise women of childbearing potential to avoid becoming pregnant during therapy.
• Caution women to discontinue breast-feeding while taking drug.

P

- Advise males not to father a child during therapy.
- As appropriate, review all other life-threatening and significant adverse reactions and interactions, especially those related to the tests mentioned above.

palifermin

Kepivance

Pharmacologic class: Keratinocyte growth factor (KGF) (rDNA origin)
Therapeutic class: Biologic and immunologic agent
Pregnancy risk category C

Action

Produced by recombinant DNA technology in *Escherichia coli;* binds to KGF receptor on cell surface, resulting in epithelial cell proliferation, differentiation, and migration

Pharmacokinetics

Drug's extravascular distribution and elimination half-life are similar in both healthy subjects and cancer patients; half-life averages 4.5 hours, with a range of 3.3 to 5.7 hours.

Onset	Peak	Duration
Unknown	Unknown	Unknown

How supplied

Powder for reconstitution for injection (white, lyophilized, preservative-free): 6.25 mg in single-use vials

Indications and dosages

➢ To decrease incidence and duration of severe oral mucositis in patients with hematologic cancers who are receiving myelotoxic therapy requiring hematopoietic stem cell support

Adults: 60 mcg/kg/day I.V. bolus injection for 3 consecutive days before and 3 consecutive days after myelotoxic therapy, for a total of six doses. Give first three doses before myelotoxic therapy, with third dose administered 24 to 48 hours before such therapy. Give last three doses after myelotoxic therapy, with first of these given after (but on same day of) hematopoietic stem cell infusion and at least 4 days after most recent palifermin dose.

Administration

Dilution and compatibility

- Reconstitute powder with 1.2 mL sterile water for injection to yield a final concentration of 5 mg/mL.
- Swirl vial gently during dissolution; do not shake or vigorously agitate.
- Do not filter reconstituted solution during preparation or administration.
- Use immediately (within 1 hour) after reconstituting; protect from light.
- Know that reconstituted solution should be clear and colorless.

Infusion considerations

- When heparin is used to maintain I.V. line, use normal saline solution to flush line before and after palifermin administration. (Drug may bind to heparin.)
- Administer by I.V. bolus injection.

Monitoring

- Monitor serum amylase and lipase levels frequently.

Storage

- Refrigerate in carton at 2° to 8°C (36° to 46°F).

Contraindications and precautions

Contraindicated in hypersensitivity to drug, its components, or *E. coli*–derived proteins.

Use cautiously in nonhematologic cancers, ***elderly patients,*** pregnant or breastfeeding patients, and ***children*** (safety and efficacy not established).

Adverse reactions

CNS: dysesthesia
CV: hypertension
EENT: tongue discoloration or thickening
GU: proteinuria
Musculoskeletal: pain, arthralgia
Skin: rash, pruritus, skin toxicities, erythema
Other: altered taste, edema, fever

Interactions

Drug-drug. *Heparin:* possible binding
Drug-diagnostic tests. *Amylase, lipase, protein:* increased

Toxicity and overdose

- Maximum amount that can be safely given in a single dose is undetermined. In overdose, expect signs and symptoms that resemble adverse reactions but may be more severe.
- Provide symptomatic and supportive therapy.

Patient teaching

- Instruct patient to report adverse reactions, including rash, itching, skin redness, swelling, discolored tongue, and altered taste.
- As appropriate, review all other significant adverse reactions and interactions, especially those related to the drugs and tests mentioned above.

palonosetron hydrochloride

Aloxi

Pharmacologic class: Selective serotonin subtype 3 ($5\text{-}HT_3$) receptor antagonist
Therapeutic class: Antiemetic
Pregnancy risk category B

Action

Selectively binds to and antagonizes $5\text{-}HT_3$ receptors on vagal nerve terminals and chemoreceptor trigger zone. This action blocks serotonin release, reducing the vomiting reflex.

Pharmacokinetics

Drug is partially metabolized, approximately 62% protein-bound, and slowly eliminated in urine. Mean terminal elimination half-life is approximately 40 hours.

Onset	Peak	Duration
Unknown	Unknown	Unknown

How supplied

Solution for injection (clear, colorless): 0.25 mg (free base) in 5-mL single-use vial

Indications and dosages

➤ To prevent nausea and vomiting caused by moderately and highly emetogenic cancer chemotherapy; to prevent delayed nausea and vomiting associated with initial and repeat courses of moderately emetogenic cancer chemotherapy
Adults: 0.25 mg I.V. as a single dose 30 minutes before chemotherapy.

Administration

Dilution and compatibility

- Be aware that drug requires no dilution.
- Do not mix with other drugs.

Infusion considerations

- Give 30 minutes before start of chemotherapy.
- Administer directly into I.V. line over 30 seconds.
- Flush I.V. line with normal saline solution before and after giving drug.

Monitoring

- Monitor vital signs and ECG. Watch closely for tachycardia, bradycardia, and hypotension.

• Monitor electrolyte levels for fluctuations (especially hyperkalemia and metabolic acidosis).
• Evaluate temperature; stay alert for flulike signs and symptoms.
• Closely monitor blood and urine glucose levels in diabetic patients. Check for hyperglycemia.

Storage
• Store at controlled room temperature of 20° to 25°C (68° to 77°F); excursions permitted from 15° to 30°C (59° to 86°F). Protect from light and freezing.

Contraindications and precautions

Contraindicated in hypersensitivity to drug or its components.

Use cautiously in hypersensitivity to other 5-HT_3 receptor antagonists, diabetes mellitus, hepatic dysfunction, pregnant or breastfeeding patients, and ***children.***

Adverse reactions

CNS: headache, fatigue, insomnia, dizziness, anxiety
CV: hypotension, vein discoloration and distention, nonsustained tachycardia, bradycardia
GI: constipation, diarrhea, abdominal pain, anorexia
GU: glycosuria
Metabolic: fluctuating electrolyte levels, hyperglycemia, **metabolic acidosis, hyperkalemia**
Musculoskeletal: joint pain
Other: fever, flulike symptoms

Interactions

Drug-diagnostic tests: *Alanine aminotransferase, aspartate aminotransferase, bilirubin, blood glucose, potassium, urine glucose:* increased

Toxicity and overdose

• Overdose signs and symptoms include pallor, cyanosis, gasping, seizures, and collapse.
• No known antidote exists. Provide symptomatic and supportive therapy. Be aware that dialysis may not remove drug.

Patient teaching

• Explain that drug helps prevent nausea and vomiting caused by chemotherapy.
• Teach patient to recognize and promptly report signs and symptoms of hyperkalemia and metabolic acidosis.
• Advise patient to report flulike symptoms.
• Instruct diabetic patient to closely monitor blood and urine glucose levels.
• Advise female patient to notify prescriber if she becomes pregnant, is planning pregnancy, or is breastfeeding during therapy.
• As appropriate, review all other significant and life-threatening adverse reactions and interactions, especially those related to the tests mentioned above.

[redacted]

pamidronate disodium

Aredia

Pharmacologic class: Bisphosphonate, hypocalcemic
Therapeutic class: Bone resorption inhibitor
Pregnancy risk category D

Action

Inhibits normal and abnormal bone resorption and decreases calcium levels

Pharmacokinetics

Drug is not metabolized. It is eliminated exclusively by the kidneys, with most of dose excreted as unchanged drug in urine in 24 hours.

Onset	Peak	Duration
Unknown	Unknown	Unknown

How supplied

Powder for reconstitution for injection (white to off-white, lyophilized): 30 mg/vial, 90 mg/vial

Indications and dosages

➣ Hypercalcemia caused by cancer
Adults: For moderate hypercalcemia, 60 to 90 mg as a single-dose I.V. infusion over 2 to 24 hours. For severe hypercalcemia, 90 mg as a single-dose I.V. infusion over 2 to 24 hours.

➣ Osteolytic lesions caused by multiple myeloma
Adults: 90 mg I.V. as a 4-hour infusion q month

➣ Osteolytic bone metastases of breast cancer
Adults: 90 mg I.V. as a 2-hour infusion q 3 to 4 weeks

➣ Paget's disease
Adults: 30 mg I.V. daily as a 4-hour infusion for 3 days

Administration

Preparation

• Hydrate patient with normal saline solution for injection before starting therapy, as needed.

Because of risk of renal failure, do not give single doses exceeding 90 mg.

Dilution and compatibility

• Reconstitute vial using 10 mL sterile water for injection. When completely dissolved, further dilute in 250 to 1,000 mL half-normal saline solution, normal saline solution, or D_5W.

• Do not mix with solutions containing calcium, such as lactated Ringer's injection.

Infusion considerations

• Give through separate I.V. line from other drugs and fluids.

• Administer as a 2- to 24-hour infusion, as prescribed.

Monitoring

• Monitor hydration status carefully.

• Assess vital signs and ECG; evaluate cardiovascular and respiratory status closely.

• Assess hematologic studies and creatinine level before each treatment.

• Monitor electrolyte levels, especially calcium, magnesium, and phosphorus.

• Closely monitor fluid intake and output; watch for signs and symptoms of urinary tract infection.

• Monitor for signs of symptoms of jaw osteonecrosis. Be aware that dental examination with appropriate preventive dentistry should be considered before therapy begins if patient has concomitant risk factors (such as cancer, chemotherapy, corticosteroid therapy, or poor oral hygiene).

Storage

• When reconstituted with sterile water for injection, drug may be refrigerated at 2° to 8°C (36° to 46°F) for up to 24 hours.

Contraindications and precautions

Contraindicated in hypersensitivity to drug, its components, or other bisphosphonates.

Use cautiously in renal impairment; patients who will undergo major dental procedures (especially cancer patients), who are at risk for jaw osteonecrosis during therapy; pregnant or breastfeeding patients; and ***children*** (safety not established).

Adverse reactions

CNS: anxiety, headache, insomnia, psychosis, drowsiness, weakness
CV: hypertension, syncope, atrial flutter, tachycardia, **arrhythmias, heart failure**
EENT: sinusitis

P

GI: nausea, vomiting, diarrhea, abdominal pain, constipation, dyspepsia, stomatitis, anorexia, **GI hemorrhage**
GU: urinary tract infection
Hematologic: anemia, **neutropenia, leukopenia, granulocytopenia, thrombocytopenia**
Metabolic: hypothyroidism
Musculoskeletal: bone pain, joint pain, myalgia, osteonecrosis (primarily of jaw)
Respiratory: crackles, coughing, dyspnea, pleural effusion, upper respiratory tract infection
Other: fever, generalized pain, injection site reaction

Interactions

Drug-diagnostic tests. *Calcium, hemoglobin, magnesium, phosphate, platelets, potassium, red blood cells, white blood cells:* decreased
Creatinine: increased

Toxicity and overdose

- Overdose signs and symptoms may include fever, hypotension, transient taste perversion, and hypocalcemia.
- Provide symptomatic and supportive therapy, including steroids for fever and hypotension and calcium I.V. for symptomatic hypocalcemia, as ordered.

Patient teaching

- Advise patient to promptly report significant respiratory problems, peripheral edema, and GI bleeding.
- Inform patient that drug lowers resistance to some infections. Advise patient to immediately report fever and other infection signs and symptoms.
- Teach patient to avoid invasive dental procedures, if possible, during therapy.
- Instruct patient to weigh himself regularly and report sudden gain.
- Explain importance of undergoing laboratory tests before, during, and after therapy.
- Caution patient to avoid driving and other hazardous activities until drug's effects on concentration, cognition, and alertness are known.
- Teach patient to minimize GI upset by eating small, frequent servings of healthy food and drinking plenty of fluids.
- As appropriate, review all other significant and life-threatening adverse reactions and interactions, especially those related to the tests mentioned above.

pancuronium bromide

Pavulon

Pharmacologic class: Nondepolarizing neuromuscular blocker
Therapeutic class: Muscle relaxant, adjunct to anesthesia
Pregnancy risk category C

FDA BOXED WARNING

- Drug should be given by adequately trained individuals who are familiar with its actions, characteristics, and hazards.

Action

Inhibits action of acetylcholine at motor endplate receptor sites, blocking neuromuscular transmission

Pharmacokinetics

Drug is approximately 87% protein-bound, and is excreted in urine unchanged and as metabolites.

Onset	Peak	Duration
2-3 min	Unknown	22-65 min

How supplied

Solution for injection (clear, colorless): 1 mg/mL, 2 mg/mL

Indications and dosages

➢ Adjunct to balanced anesthesia to relax skeletal muscles for intubation

Adults and children age 1 month and older: Initially, 0.04 to 0.1 mg/kg I.V.; may follow with 0.01 mg/kg q 25 to 60 minutes if needed. (Dosage and infusion rates are based on type of anesthesia used and patient needs and response. Dosages given here are typical.)

Administration

Preparation

- Be aware that dosages are highly individualized.
- Make sure patient's analgesic and sedative needs are met; drug does not relieve pain or provide sedation.

Dilution and compatibility

- Know that drug is compatible with normal saline solution, lactated Ringer's solution, D_5W, and dextrose 5% in normal saline solution.

Infusion considerations

- Administer at prescribed rate through established I.V. line containing compatible solution.

Monitoring

- Monitor heart rhythm, vital signs, and pulse oximetry during and after administration.
- Assess patient's sedation level.
- Evaluate fluid intake and output and potassium level.
- Assess muscle recovery using peripheral nerve stimulator and train-of-four monitoring.

Storage

- Refrigerate at 2° to 8°C (36° to 46°F).

Contraindications and precautions

Contraindicated in hypersensitivity to drug.

Use cautiously in cardiac, hepatic, neuromuscular, renal, or respiratory disease; electrolyte imbalances; severe obesity; concurrent use of tricyclic antidepressants; pregnant or breastfeeding patients; and ***neonates.***

Adverse reactions

CV: increased mean arterial pressure, increased cardiac output, tachycardia
GI: salivation
Musculoskeletal: prolonged weakness, prolonged skeletal muscle relaxation
Respiratory: cyanosis, **prolonged apnea, bronchospasm, respiratory insufficiency**
Skin: rash
Other: altered neuromuscular blockade in patients with electrolyte imbalances, hypersensitivity reaction

Interactions

Drug-drug. *Aminoglycosides (such as dihydrostreptomycin, gentamicin, kanamycin, neomycin, streptomycin), colistin, magnesium salts, polymyxin B, potassium-depleting drugs, sodium colistimethate, tetracyclines:* prolonged neuromuscular blockade

Enflurane, halofluorane, isoflurane, succinylcholine: enhanced neuromuscular blockade

Opioid analgesics: additive respiratory depression

Quinidine: recurrent paralysis

Tricyclic antidepressants (when given with both halothane and pancuronium): severe ventricular arrhythmias

Toxicity and overdose

- Overdose signs and symptoms include prolonged respiratory depression, apnea, and cardiovascular collapse.
- Maintain adequate airway and provide manual or mechanical ventilation, as indicated, until patient can maintain unassisted ventilation. Know that neostigmine can reverse drug effects.

P

Patient teaching

- Explain all procedures to patient as appropriate.

pantoprazole sodium

Protium, Protonix IV

Pharmacologic class: Proton pump inhibitor

Therapeutic class: GI antisecretory agent

Pregnancy risk category B

Action

Suppresses gastric acid production and secretion and increases gastric mucus and bicarbonate production, creating a protective coating on gastric mucosa

Pharmacokinetics

Drug is extensively metabolized in the liver to several metabolites with little or no antisecretory activity. It is about 98% protein-bound. Approximately 71% of dose is excreted in urine; remainder is excreted in feces.

Onset	Peak	Duration
15 min	Unknown	>24 hr

How supplied

Powder for reconstitution for injection (freeze-dried): 40 mg/vial

Indications and dosages

➤ Short-term treatment of erosive esophagitis caused by gastroesophageal reflux disease (GERD)

Adults: 40 mg I.V. daily for 7 to 10 days

➤ Pathologic hypersecretory conditions, short-term treatment of GERD in patients with a history of erosive esophagitis as an alternative to oral therapy

Adults:, 80 mg I.V. q 12 hours, up to a maximum of 240 mg/day (80 mg q 8 hours)

Administration

Dilution and compatibility

- For 15-minute infusion, reconstitute with 10 mL normal saline solution for injection; then further dilute in D_5W, normal saline solution, or lactated Ringer's solution, to a final concentration of approximately 0.4 mg/mL.
- For 2-minute infusion, reconstitute with 10 mL normal saline solution for injection to a final concentration of approximately 4 mg/mL.

Infusion considerations

Do not administer through same line with other I.V. solutions.

Know that inline filter (provided) must be used to remove precipitate that may form when reconstituted drug is mixed with I.V. solutions.

- Administer 15-minute I. V. infusion at a rate of approximately 7 mL/minute.

If Y-site is used, place filter below Y-site closest to patient. When administering through Y-site, immediately stop infusion if precipitation or discoloration occurs.

- Flush I.V. line before and after administration with either D_5W, normal saline solution, or lactated Ringer's solution.

Monitoring

- Assess patient for symptomatic improvement.
- Monitor blood glucose level in diabetic patient.

Storage

- Refrigerate at 2° to 8°C (36° to 46°F); protect from light.
- Know that reconstituted solution for 2-minute infusion may be stored for up to 24 hours at room temperature before I.V. infusion and does not need to be protected from light.

• Be aware that reconstituted solution for 15-minute infusion may be stored for up to 6 hours at room temperature before further dilution. Admixed solution may be stored at room temperature; it must be used within 24 hours of initial reconstitution. Neither reconstituted solution nor admixed solution need be protected from light.

Contraindications and precautions

Contraindicated in hypersensitivity to drug.

Use cautiously in severe hepatic disease, pregnant or breastfeeding patients, and ***children.***

Adverse reactions

CNS: dizziness, headache
CV: chest pain
EENT: rhinitis
GI: vomiting, diarrhea, abdominal pain, dyspepsia
Metabolic: hyperglycemia, hyperlipemia
Skin: rash, pruritus
Other: injection site reaction

Interactions

Drug-diagnostic tests. *Aspartate aminotransferase, glucose:* increased
Tetrahydrocannabinol test: false-positive result

Toxicity and overdose

• In overdose (rare), expect extension of adverse reactions.
• Know that drug is not readily dialyzable.

Patient teaching

• Instruct diabetic patient to monitor blood glucose level carefully and stay alert for signs and symptoms of hyperglycemia.
• As appropriate, review all other significant adverse reactions and interactions, especially those related to the tests mentioned above.

paricalcitol

Zemplar

Pharmacologic class: Vitamin D analogue
Therapeutic class: Hypocalcemic agent
Pregnancy risk category C

Action

Along with Vitamin D, reduces parathyroid hormone (PTH) levels by inhibiting PTH synthesis and secretion

Pharmacokinetics

Drug is extensively metabolized by hepatic and nonhepatic enzymes, and is extensively bound to plasma proteins. Most systemic exposure results from parent drug. Mean half-life is about 15 hours. It is excreted primarily by hepatobiliary excretion, with 2% of dose eliminated unchanged in feces. No parent drug is found in urine, but several unknown metabolites are.

Onset	Peak	Duration
Unknown	Unknown	Unknown

How supplied

Solution for injection (clear, colorless, aqueous): 2 mcg/mL and 5 mcg/mL in 1-mL single-dose flip-top vials, 5 mcg/mL in 2-mL fliptop vial

Indications and dosages

➤ Prevention and treatment of secondary hyperparathyroidism caused by chronic renal failure (CRF)
Adults: 0.04 mcg/kg to 0.1 mcg/kg (2.8 to 7 mcg) I.V. bolus no more frequently than every other day at any time during dialysis. If satisfactory response does not occur, dosage may be increased by 2 to 4 mcg at 2- to 4-week intervals.

Dosage adjustment

• If patient is receiving calcium-based phosphate binder (such as calcium acetate or calcium carbonate), decrease dosage or withhold dose, or expect patient to be switched to non-calcium-based phosphate binder.

• Know that dosage may need to be reduced as PTH levels decrease in response to therapy. Thus, incremental dosing must be individualized. The table below is a suggested dosage titration approach.

PTH level	Dosage
Same or increasing	Increase
Decreasing less than 30%	Increase
Decreasing between 31% and 59%	Maintain
Decreasing more than 60%	Decrease
1.5 to 3 times upper limit of normal	Maintain

• During dosage adjustment period, monitor serum calcium and phosphorus levels more frequently. If calcium level increases or the product of calcium times phosphorus exceeds 75, immediately reduce dosage or interrupt therapy until these parameters normalize. Then reinitiate drug at lower dosage.

Administration

Preparation

• Know that accepted target range for intact PTH (iPTH) levels in CRF patients is no more than 1.5 to 3 times the non-uremic upper limit of normal.

Be aware that patient should not receive phosphate or vitamin D–related compounds concomitantly with this drug.

• Obtain baseline serum calcium and phosphorus levels.

Dilution and compatibility

• Know that dilution is not required.

• Discard unused portion of drug.

Infusion considerations

• Give as I.V. bolus at any time during dialysis.

Monitoring

• Initially, monitor serum calcium and phosphorus levels at least twice weekly; after adequate dosing is established, monitor these levels monthly.

• Obtain serum iPTH assay every 3 months.

Monitor for early signs and symptoms of vitamin D intoxication associated with hypercalcemia, such as weakness, headache, somnolence, nausea, vomiting, dry mouth, constipation, muscle pain, bone pain, and metallic taste.

Be aware that late signs and symptoms of vitamin D intoxication associated with hypercalcemia include anorexia; weight loss; calcific conjunctivitis; pancreatitis; photophobia; rhinorrhea; pruritus; hyperthermia; decreased libido; hypercholesterolemia; blood urea nitrogen (BUN), alanine aminotransferase (ALT), and aspartate aminotransferase (AST) elevations; ectopic calcification; hypertension; arrhythmias; somnolence; overt psychosis (rare); and death.

Storage

• Store at 25°C (77°F); excursions permitted from 15° to 30°C (59° to 86°F).

Contraindications and precautions

Contraindicated in hypersensitivity to drug or its components, vitamin D toxicity, and hypercalcemia.

Use cautiously in ***elderly patients,*** pregnant or breastfeeding patients, and ***children.***

Adverse reactions

CNS: dizziness, light-headedness
CV: palpitations
GI: nausea, vomiting, dry mouth, bleeding
Metabolic: vitamin D intoxication

Respiratory: pneumonia
Other: chills, fever, flu, malaise, edema, **sepsis**

Interactions

Drug-drug. *Digitalis preparations:* increased risk of digitalis toxicity
Phosphate, vitamin D compounds: increased risk of hypercalcemia
Drug-diagnostic tests. *Alkaline phosphatase:* reduced
ALT, AST, BUN, cholesterol: decreased

Toxicity and overdose

• Early signs and symptoms of vitamin D intoxication associated with hypercalcemia include weakness, headache, somnolence, nausea, vomiting, dry mouth, constipation, muscle pain, bone pain, and metallic taste.
• For significant hypercalcemia, expect to reduce dosage immediately or to withhold dose, provide low calcium diet, withdraw calcium supplements, perform patient mobilization, check for fluid and electrolyte imbalances, and assess for ECG abnormalities (critical in patients receiving digitalis preparations). Patient may require hemodialysis or peritoneal dialysis against calcium-free dialysate. Monitor serum calcium levels frequently until these normalize.

Patient teaching

• Urge patient to adhere to dietary regimen of calcium supplementation and phosphorus restriction to ensure effectiveness of therapy.
• Instruct patient to avoid excessive use of aluminum-containing compounds, although some calcium forms (phosphate-binding compounds) may be needed to control serum phosphorus levels.
• Teach patient to recognize and report signs and symptoms of elevated calcium.
• As appropriate, review all other significant and life-threatening adverse reactions and interactions, especially those related to the drugs and tests mentioned above.

pemetrexed

Alimta

Pharmacologic class: Folic acid antagonist
Therapeutic class: Antineoplastic, antimetabolite
Pregnancy risk category D

Action

Disrupts folate-dependent metabolic processes essential for cell replication

Pharmacokinetics

Drug is not appreciably metabolized; it is approximately 81% protein-bound. Elimination half-life is 3.5 hours in patients with normal renal function. Drug is primarily eliminated in urine, with 70% to 90% of dose recovered unchanged within first 24 hours.

Onset	Peak	Duration
Unknown	Unknown	Unknown

How supplied

Powder for reconstitution for injection (white to light yellow or greenish yellow, lyophilized): 100 mg in 10-mL single-use vials, 500 mg in 50-mL single-use vials

Indications and dosages

➢ Malignant pleural mesothelioma in patients whose disease is unresectable or who otherwise are not eligible for curative surgery (given with cisplatin)

P

Adults: 500 mg/m^2 I.V. infusion over 10 minutes on day 1 of each 21-day cycle (given in combination with cisplatin infused over 2 hours, starting approximately 30 minutes after pemetrexed administration ends)

➢ Non-small-cell lung cancer

Adults: 500 mg/m^2 I.V. infusion over 10 minutes on day 1 of each 21-day cycle

Dosage adjustment

• Do not start new treatment cycle unless absolute neutrophil count (ANC) is 500/mm^3 or higher, platelet count is 100,000/mm^3 or higher, and creatine clearance is 45 mL/minute or higher.

• At start of subsequent cycle, base dosage adjustment on nadir hematologic counts or maximum nonhematologic toxicity from preceding cycle. Treatment may be delayed to allow sufficient recovery time. On recovery, patients should be retreated according to the following guidelines (which apply to both single-agent use and combination therapy with cisplatin).

Dosage reduction in hematologic toxicities (single-agent use or combination therapy)

ANC nadir below 500/mm^3, platelet nadir 50,000/mm^3 or higher	75% of previous dosage (both drugs)
Platelet nadir below 50,000/mm^3 (regardless of ANC nadir)	50% of previous dosage (both drugs)

• If patient develops nonhematologic toxicities (excluding neurotoxicity) of Grade 3 or higher (except Grade 3 transaminase elevations), withhold drug until these resolve to less than or equal to patient's pretherapy values; then resume drug according to guidelines in table below.

Dosage reduction in nonhematologic toxicities (single-agent use or combination therapy*, †)

	Pemetrexed (mg/m^2)	Cisplatin (mg/m^2)
Any Grade 3‡ or 4 toxicity except mucositis	75% of previous dosage	75% of previous dosage
Any diarrhea requiring hospitalization irrespective of grade, or Grade 3 or 4 diarrhea	75% of previous dosage	75% of previous dosage
Grade 3 or 4 mucositis	50% of previous dosage	100% of previous dosage

*NCI Common Toxicity Criteria; †excluding neurotoxicity; ‡except Grade 3 transaminase elevation

• If neurotoxicity occurs, adjust pemetrexed and cisplatin dosages as described in table below. Discontinue therapy if Grade 3 or 4 neurotoxicity develops.

NCI common toxicity grade	Pemetrexed dosage (mg/m^2)	Cisplatin dosage (mg/m^2)
0 to 1	100% of previous dosage	100% of previous dosage
2	100% of previous dosage	50% of previous dosage

• Discontinue drug if patient experiences any hematologic or nonhematologic Grade 3 or 4 toxicity after two dosage reductions (except Grade 3 transaminase elevations), or immediately if Grade 3 or 4 neurotoxicity develops.

Administration

Preparation

Follow hazardous drug guidelines on page S19 for handling, preparation, and administration.

• When administering pemetrexed with cisplatin, hydrate patient with 1 to 2 L fluid infused over 8 to 12 hours, before and after cisplatin administration. Maintain adequate hydration and urine output for 24 hours.
• Know that patients with mild to moderate renal insufficiency should avoid taking nonsteroidal anti-inflammatory drugs (NSAIDs) with short elimination half-lives (such as aspirin, diclofenac, and ibuprofen) for 5 days before, on day of, and for 2 days after pemetrexed administration. If concomitant NSAID use is necessary, monitor patient closely for toxicities (especially myelosuppression and renal or GI toxicity).
• Be aware that all patients should avoid NSAIDs with long half-lives (such as diflunisal, piroxicam, and sulindac) for at least 5 days before, on day of, and for 2 days after pemetrexed administration. If concomitant NSAID use is necessary, monitor patient closely for toxicities (especially myelosuppression and renal or GI toxicity).
• To minimize cutaneous reaction, pretreat with dexamethasone (or equivalent) 4 mg P.O. twice daily on day before, day of, and day after pemetrexed administration, as prescribed.
• To reduce toxicity, ensure that patient receives at least five daily doses of low-dose folic acid or multivitamin with folic acid within 7 days before first pemetrexed dose.
• Know that patient must receive one I.M. injection of vitamin B_{12} during week before first pemetrexed dose.

Dilution and compatibility
• Reconstitute 100-mg vial and 500-mg vial with 4.2 mL and 20 mL of preservative-free normal saline solution for injection, respectively, to yield 25 mg/mL. Gently swirl vial until powder dissolves completely.
• Further dilute appropriate volume of reconstituted solution to 100 mL with preservative-free normal saline solution.
• Know that reconstituted solution should be clear and colorless to yellow or green-yellow.
• Be aware that drug is physically incompatible with diluents containing calcium, including Ringer's and lactated Ringer's solutions. Administration with other drugs and diluents is not recommended.
• Discard unused portion.

Infusion considerations
• Administer by I.V. infusion only over 10 minutes.

Monitoring
• Monitor CBBC with platelet count frequently.
• Monitor renal and liver function tests and blood chemistry results (especially serum creatinine) periodically.
• If concomitant NSAID use is necessary, monitor patient closely for toxicities (especially myelosuppression and renal or GI toxicity).
• Be aware that folic acid therapy should continue for 21 days after final dose.
• Know that patient must receive one I.M. injection of vitamin B_{12} for every three cycles.

Storage
• Store at 25°C (77°F); excursions permitted from 15° to 30°C (59° to 86°F).
• Reconstituted and infusion solutions are stable for up to 24 hours after initial reconstitution when refrigerated or stored at ambient room temperature and lighting.

Contraindications and precautions

Contraindicated in severe hypersensitivity reaction to drug or its components.

Use cautiously in hepatic or renal impairment, neurotoxicity, pregnant or breastfeeding patients, and ***children*** (safety and efficacy not established).

Adverse reactions

CNS: fatigue, sensory neuropathy, altered mood, depression
CV: thrombosis, embolism
EENT: pharyngitis
GI: nausea, vomiting, constipation, diarrhea without colostomy, dysphagia, esophagitis, pain on swallowing, stomatitis, anorexia
GU: renal failure
Hematologic: neutropenia, leukopenia, anemia, thrombocytopenia, febrile neutropenia
Hepatic: abnormal liver function
Musculoskeletal: myalgia, arthralgia
Respiratory: dyspnea
Skin: rash, desquamation, alopecia
Other: fever, dehydration, noncardiac chest pain, infection without neutropenia or with Grade 3 or Grade 4 neutropenia, edema, other constitutional symptoms, hypersensitivity reaction.

Interactions

Drug-drug. *Ibuprofen:* decreased pemetrexed clearance and increased concentration
Nephrotoxic agents: possible decrease in pemetrexed clearance
Drug-diagnostic tests. *Alanine aminotransferase, aspartate aminotransferase, serum creatinine:* increased
Creatinine clearance, hematocrit, hemoglobin, platelets, white blood cells: decreased

Toxicity and overdose

- In overdose (rare), expect diarrhea, mucositis, rash, neutropenia, thrombocytopenia, anemia, and infection with or without fever.
- Provide symptomatic and supportive therapy. Be aware that I.V. leucovorin may be indicated for Grade 4 leukopenia or Grade 4 neutropenia lasting 3 days or more, and immediately for Grade 4 thrombocytopenia, bleeding associated with Grade 3 thrombocytopenia, or Grade 3 or 4 mucositis.

Patient teaching

- Instruct patient to take folic acid and vitamin B_{12} before and during therapy, as prescribed.
- Advise patient to drink ten 8-oz glasses of fluid and to urinate frequently during first 24 hours if therapy includes cisplatin.

Teach patient to recognize signs and symptoms of anemia and to contact prescriber if temperature rises above 38°C (100.4°F).

- Instruct patient to consult prescriber before taking products containing ibuprofen.
- Advise females with childbearing potential to avoid pregnancy during therapy.
- Instruct breastfeeding patient to stop breastfeeding during therapy.
- As appropriate, review all other significant and life-threatening adverse reactions and interactions, especially those related to the drugs and tests mentioned above.

penicillin G potassium

Pfizerpen

Pharmacologic class: Penicillin
Therapeutic class: Anti-infective
Pregnancy risk category B

Action

Inhibits biosynthesis of cell-wall mucopeptide; bactericidal against penicillin-susceptible microorganisms during active multiplication stage

Pharmacokinetics
Drug distributes into pleural, pericardial, peritoneal, ascitic, synovial, and interstitial fluids; penetration into cerebrospinal fluid (CSF), eyes, and prostate is poor. In normal circumstances, it easily achieves therapeutic levels in extracellular fluid and most other body tissues. Drug binds to serum proteins, mainly albumin. It is rapidly excreted in urine (primarily unchanged) by glomerular filtration and active tubular secretion, with some secretion in breast milk.

Onset	Peak	Duration
Rapid	End of infusion	4-6 hr

How supplied
Powder for reconstitution for injection (white, crystalline): 1 million, 5 million, and 20 million units/vial
Premixed (frozen) solution for injection: 1 million, 2 million, and 3 million units/50-mL single-dose plastic containers

Indications and dosages
➢ Meningococcal meningitis
Adults: 20 to 30 million units/day by continuous I.V. infusion for 14 days or until patient is afebrile for 7 days. Alternatively, 200,000 to 300,000 units/kg/day I.V. q 2 to 4 hours in divided doses for a total of 24 doses.
➢ Meningitis caused by susceptible strains of pneumococcus or meningococcus
Children: 250,000 units/kg/day in equally divided doses by continuous I.V. infusion q 4 hours for 7 to 14 days (depending on infecting organism)
Infants older than 7 days: 200,000 to 300,000 units/kg/day I.V. in divided doses q 6 hours
Infants less than 7 days old: 100,000 to 150,000 units/kg/day I.V. in divided doses q 12 hours
➢ Actinomycosis
Adults: 1 to 6 million units/day I.V. for cervicofacial infections; 10 to 20 million units/day I.V. q 4 to 6 hours for 6 weeks for thoracic and abdominal infections
➢ Clostridial infections
Adults: 20 million units/day I.V. infusion q 4 to 6 hours, given with antitoxin therapy
➢ Fusospirochetal infections
Adults: 5 to 10 million units/day I.V. infusion q 4 to 6 hours
➢ Rat bite fever, Haverhill fever
Adults: 12 to 20 million units/day I.V. infusion q 4 to 6 hours for 3 or 4 weeks
➢ *Pasteurella* infections
Adults: 4 to 6 million units/day I.V. infusion q 4 to 6 hours for 2 weeks
➢ Erysipeloid endocarditis
Adults: 12 to 20 million units/day I.V. infusion q 4 to 6 hours for 4 to 6 weeks
➢ Diphtheria (as adjunctive therapy with antitoxin to prevent carrier state)
Adults: 2 to 3 million units/day I.V. infusion in divided doses q 4 to 6 hours for 10 to 12 days
➢ Anthrax
Adults: At least 5 million units/day I.V. infusion
➢ Serious streptococcal infections
Adults: 5 to 24 million units/day I.V. infusion in divided doses q 4 to 6 hours
➢ Neurosyphilis
Adults: 18 to 24 million units/day I.V. (given in doses of 3 to 4 million units q 4 hours) for 10 to 14 days
➢ *Listeria* infections
Adults: 15 to 20 million units/day I.V. infusion q 4 to 6 hours for 2 weeks in meningitis or 4 weeks in endocarditis
➢ Disseminated gonococcal infections
Adults: 10 million units/day I.V. (3 to 4 million units q 4 hours) for 10 to 14 days

Dosage adjustment

- Reduce dosage in severe renal impairment. Make additional adjustments when hepatic disease accompanies renal impairment.

Administration

Preparation

- Before administering, ask patient about allergy to penicillin, beta-lactamase inhibitors, and benzathine. Be aware that cross-sensitivity to imipenem and cephalosporins may occur.
- Give 20-million unit dosage only by I.V. infusion.

Keep epinephrine and emergency equipment available in case anaphylaxis occurs.

Dilution and compatibility

- Dilute in sterile water for injection, normal saline solution for injection, or D_5W for injection. Shake vigorously.
- For continuous infusion, further dilute in 1 to 2 L compatible solution as above.
- For intermittent infusion, further dilute in 50 or 100 mL normal saline solution or D_5W.
- Be aware that drug also is available as premixed solution that requires no dilution.
- Do not add other drugs to premixed solutions.
- Thaw frozen premixed containers at room temperature or in refrigerator. Do not force-thaw by immersion or microwave.
- Do not use discolored or cloudy solution.

Infusion considerations

Do not administer by I.V. bolus.

- Give by intermittent I.V. infusion over 1 to 2 hours in adults or over 15 to 30 minutes in children and infants.
- Administer by continuous I.V. infusion over 24 hours.

Know that too-rapid infusion may cause electrolyte imbalance or seizures.

Do not use plastic containers in series connections. Such use could result in air embolism due to residual air being drawn from primary container before administration of fluid from secondary container ends.

Monitoring

Watch closely for anaphylaxis and serum sickness.

Closely monitor neurologic status, especially for seizures and decreasing level of consciousness.

Stay alert for signs and symptoms of superinfection and pseudomembranous colitis.

- Be aware that in syphilis treatment, Jarisch-Herxheimer reaction (fever, chills, headache, sweating, malaise, hypotension or hypertension) may occur 2 to 12 hours after therapy starts, but usually subsides within 24 hours.
- In long-term therapy, monitor CBC with white cell differential, as well as electrolyte levels; watch for blood dyscrasias and electrolyte imbalances.

Storage

- Store dry powder below 30°C (86°F). Once reconstituted, it may be refrigerated for up to 7 days.
- Know that thawed solution is stable for 24 hours at room temperature or for 14 days when refrigerated. Do not refreeze.

Contraindications and precautions

Contraindicated in hypersensitivity to penicillins or beta-lactamase inhibitors (piperacillin/tazobactam).

Use cautiously in severe renal insufficiency, significant allergies or asthma, and pregnant or breastfeeding patients.

Adverse reactions

CNS: hyperreflexia, neuropathy, **coma, seizures**

CV: arrhythmias, cardiac arrest, heart failure (with high doses)

GI: nausea, vomiting, diarrhea, epigastric distress, abdominal pain, glossitis, colitis, blood in stool, **pseudomembranous colitis**
GU: nephropathy
Hematologic: hemolytic anemia, leukopenia, thrombocytopenia
Metabolic: hyperkalemia (with continuous high-dose infusion)
Skin: rash, urticaria, exfoliative dermatitis
Other: phlebitis at I.V. site, Jarisch-Herxheimer reaction, superinfection, **anaphylaxis, serum sickness**

Interactions

Drug-drug. *Aspirin, probenecid:* increased penicillin blood level
Erythromycins, tetracyclines: decreased antimicrobial activity of penicillin
Hormonal contraceptives: decreased contraceptive efficacy
Drug-diagnostic tests. *Alanine aminotransferase, eosinophils, granulocytes, hemoglobin, platelets, potassium, white blood cells:* increased
Direct Coombs' test: positive result
Sodium: decreased
Urine glucose, urine protein: false-positive results

Toxicity and overdose

- Adverse neurologic reactions, including neuromuscular hyperexcitability or seizures, may occur if drug achieves high CSF levels, particularly in patients with severe renal impairment. Other signs and symptoms of overdose may include agitation, confusion, asterixis, hallucinations, hyperkalemia, stupor, encephalopathy, and coma.
- Discontinue drug, provide symptomatic therapy, and institute supportive measures as indicated and ordered. Hemodialysis may be effective in removing drug.

Patient teaching

Teach patient to recognize signs and symptoms of anaphylaxis and to get immediate medical attention if these occur.

Advise patient to immediately report severe, persistent diarrhea and fever.

- Instruct patient to contact prescriber if signs and symptoms of infection worsen.
- Tell female patient that drug may make hormonal contraceptives ineffective; encourage use of barrier birth-control methods if she wishes to avoid pregnancy.
- As appropriate, review all other significant and life-threatening adverse reactions and interactions, especially those related to the drugs and tests mentioned above.

pentamidine isethionate

Pentacarinat*, Pentam

Pharmacologic class: Antiprotozoal
Therapeutic class: Anti-infective
Pregnancy risk category C

Action

Unknown. May interfere with nuclear metabolism and synthesis of DNA, RNA, and proteins.

Pharmacokinetics

Drug is excreted unchanged, primarily by the kidneys, with some elimination in feces.

Onset	Peak	Duration
Unknown	1 hr	Unknown

P

How supplied

Powder for reconstitution for injection (white, crystalline, lyophilized): 300 mg/vial

Indications and dosages

➣ *Pneumocystis jiroveci* pneumonia

Adults and children age 5 and older: 4 mg/kg I.V. daily for 14 to 21 days

Off-label uses

- Trypanosomiasis
- Visceral leishmaniasis

Administration

Preparation

Follow hazardous drug guidelines on page S19 for handling, preparation, and administration.

Dilution and compatibility

- Dilute 300 mg-vial with sterile water for injection. Withdraw prescribed dose, then dilute further in 50 to 250 mL D_5W.
- Discard unused portion.

Infusion considerations

- Administer by I.V. infusion over 60 to 120 minutes.
- Keep patient supine during administration to minimize hypotension.

Monitoring

Closely monitor blood pressure and blood glucose level. Watch for arrhythmias and signs and symptoms of pulmonary infection, blood dyscrasias, and pancreatitis during and after administration until patient is stable, because severe and possibly fatal reactions may occur.

- Assess I.V. site closely during and after administration. Be aware that sterile abscess, pain, or induration at injection site may occur.
- Evaluate neurologic status.
- Monitor CBC (including platelet count), calcium and potassium levels, and kidney and liver function test results.

Storage

- Store powder at 15° to 30°C (59° to 86°F); protect from light.

Contraindications and precautions

Contraindicated in history of anaphylactic reaction to inhaled or parenteral pentamidine isethionate. (However, no absolute contraindications exist for patients with *P. jiroveci.*)

Use cautiously in anemia, blood dyscrasias, hepatic or renal disease, diabetes mellitus, ventricular tachycardia, hypocalcemia, hypertension, hypotension, hypoglycemia, pregnant or breastfeeding patients, and ***children.***

Adverse reactions

CNS: disorientation, hallucinations, dizziness, confusion, fatigue, headache, neuralgia

CV: chest pain, ECG abnormalities, vasodilation, vasculitis, phlebitis, hypertension, palpitations, syncope, **arrhythmias, severe hypotension**

EENT: pharyngitis

GI: nausea, vomiting, diarrhea, abdominal pain, anorexia, **acute pancreatitis**

Hematologic: anemia, **leukopenia, thrombocytopenia**

Metabolic: hypoglycemia, hypocalcemia, hyperkalemia

Musculoskeletal: myalgia

Respiratory: cough, dyspnea, congestion, **pneumothorax, bronchospasm**

Skin: rash, night sweats, urticaria, sterile abscess or induration at injection site

Other: metallic or bad taste, fever, chills, pain at injection site or elsewhere, edema, allergic reactions

Interactions

Drug-diagnostic tests. *Blood urea nitrogen, creatinine, liver function tests, potassium:* increased

Calcium, glucose, hemoglobin, hematocrit, platelets, white blood cells: decreased
ECG: altered

Toxicity and overdose

- Provide symptomatic and supportive therapy.

Patient teaching

- Explain purpose of therapy, and stress importance of completing entire course.

Teach patient to recognize and immediately report serious adverse cardiovascular and neurologic effects, easy bruising or bleeding, and abdominal pain.

- Tell patient to notify prescriber if infection worsens.
- Advise patient to minimize GI upset by eating small, frequent servings of healthy food and drinking plenty of fluids.
- Caution patient to avoid driving and other hazardous activities until drug's effects on concentration and alertness are known.
- As appropriate, review all other significant and life-threatening adverse reactions and interactions, especially those related to the tests mentioned above.

pentazocine

Fortral, Talwin

Pharmacologic class: Opioid agonist-antagonist
Therapeutic class: Opioid analgesic, adjunct to anesthesia
Controlled substance schedule IV
Pregnancy risk category C

Action

Unclear. Interacts with opiate receptor sites primarily in limbic system, thalamus, and spinal cord, blocking neurotransmission of pain impulses.

Pharmacokinetics

Drug crosses placental barrier and is metabolized in the liver. Less than 5% of dose is excreted in urine unchanged, with some secretion in breast milk.

Onset	Peak	Duration
12-30 min	Unknown	3 hr

How supplied

Solution for injection: 30 mg/mL (as lactate salt)

Indications and dosages

Moderate to severe pain; preoperative or preanesthetic medication; adjunct to surgical anesthesia
Adults: 30 mg I.V. q 3 to 4 hours (not to exceed 30 mg/dose). Maximum daily dosage is 360 mg.

Labor
Adults: 20 mg I.V. for two or three doses at 2- to 3-hour intervals

Administration

Dilution and compatibility

- Know that although drug may be given undiluted, it may be preferable to dilute each 5 mg in at least 1 mL sterile water for injection.
- Do not mix in same syringe with soluble barbiturates (such as pentobarbital sodium), as precipitation will occur.

Infusion considerations

- Administer each 5 mg by slow direct I.V. infusion over 1 minute, with patient lying supine.

Monitoring

Monitor vital signs. Watch closely for evidence of shock, dyspnea, and circulatory or respiratory depression.

- Monitor drug efficacy.
- In prolonged use, assess for signs and symptoms of drug dependence.

Storage
• Store at controlled room temperature.

Contraindications
Contraindicated in hypersensitivity to drug.

Use cautiously in head trauma, increased intracranial pressure, respiratory conditions, adrenal insufficiency, seizure disorder, acute CNS manifestations, hepatic impairment, acute myocardial infarction, alcohol or opioid use, history of drug abuse, pregnant or breastfeeding patients, and ***children*** (safety not established).

Adverse reactions
CNS: dizziness, drowsiness, euphoria, hallucinations, headache, sedation, dysphoria, unusual dreams, weakness, depression, insomnia, irritability, excitement, tremor, paresthesia
CV: hypertension, hypotension, syncope, tachycardia, **circulatory depression, shock**
EENT: blurred vision, diplopia, nystagmus, miosis (with high doses), tinnitus
GI: nausea, vomiting, constipation, diarrhea, ileus, cramps, abdominal distress, dry mouth, anorexia
GU: urine retention, altered rate and strength of labor contractions
Respiratory: dyspnea, transient apnea in neonates whose mothers received pentazocine during labor, **respiratory depression**
Skin: clamminess, diaphoresis, rash, urticaria, nodules, cutaneous depression, skin and subcutaneous sclerosis, dermatitis, pruritus, flushing
Other: altered taste, chills, soft-tissue induration, facial edema, physical or psychological drug dependence, drug tolerance, **anaphylaxis**

Interactions
Drug-drug. *Barbiturates, first-generation (sedating) antihistamines, other sedating drugs:* additive CNS depression
Monoamine oxidase inhibitors: unpredictable reactions
Opioids: decreased analgesic effects
Drug-diagnostic tests. *Amylase, lipase:* increased
Granulocytes, WBCs: decreased
Drug-herb. *Chamomile, hops, kava, skullcap, valerian:* increased CNS depression
Drug-behaviors. *Alcohol use:* increased CNS depression

Toxicity and overdose
• Overdose information is limited. Expect high doses to cause marked respiratory depression and tachycardia.
• Maintain patent airway and institute assisted or controlled ventilation. Provide symptomatic and supportive therapy, including I.V. fluids, and oxygen, as indicated and ordered. Give appropriate dosage of opioid antagonist (naloxone) for severe respiratory depression with extreme care, titrating with smaller-than-usual dosages. Do not give antagonist in absence of significant respiratory or cardiovascular depression.

Patient teaching
• Inform patient that withdrawal symptoms may occur if drug is stopped suddenly after prolonged use.
• Caution patient to avoid alcohol.
• Advise patient to consult prescriber before taking other prescription drugs, over-the-counter preparations, or herbal preparations.
• Caution patient to avoid driving and other hazardous activities until drug's effects are known.
• Urge patient to have periodic eye exams.

- As appropriate, review all significant and life-threatening adverse reactions and interactions, especially those related to the drugs, tests, herbs, and behaviors mentioned above.

pentobarbital sodium

Nembutal Sodium

Pharmacologic class: Barbiturate
Therapeutic class: Sedative-hypnotic, anticonvulsant
Controlled substance schedule II
Pregnancy risk category D

Action

Depresses sensory cortex, decreases motor activity, and alters cerebellar function; may interfere with nerve impulse transmission in brain

Pharmacokinetics

Drug distributes rapidly to all body tissues and fluids and achieves high concentrations in brain, liver, and kidney. It is metabolized primarily in the liver and is highly bound to tissue and plasma proteins. Negligible amounts are excreted unchanged in urine.

Onset	Peak	Duration
Immediate	1 min	3-4 hr

How supplied

Solution for injection (clear): 50 mg/mL in 2-mL prefilled syringes

Indications and dosages

➢ Preoperative sedation

Adults: Initially, 100 mg I.V.; if indicated may give additional doses in 25 to 50 mg increments.

➢ Seizures

Adults: Initially, 100 mg. I.V.; may give additional doses after 1 minute. Maximum dosage is 500 mg.
Children: Initially, 50 mg. I.V.; may give additional doses until desired response occurs. Do not exceed 100 mg/dose.

Administration

Preparation

- Be aware that drug is meant for short-term use only, because it loses effectiveness after about 2 weeks.
- Administer by I.V. injection only if other administration routes are not feasible (either because patient is unconscious or because prompt action is imperative).

Do not give by subcutaneous or intra-arterial route, because severe reactions (including tissue necrosis and gangrene) may occur.

Make sure resuscitation equipment is available.

Dilution and compatibility

- Know that drug is given undiluted. Do not mix with other solutions.
- Do not mix in same syringe with pentazocine, as precipitation will occur.
- Use solution only if clear.

Infusion considerations

Know that slow I.V. injection is essential. Observe vital signs carefully throughout administration.

- Give I.V. by direct injection no faster than 50 mg/minute.

Monitoring

Closely monitor blood pressure and heart and respiratory rates; watch for signs and symptoms of respiratory depression.

- Monitor neurologic status before and during therapy.
- Assess CBC and kidney and liver function test results.
- In long-term therapy, monitor patient for signs of drug dependence.

P

Storage
- Store at room temperature of 30°C (86°F); brief excursions to 40°C (104°F) permitted.

Contraindications and precautions

Contraindicated in hypersensitivity to drug or other barbiturates and in manifest or latent porphyria.

Use cautiously in hepatic or renal impairment, severe respiratory disease with dyspnea or obstruction, history of sedative-hypnotic abuse, increased risk of suicide, history of drug addiction, alcohol use, labor and delivery, and ***elderly or debilitated patients.***

Adverse reactions

CNS: drowsiness, agitation, confusion, hyperkinesia, ataxia, nightmares, nervousness, hallucinations, insomnia, anxiety, abnormal thinking
CV: hypotension, syncope, **bradycardia**
GI: nausea, vomiting, constipation
Hepatic: hepatic damage
Musculoskeletal: joint pain, myalgia, neuralgia
Respiratory: laryngospasm, **bronchospasm, respiratory depression**
Skin: rash, urticaria, exfoliative dermatitis
Other: phlebitis at I.V. site, physical or psychological drug dependence, fever, hypersensitivity reactions including **angioedema**

Interactions

Drug-drug. *Acetaminophen:* increased risk of hepatotoxicity
Anticoagulants, beta blockers (except timolol), carbamazepine, clonazepam, corticosteroids, digoxin, doxorubicin, doxycycline, felodipine, fenoprofen, griseofulvin, hormonal contraceptives, metronidazole, quinidine, theophylline, verapamil: decreased efficacy of these drugs
Antihistamines (first-generation), opioids, other sedative-hypnotics: additive CNS depression
Chloramphenicol, hydantoins, opioids: increased or decreased effects of these drugs or pentobarbital
Divalproex, monoamine oxidase inhibitors, valproic acid: decreased pentobarbital metabolism, increased sedation
Rifampin: increased metabolism and decreased effects of pentobarbital
Drug-diagnostic tests. *Sulfobromophthalein:* false increase
Drug-herb. *Chamomile, hops, kava, valerian, skullcap:* increased CNS depression
St. John's wort: decreased pentobarbital effects
Drug-behaviors. *Alcohol use:* increased sedation, additive CNS depression

Toxicity and overdose

- Overdose signs and symptoms include confusion, severe drowsiness, decreased reflexes, staggering gait, slurred speech, severe weakness, fever, hypothermia, dyspnea, and bradycardia. CNS and respiratory depression also may occur, progressing to Cheyne-Stokes respiration, slight pupillary constriction (or pupil dilation in severe toxicity), oliguria, tachycardia, low body temperature, and coma. Typical shock syndrome (apnea, circulatory collapse, respiratory arrest, and death) also may occur. In extreme overdose, all electrical activity in brain may cease, although this does not necessarily indicate clinical death because effect is fully reversible (unless hypoxic damage occurs).
- Provide symptomatic and supportive therapy. Maintain patent airway and provide assisted or controlled ventilation, if indicated. Administer I.V. fluids, oxygen, and vasopressors, as ordered. Forced diuresis and urine alkalinization may help remove drug; oral activated

charcoal may enhance elimination regardless of administration route. Although hemodialysis or hemoperfusion is not recommended routinely, it may be used in severe barbiturate overdose or if patient is anuric or in shock.

Patient teaching

- Advise patient to avoid St. John's wort and other herbal supplements, alcohol, and other CNS depressants during therapy.
- Caution patient to avoid driving and other hazardous activities until drug's effects are known.
- As appropriate, review all significant and life-threatening adverse reactions and interactions, especially those related to the drugs, tests, herbs, and behaviors mentioned above.

pentostatin

Nipent

Pharmacologic class: Antimetabolite
Therapeutic class: Antineoplastic
Pregnancy risk category D

FDA BOXED WARNING

- Give under supervision of physician experienced in cancer chemotherapy, in facility with adequate diagnostic and treatment resources.
- Use of higher dosages than those specified is not recommended, as dose-limiting severe renal, liver, pulmonary, and CNS toxicities may occur.
- In study of patients with refractory chronic lymphocytic leukemia receiving drug at recommended dosage in combination with fludarabine, four of six patients had severe or fatal pulmonary toxicity. Use in combination with fludarabine is not recommended.

Action

Unclear. Inhibits adenosine deaminase, thereby increasing levels of deoxyadenosine triphosphate in cells, blocking DNA synthesis, and inhibiting ribonucleotide reductase.

Pharmacokinetics

Drug has distribution half-life of about 11 minutes. Plasma protein-binding is low. Half-life is about 6 hours in patients with normal renal function and much longer in renal impairment. Drug is eliminated unchanged primarily in urine.

Onset	Peak	Duration
Unknown	Unknown	Unknown

How supplied

Powder for reconstitution for injection: 10-mg vial

Indications and dosages

➤ Hairy cell leukemia refractory to alpha-interferon therapy
Adults: 4 mg/m^2 I.V. every other week

Administration

Preparation

Follow hazardous drug guidelines on page S19 for handling, preparation, and administration.
- Before initiating therapy, obtain serum creatinine or creatinine clearance assay.
- Before giving drug, hydrate patient with 500 to 1,000 mL D_5W or normal saline solution, or its equivalent.

Dilution and compatibility

- To reconstitute powder, inject 5 mL sterile water for injection into vial and mix thoroughly to yield 2 mg/mL solution.

P

• When giving by direct I.V. injection, drug does not require further dilution.
• For I.V. infusion, dilute with 25 to 50 mL D_5W or normal saline solution. Diluting entire contents of reconstituted vial with 25 or 50 mL yields a concentration of 0.33 mg/mL or 0.18 mg/mL, respectively.
• Know that reconstituted or diluted solution should be clear and colorless. Do not use if discolored.

Infusion considerations
• For I.V. bolus injection, administer over 1 minute.
• For I.V. infusion, administer over 20 to 30 minutes.

Monitoring
• After administering, give 500 mL D_5W or its equivalent.
Monitor CBC (including platelets); watch for signs and symptoms of blood dyscrasias. Also, know that bone marrow aspirates and biopsies may be needed at 2- to 3-month intervals to assess response to treatment.
Closely monitor vital signs and ECG, particularly for indications of life-threatening arrhythmias, heart failure, and pulmonary edema.
Monitor temperature; stay alert for signs and symptoms of bacterial and viral infections.
• Assess liver function tests; watch for signs and symptoms of hepatic dysfunction.
• Continue to monitor serum creatinine level before each dose and at appropriate times during therapy.
Know that individual doses may be withheld or drug may be discontinued if patient develops severe adverse reactions, such as rash, CNS toxicity, infection, elevated serum creatinine level, or decrease in absolute neutrophil count below 200/mm^3 if initial neutrophil count was 500/mm^3.

Storage
• Refrigerate vials at 2° to 8°C (36° to 46°F). Store reconstituted or diluted solution at room temperature under ambient light. Use within 8 hours; drug contains no preservatives.

Contraindications
Contraindicated in hypersensitivity to drug.

Use cautiously in renal disease, bone marrow depression, pregnant or breast-feeding patients, and ***children.***

Adverse reactions
CNS: headache, malaise, anxiety, confusion, depression, dizziness, insomnia, nervousness, paresthesia, drowsiness, abnormal thinking, fatigue, asthenia, hallucinations, hostility, amnesia
CV: peripheral edema, cellulitis, vasculitis, hypotension, angina, tachycardia, bradycardia, phlebitis, **thrombophlebitis, cardiac arrest, heart failure, hemorrhage, ventricular asystole, pericardial effusion, sinus arrest**
EENT: abnormal vision, nonreactive pupils, photophobia, retinopathy, eye pain, conjunctivitis, dry or watery eyes, hearing loss, tinnitus, ear pain, epistaxis, rhinitis, pharyngitis
GI: nausea, vomiting, diarrhea, constipation, dyspepsia, abdominal pain, ileus, flatulence, stomatitis, glossitis, anorexia
GU: renal calculi, renal dysfunction, renal insufficiency, amenorrhea, breast lump, erectile dysfunction, decreased libido, **renal failure**
Hematologic: ecchymosis, anemia, **hemolytic anemia, agranulocytosis, aplastic anemia, leukopenia, thrombocytopenia**
Hepatic: abnormal liver function
Metabolic: hyperuricemia, hypercalcemia, hyponatremia
Musculoskeletal: myalgia, joint pain

Respiratory: cough, dyspnea, respiratory tract infection, **pulmonary embolus**
Skin: rash, eczema, petechiae, dry skin, pruritus, skin disorder, furunculosis, acne, alopecia, diaphoresis, photosensitivity
Other: unusual taste, gingivitis, fever, chills, pain, facial edema, lymphadenopathy, herpes simplex, herpes zoster, flu-like symptoms, viral or bacterial infection, allergic reaction, **sepsis, neoplasm**

Interactions

Drug-drug. *Allopurinol:* hypersensitivity vasculitis
Carmustine, cyclophosphamide, etoposide: potentially fatal acute pulmonary edema and hypotension
Fludarabine: severe or fatal pulmonary toxicity
Vidarabine: increased risk and severity of adverse reactions
Drug-diagnostic tests. *Calcium, liver function tests, serum uric acid:* increased
Granulocytes, platelets, sodium, white blood cells: decreased

Toxicity and overdose

- Dosages higher than recommended may be fatal due to severe renal, hepatic, pulmonary, or CNS toxicity.
- No known antidote exists. In overdose, provide symptomatic and supportive therapy, possibly including administration of whole blood products and blood modifiers if ordered.

Patient teaching

- Teach patient that drug lowers resistance to infection. Instruct patient to avoid crowds and to immediately report fever, cough, breathing problems, sore throat, and other signs and symptoms of infection.
- Advise patient to minimize GI upset by eating small, frequent servings of healthy food and drinking plenty of fluids.
- Advise female patients of childbearing age to avoid pregnancy while taking drug and to seek medical advice before becoming pregnant.
- Instruct patient to avoid driving and other hazardous activities until drug's effects on concentration and alertness are known.
- As appropriate, review all other significant and life-threatening adverse reactions and interactions, especially those related to the drugs and tests mentioned above.

phenobarbital sodium

Luminal Sodium

Pharmacologic class: Barbiturate
Therapeutic class: Anticonvulsant, sedative-hypnotic, anxiolytic
Controlled substance schedule IV
Pregnancy risk category D

Action

Interferes with gamma-aminobutyric acid receptors, blocking nerve impulse transmission in CNS, which in turn reduces motor activity and increases seizure threshold

Pharmacokinetics

Drug distributes rapidly to all body tissues and fluids, achieving high concentrations in brain, liver, and kidney. It is metabolized primarily in the liver, and is slightly to moderately bound to tissue and plasma proteins. About 25% to 50% is excreted unchanged in urine.

Onset	Peak	Duration
5 min	30 min	10-16 hr

How supplied

Solution for injection: 30 mg/mL and 60 mg/mL in 1-mL prefilled syringes; 65 mg/mL in 1-mL vials; 130 mg/mL in 1-mL prefilled syringes, 1-mL vials, and 1-mL ampules

Indications and dosages

➢ Tonic-clonic (grand mal) and partial seizures; febrile seizures in children

Adults: 100 to 320 mg I.V. p.r.n. (total of 600 mg I.V. in a 24-hour period).

Infants and children: 4 to 6 mg/kg/day I.V. for 7 to 10 days to achieve drug blood level of 10 to 15 mcg/mL

➢ Status epilepticus

Adults: 200 to 320 mg I.V. over 10 to 15 minutes, repeated q 6 hours as necessary

Children: 15 to 20 mg/kg I.V. in single or divided doses over 10 to 15 minutes; usual maximum loading dose is 20 mg/kg. In selected patients, may give additional 5 mg/kg/dose q 15 to 30 minutes until seizures are controlled or a total dose of 30 mg/kg is reached.

➢ Sedation or hypnotic effect

Adults: For sedation, 30 to 120 mg/day I.V. in two or three divided doses. As hypnotic, 100 to 320 mg I.V. at bedtime. Do not exceed 400 mg in a 24-hour period.

➢ Preoperative sedative

Children: 1 to 3 mg/kg I.V. 1 to 1.5 hours before procedure

Dosage adjustment

- Reduce dosage in impaired hepatic or renal function.
- Know that elderly or debilitated patients may be more sensitive to drug and therefore require dosage reduction.

Off-label uses

- Prevention and treatment of hyperbilirubinemia

Administration

Preparation

- Use parenteral route only when oral route cannot be used.
- Be aware that when given I.V. for status epilepticus, drug may take 15 minutes to reach peak level in brain. If drug is injected continuously until seizures stop, drug brain level continues to rise and could exceed that required to control seizures. To avoid barbiturate-induced depression, give minimal dosage required and wait for anticonvulsant effect to develop before giving second dose.
- Do not give by subcutaneous route, because severe reactions (including pain and tissue necrosis) may occur.
- Be aware that drug is intended for short-term use only, because it loses effectiveness after about 2 weeks.
- Keep resuscitation equipment, including respiratory support equipment, available.

Dilution and compatibility

- Know that drug may be given undiluted. If dilution is desired, dilute with up to 10 mL sterile water for injection.
- Do not mix in same syringe with pentazocine, as precipitation may occur.
- Use solution only if clear.

Infusion considerations

- Give I.V. at a maximum rate of 60 mg/minute; titrate slowly to desired effect.
- Know that rapid injection may cause respiratory depression.
- Stop injection immediately if patient complains of pain or if circulation at injection site diminishes (possibly indicating inadvertent intra-arterial injection).

Monitoring

- Monitor vital signs; watch for bradycardia and hypotension.
- In patients with seizure disorder, be aware that drug withdrawal may cause status epilepticus.

• Assess neurologic status; institute safety measures as needed.

Closely monitor respiratory status, especially for respiratory depression and airway spasms.

• Monitor phenobarbital blood level, CBC, and kidney and liver function tests.

• Watch for signs and symptoms of hypersensitivity and drug dependence.

Storage

• Store at room temperature of approximately 25°C (77°F).

Contraindications and precautions

Contraindicated in hypersensitivity to drug or other barbiturates and in manifest or latent porphyria.

Use cautiously in hepatic dysfunction, renal impairment, severe respiratory disease with dyspnea or obstruction, history of sedative-hypnotic abuse, seizure disorder, fever, hyperthyroidism, diabetes mellitus, severe anemia, pulmonary or cardiac disease, history of suicide attempt or drug abuse, chronic phenobarbital use, ***elderly and debilitated patients,*** pregnant or breastfeeding patients, and ***children younger than age 6.***

Adverse reactions

CNS: headache, dizziness, anxiety, depression, drowsiness, excitation, delirium, lethargy, agitation, confusion, hyperkinesia, ataxia, vertigo, CNS depression, nightmares, nervousness, paradoxical stimulation, abnormal thinking, hallucinations, insomnia

CV: hypotension, syncope, **bradycardia**

GI: nausea, vomiting, constipation

Hematologic: megaloblastic anemia

Hepatic: hepatic damage

Musculoskeletal: joint pain, myalgia

Respiratory: hypoventilation, **laryngospasm, bronchospasm, apnea, respiratory depression**

Skin: rash, urticaria, exfoliative dermatitis, **Stevens-Johnson syndrome**

Other: phlebitis at I.V. site, drug dependence, hypersensitivity reactions including angioedema

Interactions

Drug-drug. *Acetaminophen:* increased risk of hepatotoxicity

Anticoagulants, beta blockers (except timolol), carbamazepine, clonazepam, corticosteroids, digoxin, doxorubicin, doxycycline, felodipine, fenoprofen, griseofulvin, hormonal contraceptives, metronidazole, quinidine, theophylline, verapamil: decreased efficacy of these drugs

Chloramphenicol, hydantoins, opioids: increased or decreased effects of either drug

Cyclophosphamide: increased risk of hematologic toxicity

Divalproex, monoamine oxidase inhibitors, valproic acid: decreased phenobarbital metabolism, increased sedative effect

Other CNS depressants (including first-generation antihistamines, opioids, other sedative-hypnotics): additive CNS depression

Rifampin: increased metabolism and decreased effects of phenobarbital

Drug-diagnostic tests. *Bilirubin:* decreased in neonates and patients with seizure disorders or congenital nonhemolytic unconjugated hyperbilirubinemia

Drug-herb. *Chamomile, hops, kava, skullcap, valerian:* increased CNS depression

St. John's wort: decreased drug effects

Drug-behaviors. *Alcohol use:* additive CNS

Toxicity and overdose

• In overdose, expect confusion, severe drowsiness, decreased reflexes, staggering gait, slurred speech, severe weakness, fever, hypothermia, dyspnea, and bradycardia. In addition, CNS and respiratory depression may occur, possibly

P

progressing to Cheyne-Stokes respiration, slight pupillary constriction (pupil dilation in severe toxicity), oliguria, tachycardia, low body temperature, and coma. Typical shock syndrome (apnea, circulatory collapse, respiratory arrest, and death) also may occur. In extreme overdose, all electrical activity in brain may cease; however, this does not necessarily indicate clinical death because effect is fully reversible (unless hypoxic damage occurs).

• Provide symptomatic and supportive therapy. Maintain patent airway and provide assisted or controlled ventilation, if indicated. Administer I.V. fluids, oxygen, and vasopressors, as ordered. Forced diuresis and urine alkalinization may help remove drug; oral activated charcoal may enhance elimination regardless of administration route. Although hemodialysis or hemoperfusion is not recommended routinely, it may be used in severe barbiturate overdose or if patient is anuric or in shock.

Patient teaching

Instruct patient to promptly report rash, facial or lip edema, syncope, dyspnea, or depression.

• Advise patient to seek medical advice before taking other prescription or over-the-counter drugs.

• Caution patient to avoid driving and other hazardous activities until drug's effects are known.

• Instruct patient to avoid herbal supplements, alcohol, and other CNS depressants.

• Advise patient taking hormonal contraceptives to use alternative birth-control method.

• Tell female patient to inform prescriber if she is breastfeeding.

• As appropriate, review all other significant and life-threatening adverse reactions and interactions, especially those related to the drugs, tests, herbs, and behaviors mentioned above.

phenylephrine hydrochloride

Neo-Synephrine

Pharmacologic class: Sympathomimetic, alpha-adrenergic agonist
Therapeutic class: Vasopressor
Pregnancy risk category C

FDA BOXED WARNING

• Make sure you are completely familiar with package insert before using injection form.

Action

Stimulates alpha-adrenergic receptors, causing pronounced vasoconstriction, increased blood pressure, and pronounced vasoconstriction in skin, mucous membranes, and mucosa

Pharmacokinetics

Drug undergoes enzymatic metabolism in the liver by monoamine oxidase (MAO).

Onset	Peak	Duration
Immediate	Unknown	15-20 min

How supplied

Solution for injection: 10 mg/mL

Indications and dosages

➤ Severe hypotension and shock

Adults: 0.1 to 0.18 mg/minute by I.V. infusion. Maintenance infusion is 40 to 60 mcg/minute.

➤ Hypotensive emergency during spinal anesthesia

Adults: 0.2 mg I.V., up to a maximum of 0.5 mg/dose

➢ Paroxysmal supraventricular tachycardia
Adults: 0.5 mg by rapid I.V. injection, not to exceed initial dosage of 0.5 mg. Subsequent dosages (determined by blood pressure) should not exceed preceding dosage by more than 0.1 to 0.2 mg; maximum dosage is 1 mg.

Administration

Dilution and compatibility

• Dilute 1 mL of a 10-mg/mL solution with 9 mL sterile water for injection for direct I.V. injection.
• Dilute 10 mg in 500 mL D_5W or normal saline solution for I.V. infusion.
• Discard unused portion.

Infusion considerations

• Know that in emergency, drug may be given by direct I.V. injection.
🔈 When giving by I.V. infusion, titrate dosage until blood pressure is slightly below patient's normal pressure or until maximum dosage is reached. Infuse I.V. in large vein (preferably through central venous catheter) using infusion pump. After condition stabilizes, taper dosage gradually. Do not withdraw abruptly.
🔈 Closely monitor I.V. site to avoid extravasation, which can cause tissue damage.

Monitoring

🔈 Monitor ECG continuously during I.V. administration; monitor blood pressure every 5 to 15 minutes until it stabilizes, and then every 30 to 60 minutes. Be aware that headache or bradycardia may indicate hypertension.
• Monitor central venous pressure and fluid intake and output; keep in mind that drug does not eliminate need for fluid resuscitation.
🔈 Closely monitor CBC; watch for signs and symptoms of blood dyscrasias.
🔈 Monitor for adverse reactions, particularly life-threatening asthmatic episodes.

Storage

• Store at controlled room temperature of 15° to 30°C (59° to 86°F); protect from light.

Contraindications and precautions

Contraindicated in hypersensitivity to drug, severe hypertension, and ventricular tachycardia.

Use cautiously in sulfite sensitivity (some products), concurrent MAO inhibitor therapy (avoid use), angle-closure glaucoma, hyperthyroidism, partial heart block, bradycardia, hypertension, cardiac disease, arteriosclerosis, unstable vasomotor syndrome, ***elderly patients*** with severe arteriosclerotic or cerebrovascular disease, pregnant or breastfeeding patients, and ***low-birth-weight infants***.

Adverse reactions

CNS: headache, weakness, anxiety, restlessness, tremor, light-headedness, dizziness, drowsiness, insomnia, hallucinations, nervousness, giddiness, prolonged psychosis, photophobia, orofacial dystonia
CV: hypertension, palpitations, tachycardia, bradycardia, **arrhythmias**
GI: nausea, vomiting, gastric irritation, anorexia
GU: urine retention (in males with prostatitis)
Hematologic: leukopenia, agranulocytosis, thrombocytopenia
Respiratory: asthmatic episodes
Skin: sweating, rash, urticaria, contact dermatitis, necrosis and sloughing (with extravasation at I.V. site)

Interactions

Drug-drug. *Beta blockers:* blocked cardiostimulatory effects of phenylephrine

P

Bretylium, sympathomimetics: serious arrhythmias
Furazolidone: excessive hypertension
Guanethidine, methyldopa: decreased antihypertensive effects
Halogenated hydrocarbon anesthetics: serious arrhythmias
MAO inhibitors: severe headache, hypertension, hyperpyrexia
Oxytocics, tricyclic antidepressants: increased pressor response
Drug-behaviors. *Sun exposure:* photophobia

Toxicity and overdose

- Overdose may cause vomiting, paresthesia, palpitations, ventricular extrasystoles, short paroxysms of ventricular tachycardia, sensation of fullness in head, and excessive blood pressure elevation.
- Discontinue drug and closely monitor vitals signs. Expect to give phentolamine to treat excessive hypertension and propranolol to treat arrhythmias.

Patient teaching

- As appropriate, review all significant and life-threatening adverse reactions and interactions, especially those related to the drugs and behaviors mentioned above.

phenytoin sodium (diphenylhydantoin sodium)

Dilantin

Pharmacologic class: Hydantoin derivative
Therapeutic class: Anticonvulsant
Pregnancy risk category D

Action

Thought to limit seizure activity by promoting sodium efflux from neurons in motor cortex and reducing activity in brainstem centers responsible for tonic phase of tonic-clonic seizures

Pharmacokinetics

Drug is hydroxylated in the liver by enzyme system that becomes saturated at high plasma levels; therefore, small incremental doses may increase half-life and raise serum levels substantially. Drug is highly protein-bound. Drug is excreted in bile and urine.

Onset	Peak	Duration
Immediate	20-25 min	12-24 hr

How supplied

Solution for injection (clear): 50 mg/ml in 2- and 5-ml ampules

Indications and dosages

➢ Status epilepticus

Adults: Loading dose of 10 to 15 mg/kg by slow I.V., followed by maintenance dosage of 100 mg I.V. q 6 to 8 hours
Neonates and children: Loading dose of 15 to 20 mg/kg I.V. in divided doses of 5 to 10 mg/kg

Off-label uses

- Arrhythmias
- Recessive dystrophic epidermolysis bullosa, junctional epidermolysis bullosa
- Severe preeclampsia
- Trigeminal neuralgia

Administration

Preparation

- Individualize dosages to provide maximum benefit. In some cases, drug blood level may need to be monitored to achieve effective level of 10 to 20 mcg/mL.

Be aware that a relatively small margin exists between full therapeutic effect and minimally toxic dosages.

Dilution and compatibility
- Know that solution is stable as long as it remains free of haziness and precipitate.
- Be aware that if solution is refrigerated or frozen, precipitate may form—but that this will dissolve when solution stands at room temperature.
- Know that solution may appear faintly yellow, but this does not affect potency.
- Use solution only if clear.
- Do not mix with other drugs.

Infusion considerations
- Before use, check patency of designated I.V. line and flush with normal saline solution.
- Administer directly into large vein through large-gauge needle or I.V. catheter no faster than 50 mg/minute in adults (1 to 3 mg/kg/minute in neonates) through Y-tube or three-way stopcock.
- After injection, flush with normal saline solution to avoid local venous irritation caused by alkaline solution.

Do not give by continuous I.V. infusion; addition of phenytoin sodium injection to I.V. infusion fluids may cause precipitation.

Be aware that hypotension may occur if drug is given rapidly I.V.

Avoid extravasation, which can cause severe tissue damage.

Do not administer I.V. into dorsal hand veins, because "purple-glove syndrome" may occur.

Monitoring

If rash occurs, withhold drug and promptly notify prescriber.
- Continue to assess blood pressure, respirations, ECG, and heart rate; also watch for adverse reactions.
- Monitor drug blood level; therapeutic range is 10 to 20 mcg/mL.
- Evaluate CBC and kidney and liver function tests.
- Closely monitor prothrombin time and International Normalized Ratio in patients receiving warfarin concurrently.

Storage
- Store at room temperature of 15° to 30° C (59° to 86° F).

Contraindications and precautions

Contraindicated in hypersensitivity to hydantoins, sinus bradycardia, sinoatrial block, second- or third-degree atrioventricular (AV) block, and Adams-Stokes syndrome.

Use cautiously in hepatic disease, rash, diabetes mellitus, porphyria, hypotension, severe myocardial insufficiency, ***elderly and gravely ill patients,*** and pregnant or breastfeeding patients.

Adverse reactions

CNS: ataxia, slurred speech, confusion, agitation, depression, dizziness, drowsiness, dysarthria, dyskinesia, extrapyramidal symptoms, fatigue, headache, insomnia, irritability, twitching, nervousness, numbness, psychotic disturbances, tremor, weakness, CNS depression, **coma**

CV: vasodilation, edema, chest pain, **bradycardia, cardiac arrest, arrhythmias, tachycardia, hypotension, cardiovascular collapse**

EENT: diplopia, amblyopia, nystagmus, visual field defect, eye pain, conjunctivitis, photophobia, mydriasis, hearing loss, tinnitus, ear pain, sinusitis, rhinitis, epistaxis, lip enlargement

GI: nausea, vomiting, diarrhea, constipation, gingival hyperplasia, dry mouth

GU: pink, red, or reddish brown urine; gynecomastia; Peyronie's disease

Hepatic: jaundice, **toxic hepatitis, hepatic damage**

Hematologic: macrocytosis, megaloblastic anemia, eosinophilia, monocytosis, leukocytosis, simple anemia, hemolytic anemia, **thrombocytopenia,**

P

agranulocytosis, granulocytopenia, leukopenia, pancytopenia
Metabolic: hypocalcemia, diabetes insipidus, hyperglycemia
Musculoskeletal: back pain, osteomalacia, pelvic pain
Respiratory: pneumonia, pharyngitis, hyperventilation, apnea, aspiration pneumonia, asthma, dyspnea, increased cough and sputum, hypoxia, hemoptysis, bronchitis, chest pain, **pulmonary fibrosis, atelectasis, pneumothorax**
Skin: hypertrichosis, rash, pruritus, hirsutism, alopecia, bruising, exfoliative dermatitis
Other: altered taste, fever, lymphadenopathy, weight gain or loss, coarsened facial features, lupus erythematosus syndrome, allergic reactions, injection site reactions, **Stevens-Johnson syndrome**

Interactions

Drug-drug. *Acetaminophen, amiodarone, amprenavir, aprepitant, atorvastatin, bupropion, busulfan, carbamazepine, cardiac glycosides, caspofungin, clozapine, corticosteroids, dicumarol, disopyramide, doxycycline, estrogens, fentanyl, haloperidol, hormonal contraceptives, itraconazole, levothyroxine, lopinavir, methadone, metapyrone, mexiletine, midazolam, quetiapine, quinidine, simvastatin, tacrolimus, theophylline, valproic acid:* increased metabolism and decreased effects of these drugs
Activated charcoal, acyclovir, antacids, aprepitant, ciprofloxacin, sucralfate: decreased phenytoin absorption
Allopurinol, amiodarone, benzodiazepines, chloramphenicol, cimetidine, disulfiram, fluconazole, isoniazid, metronidazole, miconazole, omeprazole, phenacemide, phenylbutazone, succinimides, sulfonamides, trimethoprim, valproic acid: inhibited metabolism and increased effects of phenytoin
Antineoplastics, folic acid, influenza vaccine, loxapine, nitrofurantoin, pyridoxine: decreased phenytoin effects
Barbiturates, carbamazepine, diazoxide, rifampin, theophylline: increased metabolism and decreased effects of phenytoin
Capecitabine, chloramphenicol, chlorpheniramine, ciprofloxacin, clarithromycin, clopidogrel, diltiazem, disulfiram, doxorubicin, felbamate, fluconazole, fluoxetine, folic acid, ibuprofen, nifedipine, phenothiazines, tacrolimus: increased phenytoin effects
Cyclosporine, dopamine, furosemide, levodopa, levonorgestrel, mebendazole, muscle relaxants, nondepolarizing phenothiazines, sulfonylureas: decreased effects of these drugs
Salicylates, tricyclic antidepressants, valproic acid: phenytoin displacement, increased phenytoin effects
Drug-diagnostic tests. *Free thyroxine and serum thyroxine:* decreased

Toxicity and overdose

- Initial signs and symptoms of overdose include nystagmus, ataxia, and dysarthria. Patient may become comatose and hypotensive with unresponsive pupils; respiratory and circulatory depression may lead to death. Estimated lethal dosage for adults is 2 to 5 g; lethal dosage in children is unknown.
- No specific antidote exists. Provide symptomatic and supportive therapy. Hemodialysis may be beneficial.

Patient teaching

Instruct patient to immediately report signs or symptoms of hypersensitivity reactions (especially first sign of rash) or liver impairment (such as unusual tiredness, weakness, nausea, yellowing of skin or eyes, tenderness on right upper abdomen, and flulike symptoms).

- Explain drug therapy and the need for follow-up tests.
- As appropriate, review all other significant and life-threatening adverse reactions and interactions, especially those related to the drugs and tests mentioned above.

phosphates

sodium and potassium phosphates

Pharmacologic class: Phosphoric acid salt
Therapeutic class: Mineral supplements
Pregnancy risk category C

Action

Participate in bone deposition, regulation of calcium metabolism, and buffering effects on acid-base equilibrium and various enzyme systems

Pharmacokinetics

Plasma phosphates are filtered by renal glomeruli and excreted in urine.

Onset	Peak	Duration
Unknown	Unknown	Unknown

How supplied

Injection (potassium): 3 mM phosphate, 4.4 mEq postassium/mL
Injection (sodium): 3 mM phosphate, 4 mEq sodium/mL

Indications and dosages

➤ To prevent or correct hypophosphatemia in patients with restricted oral intake
Adults and children: Individualized dosage; approximately 10 to 15 mM phosphorus solution (equivalent to 310 to 464 mg elemental phosphorus) added to I.V. solution
Infants: Individualized dosage; approximately 1.5 to 2 mM/kg/day phosphorus solution added to I.V. solution

Administration

Preparation

- Consider amount of potassium or sodium in prescribed dosage, especially in potassium- or sodium-restricted patients.

Dilution and compatibility

Be sure to dilute drug in large volume of compatible I.V. solution.
Know that if drug must be added to total parenteral nutrition solution, pharmacist must perform admixture to avoid precipitation.

Infusion considerations

Infuse I.V. slowly to avoid potassium or sodium intoxication.
- Administer over 2 to 6 hours, as prescribed.

Monitoring

Closely monitor fluid balance and electrolyte levels; watch for electrolyte imbalances, including hyperkalemia and hypernatremia.
Closely monitor for hypocalcemia, which may result from high phosphate concentrations.
- Monitor cardiovascular, hepatic, and renal status.

Contraindications and precautions

Contraindicated in hyperphosphatemia, hypocalcemia, hyperkalemia (potassium form), and hypernatremia (sodium form).

Use cautiously in adrenal insufficiency, renal impairment, cirrhosis, cardiac failure, cardiac disease (especially in patients receiving digitalis preparations), patients receiving edematous or sodium-retaining drugs, and pregnant or breastfeeding patients.

P

Adverse reactions

CV: hypotension, **arrhythmias** (with high potassium concentrations)
Metabolic: fluid and electrolyte disturbances (such as hypernatremia, hyperphosphatemia, hypercalcemic tetany)

Interactions

Drug-drug. *Thiazide diuretics:* possible renal damage
Drug-diagnostic tests. *Calcium:* decreased
Phosphates, potassium, sodium: increased

Toxicity and overdose

- Potassium phosphate overdose may cause combined potassium and phosphate toxicity. Signs and symptoms include listlessness, confusion, weakness and heaviness in legs, hypotension, ECG abnormalities, arrhythmias, heart block, paresthesia, flaccid paralysis, and cardiac arrest. Signs and symptoms of sodium phosphate overdose include sodium overload and edema.
- Immediately discontinue I.V. infusion. As indicated and prescribed, restore decreased serum calcium levels by giving calcium gluconate or calcium chloride, and reduce elevated potassium levels by giving 10% or 20% dextrose with insulin. To reduce sodium level, physician may order diuretics, sodium restriction, or hemodialysis. For other clinical manifestations, intervene as appropriate.

Patient teaching

- Teach patient to recognize and report signs and symptoms of fluid and electrolyte imbalances.
- As appropriate, review all other significant and life-threatening adverse reactions and interactions, especially those related to the drugs and tests mentioned above.

physostigmine salicylate

Antilirium

Pharmacologic class: Cholinesterase inhibitor
Therapeutic class: Antimuscarinic antidote
Pregnancy risk category C

Action

Increases acetylcholine concentration at cholinergic transmission sites. Inhibits destructive action of acetylcholinesterase, thereby prolonging and exaggerating acetylcholine actions; reverses both central and peripheral anticholinergic states.

Pharmacokinetics

Drug distributes widely and easily penetrates blood-brain barrier. It has a half-life of approximately 1 to 2 hours, is hydrolyzed by acetylcholinesterase, and is excreted in urine in small amounts.

Onset	Peak	Duration
3-8 min	Unknown	45-60 min

How supplied

Solution for injection: 1 mg/mL in 2-mL ampules

Indications and dosages

➣ Anticholinergic toxicity
Adults: 2 mg by slow I.V. injection; may repeat dose at 10- to 30-minute intervals if desired response does not occur or until adverse cholinergic effects develop
Children: In life-threatening situations only, 0.02 mg/kg by slow I.V. injection. If toxic effects persist and no signs of cholinergic effects occur, may repeat dose at 5- to 10-minute intervals until

therapeutic effect occurs, a maximum of 2 mg has been given, or adverse cholinergic effects develop.

➤ Post-anesthesia care

Adults: 0.5 to 1 mg by slow I.V. injection; may repeat dose if life-threatening signs (such as arrhythmia, seizures, or coma) occur. May repeat dose q 10 to 30 minutes if desired response does not occur.

Off-label uses

- Alzheimer's disease
- Antagonism of CNS depression caused by diazepam
- Delirium tremens

Administration

Preparation

Know that some drugs and plant products can cause potentially dangerous anticholinergic syndrome either at therapeutic dosages or in overdose.

Keep atropine sulfate injection available as physostigmine antagonist and antidote in case hypersensitivity occurs.

Dilution and compatibility

- Know that drug does not require dilution.

Do not add to I.V. solutions.

- Do not use if solution has darkened.

Infusion considerations

- Give through Y-tube or three-way stopcock of infusion set.
- Administer by slow I.V. injection at controlled rate of no more than 1 mg/minute in adults and 0.5 mg/minute in children.

Know that rapid injection may cause hypersalivation, bradycardia, respiratory distress, and seizures.

Monitoring

Discontinue drug if excessive salivation, emesis, urination, or defecation occurs. Reduce dosage if excessive sweating or nausea occurs.

- Closely monitor vital signs.

Storage

- Store at controlled room temperature of 15° to 25°C (59° to 77°F).

Contraindications and precautions

Contraindicated in asthma, gangrene, diabetes mellitus, cardiovascular disease, mechanical obstruction of intestinal or urogenital tract, vagotonic state, concurrent atropine use (post-anesthesia), and in patients receiving choline esters or depolarizing neuromuscular blocking agents (such as succinylcholine).

Use cautiously in sulfite sensitivity, ***elderly patients,*** pregnant or breastfeeding patients, and ***children.***

Adverse reactions

CNS: seizures (with too-rapid administration)

CV: bradycardia (with too-rapid administration), **asytole, arrhythmias**

GI: nausea, vomiting, diarrhea, hyperperistalsis

Metabolic: cholinergic crisis

Musculoskeletal: muscle weakness

Respiratory: increased respiratory secretions, **bronchospasm**

Other: excessive salivation, hypersensitivity

Interactions

Drug-drug. *Antidepressants, antihistamines, atropine, other belladonna alkaloid derivatives, phenothiazines:* increased risk of anticholinergic syndrome

Cholinergic agents: additive toxicity

Choline esters (such as bethanechol, methacholine), depolarizing neuromuscular blockers (such as decamethonium, succinylcholine): prolonged respiratory depression

Drug-herb. *Black henbane, deadly nightshade, devil's apple, jimsonweed, loco seeds or weeds, matrimony vine, night-blooming jessamine, stinkweed:* increased risk of anticholinergic syndrome

Toxicity and overdose

- Overdose may cause cholinergic crisis that manifests as excessive salivation and sweating, miosis, nausea, vomiting, diarrhea, bradycardia or tachycardia, hypotension or hypertension, confusion, seizures, coma, severe muscle weakness, and paralysis.
- Discontinue drug immediately. Give atropine sulfate (antagonist and antidote), as ordered, but avoid atropine overdose because it may cause bronchial plug formation and anticholinergic syndrome. Otherwise, provide symptomatic and supportive therapy.

Patient teaching

- As appropriate, review all significant and life-threatening adverse reactions and interactions, especially those related to the drugs and herbs mentioned above.

phytonadione (phytomenadione ❉)

Aquamephyton

Pharmacologic class: Vitamin K_1
Therapeutic class: Antihemorrhagic
Pregnancy risk category C

FDA BOXED WARNING

- Severe reactions, including deaths, have occurred during and immediately after parenteral administration. Typically, these reactions resemble hypersensitivity or anaphylaxis, including shock and cardiac arrest, respiratory arrest, or both. Some patients have experienced such reactions on receiving drug for first time. Most events followed I.V. administration, even when precautions were taken to dilute drug and avoid rapid infusion. Therefore, reserve I.V. route for situations in which another route is not feasible and increased risk is justified.

Action

Exerts same type and degree of activity as naturally ocurring vitamin K, which promotes hepatic biosynthesis of vitamin K–dependent clotting factors needed by the liver to produce active prothrombin (factor II), proconvertin (factor VII), plasma thromboplastin component (factor IX), and Stuart factor (factor X).

Pharmacokinetics

Drug initially concentrates in the liver, but concentration declines rapidly. Little vitamin K accumulates in tissues. Drug is secreted in breast milk; almost no free, unmetabolized vitamin K appears in bile or urine.

Onset	Peak	Duration
1-2 hr	3-6 hr	12 to 24 hr

How supplied

Solution for injection (clear, yellow to amber, viscous): 2-mg/mL and 10-mg/mL ampules or prefilled syringes

Indications and dosages

➢ Oral anticoagulant-induced prothrombin deficiency

Adults: Initially, 2.5 to 10 mg, or up to 25 mg I.V. (In rare cases, 50 mg may be required.) Base amount and frequency of subsequent dosages on prothrombin time (PT) response or clinical condition. If PT does not shorten adequately within 6 to 8 hours of parenteral administration, repeat dose.

➢ Hypoprothrombinemia secondary to other causes
Adults: 2 to 25 mg or more I.V. (rarely, up to 50 mg)

Administration

Preparation

- Be aware that drug does not counteract anticoagulant action of heparin.
- Know that before phytonadione is prescribed, drugs that interfere with coagulation (such as salicylates) should be reduced in dosage or discontinued.
- Whenever possible, give drug by subcutaneous or I.M. route. Be aware that drug is given I.M., not I.V., in prophylaxis and treatment of hemorrhagic disease of newborn.
- Do not expect immediate coagulant effect. Whole blood or component therapy also may be necessary if bleeding is severe.

Dilution and compatibility

- Dilute with normal saline solution for injection, dextrose 5% injection, or dextrose 5% and normal saline solution for injection. Do not use other solutions.
- When dilution is indicated, start administration immediately after mixture with diluent. Discard unused diluted drug and unused ampule contents.
- Do not use solution unless clear and yellow to amber in color.

Infusion considerations

When I.V. administration is unavoidable, inject drug very slowly (no faster than 1 mg/minute).

Monitoring

Monitor for hypersensitivity reaction, especially after first dose; be prepared to intervene appropriately.

Storage

- Store container in closed original carton and protect from light at all times.

Contraindications and precautions

Contraindicated in hypersensitivity to drug or its components.

Use cautiously in hepatic disease (with repeated large doses), ***elderly patients,*** pregnant or breastfeeding patients, and ***children.***

Adverse reactions

CV: cardiac arrest
Respiratory: respiratory arrest
Skin: lesions
Other: transient flushing sensations, peculiar taste sensations, hypersensitivity reactions including **anaphylaxis**

Interactions

Drug-drug. *Prothrombin-depressing oral anticoagulants (such as warfarin):* temporary resistance to phytonadione
Drug-diagnostic tests. *International Normalized Ratio, PT:* decreased

Toxicity and overdose

- No information on overdose is available.
- Provide symptomatic and supportive therapy.

Patient teaching

- As appropriate, review all significant adverse reactions and interactions, especially those related to the drugs and tests mentioned above.

P

piperacillin sodium and tazobactam sodium

Tazocin ✤ ❉, Zosyn

Pharmacologic class: Penicillin (extended-spectrum), beta-lactamase inhibitor

Therapeutic class: Anti-infective

Pregnancy risk category B

Action

Inhibits bacterial cell-wall synthesis, resulting in cell death; tazobactam increases piperacillin efficacy by inhibiting penicillinases that can inactivate penicillin.

Pharmacokinetics

Piperacillin and tazobactam distribute widely into body tissues and fluids, including intestinal mucosa, gallbladder, lung, female reproductive tissues, interstitial fluid, and bile. Distribution into cerebrospinal fluid is low unless patient has inflamed meninges. Drug is approximately 30% bound to plasma proteins. Both drugs are eliminated by the kidneys. Piperacillin is excreted rapidly as unchanged drug, with 68% of dose excreted in urine; tazobactam and its metabolite are eliminated primarily by renal excretion, with 80% of dose excreted unchanged and remainder as single metabolite.

Onset	Peak	Duration
Immediate	Immediate	Unknown

How supplied

Powder for reconstitution for injection (white to off-white): 2 g piperacillin and 0.25 g tazobactam/vial, 3 g piperacillin and 0.375 g tazobactam/vial, 4 g piperacillin and 0.5 g tazobactam/vial

Solution for injection (premixed, frozen): 2.25 g (piperacillin sodium equivalent to 2 g piperacillin/tazobactam sodium equivalent to 0.25 g tazobactam) in 50 mL; 3.375 g (piperacillin sodium equivalent to 3 g piperacillin/tazobactam sodium equivalent to 0.375 g tazobactam) in 50 mL; 4.5 g (piperacillin sodium equivalent to 4 g piperacillin/tazobactam sodium equivalent to 0.5 g tazobactam) in 100 mL in single-dose plastic containers

Indications and dosages

➤ Community-acquired pneumonia, ruptured appendix, peritonitis, pelvic inflammatory disease, skin and skin-structure infections

Adults and children older than age 12: 3.375 g (3 g piperacillin, 0.375 g tazobactam) I.V. q 6 hours for 7 to 10 days

Dosage adjustment

- Adjust dosage for creatinine clearance below 40 mL/minute. In patients with nosocomial pneumonia who are receiving concomitant aminoglycosides, adjust aminoglycoside dosage according to manufacturer's recommendations. For recommended dosages and dosing frequency, see the table below. (*Note:* Dosages are given as total grams of piperacillin/tazobactam).

CrCl (mL/min)	All indications (except nosocomial pneumonia)	Nosocomial pneumonia
Above 40	3.375 q 6 hr	4.5 q 6 hr
20 to 40*	2.25 q 6 hr	3.375 q 6 hr
Below 20*	2.25 q 8 hr	2.25 q 6 hr
Hemodialysis†	2.25 q 12 hr	2.25 q 8 hr
CAPD‡	2.25 q 12 hr	2.25 q 8 hr

*Patients not receiving hemodialysis

†Give 0.75 g after each hemodialysis session on hemodialysis days.

‡Continuous ambulatory peritoneal dialysis

• Be aware that for hemodialysis patients, maximum dosage is 2.25 g every 12 hours for all indications other than nosocomial pneumonia, and 2.25 g every 8 hours for nosocomial pneumonia. Hemodialysis removes 30% to 40% of administered dose, so give additional dose of 0.75 g after each dialysis period on hemodialysis days. No additional dose is necessary for patients on continuous ambulatory peritoneal dialysis.

Administration

Preparation

Before administering, ask patient about allergy to penicillins, cephalosporins, imipenems, or beta-lactamase inhibitors.

Dilution and compatibility

• Know that drug in plastic containers does not require dilution. Do not add other drugs or solutions to plastic bags.
• Dilute each gram in vial with 5 mL diluent, such as sterile or bacteriostatic water for injection, normal saline solution, D_5W, dextrose 5% in normal saline solution, or 6% dextran in normal saline solution.

Do not use lactated Ringer's solution.

• Shake vial until drug dissolves. Further dilute with 50 mL compatible solution.
• Do not mix with other drugs.
• Do not mix in same container with aminoglycosides, which are chemically incompatible with piperacillin.
• Know that drug is chemically unstable in solutions containing only sodium bicarbonate and solutions that significantly alter pH.
• Do not add drug to blood products or albumin hydrolysates.
• Use immediately after reconstitution.
• Discard unused portion after 24 hours if stored at room temperature.

Infusion considerations

• Administer by I.V. infusion over 30 minutes.
• Discontinue primary infusion solution while drug is infusing.

Do not use plastic containers in series connections. Such use could result in air embolism due to residual air being drawn from primary container before administration of fluid from secondary container ends.

Monitoring

• Assess neurologic status, especially for seizures.
• Monitor vital signs and fluid intake and output.

Evaluate electrolyte levels, CBC with white cell differential, and culture and sensitivity test results. Watch for hypokalemia and blood dyscrasias.

• In patients receiving high doses or prolonged therapy, monitor for signs and symptoms of bacterial or fungal superinfection and pseudomembranous colitis.
• Monitor patient's dietary sodium intake (drug has high sodium content).

Immediately report rash, hives, severe diarrhea, black tongue, sore throat, fever, unusual bleeding, or bruising.

Storage

• Know that drug is stable for 24 hours when stored at room temperature of 20° to 25°C (68° to 77°F) and for 48 hours when refrigerated at 2° to 8°C (36° to 46°F).

Contraindications and precautions

Contraindicated in hypersensitivity to penicillins, cephalosporins, imipenems, or beta-lactamase inhibitors.

Use cautiously in heart failure, renal insufficiency (in children), seizures, bleeding disorders, uremia, hypokalemia, cystic fibrosis, patients with dietary sodium restrictions, pregnant or

P

breastfeeding patients, and ***children younger than age 12*** (safety and efficacy not established).

Adverse reactions

CNS: headache, insomnia, agitation, dizziness, anxiety, lethargy, hallucinations, depression, twitching, **coma, seizures**
CV: hypertension, chest pain, tachycardia
EENT: rhinitis, glossitis
GI: nausea, vomiting, diarrhea, constipation, dyspepsia, abdominal pain, **pseudomembranous colitis**
GU: interstitial nephritis, glomerulonephritis, oliguria, proteinuria, hematuria, vaginal candidiasis, vaginitis
Hematologic: anemia, eosinophilia, increased bleeding, **bone marrow depression, leukopenia, thrombocytopenia**
Metabolic: hypokalemia, hypernatremia
Respiratory: dyspnea
Skin: rash, pruritus
Other: fever; pain, edema, inflammation, or phlebitis at I.V. site; superinfection; hypersensitivity reactions including serum sickness and **anaphylaxis**

Interactions

Drug-drug. *Aminoglycosides:* aminoglycoside inactivation
Aspirin, probenecid: increased piperacillin blood level
Hormonal contraceptives: decreased contraceptive efficacy
Methotrexate: increased risk of methotrexate toxicity
Tetracyclines: decreased piperacillin efficacy
Vecuronium: prolonged neuromuscular blockade
Drug-diagnostic tests. *Coombs' test, urine glucose tests using copper-reduction method (Clinitest, Benedict's solution, or Fehling solution), urine protein:* false-positive results
Eosinophils: increased
Granulocytes, hemoglobin, platelets, white blood cells: decreased

Toxicity and overdose

- Overdose signs and symptoms include nausea, vomiting, diarrhea, and possible neuromuscular excitability or seizures (particularly in patients with renal failure).
- Provide supportive and symptomatic therapy, as indicated. Hemodialysis may reduce excessive serum concentrations of piperacillin or tazobactam.

Patient teaching

- Teach patient to monitor urine output and report significant changes.
- Instruct patient to report unusual pain, redness, swelling, or other changes at infusion site.
- As appropriate, review all other significant and life-threatening adverse reactions and interactions, especially those related to the drugs and tests mentioned above.

plasma protein fraction

Plasmanate

Pharmacologic class: Human plasma protein
Therapeutic class: Plasma expander
Pregnancy risk category C

Action

Maintains plasma colloid osmotic pressure, enhancing movement of fluid from interstitial tissues into circulatory system and thereby regulating blood volume

Pharmacokinetics

No information available

Onset	Peak	Duration
Immediate	Immediate	Unknown

How supplied

Solution for injection: 5% in 50-mL, 250-mL, and 500-mL vials

Indications and dosages

➢ Hypovolemic shock

Adults: Initially, 250 to 500 mL (12.5 to 25 g protein) by I.V. infusion, administered at a rate of up to 10 mL/minute

Infants and young children: 6.6 to 33 mL/kg (0.33 to 1.65 g/kg protein) administered at a rate of up to 5 to 10 mL/minute. May repeat dose if needed, depending on patient condition and response.

Administration

Preparation

- Ensure that patient is adequately hydrated before administering.

Dilution and compatibility

- Be aware that drug is ready for use without further preparation.
- Know that drug is compatible with usual I.V. solutions of carbohydrates or electrolytes, as well as whole blood and packed red blood cells.
- Discard unused portion.

Infusion considerations

- Know that dosage and infusion rate depend on patient's condition and response.
- Do not infuse through same I.V. line with solutions containing amino acids or alcohol.
- Do not use infusion that has been frozen or contains visible sediment.
- Infuse at site distant from infection or trauma, usually at a rate no faster than 10 mL/minute.

Be aware that rapid infusion (especially in normovolemic patients) may cause vascular overload, dyspnea, and pulmonary edema.

- Monitor blood pressure; slow infusion rate if hypotension occurs.

Monitoring

Assess for signs and symptoms of vascular overload, including heart failure and pulmonary edema.

- Monitor vital signs hourly; expect gradual return to normal during and after drug therapy.
- Monitor fluid intake and output.

Storage

- Store at room temperature no higher than 30°C (86°F).

Contraindications and precautions

Contraindicated in hypersensitivity to drug or albumin, heart failure, severe anemia, normal or increased intravascular volume, and during cardiopulmonary bypass.

Use cautiously in hepatic or renal impairment, reduced cardiac reserve, decreased sodium intake, and pregnant patients.

Adverse reactions

CNS: headache, paresthesia

CV: hypotension, tachycardia, **vascular overload and heart failure** (with rapid I.V. infusion)

GI: nausea, vomiting, increased salivation

Respiratory: dyspnea, **pulmonary edema** (with rapid I.V. infusion)

Skin: rash, flushing

Other: fever, chills

Interactions

None significant

Toxicity and overdose

- No information on overdose is available.
- Provide symptomatic and supportive therapy.

P

Patient teaching

- Instruct patient to report difficulty breathing.
- Tell patient to report such adverse effects as headache, nausea, and vomiting.
- Inform patient about the need for regular blood tests.
- As appropriate, review all other significant and life-threatening adverse reactions mentioned above.

polymyxin B sulfate

Pharmacologic class: Polypeptide antibiotic
Therapeutic class: Anti-infective
Pregnancy risk category B

FDA BOXED WARNING

- Renal function should be evaluated carefully; decrease dosage in patients with renal damage and nitrogen retention. Patients with nephrotoxicity caused by this drug usually have albuminuria, cellular casts, and azotemia. Withdraw drug if urine output diminishes and blood urea nitrogen (BUN) rises.
- Neurotoxic reactions may produce irritability, weakness, drowsiness, ataxia, perioral paresthesia, numbness of extremities, and blurred vision. Usually, these symptoms are associated with high serum levels in patients with impaired renal function or nephrotoxicity.
- Avoid concurrent or sequential use of this drug with other neurotoxic or nephrotoxic drugs, especially amikacin, bacitracin, cephaloridine, colistin, gentamicin, kanamycin, neomycin, paromomycin, streptomycin, tobramycin, and viomycin.
- Neurotoxicity may lead to respiratory paralysis from neuromuscular blockade, especially when drug is given soon after anesthetics or muscle relaxants.
- Safety of this drug in pregnancy has not been established.

Action

Interferes with bacterial cell-wall synthesis, causing cell to rupture and die; bactericidal against almost all gram-positive organisms except *Proteus* group

Pharmacokinetics

Active blood levels are low because drug loses 50% of its activity in serum; repeated injections may provide cumulative effect. Levels tend to be higher in infants and children. Tissue diffusion is poor; drug does not cross blood-brain barrier. It is excreted slowly by the kidneys.

Onset	Peak	Duration
Unknown	Unknown	Unknown

How supplied

Powder for reconstitution for injection: 500,000 units/vial

Indications and dosages

➤ Acute urinary tract and bloodstream infections caused by susceptible strains of *Pseudomonas aeruginosa;* mild to severe infections caused by susceptible strains of *Escherichia coli* (specifically urinary tract infections), *Aerobacter aerogenes* (specifically bacteremia), and *Klebsiella pneumoniae* (specifically bacteremia) when less potentially toxic drugs are ineffective or contraindicated

Adults and children older than age 2: 15,000 to 25,000 units/kg/day I.V. (may be divided and given q 12 hours) in patients with normal renal function. Maximum dosage is 25,000 units/kg.

Infants: Up to 40,000 units/kg/day I.V. in infants with normal renal function

Dosage adjustment

• In renal impairment, reduce adult dosage from 15,000 units/kg. Infusions may be given every 12 hours; however, total daily dosage must not exceed 25,000 units/kg.

Administration

Preparation

• Assess baseline renal function before starting drug.

• Avoid concurrent use of curariform muscle relaxants and other neurotoxic drugs (ether, tubocurarine, succinylcholine, gallamine, decamethonium, and sodium citrate), as respiratory depression may occur.

• Ensure adequate fluid intake before and during therapy.

Dilution and compatibility

• Dissolve 500,000 units in 300 to 500 mL D_5W.

• Discard unused portion after 72 hours.

Infusion considerations

• Administer by continuous I.V. infusion at rate prescribed.

Monitoring

Monitor for hypersensitivity reaction; be prepared to intervene appropriately.

Continue frequent monitoring of renal function and drug blood levels during therapy to avoid nephrotoxicity. Withdraw drug if nephrotoxicity occurs.

If signs or symptoms of respiratory paralysis appear, assist with respiratory support as required and withdraw drug.

Watch for neurotoxic reactions, such as irritability, weakness, drowsiness, dizziness, and ataxia; be prepared to intervene appropriately. Withdraw drug if neurotoxicity occurs.

• If superinfection occurs, provide appropriate therapy.

Storage

• Refrigerate drug.

Contraindications and precautions

Contraindicated in hypersensitivity to polymyxins.

Use cautiously in such neuromuscular diseases as myasthenia gravis, renal impairment, pregnant patients (safety not established), breastfeeding patients, and ***children.***

Adverse reactions

CNS: neurotoxicity (dizziness progressing to ataxia, drowsiness, perioral and stocking-glove paresthesias)

GU: nephrotoxicity (albuminuria, cylindruria, azotemia, rising blood levels without dosage increase)

Respiratory: respiratory paralysis

Skin: urticarial rash

Other: facial flushing, drug fever, superinfection, thrombophlebitis at injection site, hypersensitivity reaction including **anaphylaxis**

Interactions

Drug-drug. *Aminoglycosides:* increased risk of respiratory paralysis and renal dysfunction

Nondepolarizing muscle relaxants: enhanced neuromuscular blockade

Drug-diagnostic tests. *BUN, serum creatinine:* increased

Toxicity and overdose

• Overdose signs and symptoms may include neurologic, renal, and respiratory dysfunction, manifested as dizziness, drowsiness, albuminuria, and respiratory paralysis with apnea.

• Be aware that respiratory paralysis may not improve with neostigmine or edrophonium. If ordered, administer calcium chloride. Provide supportive

P

therapy until muscle function returns. Dialysis does not remove drug.

Patient teaching

Instruct patient to immediately report signs and symptoms of hypersensitivity reaction, such as rash or difficulty breathing.

- As appropriate, review all other significant and life-threatening adverse reactions and interactions, especially those related to the drugs and tests mentioned above.

[redacted]

potassium acetate

Pharmacologic class: Mineral, electrolyte
Therapeutic class: Electrolyte replacement, nutritional supplement
Pregnancy risk category C

Action

Maintains acid-base balance, isotonicity, and electrophysiologic balance throughout body tissues; crucial to nerve impulse transmission and contraction of cardiac, skeletal, and smooth muscle. Also essential for normal renal function and carbohydrate metabolism.

Pharmacokinetics

Drug appears in low concentrations in plasma and extracellular fluids. Acetate ion is completely metabolized in body, providing source of hydrogen ion acceptors. Most of dose is excreted in urine; consequently, kidney normally determines potassium balance.

Onset	Peak	Duration
Rapid	End of infusion	Unknown

How supplied

Concentrate for injection: 2 mEq/mL in 20-, 50-, and 100-mL single-dose vials

Indications and dosages

To prevent or treat potassium depletion; diabetic acidosis (especially during vigorous insulin and dextrose treatment); metabolic alkalosis; arrhythmias (especially those caused by cadiac glycosides); attacks of hereditary or familial periodic paralysis; hyperadrenocorticism; primary aldosteronism; overmedication with adrenocortical steroids, testosterone, or corticotropin; healing phase of scalds or burns

Adults: Dosage highly individualized. If potassium level is above 2.5 mEq/L, give 40 mEq/L as additive to I.V. infusion at a maximum rate of 20 mEq/hour; maximum daily dosage is 200 mEq. If potassium level is below 2 mEq/L, give 80 mEq/L as additive to I.V. infusion at a maximum rate of 40 mEq/hour (with cardiac monitoring); maximum daily dosage is 400 mEq.

Children: Dosage highly individualized; up to 3 mEq/kg or 40 mEq/m^2/day as additive to I.V. infusion.

Administration

Preparation

- Be aware that potassium preparations are not interchangeable.
- Know that dosages are expressed in milliequivalents (mEq) of potassium and that potassium acetate contains 10.2 mEq/g.
- Ensure that patient is well-hydrated and urinating before starting therapy.

Dilution and compatibility

Dilute in large volume of compatible I.V. solution according to manufacturer's instructions.

To make sure potassium is well-mixed in compatible solution, do not add it to I.V. bag in hanging position.

• Use solution only if clear.

Infusion considerations

Clinical alert: Never administer undiluted.

Clinical alert: Give as additive to large volume of solution by I.V. infusion only. Never give by I.V. push or I.M. route. Direct injection can be instantly fatal.

Clinical alert: Use peripheral I.V. line with a maximum rate of 40 mEq/hour (with cardiac monitoring).

Clinical alert: Administer slowly to reduce risk of fatal hyperkalemia.

Clinical alert: Be aware that maximum infusion rate without cardiac monitoring is 20 mEq/hour. Infusion rates above 20 mEq/hour necessitate cardiac monitoring.

• If patient complains of burning with I.V. administration, decrease flow rate.

Monitoring

• Monitor renal function, fluid intake and output, and potassium, creatinine, and blood urea nitrogen levels.

Clinical alert: Know that drug is contraindicated in severe renal impairment and must be used with extreme caution (if at all) in patients with any degree of renal impairment, due to risk of life-threatening hyperkalemia.

• Assess vital signs and ECG; watch for arrhythmias.

• Evaluate patient's neurologic status; watch for neurologic complications.

• Monitor I.V. site for signs and symptoms of irritation.

Storage

• Store at controlled room temperature of 15° to 30°C (59° to 86°F).

Contraindications and precautions

Contraindicated in acute dehydration, heat cramps, hyperkalemia, hyperkalemic familial periodic paralysis, severe renal impairment, severe hemolytic reactions, untreated Addison's disease, severe tissue trauma, concurrent use of potassium-sparing diuretics, angiotensin-converting enzyme (ACE) inhibitors, and salt substitutes containing potassium.

Use cautiously in cardiac disease, slight to moderate renal impairment, diabetes mellitus, hypomagnesemia, pregnant or breastfeeding patients, and ***children*** (safety and efficacy not established).

Adverse reactions

CNS: confusion, unusual fatigue, restlessness, asthenia, flaccid paralysis, paresthesia, absent reflexes

CV: ECG changes, hypotension, **arrhythmias, heart block, cardiac arrest**

GI: nausea, vomiting, diarrhea, abdominal discomfort, flatulence

Metabolic: hyperkalemia

Musculoskeletal: weakness and heaviness of legs

Respiratory: respiratory paralysis

Other: irritation at I.V. site

Interactions

Drug-drug. *ACE inhibitors, potassium-sparing diuretics, other potassium-containing preparations:* increased risk of hyperkalemia

Drug-diagnostic tests. *Potassium:* increased

Drug-foods. *Salt substitutes containing potassium:* increased risk of hyperkalemia

Drug-herb. *Dandelion:* increased risk of hyperkalemia

Licorice: decreased response to potassium

Toxicity and overdose

• Mild hyperkalemia (potassium level of 5.6 to 6.5 mEq/L) to moderate hyperkalemia (6.6 to 8 mEq/L) may be asymptomatic, causing only increased potassium level and ECG changes. When potassium level exceeds 8 mEq/L, other toxicity signs and symptoms

P

include dangerous arrhythmias, muscle weakness progressing to flaccid muscle paralysis, respiratory paralysis, and death. Be aware that hyperkalemia paradoxically produces symptoms similar to those of hypokalemia.
• Discontinue infusion immediately, monitor ECG constantly, and institute intensive corrective therapy to reduce serum potassium level and restore acid-base balance, if necessary. As ordered, give dextrose and insulin by I.V. infusion to shift potassium into cells, and sodium bicarbonate I.V. to reverse acidosis and produce intracellular shift. Calcium gluconate or calcium chloride 10% may reverse ECG changes. Dialysis may help remove drug.

Patient teaching

• Teach patient to report unusual pain, redness, swelling, or other reactions at infusion site.
• Advise patient to report nausea, vomiting, confusion, numbness and tingling, unusual tiredness or weakness, or heavy feeling in legs.
• Instruct patient to avoid salt substitutes.
• As appropriate, review all other significant and life-threatening adverse reactions and interactions, especially those related to the drugs, tests, foods, and herbs mentioned above.

potassium chloride

Pharmacologic class: Mineral, electrolyte
Therapeutic class: Electrolyte replacement, nutritional supplement
Pregnancy risk category C

Action

Maintains acid-base balance, isotonicity, and electrophysiologic balance throughout body tissues; crucial to nerve impulse transmission and contraction of cardiac, skeletal, and smooth muscle. Also essential for normal renal function and carbohydrate metabolism.

Pharmacokinetics

Drug appears in low concentration in plasma and extracellular fluids. Most of dose is excreted in urine; consequently, the kidneys normally determine potassium balance.

Onset	Peak	Duration
Rapid	End of infusion	Unknown

How supplied

Parenteral injection (concentrate): 2 mEq/mL
Parenteral injection (for I.V. infusion): 0.1 mEq/mL, 0.2 mEq/mL, 0.3 mEq/mL, 0.4 mEq/mL
Potassium chloride in 5% dextrose injection: 10 mEq/L, 20 mEq/L, 30 mEq/L, 40 mEq/L
Potassium chloride in 0.9% sodium chloride injection: 20 mEq/L, 40 mEq/L
Potassium chloride in dextrose and lactated Ringer's injection: various strengths
Potassium chloride in dextrose and sodium chloride injection: various strengths in plastic containers

Indications and dosages

➤ Potassium depletion; diabetic acidosis; metabolic alkalosis; arrhythmias; periodic paralysis attacks; hyperadrenocorticism; primary aldosteronism; healing phase of scalds or burns; overmedication with adrenocorticoids, testosterone, or corticotropin
Adults: Dosage highly individualized. If serum potassium level is above

2.5 mEq/L, give 40 mEq/L as additive to I.V. infusion at a rate of 10 to 20 mEq/hour; maximum daily dosage is 200 mEq. If potassium level is below 2 mEq/L, give 80 mEq/L as additive to I.V. infusion at a maximum rate of 40 mEq/hour (with cardiac monitoring); maximum daily dosage is 400 mEq.
Children: Dosage highly individualized; up to 3 mEq/kg or 40 mEq/m^2/day as additive to I.V. infusion.

Administration

Preparation

- Be aware that potassium preparations are not interchangeable.
- Know that dosages are expressed in milliequivalents (mEq) of potassium and that potassium chloride contains 13.4 mEq potassium/g.
- Make sure patient is well-hydrated and urinating before starting therapy.

Dilution and compatibility

Clinical alert: Dilute in large volume of compatible I.V. solution according to manufacturer's instructions.

Clinical alert: To make sure potassium is well-mixed in compatible solution, do not add drug to I.V. bag in hanging position.

- Use solution only if clear.

Infusion considerations

Clinical alert: Never give undiluted.

Clinical alert: Give as additive to large volume of solution by I.V. infusion only; never give by I.V. push or I.M. route. Direct injection can be instantly fatal.

Clinical alert: Administer slowly to reduce risk of fatal hyperkalemia.

Clinical alert: Be aware that maximum infusion rate without cardiac monitoring is 20 mEq/hour. Infusion rates above 20 mEq/hour necessitate cardiac monitoring.

- If patient complains of burning with I.V. administration, decrease flow rate.

Clinical alert: Do not use plastic containers in series connections. Such use could result in air embolism due to residual air being drawn from primary container before administration of fluid from secondary container ends.

Monitoring

- Assess vital signs and ECG; stay alert for arrhythmias.
- Monitor neurologic status; watch for neurologic complications.
- Monitor I.V. site for signs and symptoms of irritation.

Clinical alert: Know that potassium is contraindicated in severe renal impairment and must be used with extreme caution (if at all) in patients with any degree of renal impairment due to risk of life-threatening hyperkalemia.

- Monitor renal function, fluid intake and output, and potassium, creatinine, and blood urea nitrogen levels.

Storage

- Store at controlled room temperature.

Contraindications and precautions

Contraindicated in hypersensitivity to tartrazine or alcohol (some products); hyperkalemia; hyperkalemic familial periodic paralysis; acute dehydration; heat cramps; severe renal impairment; severe hemolytic reactions; severe tissue trauma; untreated Addison's disease; and concurrent use of potassium-sparing diuretics, angiotensin-enzyme converting (ACE) inhibitors, or salt substitutes containing potassium.

Use cautiously in cardiac disease, slight to moderate renal impairment, diabetes mellitus, hypomagnesemia, pregnant or breastfeeding patients, and ***children*** (safety and efficacy not established).

Adverse reactions

CNS: confusion, unusual fatigue, restlessness, asthenia, flaccid paralysis, paresthesia, absent reflexes
CV: ECG changes, hypotension, **arrhythmias, heart block, cardiac arrest**

GI: nausea, vomiting, diarrhea, abdominal discomfort, flatulence
Metabolic: hyperkalemia
Musculoskeletal: weakness and heaviness of legs
Respiratory: respiratory paralysis
Other: irritation at I.V. site

Interactions

Drug-drug. *ACE inhibitors, potassium-sparing diuretics, other potassium-containing preparations:* increased risk of hyperkalemia
Drug-diagnostic tests. *Potassium:* increased
Drug-foods. *Salt substitutes containing potassium:* increased risk of hyperkalemia
Drug-herb. *Dandelion:* increased risk of hyperkalemia
Licorice: decreased response to potassium

Toxicity and overdose

• Mild hyperkalemia (potassium level of 5.6 to 6.5 mEq/L) to moderate hyperkalemia (6.6 to 8 mEq/L) may be asymptomatic and cause only increased potassium concentration and ECG changes. When potassium concentration exceeds 8 mEq/L, other toxicity signs and symptoms include dangerous arrhythmias, muscle weakness progressing to flaccid muscle paralysis, respiratory paralysis, and death. Be aware that hyperkalemia paradoxically produces symptoms similar to those of hypokalemia.
• Discontinue infusion immediately, monitor ECG constantly, and institute intensive corrective therapy to reduce serum potassium level and restore acid-base balance, if necessary. As ordered, give dextrose and insulin by I.V. infusion to shift potassium into cells, and sodium bicarbonate I.V. to reverse acidosis and produce intracellular shift. Calcium gluconate or calcium chloride 10% may reverse ECG changes. Dialysis may help remove potassium.

Patient teaching

• Advise patient to report nausea, vomiting, confusion, numbness and tingling, unusual fatigue or weakness, or heavy feeling in legs.
• Teach patient not to use salt substitutes.
• As appropriate, review all other significant and life-threatening adverse reactions and interactions, especially those related to the drugs, tests, foods, and herbs mentioned above.

procainamide hydrochloride

Pronestyl

Pharmacologic class: Membrane stabilizer
Therapeutic class: Antiarrhythmic (class IA)
Pregnancy risk category C

FDA BOXED WARNING

• Prolonged use commonly leads to positive antinuclear antibody (ANA) test, with or without symptoms of lupus erythematosus–like syndrome. If ANA titer is positive, clinician must weigh benefits vs. risks of continued therapy.
• In National Heart, Lung and Blood Institute's Cardiac Arrhythmia Suppression Trial, excessive mortality or nonfatal cardiac arrest rate (7.7%) occurred in patients who received encainide or flecainide. Considering procainamide's known proarrhythmic properties and lack of evidence that any antiarrhythmic improves survival in patients without life-threatening arrhythmias, use of this drug and other antiarrhythmics

should be reserved for patients with life-threatening ventricular arrhythmias.
• Agranulocytosis, bone marrow depression, neutropenia, hypoplastic anemia, and thrombocytopenia occur in approximately 0.5% of patients receiving drug (most of whom received recommended dosages). Deaths have occurred; in agranulocytosis, mortality was approximately 20% to 25%. Because most such events occurred during first 12 weeks of therapy, CBCs with white cell differential and platelets should be performed weekly for first 3 months of therapy and then periodically. Obtain CBC promptly if patient develops signs or symptoms of infection (such as fever, chills, sore throat. or stomatitis), bruising, or bleeding. If a hematologic disorder occurs, withdraw drug; blood counts usually return to normal within 1 month of withdrawal. Use caution when administering to patients with preexisting marrow failure or cytopenia.

Action
Decreases myocardial excitability by inhibiting conduction velocity; also depresses myocardial contractility

Pharmacokinetics
Drug reversibly binds to plasma proteins (15% to 20%); considerable amounts are more slowly and reversibly bound to heart, liver, lung, and kidney tissue. Elimination half-life is 3 to 4 hours in patients with normal renal function, but longer in patients with reduced creatinine clearance and advancing age. Significant amount of circulating drug may be metabolized in the liver to *N*-acetylprocainamide (NAPA), drug's active metabolite. Hepatic acetylation, renal function, and age significantly influence effective biologic half-life of parent drug and its derivative. Trace amounts may be excreted in urine as free and conjugated p-aminobenzoic acid, 30% to 60% as unchanged drug, and 6% to 52% as NAPA. Both procainamide and NAPA are eliminated by active tubular secretion and glomerular filtration.

Onset	Peak	Duration
Immediate	Immediate	Unknown

How supplied
Solution for injection (aqueous): 100 mg/mL in 10-mL multidose vials, 500 mg/mL in 2-mL multidose vials

Indications and dosages
➤ Life-threatening ventricular arrhythmias
Adults: 100 mg by slow I.V. push at a rate of 50 mg/minute, repeated q 5 minutes until arrhythmia subsides, up to a maximum advisable dosage of 1 g. Alternatively, loading dose of 500 to 600 mg by I.V. infusion over 25 to 30 minutes. With either method, maximum loading dose is 1 g. When arrhythmia subsides, give continuous I.V. infusion of 2 to 6 mg/minute. For long-term maintenance, oral therapy is recommended.
Children: 2 to 6 mg/kg (maximum 100 mg) I.V. as loading dose over 5 minutes, repeated q 5 to 10 minutes; maximum loading dose is 15 mg/kg or 500 mg in 30-minute period. For maintenance, I.V. infusion of 0.02 to 0.08 mg/kg/minute, up to a total maintenance infusion of 2 g/24 hours.

Dosage adjustment
• Adjust dosage individually in renal impairment, which may cause accumulation of high drug blood levels.

P

Administration

Preparation

Ask patient about procaine sensitivity before giving drug (cross-sensitivity may occur).

Dilution and compatibility

- For direct I.V. injection, dilute with 5 to 10 mL D_5W for injection to help control dosage rate.
- For I.V. infusion, dilute 1 g with 50, 250, or 500 mL D_5W to yield a concentration of 20 mg/mL, 4 mg/mL, or 2 mg/mL, respectively. Use 20 mg/mL as loading dose and 4 mg/mL or 2 mg/mL as maintenance dose.
- Discard solution if darker than slightly yellow or otherwise discolored.

Infusion considerations

- Monitor blood pressure and ECG during administration to avoid transient increases in drug blood levels and possible hypotension.
- Administer I.V. with patient in supine position to avoid hypotensive effects.
- Give loading dose by slow direct I.V. injection into vein or into tubing of established infusion line, at a rate not exceeding 50 mg/minute.
- When administering loading dose by I.V. infusion, use infusion pump to ensure that drug infuses at 1 mL/minute for 25 to 30 minutes.
- Give maintenance dose by I.V. infusion. Use infusion pump to ensure drug infuses at 1 to 3 mL/minute for 2 mg/mL concentration or at 0.5 to 1.5 mL/minute for 4 mg/mL concentration.

Do not leave patient's bedside during I.V. administration.

Monitoring

Monitor blood pressure and ECG continuously.

If ECG shows prolonged QT intervals and QRS complexes, heart block, or worsening arrhythmia, stop drug administration, run rhythm strip, and contact prescriber immediately.

- Assess blood levels of procainamide and NAPA.

Monitor electrolyte levels, CBC, and ANA titer; watch for signs and symptoms of blood dyscrasias.

- Evaluate patient for signs and symptoms of lupuslike syndrome.

Storage

- Store at controlled room temperature of 15° to 30°C (59° to 86°F).

Contraindications and precautions

Contraindicated in hypersensitivity to drug, tartrazine, procaine, or sulfites; complete heart block; lupus erythematosus; and torsades de pointes.

Use cautiously in procaine hypersensitivity, renal impairment, ischemic heart disease, heart failure, first-degree heart block, atypical ventricular tachycardia, myasthenia gravis, systemic lupus erythematosus, cytopenia, concurrent use of other antiarrhythmics, pregnant or breastfeeding patients, and ***children.***

Adverse reactions

CNS: headache, dizziness, confusion, psychosis, restlessness, asthenia, depression, neuropathy, **seizures**

CV: hypotension, bradycardia, **atrioventricular block, ventricular fibrillation, ventricular asystole, cardiovascular collapse, cardiac arrest**

GI: nausea, vomiting, diarrhea, anorexia

Hematologic: hemolytic anemia, agranulocytosis, thrombocytopenia, neutropenia

Skin: rash, urticaria, pruritus, flushing

Other: bitter taste, lupuslike syndrome, edema

Interactions

Drug-drug. *Amiodarone:* increased procainamide blood level and risk of toxicity

Anticholinesterase drugs: decreased anticholinesterase effects

Antihypertensives: additive hypotension

Beta-adrenergic blockers, cimetidine, ranitidine, trimethoprim: increased procainamide blood level
Lidocaine: additive cardiodepressant action, conduction abnormalities
Neuromuscular blockers: increased skeletal muscle relaxation
Other antiarrhythmics: additive or antagonistic effects, additive toxicity
Trimethoprim: increased pharmacologic effects of procainamide
Drug-herb. *Henbane:* increased anticholinergic activity
Jimsonweed: adverse cardiovascular effects
Licorice: prolonged QT interval
Drug-behaviors. *Alcohol use:* altered drug blood level

Toxicity and overdose

- Excessive doses may cause progressive widening of QRS complex, prolonged QT and PR intervals, lowered R and T waves, and increasing atrioventricular block. Increased ventricular extrasystoles, ventricular tachycardia, or ventricular fibrillation also may occur. Transient high drug blood level may induce hypotension, affecting systolic more than diastolic pressure (especially in hypertensive patients). Such high blood levels also may cause CNS depression, tremor, and respiratory depression. Drug blood levels above 10 mcg/mL are increasingly associated with toxic findings, which occur occasionally in 10- to 12-mcg/mL range but more often in 12- to 15-mcg/mL range and commonly in patients with levels above 15 mcg/mL.
- No specific antidote exists. Provide supportive measures, observe closely, monitor vital signs, give I.V. pressor agents if ordered, and provide mechanical cardiorespiratory support. If available, procainamide and NAPA blood levels may help assess degree of toxicity and response to therapy. Hemodialysis (but not peritoneal dialysis) removes procainamide and NAPA.

Patient teaching

Advise patient to immediately report cardiovascular symptoms or bleeding tendency.
- As appropriate, review all other significant and life-threatening adverse reactions and interactions, especially those related to the drugs, herbs, and behaviors mentioned above.

prochlorperazine edisylate

Compazine

Pharmacologic class: Phenothiazine
Therapeutic class: Antiemetic, antipsychotic, anxiolytic
Pregnancy risk category C

Action

Exerts anticholinergic, CNS depressant, and antihistaminic effects. Depresses release of hypothalamic and hypophyseal hormones, decreases sensitivity of middle-ear labyrinth, and reduces conduction in vestibular-cerebellar pathways.

Pharmacokinetics

Drug distributes widely into tissues. It is metabolized in the liver, highly bound to proteins, and eliminated in urine (with less than 1% excreted unchanged).

Onset	Peak	Duration
Rapid (min)	10-30 min	3-4 hr

How supplied

Solution for injection (aqueous): 5 mg/mL

Indications and dosages

➢ Nausea

Adults: 2.5 to 10 mg I.V., not to exceed 40 mg/day

➢ Nausea and vomiting associated with surgery

Adults: 5 to 10 mg I.V. 15 to 30 minutes before anesthesia induction, repeated once if necessary

Off-label uses

- Migraine

Administration

Preparation

- Know that injection solution may cause contact dermatitis; do not get it on hands or clothing.
- Be aware that once desired response occurs, patient should be switched to oral form at same or higher dosage.

Dilution and compatibility

- For I.V. injection, drug may be given undiluted, or each 5 mg (1 mL) may be diluted in 9 mL isotonic solution, such as normal saline solution for injection.
- For I.V. infusion, dilute dosages above 10 mg in at least 1,000 mL of compatible isotonic I.V. solution, such as normal saline solution, D_5W, dextrose 5% in half-normal saline solution, Ringer's solution, or lactated Ringer's solution.
- Do not mix in same syringe with other drugs.
- Know that slight yellowish discoloration does not alter potency. Discard solution if markedly discolored.

Infusion considerations

Do not give by bolus injection.

- For slow I.V. injection, do not exceed 10 mg as a single dose, and do not exceed a rate of 5 mg/mL/minute.
- For I.V. infusion, administer by slow intermittent or prolonged infusion at no more than 5 mg/mL/minute.

Monitoring

Monitor neurologic status, especially for signs and symptoms of neuroleptic malignant syndrome (high fever, sweating, unstable blood pressure, stupor, muscle rigidity, and autonomic dysfunction).

- In long-term therapy, assess for other adverse CNS effects, including extrapyramidal symptoms and tardive dyskinesia.
- Watch for hypotension; keep patient supine for 30 minutes after infusion.
- Evaluate CBC and liver function test results.

Storage

- Store at controlled room temperature of 15° to 30°C (59° to 86°F). Do not freeze; protect from light.

Contraindications and precautions

Contraindicated in hypersensitivity to drug or other phenothiazines, coma, concurrent use of large amounts of CNS depressants, pediatric surgery, and ***children younger than age 2 or weighing less than 9 kg (20 lb).***

Use cautiously in cardiovascular or hepatic disease, glaucoma, seizures, patients who expect to be exposed to extreme heat, and ***children with acute illness.***

Adverse reactions

CNS: extrapyramidal reactions, sedation, tardive dyskinesia, **neuroleptic malignant syndrome**

CV: ECG changes, orthostatic hypotension, tachycardia

EENT: blurred vision, lens opacities, pigmentary retinopathy, dry eyes

GI: constipation, ileus, dry mouth, anorexia

GU: pink or reddish brown urine, urine retention, galactorrhea

Hematologic: agranulocytosis, leukopenia
Hepatic: cholestatic jaundice, **hepatitis**
Metabolic: hyperthermia
Skin: photosensitivity, pigmentation changes, rash
Other: allergic reactions

Interactions

Drug-drug. *Anticonvulsants:* reduced seizure threshold
Antineoplastics: masking of toxicity caused by antineoplastics
CNS depressants (including antihistamines, anticholinergics, opioid analgesics, other phenothiazines, sedative-hypnotics): additive CNS depression
Guanethidine: inhibition of antihypertensive effects
Oral anticoagulants: decreased anticoagulant effect
Phenytoin: increased or decreased phenytoin blood level
Propranolol: increased blood levels of both drugs
Thiazide diuretics: increased risk of orthostatic hypotension
Drug-diagnostic tests. *Liver function tests:* abnormal results
Phenylketonuria test: false-positive result
Drug-herb. *Betel nut:* increased risk of extrapyramidal reactions
Evening primrose oil: increased risk of seizures
Kava: increased risk of drug-related adverse reactions
Drug-behaviors. *Alcohol use:* additive CNS depression

Toxicity and overdose

- Overdose causes mainly dystonic adverse reactions, such as neck spasm, back muscle rigidity possibly progressing to opisthotonus, carpopedal spasm, trismus, difficulty swallowing, and tongue protrusion. Other manifestations may include somnolence, coma, agitation, restlessness, seizures, ECG changes, arrhythmias, fever, and autonomic reactions (such as hypotension and ileus).
- Provide symptomatic and supportive therapy. Maintain open airway. If ordered, give antiparkinsonian drugs, barbiturates, or diphenhydramine hydrochloride—but take care to avoid increasing respiratory depression with these drugs. If giving stimulants, use caution because some may cause seizures. For hypotension, expect to give norepinephrine bitartrate and phenylephrine hydrochloride. Know that other pressor agents, including epinephrine, are not recommended because they may lower blood pressure further. Dialysis does not remove drug.

Patient teaching

- (Clinical alert) Teach patient to recognize and immediately report signs and symptoms of allergic reaction or neuroleptic malignant syndrome.
- Inform patient about drug's other CNS effects; instruct patient to contact prescriber if these occur.
- Advise patient to avoid driving and other hazardous activities until drug's effects on concentration, vision, alertness, and motor skills are known.
- Caution patient to avoid alcohol and herbal products.
- Tell patient that drug may turn urine pink or reddish brown.
- As appropriate, review all other significant and life-threatening adverse reactions and interactions, especially those related to the drugs, tests, herbs, and behaviors mentioned above.

P

promethazine hydrochloride

Pharmacologic class: Phenothiazine (nonselective)
Therapeutic class: Antihistamine, antiemetic, sedative-hypnotic
Pregnancy risk category C

FDA BOXED WARNING

- Use caution when administering to pediatric patients age 2 and older. Preferably, use lowest effective dosage in these patients and avoid concurrent use of other drugs with respiratory depressant effects.

Action

Blocks effects (but not release) of histamine, exerts strong alpha-adrenergic effect, inhibits chemoreceptor trigger zone in medulla, and alters dopamine effects by indirectly reducing reticular stimulation in CNS

Pharmacokinetics

Drug is metabolized by the liver to various compounds; sulfoxides of promethazine and *N*-demethylpromethazine are predominant metabolites appearing in urine.

Onset	Peak	Duration
3-5 min	Unknown	4-12 hr

How supplied

Solution for injection: 25 mg/mL and 50 mg/mL in 1-mL ampules and 1-mL and 10-mL vials

Indications and dosages

➢ Type 1 hypersensitivity reaction
Adults: 25 mg I.V.; may repeat in 2 hours

➢ Sedation
Adults: 25 to 50 mg I.V. at bedtime

➢ Adjunct to preoperative or postoperative analgesia
Adults: 25 to 50 mg I.V. given with appropriately reduced dosage of opioid or barbiturate and required amount of belladonna alkaloid
Children older than age 2: 0.5 mg/kg I.V., given with appropriately reduced dosage of opioid or barbiturate and required amount of belladonna alkaloid

➢ Nausea
Adults: 12.5 to 25 mg I.V.; may repeat q 4 hours p.r.n.
Children older than age 2: I.V. dosages no larger than 50% of adult I.V. dosage. Do not administer if cause of vomiting is unknown.

Administration

Preparation

- Make sure ampule indicates "for I.V. use."

Dilution and compatibility

- Know that drug may be given undiluted. Or, if desired, dilute 1 mL (25 or 50 mg) with 9 mL normal saline solution for injection to yield 2.5 to 5 mg/mL, respectively.
- Know that slightly yellow color of solution does not alter potency. Discard if significantly discolored.

Infusion considerations

- Because drug may form precipitate with heparin, flush heparinized infusion set with sterile water for injection or normal saline solution before and after administration.
- Monitor blood pressure and pulse before giving, and keep patient in supine position during administration.
- Administer I.V. through Y-tube or three-way stopcock of free-flowing I.V. line.

• Do not give I.V. at concentrations above 25 mg/mL or faster than 25 mg/minute.

Know that inadvertent intra-arterial injection or I.V. extravasation may cause gangrene of affected extremity.

Monitoring

Monitor neurologic status; stay alert for signs and symptoms of neuroleptic malignant syndrome (high fever, sweating, unstable blood pressure, stupor, muscle rigidity, and autonomic dysfunction).

• In long-term therapy, assess for other adverse CNS effects, including extrapyramidal reactions. Be aware that dehydrated children are at increased risk for dystonic reactions.

• Watch for hypotension.

• Monitor CBC and liver function test results.

Storage

• Store at controlled room temperature of 15° to 30°C (59° to 86°F); protect from light. Keep in carton until use.

Contraindications and precautions

Contraindicated in hypersensitivity to drug, previous idiosyncratic reaction to phenothiazines, intra-arterial or subcutaneous use, coma, asthma, chronic obstructive pulmonary disease, sleep apnea, and ***children younger than age 2*** (safety and efficacy not established).

Use cautiously in cardiovascular or hepatic disease, seizures, bone marrow depression, angle-closure glaucoma, prostatic hypertrophy, stenosing peptic ulcer, pyloroduodenal or bladder neck obstruction, CNS depression (related to barbiturates, general anesthesia, tranquilizers, alcohol, or opioids), and pregnant or breastfeeding patients.

Adverse reactions

CNS: confusion, disorientation, marked drowsiness, sedation, dizziness, extrapyramidal reactions, fatigue, insomnia, nervousness, **neuroleptic malignant syndrome**

CV: hypertension, hypotension, bradycardia, tachycardia

EENT: blurred vision, diplopia, tinnitus, dry mouth

GI: constipation

Hematologic: blood dyscrasias

Hepatic: cholestatic jaundice

Respiratory: respiratory depression

Skin: photosensitivity, rash

Other: hypersensitivity reaction

Interactions

Drug-drug. *Anticholinergics:* additive anticholinergic effects

CNS depressants: additive CNS depression

Epinephrine: reversal of epinephrine's vasopressor effects

Monoamine oxidase inhibitors: increased extrapyramidal reactions

Drug-diagnostic tests. *Glucose:* increased

Granulocytes, platelets, white blood cells: decreased

Pregnancy test: false-positive or false-negative result

Skin tests using allergen extracts: false-negative result

Drug-herb. *Betel nut:* increased risk of extrapyramidal reactions

Evening primrose oil: increased risk of seizures

Kava: increased risk of adverse drug effects

Drug-behaviors. *Alcohol use:* additive CNS depression

Sun exposure: increased risk of photosensitivity

Toxicity and overdose

• Overdose signs and symptoms may include mild CNS depression (such as reduced mental status and sedation), cardiovascular depression (including

P

profound hypotension), respiratory depression (including apnea), and unconsciousness. However, CNS stimulation (tremors, insomnia, hallucinations, or seizures) also may occur, especially in elderly patients and children. In addition, atropine-like signs and symptoms (dry mouth, fixed dilated pupils, flushing) and GI effects may develop, particularly in children.
• Provide symptomatic and supportive therapy. Administer I.V. fluids and reposition hypotensive patient. If vasopressors are needed to manage severe hypotension unresponsive to I.V. fluids and repositioning, norepinephrine or phenylephrine may be ordered. Do not give epinephrine; in patients with partial adrenergic blockade, this drug may further lower blood pressure. For extrapyramidal reactions, expect to give anticholinergic antiparkinsonian agents, diphenhydramine, or barbiturates. Diazepam may be used to control seizures. Correct acidosis and electrolyte imbalances as indicated. Know that naloxone does not reverse depressant effects of promethazine. Avoid analeptics, which may cause seizures. Urine acidification may promote excretion; dialysis does not remove drug.

Patient teaching

Teach patient to recognize and immediately report signs and symptoms of hypersensitivity reaction or neuroleptic malignant syndrome.
• Inform patient of drug's other significant neurologic effects; tell patient to contact prescriber if these occur.
• Instruct patient to avoid driving and other hazardous activities until drug's effects on concentration, vision, alertness, and motor skills are known.
• As appropriate, review all other significant and life-threatening adverse reactions and interactions, especially those related to the drugs, tests, herbs, and behaviors mentioned above.

propofol

Diprivan

Pharmacologic class: General anesthetic
Therapeutic class: Sedative-hypnotic
Pregnancy risk category B

Action

Unclear; thought to inhibit sympathetic nerve impulse transmission, causing CNS depression

Pharmacokinetics

Drug distributes rapidly, although distribution is not constant over time and decreases as body tissues equilibriate with plasma and become saturated. Drug withdrawal after anesthesia maintenance for approximately 1 hour or for sedation in intensive care unit (ICU) for 1 day results in rapid decrease in propofol blood level and rapid awakening. Longer infusions (10 days of ICU sedation) cause build-up of significant tissue drug stores, resulting in slower reduction in circulating drug levels and increased time to awakening. Drug is eliminated primarily by hepatic conjugation to inactive metabolites, which are excreted by the kidneys. It is also secreted in breast milk.

Onset	Peak	Duration
<40 sec	Unknown	10-15 min

How supplied

Emulsion for injection (white, oil in water): 10 mg/mL in 20-mL, 50-mL, and 100-mL infusion vials

Indications and dosages

➢ General anesthesia induction

Healthy adults younger than age 55: 40 mg or 2 to 2.5 mg/kg I.V. q 10 seconds until induction onset. In neurosurgical patients, 20 mg or 1 to 2 mg/kg q 10 seconds until induction onset. In cardiac anesthesia, 20 mg or 0.5 to 1.5 mg/kg q 10 seconds until induction onset.

Adults age 55 or older or debilitated patients: 20 mg or 1 to 1.5 mg/kg I.V. q 10 seconds until induction onset

Healthy children ages 3 to 16: 2.5 to 3.5 mg/kg I.V. administered over 20 to 30 seconds

➢ General anesthesia maintenance

Healthy adults younger than age 55: 100 to 200 mcg/kg/minute (6 to 12 mg/kg/hour) by I.V. infusion, given with nitrous oxide and oxygen; or 25 to 50 mg (2.5 to 5 mL) by intermittent I.V. bolus, given with nitrous oxide

Adults age 55 or older or debilitated patients: 50 to 100 mcg/kg/minute (3 to 6 mg/kg/hour) I.V., given with nitrous oxide

Healthy children ages 2 months to 16 years: 125 to 300 mcg/kg/minute (7.5 to 18 mg/kg/hour) I.V., given with nitrous oxide. After first half-hour of maintenance therapy, decrease infusion rate if patient does not show clinical signs of light anesthesia.

➢ Patients undergoing cardiac surgery

Adults: For induction, 20 mg (0.5 to 1.5 mg/kg) I.V. q 10 seconds, given by slow I.V. injection until induction onset. For maintenance, continuous I.V. infusion at a rate of 100 to 150 mcg/kg/minute, supplemented with continuous infusion of opioid agonist.

➢ Patients undergoing neurosurgery

Adults: For induction, 20 mg (1 to 2 mg/kg) I.V. q 10 seconds until induction onset. For maintenance, 100 to 200 mcg/kg/minute (6 to 12 mg/kg/hour).

➢ To initiate monitored anesthesia care (MAC) sedation

Healthy adults younger than age 55: 100 to 150 mcg/kg/minute by I.V. infusion for 3 to 5 minutes, titrated to desired effect; or approximately 0.5 mg/kg by slow I.V. injection over 3 to 5 minutes, titrated to desired effect. If procedure is longer than anticipated or deeper anesthesia is required, may increase rate or give incremental boluses.

➢ To maintain MAC sedation

Healthy adults younger than age 55: 25 to 75 mcg/kg/minute (1.5 to 4.5 mg/kg/hour) by slow I.V. infusion for 10 to 15 minutes, decreased to 25 to 50 mcg/kg/minute

Adults age 55 or older or debilitated patients: Decrease usual adult maintenance dosage by 20%. Do not give rapid (single or repeated) bolus dose.

➢ To initiate and maintain sedation in mechanically ventilated ICU patients

Healthy adults younger than age 55: Initially, slow I.V. infusion of 5 mcg/kg/minute (0.3 mg/kg/hour) for at least 5 minutes with highly individualized dosage; may increase at 5- to 10-minute intervals in increments of 5 to 10 mcg/kg/minute until desired sedation level is reached. Maintenance rates of 5 to 50 mcg/kg/minute (0.3 to 3 mg/kg/ hour) or higher may be needed.

Dosage adjustment

- Consider that with increasing patient age, higher peak plasma levels occur for a given I.V. bolus dose; therefore, dosage requirement decreases. These higher levels can predispose elderly patients to cardiorespiratory effects, including hypotension, apnea, airway obstruction, and oxygen desaturation.
- Reduce dosage in debilitated patients, those who have received large opioid doses, and American Society of

P

Anesthesiologists Class III or IV (ASA III/IV) patients.

Administration

Preparation

Be aware that drug should be given only by individuals trained in general anesthesia administration who are not involved in surgical or diagnostic procedure.

Ask patient about allergy to eggs, soybean oil, or glycerol before administration.

- When used in cardiac anesthesia, correct fluid deficits before administration.
- Know that dosages should be individualized based on patient's condition, response, blood lipid profile, and vital signs.

Dilution and compatibility

- Drug usually does not require dilution. However, if ordered, dilute only with D_5W for injection, to a concentration of no less than 2 mg/mL.
- Know that drug is compatible with D_5W, lactated Ringer's solution, D_5W and lactated Ringer's, D_5W and 0.45% sodium chloride, and D_5W and 0.2% sodium chloride injection when using Y-type infusion set.

Do not use drug if emulsion phases have separated.

- Shake well before use.
- Do not use filter with pores smaller than 5 microns.
- Do not mix with other drugs before infusing.

Infusion considerations

- Do not deliver through same I.V. line as blood or plasma.
- Shield drug from light.

Know that bolus administration of 10 or 20 mg should be given only to deepen sedation rapidly in patients unlikely to experience hypotension. Patients with compromised myocardial function, intravascular volume depletion, or abnormally reduced vascular tone (as from sepsis) may be more susceptible to hypotension.

Be aware that rapid bolus doses should not be given to elderly, debilitated, or ASA III/IV patients.

- Monitor vital signs and ECG continuously.
- In ICU patients, evaluate sedation level and neurologic status frequently to help determine minimal dosage required.

Do not stop administering drug abruptly; dosage must be tapered.

- After 12 hours, discard unused portion of drug, along with tubing.

Monitoring

- Monitor arterial blood gas results and respiratory status.
- Continue to assess blood lipid levels.
- Know that drug should not be infused longer than 5 days without providing drug holiday to safely replace possible urinary zinc losses.

Storage

- Store between 4° and 22°C (39° and 72°F). Protect from light; do not freeze.

Contraindications and precautions

Contraindicated in hypersensitivity to drug, its components, eggs, soybean oil, or glycerol and when general anesthesia or sedation is contraindicated.

Use cautiously in sulfite sensitivity (some products), renal or hepatic disease, heart failure, arrhythmias, hypertension, respiratory disorders, hyperlipidemia, seizures, ***elderly patients,*** pregnant or breastfeeding patients, patients in labor and delivery (use not recommended), and ***children.***

Adverse reactions

CNS: headache, abnormal movements, dizziness, shivering, tremor, confusion,

drowsiness, paresthesia, agitation, abnormal dreams, euphoria, fatigue, **perioperative myoclonia** including seizures and opisthotonus (rare)
CV: hypotension, hypertension, premature ventricular or atrial contractions, abnormal ECG, ST-segment depression, tachycardia, bradycardia, phlebitis, **asystole**
EENT: blurred vision, eye pain, tinnitus, sneezing
GI: nausea, vomiting, abdominal pain, dry mouth
GU: urine retention, green urine
Musculoskeletal: myalgia
Respiratory: cough, hiccups, dyspnea, hypoventilation, wheezing, tachypnea, hypoxia, **apnea**
Skin: flushing, urticaria
Other: strange taste, fever, burning or stinging sensation at injection site, hypersensitivity reaction

Interactions

Drug-drug. *Inhalation anesthetics, opioids, sedative-hypnotics, skeletal muscle relaxants:* increased CNS depression
Drug-behaviors. *Alcohol use:* increased CNS depression

Toxicity and overdose

- Overdose is likely to cause cardiorespiratory depression.
- Immediately discontinue drug. For respiratory depression, provide artificial ventilation with oxygen, as ordered. For cardiovascular depression, expect to elevate patient's legs, increase I.V. fluid flow rate, and give pressor agents, anticholinergics, or both.

Patient teaching

- Inform patient that drug may impair mental alertness briefly after therapy ends.
- Assure patient that he will be monitored continuously.
- Tell patient that drug normally turns urine green.

propranolol hydrochloride

Pharmacologic class: Beta-adrenergic blocker (nonselective)
Therapeutic class: Antianginal, antiarrhythmic (class II), antihypertensive
Pregnancy risk category C

Action

Blocks stimulation of $beta_1$-adrenergic (myocardial) and $beta_2$-adrenergic (pulmonary, vascular, and uterine) receptor sites. This action leads to decreased cardiac output, slowing of heart rate, and blood pressure reduction.

Pharmacokinetics

Drug crosses blood-brain and placental barriers. It is extensively metabolized and approximately 90% bound to plasma proteins. Some drug is excreted in breast milk; most metabolites appear in urine.

Onset	Peak	Duration
Immediate	1 min	4-6 hr

How supplied

Solution for injection: 1 mg/mL

Indications and dosages

➤ Life-threatening arrhythmias, arrhythmias that occur during anesthesia
Adults: 1 to 3 mg slow I.V. injection under careful monitoring. If necessary, give second dose after 2 minutes and give additional doses at intervals of no

less than 4 hours until desired response occurs.

Administration

Preparation

- Be aware that I.V. administration usually is reserved for arrhythmias that are life-threatening or occur during anesthesia.

Know that propranolol is not indicated for hypertensive emergencies.

Take apical pulse for 1 full minute; if patient has bradycardia or tachycardia, withhold dose and notify prescriber.

Keep I.V. isoproterenol, atropine, or glucagon available in case of emergency.

Dilution and compatibility

- Know that compatible I.V. solutions are D_5W, normal or half-normal saline solution, and lactated Ringer's solution.
- For intermittent I.V. infusion, dilute with normal saline solution.

Infusion considerations

- Inject I.V. dose directly into large vein or into tubing of compatible I.V. solution.

Do not exceed administration rate of 1 mg/minute, to avoid hypotension and cardiac standstill.

Do not administer as continuous I.V. infusion.

- For intermittent I.V. infusion, administer in 0.1- to 0.2-mg increments over 10 to 15 minutes.

Do not stop giving drug suddenly. Dosage must be tapered.

Monitoring

- Monitor vital signs, ECG, and central venous pressure.
- Assess fluid balance; check for signs and symptoms of heart failure.
- Monitor CBC and liver and thyroid function test results.
- Watch closely for signs and symptoms of hypoglycemia (drug may mask these).
- Monitor blood glucose levels in diabetic patients to identify need to adjust insulin or oral hypoglycemic dosage. Be aware that in labile diabetes, steep blood pressure rise may accompany hypoglycemia.

Storage

- Store at controlled room temperature of 25°C (77°F). Protect from light, freezing, or excessive heat.

Contraindications and precautions

Contraindicated in hypersensitivity to drug, its components, or other beta blockers; uncompensated heart failure; cardiogenic shock; sinus bradycardia; heart block greater than first degree; bronchospastic disease; and congestive heart failure (unless secondary to tachyarrthymias treatable with propranolol).

Use cautiously in renal or hepatic impairment, sinus node dysfunction, pulmonary disease, diabetes mellitus, hyperthyroidism, Raynaud's syndrome, myasthenia gravis, history of severe allergic reactions, concurrent thioridazine use, ***elderly patients,*** pregnant or breastfeeding patients, and ***children*** (safety not established).

Adverse reactions

CNS: fatigue, asthenia, anxiety, dizziness, drowsiness, insomnia, memory loss, depression, mental status changes, nervousness, paresthesia, nightmares
CV: peripheral vasoconstriction, orthostatic hypotension, bradycardia, **arrhythmias, heart failure**
EENT: blurred vision, dry eyes, nasal congestion, rhinitis, sore throat
GI: nausea, vomiting, diarrhea, constipation, dry mouth
GU: erectile dysfunction, decreased libido
Hematologic: purpura, **thrombocytopenic purpura**

Metabolic: fluid retention, hyperglycemia
Musculoskeletal: joint pain, back pain, myalgia, muscle cramps
Respiratory: wheezing, **bronchospasm, pulmonary edema**
Skin: pruritus, rash
Other: fever

Interactions

Drug-drug. *Anticholinergics, tricyclic antidepressants:* antagonism of myocardial beta-adrenergic blocking effect
Chlorpromazine: additive hypotension
Cimetidine: increased propranolol blood level and risk of toxicity
Digoxin: additive bradycardia
Diuretics, other antihypertensives: increased hypotensive effect
Fluoxetine: decreased propranolol metabolism, heart block
Glucagon, isoproterenol: antagonism of propranolol's effects
Insulin, oral hypoglycemics: impaired glucose tolerance, increased risk of hypoglycemia
Neuromuscular blockers: increased neuromuscular blockade (with high propranolol doses)
Nonsteroidal anti-inflammatory drugs: decreased hypotensive effect
Theophylline: decreased theophylline clearance, antagonism of theophylline's bronchodilating effect
Thioridazine: increased thioridazine blood level, leading to prolonged QT interval
Drug-diagnostic tests. *Alanine aminotransferase, blood urea nitrogen, eosinophils, glucose, lactate dehydrogenase, serum transaminases, thyroxine:* increased
Eosinophils: transient increase
Platelets, triiodothyronine: decreased
Drug-behaviors. *Acute alcohol ingestion:* additive hypotension

Toxicity and overdose

• Overdose may cause hypotension, bradycardia, respiratory depression, bronchospasm, low-output cardiac failure, and cardiogenic shock.
• In overdose or exaggerated response, provide symptomatic and supportive therapy. Know that glucagon (50 to 150 mcg/kg I.V. followed by continuous drip of 1 to 5 mg/hour) may be useful in treating hypotension or depressed myocardial function; isoproterenol, dopamine, or phosphodiesterase inhibitors also may be ordered. However, epinephrine may provoke uncontrolled hypertension. For bradycardia, expect to give atropine or isoproterenol; for bronchospasm, isoproterenol and aminophylline. Serious bradycardia may warrant temporary cardiac pacing. Monitor ECG, blood pressure, neurobehavioral status, and fluid intake and output. Dialysis has little value in removing drug.

Patient teaching

• Instruct patient to avoid driving and other hazardous activities until drug's effects on concentration, vision, and alertness are known.
• As appropriate, review all other significant and life-threatening adverse reactions and interactions, especially those related to the drugs, tests, and behaviors mentioned above.

[redacted]

protamine sulfate

Prosulf

Pharmacologic class: Low-molecular-weight protein
Therapeutic class: Heparin antagonist
Pregnancy risk category C

P

FDA BOXED WARNING

- Drug may cause severe hypotension, cardiovascular collapse, noncardiogenic pulmonary edema, catastrophic pulmonary vasoconstriction, and pulmonary hypertension. Risk factors include high dosage or overdose, rapid administration, repeated doses, previous protamine administration, and current or previous use of protamine-containing drugs (such as NPH insulin, protamine zinc insulin, and certain beta blockers). Other risk factors may include allergy to fish, previous vasectomy, and severe left ventricular dysfunction and abnormal preoperative pulmonary hemodynamics. In patients with risk factors, clinicians must carefully weigh drug's risks against benefits. Keep vasopressors and resuscitation equipment at hand in case a severe reaction occurs.
- Do not give drug if bleeding occurs without previous heparin use.

Action

Binds with heparin, immediately neutralizing its anticoagulant activity

Pharmacokinetics

Drug has a shorter half-life than heparin.

Onset	Peak	Duration
5 min	Unknown	2 hr

How supplied

Solution for injection: 10 mg/mL in 5-mL and 25-mL vials

Indications and dosages

➤ Heparin overdose

Adults and children: Base dosage on heparin dosage and administration route, time elapsed since heparin dose, and partial thromboplastin time (PTT). For each 100 units heparin, give 1 to 1.5 mg protamine by slow I.V. over 10 minutes in doses not exceeding 50 mg if heparin administration occurred less than 30 minutes earlier; give 0.5 mg/100 units if heparin was given more than 30 minutes but less than 2 hours earlier; give 0.25 to 0.375/100 units if heparin was given 2 or more hours earlier.

Administration

Preparation

Be aware that 1 mg protamine neutralizes approximately 90 USP units of heparin activity (derived from lung tissue) or 115 USP units of heparin activity (derived from intestinal mucosa). Because heparin disappears rapidly from circulation, protamine requirement also decreases rapidly with time elapsed since heparin injection. (For example, if protamine is given 30 minutes after heparin, half of usual protamine dosage may be sufficient.)

Before giving drug, ask patient about fish allergies; hypersensitivity reaction may occur (however, no true relationship has been established).

Ensure that emergency equipment is available in case of anaphylaxis or sudden hypotension.

Dilution and compatibility

- Be aware that drug is ready to use and usually does not require dilution. If dilution is desired, use only D_5W for injection or normal saline solution for injection.
- Know that drug is incompatible with some anti-infectives, including cephalosporins and penicillins.

Infusion considerations

Give slowly by direct I.V. injection over 10 minutes. Rapid administration exacerbates adverse cardiovascular and respiratory effects.

Monitoring

- Monitor vital signs and ECG continuously.
- Watch closely for signs and symptoms of hypersensitivity reaction. Know that vasectomized or infertile men, patients with fish allergies, and those taking protamine-insulin products are at increased risk for hypersensitivity.

Check for spontaneous bleeding from heparin rebound, particularly after cardiac surgery or dialysis.

- Monitor activated PTT (APTT) 15 minutes after administration.

Storage

- Store at 2° to 8°C (36° to 46°F).
- Do not store diluted solution.

Contraindications and precautions

Contraindicated in hypersensitivity to drug.

Use cautiously in fish allergy, pregnant or breastfeeding patients, and ***children.***

Adverse reactions

CNS: lassitude

CV: hypotension, bradycardia, **circulatory collapse**

GI: nausea, vomiting, anorexia

Hematologic: bleeding

Respiratory: dyspnea, **pulmonary edema, severe respiratory distress**

Skin: rash, dermatitis, angioedema

Other: anaphylaxis

Interactions

None significant

Toxicity and overdose

- Bleeding may result from interaction with platelets and such proteins as fibrinogen. Rapid administration is more likely to cause bradycardia, warm sensation, flushing, dyspnea, and severe hypotension.
- Replace lost blood with blood transfusions or fresh frozen plasma, as ordered.

For hypotension, expect to give fluids, epinephrine, dobutamine, or dopamine.

Patient teaching

- Teach patient about drug's purpose and its common adverse effects.

Instruct patient to notify nurse immediately of adverse effects, especially respiratory distress or abnormal bleeding or bruising.

pyridostigmine bromide

Mestinon, Regonol

Pharmacologic class: Anticholinesterase

Therapeutic class: Muscle stimulant, antimyasthenic

Pregnancy risk category C

Action

Prevents acetylcholine destruction, leading to stronger contractions of muscles weakened by myasthenia gravis or curare-like neuromuscular blockers

Pharmacokinetics

Drug is excreted primarily unchanged by the kidneys.

Onset	Peak	Duration
2-5 min	Unknown	2-4 hr

How supplied

Solution for injection: 5 mg/mL

Indications and dosages

➤ Myasthenic crisis

Adults: 2 mg given by very slow I.V. injection q 2 to 3 hours

➤ Reversal of nondepolarizing neuromuscular blockers after surgery

Adults: 10 to 20 mg slow I.V. injection (range, 0.1 to 0.25 mg/kg) with or immediately after 0.6 to 1.2 mg atropine sulfate I.V.

Dosage adjustment
- Be aware that patients with renal impairment may require reduced dosage.

Off-label uses
- Nerve agent prophylaxis

Administration
Preparation

Keep atropine available for use in emergencies.

Infusion considerations

Do not exceed I.V. injection rate of 1 mg/minute.

Do not give concurrently with other anticholinesterase drugs.

Monitoring
- Assess patient's response to each dose.
- Monitor vital signs, ECG, and cardiovascular and respiratory status.

Contraindications and precautions
Contraindicated in hypersensitivity to drug or bromides and in mechanical intestinal or urinary tract obstruction.

Use cautiously in seizure disorders, bronchial asthma, coronary occlusion, hyperthyroidism, arrhythmias, peptic ulcer, vagotonia, bradycardia, pregnant or breastfeeding patients, and ***children*** (safety and efficacy not established).

Adverse reactions
CNS: headache, dysarthria, dysphoria, drowsiness, dizziness, headache, syncope, **loss of consciousness, seizures**
CV: nodal rhythm, decreased cardiac output leading to hypotension, bradycardia, **atrioventricular block, cardiac arrest, arrhythmias**
EENT: diplopia, lacrimation, miosis, spasm of accommodation, conjunctival hyperemia
GI: nausea, vomiting, diarrhea, abdominal cramps, flatulence, increased peristalsis, dysphagia, increased salivation
GU: urinary frequency, urgency, or incontinence
Musculoskeletal: muscle weakness, fasciculations, and cramps; joint pain
Respiratory: increased pharyngeal and tracheobronchial secretions, dyspnea, **central respiratory paralysis, respiratory muscle paralysis, laryngospasm, bronchospasm, bronchiolar constriction**
Skin: diaphoresis, flushing, rash, urticaria
Other: thrombophlebitis at I.V. site, cholinergic crisis, anaphylaxis

Interactions
Drug-drug. *Aminoglycosides:* potentiation of neuromuscular blockade
Anesthetics (general and local), antiarrhythmics: decreased anticholinesterase effects
Atropine, belladonna derivatives: suppression of parasympathomimetic GI symptoms (leaving only fasciculation and voluntary muscle paralysis as signs of anticholinesterase overdose)
Corticosteroids: decreased anticholinesterase effects; after corticosteroid withdrawal, increased anticholinesterase effects
Ganglionic blockers (such as mecamylamine): increased anticholinesterase effects
Magnesium: antagonism of beneficial anticholinesterase effects
Nondepolarizing neuromuscular blockers (atropine, pancuronium, tubocurarine): antagonism of neuromuscular blockade and reversal of muscle relaxation after surgery (with parenteral pyridostigmine)
Other anticholinesterase drugs: in myasthenia gravis patients, symptoms of

anticholinesterase overdose that mimic underdose, causing condition to worsen
Succinylcholine: increased and prolonged neuromuscular blockade (including respiratory depression)

Toxicity and overdose

- Overdose signs and symptoms reflect cholinergic crisis and include nausea; vomiting; blurred vision; constricted pupils; excessive tearing, salivation, and sweating; muscle weakness, fasciculations, and cramps; restlessness or agitation; bradycardia or tachycardia; respiratory paralysis; and death.
- Immediately withdraw drug. Support respiration with artificial ventilation, if required. Provide bronchial suctioning for excessive secretions. Administer atropine, as ordered, to block muscarinic effects, but use atropine cautiously to avoid bronchial plug formation.

Patient teaching

- Inform patient that drug may cause headache and muscle cramps. Encourage patient to discuss activity recommendations and pain management with prescriber.
- As appropriate, review all other significant and life-threatening adverse reactions and interactions, especially those related to the drugs mentioned above.

[redacted]

pyridoxine hydrochloride

Pharmacologic class: Vitamin B_6
Therapeutic class: Nutritional supplement
Pregnancy risk category A

Action

Acts as a coenzyme in metabolism of protein, carbohydrate, and fat

Pharmacokinetics

Drug degrades to 4-pyridoxic acid in the liver; it is not protein-bound. Half-life appears to be 15 to 20 days. Metabolites are excreted in urine.

Onset	Peak	Duration
Unknown	Unknown	Unknown

How supplied

Solution for injection: 100 mg/mL in 1-mL vial

Indications and dosages

➤ Dietary-induced pyridoxine deficiency
Adults: 10 to 20 mg I.V. daily for 3 weeks, with follow-up treatment with oral multivitamins containing pyridoxine
➤ Vitamin B_6 dependency syndrome
Adults: Up to 600 mg I.V. daily and 30 mg daily intake for life
➤ Drug-induced pyridoxine deficiency, as from isoniazid (INH) or hormonal contraceptives
Adults: 100 mg I.V. daily for 3 weeks followed by maintenance dosage of 30 mg daily
➤ INH poisoning (more than 10 g INH)
Adults: 4 g I.V. followed by I.M. injections q 30 minutes, as prescribed. Total dosage should equal ingested INH dosage.

Administration

Preparation

- Know that parenteral route is indicated when oral administration is not feasible.
- Be aware that some drug products contain aluminum, which may accumulate

and lead to CNS and bone toxicity, especially in patients with impaired renal function.

Be aware that vitamin B_6 deficiency alone is rare; assess for other vitamin deficiencies.

- Assess dietary habits. Know that poor dietary habits should be corrected and an adequate, well-balanced diet should be prescribed.

Dilution and compatibility

- Be aware that drug may be given undiluted or added to most I.V. solutions.
- Use solution only if clear.

Infusion considerations

- Administer I.V. injection at 50 mg or fraction thereof over 1 minute.
- Know that drug also may be given as I.V. infusion.

Monitoring

- Monitor for drug dependence followed by withdrawal, which may occur in patients receiving dosages as low as 200 mg/day.

Storage

- Store at controlled room temperature of 20° to 25°C (68° to 77°F); protect from light.

Contraindications and precautions

Contraindicated in hypersensitivity to drug or its components.

Use cautiously in ***elderly patients,*** pregnant or breastfeeding patients, and ***children*** (safety and efficacy not established in doses exceeding nutritional requirements).

Adverse reactions

CNS: headache, paresthesia, somnolence, sensory neuropathy

Interactions

Drug-drug. *Anticonvulsants:* decreased anticonvulsant blood level

Hormonal contraceptives: increased pyridoxine requirements

Levodopa: antagonized effects of levodopa

Drug-diagnostic tests. *Aspartate aminotransferase:* increased

Serum folic acid: decreased

Urobilinogen test using Ehrlich's reagent: possible false-positive result

Toxicity and overdose

- In overdose, expect CNS manifestations, including ataxia and sensory neuropathy.
- Discontinue drug.

Patient teaching

- Teach patient about proper dietary habits during treatment so that relapse is less likely to occur with dosage reduction or cessation of injection therapy.
- Advise patient taking levodopa to avoid supplemental vitamins containing more than 5 mg pyridoxine in daily dose.
- As appropriate, review all other significant adverse reactions and interactions, especially those related to the drugs and tests mentioned above.

quinidine gluconate

Pharmacologic class: Cinchona alkaloid

Therapeutic class: Antiarrhythmic (class IA), antimalarial

Pregnancy risk category C

FDA BOXED WARNING

- In many trials of antiarrhythmic therapy for non-life-threatening arrhythmias, active antiarrhythmic therapy has led to increased deaths. Risk is probably greatest in patients with structural heart disease. Deaths associated with drug were more than three times as high as those in placebo group. Another analysis showed that in patients with non-life-threatening ventricular arrhythmias, quinidine-associated deaths were consistently higher than those linked to various alternative antiarrhythmics.

Action

Slows conduction and prolongs refractory period, reducing myocardial irritability, thereby interrupting or preventing certain arrhythmias. As antimalarial, acts primarily as intraerythrocytic schizonticide.

Pharmacokinetics

Drug has several hydroxylated metabolites, some with antiarrhythmic activity. Serum levels may rise steeply in stressful situations (such as acute myocardial infarction), even though serum content of unbound (active) drug may remain normal. Drug is largely protein-bound in adults and older children, but to a lesser extent in pregnant women, infants, and neonates. Protein binding also increases in chronic renal failure, but abruptly decreases toward or below normal when heparin is given for hemodialysis. Most of dose is eliminated hepatically via cytochrome P450IIIA4. When urine pH is below 7, about 20% of dose appears unchanged in urine; in more alkaline urine, as little as 5% may appear unchanged in urine. Renal clearance involves both glomerular filtration and active tubular secretion, moderated by tubular reabsorption.

Onset	Peak	Duration
Immediate	Immediate	Unknown

How supplied

Solution for injection: 80 mg/mL in 10-mL multidose vial

Indications and dosages

➢ Paroxysmal supraventricular tachycardia (PSVT)

Adults: After test dose, 330 mg I.V. (up to 750 mg) in diluted solution infused no faster than 1 mL/minute

➢ Static atrial fibrillation or flutter

Adults: After test dose, initially give up to 0.25 mg/kg/minute I.V. of 16-mg/mL dilution. Discontinue if QRS complex or QT interval widens to 130% of pretreatment duration or QT interval exceeds 500 msec; P wave disappears; severe hypotension, substantial tachycardia, or symptomatic bradycardia occurs; normal sinus rhythm is restored; or severe adverse reactions occur. Total I.V. dosage is less than 5 mg/kg, although 10 mg/kg may be required.

➢ Severe, life-threatening *Plasmodium falciparum* malaria

Adults: After test dose, loading dose of 10 mg/kg I.V. diluted in 5 mL/kg normal saline solution for injection (250 mL normal saline solution for injection in otherwise healthy, 50-kg [110-lb] patient) by continuous infusion over 1 to 2 hours, followed by continuous maintenance infusion of 0.02 mg/kg/ minute for 72 hours or until parasitemia decreases to less than 1% or oral therapy can begin. Or give a loading dose of 24 mg/kg I.V. diluted in 250 mL normal saline solution for injection given by intermittent infusion over 4 hours, followed by maintenance dosage of 12 mg/kg I.V. at 8-hour intervals, starting 8 hours after loading dose, infused over 4 hours for 7 days or until patient can tolerate oral therapy.

Off-label uses

- Myocardial infarction

Administration

Preparation

🔊 Before first dose, assess apical pulse and blood pressure. For bradycardia or

tachycardia, withhold dose and contact prescriber.
Administer test dose, as prescribed, to check for idiosyncratic reaction.
• For atrial fibrillation, expect to give digoxin, calcium channel blocker, beta-adrenergic blocker, and possibly anticoagulant before administering quinidine.
• Know that drug is the only parenteral cinchona alkaloid antimalarial commercially available in the United States. Because newer antiarrhythmics have replaced it for many cardiac uses, it may not be readily available and prescribers may be unfamiliar with its use. For information on availability or use, contact manufacturer.
Dilution and compatibility
• To prepare infusion, dilute contents of supplied vial (80 mg/mL) to 50 mL (16 mg/mL) with D_5W for injection.
• Minimize tubing length, as drug may be adsorbed to polyvinyl chloride tubing.
Infusion considerations
Administer by slow I.V. infusion, preferably using volumetric pump, no faster than 0.25 mg/kg/minute (1 mL/kg/hour).
Know that too-rapid infusion may cause peripheral vascular collapse and severe hypotension.
During first few minutes of infusion, monitor patient closely, especially for hypersensitive or idiosyncratic reaction.
Monitoring
• If sinus rhythm does not resume after total dosage of 10 mg/kg has been given, know that clinician should consider other means of cardioversion.
Monitor ECG and vital signs closely; assess for worsening heart failure.
• Assess kidney and liver function test results, CBC, and quinidine blood level.
• Watch for signs and symptoms of blood dyscrasias.
• Closely monitor respiratory status; stay alert for asthma attacks and impending respiratory arrest.
• Monitor for adverse GI effects, which may signify drug toxicity.
Storage
• Store at 25°C (77°F); excursions permitted from 15° to 30°C (59° to 86°F).
• Know that diluted solution may be stored for up to 24 hours at room temperature or refrigerated for up to 48 hours at 4°C (39°F).

Contraindications and precautions

Contraindicated in hypersensitivity to drug or related cinchona derivatives, thrombocytopenia with previous quinidine therapy, complete heart block, left bundle-branch block or other severe intraventricular conduction defects, aberrant ectopic impulses and abnormal rhythm, history of prolonged QT interval or drug-induced torsades de pointes, digoxin toxicity, absence of functioning artificial pacemaker in patients whose heart rhythm depends on junctional or idioventricular pacemaker (including those in complete atrioventricular [AV] block), and patients who might be adversely affected by anticholinergics (such as those with myasthenia gravis).

Use cautiously in potassium imbalance, renal or hepatic disease, heart failure, respiratory depression, ***elderly patients,*** pregnant or breastfeeding patients, and ***children.***

Adverse reactions

CNS: vertigo, headache, ataxia, apprehension, excitement, delirium, syncope, confusion, depression, dementia
CV: ECG changes, hypotension, vasculitis, tachycardia, premature ventricular contractions, paradoxical tachycardia, **ventricular tachycardia, ventricular fibrillation, ventricular flutter, ventricular ectopy, torsades de pointes, complete**

AV block, widened QRS complex, prolonged QT interval, asystole, aggravated heart failure, arterial embolism, vascular collapse
EENT: diplopia, blurred vision, mydriasis, abnormal color perception, scotoma, photophobia, night blindness, optic neuritis, decreased hearing, tinnitus
GI: nausea, vomiting, diarrhea, abdominal pain, increased salivation, anorexia
GU: lupus nephritis
Hematologic: purpura, **hemolytic anemia, hypothrombinemia, leukocytosis, shift to left in white blood cell differential, neutropenia, thrombocytopenia, thrombocytopenic purpura, agranulocytosis**
Hepatic: hepatotoxicity
Respiratory: acute asthma attack, respiratory arrest
Skin: rash, pruritus, urticaria, photosensitivity, angioedema
Other: fever, cinchonism, lupuslike syndrome, hypersensitivity reaction

Interactions

Drug-drug. *Amiodarone:* increased quinidine blood level, causing potentially fatal arrhythmia
Anticholinergics: additive vagolytic effect
Anticoagulants, beta-adrenergic blockers (such as metoprolol, propranolol), procainamide, propafenone, tricyclic antidepressants: increased effects of these drugs
Barbiturates, hydantoins, nifedipine, rifampin, sucralfate: decreased therapeutic effect of quinidine
Cardiac glycosides: increased cardiac glycoside blood level, greater risk of toxicity
Cholinergics: decreased quinidine effect (possibly causing failure to terminate PSVT)
Cimetidine: increased quinidine blood level
Depolarizing (decamethonium, succinylcholine) and nondepolarizing (pancuronium, tubocurarine) neuromuscular blockers: potentiation of neuromuscular blockade
Diltiazem, verapamil: decreased quinidine clearance, resulting in hypotension, bradycardia, ventricular tachycardia, AV block, or pulmonary edema
Disopyramide: increased disopyramide or decreased quinidine blood level
Potassium, urinary alkalinizers: increased blood level and effects of quinidine
Drug-diagnostic tests. *Creatine kinase, hepatic enzymes:* increased
Granulocytes, hemoglobin, platelets: decreased
Renal function tests: altered
Drug-foods. *Reduced sodium intake:* increased quinidine blood level
Drug-herb. *Jimsonweed:* adverse cardiovascular effects
Licorice: additive effects

Toxicity and overdose

- Overdose may cause ventricular arrhythmias, hypotension, vomiting, diarrhea, tinnitus, high-frequency hearing loss, vertigo, blurred vision, diplopia, photophobia, headache, cinchonism, confusion, and delirium.
- Withdraw drugs that delay quinidine elimination (such as cimetidine), unless these are absolutely required. Although quinidine blood levels can be assayed and monitored, QT interval is better predictor of drug-induced ventricular arrhythmias. Hemodynamically unstable polymorphic ventricular tachycardia (including torsades de pointes) requires quinidine withdrawal and either immediate cardioversion or immediate overdrive pacing (if cardiac pacemaker is in place or immediately available). After pacing or cardioversion, further management depends on QT-interval length.

Q

Simple repletion of central volume (with Trendelenburg positioning and infusion of normal saline solution) may be sufficient; other interventions may include those that increase peripheral vascular resistance, including administration of alpha-agonist catecholamines (norepinephrine, metaraminol) and military antishock trousers. Although urine acidification theoretically might speed renal elimination of drug, this measure is potentially hazardous and lacks demonstrated benefits. Dialysis does not remove drug.

Patient teaching

Teach patient to recognize and immediately report signs and symptoms of toxicity, including nausea, headache, dizziness, visual disturbances, and tinnitus.

• As appropriate, review all other significant and life-threatening adverse reactions and interactions, especially those related to the drugs, tests, foods, and herbs mentioned above.

quinupristin and dalfopristin

Synercid

Pharmacologic class: Streptogramin
Therapeutic class: Anti-infective
Pregnancy risk category B

FDA BOXED WARNING

• Drug combination is approved for treating serious or life-threatening infections related to vancomycin-resistant *Enterococcus faecium* bacteremia under the Food and Drug Administration's accelerated approval regulations that allow marketing of products for use in life-threatening conditions when other therapies are not available.

Action

Synergistic effects of drug combination interfere with bacterial cell-wall synthesis by disrupting DNA and RNA transcription.

Pharmacokinetics

Both drugs are converted to several active major metabolites: two conjugated metabolites for quinupristin, one nonconjugated metabolite for dalfopristin. Protein binding is moderate. Elimination half-life is approximately 0.85 and 0.7 hours, respectively. Penetration of unchanged drug in noninflammatory blister fluid corresponds to about 19% and 11% of that estimated in plasma, respectively. Fecal excretion is the main elimination route for both parent drugs and their metabolites (75% to 77% of dose). Approximately 15% of quinupristin and 19% of dalfopristin dose is excreted in urine.

Onset	Peak	Duration
Unknown	Unknown	Unknown

How supplied

Powder for reconstitution for injection (white to very slightly yellow): 500 mg/10 mL (150 mg quinupristin, 350 mg dalfopristin), 600 mg/10 mL (180 mg quinupristin, 420 mg dalfopristin)

Indications and dosages

➤ Serious or life-threatening infections caused by vancomycin-resistant *Enterococcus faecium*

Adults and adolescents age 16 and older: 7.5 mg/kg by I.V. infusion over 1 hour q 8 hours

➤ Complicated skin and skin-structure infections caused by *Staphylococcus*

aureus (methicillin-susceptible) or *Streptococcus pyogenes*
Adults and adolescents age 16 and older: 7.5 mg/kg by I.V. infusion over 1 hour q 12 hours for at least 7 days
Dosage adjustment
• Dosage adjustment may be required in hepatic impairment.

Administration
Preparation
• Know that drug has been given to a limited number of children younger than age 16 in emergency circumstances at dosage of 7.5 mg/kg I.V. every 8 or 12 hours.
Dilution and compatibility
Clinical alert: Do not mix with other drugs or normal saline solution.
• Add 5 mL sterile water or D_5W for injection to powdered drug in vial; swirl gently by hand until powder dissolves. Do not shake vial. Solution should be clear.
• Within 30 minutes of first dilution, draw up prescribed dosage and dilute further in D_5W to a final concentration of 2 mg/mL or less.
• Know that for fluid-restricted patient with central venous catheter, drug may be given in 100 mL D_5W.
• If significant peripheral vein irritation occurs, dilute in 500 to 750 mL D_5W for injection.
Infusion considerations
• For intermittent infusion through common I.V. line, flush line with D_5W for injection before and after giving drug.
• Administer by infusion pump over 60 minutes.
Monitoring
• Be aware that duration of therapy depends on infusion site and severity.
• Monitor closely for infusion site reactions and thrombophlebitis. If these problems occur, consider increasing infusion volume, changing infusion site, or infusing through peripherally inserted central catheter or central venous catheter.
• Assess weight and fluid intake and output, to help detect edema.
• Monitor bilirubin level.
Storage
• Refrigerate unopened vials at 2° to 8°C (36° to 46°F). Diluted solution is stable for 5 hours at room temperature and for 54 hours when refrigerated at 2° to 8°C.

Contraindications and precautions
Contraindicated in hypersensitivity to drug or other streptogramins.

Use cautiously in hepatic impairment, breastfeeding patients, and ***children younger than age 16*** (safety and efficacy not established).

Adverse reactions
CNS: headache
CV: thrombophlebitis
GI: nausea, vomiting, diarrhea
Musculoskeletal: joint pain, myalgia
Skin: rash, pruritus
Other: inflammation, pain, or edema at infusion site

Q

Interactions
Drug-drug. *Drugs metabolized by CYP450-3A4 (antineoplastics, such as vinca alkaloids, docetaxel, and paclitaxel; antiretrovirals; astemizole; benzodiazepines; calcium channel blockers; carbamazepine; cisapride; corticosteroids; disopyramide; HMG-CoA reductase inhibitors; immunosuppressants, such as cyclosporine and tacrolimus; lidocaine; quinidine; and terfenadine):* increased therapeutic and adverse effects of these drugs
Drug-diagnostic tests. *Alanine aminotransferase, aspartate aminotransferase, bilirubin:* increased

Toxicity and overdose

- No adverse effects have been reported in overdose. Signs and symptoms of overdose may include dyspnea, vomiting, emesis, tremors, and ataxia.
- Observe patient closely and provide supportive treatment. Dialysis does not remove drug.

Patient teaching

Instruct patient to immediately report pain or redness at infusion site.

- Advise patient to report muscle aches and pains.
- As appropriate, review all other significant and life-threatening adverse reactions and interactions, especially those related to the drugs and tests mentioned above.

[redacted]

ranitidine hydrochloride

Zantac

Pharmacologic class: Histamine$_2$ (H_2)-receptor antagonist
Therapeutic class: Antiulcer drug
Pregnancy risk category B

Action

Reduces gastric acid secretion and increases gastric mucus and bicarbonate production, creating protective coating on gastric mucosa

Pharmacokinetics

Drug distributes into many body tissues. It is metabolized in the liver; serum protein binding averages 15%. Main excretion route is urinary.

Onset	Peak	Duration
Unknown	15 min	8-12 hr

How supplied

Solution for injection (clear, colorless to yellow): 25 mg/mL in 2-, 6-, and 40-mL vials
Solution for injection (clear, colorless to yellow, premixed): 50 mg/50 mL in 0.45% sodium chloride in single-dose plastic containers

Indications and dosages

➢ Hospitalized patients with pathologic hypersecretory conditions, including Zollinger-Ellison syndrome; intractable duodenal ulcers; patients who cannot receive oral drugs
Adults: 50 mg I.V bolus injection or intermittent I.V. infusion q 6 to 8 hours. For continuous I.V. infusion, 6.25 mg/hour. For Zollinger-Ellison syndrome, initial infusion rate of 1 mg/kg/hour.
➢ Duodenal ulcer
Children ages 1 month to 16 years: 2 to 4 mg/kg/day I.V. in divided doses q 6 to 8 hours, up to a maximum of 50 mg q 6 to 8 hours
➢ To increase gastric pH in neonates younger than 1 month who are undergoing extracorporeal membrane oxygenation and are at increased risk for GI hemorrhage
Neonates younger than 1 month: 2 mg/kg I.V. q 12 to 24 hours or as a continuous I.V. infusion
Dosage adjustment

- Reduce dosage to 50 mg every 18 to 24 hours in renal impairment.

Administration

Dilution and compatibility

- Be aware that premixed solution of 50 mg in half-normal saline solution for injection (50 mL) does not require dilution. Do not add other drugs or solutions.

- Know that drug in vial is compatible with most commonly used I.V. solutions, such as normal saline solution, D_5W, dextrose 10% in water, lactated Ringer's solution, and 5% sodium bicarbonate solution.
- For I.V. bolus injection, dilute 50 mg in normal saline solution or other compatible solution to a concentration not exceeding 2.5 mg/mL.
- For intermittent I.V. infusion, dilute in D_5W or other compatible solution to a concentration not exceeding 0.5 mg/mL.
- For continuous I.V. infusion for other than Zollinger-Ellison syndrome, add to D_5W or other compatible solution.
- For continuous I.V. infusion for Zollinger-Ellison syndrome, add to D_5W or other compatible solution; dilute to a concentration not exceeding 2.5 mg/mL.
- Know that I.V. ranitidine may be added to total parenteral nutrition solutions.
- Do not use solution unless clear.

Infusion considerations

- For I.V. injection, give dose over 5 minutes but inject no faster than 4 mL/minute.
- For intermittent I.V. infusion, administer over 15 to 20 minutes but no faster than 7 mL/minute.
- For continuous I.V. infusion for other than Zollinger-Ellison syndrome, administer at 6.25 mg/hour.
- For continuous I.V. infusion for Zollinger-Ellison syndrome, start infusion at 1 mg/kg/hour. After 4 hours, if measured gastric acid output exceeds 10 mEq/hour or symptoms occur, increase dosage in increments of 0.5 mg/kg/hour, and remeasure acid output.
- For premixed solution in plastic container, administer only by slow I.V. drip over 15 to 20 minutes. If used with primary I.V. line, discontinue primary solution during ranitidine administration.

Clinical alert: Do not use plastic containers in series connections. Such use could result in air embolism due to residual air being drawn from primary container before administration of fluid from secondary container ends.

Monitoring

- Assess vital signs.
- Monitor CBC and liver function tests.

Storage

- Store vials at 4° to 25°C (39° to 77°F); excursions permitted to 30°C (86°F). Protect from light.
- Store premixed containers at 2° to 8°C (36° to 46°F). Protect from light.

Contraindications and precautions

Contraindicated in hypersensitivity to drug or its components and in history of acute porphyria.

Use cautiously in renal or hepatic impairment, heart rhythm disturbances, ***elderly patients,*** and pregnant or breastfeeding patients.

Adverse reactions

CNS: headache, agitation, anxiety
GI: nausea, vomiting, diarrhea, constipation, abdominal discomfort or pain
Hematologic: reversible **granulocytopenia** and **thrombocytopenia**
Hepatic: hepatitis
Skin: rash
Other: burning or itching at I.V. site, hypersensitivity reaction

Interactions

Drug-diagnostic tests. *Creatinine:* slight increase
Hepatic enzymes: increased

R

Urine protein tests using Multistix: false-negative results
Drug-herb. *Yerba maté:* decreased drug clearance
Drug-behaviors. *Smoking:* decreased ranitidine effects

Toxicity and overdose

• Overdose experience is limited. Signs may include abnormal gait and hypotension.
• Provide close monitoring and supportive therapy. Hemodialysis may help remove drug.

Patient teaching

• Caution patient to avoid driving and other hazardous activities until effects of drug on concentration and alertness are known.
• Tell patient that smoking may decrease drug's effects.
• As appropriate, review all other significant and life-threatening adverse reactions and interactions, especially those related to the tests, herbs, and behaviors mentioned above.

rasburicase

Elitek, Fasturtec❉

Pharmacologic class: Recombinant urate oxidase enzyme
Therapeutic class: Antimetabolite
Pregnancy risk category C

FDA BOXED WARNING

• Drug may cause severe hypersensitivity reactions (including anaphylaxis), severe hemolysis in patients with glucose-6-phosphate dehydrogenase (G6PD) deficiency, and methemoglobinemia. Withdraw immediately and permanently if patient shows evidence of these problems. Before starting therapy, screen patients at higher risk for G6PD deficiency (those of African or Mediterranean ancestry).
• Drug causes spuriously low uric acid levels.

Action

Catalyzes oxidation of uric acid into inactive soluble metabolite

Pharmacokinetics

Insufficient data available.

Onset	Peak	Duration
4 hr	96 hr	Unknown

How supplied

Powder for reconstitution for injection (white to off-white, lyophilized): 1.5-mg single-use vial with 1 mL diluent

Indications and dosages

➤ Chemotherapy-induced hyperuricemia in children with leukemia, lymphoma, or solid-tumor cancers
Children: 0.15 to 0.2 mg/kg by I.V. infusion over 30 minutes as a single daily dose for 5 days

Off-label uses

• Chemotherapy-induced hyperuricemia in adults with leukemia, lymphoma, or solid-tumor cancers

Administration

Preparation

Follow hazardous drug guidelines on page S19 for handling, preparation, and administration.
• Be aware that chemotherapy should begin 4 to 24 hours after first rasburicase dose.

• Prescreen patients for G6PD deficiency before initiating therapy.
• Know that more than one course of treatment is not recommended.

Dilution and compatibility
• Do not use I.V. filters.
• Do not mix with other drugs.
• Dilute only by adding 1-mL vial of diluent provided. Swirl gently; do not shake. Dilute further by injecting diluted dose into infusion bag containing appropriate volume of normal saline solution to yield final volume of 50 mL.
• Do not use resulting solution if discolored.
• Use reconstituted or diluted solution within 24 hours. Discard unused portion.

Infusion considerations
Clinical alert: Do not give as I.V. bolus.
• Use separate I.V. line, or flush line with 15 mL normal saline solution for injection before and after infusing rasburicase.
• Administer daily by I.V. infusion over 30 minutes.

Monitoring
• Monitor for signs and symptoms of hypersensitivity reaction.
• Assess for respiratory distress and signs and symptoms of infection.
• Monitor CBC and uric acid level frequently.
Clinical alert: Watch closely for signs and symptoms of hemolysis, especially in patients of African or Mediterranean descent.

Storage
• Store powder and diluent at 2° to 8°C (36° to 46°F). Do not freeze; protect from light.

Contraindications and precautions

Contraindicated in hypersensitivity to drug or its components, G6PD deficiency, or history of anaphylaxis, hemolytic anemia, or methemoglobinemia in reaction to rasburicase.

Use cautiously in pregnant or breastfeeding patients and ***children younger than age 2.***

Adverse reactions

CNS: headache
GI: nausea, vomiting, diarrhea, constipation, abdominal pain
Hematologic: neutropenia, methemoglobinemia, severe hemolysis (in patients with G6PD deficiency)
Respiratory: respiratory distress
Skin: rash
Other: fever, mucositis, hypersensitivity reactions including **anaphylaxis, sepsis**

Interactions

Drug-diagnostic tests. *Neutrophils:* decreased
Uric acid: interference with measurement (if blood is at room temperature)

Toxicity and overdose

• No overdoses have been reported. Theoretically, overdose should cause low or undetectable plasma uric acid concentration, which has no known clinical consequences.
• No specific antidote exists. Monitor patient and initiate general supportive measures.

Patient teaching

Clinical alert: Teach parents and patient (as appropriate) to recognize and immediately report adverse effects, including hypersensitivity reaction.
Clinical alert: Inform parents that drug may cause sepsis. Instruct them to monitor child's temperature and immediately report fever and other signs and symptoms of infection.
• As appropriate, review all other significant and life threatening adverse reactions and interactions, especially those related to the tests mentioned above.

R

remifentanil hydrochloride
Ultiva

Pharmacologic class: Opioid agonist
Therapeutic class: Opioid analgesic, anesthesia adjunct
Controlled substance schedule II
Pregnancy risk category C

Action
Unclear. Thought to bind to mu-opioid receptors in CNS, altering perception of and emotional response to pain. Also inhibits ascending pain pathways in limbic system, thalamus, midbrain, and hypothalamus.

Pharmacokinetics
After I.V. dose given over 60 seconds, initial distribution half-life is rapid (1 minute), followed by slower distribution half-life of 6 minutes and terminal elimination half-life of 10 to 20 minutes. Drug distributes throughout the blood and into rapidly perfused tissues. It is metabolized by specific esterases; approximately 70% is bound to plasma proteins. High clearance combined with relatively small volume of distribution produces short elimination half-life (approximately 3 to 10 minutes).

Onset	Peak	Duration
Immediate	Unknown	5-10 min

How supplied
Powder for reconstitution for injection (white to off-white, lyophilized) 1 mg in 3-mL vial, 2 mg in 5-mL vial, 5 mg in 10-mL vial

Indications and dosages
➢ Adjunct to induce anesthesia through intubation
Adults: 0.5 to 1 mcg/kg/minute I.V. given with hypnotic or volatile drug. May give 1 mcg/kg I.V. over 30 to 60 seconds if endotracheal intubation will occur less than 8 minutes after drug infusion starts.
Children age 2 and older: 0.5 to 1 mcg/kg/minute; if endotracheal intubation will occur less than 8 minutes after drug infusion starts, give 1 mcg/kg over 30 to 60 seconds.
➢ Adjunct to maintain anesthesia
Adults and children age 2 and older: 0.25 to 0.4 mcg/kg/minute I.V. Increase dosage by 25% to 100% or decrease by 25% to 50% q 2 to 5 minutes, as needed. If rate exceeds 1 mcg/kg/minute, anesthetic doses may be increased. May give supplemental I.V. bolus of 1 mcg/kg.
➢ To extend analgesic effect during immediate postoperative period
Adults and children age 2 and older: Initially, 0.1 mcg/kg/minute I.V. Adjust in increments of 0.025 mcg/kg/minute q 5 minutes p.r.n.
➢ Monitored anesthesia care
Adults: 0.5 to 1 mcg/kg I.V. over 30 to 60 seconds given 90 seconds before anesthetic is given. As a continuous infusion, 0.05 to 0.1 mcg/kg/minute I.V. 5 minutes before anesthetic is given; after anesthetic is given, titrate rate to 0.025 to 0.05 mcg/kg/minute; then adjust rate by 0.025 mcg/kg/minute q 5 minutes p.r.n.

Dosage adjustment
- Decrease starting dosage by 50% in patients older than age 65; then titrate cautiously to response.
- Base starting dosage on ideal body weight (IBW) in obese patients (those more than 30% above IBW).

Off-label uses
- Peripartum anesthesia

Administration

Preparation

Clinical alert: In patients receiving anesthetic (induction) dosages, ensure that qualified personnel, opioid antagonist, resuscitative and intubation equipment, and adequate facilities are available to manage intraoperative and postoperative respiratory depression.

Clinical alert: Be aware that drug is not recommended as sole agent in general anesthesia, as loss of consciousness cannot be assured and because of high incidence of apnea, muscle rigidity, and tachycardia.

Dilution and compatibility

- Do not administer without diluting.
- Add 1 mL diluent per milligram of drug. Shake well to create clear, colorless solution of 1 mg/mL.
- Further dilute in normal or half-normal saline solution, D_5W, dextrose 5% in normal saline solution, or dextrose 5% in lactated Ringer's solution to a final concentration of 25, 50, or 250 mcg/mL before administration as shown in the table below:

Final concentration	Amount of drug/vial	Final volume after reconstitution and dilution
25 mcg/mL	1 mg	40 mL
	2 mg	80 mL
	5 mg	200 mL
50 mcg/mL	1 mg	20 mL
	2 mg	40 mL
	5 mg	100 mL
250 mcg/mL	5 mg	20 mL

Infusion considerations

- Do not administer with blood products.
- Use infusion control pump for continuous infusion. Choose site close to venous cannula. After administering, flush I.V. tubing to clear.

Clinical alert: Know that delivery rate exceeding 0.2 mcg/kg/minute may cause respiratory depression.

Monitoring

Clinical alert: When giving high doses, assess for muscle rigidity; be prepared to stop therapy.

- Continuously monitor respiratory and cardiovascular function, oxygenation, and vital signs.
- Assess fluid intake and output. Watch for urine retention.

Storage

- Store at 2° to 25°C (36° to 77°F).

Contraindications and precautions

Contraindicated in hypersensitivity to drug or other opioid analgesics, acute or severe bronchial asthma, upper airway obstruction, significant respiratory depression, during labor when delivery of premature neonate is anticipated, and with epidural or intrathecal administration.

Use cautiously in bradycardia, heart failure, pulmonary disease, hypothyroidism, ***elderly patients,*** and pregnant or breastfeeding patients.

Adverse reactions

CNS: headache, agitation, dizziness, confusion, sedation, euphoria, delirium, anxiety

CV: hypertension, hypotension, palpitations, tachycardia, bradycardia, **asystole**

EENT: blurred vision, miosis, diplopia, tinnitus

GI: nausea, vomiting, diarrhea, constipation, abdominal cramps, anorexia, dry mouth

GU: urine retention, dysuria

Musculoskeletal: muscle rigidity

Respiratory: respiratory depression, apnea

Skin: flushing, rash, urticaria, bruising, pruritus, diaphoresis

R

Interactions

Drug-drug. *Benzodiazepines, hypnotics, inhalation anesthetics:* synergistic effects
Centrally acting muscle relaxants, other opioid analgesics: increased risk of respiratory depression
Drug-herb. *Kava:* increased CNS depression

Toxicity and overdose

- Overdose manifests as extension of drug actions. Expected signs and symptoms include apnea, chest-wall rigidity, seizures, hypoxemia, hypotension, and bradycardia.
- Discontinue drug, maintain patent airway, initiate assisted or controlled ventilation with oxygen, and maintain adequate cardiovascular function, as ordered. If depressed respiration is associated with muscle rigidity, neuromuscular blocking agent or mu-opioid antagonist may be needed to promote assisted or controlled respiration. I.V. fluids and vasopressors and other supportive measures may be used to treat hypertension; glycopyrrolate or atropine, to treat bradycardia or hypotension; and I.V. opioid antagonist such as naloxone, as specific antidote to manage severe respiratory depression or muscle rigidity. Be aware that reversal of opioid effects may lead to acute pain and sympathetic hyperactivity.

Patient teaching

- Tell patient he will be monitored closely throughout anesthesia period.
- Reassure patient that drugs will be given to control pain before remifentanil is discontinued.

respiratory syncytial virus immune globulin intravenous (RSV-IGIV)

RespiGam

Pharmacologic class: Immune globulin
Therapeutic class: Antibody production stimulator
Pregnancy risk category C

Action

Contains high concentration of neutralizing and protective antibodies directed against respiratory syncytial virus (RSV) that provide passive immunity

Pharmacokinetics

Mean half-life of serum RSV neutralizing antibodies is 22 to 28 days.

Onset	Peak	Duration
Rapid	Unknown	Unknown

How supplied

Solution for injection: 50 mg/mL

Indications and dosages

➤ To prevent serious lower respiratory tract infection caused by RSV in children with bronchopulmonary dysplasia (BPD) or a history of premature birth (35 weeks' gestation or less)
Children younger than 24 months: Maximum recommended total monthly dosage is 750 mg/kg I.V.; follow infusion rate guidelines.

Administration

Preparation

- Administer first dose before RSV season starts; give subsequent doses monthly throughout RSV season to maintain protection. In northern hemisphere, RSV season typically starts in

November and runs through April. Drug should be given from early November through April, unless RSV activity begins earlier or persists later in local area.

• Know that drug has not been proven effective in treating RSV infection; however, children infected with RSV should continue to receive monthly doses for duration of RSV season.

Keep loop diuretics available to manage patients at risk for fluid overload.

Keep epinephrine and diphenhydramine available to treat acute systemic allergic reaction (rare).

Dilution and compatibility

• Know that predilution is not recommended.

• Be aware that drug is compatible with dextrose 2.5%, 5% dextrose, 10% dextrose, and 20% dextrose solutions (with or without sodium chloride).

• Do not use solution if turbid.

Infusion considerations

• Give drug within 6 hours after single-use vial is entered, and complete administration within 12 hours.

• Administer separately from other drugs.

• Know that filters are not necessary, but inline filter with pores larger than 15 microns may be used for infusion.

• Administer through I.V. line using constant infusion pump. If possible, give through separate I.V. line or piggyback into preexisting line containing compatible solution. If preexisting line must be used, dilution must not exceed 1 part drug to 2 parts solution.

• Administer initially at 1.5 mL/kg/hour for 15 minutes. If indicated, may increase to 3 mL/kg/hour for 15 minutes and finally, to a maximum rate of 6 mL/kg/hour for 30 minutes.

Do not exceed 6 mL/kg/hour. In especially ill children with BPD, slower infusion rate may be indicated.

Closely monitor vital signs and cardiopulmonary status before infusion, before each rate increase, and then every 30 minutes, until 30 minutes after infusion ends. Stay alert for increased heart or respiratory rate, retractions, and crackles.

• Be aware that except for hypersensitivity reactions, adverse reactions may be associated with administration rate.

Monitoring

Know that patients with selective immunoglobulin (Ig) A deficiency may develop antibodies to IgA, leading to anaphylactic or allergic reactions to subsequent administration of blood products containing IgA (including RSV-IGIV). If hypotension, anaphylaxis, or severe allergic reaction occurs, discontinue infusion and give epinephrine, as prescribed.

Monitor for fluid overload, especially in patients with underlying pulmonary disease. Do not give to children with clinically apparent fluid overload.

Rarely, IGIV therapy leads to aseptic meningitis syndrome (AMS). Syndrome usually begins within several hours to 2 days after treatment and causes severe headache, drowsiness, fever, photophobia, painful eye movements, muscle rigidity, nausea, and vomiting. Cerebrospinal fluid studies typically show pleocytosis (predominantly granulocytic) and elevated protein levels. Drug discontinuation has led to AMS remission within several days without sequelae.

Storage

• Store between 2° and 8°C (36° and 46°F). Do not freeze.

Contraindications and precautions

Contraindicated in history of severe prior reaction to RSV-IGIV or other human immunoglobulin preparations.

Use cautiously in renal impairment, diabetes mellitus, and pulmonary disease.

R

Adverse reactions

CNS: dizziness, **aseptic meningitis syndrome** (with high doses)
CV: tachycardia, hypertension
GI: vomiting, diarrhea, gastroenteritis
Metabolic: fluid overload
Respiratory: tachypnea, crackles, **respiratory distress**
Other: fever, infusion-related reactions (including dizziness, flushing, blood pressure changes, anxiety, palpitations, chest tightness, dyspnea, abdominal cramps, pruritus, myalgia or arthralgia), theoretical risk of **viral transmission** (including **hepatitis** C), hypersensitivity reactions including **angioneurotic edema and anaphylaxis**

Interactions

Drug-drug. *Live-virus vaccines:* interference with antibodies in RSV-IGIV

Toxicity and overdose

• In overdose, expect major manifestations to reflect those of fluid volume overload.
• Discontinue drug if fluid overload occurs. Provide supportive therapy.

Patient teaching

Instruct parents or caregiver to immediately report severe headache, drowsiness, fever, photophobia, painful eye movements, muscle rigidity, nausea and vomiting, difficulty breathing, and other unusual signs or symptoms after monthly infusions.
• Inform parents or caregiver that drug may interfere with immune response to live-virus vaccines, such as mumps, rubella, and particularly measles vaccines. If these vaccines are given during or within 10 months after RSV-IGIV infusion, reimmunization is recommended, if appropriate.
• As appropriate, review all other significant and life-threatening adverse reactions and interactions, especially those related to the drugs mentioned above.

reteplase, recombinant

Rapilysin, Retavase

Pharmacologic class: Tissue plasminogen activator
Therapeutic class: Thrombolytic enzyme
Pregnancy risk category C

Action

Converts plasminogen to plasmin, which in turn breaks down fibrin and fibrinogen, thereby dissolving thrombus

Pharmacokinetics

Drug clears from plasma at a rate of 250 to 450 mL/minute; effective half-life is 13 to 16 minutes. It is cleared primarily by the liver and kidneys.

Onset	Peak	Duration
Immediate	End of infusion	Variable

How supplied

Powder for reconstitution for injection: Retavase Half-Kit—one vial of 10.4 units (18.1 mg)/vial; Retavase Kit—two vials of 10.4 units (18.1 mg)/vial

Indications and dosages

➤ Acute myocardial infarction
Adults: 10 units by I.V. bolus over 2 minutes, repeated in 30 minutes

Off-label uses

• Pulmonary embolism

Administration

Preparation

• Before administering, assess baseline ECG, CBC with white cell differential, and clotting factors.

Dilution and compatibility

• Use only diluent supplied (preservative-free sterile water for injection) and dispensing pin to reconstitute drug into colorless solution of 1 unit/mL.
• If drug foams, let it sit until foam subsides. Do not shake.
• Do not use solution if discolored.
• Know that drug is incompatible with heparin.
• After withdrawing prescribed dose, small amount of solution will remain in vial due to overfill. Discard unused solution.
• Use immediately after reconstitution, or store according to manufacturer's direction.

Infusion considerations

• Do not give with other drugs in same I.V. line.
• If drug is given through I.V. line containing heparin, flush line with normal saline solution or D_5W for injection before and after administering reteplase.
• Give by I.V. bolus injection over 2 minutes.

Monitoring

If patient shows signs or symptoms of bleeding or anaphylaxis after first bolus dose, withhold second bolus and contact prescriber immediately.

Check closely for signs and symptoms of bleeding in all body systems. Monitor coagulation studies and CBC.

Monitor ECG for arrhythmias caused by coronary thrombolysis.

Assess neurologic status to detect early signs and symptoms of intracranial hemorrhage.

• Continue to monitor CBC with differential and clotting factors.

Storage

• Store at 2° to 25°C (36° to 77°F). Keep in sealed box until use to protect from light.
• When reconstituted as directed, solution may be used within 4 hours when stored at 2° to 30°C (36° to 86°F).

Contraindications and precautions

Contraindicated in hypersensitivity to drug or alteplase, active internal bleeding, bleeding diathesis, recent intracranial or intraspinal surgery or trauma, intracranial neoplasm, arteriovenous malformation or aneurysm, severe uncontrolled hypertension, and history of cerebrovascular accident.

Use cautiously in previous puncture of noncompressible vessels, major surgery, organ biopsy, trauma, hypertension, conditions that may cause left-sided heart thrombus (including mitral stenosis), acute pericarditis, subacute bacterial endocarditis, hemostatic defects, diabetic hemorrhagic retinopathy, cerebrovascular disease, severe hepatic or renal dysfunction, septic thrombophlebitis or occluded atrioventricular cannula at seriously infected site, other conditions in which bleeding poses significant hazard, concurrent use of oral anticoagulants (such as warfarin), ***patients older than age 75,*** obstetric delivery, and pregnant or breastfeeding patients.

Adverse reactions

CNS: intracranial hemorrhage
CV: arrhythmias, hemorrhage
GI: nausea, vomiting, **GI bleeding**
GU: hematuria
Hematologic: anemia, **bleeding tendency**
Other: fever, bleeding at puncture sites

Interactions

Drug-drug. *Anticoagulants, indomethacin, phenylbutazone, platelet aggregation inhibitors (such as abciximab, aspirin, dipyridamole):* increased risk of bleeding

Drug-diagnostic tests. *Hemoglobin:* decreased
International Normalized Ratio, partial thromboplastin time, prothrombin time: increased

R

Drug-herb. *Ginkgo, many other herbs:* increased risk of bleeding

Toxicity and overdose

- In overdose, expect bleeding.
- Discontinue drug if second dose has not been given. Be prepared to administer whole blood, packed red blood cells, platelets, or fresh frozen plasma. For arrhythmias, expect to give lidocaine or procainamide or assist with cardioversion, as indicated.

Patient teaching

- Teach patient about drug's anticoagulant effect. Review safety measures to avoid injury, which can cause uncontrolled bleeding.

Instruct patient to immediately report signs and symptoms of bleeding problems.

- Tell patient about the need for frequent blood testing during therapy.

rifampin (rifampicin, rifampicin)

Rifadin

Pharmacologic class: Rifamycin derivative
Therapeutic class: Antitubercular
Pregnancy risk category C

Action

Inhibits RNA synthesis by blocking RNA transcription in susceptible organisms (mycobacteria and some gram-positive and gram-negative bacteria)

Pharmacokinetics

Drug distributes widely throughout body, including cerebrospinal fluid. (Serum levels do not differ in patients with renal failure.) It is about 80% protein-bound, and undergoes progressive enterohepatic circulation and deacetylation to 25-desacetyl-rifampin (microbiologically active primary metabolite). Drug is rapidly eliminated in bile; less than 30% of dose is excreted in urine as rifampin or metabolites.

Onset	Peak	Duration
Rapid	End of infusion	12-24 hr

How supplied

Powder for reconstitution for injection: 600 mg/vial

Indications and dosages

➢ Tuberculosis

Adults: 10 mg/kg/day (up to 600 mg/day) I.V. infusion as a single dose
Children: 10 to 20 mg/kg/day (up to 600 mg/day) I.V. infusion as a single dose

➢ Asymptomatic *Neisseria meningitidis* carriers

Adults: 600 mg I.V. infusion b.i.d. for 2 days
Children 1 month and older: 10 mg/kg/day I.V. infusion (up to 600 mg/day) q 12 hours for 2 days
Infants younger than 1 month: 5 mg/kg I.V. infusion q 12 hours for 2 days

Off-label uses

- Anthrax
- Brucellosis
- *Haemophilus influenzae* type B
- Leprosy
- *Mycobacterium avium intracellulare* complex infection
- Prophylaxis in high-risk close contacts of patients with *N. meningitidis* infections
- Prosthetic valve endocarditis caused by coagulase-negative staphylococci
- Severe staphylococcal bone and joint infections

Administration

Dilution and compatibility

- Add 10 mL sterile water to vial to yield 60-mg/mL solution for I.V. infusion.
- Further dilute in 100 mL or 500 mL of D_5W.
- If patient cannot receive dextrose, dilute with normal saline solution. Do not use other I.V. solutions.

Infusion considerations

Clinical alert: Give by I.V. infusion only. Do not use I.M. or subcutaneous route.

- Administer by I.V. infusion over 30 minutes when diluted in 100-mL solution, or over 3 hours when diluted in 500-mL solution.

Clinical alert: Avoid extravasation, as local irritation and inflammation may occur. In extravasation, discontinue infusion and restart at another site.

Monitoring

- Monitor kidney and liver function tests, CBC, and uric acid level.

Clinical alert: Watch for signs and symptoms of bleeding tendency, especially disseminated intravascular coagulation (DIC).

- Assess for signs and symptoms of hepatic impairment.
- Monitor bowel movements for diarrhea, which may signal pseudomembranous colitis.

Storage

- Avoid temperatures above 40°C (104°F). Protect from light.
- Solution is stable at room temperature for up to 4 hours when reconstituted with D_5W and for up to 24 hours when reconstituted with normal saline solution for injection.

Contraindications and precautions

Contraindicated in hypersensitivity to drug or other rifamycin derivatives.

Use cautiously in history of sulfite allergy or hepatic disease, porphyria, concurrent use of other hepatotoxic drugs, and pregnant or breastfeeding patients.

Adverse reactions

CNS: ataxia, confusion, drowsiness, fatigue, headache, asthenia, psychosis, generalized numbness

EENT: conjunctivitis; discolored tears, saliva, and sputum

GI: nausea, vomiting, diarrhea, abdominal cramps, dyspepsia, epigastric distress, flatulence, discolored feces, sore mouth and tongue, anorexia, **pseudomembranous colitis**

GU: discolored urine

Hematologic: eosinophilia, transient **leukopenia**, **hemolytic anemia, hemolysis, DIC, thrombocytopenia**

Hepatic: jaundice

Metabolic: hyperuricemia

Musculoskeletal: myalgia, joint pain

Respiratory: dyspnea, wheezing

Skin: flushing, rash, pruritus, discolored sweat, **erythema multiforme, toxic epidermal necrolysis, Stevens-Johnson syndrome**

Other: flulike symptoms, local irritation and inflammation with extravasation, hypersensitivity reactions including vasculitis

Interactions

Drug-drug. *Barbiturates, beta-adrenergic blockers, cardiac glycosides, clarithromycin, clofibrate, cyclosporine, dapsone, diazepam, doxycycline, fluoroquinolones (such as ciprofloxacin), haloperidol, levothyroxine, methadone, progestins, quinine, tacrolimus, theophylline, tricyclic antidepressants (such as amitriptyline, nortriptyline), zidovudine:* increased metabolism of these drugs

Chloramphenicol, corticosteroids, disopyramide, efavirenz, estrogens, fluconazole, hormonal contraceptives, itraconazole, ketoconazole, nevirapine, quinidine,

R

opioid analgesics, oral hypoglycemics, phenytoin, quinidine, ritonavir, theophylline, tocainide, verapamil, warfarin: decreased efficacy of these drugs
Delavirdine, indinavir, nelfinavir, saquinavir: decreased blood levels of these drugs
Hepatotoxic drugs (including isoniazid, ketoconazole, pyrazinamide): increased risk of hepatotoxicity
Drug-diagnostic tests. *Alanine aminotransferase, alkaline phosphatase, aspartate aminotransferase, bilirubin, blood urea nitrogen, uric acid:* increased
Dexamethasone suppression test: interference with results
Direct Coombs' test: false-positive result
Folate, vitamin B_{12} assay: interference with standard assays
Hemoglobin: decreased
Liver function studies: abnormal values (transient)
Sulfobromophthalein uptake and excretion test: delayed hepatic uptake and excretion
Drug-behaviors. *Alcohol use:* increased risk of hepatotoxicity

Toxicity and overdose

• Fatal acute overdoses in adults have occurred at doses ranging from 14 to 60 g. In pediatric patients ages 1 to 4, nonfatal overdoses of 100 mg/kg for one to two doses have been reported. Nausea, vomiting, abdominal pain, pruritus, headache, and increasing lethargy usually develop shortly after ingestion; patient with severe hepatic disease may become unconscious. Liver enzyme or bilirubin levels may show transient increase. Skin, urine, sweat, saliva, tears, and feces turn brownish red or orange, with color intensity proportional to degree of overdose. Facial or periorbital edema also may occur in pediatric patients. Some patients may experience hypotension, sinus tachycardia, ventricular arrhythmias, seizures, or cardiac arrest.

• Institute intensive support measures, as ordered, and intervene for individual symptoms as they arise. If indicated and ordered, give antiemetics to control severe nausea and vomiting. Active diuresis (with measured fluid intake and output) promotes drug excretion. Hemodialysis may benefit some patients.

Patient teaching

Instruct patient to immediately report easy bruising or bleeding, fever, malaise, appetite loss, nausea, vomiting, or yellowing of skin or eyes.

• Tell patient drug may color tears, urine, and other body fluids reddish or brownish orange. Instruct patient not to wear contact lenses during therapy, because drug may stain them permanently.

• Advise patient not to drink alcohol during therapy.

• Caution patient to avoid driving and other hazardous activities until drug's effects on concentration and alertness are known.

• As appropriate, review all other significant and life-threatening adverse reactions and interactions, especially those related to the drugs, tests, and behaviors mentioned above.

rituximab

Rituxan, Rituxan Mab Thera

Pharmacologic class: Murine/human monoclonal antibody
Therapeutic class: Antineoplastic
Pregnancy risk category C

FDA BOXED WARNING

- Deaths from infusion reactions have occurred within 24 hours of infusion. Approximately 80% of fatal reactions were linked to first infusion. If severe infusion reaction develops, discontinue infusion and intervene appropriately.
- Acute renal failure requiring dialysis, severe mucocutaneous reactions, and progressive multifocal leukoencephalopathy have been reported.

Action

Binds to CD20 antigen on malignant B lymphocytes and recruits immune effector functions to mediate B-cell lysis (possibly through complement-dependent cytotoxicity and antibody-dependent cell-mediated cytotoxicity)

Pharmacokinetics

Drug has wide range of half-lives, which may reflect variable tumor burden among patients and changes in CD20-positive (normal and malignant) B-cell populations with repeated administration. Peak and trough serum levels correlate inversely with baseline values for number of circulating CD20-positive B cells and measures of disease burden.

Onset	Peak	Duration
Variable	Variable	6-12 mo

How supplied

Solution for injection (clear, colorless liquid concentrate): 10 mg/mL in 10-mL (100-mg) and 50-mL (500-mg) vials

Indications and dosages

➤ Low-grade or follicular CD20-positive B-cell non-Hodgkin's lymphoma

Adults: Initially, 375 mg/m^2 by I.V. infusion once weekly for four or eight doses at 50 mg/hour; increase rate by 50 mg/hour q 30 minutes to a maximum of 400 mg/hour. If patient tolerates first infusion, subsequent infusions may begin at 100 mg/hour; then increase by 100 mg/hour q 30 minutes to a maximum of 400 mg/hour as tolerated. When given as required component of ibritumomab tiuxetan (Zevalin) therapeutic regimen, rituximab dosage is 250 mg/m^2. (See ibritumomab tiuxetan monograph.)

➤ Moderately to severely active rheumatoid arthritis in patients with inadequate response to one or more tumor necrosis factor antagonist therapies

Adults: Two doses of 1 g each by I.V. infusion given 2 weeks apart in combination with methotrexate. Safety and efficacy of retreatment have not been established.

Off-label uses

- Waldenström's macroglobulinemia

Administration

Preparation

- Premedicate with diphenhydramine and acetaminophen, as prescribed.
- Know that in rheumatoid arthritis patients, glucocorticoids are recommended 30 minutes before each infusion to reduce incidence and severity of infusion reactions.
- Consider withholding antihypertensive drugs 12 hours before infusion, as transient hypotension may occur during infusion.

Dilution and compatibility

- Dilute in D_5W or normal saline solution to a concentration of 1 to 4 mg/mL.
- Invert bag gently to mix solution. Do not shake.
- Discard unused portion of solution left in vial.

Infusion considerations

- Administer by I.V. infusion at 50 mg/hour or at prescribed rate.

R

Never give as I.V. bolus or I.V. push.

- If hypersensitivity reaction (non-immunoglobulin E–mediated) or infusion reaction occurs, interrupt or temporarily slow infusion. When symptoms improve, resume infusion at half of previous rate, as ordered.

Monitoring

- Monitor closely for signs and symptoms of hypersensitivity reaction.

Stop drug immediately and notify prescriber if patient develops signs or symptoms of Stevens-Johnson syndrome or other severe mucocutaneous reaction (including severe rash).

Monitor pulse and blood pressure throughout infusion. Stop infusion if hypotension, bronchospasm, or angioedema occurs. Consult prescriber about restarting infusion at half of previous rate.

Monitor ECG throughout infusion. Stop infusion if serious arrhythmia develops.

- Monitor CBC and blood glucose and electrolyte levels.
- Assess for signs and symptoms of infection, including fever.

Storage

- Solutions for infusion may be stored at 2° to 8°C (36° to 46°F) for 24 hours. Do not freeze; protect from direct sunlight.

Contraindications and precautions

Contraindicated in hypersensitivity to drug, its components, or murine products.

Use cautiously in history of drug allergy or sensitivity, previous exposure to murine-based monoclonal antibodies, high level of circulating cancer cells, cardiac or pulmonary conditions, pregnant or breastfeeding patients, and ***children.***

Adverse reactions

CNS: dizziness, headache, nervousness, hypertonia, hyperesthesia, insomnia, agitation, malaise, paresthesia, asthenia, fatigue, tremor, rigors
CV: hypotension, hypertension, peripheral edema, chest pain, tachycardia, bradycardia, angina, **arrhythmias**
EENT: conjunctivitis, lacrimation disorders, rhinitis, sinusitis, pharyngitis
GI: nausea, vomiting, diarrhea, constipation, abdominal pain, dyspepsia, anorexia
GU: renal toxicity
Hematologic: anemia, **neutropenia, leukopenia, thrombocytopenia**
Metabolic: hyperglycemia, hypocalcemia
Musculoskeletal: myalgia, back pain
Respiratory: dyspnea, cough, bronchitis, **bronchospasm**
Skin: pruritus, rash, urticaria, flushing, dermatitis, angioedema, **toxic epidermal necrolysis, Stevens-Johnson syndrome**
Other: altered taste, fever, chills, pain at injection site, hypersensitivity reactions including **sepsis, severe infusion reaction**

Interactions

Drug-drug. *Cisplatin:* increased risk of renal failure
Live-virus vaccines: increased risk of infection from vaccine
Drug-diagnostic tests. *Calcium, hemoglobin, neutrophils, platelets, white blood cells:* decreased
Glucose, lactate dehydrogenase: increased

Toxicity and overdose

- Overdose has not been reported. In dose-escalation clinical trials, single doses of up to 500 mg/m^2 were given.
- Provide supportive and symptomatic therapy.

Patient teaching

Tell patient to immediately report signs and symptoms of hypersensitivity reaction or severe skin reaction.

Instruct patient to take temperature every day and immediately report fever and other signs or symptoms of infection.

Instruct patient to immediately report unusual bleeding or bruising.

- Advise patient to minimize GI upset by eating small, frequent servings of food and drinking plenty of fluids.
- As appropriate, review all other significant and life-threatening adverse reactions and interactions, especially those related to the drugs and tests mentioned above.

sargramostim (GM-CSF)

Leukine

Pharmacologic class: Granulocyte-macrophage colony stimulating factor
Therapeutic class: Hematopoietic agent
Pregnancy risk category C

Action

Stimulates proliferation and differentiation of hematopoietic cells that activate mature granulocytes and macrophages of target cells

Pharmacokinetics

Drug degrades throughout the body, but mostly in the liver and kidneys. Mean beta half-life is approximately 60 minutes. Elimination route is unknown; drug is not appreciably excreted.

Onset	Peak	Duration
Immediate	2 hr	3-6 hr

How supplied

Powder for reconstitution for injection (white): 250 mcg

Indications and dosages

➢ Post peripheral blood progenitor cell (PBPC) transplantation

Adults: 250 mcg/m²/day I.V. over 24 hours, starting immediately after infusion of progenitor cells

➢ Mobilization of PBPCs into peripheral blood for collection by leukapheresis

Adults: 250 mcg/m²/day I.V. over 24 hours, continued throughout harvesting

➢ Neutrophil recovery after chemotherapy in acute myelogenous leukemia

Adults: 250 mcg/m²/day I.V. over 4 hours, starting 4 days after completion of chemotherapy induction

➢ Bone marrow transplantation failure or engraftment delay

Adults: 250 mcg/m²/day as 2-hour I.V. infusion for 14 days. If engraftment does not occur, may repeat after 7 days of drug hiatus.

➢ Myeloid reconstitution after autologous or allogeneic bone marrow transplantation

Adults: 250 mcg/m²/day as a 2-hour I.V. infusion, starting 2 to 4 hours after autologous bone marrow infusion and at least 24 hours after last chemotherapy or radiotherapy dose

Off-label uses

- Crohn's disease
- Melanoma
- Mucositis
- Stomatitis
- Vaccine adjuvant
- Wound healing

Administration

Preparation

Do not give within 24 hours of chemotherapy or radiation therapy.

S

Dilution and compatibility
- Add 1 mL sterile water to powder for injection by directing water stream against side of vial and swirling vial gently to disperse contents.
- Avoid shaking or agitating solution.
- To obtain a final concentration of less than 10 mcg/mL, add human albumin 0.1% to normal saline solution for injection before adding drug (to prevent drug adsorption into delivery system). To obtain a final concentration of 0.1% albumin, add 1 mg albumin per 1 mL normal saline solution; for example, use 1 mL 5% albumin human in 50 mL normal saline solution.
- Know that reconstituted solution should be clear and colorless.
- Infuse as soon as possible after reconstituting but no more than 6 hours after mixing.
- Do not add other drugs to infusion; do not use inline filter.
- Discard reconstituted solution after 20 days.

Infusion considerations
- Administer by I.V. infusion at prescribed rate.
- Monitor for dyspnea. If dyspnea occurs, halve dosage and contact prescriber.

Monitoring
- Assess CBC with white cell differential. Check for blast cells, and watch for signs and symptoms of blood dyscrasias.
- Closely monitor vital signs and fluid intake and output. Stay alert for signs and symptoms of fluid overload.

Monitor liver function tests. Watch for evidence of hepatic damage and bleeding (especially GI hemorrhage).

Storage
- Store at 2° to 8°C (36° to 46°F). Do not freeze.

Contraindications and precautions

Contraindicated in hypersensitivity to drug, its components, or yeast products; excessive leukemic myeloid blasts in bone marrow or peripheral blood (10% or more); and within 24 hours before or after chemotherapy or radiation therapy.

Use cautiously in renal or hepatic insufficiency, fluid retention, pulmonary disorders, pulmonary infiltrates, heart failure, leukocytosis, transient supraventricular arrhythmias, cancer patients undergoing sargramostim-mobilized PBPC collection, patients receiving purged bone marrow or previously exposed to intensive chemotherapy or radiation therapy, pregnant or breastfeeding patients, and ***children.***

Adverse reactions

CNS: malaise, asthenia
CV: peripheral edema, tachycardia, hypotension, transient supraventricular tachycardia, **pericardial effusion**
GI: nausea, vomiting, diarrhea, anorexia, stomatitis, **GI hemorrhage**
GU: urinary tract disorder, **abnormal renal function**
Hematologic: blood dyscrasias, hemorrhage
Hepatic: hepatic damage
Musculoskeletal: joint pain, myalgia, bone pain
Respiratory: dyspnea, lung disorder
Skin: rash, alopecia
Other: fever, chills, sepsis, edema, first-dose reaction (respiratory distress, hypoxia, syncope, tachycardia, hypotension, flushing)

Interactions

Drug-drug. *Corticosteroids, lithium:* potentiation of myeloproliferative effects
Vincristine: severe peripheral neuropathy

Toxicity and overdose

• Maximum amount that can be given safely in single or multiple doses has not been determined. Increased white blood cell (WBC) count, dyspnea, malaise, nausea, fever, rash, sinus tachycardia, headache, and chills may occur.
• Withdraw drug and monitor carefully for WBC increase and respiratory symptoms.

Patient teaching

Tell patient sargramostim is a powerful drug that can cause significant adverse reactions. Teach patient to recognize and report serious reactions at once.
Instruct patient to immediately report unusual bleeding or bruising or yellowing of skin or eyes.
• Tell patient drug may cause weakness and musculoskeletal pain.
• Inform patient about the need for regular blood testing during therapy.
• As appropriate, review all other significant and life-threatening adverse reactions and interactions, especially those related to the drugs mentioned above.

scopolamine hydrobromide (hyoscine hydrobromide)

Buscopan✦

Pharmacologic class: Antimuscarinic, belladonna alkaloid
Therapeutic class: Antiemetic, antivertigo agent, anticholinergic
Pregnancy risk category C

Action

Acts as a competitive inhibitor at postganglionic muscarinic receptor sites of parasympathetic nervous system and on smooth muscles that respond to acetylcholine but lack cholinergic innervation. May block cholinergic transmission from vestibular nuclei to higher CNS centers and from reticular formation to vomiting center.

Pharmacokinetics

Drug distributes widely throughout body. Exact metabolic fate is unknown, but drug may undergo hepatic metabolism. Half-life elimination is 4.8 hours. Drug is excreted in urine as parent drug and metabolites.

Onset	Peak	Duration
10-15 min	1 hr	2-4 hr

How supplied

Solution for injection: 0.3 mg/mL and 1 mg/mL in 1-mL vials, 0.4 mg/mL in 0.5-mL ampules and 1-mL vials, 0.86 mg/mL in 0.5-mL ampules

Indications and dosages

➢ Preanesthetic sedation and obstetric amnesia
Adults: 0.3 to 0.6 mg I.V. given 45 to 60 minutes before anesthesia, usually administered with analgesics
➢ Sedative or tranquilizing effect
Adults: 0.6 mg I.V. t.i.d. to q.i.d.

Dosage adjustment

• Know that elderly and debilitated patients may respond to usual doses with excitement, agitation, drowsiness, or confusion and therefore may require lower dosages.

Administration

Dilution and compatibility
• Dilute with sterile water for injection.
• Use solution only if clear.
Infusion considerations
• Give by direct I.V. injection over 2 to 3 minutes or at prescribed rate.

S

Monitoring
- Assess vital signs and neurologic, cardiovascular, and respiratory status.
- Monitor patient for urinary hesitancy or urine retention.

Storage
- Store at controlled room temperature of 15° to 30°C (58° to 86°F). Protect from light.

Contraindications and precautions

Contraindicated in hypersensitivity to scopolamine, other belladonna alkaloids, barbiturates, or bromides; known idiosyncratic reaction to anticholinergics; angle-closure glaucoma; acute hemorrhage; myasthenia gravis; obstructive uropathy (including prostatic hypertrophy); obstructive GI disease; paralytic ileus or intestinal atony; reflux esophagitis; ulcerative colitis or toxic megacolon; hepatic or renal impairment; chronic lung disease (with repeated doses); and tachycardia secondary to cardiac insufficiency or thyrotoxicosis.

Use cautiously in history of seizures or psychosis, suspected intestinal obstruction, pulmonary or cardiac disease, tachyarrhythmia or tachycardia, open-angle glaucoma, autonomic neuropathy, hypertension, hyperthyroidism, ileostomy or colostomy, ***elderly or debilitated patients,*** pregnant or breastfeeding patients (safety not established), and ***children.***

Adverse reactions

CNS: drowsiness, dizziness, confusion, restlessness, fatigue
CV: tachycardia, palpitations, hypotension, transient heart-rate changes
EENT: blurred vision, mydriasis, photophobia, conjunctivitis
GI: constipation, dry mouth
GU: urinary hesitancy, urine retention
Skin: decreased sweating, rash

Interactions

Drug-drug. *Antidepressants, antihistamines, disopyramide, quinidine:* additive anticholinergic effects
Antidepressants, antihistamines, opioid analgesics, sedative-hypnotics: additive CNS depression
Oral drugs: altered absorption of these drugs
Wax-matrix potassium tablets: increased GI mucosal lesions
Drug-herb. *Angel's trumpet, jimsonweed, scopolia:* increased anticholinergic effects
Drug-behaviors. *Alcohol use:* increased CNS depression

Toxicity and overdose

- Overdose signs and symptoms include dilated pupils, flushed skin, tachycardia, hypertension, and ECG abnormalities. CNS manifestations (including seizures, acute psychotic reactions, CNS depression), circulatory collapse, hyperpyrexia, respiratory failure, and death also may occur.
- Artificial respiration with oxygen may be necessary. For severe life-threatening symptoms, give physostigmine 1 to 2 mg subcutaneously or I.V. slowly, as ordered, to reverse toxic effects; repeat dose after 2 hours if necessary. If marked excitement occurs and more specific treatment is unavailable, diazepam is most suitable for sedation and seizure control. (However, avoid high diazepam dosages because central depressant action may coincide with depression occurring late in belladonna poisoning.) Do not give phenothiazines because their antimuscuranic action may intensify toxicity and lead to coma. Other therapy is symptomatic and supportive.

Patient teaching

- Caution patient to avoid alcohol during therapy because it may increase CNS depression.
- As appropriate, review all other significant adverse reactions and interactions, especially those related to the drugs, herbs, and behaviors mentioned above.

sodium acetate

Pharmacologic class: Fluid and electrolyte agent
Therapeutic class: Alkalinizer
Pregnancy risk category C

Action

Plays a primary role in controlling total body water and its distribution

Pharmacokinetics

Sodium is a major cation of extracellular fluid. Acetate, a hydrogen ion acceptor, is metabolized in the liver and serves as alternate bicarbonate source. Drug is excreted by the kidneys.

Onset	Peak	Duration
Unknown	Unknown	Unknown

How supplied

Solution (concentrate) for injection: 100 mEq in 50 mL, 200 mEq in 100 mL

Indications and dosages

➤ To prevent or correct hyponatremia in patients with restricted or no oral intake
Adults: Dosage individualized according to patient's condition and degree of hyponatremia
Children: Dosage individualized

Administration

Preparation

- Know that solution is used as alternative to sodium chloride to provide sodium ion for addition to large-volume infusion fluids for I.V. use.
- Assess electrolyte levels, especially serum sodium, before giving.

Dilution and compatibility

[Clinical alert] Know that drug must be diluted before use.
- Do not administer solution unless clear.
- Discard unused portion.

Infusion considerations

[Clinical alert] Give only by slow I.V infusion in larger fluid volume.
[Clinical alert] Avoid rapid administration to prevent sodium overload and water retention.
- Know that administration rate depends on patient's needs.

Monitoring

[Clinical alert] Closely monitor fluid and electrolyte balance. Be aware that drug can cause fluid or solute overload, resulting in dilution of other serum electrolytes, metabolic alkalosis, overhydration, congested states, or pulmonary edema. Also, excessive administration of potassium-free solutions may result in significant hypokalemia.

Storage

- Store at controlled room temperature of 15° to 30°C (59° to 86°F).

Contraindications and precautions

Contraindicated in hypernatremia or fluid retention.

Use with extreme caution, if at all, in congestive heart failure, severe hepatic or renal insufficiency, edema with sodium retention, and metabolic or respiratory alkalosis. Use cautiously in cirrhosis, patients receiving corticosteroids or corticotropin, ***elderly patients,*** pregnant patients, and ***children.***

Adverse reactions

CV: congestive heart failure (with rapid administration or excessive use)
Metabolic: hypernatremia, water overload, metabolic alkalosis, hypokalemia (with rapid administration or excessive use)
Respiratory: pulmonary edema (with rapid administration or excessive use)
Skin: extravasation

Interactions

Drug-diagnostic tests. *Electrolytes:* imbalances

Toxicity and overdose

- Overdose may lead to hypernatremia resulting in dizziness, edema, headache, hypotension, oliguria, restlessness, pulmonary edema, heart failure, metabolic alkalosis, and delirium.
- Discontinue infusion immediately and use corrective measures to reduce elevated serum sodium levels and restore acid-base balance, as needed.

Patient teaching

- As appropriate, review all significant and life-threatening adverse reactions and interactions, especially those related to the tests mentioned above.

sodium bicarbonate

Pharmacologic class: Fluid and electrolyte agent
Therapeutic class: Alkalinizer
Pregnancy risk category C

Action

Restores body's buffering capacity; neutralizes excess acid

Pharmacokinetics

Sodium is principal cation of extracellular fluid. At proper concentration of hydrogen ion, bicarbonate anion may be converted to carbonic acid and then to its volatile form, carbon dioxide, which is excreted by the lungs. Normally, extracellular fluid has a carbonic acid:bicarbonate ratio of 1:20. Blood drug level is regulated by the kidneys through urine acidification or by urine alkalinization. In healthy adult with normal renal function, nearly all glomerular-filtered bicarbonate ion is reabsorbed; less than 1% is excreted in urine.

Onset	Peak	Duration
Immediate	Immediate	Unknown

How supplied

Solution for injection (hypertonic): 4% (2.4 mEq/5 mL), 4.2% (5 mEq/10 mL), 5% (297.5 mEq/500 mL), 7.5% (8.92 mEq/10 mL and 44.6 mEq/50 mL), 8.4% (10 mEq/10 mL and 50 mEq/50 mL) in syringes and vials

Indications and dosages

➤ Metabolic acidosis

Adults and children: 2 to 5 mEq/kg by I.V. infusion over 4 to 8 hours. However, dosage is highly individualized based on patient's condition and blood pH and carbon dioxide content.

Administration

Preparation

- Assess electrolyte levels.

Dilution and compatibility

- For I.V. infusion, dilute with sterile water for injection, normal saline solution, D_5W, or other common I.V. solution to a suitable concentration, depending on patient condition and requirements.
- Use solution only if clear.
- Do not mix with other drugs.

Infusion considerations

• Administer by slow I.V. infusion at prescribed rate, using controlled infusion device.

Clinical alert: In children, do not administer more than 8 mEq/kg/day.

Clinical alert: Avoid rapid infusion, which may cause tetany; in children, it may decrease cerebrospinal fluid pressure and cause intracranial hemorrhage.

Clinical alert: Do not give concurrently with calcium or catecholamines (such as norepinephrine, dobutamine, or dopamine). If patient is receiving any of these drugs, flush I.V. line thoroughly after each dose to prevent contact between these drugs and sodium bicarbonate.

Monitoring

Clinical alert: Closely monitor arterial blood gas results and electrolyte levels.

Clinical alert: Stay alert for signs and symptoms of metabolic alkalosis and electrolyte imbalances.

• Monitor fluid intake and output. Assess for fluid overload.

• Watch for inflammation at I.V. site.

Storage

• Store at 15° to 30°C (59° to 86°F); brief excursions permitted to 40°C (104°F). Do not freeze.

Contraindications and precautions

Contraindicated in metabolic or respiratory alkalosis, hypocalcemia, hypernatremia, hypokalemia, severe pulmonary edema, seizures, vomiting resulting in chloride loss, and diuretic use resulting in hypochloremic alkalosis.

Use cautiously in renal insufficiency, heart failure, hypertension, peptic ulcer, cirrhosis, toxemia, and pregnant patients.

Adverse reactions

CNS: headache, irritability, confusion, stimulation, tremors, twitching, hyperreflexia, weakness, **seizures of alkalosis, tetany**

CV: irregular pulse, edema, **cardiac arrest**

GI: gastric distention, belching, flatulence, acid reflux, **paralytic ileus**

GU: renal calculi

Metabolic: hypokalemia, fluid retention, hypernatremia, **hyperosmolarity** (with overdose), **metabolic alkalosis**

Respiratory: slow and shallow respirations, **cyanosis, apnea**

Other: weight gain, pain and inflammation at I.V. site

Interactions

Drug-drug. *Anorexiants, flecainide, mecamylamine, methenamine, quinidine, sympathomimetics:* increased urinary alkalization, decreased renal clearance of these drugs

Chlorpropamide, lithium, methotrexate, salicylates, tetracycline: increased renal clearance and decreased efficacy of these drugs

Enteric-coated tablets: premature gastric release of these drugs

Drug-diagnostic tests. *Lactate, potassium, sodium:* increased

Drug-herb. *Oak bark:* decreased sodium bicarbonate action

Toxicity and overdose

• Excessive or too-rapid administration may cause alkalosis with hyperirritability or tetany.

• In alkalosis, discontinue infusion and provide care according to degree of alkalosis, such as I.V. administration of normal saline solution for injection. As ordered and needed, give potassium chloride for hypokalemia, calcium gluconate for hyperirritability or tetany, and acidifying agent (such as ammonium chloride) for severe alkalosis.

Patient teaching

• As appropriate, review all significant and life-threatening adverse reactions and interactions, especially those related to the drugs, tests, and herbs mentioned above.

S

sodium chloride

Pharmacologic class: Electrolyte supplement
Therapeutic class: Sodium replacement
Pregnancy risk category C

Action

Replaces sodium and chloride deficiencies and maintains these electrolytes at adequate levels

Pharmacokinetics

Sodium (a principal cation of extracellular fluid) in combination with chloride is widely distrubuted. Metabolism is insignificant. Excess is eliminated in urine, sweat, tears, and saliva.

Onset	Peak	Duration
Immediate	Immediate	Unknown

How supplied

Injection: 0.45% sodium chloride (hypotonic)—25 mL, 50 mL, 150 mL, 250 mL, 500 mL, 1,000 mL
0.9% sodium chloride (isotonic)—2 mL, 3 mL, 5 mL, 10 mL, 20 mL, 25 mL, 30 mL, 50 mL, 100 mL, 150 mL, 250 mL, 500 mL, 1,000 mL
3% sodium chloride (hypertonic)—500 mL
5% sodium chloride—500 mL
14.6% sodium chloride (concentrated)—20 mL, 40 mL, 200 mL
23.4% sodium chloride—30 mL, 50 mL, 100 mL, 200 mL

Indications and dosages

➤ Water and sodium chloride replacement; metabolic alkalosis; to dilute or dissolve drugs for I.V., I.M., or subcutaneous use; to flush I.V. catheters; as priming solution in hemodialysis; to initiate or terminate blood transfusions
Adults: 0.9% sodium chloride (isotonic solution) at individualized dosage

➤ Hydrating solution; hyperosmolar diabetes
Adults: 0.45% sodium chloride (hypotonic solution) at individualized dosage

➤ Rapid fluid and electrolyte replacement in hyponatremia and hypochloremia; severe sodium depletion; drastic body water dilution after excessive water intake
Adults: 3% or 5% sodium chloride (hypertonic solution) at individualized dosage given by slow I.V. with close electrolyte monitoring

Administration

Preparation

- Assess electrolyte levels.

Do not confuse normal saline solution for injection with concentrates meant for use in total parenteral nutrition.

- High-alert drug designation applies to concentration of 9% and above.

Dilution and compatibility

Be aware that concentrated solution of 14.6 % must be diluted before use.

- Dilute I.V. doses according to product label.

Infusion considerations

Do not use preparation in plastic containers in series connections. Such use could result in air embolism due to residual air being drawn from primary container before administration of fluid from secondary container ends.

Infuse slow I.V. to minimize risk of pulmonary edema.

Monitoring

- Monitor electrolyte levels and blood chemistry results.

Watch for signs and symptoms of pulmonary edema or worsening heart failure.

• Carefully monitor vital signs, fluid balance, weight, and cardiovascular status.
• Assess injection site closely to help prevent tissue necrosis and thrombophlebitis.

Storage

• Store at controlled room temperature of 15° to 30°C (59° to 86°F); brief excursions permitted to 40°C (104°F). Do not freeze.

Contraindications and precautions

Contraindicated in normal or above-normal electrolyte levels (3% and 5% solutions) and fluid retention.

Use with extreme caution, if at all, in congestive heart failure, severe hepatic or renal insufficiency, and edema with sodium retention. Use cautiously in renal impairment, hypoproteinemia, surgical patients, patients receiving corticosteroids or corticotrophin, ***elderly patients,*** pregnant or breastfeeding patients, and ***children.***

Adverse reactions

CV: edema (when given too rapidly or in excess), **thrombophlebitis, heart failure exacerbation**
Metabolic: fluid and electrolyte disturbances (such as hypernatremia, hyperphosphatemia), **aggravation of existing metabolic acidosis** (with excessive infusion)
Respiratory: pulmonary edema
Other: pain, swelling, local tenderness, abscess, or tissue necrosis at I.V. site

Interactions

Drug-diagnostic tests. *Phosphate, potassium, sodium:* increased

Toxicity and overdose

• Excessive administration may lead to serious electrolyte imbalances resulting in water retention, edema, hypokalemia, and aggravation of existing acidosis.
• Discontinue infusion and provide symptomatic and supportive therapy.

Patient teaching

[Clinical alert] Teach patient to recognize and immediately report serious adverse reactions, such as breathing problems or swelling.
• Instruct patient to report pain, tenderness, or swelling at injection site.
• As appropriate, review all other significant and life-threatening adverse reactions and interactions, especially those related to the tests mentioned above.

sodium ferric gluconate complex

Ferrlecit

Pharmacologic class: Trace element
Therapeutic class: Iron supplement, hematinic
Pregnancy risk category B

Action

Critical in normal hemoglobin synthesis to maintain oxygen transport; additionally, iron is necessary for metabolism and various enzymatic processes.

Pharmacokinetics

Pharmacokinetic studies have not been performed in humans.

Onset	Peak	Duration
Unknown	Unknown	Unknown

How supplied

Solution for injection (dark red): 62.5 mg (12.5 mg/mL) of elemental iron in 5-mL ampules with 20% sucrose and 9 mg benzyl alcohol

S

Indications and dosages

➤ Iron deficiency in patients undergoing chronic hemodialysis who are receiving supplemental erythropoietin
Adults: 10 mL (125 mg of elemental iron) I.V. infusion over 1 hour (typically 1,000 mg elemental iron given over eight sequential dialysis sessions)
Children: 1.5 mg/kg (up to 125 mg/dose) diluted in normal saline solution and given I.V. over 1 hour during eight sequential dialysis sessions

Administration

Preparation

- If ordered, give I.V. test dose of 2 mL (25 mg elemental iron) before starting therapy. Dilute test dose in 50 mL normal saline solution and administer over 60 minutes.
- Be aware that most patients need minimum cumulative dosage of 1 g elemental iron given over eight sequential dialysis sessions to achieve favorable hemoglobin or hematocrit response. Patients may continue to require therapy with this drug or other I.V. iron preparations at lowest dosage that maintains target levels of hemoglobin, hematocrit, and laboratory parameters of iron storage within acceptable limits.
- Know that drug has been given at sequential dialysis sessions by infusion during dialysis session itself.
- Assess hemoglobin, hematocrit, and serum iron levels.

Dilution and compatibility

- Dilute 10 mL in 100 mL normal saline solution for injection.

Do not mix with other medications or solutions or add to parenteral nutrition solutions for I.V. infusion.

- Use immediately after dilution.

Infusion considerations

- Administer by slow I.V. infusion over 1 hour.

Do not exceed infusion rate of 2.1 mg/minute.

- Keep patient in recumbent position to help relieve hypotension.

Monitoring

Know that drug has caused potentially fatal hypersensitivity reactions characterized by cardiovascular collapse, cardiac arrest, bronchospasm, oral or pharyngeal edema, dyspnea, angioedema, urticaria, or pruritus (sometimes associated with pain and muscle spasm of chest or back), which could result in death. Be prepared to intervene appropriately.

Be aware that flushing, hypotension, light-headedness, malaise, fatigue, weakness, or severe pain in chest, back, flank, or groin may result from rapid I.V. iron administration, but usually resolve within 1 or 2 hours.

- Continue to monitor hemoglobin, hematocrit, and serum iron levels.
- Monitor vital signs.

Storage

- Store at 20° to 25°C (68° to 77°F).

Contraindications and precautions

Contraindicated in hypersensitivity to drug or its components and in anemias not associated with iron deficiency.

Use cautiously in hemoglobinopathies and other refractory anemias, iron overload (do not administer), ***elderly patients***, pregnant or breastfeeding patients, and ***children*** (safety and efficacy not established).

Adverse reactions

CNS: dizziness, light-headedness, malaise, weakness
CV: flushing, hypotension
EENT: diplopia
GI: vomiting, severe epigastric pain

Other: sensation of heat, loin pain, hypersensitivity including **anaphylaxis**

Interactions

Drug-drug. *Angiotensin-converting enzyme inhibitors:* potentiation of adverse effects of I.V. iron

Oral iron preparations: decreased absorption of these preparations

Toxicity and overdose

- Dosages above patient's iron needs may cause iron accumulation in iron storage sites and hemosiderosis. Serum iron levels above 300 mcg/dL (combined with transferrin oversaturation) may indicate iron poisoning, characterized by abdominal pain, diarrhea, or vomiting, which progresses to pallor or cyanosis, lassitude, drowsiness, hyperventilation, and cardiovascular collapse. Some patients have experienced signs and symptoms attributed to transferrin oversaturation after rapid I.V. infusion.
- To detect iron accumulation, periodically monitor laboratory parameters of iron. In overdose, discontinue infusion and provide supportive therapy. Drug is not dialyzable.

Patient teaching

- As appropriate, review all significant adverse reactions.

streptokinase

Streptase

Pharmacologic class: Group C beta-hemolytic streptococcal nonenzymatic protein

Therapeutic class: Thrombolytic

Pregnancy risk category C

Action

Converts plasminogen to plasmin, an enzyme that degrades fibrin clots and lyses thrombi and emboli

Pharmacokinetics

Drug is inactivated partly by antistreptococcal antibodies. No metabolites have been identified. Half-life is about 23 minutes.

Onset	Peak	Duration
Immediate	1 hr	4 hr

How supplied

Powder for reconstitution for injection (white): 250,000, 750,000, and 1.5 million international units/vial

Indications and dosages

➢ Acute evolving transmural myocardial infarction

Adults: 1.5 million international units by I.V. infusion over 1 hour as soon as possible after symptom onset

➢ Deep vein thrombosis (DVT)

Adults: Loading dose of 250,000 international units by I.V. infusion over 30 minutes, followed by 100,000 international units/hour I.V. for 72 hours. Start therapy as soon as possible after thrombotic symptoms begin (preferably within 7 days).

➢ Pulmonary embolus

Adults: Loading dose of 250,000 international units by I.V. infusion over 30 minutes, followed by 100,000 international units/hour I.V. for 24 hours (or 72 hours in suspected concurrent DVT). Start therapy as soon as possible after thrombotic symptoms begin (preferably within 7 days).

➢ Arterial thrombosis or embolus

Adults: Loading dose of 250,000 international units by I.V. infusion over 30 minutes, followed by 100,000

international units/hour I.V. for 24 to 72 hours. Start therapy as soon as possible after thrombotic symptoms begin (preferably within 7 days).

Administration

Preparation

Before giving, make sure hydrocortisone is available to treat allergic reaction and aminocaproic acid is available to treat excessive bleeding.

As prescribed, give test dose of 100 international units intradermally to check for hypersensitivity. Wheal-and-flare response within 20 minutes indicates probable allergy.

Dilution and compatibility

- To reconstitute, slowly add 5 mL normal saline solution or D_5W to each vial by directing diluent at side of vial (not powder); then dilute again to 45 mL. Roll vial gently between hands; do not shake.
- If necessary, further dilute to 50 mL in plastic container or to 500 mL in glass bottle.
- Know that reconstituted solution may be slightly yellow.
- Do not mix with other drugs or give other drugs through same I.V. line.
- Discard unused reconstituted drug.
- Use within 8 hours or store according to manufacturer's directions.

Infusion considerations

- Use infusion pump to administer by I.V. infusion at prescribed rate.
- Know that reconstituted solution can be filtered through 0.8-micron filter.

Monitoring

- Monitor vital signs and neurologic status carefully after test dose and throughout therapy.

Watch for signs and symptoms of hypersensitivity reaction. Stop drug if these occur.

- Check for bleeding every 15 minutes for first hour, every 30 minutes for next 7 hours, and then every 4 hours.

Stop therapy and contact prescriber immediately if excessive bleeding occurs.

Assess neurologic status closely. Watch for indications of intracranial bleeding.

- Handle patient gently and sparingly. If necessary, pad bed rails to prevent injury.
- Monitor pulse hourly. Also monitor distal circulation and sensation to extremities.
- Monitor partial thromboplastin time (PTT), prothrombin time (PT), plasma thrombin time, hemoglobin, hematocrit, and platelet count.
- Avoid giving I.M. injections during therapy.

Storage

- Store unopened vials at controlled room temperature of 15° to 30°C (59° to 86°F).
- Store reconstituted solution at 2° to 8°C (36° to 46°F).

Contraindications and precautions

Contraindicated in hypersensitivity to drug or anistreplase, cerebrovascular accident, intracranial or intraspinal surgery within past 2 months, active internal bleeding, intracranial neoplasm, or severe, uncontrolled hypertension (systolic pressure above 180 mm Hg or diastolic pressure above 110 mm Hg).

Use cautiously in severe hepatic or renal disease, recent major surgery or trauma, obstetric delivery, acute pericarditis, infectious endocarditis, atrioventricular malformation or aneurysm, suspected thrombus in left side of heart, septic thrombophlebitis or occluded arteriovenous cannula at seriously infected site, conditions in which bleeding may be hard to manage (such as organ biopsy, peptic ulcer, and previous puncture of noncompressible blood vessel), history of cerebrovascular disease, use of drug within past 2 years, concurrent anticoagulant use, ***elderly patients,*** pregnant or breastfeeding patients, and ***children*** (safety and efficacy not established).

Adverse reactions

CNS: headache, **intracranial hemorrhage**
CV: hypotension, **arrhythmias**
EENT: periorbital swelling
GI: nausea, vomiting, **GI hemorrhage**
GU: hematuria
Hematologic: anemia, **bleeding tendency**
Musculoskeletal: musculoskeletal pain
Respiratory: minor breathing difficulties, **bronchospasm, apnea**
Skin: urticaria, itching, flushing
Other: bleeding at puncture sites, hypersensitivity reactions including fever, shivering, and **anaphylaxis**

Interactions

Drug-drug. *Anticoagulants, aspirin, dipyridamole, indomethacin, phenylbutazone:* increased risk of bleeding
Drug-diagnostic tests. *Hemoglobin:* decreased
International Normalized Ratio, transaminases: increased
PT, PTT: prolonged

Toxicity and overdose

- In overdose, serious bleeding may occur, manifested by epistaxis, bleeding gums, spontaneous ecchymosis, and oozing at I.V. site. Increased pulse rate and pain (from internal bleeding) also may occur.
- Discontinue infusion immediately. If necessary, manage blood loss and reverse bleeding tendency by administering whole blood, packed red cells, and cryoprecipitate or fresh frozen plasma, as prescribed. Restart infusion when bleeding subsides, as ordered.

Patient teaching

- Tell patient why drug is necessary.
- Teach patient to recognize and immediately report signs or symptoms of hypersensitivity reaction or excessive bleeding.
- Instruct patient to report unusual bruising or bleeding, and teach about safety measures to avoid bruising and bleeding.
- Advise patient about the need for regular blood tests during therapy.
- As appropriate, review all other significant and life-threatening adverse reactions and interactions, especially those related to the drugs and tests mentioned above.

[redacted]

succinylcholine chloride

Anectine, Quelicin

Pharmacologic class: Depolarizing neuromuscular blocker
Therapeutic class: Skeletal muscle relaxant
Pregnancy risk category C

FDA BOXED WARNING

- In rare cases, drug has caused acute rhabdomyolysis with hyperkalemia followed by ventricular arrhythmias, cardiac arrest, and death in apparently healthy children (later found to have undiagnosed skeletal muscle myopathy). This syndrome commonly presents as peaked T waves and sudden cardiac arrest within minutes after administration in children (usually males age 8 or younger); some cases have occurred in adolescents. When healthy-seeming infant or child develops cardiac arrest (not thought to stem from inadequate ventilation, oxygenation, or anesthetic overdose) soon after administration, start immediate treatment for hyperkalemia, including I.V. calcium, bicarbonate, glucose with insulin, and hyperventilation, as ordered. Although routine resuscitative measures are likely to fail because of syndrome's abrupt onset, extraordinary and prolonged resuscitative efforts have produced successful resuscitation in some cases. Also, if patient has signs of malignant hyperthermia, begin appropriate treatment concurrently. Patients may lack signs or symptoms to alert clinicians that they are at risk; therefore, reserve use of this drug in children for emergency intubation or when airway must be secured immediately or for I.M. use when suitable vein is inaccessible.

Action

Relaxes skeletal muscles by decreasing response of nerve-impulse transmission at cholinergic receptor sites and decreasing action of acetylcholine

Pharmacokinetics

Drug distributes in extracellular fluid. It is rapidly hydrolyzed by plasma cholinesterase to succinylmonocholine, and then more slowly to succinic acid and choline. Because it is highly ionized with low fat solubility, it does not readily cross the placenta. About 10% of dose is excreted unchanged in urine.

Onset	Peak	Duration
0.5-1 min	1-2 min	4-10 min

How supplied

Powder for reconstitution for injection (white): 500-mg vial, 1-g vial

Solution for injection: 20 mg/mL, 100 mg/mL

Indications and dosages

➤ Adjunct to anesthesia to produce skeletal muscle relaxation during short surgical procedures; endotracheal intubation with mechanical ventilation; electrically induced convulsive therapy

Adults: 0.6 mg/kg I.V. over 10 to 30 seconds, or continuous I.V. infusion at 0.5 to 10 mg/minute, or 0.04 to 0.07 mg/kg I.V. intermittently p.r.n.

➤ For emergency tracheal intubation or when airway must be secured immediately

Older children and adolescents: 1 mg/kg I.V. over 10 to 30 seconds

Infants and young children: 2 mg/kg I.V. over 10 to 30 seconds

Administration

Preparation

Know that drug should be used only by personnel familiar with its actions, characteristics, and hazards.

Make sure patient has received sedatives or general anesthesia before administering.

Verify that emergency resuscitation equipment is at hand before giving drug.

As prescribed, give test dose of 5 to 10 mg I.V. after anesthesia administration. Drug may be administered if patient experiences no respiratory depression or transient (up to 5 minutes) respiratory depression. Do not give drug if patient develops respiratory paralysis sufficient to necessitate endotracheal intubation.

• Know that drug has no effect on consciousness, pain threshold, or cerebration. It should be used only with adequate anesthesia.

In children, pretreat with atropine, if prescribed, to reduce bradyarrhythmias.

Dilution and compatibility

- Reconstitute with D_5W or normal saline solution.
- Do not mix with alkaline solutions, such as sodium bicarbonate, barbiturates, or thiopental sodium.
- Use only freshly prepared solutions.
- Discard unused portion of diluted drug.

Infusion considerations

- Administer by intermittent or continuous I.V. infusion at prescribed rate.
- Be aware that continuous I.V. infusion is not recommended for children or adolescents.

Know that in rare cases, direct I.V. injection administration in infants and children leads to malignant ventricular arrhythmias and cardiac arrest secondary to acute rhabdomyolysis with hyperkalemia. In such situations, suspect underlying myopathy.

Be aware that administration by direct I.V. injection in infants or children may cause profound bradycardia or asystole (rare). Bradycardia incidence is higher after second dose.

Monitoring

Watch for potentially fatal adverse reactions, including anaphylaxis, malignant hyperthermia, and hypersensitivity reactions.

- Monitor ECG and vital signs (especially respirations) until patient recovers fully from neuromuscular blockade.
- Assess recovery from neuromuscular blockade by checking hand grip, head lift, and voluntary cough response.

Storage

- Refrigerate at 2° to 8°C (36° to 46°F).
- Know that multidose vials are stable for up to 14 days at room temperature without significant potency loss.

Contraindications and precautions

Contraindicated in hypersensitivity to drug or its components, genetic plasma pseudocholinesterase disorders, acute angle-closure glaucoma, myopathies associated with creatine kinase elevation, penetrating eye injury, personal or family history of malignant hyperthermia, acute phase of major trauma or burn, and extensive denervation of skeletal muscle.

Use cautiously in renal, hepatic, or pulmonary impairment; severe burns or trauma; electrolyte imbalances; spinal injury; cerebrovascular accident; neuromuscular disease; myasthenic syndrome related to lung cancer; dehydration; thyroid disorders; collagen disease; porphyria; pheochromocytoma; eye surgery; cesarean delivery; ***elderly or debilitated patients;*** pregnant or breastfeeding patients; and ***children.***

Adverse reactions

CV: flushing, tachycardia, hypertension, hypotension, bradycardia, **arrhythmias, cardiac arrest**
EENT: increased intraocular pressure
GI: excessive salivation
Hematologic: myoglobulinemia
Musculoskeletal: muscle fasciculations, postoperative muscle pain
Respiratory: prolonged respiratory depression, apnea, bronchoconstriction
Skin: rash, flushing, pruritus, urticaria
Other: hypersensitivity reaction, **anaphylaxis, malignant hyperthermia**

Interactions

Drug-drug. *Aminoglycosides, anticholinesterases, general anesthetics, polymyxin antibiotics:* increased neuromuscular blockade
Amphotericin B, thiazide diuretics: increased succinylcholine effects

S

Aprotinin, beta-adrenergic blockers, chloroquine, diethylether, desflurane, isoflurane, lidocaine, magnesium sulfate (parenteral), methotrimeprazine, metoclopramide, opioid analgesics, oxytocin, procainamide, promazine, quinidine, quinine, terbutaline, trimethaphan: increased neuromuscular blockade, leading to skeletal muscle relaxation and possible respiratory paralysis
Cardiac glycosides: arrhythmias
Cyclophosphamide, lithium, monoamine oxidase inhibitors: prolonged apnea
Diazepam: prolonged neuromuscular blockade
Opioid analgesics: increased risk of bradycardia and sinus arrest
Drug-diagnostic tests. *Myoglobin, potassium:* increased
Drug-herb. *Melatonin:* potentiation of neuromuscular blockade

Toxicity and overdose

• Overdose may cause neuromuscular blockade beyond time needed for surgery and anesthesia, which may manifest as skeletal muscle weakness, decreased respiratory reserve, and low tidal volume. Depending on dosage and duration of succinylcholine administration, depolarizing neuromuscular block may change to a block that superficially resembles nondepolarizing block, manifesting as prolonged respiratory depression and apnea.
• Maintain patent airway and provide respiratory support until recovery of normal respiration is assured.

Patient teaching

• Explain why drug is given. Provide reassurance that patient will be monitored closely until full recovery from neuromuscular blockade occurs.

sufentanil citrate

Sufenta

Pharmacologic class: Opioid agonist
Therapeutic class: Opioid agonist, analgesic, anesthesia adjunct
Controlled substance schedule II
Pregnancy risk category C

Action

Acts on selective opioid receptors, causing respiratory and CNS depression

Pharmacokinetics

Drug has extensive, rapid (1.4 minutes) distribution, redistribution of 17.1 minutes, and elimination half-life of 164 minutes. The liver and small intestine are major biotransformation sites. Drug is highly lipophilic, with plasma-protein binding of approximately 93% in healthy males, 91% in females, and 79% in neonates. Approximately 80% of dose is excreted within 24 hours, with 2% eliminated unchanged.

Onset	Peak	Duration
Immediate	Unknown	Unknown

How supplied

Solution for injection (aqueous): 50-mcg/mL ampules

Indications and dosages

➤ As primary anesthetic for induction and maintenance of anesthesia
Adults: Initially, 8 to 30 mcg/kg I.V. with oxygen and a muscle relaxant; maintenance dosage is 0.5 to 10 mcg/kg p.r.n. Maximum dosage is 30 mcg/kg.
Children younger than age 12: 10 to 25 mcg/kg I.V. given with oxygen. Maintenance dosage is 25 to 50 mcg.

➢ Analgesic adjunct to maintain balanced general anesthesia
Adults: 1 to 8 mcg/kg I.V. Give 75% of dose immediately before intubation; remainder can be given as 10- to 50-mcg bolus doses to maintain analgesia.
➢ Analgesic adjunct or maintenance of conscious sedation for bedside procedures in sedated, responsive, and spontaneously breathing patients
Adults: Initially, 0.25 to 0.75 mcg/kg I.V., followed by a continuous infusion of 0.005 to 0.02 mcg/kg/minute I.V.

Dosage adjustment
• Base dosage on ideal body weight (IBW) in obese patients (those more than 20% above IBW).
• Reduce dosage in elderly and debilitated patients.
• When using as analgesic adjunct or to maintain conscious sedation, reduce loading dosages by 25% to 50% in elderly and hemodynamically compromised patients.
• Reduce dosages of sufentanil and concomitantly used benzodiazepines, barbiturates, inhalation agents, other opioids, or other CNS depressants.

Administration
Preparation
🔈 Know that drug should be given only by healthcare professionals specifically trained in using I.V. anesthetics and managing respiratory effects of potent opioids.
🔈 Keep resuscitative and intubation equipment and oxygen at hand.
• Be aware that dosages are based on mean body weight.
• Know that selection of preanesthetic medications should be based on individual patient needs.

Dilution and compatibility
• For I.V. infusion, use compatible I.V. solution according to manufacturer's direction.
Infusion considerations
• Administer before intubation by slow I.V. injection or intermittent I.V infusion, titrated to response.
Monitoring
🔈 Monitor ECG and vital signs. Stay alert for signs and symptoms of shock and impending cardiac arrest.
🔈 Assess airway patency closely. Watch for respiratory depression and airway spasms.
• Monitor neurologic status during and after administration. Institute safety measures as needed to prevent injury.
• Monitor fluid intake and output and vital signs frequently.
Storage
• Store at room temperature of 15° to 30° C (59° to 86° F).

Contraindications and precautions
Contraindicated in hypersensitivity to drug or other opioids, acute or severe bronchial asthma, upper airway obstruction, significant respiratory depression, during labor when delivery of premature neonate is anticipated, and premature neonates.

Use cautiously in hepatic disease, head injury, diabetes mellitus, arrhythmias, renal or pulmonary disease, obesity, ***elderly patients,*** pregnant or breastfeeding patients, and ***children.***

Adverse reactions
CNS: sedation, headache, vertigo, floating feeling, dizziness, lethargy, confusion, light-headedness, nervousness, insomnia, unusual dreams, agitation, euphoria, hallucinations, delirium, anxiety, fear, disorientation, impaired mental and physical performance, mood changes, weakness, tremor

S

CV: palpitations, blood pressure changes, tachycardia, bradycardia, **arrhythmias, cardiac arrest, circulatory depression, shock**
EENT: diplopia, blurred vision
GI: nausea, vomiting, constipation, biliary tract spasm, dry mouth, anorexia
GU: urine retention, ureteral spasm, vesical sphincter spasm, antidiuretic effect, reduced libido, erectile dysfunction
Musculoskeletal: intraoperative muscle movement, skeletal muscle rigidity
Respiratory: slow and shallow respirations, suppressed cough reflex, **apnea, laryngospasm, bronchospasm**
Skin: clammy skin, sweating, erythema
Other: hypersensitivity reaction

Interactions

Drug-drug. *Barbiturate anesthetics:* enhanced barbiturate effects
Beta-adrenergic blockers, calcium channel blockers: increased risk of hypotension, bradycardia
CNS depressants: additive CNS depression
Drug-diagnostic tests. *Amylase, lipase:* increased
Liver function tests: abnormal results

Toxicity and overdose

• Overdose signs and symptoms are extension of drug's potent opioid actions. Most serious and significant effect is respiratory depression.
• As prescribed, give opioid antagonist such as naloxone I.V. as specific antidote to manage respiratory depression. Be aware that duration of respiratory depression after overdose may be longer than antagonist's duration of action. Do not give antagonist in absence of significant respiratory or cardiovascular depression. For hypoventilation or apnea, administer oxygen and provide assisted or controlled ventilation, as indicated and ordered. Maintain patent airway with nasopharyngeal airway or endotracheal tube, as indicated. If depressed respiration is associated with muscular rigidity, neuromuscular blocker may be needed to promote assisted or controlled respiration. Give I.V. fluids and vasopressors for hypotension, as ordered, and provide other supportive measures, as required.

Patient teaching

• Explain use of drug. Reassure patient that he will be monitored closely.

sulfamethoxazole-trimethoprim (co-trimoxazole), SMZ-TMP

Bactrim, Septra

Pharmacologic class: Sulfonamide
Therapeutic class: Anti-infective
Pregnancy risk category C

Action

Sulfamethoxazole inhibits bacterial synthesis of dihydrofolic acid by competing with para-aminobenzoic acid (PABA). Trimethoprim inhibits enzymes of folic acid pathways.

Pharmacokinetics

Drug distributes to sputum and vaginal fluid; trimethoprim also distributes to bronchial secretions. Both components cross placental barrier and are excreted in breast milk. Sulfamethoxazole is metabolized predominately by N_4-acetylation. Approximately 44% of trimethoprim and 70% of sulfamethoxazole are bound to plasma proteins.

Excretion occurs primarily by the kidneys; urine concentration is considerably higher than blood level. Urinary excretion ranges from 17% to 42% as free trimethoprim, 7% to17% as free sulfamethoxazole, and 36% to 56% as total sulfamethoxazole. Both components have longer half-life in severely impaired renal function.

Onset	Peak	Duration
Rapid	1 hr	Unknown

How supplied

Solution for injection: 80 mg/mL sulfamethoxazole and 16 mg/mL trimethoprim in multidose vials

Indications and dosages

➤ Severe or complicated urinary tract infections caused by susceptible strains of *Escherichia coli, Klebsiella* species, *Enterobacter* species, *Morganella morganii,* and *Proteus* species when oral administration is not feasible and organism is not susceptible to single-agent anti-infectives

Adults and children age 2 months and older: 8 to 10 mg/kg (based on trimethoprim component) I.V. q 6, 8, or 12 hours for up to 14 days

➤ Shigellosis caused by susceptible strains of *Shigella flexneri* or *Shigella sonnei*

Adults: 8 to 10 mg/kg (based on trimethoprim component) I.V. q 6, 8, or 12 hours for 5 days

Children age 2 months and older: 8 to 10 mg/kg (based on trimethoprim component) I.V. q 6, 8, or 12 hours for up to 5 days

➤ Treatment of *Pneumocystis jiroveci* pneumonia

Adults and children older than 2 months: 15 to 20 mg/kg (based on trimethoprim component) I.V. q 6 to 8 hours for up to 14 days

Dosage adjustment

- As needed, adjust dosage in severely impaired renal function.

Administration

Preparation

- Before administering drug, assess CBC with white cell differential, fluid intake and output, and renal function tests.

Dilution and compatibility

- (Clinical alert) Dilute each 5 mL in 125 mL D_5W for infusion.
- In fluid-restricted patients, dilute each 5 mL in 75 mL D_5W.
- (Clinical alert) Do not mix with other drugs or solutions.
- Discard solution if cloudy or if crystallization appears.
- Use within 6 hours after dilution.

Infusion considerations

- Infuse slowly over 60 to 90 minutes.
- (Clinical alert) Avoid rapid infusion or bolus injection.
- Flush I.V. line to remove residual drug after administration.

Monitoring

- (Clinical alert) Monitor CBC with white cell differential. Watch for evidence of blood dyscrasias.
- (Clinical alert) Stay alert for erythema multiforme. Report early signs before condition can progress to Stevens-Johnson syndrome.
- Monitor for signs and symptoms of superinfection, including fever, tachycardia, and chills.
- (Clinical alert) Monitor liver function test results and assess for evidence of hepatitis.
- (Clinical alert) Check kidney function test results weekly. Evaluate fluid intake, urine output, and urine pH. Maintain adequate hydration to prevent crystalluria. Report hematuria, oliguria, or anuria right away.
- Monitor neurologic status. Report seizures, hallucinations, or depression.

S

Storage

• Store at controlled room temperature of 15° to 30°C (59° to 86°F). Do not refrigerate; protect from light.

Contraindications and precautions

Contraindicated in hypersensitivity to sulfonamides, trimethoprim, sulfonylureas, thiazides, or loop diuretics; porphyria; marked renal or hepatic impairment; megaloblastic anemia caused by folate deficiency; pregnant women at term or when possibility of premature birth exists; and ***infants younger than 2 months.***

Use cautiously in urinary obstruction, renal or hepatic disease, bronchial asthma, glucose-6-phosphate dehydrogenase deficiency, group A beta-hemolytic streptococcal infection, blood dyscrasias, history of multiple allergies, ***elderly patients,*** pregnant or breastfeeding patients, and ***children.***

Adverse reactions

CNS: headache, depression, hallucinations, insomnia, drowsiness, vertigo, fatigue, apathy, anxiety, ataxia, polyneuritis, peripheral neuropathy, **seizures**

CV: allergic myocarditis or pericarditis

EENT: periorbital edema, optic neuritis, transient myopia, tinnitus

GI: nausea, vomiting, abdominal pain, stomatitis, glossitis, dry mouth, anorexia, pancreatitis, **pseudomembranous colitis**

GU: hematuria, proteinuria, crystalluria, **toxic nephrosis with oliguria and anuria, renal failure**

Hematologic: megaloblastic anemia, agranulocytosis, aplastic anemia, thrombocytopenia, leukopenia, hemolytic anemia

Hepatic: jaundice, **hepatitis, hepatocellular necrosis**

Respiratory: shortness of breath, pleuritis, **allergic pneumonitis, pulmonary infiltrates, fibrosing alveolitis**

Skin: generalized skin eruption, urticaria, pruritus, alopecia, local irritation, exfoliative dermatitis, photosensitivity reaction, **epidermal necrolysis, erythema multiforme, Stevens-Johnson syndrome**

Other: irritation at I.V. site, chills, drug fever, hypersensitivity reactions including **anaphylaxis, serum sickness, lupus-like syndrome**

Interactions

Drug-drug. *Cyclosporine:* increased nephrotoxicity

Dapsone: increased blood levels of both drugs

Hydantoins, zidovudine: increased blood levels of these drugs

Indomethacin, probenecid: increased sulfamethoxazole blood level

Methotrexate: increased risk of bone marrow suppression

Oral anticoagulants: increased anticoagulant effect

PABA, PABA-derived local anesthetics: inhibited sulfamethoxazole action

Sulfonylureas: increased risk of hypoglycemia

Thiazide diuretics: increased thrombocytopenic effects

Uricosuric drugs: increased uricosuric effects

Drug-diagnostic tests. *Bilirubin, blood urea nitrogen, creatinine, eosinophils, transaminases:* increased

Granulocytes, hemoglobin, platelets, white blood cells: decreased

Urine glucose test: false-positive result

Drug-herb. *Dong quai, St. John's wort:* increased risk of photosensitivity

Drug-behaviors. *Sun exposure:* increased risk of photosensitivity

Toxicity and overdose

- Overdose signs and symptoms include anorexia, nausea, vomiting, dizziness, headache, drowsiness, pyrexia, hematuria, crystalluria, depression, confusion, unconsciousness, blood dyscrasias, and jaundice. High doses or prolonged use also may cause bone marrow depression manifested by megaloblastic anemia, thrombocytopenia, or leukopenia.
- Provide supportive therapy as ordered, including I.V. fluids if urine output is low, and urine acidification to increase renal elimination of drug. Closely monitor renal function tests, CBC with differential, and blood chemistries (including electrolytes). Peritoneal dialysis is ineffective in removing drug, but hemodialysis is moderately effective in removing both components.

Patient teaching

Teach patient to recognize and immediately report signs and symptoms of hypersensitivity reaction, especially rash.

Inform patient that drug can cause blood disorders, GI and liver problems, serious skin reactions, and other infections. Instruct patient to immediately report key warning signs and symptoms, such as easy bruising or bleeding, severe diarrhea, unusual tiredness, yellowing of skin or eyes, sore throat, rash, cough, mouth sores, and fever.

- Urge patient to promptly report scant or bloody urine or inability to urinate.
- Tell patient to contact prescriber if depression occurs.
- Teach patient effective ways to counteract photosensitivity effect. Advise patient not to take dong quai or St. John's wort during therapy because these herbs increase phototoxicity risk.
- Advise female patient to inform prescriber if she is pregnant. Tell her not to take drug near term.
- Caution female patient not to breastfeed, because she could pass drug effects to infant.
- As appropriate, review all other significant and life-threatening adverse reactions and interactions, especially those related to the drugs, tests, herbs, and behaviors mentioned above.

tacrolimus

Prograf

Pharmacologic class: Macrolide
Therapeutic class: Immunosuppressant
Pregnancy risk category C

FDA BOXED WARNING

- Immunosuppression caused by drug may increase patient's susceptibility to infection and lymphoma development. Give under supervision of physician experienced in immunosuppressive therapy and management of organ transplant patients, in facility with adequate diagnostic and treatment resources. Physician responsible for maintenance therapy should have complete information needed for patient follow-up.

Action

Unclear. Thought to inhibit T-lymphocyte activation.

Pharmacokinetics

Distribution between whole blood and plasma depends on such factors as hematocrit, temperature at time of plasma separation, drug concentration, and plasma-protein concentration. Drug is extensively metabolized by mixed-function oxidase system (primarily CYP450 system). Metabolic pathway leading to formation of eight possible metabolites has been proposed; major metabolite may have same activity as parent drug. Plasma-protein binding is approximately 99%. Less than 1% of dose is excreted unchanged in urine.

Onset	Peak	Duration
Rapid	1-2 hr	Unknown

How supplied

Solution for injection: 5 mg/mL in 1-mL ampules

Indications and dosages

➢ Prevention of organ rejection in patients with allogeneic liver transplants
Adults and children: 0.03 to 0.05 mg/kg/day by continuous I.V. infusion
➢ Prevention of organ rejection in patients with allogeneic kidney transplants
Adults: 0.03 to 0.05 mg/kg/day by continuous I.V. infusion

Dosage adjustment

- For all adults and patients with hepatic or renal impairment, use dosage at lower end of recommended range.
- Know that children need higher doses than adults to achieve similar drug trough levels.
- Be aware that black patients undergoing kidney transplants may require higher dosages to achieve desirable blood concentrations.

Administration

Preparation

Follow hazardous drug guidelines on page S19 for handling, preparation, and administration.

Before giving I.V., ensure that epinephrine 1:1,000 and oxygen are at hand in case of emergency.

- Start therapy within 24 hours of kidney transplantation and no earlier than 6 hours after liver transplantation. Switch to oral dosing as soon as tolerable, starting 8 to 12 hours after I.V. dosing ends.

Dilution and compatibility

Dilute with normal saline solution or D_5W to a concentration between 0.004 and 0.02 mg/mL.

Do not mix or co-infuse with alkaline solutions of pH 9 or greater (such as those containing ganciclovir or acyclovir).

Infusion considerations

- Administer single dose over 24 hours or as prescribed. Use infusion pump to control rate.

Do not administer simultaneously with cyclosporine. Discontinue either tacrolimus or cyclosporine 24 hours before administering other drug.

Monitoring

Once I.V. infusion starts, watch closely for signs and symptoms of anaphylaxis.

Monitor blood drug levels. If tacrolimus or cyclosporine blood concentration is elevated, delay dosing with other drug.

- Monitor liver and kidney function test results. Watch for signs and symptoms of nephrotoxicity and hepatic dysfunction.
- Assess neurologic status for evidence of neurotoxicity.
- Monitor potassium level closely. Stay alert for signs and symptoms of hyperkalemia.

Monitor blood glucose level closely. Watch for indications of hyperglycemia; be aware that Black and Hispanic kidney-transplant patients are at increased risk for type 1 posttransplant diabetes mellitus (PTDM).

- Evaluate respiratory status regularly.

Storage

• Store at controlled room temperature before dilution.

• Store diluted infusion in glass or polyethylene container; discard after 24 hours. Do not store diluted infusion in polyvinyl chloride container, due to decreased stability and potential extraction of phthalates.

Contraindications and precautions

Contraindicated in hypersensitivity to drug or its components (including castor oil derivatives).

Use cautiously in severe hepatic disease, renal impairment, diabetes mellitus, hypertension, hyperkalemia, hyperuricemia, lymphoma, pregnant or breastfeeding patients, and ***children younger than age 12.***

Adverse reactions

CNS: tremor, headache, insomnia, paresthesia, delirium, asthenia, **coma**
CV: hypertension, peripheral edema
GI: nausea, vomiting, diarrhea, constipation, abdominal pain, ascites, anorexia
GU: hematuria, proteinuria, urinary tract infection, albuminuria, abnormal renal function, **oliguria, renal failure**
Hematologic: anemia, **leukocytosis, thrombocytopenia**
Metabolic: hyperglycemia, type 1 PTDM, hypomagnesemia, hypokalemia, **hyperkalemia**
Musculoskeletal: back pain
Respiratory: dyspnea, **pleural effusion, atelectasis**
Skin: rash, flushing, pruritus, alopecia, pruritus
Other: pain, fever, chills, **anaphylaxis**

Interactions

Drug-drug. *Bromocriptine, chloramphenicol, cimetidine, clarithromycin, clotrimazole, cyclosporine, danazol, diltiazem, erythromycin, fluconazole, itraconazole, ketoconazole, methylprednisolone, metoclopramide, metronidazole, nicardipine, omeprazole, protease inhibitors, verapamil:* increased tacrolimus blood level
Cyclosporine: increased risk of nephrotoxicity
CYP450 inducers (such as carbamazepine, phenobarbital, phenytoin, rifampin): decreased tacrolimus metabolism
Immunosuppressants (except adrenocorticoids): immunologic oversuppression
Live-virus vaccines: interference with immune response to vaccine
Mycophenolate mofetil: increased mycophenolate blood level
Nephrotoxic drugs (such as aminoglycosides, amphotericin B, cisplatin, cyclosporine): additive or synergistic effects
Drug-diagnostic tests. *Blood urea nitrogen, creatinine, glucose:* increased
Hemoglobin, magnesium, platelets, white blood cells: decreased
Liver function tests: abnormal values
Potassium: increased or decreased
Drug-herb. *Astragalus, echinacea, melatonin:* decreased immunosuppression
St. John's wort: decreased tacrolimus blood level

Toxicity and overdose

• Inadvertent overdoses have not caused untoward effects. However, expect extension of pharmacologic effects and adverse reactions.

• Provide symptomatic and supportive therapy. Drug is not significantly dialyzable.

Patient teaching

Teach patient to recognize and immediately report serious adverse reactions.

• Tell diabetic patient to expect increased blood glucose level, which may warrant further antidiabetic therapy.

Advise patient to monitor glucose level carefully.

- As appropriate, review all other significant and life-threatening adverse reactions and interactions, especially those related to the drugs, tests, and herbs mentioned above.

tenecteplase

Metalyse, TNKase

Pharmacologic class: Tissue plasminogen activator

Therapeutic class: Thrombolytic enzyme

Pregnancy risk category C

Action

Binds to fibrin and converts plasminogen to plasmin, which breaks down fibrin clots and lyses thrombi and emboli. Causes systemic fibrinolysis.

Pharmacokinetics

Drug has biphasic disposition from plasma. It clears plasma with an initial half-life of 20 to 24 minutes; terminal-phase half-life is 90 to 130 minutes. Initial volume of distribution is weight-related and approximates plasma volume. Drug is eliminated primarily by hepatic metabolism.

Onset	Peak	Duration
Immediate	Unknown	Unknown

How supplied

Powder for reconstitution for injection: 50 mg/vial with 10-mL syringe, TwinPak Dual Cannula Device, and 10-mL vial of sterile water for injection

Indications and dosages

➢ To reduce mortality associated with acute myocardial infarction

Adults weighing 90 kg (198 lb) or more: 50 mg I.V. bolus given over 5 seconds

Adults weighing 80 kg to 89 kg (176 to 197 lb): 45 mg I.V. bolus given over 5 seconds

Adults weighing 70 kg to 79 kg (154 to 175 lb): 40 mg I.V. bolus given over 5 seconds

Adults weighing 60 to 69 kg (132 to 153 lb): 35 mg I.V. bolus given over 5 seconds

Adults weighing less than 60 kg: 30 mg I.V. bolus given over 5 seconds

Administration

Dilution and compatibility

- Reconstitute by using supplied syringe to mix vial contents with 10 mL sterile water for injection. Swirl gently; do not shake. Let drug stand a few minutes. Draw up prescribed dosage from vial, then discard remainder.
- Do not use bacteriostatic water for injection.
- Know that reconstituted solution should be colorless to pale yellow.
- Use immediately after reconstitution, or refrigerate for up to 8 hours.

Infusion considerations

- Administer I.V. over 5 seconds through designated line. Flush I.V.
- Give with heparin if prescribed, but not through same I.V. line.

Do not deliver in same I.V. line with dextrose solutions. If patient has been receiving dextrose, flush I.V. line with normal saline solution before giving drug.

Monitoring

Closely monitor ECG. Stay alert for reperfusion arrhythmias.

Monitor vital signs carefully. Watch for signs and symptoms of respiratory depression and reinfarction.

Evaluate all body systems closely for signs and symptoms of bleeding. If bleeding occurs, stop drug and give antiplatelet agents, as prescribed.
• Monitor coagulation studies and CBC. However, know that drug may skew coagulation results.

Storage

• Store powder at controlled room temperature not exceeding 30°C (86°F), or refrigerate at 2° to 8°C (36° to 46°F).

Contraindications and precautions

Contraindicated in hypersensitivity to drug or other tissue plasminogen activators, active internal bleeding, bleeding diathesis, recent intracranial or intraspinal surgery or trauma, severe uncontrolled hypertension, intracranial neoplasm, arteriovenous malformation or aneurysm, or history of cerebrovascular accident (CVA).

Use cautiously in previous puncture of noncompressible vessels, organ biopsy, hypertension, acute pericarditis, high risk of left ventricular thrombosis, subacute bacterial endocarditis, hemostatic defects, diabetic hemorrhagic retinopathy, septic thrombophlebitis, obstetric delivery, patients taking warfarin concurrently, ***patients older than age 75,*** and pregnant or breastfeeding patients.

Adverse reactions

CNS: intracranial hemorrhage, CVA
CV: hypotension, **arrhythmia, myocardial rupture, myocardial reinfarction, cardiogenic shock, atrioventricular block, cardiac arrest, cardiac tamponade, heart failure, pericarditis, pericardial effusion, mitral regurgitation, thrombosis, embolism**
EENT: epistaxis, minor pharyngeal bleeding
GI: nausea, vomiting, **GI hemorrhage**
GU: hematuria
Hematologic: anemia, **bleeding tendency**
Respiratory: respiratory depression, pulmonary edema, apnea
Skin: bleeding at puncture sites, hematoma

Interactions

Drug-drug. *Anticoagulants, aspirin, dipyridamole, indomethacin, phenylbutazone:* increased bleeding risk
Drug-diagnostic tests. *Coagulation tests:* fibrinogen degradation in blood sample

Toxicity and overdose

• In overdose, expect bleeding and possibly hypotension, bradycardia, and arrhythmias.
• Withhold drug and obtain prothrombin time, partial thromboplastin time, CBC with white cell differential, platelet count, fibrinogen, and blood for typing and crossmatching. Administer whole blood, packed red blood cells, fresh frozen plasma, desmopressin, or aminocaproic, as needed and prescribed. For hypotension, use positioning and possibly vasopressors; for bradycardia, atropine; for reperfusion arrhythmias, procainamide or other standard antiarrhythmics, as prescribed.

Patient teaching

Inform patient that drug increases risk of bleeding. Advise patient to immediately report signs and symptoms of bleeding.
• Teach patient safety measures to avoid bruising and bleeding.
• Tell patient about the need for regular blood tests during therapy.
• As appropriate, review all other significant and life-threatening adverse reactions and interactions, especially those related to the drugs and tests mentioned above.

T

thiamine hydrochloride

Pharmacologic class: Vitamin B_1
Therapeutic class: Nutritional supplement
Pregnancy risk category A

Action

Water-soluble vitamin; combines with adenosine triphosphate and thiamine diphosphokinase to form thiamine pyrophosphate, a coenzyme essential for normal growth and aerobic metabolism, nerve impulse transmission, and acetylcholine synthesis.

Pharmacokinetics

Drug distributes to all tissues. Concentration is highest in the liver, but some drug is stored in the brain, kidneys, intestine, lung, spleen, muscle, and heart. Metabolism is rapid; excess is excreted in urine.

Onset	Peak	Duration
Unknown	Unknown	Unknown

How supplied

Solution for injection (clear): 100 mg/mL in syringes and vials

Indications and dosages

➢ Wernicke's encephalopathy
Adults: Initially, 100 mg I.V., followed by I.M. dosing until patient can consume a regular balanced diet

➢ Prevention of thiamine deficiency in patients receiving total parenteral nutrition (TPN)
Adults: 3 mg I.V. daily admixed with TPN

➢ Beriberi
Adults: 5 to 30 mg I.V. daily or in three divided doses daily for up to 2 weeks

➢ Infantile beriberi
Infants: If infantile beriberi does not respond to oral therapy and collapse occurs, 25 mg I.V. daily, as needed and administered cautiously

Administration

Preparation

• Know that parenteral administration is indicated when oral route is not feasible (as in anorexia, nausea, vomiting, or preoperative and postoperative conditions) or GI absorption is impaired (as in malabsorption syndrome).

Be aware that intradermal test dose is recommended in patients with suspected sensitivity to drug.

Assess for additional vitamin deficiences, because vitamin B_1 deficiency rarely occurs alone.

• Correct poor dietary habits or other underlying conditions (such as alcoholism, anorexia nervosa), as ordered, and provide adequate, well-balanced diet.

Dilution and compatibility

• Drug may be given undiluted by I.V. injection or added to most commonly used I.V. solutions for infusion or TPN.
• Do not mix with alkaline solutions (such as barbiturates or carbonates) or solutions containing sulfites.
• Use solution only if clear.

Infusion considerations

• Administer by direct I.V. injection as 100 mg or fraction thereof over 5 minutes.
• Give by I.V. infusion over prescribed time.

Know that thiamine-deficient patients may experience sudden onset or worsening of Wernicke's encephalopathy after glucose administration. Administer thiamine before or with glucose-containing fluids.

Monitoring

Watch for hypersensitivity reactions; be prepared to intervene appropriately.

Storage

- Store at controlled room temperature of 15° to 30°C (59° to 86°F); protect from light. Keep in carton until use.

Contraindications and precautions

Contraindicated in hypersensitivity to drug or its components.

Use cautiously in pregnant or breast-feeding patients.

Adverse reactions

CNS: weakness, restlessness
CV: cyanosis, **cardiovascular collapse**
GI: nausea, **GI hemorrhage**
Respiratory: pulmonary edema
Skin: pruritus, urticaria
Other: sensation of warmth, sweating, hypersensitivity reactions including tightness of throat, angioneurotic edema, **anaphylaxis, shock, and death**

Interactions

None significant

Toxicity and overdose

- Parenteral doses of 100 to 500 mg (single or repeated) have been given without toxic effects. However, dosages exceeding 30 mg three times daily are not used effectively by the body. When body tissues become saturated with thiamine, drug is excreted in urine as pyrimidine; as thiamine intake increases further, it appears unchanged in urine in amounts exceeding 100 mcg/24 hours.
- Withdraw drug and provide supportive therapy.

Patient teaching

- Teach patient about proper dietary habits to help prevent relapse after dosage reduction or cessation of injection therapy.
- As appropriate, review all other significant and life-threatening adverse reactions.

[redacted]

thiopental sodium

Pentothal

Pharmacologic class: Barbiturate
Therapeutic class: Anesthetic
Controlled substance schedule III
Pregnancy risk category C

Action

Inhibits ascending nerve impulse transmission in reticular formation and depresses CNS; may enhance or mimic inhibitory action of gamma-aminobutyric acid, causing sedation, hypnosis, and anticonvulsant effect. Increases cerebrovascular resistance, which reduces intracranial pressure (ICP).

Pharmacokinetics

Distribution and fate are influenced mainly by drug's lipid solubility, protein binding, and extent of ionization. Spinal fluid level is slightly lower than plasma level. Drug is degraded largely in the liver and to a smaller extent in other tissues (especially kidney and brain). Approximately 80% is bound to plasma proteins. Biotransformation products are pharmacologically inactive and excreted mostly in urine. Elimination half-life is 3 to 8 hours.

Onset	Peak	Duration
10-40 sec	Unknown	10-30 min

How supplied

Powder for reconstitution for injection: 2% (400 mg), 2.5% (500 mg) in Thiopental Kits, Thiopental Ready-to-Mix Syringes, and vials with diluent

Indications and dosages

➤ Slow induction and maintenance of anesthesia

Adults: 50 to 75 mg I.V. given slowly at 20- to 40-second intervals, based on response. May give additional doses of 25 to 50 mg I.V. p.r.n.

➢ Rapid induction and maintenance of anesthesia before other general anesthestics are given

Adults: 210 to 280 mg (3 to 4 mg/kg) I.V. in two to four divided doses

➢ Maintenance of anesthesia without other general anesthetics for short procedures

Adults: 0.2% or 0.4% solution by intermittent I.V. injection or continuous I.V. infusion

➢ Seizures associated with anesthesia or other causes in mechanically ventilated patients

Adults: 75 to 125 mg I.V. infusion as soon as possible after seizure onset

➢ Increased ICP

Adults: 1.5 to 3.5 mg/kg intermittent I.V. infusion

➢ To promote narcoanalysis or narcosynthesis in psychiatric patients

Adults: Test dose of 25 to 75 mg after anticholinergic administration (with dosage based on patient's age, sex, and weight). Give by slow I.V. injection at 100 mg/minute with patient counting backwards from 100. Just after patient becomes confused with counting but before he falls asleep, discontinue drug; this allows patient to return to semidrowsy state in which conversation is coherent.

Administration

Preparation

Know that drug should be given by healthcare professionals qualified in use of I.V. anesthetics. Keep resuscitative equipment on hand.

- Give test dose of 25 to 75 mg I.V. as prescribed; assess tolerance and monitor for hypersensitivity reaction for 1 minute.
- Premedicate patient with atropine or scopolamine to suppress vagal reflexes and inhibit secretions, as prescribed. Barbiturate or opioid also may be given.

Dilution and compatibility

- Reconstitute drug according to manufacturer's directions.
- Know that diluent choice and volume depend on concentration and vehicle desired. Thiopental Kits provide only sterile water for injection as diluent for individual or multipatient use; Thiopental Ready-to-Mix Syringes provide only normal saline solution for injection; vials provide only sterile water for injection.
- Do not mix with solutions of succinylcholine, tubocurarine, or other drugs with acidic pH. Thiopental solution is most stable when reconstituted in sterile water for injection or normal saline solution for injection, kept under refrigeration, and tightly stoppered.
- Use only freshly prepared, clear solutions.
- Discard unused portion after 24 hours.

Infusion considerations

- Administer I.V. injection over 20 to 30 seconds or by continuous I.V. infusion using infusion pump.
- Know that when drug is used as sole anesthetic, desired anesthesia level can be maintained by injecting small repeated doses as needed or by using continuous I.V. drip with 0.2% or 0.4% concentration. Do not use sterile water for injection as diluent in these concentrations, as hemolysis will occur. With continuous drip, anesthesia depth is controlled by adjusting infusion rate.
- Avoid extravasation to prevent severe tissue reaction (necrosis, sloughing). If extravasation occurs, stop infusion immediately, contact prescriber, apply moist heat, and inject 1% procaine hydrochloride, as prescribed.

Monitoring
- Monitor vital signs and ECG carefully.

Closely monitor respiratory status, particularly for respiratory depression.

Assess patient carefully to detect early signs and symptoms of shock; stop drug and contact prescriber immediately if these occur.
- Monitor neurologic status; institute safety measures if seizures, agitation, or anxiety occurs.
- Continue to assess injection site closely and frequently to prevent extravasation and detect thrombophlebitis.

Storage
- Do not store reconstituted solutions.

Contraindications and precautions

Contraindicated in hypersensitivity to drug, its components, or other barbiturates; hepatic or renal impairment; and porphyria.

Use cautiously in severe cardiovascular disease, hypotension, shock, status asthmaticus, Addison's disease, myxedema, myasthenia gravis, increased blood urea concentration, severe anemia, ***elderly patients,*** pregnant or breastfeeding patients, and ***children.***

Adverse reactions

CNS: anxiety, agitation, prolonged drowsiness, confusion, amnesia, headache, myoclonus, postoperative shivering
CV: bradycardia, tachycardia
Musculoskeletal: twitching
Respiratory: wheezing, cough, **laryngospasm, apnea, respiratory depression**
Skin: rash, hives
Other: pain, venous thrombosis, phlebitis, and thrombophlebitis at I.V. site; hiccups; hypersensitivity reaction

Interactions

Drug-drug. *Aminophylline (low-dose I.V. use):* partial reversal of sedation during early recovery phase
Clonidine, metoclopramide: enhanced thiopental effects
CNS depressants: additive CNS depression
Highly protein-bound drugs (such as diazoxide): hypotension
Protein-bound drugs (such as aspirin, meprobamate, probenecid, sulfisoxazole): potentiation of thiopental's hypnotic effects
Drug-herb. *Valerian:* increased sedation
Drug-behaviors. *Alcohol use:* additive CNS depression
Chronic alcohol use: decreased thiopental efficacy, necessitating dosage increase

Toxicity and overdose

- Overdose may result from too-rapid or repeated injections. Apnea, occasional laryngospasm, coughing, and other respiratory problems may follow excessive dosage or too-rapid injection. Too-rapid injection may cause steep blood pressure drop, even to shock levels. Lethal blood levels may be as low as 1 mg/ 100 mL for short-acting barbiturates; lower if another depressant drug or alcohol is also present.
- Discontinue drug, establish or maintain patent airway, and administer oxygen with assisted ventilation if necessary and ordered. Respiratory depression or arrest caused by overdose or unusual drug sensitivity is easily managed in patient without concomitant respiratory obstruction. If airway is patent, any method of ventilating lungs and preventing hypoxia should effectively maintain other vital functions. Observe respirations closely, as respiratory depression is a characteristic drug effect. If laryngeal spasm occurs, expect to give relaxant drug or positive-pressure oxygen. Endotracheal intubation may be indicated in difficult cases. Administer vasopressors to maintain blood pressure, as indicated and prescribed.

T

Patient teaching

- Explain why drug is being used; reassure patient he will be closely monitored.

ticarcillin disodium and clavulanate potassium/ clavulanic acid

Timentin

Pharmacologic class: Penicillin (extended-spectrum)

Therapeutic class: Anti-infective

Pregnancy risk category B

Action

Ticarcillin inhibits cell-wall synthesis during microorganism replication; clavulanic acid extends ticarcillin's antibiotic spectrum by inactivating beta-lactamase enzymes (which otherwise would degrade ticarcillin).

Pharmacokinetics

Drug distributes widely into most body tissues, but minimally penetrates cerebrospinal fluid (CSF). Neither component is highly protein-bound (ticarcillin, approximately 45%; clavulanic acid, 25%). Roughly 13% of ticarcillin undergoes metabolism; clavulanic acid may be extensively metabolized. Elimination half-life of both components is about 1 hour, but lengthens in severe renal failure. Both components are excreted primarily in urine, with some excretion in breast milk and bile.

Onset	Peak	Duration
Immediate	Immediate	Unknown

How supplied

Powder for reconstitution for injection (white to pale yellow): 3 g ticarcillin and 100 mg clavulanic acid in 3.1-g vials

Indications and dosages

➢ Systemic and urinary tract infections caused by susceptible organisms, including beta-lactamase-producing strains of *Escherichia coli, Klebsiella* species, *Pseudomonas aeruginosa* (or other *Pseudomonas* species), *Citrobacter* species, *Enterobacter cloacae, Serratia marcescens, Bacteroides* species, and *Staphylococcus aureus*

Adults weighing more than 60 kg (132 lb): 3.1-g (30:1 fixed-ratio combination of 3 g ticarcillin and 100 mg clavulanic acid) I.V. infusion q 4 to 6 hours

Adults weighing less than 60 kg: 200 to 300 mg/kg/day (based on ticarcillin content) by I.V. infusion in divided doses q 4 to 6 hours

➢ Gynecologic infections caused by susceptible organisms, including beta-lactamase-producing strains of *Prevotella melaninogenica, Enterobacter* species (including *E. cloacae*), *E. coli, Klebsiella pneumoniae, S. aureus,* and *Staphylococcus epidermidis*

Adults weighing more than 60 kg (132 lb): For moderate infections, 200 mg/kg/day (based on ticarcillin content) I.V. infusion in divided doses q 6 hours. For severe infections, 300 mg/kg/day (based on ticarcillin content) I.V. infusion in divided doses q 4 hours.

Adults weighing less than 60 kg: 200 to 300 mg/kg/day I.V. infusion q 4 to 6 hours

➢ Mild to moderate or severe infections in children caused by susceptible organisms, including beta-lactamase-producing strains of *E. coli, Klebsiella* species, *P. aeruginosa* (or other *Pseudomonas* species), *Citrobacter* species, *E. cloacae, S. marcescens, Bacteroides* species, and *S. aureus*

Children weighing more than 60 kg (132 lb): For mild to moderate infections, 3.1-g (30:1 fixed-ratio combination of 3 g ticarcillin and 100 mg clavulanic acid) I.V. infusion q 6 hours. For severe infections, 3.1-g (30:1 fixed-ratio combination of 3 g ticarcillin and 100 mg clavulanic acid) I.V. infusion q 4 hours.
Children ages 3 months to 16 years weighing less than 60 kg: For mild to moderate infections, 200 mg/kg/day (based on ticarcillin content) I.V. infusion in divided doses q 6 hours. For severe infections, 300 mg/kg/day (based on ticarcillin content) I.V. infusion in divided doses q 4 hours.

Dosage adjustment

• Adjust dosage in severe renal impairment, as shown in the table below:

CrCl (mL/min)	Dosage
Greater than 60	3.1 g q 4 hr
30 to 60	2 g q 4 hr
10 to 30	2 g q 8 hr
Less than 10	2 g q 12 hr
Less than 10, with hepatic dysfunction	2 g q 24 hr
Patients on peritoneal dialysis	3.1 g q 12 hr
Patients on hemodialysis	2 g q 12 hr, supplemented with 3.1 g after each dialysis session

Administration

Preparation
• Ask patient about penicillin allergy before giving.
Dilution and compatibility
• Add 13 mL sterile water or normal saline solution for injection to vial; shake gently.
• Dilute further with 50 to 100 mL of normal saline solution, D_5W, or lactated Ringer's solution, as prescribed.
• Know that reconstituted solution should be clear, colorless, or pale yellow.
• Do not mix with sodium bicarbonate.
Infusion considerations
• Infuse I.V. over 30 minutes.
• If infusing through Y-type administration set, temporarily discontinue other solutions.
• Give at least 1 hour before I.V. aminoglycosides (such as amikacin or gentamicin).
Monitoring
Closely monitor for severe allergic reactions.
• Monitor liver function tests and CBC with white cell differential.
• Watch for signs and symptoms of superinfection.
• Assess neurologic status; stay alert for seizures.
• Monitor I.V. site closely for thrombophlebitis.
Storage
• Store 200-mg/mL solution at controlled room temperature of 21° to 23°C (70° to 74°F) for up to 6 hours, or refrigerate at 4°C (40°F) for up to 72 hours.
• If further diluted to 10 to 100 mg/mL with normal saline solution, D_5W, or lactated Ringer's solution, solution may be stored for 24 hours at controlled room temperature. If further diluted with normal saline solution or lactated Ringer's solution, it may be refrigerated for up to 3 days; if further diluted with D_5W, it may be refrigerated for up to 7 days.

Contraindications and precautions

Contraindicated in hypersensitivity to drug or other penicillins.

Use cautiously in cystic fibrosis, renal or hepatic disease, and pregnant or breastfeeding patients.

T

Adverse reactions

CNS: headache, giddiness, dizziness, lethargy, fatigue, hyperreflexia, neuromuscular excitability, asterixis, hallucinations, stupor, **seizures**
GI: nausea, vomiting, diarrhea, flatulence, **pseudomembranous colitis**
Hematologic: eosinophilia, transient **neutropenia** and **leukopenia** (with high doses)
Skin: urticaria, rash
Other: unpleasant taste; fever; overgrowth of nonsusceptible organisms; pain, vein irritation, erythema, phlebitis, and **thrombophlebitis** at I.V. site; hypersensitivity reactions including **anaphylaxis**

Interactions

Drug-drug. *Aminoglycosides:* physical incompatibility, causing aminoglycoside inactivation when mixed in same I.V. solution
Aminoglycosides, tetracyclines: additive activity against some bacteria
Lithium: altered lithium elimination
Probenecid: increased ticarcillin blood level
Drug-diagnostic tests. *Alanine aminotransferase, alkaline phosphatase, aspartate aminotransferase, eosinophils, lactate dehydrogenase, sodium:* increased
Bleeding time: prolonged
Granulocytes, hemoglobin, platelets, white blood cells: decreased
Liver function test results: transient increases
Urine glucose, urine protein: false-positive results

Toxicity and overdose

• High doses may lead to neurotoxic reactions, especially in impaired renal function. If CSF drug level is high, neurologic adverse reactions (including neuromuscular hyperexcitability or seizures) may develop. Other effects of toxicity may include agitation, confusion, asterixis, hallucinations, stupor, encephalopathy, hyperkalemia, and coma.
• Discontinue drug, provide symptomatic therapy, and institute supportive measures as indicated and ordered. Hemodialysis removes both ticarcillin and clavulanic acid; peritoneal dialysis removes only slight amounts.

Patient teaching

Advise patient to report skin reactions and severe diarrhea right away.
Tell patient drug may increase risk of other infections. Advise patient to promptly report signs and symptoms of new infection.
• Instruct patient to limit sodium intake (drug contains sodium).
• As appropriate, review all other significant and life-threatening adverse reactions and interactions, especially those related to the drugs and tests mentioned above.

tigecycline

Tygacil

Pharmacologic class: Glycylcycline antibiotic
Therapeutic class: Anti-infective
Pregnancy risk category D

Action

Inhibits protein translation in bacteria by binding to 30S ribosomal subunit and blocking entry of amino-acyl tRNA molecules into ribosomal A site, which in turn prevents incorporation of amino acid residues into elongating peptide chains

Pharmacokinetics

Drug distributes extensively beyond plasma volume and into tissues. It is not extensively metabolized; 71% to 89% is protein-bound. Overall, primary elimination route is biliary excretion of unchanged drug and its metabolites; approximately 22% of dose is excreted unchanged in urine. Glucuronidation and renal excretion of unchanged drug are secondary elimination routes. About 59% of dose is eliminated by biliary-fecal excretion and 33% is excreted in urine.

Onset	Peak	Duration
Unknown	Unknown	Unknown

How supplied

Powder for reconstitution for injection (lyophilized): 50 mg/5 mL in single-dose vial

Indications and dosages

➢ Skin and skin-structure infections caused by susceptible strains of *Escherichia coli*, *Enterococcus faecalis* (vancomycin-susceptible isolates only), *Staphylococcus aureus* (methicillin-susceptible and -resistant isolates), *Streptococcus agalactiae*, *Streptococcus anginosus* group, *Streptococcus pyogenes*, and *Bacteroides fragilis;* complicated intra-abdominal infections caused by *Citrobacter freundii*, *E. coli*, *Enterobacter cloacae*, *E. faecalis* (vancomycin-susceptible isolates only), *Klebsiella oxytoca*, *Klebsiella pneumoniae*, *S. aureus* (methicillin-susceptible isolates only), *S. anginosus* group, *S. pyogenes*, *B. fragilis*, *Bacteroides thetaiotaomicron*, *Bacteroides uniformis*, *Bacteroides vulgatus*, *Clostridium perfringens*, and *Peptostreptococcus micros*

Adults age 18 and older: Initially, 100 mg I.V., followed by 50 mg I.V. q 12 hours for 5 to 14 days, depending on infection site and severity and patient's clinical and bacteriologic process

Dosage adjustment

• In severe hepatic impairment, administer 100 mg initially, then give maintenance dosage of 25 mg q 12 hours.

Administration

Dilution and compatibility

• Reconstitute with 5.3 mL normal saline solution for injection or 5% dextrose injection to yield a concentration of 10 mg/mL (50 mg).

• Swirl vial gently until drug dissolves. Immediately withdraw 5 mL of reconstituted solution from vial and add to 100-mL I.V. bag of D_5W or normal saline solution for infusion. Maximum concentration in I.V. bag should be 1 mg/mL.

• Discard reconstituted solution that is not yellow or orange.

Infusion considerations

• Administer through dedicated I.V. line or Y-site. If same I.V. line is used for sequential infusion of several drugs, flush before and after infusion, using either normal saline solution or 5% dextrose injection. Use infusion solution compatible with tigecycline and other drugs given through same line.

• Do not give amphotericin B, chlorpromazine, methylprednisolone, or voriconazole simultaneously through same Y-site.

• Administer over 30 to 60 minutes.

Monitoring

• Monitor prothrombin time or other suitable anticoagulation tests if patient is receiving warfarin concomitantly.

• Closely monitor patient with severe hepatic impairment.

Storage

• Before reconstitution, store at 20° to 25°C (68° to 77°F); excursions permitted from 15° to 30°C (59° to 86°F).

T

• Know that reconstituted solution may be stored in I.V. bag at room temperature for up to 6 hours, or refrigerated at 2° to 8°C (36° to 46°F) for up to 24 hours.

Contraindications and precautions

Contraindicated in hypersensitivity to drug or its components.

Use cautiously in hepatic impairment, complicated intra-abdominal infections secondary to perforation, pregnant and breastfeeding patients, and ***children younger than age 18.***

Adverse reactions

CNS: headache, dizziness, insomnia, asthenia
CV: hypertension, hypotension, phlebitis
GI: nausea, vomiting, diarrhea, constipation, abdominal pain, dyspepsia, increased GI enzymes, **pseudomembranous colitis**
Hematologic: anemia, leukocytosis, thrombocytopenia
Musculoskeletal: back pain
Respiratory: increased cough, dyspnea
Skin: pruritus, rash, sweating, photosensitivity
Other: abscess, fever, infection, pain, peripheral edema, abnormal healing, superinfection, allergic reaction

Interactions

Drug-drug. *Hormonal contraceptives:* reduced contraceptive efficacy
Drug-diagnostic tests. *Alanine aminotransferase, alkaline phosphatase, amylase, aspartate aminotransferase, bilirubin, blood glucose, blood urea nitrogen:* increased
Blood protein, potassium, white blood cells: decreased

Toxicity and overdose

• In overdose, expect increased nausea and vomiting and possibly other adverse reactions.
• Provide supportive therapy. Hemodialysis does not remove significant amounts of drug.

Patient teaching

• Instruct patient to report rash and other signs or symptoms of allergic reaction.
• Advise patient taking oral hormonal contraceptives to use alternative birth control method during therapy.
• Caution female with childbearing potential to avoid pregnancy, as drug may harm fetus.
• As appropriate, review all other significant and life-threatening adverse reactions and interactions, especially those related to the drugs and tests mentioned above.

tirofiban hydrochloride

Aggrastat

Pharmacologic class: Glycoprotein (GP IIb/IIIa)-receptor inhibitor
Therapeutic class: Platelet aggregation inhibitor
Pregnancy risk category B

Action

Inhibits reversible platelet aggregation by binding to GP IIb/IIIa receptor on platelets

Pharmacokinetics

Drug has limited metabolism; unbound fraction in plasma is 35%. Half-life is approximately 2 hours. It is eliminated largely unchanged by renal excretion, with some excretion in feces.

Onset	Peak	Duration
Immediate	Immediate	4-6 hr

How supplied

Concentrate for dilution for injection (clear, colorless): 250 mcg/mL in 25-mL and 50-mL vials
Solution for injection (clear): 50 mcg/mL in 100-mL and 250-mL premixed plastic containers with normal saline solution injection

Indications and dosages

➣ Acute coronary syndrome (given with heparin); patients undergoing percutaneous transluminal coronary angioplasty (PTCA) or atherectomy
Adults: Loading dose of 0.4 mcg/kg /minute I.V. for 30 minutes, followed by continuous I.V. infusion of 0.1 mcg/kg/ minute for 48 to 108 hours in patients being managed medically. Continue infusion for 12 to 24 hours after PTCA or atherectomy.

Dosage adjustment

- Reduce infusion rate 50% in severe renal insufficiency.

Administration

Dilution and compatibility

Know that drug is available in injection concentrate in vials and in premixed (ready-to-use) plastic containers.

When using drug in vial, first dilute to same strength as premixed drug using one of these methods:

– If using 500-mL bag of normal saline solution or D_5W, withdraw and discard 100 mL from bag and replace this volume with 100 mL tirofiban (from four 25-mL vials or two 50-mL vials).

– If using 250-mL bag of normal saline solution or D_5W, withdraw and discard 50 mL from bag and replace this volume with 50 mL tirofiban (from two 25-mL vials or one 50-mL vial).

– If using 100-mL bag of normal saline solution or D_5W, add contents of 25-mL vial to bag.

Do not add other drugs to plastic bags containing tirofiban.

- Do not use solution unless clear.

Infusion considerations

- For infusion rates in patients without renal insufficiency, use the table below:

Patient weight (kg)	30-min loading infusion rate (mL/hr)	Maintenance infusion rate (mL/hr)
30 to 37	16	4
38 to 45	20	5
46 to 54	24	6
55 to 62	28	7
63 to 70	32	8
71 to 79	36	9
80 to 87	40	10
88 to 95	44	11
96 to 104	48	12
105 to 112	52	13
113 to 120	56	14
121 to 128	60	15
129 to 137	64	16
138 to 145	68	17
146 to 153	72	18

- For patients with renal insufficiency, adjust dose downward as appropriate.

Do not use plastic containers in series connections. Such use could result in air embolism due to residual air being drawn from primary container before administration of fluid from secondary container ends.

T

Do not administer in same I.V. line as diazepam.

Monitoring

Monitor CBC, platelet count, and coagulation studies. Assess stool for occult blood.

- Watch for bleeding at puncture sites, especially at cardiac catheterization access site. Immobilize access site to reduce bleeding risk.

Monitor for signs and symptoms of bleeding in cranium and other body systems (especially respiratory, GI, and GU).

- Monitor vital signs and ECG.

Assess cardiovascular status. Stay alert for signs and symptoms of coronary artery dissection or hemopericardium.

Storage

- Store at 25°C (77°F); excursions permitted from 15° to 30°C (59° to 86°F). Do not freeze. Protect from light.

Contraindications and precautions

Contraindicated in hypersensitivity to drug or its components; active internal bleeding or history of bleeding diathesis within past 30 days; cerebrovascular accident (CVA) within past 30 days or history of hemorrhagic CVA; history of intracranial hemorrhage, intracranial neoplasm, arteriovenous malformation, aneurysm, or thrombocytopenia after previous tirofiban use; history, symptoms, or findings that suggest aortic dissection; major surgery or severe trauma within past 30 days; severe hypertension; concurrent use of other parenteral GP IIb/IIIa inhibitors; and acute pericarditis.

Use cautiously in renal disease, ***elderly patients,*** pregnant or breastfeeding patients, and ***children younger than age 18*** (safety not established).

Adverse reactions

CNS: headache, dizziness, **spinal-epidural hematoma, intracranial hemorrhage**

CV: vasovagal reaction, bradycardia, **hemopericardium, coronary artery dissection**

GI: nausea, vomiting, occult bleeding, hematemesis, **retroperitoneal hemorrhage**

GU: pelvic pain, hematuria

Hematologic: bleeding, **thrombocytopenia**

Musculoskeletal: leg pain

Respiratory: pulmonary hemorrhage

Skin: diaphoresis

Other: infusion site bleeding, chills, fever, edema, allergic reactions, **anaphylaxis**

Interactions

Drug-drug. *Clopidogrel, dipyridamole, nonsteroidal anti-inflammatory drugs, oral anticoagulants (such as thrombolytics, ticlopidine, warfarin), other drugs affecting hemostasis:* increased risk of bleeding

Levothyroxine, omeprazole: increased renal clearance of tirofiban

Vitamin A: increased risk of bleeding

Drug-diagnostic tests. *Hematocrit, hemoglobin, platelets:* decreased

Drug-herb. *Alfalfa, anise, arnica, astragalus, bilberry, black currant seed oil, bladderwrack, bogbean, boldo (with fenugreek), borage oil, buchu, capsaicin, cat's claw, celery, chaparral, chincona bark, clove oil, dandelion, dong quai, evening primrose oil, fenugreek, feverfew, garlic, ginger, ginkgo, guggul, papaya extract, red clover, rhubarb, safflower oil, skullcap, tan-shen:* increased risk of bleeding

Toxicity and overdose

- Most common signs and symptoms of overdose are minor mucocutaneous bleeding and minor bleeding at cardiac catheterization sites.

• Closely monitor patient's clinical condition; adjust infusion rate or stop drug if indicated. Provide supportive therapy. Hemodialysis removes drug.

Patient teaching

🔈 Teach patient to recognize and immediately report serious adverse reactions.

• Tell patient he will be closely monitored and undergo regular blood testing during therapy.

• As appropriate, review all other significant and life-threatening adverse reactions and interactions, especially those related to the drugs, tests, and herbs mentioned above.

[redacted]

tobramycin sulfate

Nebcin

Pharmacologic class: Aminoglycoside
Therapeutic class: Anti-infective
Pregnancy risk category D

FDA BOXED WARNING

• When giving drug by injection, observe patient closely for potential ototoxicity and nephrotoxicity. Rarely, nephrotoxicity does not emerge until first few days after therapy ends.

• Neurotoxicity, manifested as both auditory and vestibular ototoxicity, may occur. Auditory changes are irreversible and usually bilateral. Eighth-nerve impairment and nephrotoxicity also may develop, mainly in patients with preexisting renal damage and in those with normal renal function who receive drug for longer periods or in doses higher than recommended. Other neurotoxicity manifestations may include numbness, skin tingling, muscle twitching, and seizures. Risk of drug-induced hearing loss increases with degree of exposure to high peak or high trough blood levels. Patients who develop cochlear damage may lack symptoms during therapy to warn of eighth-nerve toxicity, and partial or total irreversible bilateral deafness may continue to develop after drug withdrawal.

• Monitor renal and eighth-nerve function closely in patients with known or suspected renal impairment and in those whose renal function initially is normal but who develop signs of renal dysfunction during therapy. Monitor peak and trough drug blood levels periodically during therapy; avoid levels above 12 mcg. Rising trough levels (above 2 mcg) may indicate tissue accumulation. Such accumulation, excessive peak levels, advanced age, and cumulative dose may contribute to ototoxicity and nephrotoxicity. Examine urine for decreased specific gravity and increased protein, cells, and casts. Measure blood urea nitrogen (BUN), serum creatinine, and creatinine clearance periodically. When feasible, obtain serial audiograms. Evidence of impairment of renal, vestibular, or auditory function warrants drug withdrawal or dosage adjustment.

• Avoid concurrent or sequential use of other neurotoxic or nephrotoxic antibiotics, especially other aminoglycosides (such as amikacin, gentamicin, kanamycin, neomycin, and streptomycin), cephaloridine, cisplatin, colistin, polymyxin B, vancomycin, and viomycin. Advanced age and dehydration also increase risk.

• Do not give concurrently with potent diuretics (such as furosemide and ethacrynic acid), because these drugs are also ototoxic. Also, I.V. diuretics may

increase tobramycin toxicity by altering antibiotic serum and tissue levels.
- Use drug cautiously in premature infants and neonates.
- Drug may harm fetus when given to pregnant women.

Action
Interferes with protein synthesis in bacterial cell by binding to 30S ribosomal subunit

Pharmacokinetics
Drug distributes to tissues and body fluids, including sputum, peritoneal fluid, synovial fluid, and abscess fluids. Cerebrospinal fluid concentration is low; drug crosses placental barrier. Therapeutic serum level ranges from 4 to 6 mcg/mL. Virtually no serum protein binding occurs. With parenteral administration, little if any metabolic transformation occurs. Drug is eliminated almost exclusively by glomerular filtration. When renal function is impaired, excretion slows and drug accumulation may cause toxic blood levels. In patients with normal renal function, up to 84% of dose is recoverable from urine in 8 hours and up to 93% in 24 hours. Concentration in bile and stool normally is low, suggesting minimum biliary excretion.

Onset	Peak	Duration
Rapid	15-30 min	Unknown

How supplied
Pediatric solution for injection (clear and colorless): 20 mg/2 mL
Solution for injection (clear and colorless): 10 mg/mL, 40 mg/mL, 1.2-g vial

Indications and dosages
➤ Serious infections caused by susceptible organisms
Adults: 3 mg/kg/day I.V. in evenly divided doses q 8 hours. For life-threatening infections, may increase up to 5 mg/kg/day I.V. in three or four evenly divided doses, then reduce to 3 mg/kg/day as soon as possible.
Children older than 1 week: 6 to 7.5 mg/kg/day in three or four evenly divided doses, such as 2 to 2.5 mg/kg I.V. q 8 hours or 1.5 to 1.9 mg/kg I.V. q 6 hours
Neonates younger than 1 week: Up to 4 mg/kg/day I.V. in evenly divided doses q 12 hours

Dosage adjustment
- In neonates and patients with reduced renal function, serum level usually is higher and can be measured for longer periods than in normal adults. Adjust dosage for such patients accordingly.
- For obese patients, calculate appropriate dosage (mg/kg) by using estimated lean body weight plus 40% of excess as basic weight.

Administration
Dilution and compatibility
- Dilute I.V. dose in 50 to 100 mL normal saline solution or D_5W. For children, use smaller volumes.
- Do not mix with other drugs.

Infusion considerations
- Give cephalosporins or penicillins 1 hour before or after tobramycin to avoid inactivation of tobramycin.
- Infuse over at least 20 to 60 minutes. Infusions of less than 20 minutes are not recommended because peak serum levels may exceed 12 mcg/mL.
- Flush line after administration.

Monitoring
- Draw sample for peak drug level 30 minutes after administration; draw sample for trough level just before next dose.
- Assess liver and kidney function tests.

• Monitor CBC with white cell differential.
• Closely monitor patient's hearing.
Storage
• Store at controlled room temperature.

Contraindications and precautions

Contraindicated in hypersensitivity to drug, other aminoglycosides, bisulfites (with some products), or benzyl alcohol (in neonates, with some products).

Use cautiously in renal or hearing impairment, neuromuscular diseases, obesity, ***elderly patients,*** pregnant or breastfeeding patients, and ***neonates and premature infants.***

Adverse reactions

CNS: confusion, lethargy, headache, delirium, dizziness, vertigo
EENT: totoxicity, hearing loss, roaring in ears, tinnitus
GI: nausea, diarrhea, stomatitis
GU: proteinuria, **oliguria, nephrotoxicity**
Hematologic: anemia, eosinophilia, **leukocytosis, leukopenia, thrombocytopenia, granulocytopenia**
Metabolic: hypocalcemia, hyponatremia, hypokalemia, hypomagnesemia
Musculoskeletal: muscle weakness
Respiratory: apnea
Skin: rash, urticaria, itching
Other: superinfection, fever, pain and irritation at injection site, hypersensitivity reaction

Interactions

Drug-drug. *Cephalosporins, vancomycin:* increased risk of nephrotoxicity
Dimenhydrinate: masking of ototoxicity symptoms
General anesthetics, neuromuscular blockers: increased neuromuscular blockade and respiratory depression
Indomethacin: increased tobramycin trough and peak levels
Loop diuretics: increased risk of ototoxicity
Penicillins: physical incompatibility, tobramycin inactivation when mixed in same I.V. solution
Polypeptide anti-infectives: increased risk of respiratory paralysis and renal dysfunction
Drug-diagnostic tests. *Alanine aminotransferase, aspartate aminotransferase, bilirubin, BUN, creatinine, lactate dehydrogenase, nonprotein nitrogen, urine protein:* increased
Calcium, granulocytes, hemoglobin, magnesium, platelets, potassium, sodium, white blood cells: decreased

Toxicity and overdose

• Severity of overdose signs and symptoms depend on dosage; patient's renal function, hydration, and age; and whether other drugs with similar toxicities are being administered concurrently. Toxicity may occur in patients treated for more than 10 days, adults given more than 5 mg/kg/day, children given more than 7.5 mg/kg/day, and patients with impaired renal function if dosage has not been adjusted appropriately. Auditory and vestibular toxicities may be asymptomatic or may cause dizziness, tinnitus, vertigo, and loss of high-tone acuity as ototoxicity progresses. Ototoxicity signs and symptoms may not begin until long after drug withdrawal. Neuromuscular blockade or respiratory paralysis also may occur. Prolonged respiratory paralysis may develop in patients receiving decamethonium, tubocurarine, or succinylcholine.
• Establish airway and ensure oxygenation and ventilation. Initiate resuscitative measures promptly if respiratory paralysis occurs. If patient has normal renal function, hydrate adequately to maintain urine output of 3 to 5 mL/kg/hour. Carefully monitor fluid

T

balance, creatinine clearance, and tobramycin plasma level until this level falls below 2 mcg/mL. Patients with elimination half-life exceeding 2 hours and those with abnormal renal function may need more aggressive therapy; in such patients, hemodialysis may be helpful. Consider exchange transfusions for newborns. To reverse neuromuscular blockade, calcium salts may be used, but mechanical assistance may be necessary.

Patient teaching

Tell patient drug may cause hearing impairment, urinary difficulties, and other serious adverse reactions, such as unusual bleeding or bruising. Instruct patient to report these reactions at once.
- Advise patient to report new signs or symptoms of infection.
- As appropriate, review all other significant and life-threatening adverse reactions and interactions, especially those related to the drugs and tests mentioned above.

topotecan hydrochloride

Hycamtin

Pharmacologic class: DNA topoisomerase inhibitor
Therapeutic class: Antineoplastic
Pregnancy risk category D

FDA BOXED WARNING

- Give under supervision of physician experienced in cancer chemotherapy, in facility with adequate diagnostic and treatment resources.
- Do not administer to patients with baseline neutrophil counts below 1,500/mm^3. Obtain frequent peripheral blood cell counts on all patients to monitor for bone marrow depression.

Action

Regulates DNA replication and repair of broken DNA strands, relieving torsional strain; exerts cytoxic effects during DNA synthesis

Pharmacokinetics

Drug is not extensively metabolized. Terminal half-life is approximately 2 to 3 hours. About 30% of dose is excreted in urine.

Onset	Peak	Duration
Unknown	Unknown	Unknown

How supplied

Powder for reconstitution for injection (lyophilized): 4 mg in single-dose vials

Indications and dosages

➢ Metastatic ovarian cancer or small-cell lung cancer after first-line chemotherapy fails

Adults: 1.5 mg/m^2 I.V. infusion daily given over 30 minutes for 5 consecutive days, starting on day 1 of 21-day cycle

➢ Cervical cancer

Adults: 0.75 mg/m^2 by I.V. infusion over 30 minutes daily on days 1, 2, and 3, followed by prescribed cisplatin dosage by I.V. infusion on day 1; repeat q 21 days (21-day course)

Dosage adjustment

- Reduce dosage to 0.75 mg/m^2 in moderate renal impairment.
- Be aware that drug is likely to cause greater myelosuppression when given with other cytotoxic agents, necessitating dosage reduction.
- Know that patients should not receive subsequent courses until neutrophil count recovers to above 1,000/mm^3,

platelet count to 100,000/mm^3 or higher, and hemoglobin to 9 g/dL or higher (with transfusions, if necessary).

Administration

Preparation

Follow hazardous drug guidelines on page S19 for handling, preparation, and administration.

Before starting therapy, check blood counts. Patient must have baseline neutrophil count above 1,500/mm^3 and platelet count above 100,000/mm^3 to receive drug.

Dilution and compatibility

- To reconstitute, add 4 mL sterile water to 4-mg vial. Dilute further in normal saline solution or D_5W.

Infusion considerations

- Give immediately after reconstitution over 30 minutes, using infusion pump.
- Avoid extravasation, which may cause mild erythema and bruising.

Monitoring

- Closely monitor CBC with white cell differential.
- Monitor closely for sepsis, other infections, and increased hepatic enzyme levels.
- Monitor renal and hepatic function, especially in elderly patients.
- Assess for signs and symptoms of bleeding tendency.

Storage

- Store in original carton at controlled temperature of 20° to 25°C (68° to 77°F). Protect from light.
- Reconstituted vials are stable for 24 hours when stored at approximately 20° to 25°C (68° to 77°F) in ambient lighting conditions.

Contraindications and precautions

Contraindicated in hypersensitivity to drug or its components, severe bone marrow depression, and pregnancy or breastfeeding.

Use cautiously in ***children*** (safety and efficacy not established).

Adverse reactions

CNS: asthenia, headache, fatigue, paresthesia
GI: nausea, vomiting, diarrhea, constipation, abdominal pain, stomatitis, anorexia
Hematologic: anemia, **leukopenia, thrombocytopenia, neutropenia**
Musculoskeletal: back pain, skeletal pain
Respiratory: coughing, dyspnea
Skin: erythematous or maculopapular rash, pruritus, urticaria, dermatitis, bullous eruption, alopecia
Other: fever, body pain, **sepsis**

Interactions

Drug-drug. *Cisplatin:* severe bone marrow depression
Granulocyte colony-stimulating factor: prolonged neutropenia
Live-virus vaccines: increased risk of infection from vaccine
Drug-diagnostic tests. *Alanine aminotransferase, aspartate aminotransferase, bilirubin:* increased

Toxicity and overdose

- In overdose, expect bone marrow depression, including severe neutropenia.
- No known antidote exists. Provide supportive thearpy. In severe toxicity, withhold drug.

Patient teaching

Advise patient to immediately report unusual bleeding or bruising, sore throat, fever, or chills.

- Teach patient safety measures to avoid bruising and bleeding.
- Advise patient to minimize GI upset by eating small, frequent servings of food and drinking plenty of fluids.

T

Instruct female patient to notify prescriber of suspected pregnancy. Caution her not to breastfeed during therapy.

- Inform patient that drug may cause hair loss.
- Emphasize the need for regular blood testing during therapy.
- As appropriate, review all other significant and life-threatening adverse reactions and interactions, especially those related to the drugs and tests mentioned above.

[redacted]

torsemide (torasemide❋)

Demadex

Pharmacologic class: Loop diuretic
Therapeutic class: Diuretic, antihypertensive
Pregnancy risk category B

Action

Inhibits sodium and chloride reabsorption from ascending loop of Henle and distal renal tubule; increases renal excretion of water, sodium, chloride, magnesium, hydrogen, and calcium. Also may exert renal and peripheral vasodilatory effects. Net effect is natriuretic diuresis.

Pharmacokinetics

Major metabolite, carboxylic acid derivative, is biologically inactive. Two lesser metabolites possess some diuretic activity, but metabolism practically ends drug activity. Drug is more than 90% bound to plasma protein, so little enters tubular urine via glomerular filtration. Drug clears from circulation by both hepatic metabolism and excretion into urine. Most renal clearance occurs via active secretion by proximal tubules into tubular urine.

Onset	Peak	Duration
Within 10 min	Within 1 hr	6-8 hr

How supplied

Solution for injection (clear): 10 mg/mL in ampules

Indications and dosages

➢ Heart failure

Adults: 10 to 20 mg I.V. daily. For inadequate response, double dosage until desired response occurs. Do not exceed 200 mg as a single dose.

➢ Chronic renal failure

Adults: 20 mg I.V. daily. For inadequate response, double dosage until desired response occurs. Do not exceed 200 mg as a single dose.

➢ Hepatic cirrhosis

Adults: 5 or 10 mg I.V. daily, given with aldosterone antagonist or potassium-sparing diuretic. For inadequate response, double dosage. Do not exceed 40 mg as a single dose.

➢ Hypertension

Adults: 5 mg I.V. once daily. If 5-mg dose does not adequately reduce blood pressure within 4 to 6 weeks, increase dosage to 10 mg daily. If response to 10 mg is insufficient, add another antihypertensive agent to regimen.

Administration

Dilution and compatibility

- Know that drug may be given undiluted or diluted in compatible I.V. infusion solution, such as D_5W or normal saline.
- Do not use if discolored.

Infusion considerations

- Give by direct I.V. injection over at least 2 minutes, or by continuous I.V. infusion over 24 hours.
- Flush I.V. line with normal saline solution before and after administering.

Monitoring
- Monitor vital signs, especially for hypotension.
- Assess ECG for arrhythmias and other changes.
- Monitor weight and fluid intake and output to assess drug efficacy.

🔈 Monitor electrolyte levels, particularly potassium. Stay alert for signs and symptoms of hypokalemia.
- Assess hearing for signs and symptoms of ototoxicity.
- Monitor blood glucose level carefully in diabetic patient.

Storage
- Store at room temperature of 15° to 30°C (59° to 86°F). Do not freeze.

Contraindications and precautions

Contraindicated in hypersensitivity to drug, thiazides, or sulfonylureas and in anuria.

Use cautiously in severe hepatic disease accompanied by cirrhosis or ascites, preexisting uncorrected electrolyte imbalances, diabetes mellitus, worsening azotemia, ***elderly patients,*** pregnant or breastfeeding patients, and ***children younger than age 18.***

Adverse reactions

CNS: dizziness, headache, asthenia, insomnia, nervousness, syncope
CV: hypotension, ECG changes, chest pain, volume depletion, **atrial fibrillation, ventricular tachycardia, shunt thrombosis**
EENT: rhinitis, sore throat
GI: nausea, diarrhea, vomiting, constipation, dyspepsia, anorexia, rectal bleeding, **GI hemorrhage**
GU: excessive urination
Metabolic: hyperglycemia, hyperuricemia, hypokalemia
Musculoskeletal: joint pain, myalgia
Respiratory: increased cough
Skin: rash
Other: edema

Interactions

Drug-drug. *Aminoglycosides, cisplatin:* increased risk of ototoxicity
Amphotericin B, corticosteroids, mezlocillin, piperacillin, potassium-wasting diuretics, stimulant laxatives: additive hypokalemia
Antihypertensives, nitrates: additive hypotension
Lithium: increased lithium blood level and toxicity
Neuromuscular blockers: prolonged neuromuscular blockade
Nonsteroidal anti-inflammatory drugs, probenecid: inhibited diuretic response
Sulfonylureas: decreased glucose tolerance, hyperglycemia in patients with previously well-controlled diabetes
Drug-diagnostic tests. *Glucose, uric acid:* increased
Potassium: decreased
Drug-herb. *Dandelion:* interference with diuresis
Ephedra (ma huang): reduced hypotensive effect of torsemide
Geranium, ginseng: increased risk of diuretic resistance
Licorice: rapid potassium loss
Drug-behaviors. *Acute alcohol ingestion:* additive hypotension

Toxicity and overdose

- In ovedose, expect signs and symptoms to reflect excessive pharmacologic actions, such as dehydration, hypovolemia, hypotension, hyponatremia, hypokalemia, hypochloremic alkalosis, and hemoconcentration.
- Replace fluids and electrolytes, as ordered and needed. Know that serum levels of torsemide and its metabolites are not widely available. Provide symptomatic and supportive therapy. Drug is not dialyzable.

T

Patient teaching

- Instruct patient to move slowly when sitting up or standing, to avoid dizziness from sudden blood pressure decrease.
- Advise patient to monitor weight and report sudden increase.
- Instruct diabetic patient to monitor blood glucose level carefully.
- Caution patient to avoid alcohol during therapy.
- Advise patient to consult prescriber before using herbs.
- As appropriate, review all other significant and life-threatening adverse reactions and interactions, especially those related to the drugs, tests, herbs, and behaviors mentioned above.

tositumomab and iodine^{131} tositumomab

Bexxar Dosimetric, Bexxar ^{131}I Dosimetric, Bexxar ^{131}I Therapeutic, Bexxar Therapeutic

Pharmacologic class: Monoclonal antibody

Therapeutic class: Antineoplastic

Pregnancy risk category X

FDA BOXED WARNING

- Serious hypersensitivity reactions, some of them fatal, have occurred with Bexxar therapeutic regimen. Keep appropriate drugs immediately available to treat hypersensitivity reactions. If such reactions develop, discontinue regimen and provide interventions as needed.
- Most patients who receive regimen experience severe thrombocytopenia and neutropenia. Do not administer if patient has more than 25% lymphoma marrow involvement, impaired bone marrow reserve, or both.
- Regimen can cause fetal harm when given to pregnant women.
- Because of radioactive component, regimen should be administered only by clinicians qualified in safe use and handling of therapeutic radionuclides and who have been certified (or are in process of getting certified) by Corixa Corp. in calculating dosage and administering regimen.

Action

May induce apoptosis, complement-dependent cytotoxicity, and antibody-dependent cellular cytotoxicity mediated by antibody. Additionally, ionizing radiation from radioisotope leads to cell death.

Pharmacokinetics

Tositumomab and iodine^{131} tositumomab 475 mg predose of unlabeled antibody decrease splenic targeting and increase terminal half-life of radiolabeled antibody. Median blood clearance of tositumomab in patients with non-Hodgkin's lymphoma is 68.2 mg/hour. Patients with high tumor burden, splenomegaly, or bone marrow involvement typically have faster clearance, shorter terminal half-life, and larger distribution volume. Total-body clearance depends on same factors as blood clearance. Median total-body effective half-life in patients with non-Hodgkin's lymphoma is 67 hours. Elimination of ^{131}I results from decay and urinary excretion.

Onset	Peak	Duration
Unknown	Unknown	Unknown

How supplied

Tositumomab is supplied as sterile, pyrogen-free, clear to opalescent, colorless to

slightly yellow, preservative-free liquid concentrate.
Bexxar Dosimetric packaging: two single-use 225-mg vials and one single-use 35-mg vial of tositumomab; one single-use vial of ^{131}I tositumomab (0.61 mCi/mL at calibration)
Bexxar Therapeutic packaging: two single-use 225-mg vials and one single-use 35-mg vial of tositumomab; one or two single-use vials of ^{131}I tositumomab (5.6 mCi/mL at calibration)

Indications and dosages

➤ CD20-positive, follicular non-Hodgkin's lymphoma (with and without transformation) in patients whose disease is refractory to rituximab and has relapsed after chemotherapy
Adults: Bexxar therapeutic regimen is given in two steps—dosimetric and therapeutic. Each step consists of sequential tositumomab infusion followed by ^{131}I tositumomab. Administer therapeutic step 7 to 14 days after dosimetric step.
Dosimetric step: (1) Tositumomab 450 mg I.V. in 50 mL normal saline solution over 60 minutes. (2) ^{131}I tositumomab (containing 5 mCi ^{131}I and 35 mg tositumomab) I.V. in 30 mL normal saline solution over 20 minutes.
Therapeutic step: Do not administer this step if ^{131}I tositumomab biodistribution is altered. See manufacturer's prescribing information on assessing biodistribution. (1) Tositumomab 450 mg I.V. in 50 mL normal saline solution over 60 minutes. (2) ^{131}I tositumomab: See manufacturer's prescribing information for calculating ^{131}I activity.

Dosage adjustment

- Be aware that in patients with platelet count of 150,000/mm^3 or higher, recommended dosage is ^{131}I activity calculated to deliver 75 cGy total body irradiation and 35 mg tositumomab, given I.V. over 20 minutes.
- Know that in patients with National Cancer Institute Grade 1 thrombocytopenia (platelet count of 100,000/mm^3 or higher but below 150,000/mm^3), recommended dosage is ^{131}I activity calculated to deliver 65 cGy total body irradiation and 35 mg tositumomab, given I.V. over 20 minutes.
- Reduce infusion rate 50% for mild to moderate infusional toxicity; interrupt infusion for severe infusional toxicity. After severe infusional toxicity resolves completely, infusion may be resumed at 50% of previous infusion rate.

Administration

Preparation

🔊 Follow hazardous drug guidelines on page S19 for handling, preparation, and administration.
🔊 Be aware that Bexxar therapeutic regimen contains radioactive component.
🔊 Know that Bexxar therapeutic regimen is not indicated for initial treatment of CD20-positive non-Hodgkin's lymphoma and is intended as a single course of treatment. Safety of multiple courses of ^{131}I tositumomab, tositumomab therapeutic regimen, or combination of this regimen with other forms of irradiation or chemotherapy has not been evaluated.
🔊 Keep in mind that highly specific guidelines exist for preparation and administration. See manufacturer's prescribing information for more guidelines on administration qualifications, radiation precautions, preparation, and dosage calibrations. Regimen components are shipped only to individuals who participate in certification program or have been certified in preparation and administration of

T

Bexxar therapeutic regimen. Components are shipped separately; when ordering, make sure components are scheduled to arrive on same day.
• Obtain CBC with white cell differential and platelet count before administration.
• Check results of serum creatinine and thyroid-stimulating hormone (TSH) tests immediately before administering.
• Because kidney excretes both components, impaired renal function may reduce ^{131}I excretion rate and increase exposure to radioactive component. No data exist on safety of regimen in patients with impaired renal function.
Keep appropriate drugs available for immediate use in case of severe hypersensitivity reaction.
Know that patients should not receive dosimetric dose if they have not received the following medications:

Thyroid-protective agents—saturated solution of potassium iodide, four drops P.O. t.i.d.; Lugol's solution, 20 drops P.O. t.i.d.; or potassium iodide tablets, 130 mg P.O. daily. Start thyroid-protective agents at least 24 hours before dosimetric dose and continue until 2 weeks after administration of therapeutic dose. All patients must receive thyroid-blocking agents; those who cannot tolerate these agents should not receive regimen.

Acetaminophen 650 mg P.O. and *diphenhydramine* 50 mg P.O. 30 minutes before tositumomab administration in dosimetric and therapeutic steps.

Dilution and compatibility

Be aware that for dosimetric and therapeutic steps, all supplies, calibration, confirmation of radiochemical purity, and preparation techniques must be provided by personnel authorized to handle radiopharmaceuticals.
• Discard unused portions of tositumomab left in vial, according to manufacturer's instructions.
• Discard unused portion of ^{131}I according to federal and state laws.

Infusion considerations

• Administer through I.V. tubing set with inline 0.22-micron filter.
• Use same I.V. tubing set and filter throughout both administration steps. (Filter change could cause drug loss.)
• For dosimetric step, administer tositumomab I.V. over 60 minutes and ^{131}I tositumomab I.V. over 20 minutes.
• For therapeutic step, administer tositumomab I.V. over 60 minutes and ^{131}I tositumomab I.V. according to manufacturer's prescribing information.

Monitoring

Monitor closely for allergic reactions, including bronchospasm and angioedema; be prepared to intervene appropriately.
Monitor for infusion reactions, including fever, sweating, rigors, chills, hypotension, dyspnea, bronchospasm, and nausea. These may occur within 48 hours of infusion. Slow or temporarily interrupt infusion.
Continue weekly monitoring of CBC with differential and platelet count for at least 10 weeks, or until persistent cytopenias resolve completely. Be aware that patients with moderate or more severe cytopenias require more frequent monitoring, especially for infection and in thrombocytopenic patients, for hemorrhage.
• Know that after therapy, patient should have TSH level measured yearly to check for hypothyroidism.

Storage

• Refrigerate tositumomab vials at 2° to 8°C (36° to 46°F) before dilution. Diluted tositumomab solutions are stable for up to 24 hours when refrigerated at 2° to 8° C and for up to 8 hours at room temperature. Refrigerate diluted solution at 2° to 8°C before use. Do not freeze; protect from strong light.

• Store frozen ^{131}I in original lead pot in freezer at –20°C (–36°F) or below until removal for thawing before administration. Thawed doses are stable for up to 8 hours at 2° to 8°C (36° to 46°F). Refrigerate diluted solution before use. Do not freeze.

Contraindications and precautions

Contraindicated in hypersensitivity to murine proteins or other components of Bexxar therapeutic regimen, intolerance to thyroid-blocking agents, females with childbearing potential, and pregnancy.

Use cautiously when handling radioactive material and in cytopenia or impaired renal function; concurrent use of drugs that interfere with platelet function or anticoagulation; breastfeeding patients; ***elderly patients;*** and ***children*** (safety and efficacy not established).

Adverse reactions

CNS: asthenia, headache, dizziness, somnolence
CV: hypotension, vasodilation
EENT: rhinitis, pharyngitis
GI: nausea, vomiting, abdominal pain, diarrhea, constipation, dyspepsia, decreased appetite
Hematologic: anemia, **thrombocytopenia, neutropenia**
Metabolic: hypothyroidism
Musculoskeletal: back pain, neck pain, arthralgia, myalgia
Respiratory: cough, dyspnea, pleural effusion, bronchitis, pneumonia
Skin: infection, herpes simplex, rash, pruritus, sweating
Other: fever, flulike symptoms, shivering, pain, antibody development, dehydration, peripheral edema, weight loss, chest pain, infusion reactions, **sepsis** (with severe cytopenia), **secondary cancers,** hypersensitivity reactions including serum sickness and **anaphylaxis**

Interactions

Drug-diagnostic tests. *Platelets, red blood cells, TSH, white blood cell count with differential:* decreased
Tests using murine antibody technology: possible alterations if human antimouse antibodies immune response develops

Toxicity and overdose

• In overdose, expect hematologic and radiation-related toxicities. (In clincal trials, maximum dosage of therapeutic regimen was 88 cGy.)
• In accidental overdose, monitor patient closely. Effectiveness of hematopoietic stem-cell transplantation for marrow injury has not been studied. However, when timing such measures, consider pharmacokinetics of regimen and decay rate of ^{131}I to minimize possibility of irradiating infused hematopoietic stem cells.

Patient teaching

• Inform patient that radioactive material remains in body for several days after discharge. At discharge, provide oral and written instructions to minimize exposure of family and others.
• Urge patient to comply with thyroid-blocking therapy, and stress the need for lifelong thyroid monitoring.
• Explain risks of blood-cell disorders and associated symptoms, the need for frequent monitoring for up to 12 weeks after treatment, and risk of such disorders lasting beyond 12 weeks.
• Inform patient of risk of secondary cancers.
• Tell patient drug therapy may interfere with some tests results.

- Caution females of childbearing potential to avoid pregnancy during therapy.
- Instruct breastfeeding patient to discontinue breastfeeding because of potential harm to infant.
- Advise male patients of potential risk of toxic effects on gonads. Teach them to use effective contraceptive methods during treatment and for 12 months afterward.
- As appropriate, review all other significant and life-threatening adverse reactions and interactions, especially those related to the tests mentioned above.

trace metals

Multitrace-4 Concentrate, Multitrace-4 Neonatal, Multitrace-4 Pediatric, Multitrace-5 Concentrate

Pharmacologic class: Trace elements
Therapeutic class: Nutritional supplement
Pregnancy risk category C

Action

Of the many trace elements essential for body functions, only five are routinely added to total parenteral nutrition (TPN) solutions. *Chromium* helps maintain normal glucose and peripheral nerve function. *Copper* is a cofactor for serum ceruloplasmin (an oxidase needed for proper formation of iron carrier protein). *Manganese* is an activator for several enzymes, such as polysaccharide polymerase, liver arginase, cholinesterase, and pyruvate carboxylase. *Selenium* is part of glutathione peroxidase, which protects cell components from oxidative damage caused by peroxides produced in cellular metabolism. *Zinc* is a cofactor for more than 70 enzymes; it promotes wound healing and helps maintain normal growth rates, normal skin hydration, and taste and smell sensation. *Iodine* and *molybdenum* are other trace-element TPN additives.

Pharmacokinetics

Chromium binds to transferrin and is excreted in urine and bile. *Copper* is excreted primarily in bile, with some excretion in the intestinal wall and urine. *Manganese* distributes widely, concentrating in the brain, kidney, pancreas, and liver; it binds to specific transport protein. *Selenium* may cross placental barrier and is excreted in urine, feces, lungs, and skin. *Zinc* concentrates in muscle, bone, skin, kidneys, liver, pancreas, retina, prostate, and particularly in red and white blood cells; protein-bound, it is excreted primarily in stools, with some excretion in urine and perspiration. *Iodine* concentrates primarily in the thyroid gland, with some uptake by the salivary glands, gastric mucosa, choroid plexus, skin, hair, mammary glands, and placenta; it is excreted in urine and bile. *Molybdenum* is stored in the liver, kidney, and adrenal cortex; it crosses placental barrier, and is excreted mainly in urine, with some excretion in bile.

Onset	Peak	Duration
Unknown	Unknown	Unknown

How supplied

Solution for injection: Various products as single elements, combination products, and in combination with electrolyte solutions

Indications and dosages

➤ Supplement to I.V. solutions given for TPN

Adults and children: Individualized dosage according to product and manufacturer's directions

Dosage adjustment
• Adjust, reduce, or omit copper and manganese in patients with renal dysfunction or GI malfunction.

Administration
Preparation
• Know that normal plasma levels are chromium, 1 to 5 mcg/dL; copper, 80 to 163 mcg/dL; manganese, 6 to 12 mcg/L in whole blood; zinc, 88 to 112 mcg/dL; and iodine, 0.5 to 1.5 mcg/dL. No data are available on molybdenum and selenium.

🔈 Be aware that some products contain aluminum, which may be toxic with prolonged administration.

🔈 Know that some products contain benzyl alcohol, associated with fatal gasping syndrome in premature infants.

Dilution and compatibility
🔈 Add trace metals to daily volume of TPN solution.

🔈 Do not use syringes with aluminum needles, because formulations are acidic.

Infusion considerations
🔈 Do not give drug undiluted into peripheral vein, because of risk of infusion phlebitis, tissue irritation, and increased renal loss of minerals (with bolus injection).

Monitoring
🔈 Monitor for hypersensitivity reactions to iodine. If these occur, immediately discontinue infusion and intervene as appropriate.

• Know that other adverse reactions are unlikely at recommended dosages.

• Frequently monitor blood levels of all trace elements administered, to aid dosage adjustment.

Storage
• Store at room temperature.

Contraindications and precautions
Contraindicated in hypersensitivity to iodine, direct injection into peripheral vein, and molybdenum administration without copper supplementation in copper-deficient patients.

Use cautiously in renal failure, biliary tract obstruction, Wilson's disease (avoid copper supplements), ***elderly patients,*** pregnant or breastfeeding patients, and ***children.***

Adverse reactions
Other: hypersensitivity reactions including **anaphylaxis** (to iodine)

Interactions
No information available

Toxicity and overdose
• Overdose may occur if patient's requirement for one trace element is much higher than for others in formulation. *Chromium* overdose may cause nausea, vomiting, GI ulcers, renal and hepatic damage, seizures, and coma. *Copper* overdose may lead to prostration, behavior changes, diarrhea, progressive marasmus, hypotonia, photophobia, hepatic damage, and peripheral edema (with serum copper levels of 286 mcg/dL). *Manganese* overdose may cause "manganese madness" (irritability, speech disturbances, abnormal gait, headache, anorexia, apathy, and erectile dysfunction). In *selenium* toxicity, expect metallic taste, vomiting, garlic breath and sweat odor, hair loss, weak nails, dermatitis, GI disorders, dental defects, nervousness, mental depression, and (in acute poisoning) coma and death. Acute *zinc* toxicity may manifest as profuse sweating, blurred vision, tachycardia, marked hypothermia, and

T

decreased consciousness; it may follow infusion of 10 mg zinc over 1 hour for 4 consecutive days. Very large doses of zinc may lead to death. Chronic *iodine* poisoning causes metallic taste, sore mouth, increased salivation, salivary gland tenderness, coryza, sneezing, acneiform skin lesions and eruptions, eyelid swelling, severe headache, and pulmonary edema. *Molybdenum* overdose may lead to goutlike symptoms.

• Provide symptomatic and supportive therapy. Know that penicillamine is antidote for copper overdose. No known antidote exists for selenium. Calcium supplements may be beneficial in zinc toxicity. Large volumes of fluid and sodium intake may help eliminate iodine. No information is available on treating chromium or manganese overdose.

Patient teaching

• As appropriate, review all significant and life-threatening adverse reactions.

trastuzumab

Herceptin

Pharmacologic class: Recombinant DNA-derived monoclonal antibody
Therapeutic class: Antineoplastic
Pregnancy risk category B

FDA BOXED WARNING

• Drug may cause clinical and subclinical cardiac failure manifesting as congestive heart failure and decreased left ventricular ejection fraction (LVEF). Incidence and severity of left ventricle dysfunction were highest in patients who received drug concurrently with anthracyclines and cyclophosphamide. Evaluate left ventricle function in all patients before and during therapy. Withdraw drug in patients receiving adjuvant therapy, and strongly consider withdrawal in patients with metastatic breast cancer who experience significant decrease in left ventricle function.

• Drug may lead to serious infusion reactions (possibly fatal) and pulmonary toxicity. In most cases, symptoms occur during or within 24 hours after administration. Interrupt infusion if dyspnea or significant hypotension occurs; monitor patient until signs and symptoms resolve completely. Withdraw drug for infusion reaction manifesting as anaphylaxis, angioedema, interstitial pneumonitis, or acute respiratory distress syndrome.

Action

Selectively binds to human epidermal growth factor receptor 2 (HER2), inhibiting proliferation of human tumor cells that overexpress HER2

Pharmacokinetics

Drug is minimally cleared by the kidneys and liver. Mean half-life increases and clearance decreases with increasing doses; half-life averages 1.7 and 12 days at 10- and 50-mg dosage levels, respectively. Data suggest disposition does not depend on age or serum creatinine level (up to 2 mg/dL).

Onset	Peak	Duration
Unknown	Unknown	Unknown

How supplied

Powder for reconstitution for injection (white to pale yellow, lyophilized): 440-mg vial

Indications and dosages

➢ Adjuvant treatment of metastatic breast cancer in patients whose tumors overexpress HER2

Adults: Use one of the following dosage schedules:

(1) After anthracycline therapy ends and concurrently with paclitaxel for first 12 weeks, initial dosage of 4 mg/kg as a 90-minute I.V. infusion weekly, followed by once-weekly dosage of 2 mg/kg as a 30-minute I.V. infusion, as tolerated, for a total of 52 doses

(2) Alternatively, after completion of all chemotherapy, initial dosage of 8 mg/kg as a 90-minute I.V. infusion, followed by dosage of 6 mg/kg q 3 weeks as a 90-minute I.V. infusion for 52 weeks

Metastatic breast cancer in patients whose tumors overexpress HER2

Adults: Alone or in combination with paclitaxel, initially 4 mg/kg as a 90-minute I.V. infusion, followed by once-weekly dosage of 2 mg/kg as a 30-minute I.V. infusion until disease progresses

Dosage adjustment

- Withhold dose for at least 4 weeks if patient has 16% absolute decrease in LVEF (compared to pretreatment value) or if LVEF falls below institutional limits of normal and is 10% or more lower than pretreatment value. Resume drug if, within 4 to 8 weeks, LVEF returns to normal limits and absolute decrease from baseline is 15% or less. Permanently discontinue drug if patient has persistent LVEF decrease (greater than 8 weeks) or if doses have been suspended more than three times for cardiomyopathy.

Administration

Preparation

Follow hazardous drug guidelines on page S19 for handling, preparation, and administration.

- Assess LVEF before starting therapy.
- Give antiemetic as prescribed before administering.

Dilution and compatibility

- Know that drug is supplied with diluent vial containing 20 mL bacteriostatic water for injection and 1.1% benzyl alcohol.
- To reconstitute, add 20 mL bacteriostatic water for injection to vial, pointing diluent stream at lyophilized cake. Swirl vial gently; do not shake. Withdraw prescribed dose and add to 250 mL normal saline solution for I.V. infusion.
- For patient with benzyl alcohol hypersensitivity, reconstitute with sterile water for injection. Use drug immediately after reconstitution; discard unused portion.

Do not use D_5W injection.

- After reconstituting, immediately write date on vial label after "Do not use after:"; date must be 28 days from reconstitution date.

Infusion considerations

Never administer intrathecally; doing so causes death.

Administer by I.V. infusion only. Do not give by I.V. push or bolus.

- Infuse initial dose I.V. over 90 minutes. Infuse weekly doses I.V. over 30 minutes (except all doses above 4 mg, which should be infused over 90 minutes).

Monitoring

Monitor closely for signs and symptoms of infusion reaction. Decrease infusion rate for mild to moderate reactions. Interrupt infusion if patient develops dyspnea or significant hypotension. Discontinue infusion if serious or life-threatening reactions occur.

- Monitor vital signs, especially for hypotension and bradycardia.

Use with extreme caution in patients with cardiac dysfunction.

T

Carefully assess cardiovascular status (including LVEF). Stay alert for heart failure and peripheral edema.

Monitor respiratory status closely. Report increased dyspnea or flulike symptoms.

• Assess neurologic status for depression and paresthesia.
• Watch closely for signs and symptoms of infection, including herpes simplex.
• Monitor electrolyte levels and CBC with white cell differential.

Storage

• Refrigerate unopened vials and reconstituted solution at 2° to 8°C (36° to 46°F). Solution reconstituted with bacteriostatic water for injection is stable for 28 days at this temperature.

Contraindications and precautions

Contraindicated in hypersensitivity to drug.

Use cautiously in hypersensitivity to Chinese hamster ovary cell protein or benzyl alcohol, cardiac disease, anemia, leukopenia, ***elderly patients,*** pregnant or breastfeeding patients, and ***children younger than age 18*** (safety and efficacy not established).

Adverse reactions

CNS: dizziness, headache, depression, paresthesia, insomnia, ataxia, confusion, manic reaction, **seizures**

CV: peripheral edema, hypotension, tachycardia, syncope, **arrhythmias, shock, pericardial effusion, vascular thrombosis, heart failure, cardiotoxicity, cardiac arrest, cardiomyopathy**

EENT: amblyopia, hearing loss

GI: nausea, vomiting, diarrhea, gastroenteritis, hematemesis, ileus, colitis, esophageal ulcer, stomatitis, anorexia, **intestinal obstruction, pancreatitis**

GU: urinary tract infection, hematuria, hemorrhagic cystitis, hydronephrosis, pyelonephritis, **renal failure**

Hematologic: coagulation disorder, pancytopenia, leukemia

Hepatic: ascites, **hepatitis, hepatic failure**

Metabolic: hypothyroidism, hypercalcemia, hyponatremia

Musculoskeletal: back, bone, and joint pain; myopathy; fractures; **bone necrosis**

Respiratory: upper respiratory tract infection, dyspnea, **acute respiratory distress syndrome, pulmonary toxicity**

Skin: cellulitis, rash, acne, herpes simplex, herpes zoster, skin ulcers

Other: weight loss, edema, infection, fever, chills, flulike syndrome, lymphangitis, **infusion reaction,** hypersensitivity reactions including **anaphylaxis**

Interactions

Drug-drug. *Anthracyclines, cyclophosphamide:* cardiotoxicity

Toxicity and overdose

• Single doses above 500 mg have not been tested. In overdose, expect extension of pharmacologic effects and adverse reactions.
• Provide symptomatic and supportive therapy.

Patient teaching

Instruct patient to immediately report difficulty breathing, flulike symptoms, fever, chills, and other signs and symptoms of infection.

Advise patient to monitor weight and to report sudden weight gain as well as swelling and other signs of heart failure.

Instruct patient to immediately report abdominal pain, change in bowel habits, yellowing of skin or eyes, and easy bruising or bleeding.

• Tell patient drug may cause depression. Advise patient (or significant other as appropriate) to contact prescriber if this occurs.

- As appropriate, review all other significant and life-threatening adverse reactions and interactions, especially those related to the drugs mentioned above.

tromethamine

Tham

Pharmacologic class: Protein substrate
Therapeutic class: Systemic alkalinizer
Pregnancy risk category C

Action

Combines with hydrogen ions to form bicarbonate and a buffer, correcting acidosis. Also exerts some diuretic activity.

Pharmacokinetics

Drug is rapidly eliminated by the kidneys, with 75% or more appearing in urine after 8 hours. Urinary excretion continues for 3 days.

Onset	Peak	Duration
Immediate	Immediate	Unknown

How supplied

Injection: 18 g/500 mL in single-dose container

Indications and dosages

➤ Metabolic acidosis associated with cardiac bypass surgery

Adults: 9 mL/kg (0.32 g/kg) by slow I.V. infusion; 500 mL (18 g) is usually adequate. Maximum single dose is 500 mg/kg infused over at least 1 hour.

➤ Metabolic acidosis associated with cardiac arrest

Adults: 3.6 to 10.8 g by I.V. injection into large peripheral vein if chest is not open; or 2 to 6 g I.V. directly into ventricular cavity if chest is open. After reversal of cardiac arrest, patient may need additional amounts to control persistent acidosis.

Administration

Preparation

Keep intubation equipment nearby in case respiratory depression occurs.

Dilution and compatibility

- Know that drug may be given undiluted or may be added to I.V. infusion solution.
- Discard unused solution.

Infusion considerations

- For metabolic acidosis associated with cardiac bypass surgery, give by slow I.V. infusion through large-bore I.V. catheter into large antecubital vein. Elevate arm after infusion.

If extravasation occurs, discontinue drug and infiltrate affected area with 1% procaine hydrochloride (containing hyaluronidase).

Be aware that in cardiac arrest, drug is used with standard resuscitative measures. When giving by direct I.V. injection into open chest, never inject into cardiac muscle.

- Maintain continuous cardiac monitoring during and after administration.

Monitoring

- Monitor arterial blood gas levels. Watch for alkalosis and signs and symptoms of respiratory depression.
- Assess liver function studies. Stay alert for signs and symptoms of hepatic impairment.

Monitor glucose and potassium levels. Watch for hypoglycemia and hyperkalemia.

Closely monitor fluid intake and output. Check for fluid and electrolyte imbalances and oliguria related to hyperkalemia.

Storage
- Discard 24 hours after reconstitution. Protect from freezing and extreme heat.

Contraindications and precautions
Contraindicated in hypersensitivity to drug, anuria, and uremia.

Use cautiously in renal disease, severe respiratory disease, respiratory depression, pregnant patients, and ***infants.***

Adverse reactions
GU: oliguria
Hepatic: hemorrhagic hepatic necrosis
Metabolic: metabolic alkalosis, transient hypoglycemia, fluid-solute overload, hyperkalemia
Respiratory: respiratory depression
Other: fever; I.V. site infection; extravasation with venous thrombosis or phlebitis, inflammation, necrosis, and sloughing

Interactions
Drug-diagnostic tests. *Glucose:* decreased
Potassium: increased

Toxicity and overdose
- Overdose may result from excessive drug amounts or too-rapid administration. Excessive amounts may cause alkalosis, severe and prolonged hypoglycemia, overhydration or solute overload.
- Discontinue infusion, assess patient, and provide appropriate countermeasures.

Patient teaching
- Explain drug therapy to patient. Assure patient that he will be monitored continuously.
- As appropriate, review all other significant and life-threatening adverse reactions and interactions, especially those related to the tests mentioned above.

valproate sodium
Depacon

Pharmacologic class: Carboxylic acid derivative
Therapeutic class: Anticonvulsant, mood stabilizer, antimigraine agent
Pregnancy risk category D

FDA BOXED WARNING

- Drug has led to hepatic failure resulting in death. Children younger than age 2 are at considerably increased risk for fatal hepatotoxicity, especially those receiving multiple anticonvulsants, those with congenital metabolic disorders or organic brain disease, and those with severe seizure disorders accompanied by mental retardation. In this patient group, weigh benefits against risk and use drug as sole agent and with extreme caution. Above this age-group, incidence of fatal hepatotoxicity decreases considerably in progressively older patients.
- Drug can cause teratogenic effects, such as neural tube defects. Before administering to women with childbearing potential, weigh benefits against risk of fetal injury.
- Life-threatening pancreatitis has occurred in both children and adults receiving drug. Some cases were hemorrhagic, with rapid progression from initial symptoms to death.

Action
Increases level of gamma-aminobutyric acid in brain, reducing seizure activity

Pharmacokinetics
Drug distributes rapidly. Protein binding depends on concentration; it is lower in

elderly patients, chronic hepatic disease, renal impairment, and concurrent use of other drugs (such as aspirin). Conversely, valproate may displace certain protein-bound drugs (such as phenytoin, carbamazepine, warfarin, and tolbutamide). It is metabolized primarily in the liver and excreted largely in urine.

Onset	Peak	Duration
Rapid	End of 1-hr infusion	Unknown

How supplied

Solution for injection (clear, colorless): 100 mg/mL in 5-mL single-dose vial

Indications and dosages

➤ Complex partial seizures

Adults and children older than age 10: Initially, 10 to 15 mg/kg/day I.V. May increase by 5 to 10 mg/kg/day q week until blood drug level is 50 to 100 mcg/mL or adverse reactions occur; do not exceed 60 mg/kg/day. If daily dosage exceeds 250 mg, give in two divided doses.

➤ Simple and complex absence seizures

Adults and children older than age 10: Initially, 15 mg/kg/day I.V. May increase by 5 to 10 mg/kg/day at 1-week intervals until seizures are controlled or adverse reactions preclude further increases. Maximum recommended dosage is 60 mg/kg/day. Divide daily dosages above 250 mg.

Administration

Preparation

🔊 Obtain liver function tests before starting therapy.

- Give I.V. only if oral therapy is not feasible.
- Know that I.V. and P.O. dosages and dosing frequencies are identical, and patient should be switched to oral therapy as soon as possible. However, be aware that not all oral forms are bioequivalent.

Dilution and compatibility

- Dilute in at least 50 mL D_5W, lactated Ringer's solution, or normal saline solution.
- Discard unused portion.

Infusion considerations

- Infuse over 1 hour at a rate slower than 20 mg/minute.

Monitoring

🔊 Closely monitor neurologic status. Watch for seizures.

🔊 Monitor liver function tests frequently after therapy begins, especially during first 6 months.

🔊 Stay alert for nonspecific symptoms, such as malaise, weakness, lethargy, anorexia, and vomiting; these may precede serious or fatal hepatotoxicity.

🔊 Evaluate GI status. Stay alert for signs and symptoms of pancreatitis, such as abdominal pain, nausea, vomiting, and anorexia.

🔊 Discontinue drug immediately if significant hepatic dysfunction is suspected or diagnosed or if patient has signs or symptoms of pancreatitis.

- Monitor I.V. infusion site for local reactions.
- Assess CBC (including platelet count), prothrombin time, International Normalized Ratio, and liver function tests.
- Monitor drug blood level; therapeutic range is 50 to 100 mcg/mL.

Storage

- Store at room temperature of 15° to 30°C (59° to 86°F).
- Diluted solution is stable for at least 24 hours when stored in glass or polyvinyl chloride bags at controlled room temperature.

Contraindications and precautions

Contraindicated in hypersensitivity to drug or tartrazine (some products), hepatic impairment, urea cycle disorders, and pregnancy.

Use cautiously in bleeding disorders, organic brain disease, bone marrow depression, renal impairment, posttraumatic seizures caused by head injury (use not recommended), severe seizure disorders accompanied by mental retardation, congenital metabolic disorders, history of hepatic disease, patients on multiple anticonvulsants, breastfeeding patients, and ***children younger than age 2*** (safety and efficacy not established).

Adverse reactions

CNS: confusion, dizziness, headache, sedation, ataxia, paresthesia, asthenia, tremor, drowsiness, emotional lability, abnormal thinking, amnesia
EENT: amblyopia, blurred vision, nystagmus, tinnitus, pharyngitis
GI: nausea, vomiting, diarrhea, abdominal pain, dyspepsia, anorexia, **pancreatitis**
Hematologic: leukopenia, thrombocytopenia
Hepatic: hepatotoxicity
Musculoskeletal: back pain
Respiratory: dyspnea
Skin: rash, alopecia, bruising
Other: abnormal taste, increased appetite, weight gain, flulike symptoms, infection, infusion site pain and reaction.

Interactions

Drug-drug. *Activated charcoal, cholestyramine:* decreased valproate absorption
Antiplatelet agents (including abciximab, aspirin and other nonsteroidal anti-inflammatory drugs, eptifibatide, tirofiban), cefamandole, cefoperazone, cefotetan, heparin, thrombolytics, warfarin: increased risk of bleeding
Barbiturates, primidone: decreased metabolism and greater risk of toxicity of these drugs, decreased valproate efficacy
Carbamazepine: increased carbamazepine blood level, decreased valproate blood level, poor seizure control
Carbapenem antibiotics (such as meropenem): possible subtherapeutic valproate levels
Chlorpromazine: decreased valproate clearance and increased drug trough level
Cimetidine: decreased valproate clearance
Clonazepam: absence seizures in patients with history of these seizures
CNS depressants (such as antihistamines, antidepressants, monoamine oxidase inhibitors, opioid analgesics, sedative-hypnotics): additive CNS depression
Diazepam: displacement of diazepam from binding site, inhibited diazepam metabolism
Erythromycin, felbamate: increased valproate blood level, greater risk of toxicity
Ethosuximide: inhibited ethosuximide metabolism
Lamotrigine: decreased valproate blood level, increased lamotrigine blood level
Phenytoin: increased phenytoin effects and risk of toxicity, decreased valproate effects
Salicylates (large doses in children): increased valproate effects
Tricyclic antidepressants: increased blood levels of these drugs, greater risk of adverse reactions
Zidovudine: decreased zidovudine clearance in patients with HIV
Drug-diagnostic tests. *Alanine aminotransferase, alkaline phosphatase, aspartate aminotransferase, bilirubin:* increased
Bleeding time: prolonged
Ketone bodies: false-positive results
Platelets, white blood cells: decreased
Thyroid function tests: interference with results
Drug-behaviors. *Alcohol use:* additive CNS depression

Toxicity and overdose

• Overdose may lead to somnolence, heart block, and deep coma.

• In overdose, fraction of unbound drug is high; thus, hemodialysis or tandem hemodialysis plus hemoperfusion may remove significant amounts. Provide general supportive measures; pay particular attention to maintaining adequate urine output. Naloxone may reverse CNS depressant effects; however, use this drug cautiously in patients with seizures, because theoretically it could reverse anticonvulsant effect of valproate.

Patient teaching

Advise patient to immediately report malaise, weakness, lethargy, appetite loss, nausea and vomiting, yellowing of skin or eyes, and abdominal pain.

• Instruct patient using drug for seizure control to avoid driving and other hazardous activities.

Caution patient not to stop therapy abruptly.

• Advise patient to avoid alcohol.

• Stress importance of follow-up laboratory tests.

• As appropriate, review all other significant and life-threatening adverse reactions and interactions, especially those related to the drugs, tests, and behaviors mentioned above.

vancomycin hydrochloride

Vancocin

Pharmacologic class: Tricyclic glycopeptide

Therapeutic class: Anti-infective

Pregnancy risk category C

Action

Binds to bacterial cell wall, immediately inhibiting cell-wall synthesis and causing secondary damage to bacterial membrane

Pharmacokinetics

Drug appears in urine; pleural, pericardial, ascitic, synovial, and peritoneal dialysis fluids; and atrial appendage tissue. Except in meningeal inflammation, it does not readily diffuse into spinal fluid. Drug is approximately 55% serum protein–bound. Mean elimination half-life is 4 to 6 hours in patients with normal renal function. During first 24 hours, about 75% of dose is excreted in urine by glomerular filtration. Total systemic and renal clearance may be reduced in the elderly.

Onset	Peak	Duration
Immediate	Immediate	Unknown

How supplied

Powder for reconstitution for injection: 500-mg vial, 1-g vial, 5-g vial, 10 g-vial

Indications and dosages

➤ To prevent endocarditis in penicillin-allergic patients at moderate risk who are scheduled for dental and other invasive produres

Adults: 1 g I.V. slowly over 1 to 2 hours, with infusion completed 30 minutes before invasive procedure begins

Children: 20 mg/kg I.V. over 1 to 2 hours, with infusion completed 30 minutes before invasive procedure begins

➤ Severe, life-threatening infections caused by susceptible strains of methicillin-resistant staphylococci, *Staphylococcus epidermidis, Streptococcus viridans* or *Streptococcus bovis* (alone or combined with an aminoglycoside), or

Enterococcus faecalis (combined with an aminoglycoside)
Adults: 500 mg I.V. q 6 hours or 1 g I.V. q 12 hours
Children: 10 mg/kg I.V. q 6 hours
Infants and neonates: Initially, 15 mg/kg I.V., followed by 10 mg/kg I.V. q 8 hours in infants 8 days to 1 month old or 10 mg/kg I.V. q 12 hours in infants less than 8 days old

Dosage adjustment

- Adjust dosage in impaired renal function according to the table below. However, know that initial dosage should not be less than 15 mg/kg, even in patients with mild to moderate renal insufficiency.

Creatinine clearance (mL/min)	Vancomycin dosage (mg/24 hr)
100	1,545
90	1,390
80	1,235
70	1,080
60	925
50	770
40	620
30	465
20	310
10	155

- Know that premature infants may require greater dosage reductions because of decreased renal function.

Off-label uses

- Febrile neutropenia
- Meningitis
- Peritonitis

Administration

Preparation

Know that I.V. therapy is ineffective against enterocolitis and pseudomembranous diarrhea.

Keep emergency equipment and epinephrine on hand in case of anaphylaxis.

- Perform baseline hearing test before and during therapy.

Dilution and compatibility

- Dilute by adding 10 or 20 mL sterile water for injection to vial containing 500 mg or 1 g drug, respectively, to yield a concentration of 50 mg/mL. Dilute further by adding at least 100 mL or 200 mL, respectively, of D_5W or normal saline solution.
- Know that reconstituted solution should be clear.

Infusion considerations

Do not give by I.M. route.

- Administer by intermittent I.V. infusion over at least 1 hour.

Monitoring

Monitor closely for signs and symptoms of hypersensitivity reactions, including anaphylaxis.

Monitor vital signs and cardiovascular status, especially for vascular collapse and other signs of impending cardiac arrest.

- Monitor drug blood level weekly. Therapeutic peak levels range from 30 to 40 g/L; therapeutic trough levels, from 5 to 10 mg/L.
- Assess blood urea nitrogen (BUN) and creatinine levels every 2 days, or daily in patients with unstable renal function.
- Monitor urine output daily. Weigh patient at least weekly.
- Assess hearing during therapy; stay alert for hearing loss. Patient may require weekly audiograms.
- Check I.V. site often for phlebitis.

• Watch for "red-man" syndrome, a nonallergic histamine reaction caused by rapid I.V. infusion. Signs and symptoms include hypotension, pruritus, and maculopapular rash on face, neck, trunk, and limbs.
• Monitor CBC. Watch for signs and symptoms of blood dyscrasias.
• Closely monitor respiratory status. Stay alert for wheezing and dyspnea.

Storage

• Store vials at controlled room temperature of 15° to 30°C (59° to 86°F).
• Diluted solution may be refrigerated for 14 days without significant potency loss.

Contraindications and precautions

Contraindicated in hypersensitivity to drug.

Use cautiously in renal impairment; preexisting hearing loss; concurrent use of anesthetics, immunosuppressants, or nephrotoxic or ototoxic drugs; ***elderly patients;*** pregnant or breastfeeding patients; and ***neonates.***

Adverse reactions

CV: hypotension, **cardiac arrest, vascular collapse**
EENT: permanent hearing loss, ototoxicity, tinnitus
GI: nausea, vomiting, **pseudomembranous colitis**
GU: nephrotoxicity, severe uremia
Hematologic: eosinophilia, **leukopenia, neutropenia**
Respiratory: wheezing, dyspnea
Skin: "red man" syndrome, rash, urticaria, pruritus, necrosis
Other: chills, fever, thrombophlebitis at injection site, **anaphylaxis**

Interactions

Drug-drug. *Aminoglycosides, amphotericin B, bacitracin, cephalosporins, cisplatin, colistin, nondepolarizing neuromuscular blockers, pentamidine:* increased risk of nephrotoxicity and ototoxicity
Warfarin: increased risk of bleeding
Drug-diagnostic tests. *Albumin, BUN, creatinine:* increased
Eosinophils, neutrophils: decreased

Toxicity and overdose

• In overdose, expect extension of pharmacologic effects and adverse reactions.
• Provide supportive care. Although hemodialysis and peritoneal dialysis do not remove drug, hemoperfusion and hemofiltration may be beneficial.

Patient teaching

• Explain importance of prophylactic I.V. therapy to patients scheduled for invasive procedures who are at risk for endocarditis.
[Clinical alert] Advise patient to promptly report rash, hearing loss, breathing problems, and signs and symptoms of "red-man" syndrome, nephrotoxicity, and blood dyscrasias.
• As appropriate, review all other significant and life-threatening adverse reactions and interactions, especially those related to the drugs and tests mentioned above.

vecuronium bromide

Norcuron (Canada)

Pharmacologic class: Nondepolarizing neuromuscular blocker (intermediate-acting)
Therapeutic class: Muscle relaxant
Pregnancy risk category C

FDA BOXED WARNING

• Drug should be given by adequately trained clinicians who are familiar with its actions, characteristics, and hazards.

Action

Inhibits neuromuscular depolarization by preventing acetylcholine from binding to motor end-plate receptors

Pharmacokinetics

At dosages of 0.04 to 0.1 mg/kg, drug is 60% to 80% bound to plasma protein. After single I.V. dose, distribution half-life is approximately 4 minutes. Elimination half-life over same dosage range is approximately 65 to 75 minutes in healthy surgical patients and in renal-failure patients undergoing transplant surgery. From 3% to 35% of dose appears in urine within 24 hours; 25% to 50% may be excreted in bile within 42 hours.

Onset	Peak	Duration
1 min	3-5 min	15-25 min

How supplied

Powder for reconstitution for injection (freeze-dried): 10-mg and 20-mg single-use vials

Indications and dosages

➢ Adjunct to anesthesia to aid endotracheal intubation and relax skeletal muscles during surgery or mechanical ventilation

Adults and children older than age 10: Initially, 0.08 to 0.1 mg/kg by I.V. bolus. During prolonged surgery, give maintenance dose of 0.01 to 0.015 mg/kg by continuous I.V. infusion within 25 to 40 minutes of initial dose. In patients receiving balanced anesthesia, maintenance dose may be given q 12 to 15 minutes.

Administration

Preparation

Initiate infusion only after early evidence of spontaneous recovery from bolus dose.

Make sure patient's analgesic and sedative needs are met, as drug does not relieve pain or provide sedation.

Dilution and compatibility

- Reconstitute by adding supplied bacteriostatic water for injection to yield a concentration of 1 mg/mL. For continuous I.V. infusion, dilute further with sterile water for injection, D_5W, normal saline solution, or lactated Ringer's solution.
- Use within 24 hours of dilution.
- Discard unused portion.

Infusion considerations

- Give I.V. bolus over 1 to 2 minutes.
- For maintenance infusion, adjust administration rate according to twitch response, as determined by peripheral nerve stimulation. Initial rate of 1 mcg/kg/minute is recommended, with rate adjusted to maintain 90% suppression of twitch response. Average infusion rates range from 0.8 to 1.2 mcg/kg/minute.
- Deliver continuous infusion using an infusion control device.

Monitoring

- Monitor heart rhythm, blood pressure, and pulse oximetry during and after administration.
- Assess sedation level.
- Monitor fluid intake and output, and measure temperature.
- Evaluate muscle recovery using peripheral nerve stimulator and train-of-four monitoring.

Storage

- Store at 15° to 25°C (59° to 77°F), protected from light.
- When reconstituted with bacteriostatic water for injection, use within 5 days.

Solution may be stored at room temperature or refrigerated.
• When reconstituted with sterile water for injection or other compatible I.V. solution, refrigerate vial and use within 24 hours.

Contraindications and precautions

Contraindicated in hypersensitivity to drug or other bromides.

Use cautiously in neuromuscular, respiratory, hepatic, or cardiac disease; edema; severe obesity; dehydration; electrolyte imbalance; ***elderly patients;*** pregnant or breastfeeding patients; and ***infants.***

Adverse reactions

CNS: musculoskeletal paralysis or weakness
Respiratory: respiratory paralysis, **prolonged apnea**
Other: anaphylaxis

Interactions

Drug-drug. *Aminoglycosides, anticholinesterases, general anesthetics, opioid analgesics, polymyxin anti-infectives:* enhanced neuromuscular blockade
Carbamazepine: decreased vecuronium duration
Fosphenytoin, phenytoin: altered vecuronium efficacy
Nicardipine, procainamide, verapamil: excessive neuromuscular blockade
Nitrous oxide: vecuronium toxicity
Drug-herb. *St. John's wort:* increased risk of cardiovascular collapse or delayed emergence from anesthesia

Toxicity and overdose

• Expect excessive doses to produce enhanced pharmacologic effects. Residual neuromuscular blockade beyond time required may manifest as skeletal muscle weakness, decreased respiratory reserve, low tidal volume, or apnea. However, keep in mind that respiratory depression may result wholly or partly from other drugs used for general anesthesia (such as opioids, thiobarbiturates, and other CNS depressants).
• Maintain patent airway and provide manual or mechanical ventilation, as ordered, until complete recovery of normal respiration is assured. If ordered, administer pyridostigmine bromide injection, neostigmine, or edrophonium in conjunction with atropine or glycopyrrolate to antagonize vecuronium's skeletal-muscle relaxant action; adequate skeletal muscle tone and respiration indicate satisfactory reversal. Peripheral nerve stimulator may be used to monitor twitch height restoration or to assess degree of residual neuromuscular blockade from other causes of decreased respiratory reserve. Failure of prompt reversal (within 30 minutes) may occur in extreme debilitation, carcinomatosis, or concomitant use of certain broad-spectrum antibiotics, anesthetics, and other drugs that enhance neuromuscular blockade or cause respiratory depression. In this case, management resembles that used for prolonged neuromuscular blockade. Support ventilation by artificial means until patient resumes respiratory control. Before giving reversal agent, see package insert for that agent. Effects of dialysis on drug removal are unknown.

Patient teaching

• Explain all procedures while patient's hearing is still intact.
• As appropriate, review all significant and life-threatening adverse reactions and interactions, especially those related to the drugs and herbs mentioned above.

verapamil hydrochloride

Isoptin

Pharmacologic class: Calcium channel blocker
Therapeutic class: Antianginal, antiarrhythmic (class IV), antihypertensive
Pregnancy risk category C

Action

Decreases conduction of sinoatrial and atrioventricular (AV) nodes by inhibiting calcium influx into cardiac and vascular smooth muscle cells, inhibiting excitatory contraction. These effects prolong AV node refractoriness and decrease myocardial oxygen consumption.

Pharmacokinetics

Drug crosses placental barrier, is metabolized in the liver, and is largely protein-bound. It is secreted in breast milk and excreted in urine as unchanged drug and metabolite, with some excretion in feces.

Onset	Peak	Duration
Immediate	3-5 min	2 hr

How supplied

Solution for injection: 2.5 mg/mL in 2- and 4-mL vials, ampules, and syringes

Indications and dosages

➤ Rapid conversion of paroxysmal supraventricular tachycardia to sinus rhythm; temporary control of rapid ventricular rate in atrial flutter or fibrillation

Adults: 5 to 10 mg (0.075 to 0.15 mg/kg) I.V. bolus over 2 minutes; may give additional 10 mg after 30 minutes if response is inadequate

Children ages 1 to 15: 0.1 to 0.3 mg/kg (usual single-dose range, 2 to 5 mg) as I.V. bolus over at least 2 minutes. Do not exceed 5 mg; may give additional dose after 30 minutes if response is inadequate

Children younger than age 1: 0.1 to 0.2 mg/kg (usual single-dose range, 0.75 to 2 mg) as I.V. bolus over at least 2 minutes with continuous ECG monitoring

Off-label uses

- Neurogenic bladder
- Premature labor
- Ventricular tachycardia

Administration

Preparation

Discontinue disopyramide 48 hours before starting verapamil. Do not restart disopyramide for at least 24 hours after verapamil therapy ends.

Keep resuscitative equipment available in case of life-threatening adverse reaction, such as severe hypotension or extreme bradycardia.

Dilution and compatibility

- Know that drug may be given undiluted, but is compatible with most large-volume I.V. solutions.

Do not mix with albumin, amphotericin B, hydralazine, aminophylline, or trimethoprim-sulfamethoxazole.

Do not mix with sodium lactate injection in polyvinyl chloride bags.

Know that mixing or administering through same line with sodium bicarbonate, nafcillin, or any solution with pH above 6 causes precipitation.

- Discard unused solution.

Infusion considerations

Give by slow I.V. injection over at least 2 minutes (3 minutes for elderly patients) while monitoring ECG and blood pressure.

Monitoring

Watch closely for signs and symptoms of heart failure.

Monitor for signs and symptoms of erythema multiforme (fever, rash, sore throat, mouth sores, cough, and iris lesions). Report early indications immediately, before condition can progress to Stevens-Johnson syndrome.
- Assess CBC. Watch for blood dyscrasias.
- Monitor blood glucose level. Stay alert for hyperglycemia in diabetic patients.

Storage
- Store at room temperature of 15° to 30°C (59° to 86°F); protect from light.
- Know that drug is stable in most large-volume I.V. solutions for 24 hours at 25°C (77°F).

Contraindications and precautions

Contraindicated in hypersensitivity to drug or other calcium channel blockers, sick sinus syndrome, second- or third-degree AV block (unless patient has artificial pacemaker), hypotension, heart failure, severe ventricular dysfunction, cardiogenic shock (except when associated with supraventricular tachycardias), and atrial flutter or atrial fibrillation associated with accessory bypass tracts (such as Wolff-Parkinson-White or Lown-Ganong-Levine syndrome).

Use cautiously in renal or severe hepatic impairment, first-degree AV block, idiopathic hypertrophic cardiomyopathy, neuromuscular transmission defects (such as Duchenne's muscular dystrophy), respiratory depression, digital ulcers, ischemia, gangrene, concurrent digoxin therapy, ***elderly patients,*** and pregnant or breastfeeding patients.

Adverse reactions

CNS: anxiety, confusion, dizziness, light-headedness, syncope, drowsiness, headache, jitteriness, abnormal dreams, disturbed equilibrium, psychiatric disturbances, asthenia, paresthesia, tremor, fatigue
CV: chest pain, hypotension, palpitations, peripheral edema, tachycardia, **arrhythmias, heart failure, bradycardia, AV block**
EENT: blurred vision, epistaxis, tinnitus
GI: nausea, vomiting, diarrhea, constipation, dyspepsia, dry mouth, anorexia
GU: dysuria, urinary frequency, nocturia, polyuria, sexual dysfunction, gynecomastia
Hematologic: anemia, **leukopenia, thrombocytopenia**
Metabolic: hyperglycemia
Musculoskeletal: joint stiffness, muscle cramps
Respiratory: cough, dyspnea, shortness of breath, **pulmonary edema**
Skin: dermatitis, flushing, diaphoresis, photosensitivity, pruritus, urticaria, rash, **erythema multiforme**
Other: gingival hyperplasia, edema, weight gain, **Stevens-Johnson syndrome**

Interactions

Drug-drug. *Antihypertensives:* additive hypotension
Aspirin: increased risk of bleeding
Beta-adrenergic blockers, other antiarrhythmics: additive cardiovascular adverse reactions
Carbamazepine, cyclosporine: increased blood levels of these drugs
CYP450-3A4 inducers (such as rifampin): decreased verapamil blood level
CYP450-3A4 inhibitors (such as erythromycin, ritonavir): increased verapamil blood level
Digoxin: increased digoxin blood level, greater risk of toxicity
Lithium: increased or decreased lithium blood level
Neuromuscular blockers (succinylcholine, tubocurarine, vecuronium): prolonged neuromuscular blockade
Simvastatin: increased risk of myopathy

V

Theophylline: decreased verapamil clearance, increased blood level, and possible toxicity
Drug-diagnostic tests. *Alanine aminotransferase, alkaline phosphatase, aspartate aminotransferase, blood urea nitrogen, glucose, lactate dehydrogenase:* increased
Granulocytes: decreased
Drug-foods. *Coffee, tea:* increased caffeine blood level
Grapefruit juice: increased verapamil blood level and effects
Drug-herb. *Black catechu:* increased drug effects
Cola nut, guarana: increased caffeine blood level
Ephedra (ma huang), St. John's wort: reduced hypotensive effect of verapamil
Yerba maté: decreased yerba maté clearance
Drug-behaviors. *Alcohol use:* additive hypotension

Toxicity and overdose

- Overdose may cause pronounced hypotension, bradycardia, and conduction system abnormalities (arrhythmias, junctional rhythm with AV dissociation, and high-degree AV block, including asystole). Other signs and symptoms (metabolic acidosis, hyperglycemia, hyperkalemia, renal dysfunction, decreased mental status, and seizures) may result from hypoperfusion. Noncardiogenic pulmonary edema may develop with major overdose (up to approximately 9 g).
- No specific antidote exists. Provide supportive therapy, including beta-adrenergics or parenteral administration of calcium solutions to increase calcium ion flux across slow channel. For significant hypotension or high-degree AV block, use vasopressors or cardiac pacing, respectively, as ordered. For asystole, provide cardiopulmonary resuscitation and other measures as needed. Hemodialysis does not remove drug.

Patient teaching

- As appropriate, review all significant and life-threatening adverse reactions and interactions, especially those related to the drugs, tests, foods, herbs, and behaviors mentioned above.

vinblastine sulfate (VLB)

Velbe ❁

Pharmacologic class: Vinca alkaloid
Therapeutic class: Antineoplastic
Pregnancy risk category D

FDA BOXED WARNING

- Drug should be administered only by individuals experienced in giving it. ***Make sure needle is positioned properly in vein before injecting drug.*** Leakage into surrounding tissue during I.V. administration may cause considerable irritation. If it does, discontinue injection immediately and inject remaining portion of dose into another vein. To treat extravasation, give local injection of hyaluronidase and apply moderate heat to affected area.
- Drug is fatal if given intrathecally. Administer I.V. only.

Action

Arrests mitosis and blocks cell division, interfering with nucleic acid synthesis. Cell-cycle-phase specific.

Pharmacokinetics

Drug distributes widely and is metabolized primarily in the liver to active metabolite. Elimination half-life is approximately 20 hours. Excretion is predominantly through bile.

Onset	Peak	Duration
Unknown	Unknown	Unknown

How supplied

Powder for reconstitution for injection (lyophilized): 10-mg vial

Indications and dosages

➢ Hodgkin's disease; advanced testicular cancer; lymphoma; AIDS-related Kaposi's sarcoma; bladder cancer; renal cancer; non-small-cell lung cancer; melanoma; breast cancer; choriocarcinoma; histiocytosis X; mycosis fungoides

Adults: 3.7 mg/m^2 I.V. weekly; may increase to a maximum of 18.5 mg/m^2 I.V. weekly based on response. Withhold weekly dose if white blood cell (WBC) count is less than 4,000/mm^3. May increase dosage in increments of 1.8 mg/m^2 if needed, but not after WBC count drops to approximately 3,000/mm^3.

Dosage adjustment

- Reduce dosage 50% in hepatic impairment (direct serum bilirubin level above 3 mg/dL).

Off-label uses

- Cervical and head and neck cancer
- Germ cell tumors

Administration

Preparation

Follow facility protocol for handling and preparing chemotherapeutic drugs. Take special care to avoid eye contamination.

- As ordered, premedicate with antiemetic.

Dilution and compatibility

- Reconstitute powder in 10-mg vial with 10 mL normal saline solution for injection to a concentration of 1 mg/mL.

Infusion considerations

Give by I.V. route only.

- Inject I.V. dose into tubing of running I.V. line, or inject directly into vein over about 1 minute.

Avoid extravasation, which may cause tissue necrosis. If extravasation occurs, stop injection, inject hyaluronidase locally, and apply moderate heat.

Monitoring

Assess respiratory status closely. Drug may cause acute shortness of breath and bronchospasm, especially in patients who previously received mitomycin.

- Monitor blood pressure.
- Assess CBC. Stay alert for signs and symptoms of infection.
- Monitor closely for numbness and tingling of hands or feet and other adverse reactions.

Storage

- Refrigerate unopened vials at 2° to 8°C (36° to 46°F).
- Refrigerate reconstituted solution and protect from light; discard after 28 days.

Contraindications and precautions

Contraindicated in hypersensitivity to drug, significant granulocytopenia from causes other than disease being treated, uncontrolled bacterial infections, intrathecal use, and ***elderly patients*** with cachexia or skin ulcers.

Use cautiously in hepatic or pulmonary dysfunction, renal disease with hypertension, malignant-cell infiltration of bone marrow, neuromuscular disease, females with childbearing potential, and pregnant or breastfeeding patients (use not recommended).

V

Adverse reactions

CNS: headache, malaise, depression, paresthesia, loss of deep-tendon reflexes, peripheral neuropathy and neuritis, **cerebrovascular accident, seizures**
CV: hypertension, tachycardia, **myocardial infarction**
EENT: pharyngitis
GI: nausea, vomiting, diarrhea, constipation, bleeding ulcer, abdominal pain, stomatitis, anorexia, **paralytic ileus**
GU: aspermia
Hematologic: anemia, **thrombocytopenia, leukopenia**
Metabolic: hyperuricemia, **syndrome of inappropriate antidiuretic hormone secretion** (SIADH)
Musculoskeletal: bone pain, muscle pain and weakness
Respiratory: shortness of breath, **acute bronchospasm, pulmonary infiltrates**
Skin: alopecia, skin irritation
Other: weight loss; jaw pain; tumor-site pain; phlebitis, cellulitis, and sloughing at I.V. site; tissue necrosis (with extravasation)

Interactions

Drug-drug. *Erythromycin, other CYP450 inhibitors:* increased vinblastine toxicity
Mitomycin: increased risk of bronchospasm and shortness of breath
Phenytoin: decreased phenytoin blood level

Toxicity and overdose

- Overdose may lead to potentially life-threatening myelosuppression as well as stomatitis, paresthesia, and SIADH. Toxicity may increase in patients with hepatic insufficiency (as drug is excreted mainly through biliary system).
- No specific antidote exists. Provide supportive measures, including those that prevent SIADH effects, such as fluid restriction, diuretics and anticonvulsants (if ordered), GI decompression to prevent ileus, cardiovascular monitoring, and monitoring of daily blood counts for guidance in transfusion requirements and assessing infection risk. Protect airway and support ventilation and perfusion. Meticulously monitor and maintain vital signs, blood gases, and electrolytes within acceptable limits. Dialysis is unlikely to be helpful.

Patient teaching

- Explain drug therapy to patient. Stress importance of follow-up laboratory tests.
- Advise patient to promptly report signs and symptoms of infection and to take temperature daily.
- Inform patient that drug may cause pain over tumor site.
- Instruct female with childbearing potential to avoid pregnancy. Caution her not to breastfeed during therapy.
- Encourage patient to practice good oral hygiene to help prevent infected mouth sores.
- Inform patient that hair loss is a common side effect but typically reverses after treatment ends.
- As appropriate, review all other significant and life-threatening adverse reactions and interactions, especially those related to the drugs mentioned above.

vincristine sulfate (VCR)

Oncovin ❋, Vincasar PFS

Pharmacologic class: Vinca alkaloid
Therapeutic class: Antineoplastic
Pregnancy risk category D

FDA BOXED WARNING

- Drug should be administered only by clinicians experienced in giving it. ***Make sure needle is positioned properly in vein***

before injecting drug. Leakage into surrounding tissue during I.V. administration may cause considerable irritation. If it does, discontinue injection immediately and inject remaining portion of dose into another vein. To treat extravasation, administer local injection of hyaluronidase and apply moderate heat to affected area.
• Drug is fatal if given intrathecally. Give I.V. only.

Action

Unclear. Thought to block cell division and interfere with synthesis of nucleic acid. Cell-cycle-phase specific.

Pharmacokinetics

Drug distributes rapidly and widely throughout the body, except in cerebrospional fluid. It is partially metabolized in the liver by P4503A cytochromes. Initial, middle, and terminal half-lives are 5 minutes, 2.3 hours, and 85 hours, respectively; however, terminal half-life ranges from 19 to 155 hours. Parent drug and metabolites are excreted primarily in bile and feces.

Onset	Peak	Duration
Unknown	4 days	7 days

How supplied

Solution for injection: 1 mg/mL in 1- and 2-mL vials

Indications and dosages

➢ Acute leukemia

Adults: 0.4 to 1.4 mg/m^2 I.V. weekly, not to exceed 2 mg/dose. (Dosages above 2 mg may be given depending on patient, physician, protocol, and facility.)
Children weighing more than 10 kg (22 lb): 2 mg/m^2 I.V. weekly
Children weighing 10 kg or less: 0.05 mg/kg I.V. weekly

Dosage adjustment

• Reduce dosage by 50% in hepatic impairment (direct serum bilirubin level above 3 mg/dL).

Off-label uses

• Brain, hepatic, ovarian, testicular, and other cancers
• Idiopathic thrombocytopenic purpura
• Kaposi's sarcoma
• Neuroblastoma

Administration

Preparation

Follow hazardous drug guidelines on page S19 for handling, preparation, and administration.
• Know that drug may be used with other antineoplastics for some diseases.
• As ordered, premedicate patient with antiemetic.

Dilution and compatibility

• Be aware that drug is compatible with normal saline solution and D_5W. Do not mix with other solutions.

Infusion considerations

Give by I.V. route only.
• Inject I.V. dose into tubing of running I.V. line with normal saline solution or D_5W, or inject directly into vein over about 1 minute.
Avoid extravasation, which may cause tissue necrosis. If extravasation occurs, stop injection, inject hyaluronidase locally, and apply moderate heat.

Monitoring

Assess respiratory status. Injection may cause bronchospasm, especially in patients who previously received mitomycin.
• Monitor blood pressure.
• Evaluate neurologic status. Know that neurotoxicity is a dose-limiting adverse reaction. Monitor closely for numbness and tingling of hands or feet and other adverse reactions.

V

• Monitor CBC, including platelet count. Watch for signs and symptoms of blood dyscrasias.
• Stay alert for signs and symptoms of infection.

Storage

• Refrigerate unopened vials at 2° to 8°C (36° to 46°F).
• Refrigerate reconstituted solution and protect from light; discard after 28 days.

Contraindications and precautions

Contraindicated in hypersensitivity to drug, demyelinating form of Charcot-Marie-Tooth disease, and intrathecal use.

Use cautiously in decreased bone marrow reserve, infection, hepatic impairment, acute uric acid nephropathy, neuromuscular disease, pulmonary dysfunction, other chronic debilitating illnesses, females with childbearing potential, and pregnant or breastfeeding patients (use not recommended).

Adverse reactions

CNS: agitation, insomnia, depression, mental status changes, ascending peripheral neuropathy, transient cortical blindness, **seizures, coma**
EENT: diplopia
GI: nausea, vomiting, constipation, abdominal cramps, stomatitis, anorexia, **paralytic ileus**
GU: nocturia, urine retention, gonadal suppression, **oliguria**
Hematologic: anemia, **leukopenia, thrombocytopenia** (mild and brief)
Metabolic: hyperuricemia, **syndrome of inappropriate antidiuretic hormone secretion (SIADH)**
Respiratory: bronchospasm
Skin: alopecia
Other: tissue necrosis (with extravasation), phlebitis at I.V. site

Interactions

Drug-drug. *Asparaginase:* decreased hepatic metabolism of vincristine
Live-virus vaccines: decreased antibody response to vaccine, increased risk of adverse reactions
Mitomycin: increased risk of bronchospasm and shortness of breath
Drug-diagnostic tests. *Platelets:* increased or decreased
Uric acid: increased
White blood cells: decreased (slight leukopenia) 4 days after therapy, resolving within 7 days

Toxicity and overdose

• Higher-than-recommended dosages can cause exaggerated adverse effects. In children younger than age 13, death has occurred from doses 10 times those recommended. Severe symptoms may occur in this patient group after dosages of 3 to 4 mg/m^2. In adults, expect severe signs and symptoms after single doses of 3 mg/m^2 or more. Patients with hepatic disease severe enough to decrease biliary excretion may experience more severe adverse effects.
• No specific antidote exists. Provide supportive measures, including those that prevent SIADH effects, such as fluid restriction, diuretics and anticonvulsants (if ordered), GI decompression to prevent ileus, cardiovascular monitoring, and monitoring of daily blood counts for guidance in transfusion requirements and assessing infection risk. Protect airway and support ventilation and perfusion. Meticulously monitor and maintain vital signs, blood gases, and electrolytes within acceptable limits. Dialysis is unlikely to be helpful.

Patient teaching

• Explain drug therapy to patient. Stress importance of follow-up laboratory tests.

• Advise patient to promptly report signs and symptoms of infection and to take temperature daily.
• Teach patient to practice good oral hygiene, to help prevent infected mouth sores.
• Instruct female with childbearing potential to avoid pregnancy. Caution her not to breastfeed during therapy.
• Tell patient hair loss is a common side effect but typically reverses once treatment ends.
• As appropriate, review all other significant and life-threatening adverse reactions and interactions, especially those related to the drugs and tests mentioned above.

vinorelbine tartrate

Navelbine

Pharmacologic class: Vinca alkaloid
Therapeutic class: Antineoplastic
Pregnancy risk category D

FDA BOXED WARNING

• Give under supervision of physician experienced in use of cancer chemotherapy, in facility with adequate diagnostic and treatment resources.
• ***Product is for I.V. use only.*** Intrathecal administration of other vinca alkaloids has resulted in death. Syringes containing this product should be labeled "WARNING. FOR I.V. USE ONLY. FATAL IF GIVEN INTRATHECALLY."
• Severe granulocytopenia causing increased susceptibility to infection may occur. Before starting drug, patient's granulocyte count should be at least 1,000/mm³. Adjust dosage according to CBCs with differentials obtained on day of treatment.
• ***Make sure I.V. needle or catheter is properly positioned before injecting drug.*** Administration may lead to extravasation, causing local tissue necrosis and thrombophlebitis.

Action

Blocks cell division and interferes with nucleic acid synthesis. Cell-cycle-phase specific.

Pharmacokinetics

Drug concentration in plasma decays in triphasic manner. Initial rapid decline primarily represents distribution to peripheral compartments, followed by metabolism (by hepatic CYP450 isoenzymes) and excretion during subsequent phases. Prolonged terminal-phase half-life (27.7 to 43.6 hours) results from relatively slow efflux from peripheral compartments. Drug is highly bound to platelets and lymphocytes. It is metabolized in the liver; elimination half-life is approximately 24 hours. It is excreted predominantly through bile.

Onset	Peak	Duration
Unknown	7-10 days	7-15 days

How supplied

Solution for injection (clear, colorless to pale yellow): 10 mg/mL in 1-mL and 5-mL vials

Indications and dosages

➤ Inoperable non-small-cell lung cancer

Adults: As monotherapy, 30 mg/m² I.V. weekly given over 6 to 10 minutes. In combination therapy, 25 mg/m² weekly given with cisplatin q 4 weeks. Alternatively, in combination therapy, 30 mg/m² I.V. given with cisplatin on days 1 and 29, then q 6 weeks.

V

Dosage adjustment

• In patients who develop hyperbilirubinemia during treatment, adjust dosage based on hepatic insufficiency as shown in the table below:

Total bilirubin level (mg/dL)	Percentage of starting dosage to give
2 or lower	100%
2.1 to 3	50%
Above 3	25%

• Adjust dosage according to hematologic toxicity as shown in the table below:

Granulocyte count on treatment day (cells/mm^3)	Percentage of starting dosage to give
1,500 or higher	100%
1,000 to 1,499	50%
Below 1,000	Do not administer. Repeat granulocyte count in 1 week. If three consecutive weekly doses are withheld because granulocyte count is below 1,000/mm^3, discontinue drug.

• For patients who experience fever, sepsis, or both during vinorelbine therapy while granulocytopenic or who have had two consecutive weekly doses withheld due to granulocytopenia, adjust subsequent dosage as shown in the table below:

Granulocyte count on day of treatment (cells/mm^3)	Percentage of starting dosage to give
1,500 or higher	75%
1,000 to 1,499	37.5%
Below 1,000	Do not administer. Repeat granulocyte count in 1 week. If three consecutive weekly doses are withheld because granulocyte count is below 1,000/mm^3, discontinue drug.

• For patients with both hepatic insufficiency and hematologic toxicity, administer lower of dosages based on corresponding starting dosage determined from the three tables above.

• If neurotoxicity of grade 2 or higher develops, discontinue drug.

Off-label uses

• Cervical, breast, or ovarian cancer

Administration

Preparation

Follow hazardous drug guidelines on page S19 for handling, preparation, and administration.

• As ordered, premedicate patient with antiemetic.

Dilution and compatibility

• Dilute drug in syringe with D_5W for injection or normal saline solution for injection to yield a concentration of 1.5 to 3 mg/mL.

• Dilute in I.V. bag with D_5W for injection, normal saline solution for injection, 0.45% sodium chloride injection, 5% dextrose and 0.45% sodium chloride injection, Ringer's injection, or lactated Ringer's injection to yield a concentration of 0.5 to 2 mg/mL.

• Discard solution if other than clear, colorless to pale yellow.

Infusion considerations

Give by I.V. route only.

• Administer into side port of free-flowing I.V. closest to I.V. bag or directly into large vein over 6 to 10 minutes.

• Immediately after injection, flush line with 75 to 125 mL of compatible I.V. solution.

Avoid extravasation, which may cause tissue necrosis. If extravasation occurs, immediately stop injection and administer in another vein.

Monitoring

- Monitor CBC with white cell differential (including platelet count) frequently for signs of myelosuppression during and after therapy.
- Monitor vital signs closely.
- Assess liver function tests.
- Watch for signs and symptoms of infection.
- Check closely for new or worsening signs and symptoms of neuropathy if patient has history of or preexisting neuropathy (regardless of cause).

Be aware that "radiation recall" (severe skin reaction resembling severe sunburn) may occur if drug is given to patient who has received radiation therapy.

Monitor GI function closely. Be aware that drug may cause severe constipation, paralytic ileus, intestinal obstruction, necrosis, or perforation, which may be fatal.

Closely monitor neurologic and respiratory status. Drug may cause acute pulmonary changes, including potentially fatal interstitial pulmonary changes and acute respiratory distress syndrome, especially in patients who previously received mitomycin.

Storage

- Refrigerate unopened vials in carton at 2° to 8°C (36° to 46°F). Protect from light; do not freeze. Unopened vials are stable at temperatures up to 25°C (77°F) for up to 72 hours.
- Know that diluted drug may be used for up to 24 hours under normal room lighting when stored in polypropylene syringes or polyvinyl chloride bags at 5° to 30°C (41° to 86°F).

Contraindications and precautions

Contraindicated in hypersensitivity to drug and in pretreatment granulocyte count below 1,000/mm^3.

Use cautiously in hepatic impairment, decreased bone marrow reserve, current or previous neuropathy, history of radiation therapy, females with childbearing potential, pregnant or breastfeeding patients (use not recommended), and ***children*** (safety not established).

Adverse reactions

CNS: fatigue, **neurotoxicity**
CV: chest pain, phlebitis
GI: nausea, vomiting, diarrhea, constipation, abdominal pain, anorexia, **pancreatitis, intestinal obstruction, paralytic ileus**
Hematologic: anemia, **bone marrow depression, severe granulocytopenia, neutropenia, thrombocytopenia**
Metabolic: hyponatremia
Musculoskeletal: joint, back, or jaw pain; myalgia
Respiratory: acute respiratory distress syndrome, acute shortness of breath, bronchospasm, interstitial pulmonary changes
Skin: alopecia, rash, skin reactions
Other: tumor site pain; irritation, pain, and phlebitis at I.V. site; "radiation recall," **sepsis**

Interactions

Drug-drug. *Cisplatin, other antineoplastics:* increased risk and severity of bone marrow depression
Mitomycin: increased risk of acute pulmonary reaction
Drug-diagnostic tests. *Bilirubin, hepatic enzymes, liver function tests:* increased
Granulocytes, hemoglobin, platelets, white blood cells: decreased

V

Toxicity and overdose

- Overdose may lead to death or may cause bone marrow aplasia, sepsis, paresis, paralytic ileus, stomatitis, and esophagitis.

- No known antidote exists. Provide general supportive measures, including blood transfusions, growth factors, and anti-infectives, as indicated and ordered.

Patient teaching

- Explain drug therapy to patient. Stress importance of follow-up laboratory tests.
- Advise patient to promptly report signs and symptoms of infection (such as fever or chills) and to take temperature daily.
- Tell patient to report increased shortness of breath, cough, or other new pulmonary symptoms, as well as abdominal pain or constipation.
- Tell patient hair loss is a common side effect but typically reverses once treatment ends.
- Instruct female with childbearing potential to avoid pregnancy. Caution her not to breastfeed during therapy.
- Advise patient to practice good oral hygiene, to help prevent infected mouth sores.
- As appropriate, review all other significant and life-threatening adverse reactions and interactions, especially those related to the drugs and tests mentioned above.

voriconazole

Vfend I.V.

Pharmacologic class: Triazole
Therapeutic class: Antifungal
Pregnancy risk category D

Action

Inhibits fungal cytochrome P450–mediated 14-alpha-lanosterol demethylation, preventing fungal biosynthesis and inactivating fungal cell

Pharmacokinetics

Drug is distributed extensively to tissues and metabolized by hepatic CYP450 enzymes CYP2C19, CYP2C9, and CYP3A4. Major metabolite (N-oxide) has minimal antifungal activity. Plasma-protein binding is about 58% and does not depend on plasma concentration; also, varying degrees of hepatic and renal insufficiency do not affect protein binding. Less than 2% of dose is excreted unchanged in urine.

Onset	Peak	Duration
Start of infusion	Unknown	Unknown

How supplied

Powder for reconstitution for injection (white to light-colored, lyophilized): 200 mg in single-use vials

Indications and dosages

➤ Invasive aspergillosis; serious fungal infections caused by *Scedosporium apiospermum* and *Fusarium* species

Adults and children older than age 12: Initially, 6 mg/kg I.V. q 12 hours for two doses (each dose infused over 1 to 2 hours), followed by a maintenance dose of 4 mg/kg I.V. q 12 hours given no faster than 3 mg/kg/hour. Change to oral dosing when patient can tolerate it.

➤ Candidemia and other serious *Candida* infections, such as disseminated skin infections and infections of abdomen, kidney, bladder wall, and wounds

Adults and children older than age 12: Initially, 6 mg/kg I.V. q 12 hours as an I.V. infusion for first 24 hours (day 1), followed by 3 to 4 mg/kg as I.V. infusion q 12 hours for at least 14 days and at least 7 days after symptoms resolve. Base dosage on infection nature and severity. If patient cannot tolerate 4 mg/kg I.V., reduce maintenance dosage to 3 mg/kg I.V. q 12 hours.

Dosage adjustment

- Be aware that although standard loading-dose regimen can be used, maintenance dosage should be halved in patients with mild to moderate hepatic cirrhosis.
- Know that patients with moderate or severe renal insufficiency should receive oral form unless benefit of I.V. form outweighs risk.

Off-label uses

- Febrile neutropenia (empiric therapy)

Administration

Preparation

- Correct electrolyte disturbances before therapy starts.

Clinical alert: Do not give concurrently with astemizole, cisapride, or terfenadine (no longer available in United States); carbamazepine; efavirenz; ergot alkaloids; long-acting barbiturates; pimozide; quinidine; rifabutin; rifampin; ritonavir; or sirolimus.

Dilution and compatibility

- Reconstitute powder with 19 mL sterile water for injection, to yield a volume of 20 mL. Shake vial until powder dissolves.
- Withdraw prescribed dose, then dilute further in normal saline solution, 5% dextrose and normal saline solution, 0.45% sodium chloride solution, D_5W, 5% dextrose and lactated Ringer's solution, 5% dextrose and 0.45% sodium chloride, 5% dextrose and 20 mEq potassium chloride, or lactated Ringer's solution, to yield a final concentration of 0.5 to 5 mg/mL.
- Use solution only if clear.
- Discard unused portion of vial.
- Use reconstituted solution immediately or store as recommended.

Infusion considerations

Clinical alert: Do not administer as I.V. bolus injection.

Clinical alert: Do not give through same I.V. line with other drugs, blood products, or electrolytes.

- Give by I.V. infusion over 1 to 2 hours at a rate not exceeding 3 mg/kg/hour.

Monitoring

- Monitor kidney and liver function tests. Watch for signs and symptoms of organ toxicity.
- Assess electrolyte levels and CBC, including platelet count.

Clinical alert: Monitor ECG; stay alert for prolonged QT interval.

- Check for vision problems in therapy exceeding 28 days.

Storage

- Store unopened vials at 15° to 30°C (59° to 86°F).
- If not used immediately, store reconstituted solution no longer than 24 hours at 2° to 8°C (36° to 46°F).

Contraindications and precautions

Contraindicated in hypersensitivity to drug or its components and in concurrent use of long-acting barbiturates, ergot alkaloids, rifabutin, rifampin, CYP450-3A4 substrates (such as astemizole, cisapride, pimozide, quinidine, terfenadine), sirolimus, ritonavir, efavirenz, or carbamazepine.

Use cautiously in hypersensitivity to other azoles, renal disease, mild to moderate hepatic cirrhosis, lactose or galactose intolerance, and pregnant or breastfeeding patients.

Adverse reactions

CNS: dizziness, headache, hallucinations

V

CV: hypotension, hypertension, tachycardia, chest pain, vasodilation, peripheral edema
EENT: photophobia, blurred vision, visual disturbances, eye hemorrhage, chromatopsia
GI: nausea, vomiting, diarrhea, abdominal pain, dry mouth
GU: renal dysfunction, acute renal failure
Hematologic: anemia, **pancytopenia, leukopenia, thrombocytopenia**
Hepatic: cholestatic jaundice, **hepatic failure**
Metabolic: hypomagnesemia, hypokalemia
Respiratory: respiratory disorders
Skin: pruritus, maculopapular rash, **erythema multiforme, toxic epidermal necrolysis, Stevens-Johnson syndrome**
Other: chills, fever, **sepsis, anaphylaxis**

Interactions

Drug-drug. *Barbiturates (long-acting), carbamazepine, phenytoin, rifampin:* decreased voriconazole blood level
Benzodiazepines: sedation
Calcium channel blockers, HMG-CoA reductase inhibitors: increased blood levels of these drugs
Cyclosporine, sirolimus, tacrolimus: increased blood levels of these drugs, greater risk of nephrotoxicity
CYP450-3A4 substrates (such as astemizole, cisapride, pimozide, quinidine, terfenadine): increased blood levels of these drugs, causing prolonged QT interval and risk of torsades de pointes
Ergot alkaloids: increased blood levels of these drugs, resulting in ergotism
Nonnucleoside reverse transcriptase inhibitors, protease inhibitors: inhibited voriconazole metabolism
Rifabutin: decreased voriconazole blood level, increased rifabutin blood level
Sulfonylureas: increased sulfonylurea blood level, greater risk of hypoglycemia
Vinca alkaloids: increased risk of neurotoxicity
Warfarin, other coumarin derivatives: increased partial thromboplastin time
Drug-diagnostic tests. *Alanine:* interference with alanine aminotransferase test results.

Toxicity and overdose

- Of three cases of accidental overdose seen in clinical trials (all in pediatric patients who received up to five times the recommended I.V. dosage), sole adverse event was photophobia. In overdose, expect extension of pharmacologic effects and adverse reactions.
- No known antidote exists. Provide symptomatic and supportive therapy. Hemodialysis may aid drug removal.

Patient teaching

- Explain therapy to patient. Stress the need for follow-up laboratory tests.
- Instruct patient to promptly report adverse reactions, such as rash, urinary changes, easy bruising or bleeding, signs of infection, unusual fatigue, or yellowing of skin or eyes.
- Instruct female with childbearing potential to immediately report pregnancy.
- Caution patient to avoid driving and other hazardous activities, because drug may cause visual disturbances.
- Advise patient to minimize GI upset by eating small, frequent servings of food and drinking plenty of fluids.
- As appropriate, review all other significant and life-threatening adverse reactions and interactions, especially those related to the drugs and tests mentioned above.

warfarin sodium

Coumadin

Pharmacologic class: Coumarin derivative

Therapeutic class: Anticoagulant

Pregnancy risk category X

FDA BOXED WARNING

- Drug may cause major or fatal bleeding. Bleeding is more likely during starting period and with higher dosage (resulting in higher International Normalized Ratio [INR]). Monitor INR regularly in all patients. Those at high risk for bleeding may benefit from more frequent INR monitoring, careful dosage adjustment, and shorter duration of therapy. Instruct patients about measures to minimize risk of bleeding and advise them to immediately report signs and symptoms of bleeding.

Action

Interferes with synthesis of vitamin K–dependent clotting factors (II, VII, IX, and X) and anticoagulant proteins C and S in the liver

Pharmacokinetics

Drug distributes into relatively small apparent volume of distribution. It is metabolized by hepatic microsomal enzymes (CYP450) to inactive hydroxylated metabolites and by reductases to reduced metabolites (warfarin alcohols, which have minimal anticoagulant activity). About 99% of drug is bound to plasma proteins. Elimination occurs almost entirely by metabolism. Terminal half-life after single dose is approximately 1 week; however, effective half-life ranges from 20 to 60 hours, with mean half-life of about 40 hours. Metabolites are primarily excreted in urine and to a lesser extent into bile; very little parent drug is excreted unchanged in urine.

Onset	Peak	Duration
24 hr	72-96 hr	2 to 5 days

How supplied

Powder for reconstitution for injection: 5.4 mg/vial (2 mg/mL when reconstituted)

Indications and dosages

➤ Venous thrombosis; pulmonary embolism; atrial fibrillation; myocardial infarction (MI); thromboembolic complications of cardiac valve placement

Adults: Initially, 2.5 to 10 mg I.V. daily for 2 to 4 days, then adjusted based on prothrombin time (PT) or INR. Maintenance dosages are administered orally.

Dosage adjustment

- Know that elderly or debilitated patients usually require lower dosages to produce a therapeutic level of anticoagulation.

Off-label uses

- Acute coronary syndrome
- Intracoronary stent placement
- Prevention of catheter thrombosis

Administration

Preparation

Follow hazardous drug guidelines on page S19 for handling, preparation, and administration.

- Know that I.V. form is reserved for patients who cannnot tolerate oral form. Oral dosages are identical to I.V. dosages.
- When converting to warfarin from heparin, give both drugs concomitantly for 4 to 5 days until therapeutic effect of warfarin occurs.

W

Dilution and compatibility
• Reconstitute vial with 2.7 mL sterile water for injection.
• Discard unused solution.
Infusion considerations
• Administer by bolus I.V. injection into peripheral vein over 1 to 2 minutes.
Monitoring
• Monitor PT and INR. Be aware that INR above 4.0 provides no additional therapeutic benefit in most patients and is associated with higher risk of bleeding.
• Monitor liver function tests.
Watch for signs and symptoms of bleeding and hepatitis.
Storage
• Store vial in box until use at controlled room temperature of 15° to 30°C (59° to 86°F); protect from light.
• After reconstitution, store at controlled room temperature and use within 4 hours. Do not refrigerate.

Contraindications and precautions

Contraindicated in hypersensitivity to drug; uncontrolled bleeding; open wounds; severe hepatic disease; hemorrhagic or bleeding tendency; cerebrovascular hemorrhage; cerebral aneurysm or dissecting aorta; blood dyscrasias; pericarditis or pericardial effusion; bacterial endocarditis; recent brain, eye, or spinal cord injury or surgery; lumbar puncture and other procedures that may cause uncontrollable bleeding; malignant hypertension; major regional or lumbar block anesthesia; threatened abortion; eclampsia; preeclampsia; unsupervised senile, alcoholic, or psychotic patients; pregnancy; and females who may become pregnant.

Use cautiously in cancer, heparin-induced thrombocytopenia, moderate to severe renal impairment, moderate to severe hypertension, infectious GI disease, known or suspected deficiency in protein C–mediated anticoagulant response, polycythemia vera, vasculitis, severe diabetes mellitus, indwelling catheter use, history of poor compliance, ***elderly or debilitated patients,*** breastfeeding patients, and ***children younger than age 18*** (safety and efficacy not established).

Adverse reactions

GI: nausea, vomiting, diarrhea, abdominal cramps, stomatitis, anorexia
GU: hematuria
Hematologic: eosinophilia, **bleeding, hemorrhage, agranulocytosis, leukopenia**
Hepatic: hepatitis
Skin: rash, dermatitis, urticaria, pruritus, alopecia, dermal necrosis
Other: fever, "purple toes" syndrome (bilateral painful, purple lesions on toes and sides of feet), hypersensitivity reaction

Interactions

Drug-drug. *Abciximab, acetaminophen (chronic use), androgens, aspirin, capecitabine, cefamandole, cefoperazone, cefotetan, chloral hydrate, chloramphenicol, clopidogrel, disulfiram, eptifibatide, fluconazole, fluoroquinolones, itraconazole, metronidazole (including vaginal use), nonsteroidal anti-inflammatory drugs, plicamycin, quinidine, quinine, sulfonamides, thrombolytics, ticlopidine, tirofiban, valproic acid:* increased response to warfarin, greater risk of bleeding
Barbiturates, hormonal contraceptives containing estrogen: decreased anticoagulant effect
Drug-diagnostic tests. *Alanine aminotransferase, aspartate aminotransferase, INR:* increased

Partial thromboplastin time, PT: prolonged
Drug-foods. *Vitamin K–rich foods (large amounts):* antagonism of anticoagulant effect
Drug-herb. *Angelica:* prolonged PT
Anise, arnica, asafetida, bromelain, chamomile, clove, danshen, devil's claw, dong quai, fenugreek, feverfew, garlic, ginger, ginkgo, ginseng, horse chestnut, licorice, meadowsweet, motherwort, onion, papain, parsley, passionflower, quassia, red clover, Reishi mushroom, rue, sweet clover, turmeric, white willow, others: increased risk of bleeding
Coenzyme Q10, green tea, St. John's wort: decreased anticoagulant effect
Drug-behaviors. *Alcohol use:* enhanced warfarin activity

Toxicity and overdose

• Evidence of suspected or overt abnormal bleeding (for instance, blood in stools or urine, hematuria, excessive menstrual bleeding, melena, petechiae, excessive bruising, or persistent oozing from superficial injuries) is early sign of anticoagulation beyond safe level.
• To control excessive anticoagulation with or without bleeding, discontinue drug and, if necessary and ordered, give oral or parenteral vitamin K_1. However, know that patient may return to pretreatment thrombotic status after rapid reversal of prolonged PT or INR. Warfarin resumption reverses effect of vitamin K_1; if minor bleeding progresses to major bleeding, give 5 to 25 mg (rarely up to 50 mg) parenteral vitamin K_1. In emergencies with severe hemorrhage, 200 to 500 mL of fresh whole blood or fresh frozen plasma, or commercial factor IX complex can return clotting factors to normal. Because of risk of hepatitis and other viral diseases from these blood products, use only in exceptional or life-threatening bleeding episodes secondary to warfarin overdose. In addition, factor IX complex is associated with increased thrombosis risk. Do not use purified factor IX preparations because they do not increase prothrombin levels. In significant blood loss, packed red blood cells may also be given. Carefully monitor blood or plasma infusions to avoid precipitating pulmonary edema in patients who are elderly or have heart disease.

Patient teaching

🔊 Explain therapy to patient. Stress importance of adhering to schedule for laboratory tests.
🔊 Instruct patient to promptly report unusual bleeding or bruising.
• Caution patient to consult prescriber before taking over-the-counter preparations or herbs.
• Advise patient to inform all other healthcare providers (including dentist) of warfarin therapy.
• Teach patient not to vary intake of foods containing vitamin K (such as leafy green vegetables, fish, pork, green tea, and tomatoes), to avoid changes in drug's anticoagulant effect.
• Advise patient to avoid contact sports and other activities that could cause injury and bleeding.
• Caution patient to avoid alcohol during therapy.
🔊 Instruct female with childbearing potential to report pregnancy immediately.
• As appropriate, review all other significant and life-threatening adverse reactions and interactions, especially those related to the drugs, tests, foods, herbs, and behaviors mentioned above.

zidovudine

Retrovir

Pharmacologic class: Nucleoside reverse transcriptase inhibitor
Therapeutic class: Antiretroviral
Pregnancy risk category C

FDA BOXED WARNING

- Drug has been linked to hematologic toxicity (including neutropenia and severe anemia), particularly in patients with advanced HIV infection. Prolonged use is associated with symptomatic myopathy.
- Lactic acidosis and severe hepatomegaly with steatosis (including fatal cases) have occurred with use of nucleoside analogues alone or in combination, including zidovudine and other antiretrovirals.

Action

After conversion to active metabolite, inhibits activity of HIV reverse transcriptase and terminates viral DNA growth

Pharmacokinetics

Drug achieves some cerebrospinal fluid penetration. It is rapidly metabolized to inactive metabolite; plasma-protein binding is less than 38%. Urinary recovery of drug and its metabolite accounts for 18% and 60%, respectively. Mean elimination half-life is 1.1 hour (range, 0.5 to 2.9 hours). Drug is eliminated primarily by hepatic metabolism.

Onset	Peak	Duration
Rapid	End of infusion	4 hr

How supplied

Solution for injection: 10 mg/mL in 20-mL single-use vial

Indications and dosages

➢ HIV infection

Adults and children older than age 12: 1 mg/kg I.V. five to six times daily; usually given with other antiretrovirals

➢ To prevent maternal-fetal transmission of HIV

Pregnant women: Daily divided oral doses until labor begins; then 2 mg/kg I.V. over 1 hour followed by a continuous infusion of 1 mg/kg/hour until umbilical cord is clamped

Neonates: In neonates unable to receive oral doses, 1.5 mg/kg I.V. infused over 30 minutes q 6 hours

Dosage adjustment

- Adjust dosage in hepatic impairment and in patients undergoing hemodialysis or peritoneal dialysis.

Administration

Preparation

Follow hazardous drug guidelines on page S19 for handling, preparation, and administration.

- In adults, give by I.V. route only until patient can tolerate oral dose. Do not give I.M.

Dilution and compatibility

- Dilute drug before administering.
- Remove dose from vial and add to I.V. solution containing D_5W for infusion, to yield a final concentration no greater than 4 mg/mL.

Infusion considerations

- Administer by I.V. infusion at a constant rate over 1 hour.

Avoid rapid infusion or bolus injection.

Monitoring

Closely monitor neurologic status, especially for signs and symptoms of impending seizure.

Periodically assess CBC and kidney and liver function tests. Be aware that drug can cause hepatotoxicity.

- Watch for signs and symptoms of pancreatitis.

Storage

- Store vials at 15° to 25°C (59° to 77°F); protect from light.
- After dilution, solution is stable for 24 hours at room temperature and for 48 hours when refrigerated at 2° to 8°C (36° to 46°F). Administer within 8 hours if stored at 25°C (77°F) or within 24 hours if refrigerated at 2° to 8°C.

Contraindications and precautions

Contraindicated in hypersensitivity to drug or its components and in concomitant use of Combivir or Trizivir (zidovudine-containing products).

Use cautiously in renal or hepatic impairment, decreased bone marrow reserve, hemoglobin level below 9.5 g/dL, granulocyte count below 1,000/mm^3, and pregnant or breastfeeding patients.

Adverse reactions

CNS: headache, paresthesia, malaise, insomnia, dizziness, drowsiness, asthenia, **seizures**

GI: nausea, vomiting, constipation, abdominal pain, dyspepsia, anorexia, **pancreatitis**

Hematologic: severe anemia (necessitating transfusions), **agranulocytopenia, severe bone marrow depression**

Musculoskeletal: myalgia, back pain, myopathy

Respiratory: dyspnea

Skin: diaphoresis, rash, altered nail pigmentation

Other: abnormal taste, fever

Interactions

Drug-drug. *Acetaminophen, aspirin, indomethacin:* increased risk of zidovudine toxicity

Amphotericin B, dapsone, flucytosine, pentamidine: increased risk of nephrotoxicity and bone marrow depression

Cyclosporine: extreme drowsiness, lethargy

Cytotoxic drugs, myelosuppressants, nephrotoxic drugs (such as ganciclovir, interferon alfa): increased risk of hematologic toxicity

Fluconazole, methadone, probenecid, valproic acid: increased zidovudine blood level, greater risk of toxicity

Ribavirin: antagonism of zidovudine's antiviral activity

Drug-diagnostic tests. *Granulocytes, hemoglobin, platelets:* decreased

Drug-herb. *St. John's wort:* decreased zidovudine efficacy

Toxicity and overdose

- In acute overdose, expect extension of such adverse reactions as fatigue, headache, vomiting, and possibly hematologic disturbances.
- Provide symptomatic and supportive therapyy. Hemodialysis and peritoneal dialysis have a minimal effect on removal of parent drug, but enhance elimination of primary metabolite.

Patient teaching

- Explain therapy to patient. Emphasize that drug does not cure HIV infection.

Teach patient to recognize and immediately report signs and symptoms of serious side effects such as seizures.

- Stress the need for follow-up laboratory testing.
- Advise female with childbearing potential to use effective contraception.
- Inform pregnant HIV-infected patient that drug reduces risk of, but may not prevent, HIV transmission to neonate.

Z

• As appropriate, review all other significant and life-threatening adverse reactions and interactions, especially those related to the drugs, tests, and herbs mentioned above.

zoledronic acid

Reclast, Zometa

Pharmacologic class: Third-generation bisphosphonate
Therapeutic class: Calcium regulator
Pregnancy risk category D

Action

Inhibits osteoclast-mediated bone by blocking resorption of mineralized bone and cartilage, eventually causing cell death and limiting tumor growth. Also limits calcium release from tumor.

Pharmacokinetics

Drug does not undergo biotransformation, is 22% bound to plasma proteins, and is primarily eliminated intact by the kidneys. Terminal elimination half-life is 167 hours.

	Onset	Peak	Duration
(Reclast)	Rapid	End of infusion	Short
(Zometa)	Unknown	Unknown	7-28 days

How supplied

Solution (concentrate): 4 mg/5 mL single-dose vial (Zometa)
Solution for infusion: 5 mg in 100-mL ready-to-infuse solution bottle (Reclast)

Indications and dosages

➢ Hypercalcemia caused by cancer
Adults: 4 mg (Zometa) I.V. as a single dose infused over 15 minutes. If albumin-corrected calcium level does not return to normal or stay normal, start retreatment with 4 mg I.V. no sooner than 7 days after initial treatment. For single dose, maximum recommended dosage is 4 mg.

➢ Multiple myeloma; bone metastasis from solid tumors
Adults: 4 mg I.V. (Zometa) as a single dose infused over 15 minutes q 3 to 4 weeks; may continue treatment for 9 to 15 months, depending on clinical condition

➢ Paget's disease of bone
Adults: 5 mg (Reclast) I.V. as a single dose in 100-mL of ready-to-infuse solution supplied infused over 15 minutes at a constant infusion rate by vented infusion line in patients with creatinine clearance of 35 mL/minute or higher

➢ Osteoporosis in postmenopausal women
Adults: 5 mg (Reclast) I.V. as a single 5-mg infusion over 15 minutes once yearly in patients with creatinine clearance of above 35 mL/minute or higher

Dosage adjustment

• For patients who require retreatment with Zometa for hypercalcemia caused by cancer and whose renal function decreases after receiving drug, adjust dosage as follows: (1) For patients with normal pretreatment serum creatinine whose level increases by 0.5 mg/dL within 2 weeks of next dose, withhold Zometa until creatinine level is at least within 10% of baseline value. (2) For patients with abnormal pretreatment serum creatinine whose levelsincreases 1 mg/dL within 2 weeks of next dose, withhold Zometa until serum creatinine level is at least within 10% of baseline value. Potential risk of renal failure with subsequent doses must be weighed carefully against potential benefits of this drug and other treatment options.

Administration

Preparation

• Before starting therapy, make sure patient is adequately hydrated.

• Perform standard laboratory tests and assess renal function before starting therapy.

• Be aware that patients on Zometa usually receive daily oral calcium supplements of 500 mg and a multivitamin containing 400 international units vitamin D.

• Know that patients with Paget's disease should receive 1,500 mg elemental calcium and 800 international units vitamin D daily, particularly during 2 weeks after Reclast therapy.

Dilution and compatibility

Do not let drug come in contact with calcium-containing solutions.

• Know that Reclast is available as a ready-to-infuse solution.

Dilute Zometa by immediately adding 4 mg to 100 mL normal saline solution or D_5W. To avoid inadvertent injection, do not store undiluted concentrate in syringe.

Infusion considerations

• Give Zometa by I.V. infusion over no less than 15 minutes.

• Give Reclast I.V. in 100 mL ready-to-infuse solution administered by vented infusion line. Infusion time must be no less than 15 minutes, and infusion rate must be constant.

Know that infusion times faster than 15 minutes may cause renal failure.

Be aware that a single Zometa dose should not exceed 4 mg.

Be aware that a single Reclast dose should not exceed 5 mg.

Monitoring

• Monitor electrolyte levels (especially calcium). Watch for signs and symptoms of electrolyte imbalance.

• Assess vital signs. Stay alert for hypotension, dyspnea, and pleural effusion.

Closely monitor fluid intake and output.

Closely monitor serum creatinine level before each dose. Be aware that patients with impaired renal function may experience transient increases; consider interim monitoring in these at-risk patients. Check carefully for signs and symptoms of renal toxicity.

• Monitor CBC, including platelet count.

Storage

• Store Zometa at 25°C (77°F), with excursions permitted from 15° to 30°C (59° to 86°F). If solution is not used immediately after reconstitution, refrigerate at 2° to 8°C (36° to 46°F). Total time from reconstitution, dilution, and storage to end of administration must not exceed 24 hours.

• Store Reclast at 25°C (77°F), with excursions permitted from 15° to 30°C (59° to 86°F). After opening bottle, solution is stable for 24 hours at 2° to 8°C (36° to 46°F).

Contraindications and precautions

Contraindicated in hypersensitivity to drug, its components, or other bisphosphonates; hypocalcemia (Reclast); pregnancy (Zometa); and breastfeeding (Reclast).

Use cautiously in asthma, renal dysfunction, severe renal impairment with creatinine clearance below 35 mL/minute (Reclast not recommended), hepatic insufficiency, history of hypoparathyroidism, bone metastasis with severe renal impairment, and pregnant patients (Reclast not recommended).

Adverse reactions

CNS: dizziness, lethargy, rigors, asthenia, headache, agitation, confusion, insomnia, anxiety, drowsiness, fatigue, paresthesia

CV: hypotension

Z

EENT: conjunctivitis
GI: nausea, vomiting, diarrhea, constipation, dysphagia, anorexia
GU: urinary tract infection, **renal toxicity**
Hematologic: anemia, **neutropenia**
Metabolic: dehydration, hypomagnesemia, hypocalcemia, hypophosphatemia
Musculoskeletal: myalgia, joint or bone pain, jaw osteonecrosis
Respiratory: dyspnea, cough, **pleural effusion**
Skin: rash
Other: flulike syndrome, pyrexia, peripheral edema, infection, fever, chills, infusion site pain or reactions

Interactions

Drug-drug. *Aminoglycosides, loop diuretics, other nephrotoxic agents, thalidomide:* increased risk of renal toxicity
Drug-diagnostic tests. *Calcium, hemoglobin, magnesium, phosphorus, platelets, potassium, red blood cells, white blood cells:* decreased
Creatinine: increased or decreased

Toxicity and overdose

- Overdose may cause significant hypocalcemia, hypophosphatemia, and hypomagnesemia.
- Correct significant decreases in calcium, phosphorus, and magnesium with I.V. administration of calcium gluconate, potassium or sodium phosphate, and magnesium sulfate, respectively, as ordered.

Patient teaching

- Explain therapy to patient, including associated risk of renal failure and the need for follow-up laboratory tests.
- Tell patient to immediately report shortness of breath, unusual bleeding or bruising, decreased urine output, or other significant problems.
- Instruct patient to take daily oral calcium supplement and multivitamin containing vitamin D, as prescribed.
- Advise female with childbearing potential to avoid pregnancy and breastfeeding.
- Tell patient to avoid invasive dental procedures during therapy.
- As appropriate, review all other significant and life-threatening adverse reactions and interactions, especially those related to the drugs and tests mentioned above.

Part 2

Less commonly used drugs

A

acetazolamide

Dazamide, Diamox, Storzolamide

Indications and dosages

➢ Preoperative treatment of closed-angle glaucoma (rapid relief of increased intraocular pressure)
Adults: 500 mg I.V, repeated in 2 to 4 hours; follow with oral therapy.
Children: 5 to 10 mg/kg I.V. q 6 hours
➢ Drug-induced edema or edema secondary to heart failure
Children: 150 mg/m^2 I.V. once daily in morning

Administration

🔊 Before giving, ask if patient is pregnant; drug may cause fetal toxicity.
• Know that direct I.V. administration is preferred. When giving by direct I.V., reconstitute 500-mg vial with more than 5 mL sterile water for injection; administer over 1 minute.
• When giving by intermittent I.V. infusion, further dilute with normal saline solution or dextrose solution, and infuse over 4 to 8 hours.

Patient monitoring

🔊 Evaluate for signs and symptoms of sulfonamide sensitivity; drug can cause fatal hypersensitivity.
🔊 Monitor laboratory test results for hematologic changes; blood glucose, potassium, bicarbonate, and chloride levels; and hepatic and renal function changes.
• Observe for signs and symptoms of bleeding tendency.
• Monitor fluid intake and output.

agalsidase beta

Fabrazyme, Fibrazyme

Indications and dosages

➢ Fabry disease
Adults and children: 1 mg/kg q 2 weeks as I.V. infusion

Administration

• Administer antipyretics before infusion to help prevent infusion reactions.
• To reconstitute, slowly inject 7.2 mL sterile water for injection into vial; then roll and tilt vial gently to mix drug. Do not shake; do not use filter needles.
• Dilute reconstituted solution with normal saline solution to a final volume of 500 mL.
• Infuse through separate I.V. line; do not mix with other drugs.
• Know that initial infusion rate should be no more than 0.25 mg/minute (15 mg/hour); once patient tolerance to infusion is well established, may increase infusion rate in increments of 0.05 to 0.08 mg/minute (3 to 5 mg/hour) with each subsequent infusion.
• For patients weighing less than 30 kg (66 lb), maximum infusion rate is 0.25 mg/minute.
• For patients weighing 30 kg (66 lb) or more, duration of therapy should be at least 1.5 hours.
🔊 Slow infusion rate if infusion reaction occurs.

Patient monitoring

• Monitor patient for signs and symptoms of infusion reactions, including chills, vomiting, hypotension, paresthesia, pyrexia, flushing, fatigue, headache, hypertension, extremity pain, chest pain, throat tightness, peripheral edema, myalgia, and bradycardia.

• Because patient may develop immunoglobulin (Ig) E antibodies to drug, consider IgE testing. For patients with anti-Fabrazyme IgE, weigh risks and benefits of continued treatment.

alefacept

Amevive

Indications and dosages

➢ Adults with moderate to severe chronic plaque psoriasis who are candidates for systemic therapy or phototherapy

Adults: 7.5 mg given as I.V. bolus once weekly as 12-week course of therapy

Administration

• Use only supplied diluent (6 mL sterile water for injection) to reconstitute drug. Swirl gently; do not shake or agitate. Each reconstituted solution yields 7.5 mg of drug. Use immediately after reconstitution.

• Use winged infusion set. Flush before and after injection with 3 mL normal saline solution injection.

• Attach Amevive-filled syringe to infusion set, and administer over no more than 5 seconds.

• Repeat 12-week course may be given if CD4+ T lymphocytes are within normal range and at least 12 weeks have passed since previous course.

Patient monitoring

Watch for anaphylactic reaction. If one occurs, discontinue drug immediately and institute appropriate measures.

• Monitor CD4+ T-lymphocyte level every 2 weeks during 12-week dosing period; use level as dosing guide.

If CD4+ T-lymphocyte counts fall below 250/μL, withhold doses and institute weekly monitoring.

Discontinue drug if CD4+ T-lymphocyte level remains below 250/μL for 1 month.

Discontinue drug if patient develops significant signs or symptoms of hepatic impairment.

alemtuzumab

Campath, MabCampath

FDA BOXED WARNING

• Give under supervision of physician experienced in cancer chemotherapy.

• Drug may cause hematologic toxicity. Serious and rarely fatal cases of pancytopenia, thrombocytopenia, and autoimmune hemolytic anemia have occurred. Do not give single doses exceeding 30 mg or cumulative doses exceeding 90 mg/week.

• Drug may cause serious infusion reactions. Monitor patient carefully during infusion; if indicated, discontinue drug. Escalate dosage gradually to recommended maintenance dosage when initiating therapy and if therapy is interrupted for 7 or more days.

• Serious and sometimes fatal infections have occurred. Prophylaxis against *Pneumocystis jiroveci* pneumonia and herpesvirus infections may decrease such infections.

Indications and dosages

➢ Chronic lymphocytic (B-cell) leukemia

Adults: Use dosage escalation strategy until patient receives recommended single dose of 30 mg. Initially administer

3 mg by I.V. infusion daily until tolerance occurs (infusion reactions are at or below grade 2). Then give 10 mg I.V. infusion daily until further tolerance occurs. Then give 30 mg/day I.V. infusion three times weekly on alternate days for up to 12 weeks.

Administration

Withhold drug and contact prescriber if patient has signs or symptoms of systemic infection at time of scheduled infusion and during antiviral treatment for cytomegalovirus (CMV) infection or confirmed CMV viremia.

- Premedicate with oral antihistamine and acetaminophen, as prescribed.
- Be aware that patients should receive prophylaxis for *P. jiroveci* pneumonia and herpes viral infection during therapy and for at least 2 months after completion of alemtuzumab therapy, or until CD4+ count is 200/μL or higher (whichever is later).

Do not give by I.V. push or bolus.

- Withdraw dose from ampule and filter with sterile low-protein-binding, 5-micron filter. Dilute with 100 mL normal saline solution or D$_5$W.
- Administer as I.V. infusion over 2 hours.

Interrupt therapy for infusion reactions, as needed. If therapy is interrupted for 7 days or more, reinstitute using dosage escalation schedule described above.

- Protect I.V. solution from light.

Patient monitoring

- Institute medical management (such as glucocorticoids, epinephrine, and meperidine) for infusion reactions, as needed and ordered.
- Assess for hypotension during infusion.
- Monitor vital signs frequently throughout entire course of therapy.
- Monitor CBC, CD4+ level, electrolyte levels, and platelet counts.
- Obtain CBCs with platelets weekly, and obtain CD4+ counts after therapy until recovery at or above 200/μL.

alpha$_1$-proteinase inhibitor (human)

Aralast NP, Prolastin, Zemaira

Indications and dosages

➤ Chronic replacement therapy in patients with congenital alpha$_1$-protease inhibitor (alpha$_1$-antitrypsin deficiency) with clinically evident panacinar emphysema

Adults: Recommended dosage is 60 mg/kg I.V. once weekly.

Administration

- Know that hepatitis B immunization is recommended for patient before drug therapy begins.
- Before reconstituting, warm unopened diluent and concentrate to room temperature.
- Invert diluent bottle and penetrate rubber seal on concentrate bottle by holding needle at angle; vacuum will draw diluent into concentrate bottle. For best results and to avoid foaming, hold diluent bottle at angle to concentrate bottle to direct diluent jet against wall of concentrate bottle.
- Do not mix with other drugs or solutions.
- After removing diluent bottle and transfer needle, gently swirl concentrate bottle until powder completely dissolves.
- With filter needle in place, insert syringe into reconstituted bottle of alpha$_1$-proteinase inhibitor and withdraw drug.
- To administer drug, replace filter needle with appropriate injection needle and follow procedure for I.V. administration.

• Avoid pushing I.V. administration set spike into product container stopper, as this may force stopper into vial and breach sterility.
• Administer within 3 hours after reconstitution. Do not refrigerate after reconstitution.
• Give by I.V. infusion only at 0.08 mL/kg/minute or faster over 15 to 30 minutes.

Patient monitoring

During infusion, closely monitor patients who are at risk for circulatory overload.
• Periodically monitor alpha$_1$-proteinase inhibitor blood level during therapy.

anti-thymocyte globulin (rabbit)

Thymoglobulin

FDA BOXED WARNING

• Drug should only be used by physicians experienced in immunosuppressive therapy for management of renal transplant patients.

Indications and dosages

➢ Treatment of renal transplant acute rejection in conjunction with concomitant immunosuppression
Adults and children: 1.5 mg/kg I.V. daily for 7 to 14 days

Administration

• Know that administration of antiviral prophylactic therapy is recommended.
• Premedicate with corticosteroids, acetaminophen, or antihistamine 1 hour before infusion, as prescribed, to reduce incidence and intensity of adverse reactions during infusion.
• Reconstitute using supplied diluent (sterile water for injection) as directed by manufacturer. Use immediately after reconstitution.
• Deliver through high-flow vein with inline 0.22-micron filter.
• Administer first infusion over at least 6 hours; administer subsequent infusions over 4 hours in 50 to 500 mL normal saline solution or D_5W.

Patient monitoring

• Monitor for adverse events (such as fever, chills, nausea, vomiting, malaise, and dizziness) during and after infusion.
• Monitor lymphocyte count during therapy to help assess degree of T-cell depletion.
• Monitor platelet and white blood cell counts.

anti-thymocyte globulin (equine) sterile solution

Atgam

FDA BOXED WARNING

• Drug should be given only by physicians experienced in immunosuppressive therapy for treatment of renal transplant or aplastic anemia patients, in facility with adequate laboratory and supportive resources.

Indications and dosages

➢ Adjunct to other immunosuppressive therapy to delay onset of first rejection episode in renal transplant patients
Adults and children: 15 mg/kg daily I.V. for 14 days, then every other day for 14 days, for a total of 21 doses in 28 days

➢ Treatment of rejection in renal transplant patients
Adults and children: 10 to 15 mg/kg daily I.V. for 14 days; additional alternate-day therapy may be given.
➢ Moderate to severe aplastic anemia in patients who are ineligible for bone marrow transplantation
Adults and children: 10 to 20 mg/kg daily I.V. for 8 to 14 days. Additional alternate-day therapy up to a total of 21 doses may be given.

Administration

- Know that prophylactic platelet transfusions may be necessary.
- To prevent allograft rejection, give first dose within 24 hours before or after transplantation, as ordered.
- Before first infusion, administer intradermal test dose of 0.1 mL of 1:1000 dilution in normal saline solution injection, plus a contralateral injection of normal saline solution; observe patient for reaction every 15 to 20 minutes for first hour. Local reaction of 10 mm or greater with wheal, erythema, or both (with or without pseudopod formation and itching or marked local swelling) is a positive result. However, allergic reactions such as anaphylaxis may occur even in patients with negative skin tests.
- Let diluted drug reach room temperature before infusion.
- Administer into vascular shunt, arteriovenous fistula, or high-flow central vein through inline filter with pore size of 0.2 to 1 micron.
- Administer over at least 4 hours.

Patient monitoring

- Monitor for signs and symptoms of leukopenia.
- Monitor platelet count in patients being treated for aplastic anemia.

A

asparaginase

Elspar, Kidrolase✤

FDA BOXED WARNING

- Drug may cause severe reactions (including anaphylaxis and sudden death) and should be given only in hospital setting under supervision of physician qualified to administer cancer chemotherapy. Be prepared to treat anaphylaxis at each administration.
- Carefully weigh possible benefits of therapy against risk of toxicity.

Indications and dosages

➢ As a component of multiagent chemotherapy for patients with acute lymphoblastic leukemia
Adults and children: 6,000 international units/m^2 I.V. three times weekly

Administration

- Reconstitute using 5 mL sterile water for injection or normal saline solution for injection.
- Use reconstituted drug within 8 hours.
- Administer over no less than 30 minutes through side arm of already-running infusion of normal saline solution or D_5W.

Patient monitoring

Watch for severe allergic reaction for 1 hour after administration
Check for evidence of pancreatitis if patient complains of abdominal pain.
- Monitor serum glucose level. Drug may lead to glucose intolerance (sometimes irreversible).
- Monitor coagulation parameters at baseline and periodically during and after therapy.

[redacted]

azathioprine sodium
Imuran

FDA BOXED WARNING

• Chronic immunosuppression from drug increases neoplasia risk. Clinicians who administer it should be thoroughly familiar with this risk, as well as with drug's possible hematologic toxicities and mutagenic potential in both sexes.

Indications and dosages
➢ To prevent rejection of kidney transplant
Adults: Dosage individualized. Usual initial dosage is 3 to 5 mg/kg I.V. daily, starting at time of transplant. Patient may be switched to oral therapy at same dosage postoperatively.
➢ Rheumatoid arthritis
Adults: 1 mg/kg I.V. (50 to 100 mg) as a single daily dose or on twice-daily schedule when patient cannot take tablets. Dosage may be increased starting at 6 to 8 weeks and thereafter by steps at 4-week intervals. Use dosage increments of 0.5 mg/kg/day up to a maximum of 2.5 mg/kg/day.

Administration
• Reconstitute with 10 mg sterile water for injection.
• Further dilute for infusion using normal saline solution or D_5W. Final dilution volume depends on infusion time (usually 30 to 60 minutes).
• Use reconstituted product within 24 hours.

Patient monitoring
• Monitor patient for GI toxicity.
• Obtain CBC weekly for first month of therapy, twice monthly for second and third months, and then monthly or more often if dosage adjustments or other changes to therapy are necessary.
• Monitor patient for unusual bleeding or bruising and for signs and symptoms of infection.

[redacted]

basiliximab
Simulect

FDA BOXED WARNING

• Drug should be prescribed only by physicians experienced in immunosuppressive therapy and management of organ transplantation who have complete information needed for patient follow-up. Patient should be managed in facility with adequate laboratory and supportive resources.

Indications and dosages
➢ Prophylaxis of acute organ rejection in kidney transplant, in conjunction with cyclosporine and corticosteroids
Adults and children weighing 35 kg (77 lb) or more: Two doses of 20 mg each. Give first 20-mg dose I.V. either as bolus injection or infusion 2 hours before transplantation; give second 20-mg dose 4 days after transplantation. Withhold second dose if complications, such as severe hypersensitivity reactions or graft loss, occur.
Children weighing less than 35 kg: Two doses of 10 mg each I.V. given either as bolus injection or infusion. Give first 10-mg dose 2 hours before transplantation; give second 10-mg dose 4 days after transplantation. Withhold second dose

if complications, such as severe hypersensitivity reactions or graft loss, occur.

Administration

- For I.V. bolus injection, dilute with 5 mL sterile water for injection.
- For I.V. infusion, dilute with normal saline solution or D_5W to a volume of 50 mL for adults or 25 mL for children. Administer over 20 to 30 minutes.
- Give by central or peripheral I.V. route only.
- Do not infuse other drugs simultaneously through same I.V. line.

Patient monitoring

Monitor for signs and symptoms of severe, acute hypersensitivity reactions.

[redacted]

botulism immune globulin intravenous (human) (Big-IV)

BabyBIG

Indications and dosages

➤ Infant botulism caused by toxin type A or B

Children younger than age 1: 50 mg/kg given as a single I.V. infusion as soon as diagnosis of infant botulism is made

Administration

- Reconstitute powder with 2 mL sterile water for injection. Rotate vial gently; do not shake. Allow 30-minute interval for powder to dissolve.
- Start infusion within 2 hours of reconstitution, and complete it within 4 hours.
- Infuse drug using low-volume tubing and constant infusion pump.
- Administer through separate I.V. line. If this is not possible, piggyback infusion into preexisting I.V. line that contains either normal saline solution or dextrose 2.5%, 5%, 10%, or 20% in water (with or without sodium chloride added). If preexisting line must be used, do not dilute drug more than 1:2.
- Start infusion slowly. Administer I.V. at 0.5 mL (25 mg)/kg/hour. If no untoward reactions occur after 15 minutes, increase rate to 1 mL (50 mg)/kg/hour.

Patient monitoring

- Before initial infusion, assess renal function with blood urea nitrogen or serum creatinine level.

Monitor vital signs constantly throughout infusion.

- During infusion, monitor patient with each administration rate change.
- Be sure to periodically monitor renal function and urine output in patients at risk for acute renal failure.

[redacted]

calcium gluconate injection, 10%

Indications and dosages

➤ Conditions arising from calcium deficiencies, such as hypocalcemic tetany, hypocalcemia related to hypoparathyroidism, and hypocalcemia caused by rapid growth or pregnancy; to relieve muscle cramping in black widow spider bites; as adjunct in treatment of rickets, osteomalacia, lead colic, and magnesium sulfate overdose

Adults: 500 mg to 2 g I.V. as direct injection or infusion, depending on patient's needs

Children: 200 to 500 mg I.V. as direct injection or well-diluted infusion, depending on patient's needs

Infants: Maximum of 200 mg I.V. as direct injection or well-diluted infusion, depending on patient's needs

Administration

Be aware that 100-mL pharmacy bulk package is not for direct infusion.

- When giving by I.V. bolus, inject slowly at a rate of 1.5 mL over 1 minute, using a small needle into large vein.
- Administer continuous or intermittent I.V. infusion in 500 to 1,000 mL normal saline solution or D_5W at a rate not exceeding 200 mg/minute.
- After administration, flush line with normal saline solution.

Patient monitoring

- Monitor for signs and symptoms of extravasation into local tissue.

Monitor vital signs during injection; rapid injection may cause vasodilation, decreased blood pressure, bradycardia, cardiac arrhythmias, syncope, and cardiac arrest.

capreomycin

Capastat Sulfate

FDA BOXED WARNING

- Use extreme caution when giving to patients with renal insufficiency or preexisting auditory impairment. Weigh risk of additional renal injury or eighth cranial nerve impairment against drug's benefits.
- Do not give simultaneously with other parenteral antituberculars with similar toxic effects. Use extreme caution when administering with other drugs that have ototoxic or nephrotoxic potential (polymyxin A sulfate, colistin sulfate, amikacin, gentamicin, tobramycin, vancomycin, kanamycin, and neomycin).
- Safety during pregnancy has not been determined.
- Safety and efficacy in pediatric patients have not been established.

Indications and dosages

➤ Capreomycin-susceptible strains of *Mycobacterium tuberculosis* in conjunction with other appropriate antituberculars when primary agents have been ineffective or cannot be used because of toxicity or resistant bacilli

Adults: 1 g daily (not to exceed 20 mg/kg/day) I.V. for 60 to 120 days, followed by 1 g I.V. two or three times weekly for 12 to 24 months

Administration

- Reconstitute vial in 2 mL normal saline solution for injection or sterile water for injection. Allow 2 to 3 minutes for powder to dissolve.
- For I.V. infusion, further dilute in 100 mL normal saline solution and administer over 60 minutes.
- Reduce dosage based on creatinine clearance in patients with reduced renal function.

Patient monitoring

- Perform audiometric measurements and vestibular function evaluation in elderly patients before therapy starts and at regular intervals throughout therapy.
- Monitor renal function, particularly in elderly patients, who are more likely to have decreased renal function.
- Monitor serum potassium levels frequently; be aware that drug may cause hypokalemia.

cladribine

Leustatin, Leustat, Litat

FDA **BOXED WARNING**

- Give under supervision of qualified physician experienced in antineoplastic therapy. Expect suppression of bone marrow function, which is usually reversible and apparently dose-dependent.
- Serious neurologic toxicity (including irreversible paraparesis and quadraparesis) has occurred with continuous infusion at high doses (four to nine times recommended dosage for hairy cell leukemia). Neurologic toxicity is dose-dependent; with standard dosing regimens, severe toxicity is rare.
- Acute nephrotoxicity may occur at high doses (four to nine times recommended dosage for hairy cell leukemia), especially when given with other nephrotoxic therapies.

Indications and dosages

➤ Active hairy cell leukemia

Adults: 0.09 mg/kg/day by continuous I.V. infusion for 7 consecutive days as a single course

Administration

Do not use D_5W as diluent, because of increased risk of drug degradation.

- Prepare single daily dose only with normal saline solution. Add drug to 500 mL normal saline solution in compatible Baxter Viaflex PVC infusion container; administer continuously over 24 hours.
- Prepare 7-day infusion with total volume of 100 mL bacterostatic normal saline solution for injection (0.9% benzyl alcohol preserved), using sterile 0.22-micron disposable hydrophilic syringe filter for drug and diluent. Disconnect and discard filter; infuse continuously over 7 days by compatible Sims Deltec Medication Cassette reservoir.
- Do not mix with other drugs or additives; do not infuse simultaneously through common I.V. line.
- Administer diluted solutions promptly.

Patient monitoring

- Monitor hematologic profile during and after treatment to determine degree of hematologic suppression.
- Investigate febrile events with laboratory and radiologic studies.
- Monitor renal and hepatic function, if indicated.

Know that in neurotoxicity or renal toxicity, dose should be delayed or drug should be discontinued.

cosyntropin

Cortrosyn

Indications and dosages

➤ Screening of patients with presumptive adrenocortical insufficiency

Adults: 0.25 mg in 2 to 5 mL normal saline solution injection by I.V. injection for rapid screening; or 0.25 mg added to glucose or saline solution and given by I.V. infusion

Administration

- For I.V. injection, administer over 2 minutes.
- For I.V. infusion, administer at approximately 40 mcg/hour over 6-hour period.

Patient monitoring

- Measure plasma cortisol levels before and at 30 or 60 minutes after I.V. injection.

• Measure plasma and urinary plasma cortisol levels before and at end of I.V. infusion.

daclizumab
Zenapax

FDA BOXED WARNING

• Drug should be prescribed only by physicians experienced in immunosuppressive therapy and management of organ-transplant patients who have complete information needed for patient follow-up. Drug should be given only by personnel trained in administering it, in setting with adequate laboratory and supportive resources.

Indications and dosages
➢ To prevent acute organ rejection in kidney transplantation, in conjunction with cyclosporine and steroids
Adults and children ages 11 months to 17 years: 1 mg/kg by I.V. infusion, usually for five doses. Give first dose no more than 24 hours before transplantation; give remaining doses at 14-day intervals.

Administration
Do not give by direct I.V. injection.
• Dilute dose in 50 mL normal saline solution.
• Deliver through peripheral or central vein over 15 minutes.
• Do not add or infuse other drugs through same I.V. line.
• Administer diluted drug within 4 hours of preparation if stored at room temperature or within 24 hours if refrigerated. Discard prepared solution after 24 hours.
• Shield undiluted solution from direct light.

Patient monitoring
Monitor patient for opportunistic infections and secondary cancers.
• Monitor bone marrow function and CBC (including platelet count) frequently.
• Assess cardiovascular, respiratory, and renal function during infusion and periodically between infusions.
• Monitor blood glucose level, especially in patients receiving concurrent high-dose corticosteroids.

denileukin diftitox
Ontak

FDA BOXED WARNING

• Drug should be given by physicians experienced with antineoplastic therapy and management of cancer patients, in facilities equipped and staffed for cardiopulmonary resuscitation where patients can be monitored closely.

Indications and dosages
➢ Persistent or recurrent cutaneous T-cell lymphoma in which malignant cells express CD25 component of interleukin-2 receptor
Adults: 9 or 18 mcg/kg/day I.V. for 5 consecutive days q 21 days

Administration
• Premedicate with acetaminophen, nonsteroidal anti-inflammatory drugs, and antihistamines, as prescribed, to minimize infusion-related events.
• Obtain CBC and blood chemistry panel (including liver and renal function tests) before therapy begins and weekly during therapy.

- For each 1 mL of drug from vial, add no more than 9 mL normal saline solution for injection without preservative for a concentration of at least 15 mcg/mL.
- Administer each dose over at least 15 minutes by I.V. infusion.
- Gently swirl vial to mix; avoid vigorous agitation.
- Do not mix with other drugs.
- Do not use inline filter.
- Do not give as bolus injection.
- Within 6 hours of preparing solution, infuse over at least 15 minutes using syringe pump or I.V. infusion bag.
- During infusion, observe closely for signs and symptoms of hypersensitivity; be prepared to intervene appropriately.
- During infusion, observe closely for infusion reaction (flulike syndrome). If one occurs, reduce infusion rate.
- Discard unused portion immediately.

Patient monitoring

- Continue to monitor patient closely during first infusion and for 24 hours afterward.
- Evaluate patient for vascular leak syndrome (marked by at least two of the following: edema, hypotension, hypoalbuminemia).
- Continue to monitor patient's weight, CBC, blood chemistry panel, renal and hepatic function, and albumin level.
- Stay alert for infection.

dexmedetomidine hydrochloride

Precedex

Indications and dosages

➤ Sedation of initially intubated and mechanically ventilated patients during treatment in intensive care setting

Adults: 1 mcg/kg I.V. as a loading dose, then 0.2 to 0.7 mcg/kg/hour

Administration

- Assess renal and hepatic function before starting therapy.
- Monitor for hypertension when giving loading dose.
- Administer only in continually monitored setting.
- To prepare infusion, add 2 mL drug to 48 mL normal saline solution, for a total volume of 50 mL.
- Do not infuse through same I.V. line with plasma or blood.
- Infuse I.V. loading dose over 10 minutes.
- Do not infuse longer than 24 hours.
- Use controlled infusion device for continuous infusion. Calculate infusion rate according to patient weight and desired sedation level.

Patient monitoring

- Monitor cardiovascular status continuously.
- Evaluate infusion site for burning and irritation.

dihydroergotamine mesylate

D.H.E. 45

FDA BOXED WARNING

- Concomitant use with potent CYP3A4 inhibitors (including protease inhibitors and macrolide antibiotics) may cause serious or life-threatening peripheral ischemia. Concomitant use of these drugs is contraindicated.

Indications and dosages

➢ Acute treatment of vascular headaches, including migraine and cluster headaches

Adults: 1 mg I.V.; may repeat in 1 hour (not to exceed 2 mg/day or 6 mg/week)

Administration

- Assess patient for coronary artery disease before starting therapy.
- Give at first sign of migraine or as soon as possible after symptom onset.
- Drug may be given undiluted over 1 minute.

Patient monitoring

- Monitor cardiac status, especially when giving large doses.
- Assess for and report numbness and tingling of fingers and toes, arm or leg weakness, muscle pain, or intermittent claudication.
- Monitor for dizziness, nausea, and vomiting (possible signs of drug toxicity).

[redacted]

dimenhydrinate injection

Dinate Injection, Dramamine Injection, Dramanate Injection, Dymenate Injection, Hydrate Injection

Indications and dosages

➢ Prevention and treatment of nausea, vomiting, dizziness, and vertigo caused by motion sickness when oral forms are impractical

Adults and children age 12 and older: 50 mg I.V. q 4 hours p.r.n.

Administration

- Dilute in normal saline solution for injection.
- Administer each 50-mg I.V. dose over 2 minutes.

Patient monitoring

- Assess for lethargy and drowsiness.

[redacted]

dipyridamole

Persantine IV

Indications and dosages

➢ Alternative to exercise in thallium myocardial perfusion imaging for evaluation of coronary artery disease in patients who cannot exercise adequately

Adults: 0.57 mg/kg I.V. (0.142 mg/kg/minute); maximum I.V. dosage is 60 mg.

Administration

- Dilute to at least 1:2 ratio solution with D_5W or normal or half-normal saline solution, for a total volume of 20 to 50 mL.
- Do not mix with other drugs in same syringe or infusion container.
- Give single I.V. dose over 4 minutes.
- Administer 5 minutes before thallium injection.

Patient monitoring

- Monitor ECG and vital signs, especially blood pressure, during and for 10 to 15 minutes after I.V. infusion.
- Monitor for therapeutic efficacy, including improved exercise tolerance and decreased need for nitrates.

[redacted]

edetate calcium disodium injection

Calcium Disodium Versenate

FDA BOXED WARNING

- Drug may cause toxic effects that can be fatal. Lead encephalopathy (rare in adults) may cause death in pediatric patients. Patients with lead encephalopathy and cerebral edema may experience lethal intracranial pressure increase after I.V. infusion; I.M. route is preferred for these patients. When I.V. route is necessary, avoid rapid infusion, follow dosage schedule, and never exceed recommended daily dosage.

Indications and dosages

➢ To reduce blood levels and depot stores of lead in lead poisoning (acute and chronic) and lead encephalopathy

Adults and children with blood lead levels between 21 and 69 mcg/dL (asymptomatic): 1,000 mg/m²/day I.V.

➢ Lead nephropathy

Adults: Suggested regimen is 500 mg/m² q 24 hours for 5 days in patients with serum creatinine levels of 2 to 3 mg/dL; q 48 hours for three doses in patients with creatinine levels of 3 to 4 mg/dL; and once weekly in patients with creatinine levels above 4 mg/dL. Regimen may be repeated at 1-month intervals.

Administration

Clinical alert: Do not confuse drug with edetate disodium, used to treat hypercalcemia.

- Know that acutely ill patients may be dehydrated from vomiting. Because drug is excreted almost exclusively in urine, establish urine flow with I.V. fluids before giving first dose; however, avoid excessive hydration in encephalopathic patients. Once urine flow is established, restrict further I.V. fluids to basal water and electrolyte requirements.

Clinical alert: Know that drug toxicity may develop rapidly. Stop therapy if urine output decreases or anuria occurs.

- Reduce dosage in preexisting mild renal disease.
- Be aware that when used alone, drug may aggravate symptoms in patients with very high blood lead levels. When blood lead level exceeds 70 mcg/dL or patient has symptoms of lead poisoning, give in conjunction with Bal (dimercaprol). Consult published protocols and specialized references for combination therapy dosages.
- Add each 1,000 mg/m²/day dose to 250 to 500 mL D_5W or normal saline solution.
- Administer total daily dose by I.V. infusion over 8 to 12 hours.

Clinical alert: Know that rapid infusion may be lethal. Infuse at rate suggested by manufacturer.

- After 5 days, interrupt therapy for 2 to 4 days to allow redistribution of lead and prevent severe depletion of zinc and other essential metals. Usually, two courses of treatment are used.

Patient monitoring

- Assess neurologic status frequently.
- Watch for and report febrile reactions, which may occur 4 to 8 hours after administration.
- Assess fluid intake and output; report changes.
- In severe cases, monitor urinalysis, urine sediment, other renal function tests, hepatic function, and serum electrolyte levels before each course and daily during therapy. In less serious cases, monitor these tests after days 2 and 5 of therapy.
- Stay alert for arrhythmias and other ECG changes during therapy.
- Monitor zinc, calcium, phosphate, and electrolyte levels daily.

edetate disodium
Endrate

FDA BOXED WARNING

- Drug should be used only when severity of patient's condition justifies aggressive measures associated with this drug.

Indications and dosages

➢ Hypercalcemic emergency; to control ventricular arrhythmias associated with digitalis toxicity
Adults: 50 mg/kg/day by slow I.V. infusion over at least 3 hours, up to a maximum of 3 g/day for 5 days; then skip 2 days. Repeat course as needed for up to 15 doses.

Administration

- Do not confuse this drug with edetate calcium disodium, used as lead poisoning antidote.
- Dilute in 500 mL normal saline solution or D_5W.
- Administer over 3 or more hours. Do not infuse rapidly.
- Alternate I.V. sites daily to decrease thrombophlebitis risk.

Patient monitoring

- Know that drug may cause profound hypocalcemia leading to tetany, seizures, arrhythmias, and respiratory arrest. Keep I.V. calcium readily available.
- Keep patient in bed for 15 minutes after infusion to avoid orthostatic hypotension.
- Monitor blood pressure closely.
- Obtain daily urinalysis.
- Monitor ECG and blood urea nitrogen (BUN) and creatinine levels frequently.
- Measure blood calcium level after each dose.
- Check electrolyte, BUN, and creatinine levels periodically.

enoxaparin
Lovenox

FDA BOXED WARNING

- When neuroaxial (epidural or spinal anesthesia) or spinal puncture is used, patients who are receiving or are scheduled to receive drug for thromboprophylaxis are at risk for epidural or spinal hematoma, which can lead to long-term or permanent paralysis. Risk increases with use of indwelling epidural catheter for analgesia administration and with concurrent use of drugs affecting hemostasis (such as nonsteroidal anti-inflammatory drugs [NSAIDs], platelet inhibitors, and other anticoagulants). Risk also rises with traumatic or repeated epidural or spinal puncture. Physician should weigh drug's potential benefits against risks.
- Monitor patient frequently for signs and symptoms of neurologic impairment. If these occur, provide urgent interventions.

Indications and dosages

➢ Acute ST-segment-elevation myocardial infarction (STEMI) managed medically or with subsequent percutaneous coronary intervention
Adults younger than age 75: Single I.V. bolus of 30 mg plus a subcutaneous dose, followed by another subcutaneous dose q 12 hours (maximum 100 mg for

first two doses only, followed by 1 mg/kg for each remaining dose)

Administration

- When given with fibrin-specific or nonfibrin thrombolytic, administer between 15 minutes before and 30 minutes after fibrinolytic therapy starts.
- Be aware that all patients should receive acetylsalicylic acid (ASA) as soon as they are diagnosed with STEMI and should be maintained on 75 to 325 mg ASA once daily, unless contraindicated.
- Use multidose vial for I.V. use.
- Administer through existing I.V. line.
- Flush I.V. line with normal saline solution or dextrose in water solution before and after bolus administration to clear port of drug.
- Do not mix or coadminister with other drugs.

Patient monitoring

- Monitor patient for thrombocytopenia.
- Periodically obtain CBC (including platelet count) and stool occult blood tests during therapy.
- Know that anti-factor Xa may be used to monitor anticoagulant effect in patients with significant renal impairment, abnormal coagulation parameters, or bleeding.
- Stay alert for signs and symptoms of neurologic impairment.
- Know that for patients who must take NSAIDs, close clinical laboratory monitoring is recommended.

fenoldopam mesylate
Corlopam

Indications and dosages

➤ In-hospital, short-term (up to 48 hours) management of severe hypertension in patients requiring rapid but quickly reversible emergency blood pressure reduction, including those with malignant hypertension with deteriorating end-organ function

Adults: Individualize dosage and infusion rate according to patient weight and desired rapidity and extent of pharmacodynamic effect. Consult prescribing information for complete dosing information.

➤ In-hospital, short-term (up to 4 hours) reduction in blood pressure in children

Children: Individualize dosage and infusion rate according to patient weight and desired rapidity and extent of pharmacodynamic effect. Consult prescribing information for complete dosing information.

Administration

Clinical alert: Do not give as I.V. bolus. Administer only by slow, continuous I.V. infusion using infusion pump, diluted to a concentration of 40 mcg/mL or less (60 mcg/mL or less for children).

- Each 10 mg (1 mL) of drug must be diluted in at least 250 mL of compatible solution (normal saline solution or dextrose 5% solution) and given by I.V infusion.

Patient monitoring

Clinical alert: Watch closely for signs and symptoms of anaphylaxis and severe asthma.

Clinical alert: Monitor blood pressure carefully at least every 15 minutes to detect hypotension, especially in patients with acute cerebral infarction or hemorrhage.

- When desired blood pressure decrease occurs, discontinue therapy or taper dosage, as prescribed.
- Assess respiratory and cardiac status (with ECG monitoring) regularly.
- Closely monitor serum electrolyte levels, especially potassium.

• Evaluate fluid intake and urine output.

foscarnet sodium
Foscavir

FDA BOXED WARNING

• Renal impairment is major toxicity. Frequently monitor serum creatinine level, adjusting dosage as needed for renal function changes. Ensure adequate hydration.
• Drug may cause seizures due to alterations in plasma minerals and electrolytes. Monitor patients carefully for such changes and potential sequelae. Mineral and electrolyte supplements may be required.
• Drug is indicated only in immunocompromised patients with cytomegaolvirus (CMV) retinitis and mucocutaneous acyclovir-resistant herpes simplex virus (HSV) infections.

Indications and dosages
➢ Acyclovir-resistant HSV infection in immunocompromised patients
Adults: 40 mg/kg I.V. given over 1 hour q 8 to 12 hours for 2 to 3 weeks or until infection heals
➢ CMV retinitis in AIDS patients
Adults: 90 mg/kg I.V. given over 1.5 to 2 hours q 12 hours for 2 to 3 weeks, or 60 mg/kg I.V. given over at least 1 hour q 8 hours for 2 to 3 weeks, depending on patient response. Follow with maintenance I.V. infusion of 90 to 120 mg/kg daily over 2 hours.

Administration
• Know that hydration may reduce risk of nephrotoxicity. As prescribed, give 750 to 1,000 mL D_5W or normal saline solution before first infusion to establish diuresis. With subsequent infusions, give 750 to 1,000 mL fluid with 90- to 120-mg/kg dose or 500 mL fluid with 40- to 60-mg/kg dose. Decrease fluids if warranted.
• Obtain baseline renal function tests, including calcium, magnesium, potassium, and phosphorus.
Do not give by rapid I.V. infusion or bolus injection.
• Administer by controlled I.V. infusion pump through central or peripheral line with good blood flow.
• For peripheral administration, dilute with D_5W or normal saline solution to a concentration of 12 mg/mL to avoid local irritation.
• Administer induction treatment over at least 1 hour (or 1.5 to 2 hours with 90-mg induction dose). Administer maintenance infusion over at least 2 hours.

Patient monitoring
• Monitor fluid intake and output and renal function test results (especially 24-hour creatinine clearance) and serum electrolyte levels carefully; adjust dosage as necessary.
• Assess hematocrit and hemoglobin levels.
• Monitor cardiovascular and respiratory status regularly.
• Evaluate neurologic status closely.
• Assess frequently for evidence of infection, including sepsis.

fosphenytoin sodium
Cerebyx

Indications and dosages
➢ Status epilepticus
Adults: 15 to 20 mg phenytoin sodium equivalent (PE)/kg I.V. at 100 to

150 mg PE/minute as loading dose; then 4 to 6 mg PE/kg I.V. daily as maintenance dose

➢ To prevent seizures during neurosurgery

Adults: 10 to 20 mg PE/kg I.V. as loading dose; then 4 to 6 mg PEe/kg I.V. daily as maintenance dose

➢ I.V. substitution for oral phenytoin therapy

Adults: Administer I.V. at same total daily dosage as for oral therapy.

Administration

- Know that drug is phenytoin prodrug and is given in PE units to avoid need to make molecular weight–based adjustments when converting between fosphenytoin and phenytoin sodium doses. Fosphenytoin and parenteral phenytoin have important administration differences.
- Be aware that because full anticonvulsant effect is not immediate, other measures (including concomitant I.V. benzodiazepine administration) usually are necessary to control status epilepticus.
- Before I.V. infusion, dilute in D_5W or normal saline solution to a concentration ranging from 1.5 to 25 mg PE/mL.

Because of hypotension risk, administer no faster than 150 mg PE/minute.

Patient monitoring

Check ECG, vital signs, and overall patient status continuously during infusion and for 10 to 20 minutes afterward.

Continuously monitor ECG, blood pressure, and respiratory function.

- Observe patient closely throughout period of maximal serum phenytoin levels (approximately 10 to 20 minutes after infusion ends).
- Monitor plasma phenytoin levels if drug interactions are suspected.

hydralazine hydrochloride

Indications and dosages

➢ Severe essential hypertension when drug cannot be given orally or when urgent blood pressure reduction is needed

Adults: 20 to 40 mg as rapid I.V. injection; repeat dose as necessary.

Administration

- Use drug immediately after vial is opened.

Do not add to infusion solution.

- Administer by I.V. injection directly into vein.
- Know that patients with marked renal damage may require lower dosage.
- Be aware that most patients can be converted to oral drug within 24 to 48 hours.

Patient monitoring

- Monitor blood pressure frequently.

hyoscyamine sulfate (hyoscine❋)

Levsin

Indications and dosages

➢ Adjunct in treatment of GI disorders; pain and hypersecretion in pancreatitis; cystitis; renal colic; infant colic; acute rhinitis; rigidity, tremors, and hyperhidrosis in Parkinson's disease; partial heart block associated with vagal activity

H

Adults and children age 12 and older: 0.25 to 0.5 mg I.V. two to four times daily p.r.n.

➢ Before diagnostic procedures

Adults: 0.25 to 0.5 mg I.V. 5 to 10 minutes before procedure

➢ Preoperatively to inhibit salivation and excessive respiratory secretions

Adults and children older than age 2: 5 mcg/kg I.V. 30 to 60 minutes before anesthesia induction

➢ Reversal of neuromuscular blockade

Adults: 0.2 mg I.V. for every 1 mg neostigmine or equivalent dosage of physostigmine or pyridostigmine

➢ Reduction of drug-induced bradycardia during surgery

Adults: Increments of 0.25 mL I.V., repeated as needed

Administration

• Know that drug may be given without dilution.

Patient monitoring

• Monitor blood pressure frequently.
• Watch for adverse reactions, such as mental status changes (confusion).
• Evaluate fluid intake and output.

[redacted]

indomethacin

Indocin I.V.

Indications and dosages

➢ To close hemodynamically significant patent ductus arteriosus in premature neonates weighing 500 to 1,750 g (when usual medical management is ineffective after 48 hours)

Neonates: In neonates less than 48 hours old, initial dosage of 0.2 mg/kg I.V., followed by two doses of 0.1 mg/kg I.V. at 12- to 24-hour intervals. In neonates 2 to 7 days old, initial dosage of 0.2 mg/kg I.V., followed by two doses of 0.2 mg/kg I.V. at 12- to 24-hour intervals. In neonates older than 7 days, initial dosage of 0.2 mg/kg I.V., followed by two doses of 0.25 mg/kg I.V. given at 12- to 24-hour intervals.

Administration

• Reconstitute only with 1 or 2 mL preservative-free normal saline solution for injection or preservative-free sterile water for injection. Solution made with 1 mL diluent yields a concentration of 100 mcg (0.1 mg) indomethacin/0.1 mL. Solution made with 2 mL diluent yields a concentration of 50 mcg (0.05 mg) indomethacin/0.1 mL.
• Administer each single dose immediately after reconstitution over 5 to 10 seconds or as prescribed.

If severe adverse reactions occur, discontinue drug immediately.

Patient monitoring

If urine output drops significantly, do not give additional doses until output returns to normal.

• Monitor serum electrolyte levels, because drug may suppress water excretion.
• Observe patient for signs of bleeding.

[redacted]

levocarnitine

Carnitor

Indications and dosages

➢ Acute or chronic treatment of inborn error of metabolism resulting in carnitine deficiency

Adults and children: 50 mg/kg I.V. given as slow direct injection or by infusion. Commonly, loading dose is given to patients with severe metabolic crisis, followed by equivalent dose over next 24 hours. All subsequent daily doses should be in range of 50 mg/kg, or as required.

Administration

- Obtain plasma carnitine level before starting therapy.
- For infusion administration, know that drug is compatible with normal saline solution or lactated Ringer's in concentrations ranging from 250 mg/500 mL (0.5 mg/mL) to 4,200 mg/500 mL (8 mg/mL).
- Administer by slow I.V. injection over 2 to 3 minutes. For infusion, administer at prescribed rate.

Patient monitoring

- Monitor blood chemistries, vital signs, drug plasma levels (plasma free carnitine should range between 35 and 60 µmol/L), and overall clinical condition.

levothyroxine sodium (L-thyroxine, T_4)

Synthroid

Indications and dosages

➣ Replacement therapy for reduced or absent thyroid function of any cause
Adults and children: Initially, I.V. dosage should be approximately half of previously established oral dosage. Daily maintenance dosage of 50 to 100 mcg I.V. should maintain euthyroid state, once established.

➣ Myxedema coma or stupor in patients without severe heart disease
Adults: 200 to 500 mcg I.V. as a solution containing 100 mcg/mL. If significant improvement does not occur, additional 100 to 300 mcg may be given on day 2. Convert to oral therapy when patient is clinically stable.

Administration

- Reconstitute powder for injection with 5 mL normal saline solution for injection. Shake until clear, and use immediately.
- Do not mix with other fluids.
- Administer each 100 mcg I.V. over at least 1 minute.

Patient monitoring

- Check vital signs and ECG routinely.
- Monitor thyroid and liver function test results.

Evaluate for signs and symptoms of overdose, including those of hyperthyroidism (weight loss, cardiac symptoms, abdominal cramps).

liothyronine sodium injection (T_3)

Triiodothyronine Injection ❋, Triostat

FDA BOXED WARNING

- Drugs with thyroid hormone activity, alone or with other agents, have been used to treat obesity. In euthyroid patients, dosages within range of daily hormonal requirements are ineffective for weight reduction. Larger doses may cause serious or life-threatening toxicity, particularly when given with sympathomimetic amines, such as those with anorectic effects.

Indications and dosages

➣ Myxedema coma or precoma
Adults: Initially, 25 to 50 mcg I.V.; after 4 hours, reassess need for subsequent doses (up to 65 mcg in 24 hours). In cardiovascular disease, initial dosage is 10 to 20 mcg I.V. Separate doses by at least 4 hours but no more than 12 hours.

Administration

- Be aware that no controlled clinical studies have been done with this drug. Dosing guidelines derive from data analysis; clinical experience at total daily dosages above 100 mcg is limited.
- Know that all dosages are highly individualized.
- Be aware that injectable form is for I.V. use only. Do not give I.M.
- Infuse each 10-mcg dose over 1 minute.

Patient monitoring

Monitor for evidence of overdose, including signs and symptoms of hyperthyroidism (weight loss, cardiac symptoms, and abdominal cramps).

- Monitor vital signs and ECG routinely, especially in patients with compromised cardiac function.
- Check thyroid and liver function test results regularly.

methadone hydrochloride

Dolophine

Controlled substance schedule II

FDA BOXED WARNING

- Federal law requires that when drug is used to treat opioid addiction in detoxification or maintenance program, it can be dispensed only by treatment programs certified by Substance Abuse and Mental Health Services Administration and approved by designated state authority. Certified treatment programs must dispense and use drug in oral form only and according to treatment requirements stipulated in Federal Opioid Treatment Standards. Failure to obey regulations may lead to criminal prosecution, drug seizure, revocation of program approval, and injunction precluding program operation.
- Prolonged QT intervals and torsades de pointes have occurred. Most cases involved patients being treated for pain with large, multiple daily doses.

Indications and dosages

➢ Moderate to severe pain unresponsive to nonopioid analgesics.

Adults: Optimal I.V. initiation and dosage titration for treatment of moderate to severe pain have not been determined. Dosage must be individualized. Drug is safest when given in small initial dosages and gradual dosage adjustments.

➢ To initiate pain treatment in opioid-nontolerant patients

Adults: 2.5 to 10 mg I.V. q 8 to 12 hours, slowly titrated to effect

➢ Temporary treatment of opioid dependence in patients unable to take oral medication

Adults: Use parenteral methadone only for patients unable to take oral medication, such as during hospitalization. To convert dosage from oral to parenteral methadone, initially use 2:1 ratio (for instance, 10 mg P.O. to 5 mg I.V.).

Administration

- Know that when choosing initial dosage, prescriber must consider dosage, characteristics, and potency of opioid patient was previously taking; relative potency estimate used to calculate equianalgesic dose; patient's degree of opioid tolerance; patient's age, general condition, and status; concurrent medications, particularly respiratory depressants; type, severity, and expected duration of pain; and expected balance between pain control and adverse effects.

• May be given undiluted or diluted with 1 to 5 mL of normal saline solution for each 1 mL (10 mg) of drug.

Patient monitoring

• Assess for relief of severe, chronic pain requiring around-the-clock dosing.
• Tailor dosage to patient's pain level and drug tolerance.
• Closely monitor CNS and respiratory status.
• Monitor cardiovascular status, especially in patients with history of cardiac conduction abnormalities, those taking drugs affecting cardiac conduction, and patients whose history or physical findings suggest increased arrhythmia risk.
• Watch for deepening sedation, which may increase with successive doses.
• Evaluate bowel and bladder function. Give laxatives if appropriate and ordered.

methyldopate hydrochloride

Aldomet

Indications and dosages

➢ Hypertension when parenteral medication is indicated

Adults: Usual dosage is 250 to 500 mg I.V. at 6-hour intervals, as required. Maximum recommended I.V. dosage is 1 g q 6 hours.

Children: 20 to 40 mg/kg I.V. in divided doses q 6 hours. Maximum dosage is 65 mg/kg or 3 g daily, whichever is less.

Administration

• Assess CBC, Coombs' test, and liver function tests before starting therapy.
• Add desired dosage to 100 mL dextrose 5% injection. Alternatively, administer desired dose in D_5W in a concentration of 100 mg/10 mL.
• Deliver by I.V. infusion slowly over 30 to 60 minutes.

Patient monitoring

• When giving drug concurrently with lithium, monitor patient for signs and symptoms of lithium toxicity.
• Continue to monitor CBC, Coombs' test, and liver function tests periodically.

nelarabine

Arranon

FDA BOXED WARNING

• Give under supervision of physician experienced in use of cancer chemotherapy.
• Administer I.V. only.
• Drug may cause severe neurologic events, including altered mental states (such as severe somnolence), CNS effects (such as seizures), and peripheral neuropathy. Demyelination-associated events and ascending peripheral neuropathies also may occur. Drug withdrawal does not always lead to full recovery from these events. Monitor patient closely for neurologic changes; discontinue drug for neurologic events of National Cancer Institute Common Toxicity Criteria grade 2 or greater.

Indications and dosages

➢ T-cell acute lymphoblastic leukemia and T-cell lymphoblastic lymphoma when disease has not responded to or has relapsed after treatment with at least two chemotherapy regimens

Adults: 1,500 mg/m^2 I.V. on days 1, 3, and 5, repeated q 21 days. Continue therapy until disease progresses, unacceptable toxicity occurs, patient

N

becomes eligible for bone marrow transplant, or patient no longer benefits from therapy.
Children: 650 mg/m^2 I.V. daily for 5 consecutive days, repeated q 21 days. Continue therapy until disease progresses, unacceptable toxicity occurs, patient becomes eligible for bone marrow transplant, or patient no longer benefits from therapy.

Administration
- Administer undiluted.
- Infuse over 2 hours in adults or over 1 hour in children.
- Discontinue drug if serious neurologic reactions occur.

Patient monitoring
- Monitor CBC (including platelet count) regularly.
- Closely monitor patients with renal or hepatic impairment, because of greater risk of adverse events.

pegaspargase (PEG-L-asparaginase)
Oncaspar

Indications and dosages
➢ As component of multi-agent chemotherapeutic regimen for patients with acute lymphoblastic leukemia who require l-asparaginase in regimen but are hypersensitive to native forms
Adults and children with body surface area (BSA) greater than 0.6 m^2: 2,500 international units/m^2 I.V. q 14 days
Adults and children with BSA less than 0.6 m^2: 82.5 international units/m^2 I.V. q 14 days

Administration
Keep resuscitation equipment, epinephrine, oxygen, steroids, and antihistamines readily available in case hypersensitivity reaction occurs.
- Know that drug should be used as a single agent when multi-agent chemotherapy is deemed inappropriate.
- Monitor baseline coagulation parameters.
- Dilute in 100 mL normal saline solution or D_5W.
- Administer over 1 to 2 hours through existing I.V. infusion line.

Do not administer if drug has been frozen, stored at room temperature for more than 48 hours, or shaken or vigorously agitated.

Patient monitoring
Watch for anaphylaxis and other hypersensitivity reactions, especially during first hour of therapy.
- Monitor CBC (including platelet count); fibrinogen; prothrombin and partial thromboplastin times; International Normalized Ratio; and serum amylase, lipase, and uric acid levels.

Assess neurologic status; stay alert for decreased level of consciousness and signs and symptoms of impending seizures.
- Check for signs and symptoms of bleeding, infection, and hyperglycemia.
- Monitor heart rate, blood pressure, respiratory rate, temperature, and fluid intake and output.

phentolamine
Rogitine

Indications and dosages
➢ To prevent or control hypertensive episodes before or during pheochromocytomectomy

Adults: 5 mg I.V. injection 1 to 2 hours before surgery; then 5 mg I.V. during surgery as indicated
Children: 1 mg I.V. 1 to 2 hours before surgery; then 1 mg I.V. during surgery as indicated
➢ To diagnose pheochromocytoma (phentolamine blocking test)
Adults: 5 mg dissolved in 1 mL sterile water for injection given by rapid I.V. injection. Record blood pressure at 30-second intervals for first 3 minutes, and at 60-second intervals for next 7 minutes.
➢ To prevent dermal necrosis after norepinephrine extravasation
Adults: Add 10 mg to each liter I.V. solution containing norepinephrine.

Administration

- Reconstitute powder by diluting with 1 mL sterile water for injection.
- For pheochromocytoma diagnosis, withhold sedatives, analgesics, and nonessential drugs for 24 to 72 hours before test (until blood pressure returns to hypertensive level). Keep patient supine until blood pressure stabilizes. Maximum effect usually occurs within 2 minutes of administration.
- When treating extravasation, in addition to placing drug in I.V. solution, infiltrate area with solution. Make sure treatment occurs within 12 hours of extravasation.

Patient monitoring

- For pheochromocytoma diagnosis, monitor blood pressure; in pheochromocytoma, expect immediate, steep drop in systolic and diastolic pressures. Systolic decrease of 60 mm Hg and diastolic decrease of 25 mm Hg within 2 minutes after I.V. administration indicates positive reaction for pheochromocytoma.
- When using for norepinephrine extravasation, monitor injection site closely and assess blood pressure, heart rate, and respiratory rate.

piperacillin sodium

Indications and dosages

➢ Serious infections, such as septicemia, nosocomial pneumonia, intra-abdominal infections, aerobic and anaerobic gynecologic infections, and skin and soft-tissue infections caused by piperacillin-susceptible microorganism strains
Adults: 12 to 18 g/day (200 to 300 mg/kg/day) I.V. in divided doses q 4 to 6 hours
➢ Uncomplicated urinary tract infections (UTIs) or community-acquired pneumonia caused by piperacillin-susceptible microorganism strains
Adults: 6 to 8 g/day (100 to 125 mg/kg/day) I.V. in divided doses q 6 to 12 hours
➢ Complicated UTIs caused by piperacillin-susceptible microorganism strains
Adults: 8 to 16 g/day (125 to 200 mg/kg/day) I.V. in divided doses q 6 to 8 hours

Administration

🔈 Ask patient about allergy to penicillin and cephalosporins before administering.
🔈 Keep epinephrine and emergency equipment available.
- Reconstitute each gram of drug with at least 5 mL sterile water or normal saline for injection.
- For direct I.V injection, give each single dose over 3 to 5 minutes.
- For intermittent I.V. infusion, dilute reconstituted solution in 50 mL D_5W,

P

normal saline solution, dextrose 5% in normal saline solution, or lactated Ringer's solution. Infuse over 20 to 30 minutes.
• Do not mix with aminoglycoside in syringe or infusion container, as this inactivates aminoglycoside.

Patient monitoring

Monitor for signs and symptoms of anaphylaxis or superinfection.
Be aware that high doses may cause seizures.
Watch for signs and symptoms of thrombophlebitis and deep vein thrombosis.
Assess for signs and symptoms of erythema multiforme (sore throat, rash, cough, iris lesions, mouth sores, fever). Report early indications before condition can progress to Stevens-Johnson syndrome.
• Monitor potassium level and CBC with white cell differential; check for hypokalemia and blood dyscrasias.
• Assess drug efficacy; obtain repeat cultures after therapy ends.

[redacted]

porfimer sodium

Photofrin

Indications and dosages

➣ Completely or partially obstructive esophageal cancer; completely or partially obstructive endobronchial non-small-cell lung cancer
Adults: 2 mg/kg I.V. over 3 to 5 minutes, followed 40 to 50 hours later by laser light illumination. Second laser light application may be given 96 to 120 hours after injection. A total of three courses may be given, separated by at least 30 days.

Administration

• Reconstitute with 31.8 mL 5% dextrose injection or normal saline solution injection. Shake well until dissolved. Shield from light and use immediately after reconstitution.
• Do not mix with other drugs in same syringe.
Know that drug should be given by slow I.V. push over 3 to 5 minutes by clinicians trained in photodynamic therapy.
Avoid extravasation. If it occurs, protect affected area from light.

Patient monitoring

Monitor for signs and symptoms of esophageal obstruction.
Know that patients with endobronchial lesions must be monitored closely for respiratory distress during interval between laser light therapy and mandatory debridement bronchoscopy.
Assess vital signs and cardiovascular status; watch for signs and symptoms of cardiac complications.
Monitor respiratory status, especially for difficulty breathing.
• Evaluate nutritional and hydration status.
• Watch for photosensitivity reaction; protect patient's skin and eyes from direct sunlight and bright indoor light.

[redacted]

secretin

*ChiRho*Stim (human formulation), SecreFlo (porcine preparation), SecreMax

Indications and dosages

➣ To stimulate pancreatic secretions, including bicarbonate; to aid diagnosis of exocrine pancreatic dysfunction ; to promote identification of ampulla of Vater and accessory papilla during

endoscopic retrograde cholangiopancreatography and to aid in cannulation of pancreatic duct (*ChiRhoStim* only)
Adults: 0.2 mcg/kg by I.V. injection.
➤ Stimulation of gastrin secretion to aid in diagnosis of gastrinoma
Adults: 0.4 mcg/kg I.V. injection

Administration

As ordered, administer test dose of 0.2 mcg I.V. to check for possible allergies.
- Dissolve contents of vial in 8 mL normal saline solution for injection to yield a concentration of 2 mcg/mL. Shake vigorously to ensure dissolution. Use immediately after reconstitution. Discard unused portion.
- Give by I.V. injection over 1 minute.

Patient monitoring

- Monitor patient for allergic reaction for 1 minute after test dose.

streptozocin

Zanosar

FDA BOXED WARNING

- Give under supervision of physician experienced in using cancer chemotherapy. Patients should have access to facility with laboratory and supportive resources sufficient to monitor drug tolerance and treat drug toxicity.
- Renal toxicity, which may be severe or fatal, is dose-related and cumulative.
- Drug may cause nausea and vomiting, which may be severe and treatment-limiting. Some patients have experienced hepatic dysfunction, diarrhea, and hematologic changes.
- Drug is mutagenic. In some rodents, it is tumorigenic or carcinogenic when given parenterally. Physician must weigh possible benefits against known toxic effects.

Indications and dosages

➤ Metastatic islet-cell carcinoma of the pancreas
Adults: *Daily schedule:* 500 mg/m^2 for 5 consecutive days q 6 weeks until maximum benefit or treatment-limiting toxicity occurs. Dosage escalation is not recommended. *Weekly schedule:* 1,000 mg/m^2 at weekly intervals for first 2 courses (weeks). In subsequent courses, may escalate dosage if patient has not achieved therapeutic response and did not have significant toxicity with previous course. However, do not exceed single dose of 1,500 mg/m^2, as higher dosage may cause azotemia. When given on this schedule, median time to response onset is about 17 days, and median time to maximum response is about 35 days. Median total dosage to response onset is about 2,000 mg/m^2 and median total dosage to maximum response is about 4,000 mg/m^2.

Administration

- Obtain serial urinalysis, blood urea nitrogen (BUN), plasma creatinine, serum electrolyte, and creatinine clearance levels before therapy starts. Serial urinalysis is particularly important for early proteinuria detection; if proteinuria is detected, obtain 24-hour collection.

Know that mild proteinuria is one of first signs of renal toxicity and may herald further deterioration of renal function.
- Ensure that patient is well hydrated to help reduce risk of nephrotoxicity.

Be aware that drug irritates tissues. Extravasation may cause severe tissue lesions and necrosis.

S

• Reconstitute with 9.5 mL D_5W injection or normal saline solution injection. Resulting pale-gold solution contains 100 mg drug and 22 mg citric acid per mL. For more dilute infusion solution, dilute further in D_5W or normal saline solution. Total storage time after drug has been placed in solution should not exceed 12 hours. Product contains no preservatives and is not intended as multidose vial.
• Administer as a short I.V. infusion over 10 to 15 minutes or as a prolonged infusion over 6 hours.

Patient monitoring

• Continue to monitor renal function parameters, including serial urinalysis, BUN, plasma creatinine, serum electrolytes, and creatinine clearance at least weekly during therapy and for 4 weeks afterward.
• Watch for evidence of hematopoietic and hepatic toxicities. Monitor CBC and liver function tests at least weekly.

teniposide injection

Vumon

FDA BOXED WARNING

• Drug should be given under supervision of qualified physician experienced in using cancer chemotherapy, in facility with adequate management resources.
• Severe myelosuppression with resulting infection or bleeding may occur. Hypersensitivity reactions, including anaphylaxis-like symptoms, may follow initial dose or develop on repeated drug exposure. Epinephrine, corticosteroids, and antihistamines have been used to relieve reaction.

Indications and dosages

➢ Refractory childhood acute lymphoblastic leukemia
Children: 165 mg/m² I.V. infusion in combination with cytarabine I.V. infusion twice weekly for eight or nine doses; or 250 mg/m² I.V. infusion weekly for 4 to 8 weeks in combination with oral prednisone for 28 days

Administration

• Assess CBC with white cell differential and platelets, hemoglobin, and renal and hepatic function tests before starting drug.
Administer using non-DEHP (toxic plasticizer) containers, such as glass or polyolefin plastic bags or I.V. administration sets to avoid softening, cracking, and possible drug leakage that may occur with plastic equipment.
• Dilute with 5% dextrose or normal saline solution for a final concentration of 0.1 mg/mL, 0.2 mg/mL, 0.4 mg/mL. These diluted solutions are stable at room temperature for up to 24 hours. Solutions prepared at final concentration of 1 mg/mL should be administered within 4 hours to reduce risk of precipitation. Do not refrigerate solutions.
Be aware that precipitation has occurred during 24-hour infusion of injection concentrate diluted to 0.1 to 0.2 mg/mL, causing occlusion of central venous access catheters in several patients. Because heparin solutions may cause tenoposide precipitation, flush administration apparatus thoroughly with 5% dextrose injection or normal saline solution injection before and after teniposide administration.
• Give only by slow I.V. infusion (lasting at least 30 to 60 minutes), as hypotension may occur with rapid I.V. injection.
• Know that improper administration may lead to extravasation resulting in local tissue necrosis, as well as thrombophlebitis.

Patient monitoring

Be aware that drug may cause hypersensitivity reaction manifested by chills, fever, urticaria, tachycardia, bronchospasm, dyspnea, hypertension or hypotension, and facial flushing. Reaction may occur with first dose and may be life-threatening if not treated promptly with antihistamines, corticosteroids, epinephrine, I.V. fluids, and other supportive measures.

Monitor for hypotension. If significant hypotension occurs, stop infusion and provide supportive therapy as appropriate. When restarting infusion, use slower infusion rate and monitor patient continuously.

- Continue to monitor hemoglobin and CBC with differential and platelet counts frequently for myelosuppression, both during and after therapy. Dose-limiting bone marrow suppression is most significant toxicity.
- Know that repeat bone marrow examination should be done, if necessary, to guide decision as to whether to continue therapy despite severe myelosuppression.
- Monitor plasma albumin, platelets, and renal and hepatic function tests carefully throughout therapy.
- Observe for acute CNS depression and hypotension in patients receiving high doses who were pretreated with antiemetics. In patients receiving higher-than-recommended teniposide dosages, depressant effects of antiemetics and alcohol content of teniposide may place patient at risk for CNS depression.

thiotepa

Thioplex

Indications and dosages

➢ Adenocarcinoma of breast or ovary; Hodgkin's disease; lymphomas

Adults: 0.3 to 0.4 mg/kg administered by I.V. injection at 1- to 4-week intervals

Administration

- Carefully individualize dosage. Because slow response does not necessarily indicate lack of effect, increase in dosing frequency may only increase toxicity. After initial therapy achieves maximum benefit, administer maintenance therapy at 1- to 4-week intervals. To continue optimal effect, do not give maintenance doses more often than weekly, to preserve correlation between dosage and blood counts.
- Reconstitute with 1.5 mL sterile water for injection to yield a concentration of approximately 10 mg/mL. Reconstituted solution is hypotonic; further dilute with normal saline solution before use. When solution is reconstituted with sterile water for injection, store in refrigerator and use within 8 hours. Immediately use reconstituted solutions that have been further diluted with normal saline solution.
- To eliminate haze, filter solution through 0.22-micron filter. (Filtering does not alter potency.) Reconstituted solution should be clear. Do not use solution that remains opaque or precipitates after filtration.

Patient monitoring

- Obtain weekly CBC and platelet counts during therapy and for at least 3 weeks after drug is discontinued.

T

• Carefully monitor patients with hepatic or renal impairment.

[redacted]

tranexamic acid injection

Cyklokapron

Indications and dosages

➢ Short-term use (2 to 8 days) in patients with hemophilia to reduce or prevent hemorrhage and reduce need for replacement therapy during and after tooth extraction

Adults: 10 mg/kg I.V. immediately before dental extraction, given with replacement therapy

Administration

• Mix with commonly used solution for infusion, such as electrolyte solution, carbohydrate solution, amino acid solution, or dextran solution. Prepare mixture on same day solution will be used.

• Do not mix with blood or solutions containing penicillin.

Patient monitoring

• Monitor patient for bleeding.

• Monitor renal function; drug is excreted largely by the kidneys.

[redacted]

verteporfin

Visudyne

Indications and dosages

➢ Predominantly classic subfoveal choroidal neovascularization caused by age-related macular degeneration, pathologic myopia, or presumed ocular histoplasmosis

Adults: 6 mg/m^2 I.V.

Administration

• Administer 6 mg/m^2 I.V. over 10 minutes at a rate of 3 mL/minute, using appropriate syringe pump and inline filter.

• Reconstitute each vial with 7 mL sterile water for injection to provide 7.5 mL containing 2 mg/mL. Then withdraw required volume of reconstituted drug to achieve desired dosage of 6 mg/m^2 from vial; dilute with dextrose 5% for injection for a total infusion volume of 30 mL.

• After dilution, protect drug from light and use within 4 hours.

Patient monitoring

• Avoid extravasation. Establish free-flowing I.V. line before starting infusion. Monitor line carefully throughout infusion.

Part 3

Appendix
Selected references
Index

Common laboratory values

The table below shows normal laboratory values for commonly ordered blood tests. Results may vary slightly among laboratories. Many of these values are monitored regularly to assess patient response and drug efficacy.

Hematology

White blood cell count
4,100 to 10,900/mm^3

Red blood cell count
Men: 4.5 to 6.2 million/mm^3
Women: 4.2 to 5.4 million/mm^3

Hemoglobin
Men: 14 to 18 g/dl
Women: 12 to 16 g/dl

Hematocrit
Men: 42% to 54%
Women: 38% to 46%

Platelet count
140,000 to 400,000/mm^3

Red blood cell indices
MCH: 26 to 32 pg
MCHC: 32 to 36 g/dl
MCV: 80 to 95 μm^3

Reticulocyte count
0.5% to 2% of total red blood cell count

White blood cell differential
Basophils: 0.3% to 2%
Eosinophils: 0.3% to 7%
Lymphocytes: 16.2% to 43%
Monocytes: 4% to 10%
Neutrophils: 47.6% to 76.8%

Coagulation studies

Partial thromboplastin time
60 to 70 seconds

Prothrombin time
10 to 14 seconds

International Normalized Ratio
2.0 to 3.0 in patients receiving warfarin

Bleeding time
3 to 6 minutes (template and Ivy methods)
1 to 3 minutes (Duke method)

D-Dimer
< 250 µg/L

Fibrinogen
215 to 519 mg/dl

Chemistry

Glucose
70 to 100 mg/dl

Blood urea nitrogen
8 to 20 mg/dl

Creatinine
Men: 0.8 to 1.2 mg/dl
Women: 0.6 to 1.1 mg/dl

Sodium
135 to 145 mEq/L

Potassium
3.5 to 5.0 mEq/L

Chemistry (continued)

Anion gap
8 to 16 mEq/L

Chloride
100 to 108 mEq/L

Carbon dioxide
22 to 34 mEq/L

Albumin
3.3 to 4.5 g/dl

Calcium
9 to 10.5 mg/dl

Magnesium
1.5 to 2.5 mEq/L

Phosphorus
2.5 to 4.5 mg/dl

Amylase
60 to 180 units/L

Lipase
0 to 110 units/L

Lactate dehydrogenase
48 to 115 IU/L

Lactic acid
3 to 12 mg/dl

Protein
6.0 to 8.5 g/dl

Uric acid
Men: 4.0 to 8.5 mg/dl
Women: 2.5 to 7.5 mg/dl

Erythrocyte sedimentation rate
Men: 0 to 15 mm/hour
Women: 0 to 20 mm/hour

KEY MCH: Mean corpuscular hemoglobin
MCHC: Mean corpuscular hemoglobin concentration
MCV: Mean corpuscular volume

Chemistry (continued)

Glucose-6-phosphate dehydrogenase
5 to 13 units/g hemoglobin

Hemoglobin A1c
< 6.0% of total hemoglobin

B-Type natriuretic peptide
< 100 pg/ml

Zinc
60 to 130 mcg/dl

Serotonin
Men: 21 to 321 ng/ml
Women: 0 to 420 ng/ml

Arterial blood gases

pH
7.35 to 7.45 mmHg

$Paco_2$
35 to 45 mmHg

Pao_2
75 to 100 mmHg

HCO_3^-
22 to 26 mEq/L

Sao_2
94% to 100%

Lipid studies

Low-density lipoproteins
Optimal: < 100 mg/dl
Near optimal: 100 to 129 mg/dl

High-density lipoproteins
Desirable: ≥ 60 mg/dl

Total cholesterol
Desirable: < 200 mg/dl

Triglycerides
Desirable: < 200 mg/dl

Liver function studies

Alanine aminotransferase
Men: 10 to 35 units/L
Women: 9 to 24 units/L

Alkaline phosphatase
39 to 117 units/L

Aspartate aminotransferase
Men: 8 to 20 units/L
Women: 5 to 40 units/L

Serum bilirubin
Direct: ≤ 0.4 mg/dl
Indirect: ≤ 1.3 mg/dl
Total: ≤ 1.3 mg/dl

Cardiac studies

Cardiac troponin I
< 1.0 μg/ml

Creatine kinase (CK)
Total CK—
- Men: 54 to 186 IU/L
- Women: 41 to 117 IU/L

Isoenzymes—
- CK-MM: 96% to 100% of total
- CK-MB: 0% to 4% of total
- CK-BB: 0% of total

High sensitivity C-reactive protein
Low cardiovascular risk: < 1.0 mg/L
Average cardiovascular risk: 1.0 to 3.0 mg/L

Prostate studies

Prostate-specific antigen
≤ 4 ng/ml

Prostatic acid phosphatase
< 0 to 2.7 ng/ml

Thyroid studies

Triiodothyronine (T_3)
60 to 181 ng/dl

Thyroxine (T_4)
4.5 to 12.5 mcg/dl

Thyroid-stimulating hormone
0.5 to 4.70 microIU/ml

Parathyroid hormone, intact
Ages 2 to 20 years: 9 to 52 pg/ml
Older than age 20: 8 to 97 pg/ml

Lymphocyte surface markers

CD3
Absolute: 840 to 3,060 cells/μL
Percentage: 57% to 85%

CD4
Absolute: 490 to 1,740 cells/μL
Percentage: 30% to 61%

CD8
Absolute: 180 to 1,170 cells/μL
Percentage: 12% to 42%

Helper: suppressor (CD4: CD8) ratio
0.86 to 5

(continued)

Common laboratory values (continued)

Iron studies

Serum iron
40 to 180 mcg/dl

Ferritin
Men: 18 to 270 μg/ml
Women: 18 to 160 μg/ml

Iron-binding capacity
200 to 450 mcg/dl

Transferrin
88 to 341 mg/dl

Transferrin saturation
12% to 57%

Hormone studies

Growth hormone
Age 1 day: 5 to 53 ng/ml
Age 1 week: 5 to 27 ng/ml
Age 1 to 12 months: 2 to 10 ng/ml
Age 1 year and older: < 5 ng/ml

Estradiol
Men: < 50 pg/ml
Women: Menstruating (day of cycle relative to LH peak) —
- Follicular (-12): 19 to 83 pg/ml
- Follicular (-4): 64 to 183 pg/ml
- Midcycle (-1): 150 to 528 pg/ml
- Luteal (+2): 58 to 157 pg/ml
- Luteal (+6): 60 to 211 pg/ml
- Luteal (+12): 55 to 150 pg/ml

Postmenopausal (no treatment): 0 to 31 pg/ml

Testosterone
Males > age 18: 241 to 827 ng/dl
Females > age 18: 14 to 76 ng/dl

Body surface area in adults

To estimate an adult's body surface area (BSA) with the nomogram below, use a straightedge to connect the patient's weight in the right column with height in the left column. The point of intersection in the middle column is the BSA. For example, a patient who weighs 120 lb and is 62" tall has a BSA of 1.60 m².

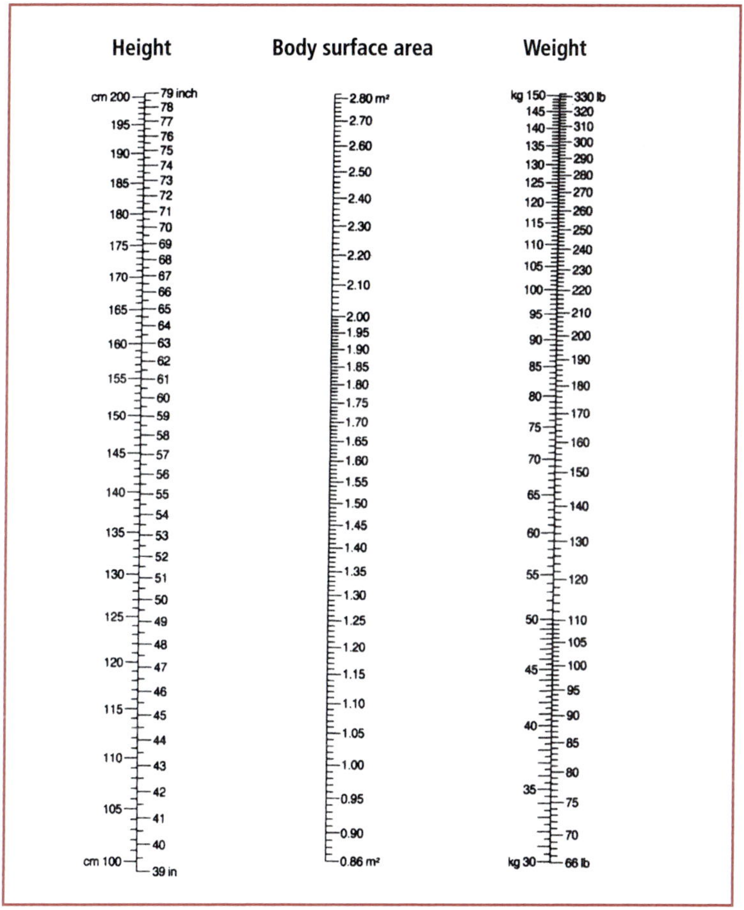

From Lentner, C. (1981). *Geigy Scientific Tables: Units of Measurement, Body Fluid, Composition of Body, and Nutrition* (8th ed.). Basel, Switzerland: Novartis Medical Education. Used with permission from Icon Learning Systems, a division of MediMedia USA, Inc.

Body surface area in children

For children of average size, you can estimate body surface area (BSA) by using the nomogram on the left. Simply find the child's weight in pounds and then read across to the corresponding BSA on the right. For other children, use the nomogram on the right. With a straightedge, connect the patient's weight in the right column with height in the left column; the point of intersection in the middle column is the BSA.

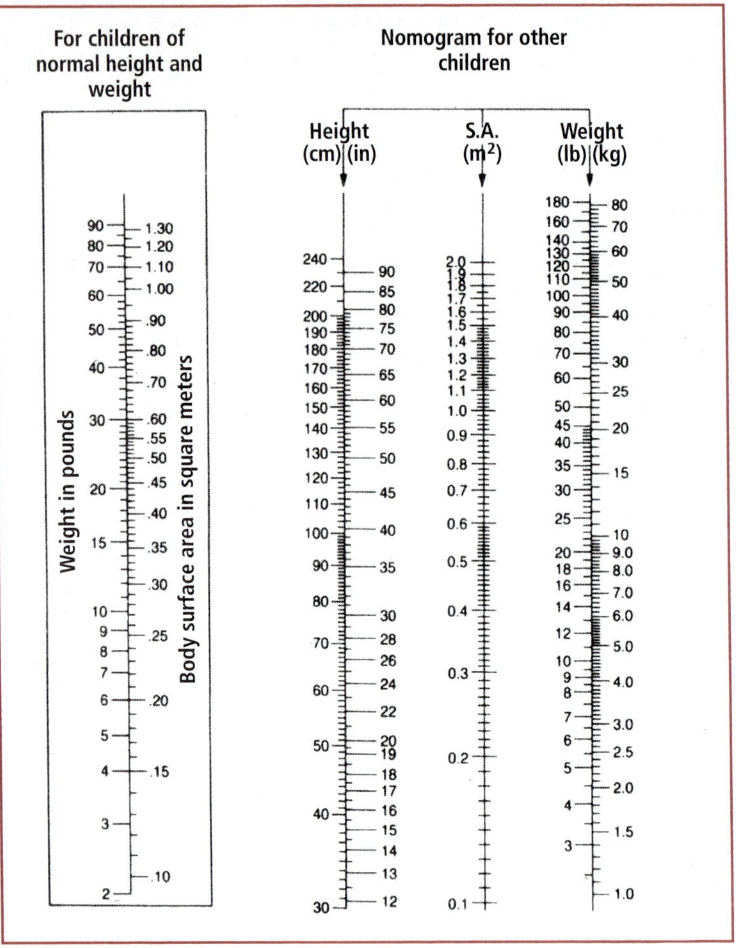

Reprinted from Behrman, R.E., Kliegman, R.M., and Jenson, H.B., eds. *Nelson Textbook of Pediatrics* (17th ed.), 2003, with permission from Elsevier.

I.V. drug and solution compatibilities

Use the table below to determine which I.V. solutions (listed in the top row) you can safely use to dilute a drug in the same syringe for I.V. injection or to dilute it for intermittent or continuous I.V. infusion.

Key:
C = compatible.
Blank = incompatible or no compatibility reported.
D = dextrose, W = water
LR = lactated Ringer's, NS = normal saline

	Fluid										
I.V. drug	D_5W	$D_{10}W$	$D_5\,^1/_4NS$	$D_5\,^1/_2NS$	D_5NS	NS	$^1/_2NS$	LR	D_5LR	Ringer's	D_5Ringer's
acyclovir sodium											
alfentanil hydrochloride	C				C	C		C			
alteplase						C					
amikacin sulfate	C	C	C	C	C	C	C	C	C	C	C
aminophylline	C	C	C	C	C		C	C	C	C	C
amiodarone											
amphotericin B	C										
amphotericin B cholesteryl sulfate	C										
amphotericin B lipid complex	C										
ampicillin sodium											
ampicillin sodium and sulbactam sodium						C					
anidulafungin	C					C					
atracurium besylate	C				C	C					
atropine sulfate						C					
azithromycin dihydrate	C			C		C	C	C			
aztreonam	C					C					
bleomycin sulfate						C					
bortezomib						C					
buprenorphine hydrochloride	C				C	C		C			
caffeine citrate	C	C	C								
calcium chloride	C										
carboplatin	C		C	C	C	C					
caspofungin acetate						C					
cefazolin	C					C		C	C		
cefepime hydrochloride	C	C			C	C			C		
cefotaxime sodium	C	C	C	C	C	C		C			
cefoxitin	C	C	C	C		C		C	C	C	
ceftazidime					C			C			
ceftizoxime sodium		C	C	C	C	C		C		C	
ceftriaxone sodium	C	C		C	C	C					
cefuroxime sodium	C	C	C	C	C	C		C		C	
cimetidine hydrochloride	C	C	C	C	C	C		C	C	C	C
ciprofloxacin	C	C	C	C		C		C		C	
cisplatin			C	C	C	C	C				

(continued)

I.V. drug and solution compatibilities (continued)

Key:
C = compatible.
Blank = incompatible or no compatibility reported.
D = dextrose, W = water
LR = lactated Ringer's, NS = normal saline

I.V. drug	Fluid										
	D_5W	$D_{10}W$	D_5 $^1/_4$NS	D_5 $^1/_2$NS	D_5NS	NS	$^1/_2$NS	LR	D_5LR	Ringer's	D_5Ringer's
clindamycin phosphate	C	C		C	C	C		C			C
diazepam											
diltiazem hydrochloride	C			C		C					
diphenhydramine hydrochloride	C	C	C	C	C	C	C	C	C	C	C
dobutamine hydrochloride	C			C	C	C	C	C	C		
doxorubicin hydrochloride	C					C		C			
doxorubicin hydrochloride liposomal	C										
doxycycline hyclate	C					C					
droperidol	C					C		C			
drotrecogin alfa						C					
enalaprilat	C				C	C			C		
ertapenem											
erythromycin lactobionate						C					
esomeprazole sodium	C					C		C			
famotidine	C	C				C		C			
fentanyl citrate	C					C					
filgrastim	C										
fluconazole	C					C		C			
fosphenytoin sodium	C	C		C		C		C	C		
furosemide	C	C				C		C	C		
gentamicin sulfate		C				C		C		C	
glycopyrrolate	C	C			C	C				C	
granisetron hydrochloride	C			C	C	C					
heparin sodium				C			C	C	C	C	C
hydrocortisone sodium succinate	C	C	C	C	C	C	C	C	C	C	C
hydromorphone hydrochloride	C			C	C	C	C	C	C	C	C
ifosfamide	C				C	C	C	C			C
imipenem and cilastatin sodium											
insulin, regular											
ketorolac tromethamine	C				C	C		C			C
levofloxacin	C				C	C		C			
lidocaine hydrochloride	C			C	C	C	C	C	C		
linezolid	C					C		C			
magnesium sulfate											
meperidine hydrochloride	C	C	C	C	C	C	C	C	C	C	C
meropenem											
metoclopramide hydrochloride				C		C		C		C	
midazolam hydrochloride	C				C	C					
morphine sulfate	C	C	C	C	C		C	C	C	C	C
nafcillin	C	C	C	C	C			C	C	C	C
nalbuphine hydrochloride		C			C	C		C			

I.V. drug and solution compatibilities (continued)

Key:
C = compatible.
Blank = incompatible or no compatibility reported.
D = dextrose, W = water
LR = lactated Ringer's, NS = normal saline

I.V. drug	Fluid										
	D_5W	$D_{10}W$	$D_5\,{}^1/_4NS$	$D_5\,{}^1/_2NS$	D_5NS	NS	${}^1/_2NS$	LR	D_5LR	Ringer's	D_5Ringer's
naloxone hydrochloride	C					C					
ofloxacin	C				C	C			C	C	
ondansetron hydrochloride	C					C		C		C	
oxytocin	C	C	C	C	C	C	C	C	C	C	C
pantoprazole sodium	C					C		C			
penicillin G potassium	C	C	C	C	C		C	C	C		C
pentobarbital sodium		C	C	C	C		C	C	C	C	C
phenylephrine hydrochloride	C	C	C	C	C	C	C	C	C	C	C
piperacillin sodium and tazobactam sodium	C					C		C			
potassium chloride	C	C	C	C	C	C	C	C	C	C	C
prochlorperazine edisylate	C	C	C	C	C	C	C	C	C	C	C
promethazine hydrochloride	C	C	C	C	C	C	C	C	C	C	C
ranitidine	C	C		C	C			C			
remifentanil hydrochloride	C				C	C	C		C		
sodium bicarbonate	C	C	C	C	C	C	C				C
streptokinase	C					C					
sufentanil citrate	C										
sulfamethoxazole/trimethoprim				C			C	C			
ticarcillin disodium and clavulanate potassium								C			
tigecycline	C				C			C	C		
tirofiban hydrochloride	C			C		C					
tobramycin sulfate	C	C			C			C		C	
topotecan hydrochloride	C					C					
vancomycin hydrochloride	C	C			C	C		C	C		
vecuronium bromide	C					C		C			
verapamil	C			C	C	C	C	C	C	C	C
vinblastine sulfate	C					C		C			
vincristine sulfate	C					C		C			
vinorelbine tartrate	C			C		C	C	C		C	
voriconazole	C					C					

Effects of dialysis on drug therapy

A patient receiving a drug that's removed by hemodialysis (HD) or peritoneal dialysis (PD) will need supplemental doses of that drug. The chart below shows which drugs are removed by dialysis and therefore will necessitate supplemental dosing during or after dialysis. Drugs listed as "unlikely" haven't been studied; however, because of their chemical properties, dialysis is unlikely to remove them.

Generic drug	Removed by HD	Removed by PD
acetaminophen	Yes	No
acyclovir	Yes	No
adenosine	Unlikely	Unlikely
albumin	Unlikely	Unlikely
alendronate	No	No data
allopurinol	Yes	No data
alprazolam	No	Unlikely
amikacin	Yes	Yes
amiodarone	No	No
amitriptyline	No	No
amlodipine	No	No
amoxicillin	Yes	No
amphotericin B	No	No
ampicillin	Yes	No
ascorbic acid	Yes	Yes
aspirin	Yes	Yes
atenolol	Yes	No
atorvastatin	No	Unlikely
aztreonam	Yes	No
bleomycin	No	No
bumetanide	No	Unlikely
bupropion	No	No
buspirone	No	No data
candesartan	No	No data
captopril	Yes	No
carbamazepine	No	No
carbenicillin	Yes	No
carboplatin	Yes	No data
carisoprodol	Yes	Yes
carmustine	No	No data
cefaclor	Yes	Yes
cefadroxil	Yes	No
cefazolin	Yes	No
cefepime	Yes	Yes
cefmetazole	Yes	No
cefonicid	No	No

Generic drug	Removed by HD	Removed by PD
cefoperazone	No	No
cefotaxime	Yes	No
cefotetan	Yes	Yes
cefoxitin	Yes	No
cefpodoxime	Yes	No
ceftazidime	Yes	Yes
ceftriaxone	No	No
cefuroxime	Yes	No
cephalexin	Yes	No
chloramphenicol	Yes	No
chlorpheniramine	Yes	No
cimetidine	No	No
ciprofloxacin	No	No
citalopram	No	Unlikely
clindamycin	No	No
clofibrate	No	No
clonazepam	No	Unlikely
clonidine	No	No
codeine	No	Unlikely
colchicine	No	No
cyclophosphamide	Yes	No data
cyclosporine	No	No
dapsone	Yes	No data
desipramine	No	No
dexamethasone	No	No
diazepam	No	Unlikely
diazoxide	Yes	Yes
dicloxacillin	No	No
digoxin	No	No
diltiazem	No	No
diphenhydramine	Unlikely	Unlikely
divalproex	No	No
dobutamine	No	No
dopamine	No	Unlikely
doxazosin	No	No

Generic drug	Removed by HD	Removed by PD
doxepin	No	No
doxycycline	No	No
drotrecogin alfa	Unlikely	Unlikely
edetate calcium	Yes	Yes
enalapril	Yes	Yes
exoxaparin	No	Unlikely
epinephrine	No data	No data
epoetin alfa	No	No
ertapenem	Yes	No data
erythromycin	No	No
esmolol	Yes	Yes
estradiol	No	No data
ethacrynic acid	No	Unlikely
etoposide	No	No
famciclovir	Yes	No data
famotidine	No	No
felodipine	No	Unlikely
fenofibrate	No	Unlikely
filgrastim	No	Unlikely
flecainide	No	Unlikely
fluconazole	Yes	Yes
flucytosine	Yes	Yes
fluoxetine	No	No
folic acid	Yes	No data
foscarnet	Yes	No data
furosemide	No	Unlikely
gabapentin	Yes	No data
ganciclovir	Yes	No data
gemfibrozil	No	No
gentamicin	Yes	Yes
glyburide	No	Unlikely
haloperidol	No	No
heparin	No	No
hydralazine	No	No
hydrochlorothiazide	No	Unlikely
hydrocodone	No data	No data
hydromorphone	No data	No data
hydroxyzine	No	No
ibuprofen	No	Unlikely
ibutilide	No data	No data
imipenem	Yes	Yes
imipramine	No	No
indomethacin	No	Unlikely
insulin	No	No
irbesartan	No	No data

Generic drug	Removed by HD	Removed by PD
isoniazid	No	No
isosorbide dinitrate	No	No
isosorbide mononitrate	Yes	No
isradipine	No	No
ketoconazole	No	No
ketoprofen	Unlikely	Unlikely
labetalol	No	No
lansoprazole	No	Unlikely
levetiracetam	Yes	No data
levofloxacin	Unlikely	Unlikely
lidocaine	No	Unlikely
linezolid	Yes	No data
lisinopril	Yes	No data
lithium	Yes	Yes
loracarbef	Yes	No data
loratadine	No	No
lorazepam	No	Unlikely
losartan	No	No
lovastatin	Unlikely	Unlikely
loxapine	No data	No data
mannitol	Yes	Yes
maprotiline	No	Unlikely
melphalan	No	No data
meperidine	No	Unlikely
mercaptopurine	Yes	No data
meropenem	Yes	No data
mesalamine	Yes	Unlikely
mesna	No data	No data
metformin	Yes	No data
methadone	No	No
methicillin	No	No
methotrexate	Yes	No
methyldopa	Yes	Yes
methylprednisolone	Yes	No data
metoclopramide	No	No
metoprolol	Yes	No data
metronidazole	Yes	No
mexiletine	Yes	No
mezlocillin	Yes	No
miconazole	No	No
midazolam	No	Unlikely
minoxidil	Yes	Yes
morphine	No data	No
		(continued)

Generic drug	Removed by HD	Removed by PD
nadolol	Yes	No data
nafcillin	No	No
nalbuphine	No data	No data
naloxone	No data	No data
naltrexone	No data	No data
naproxen	No	Unlikely
neomycin	Yes	Yes
nicardipine	No	Unlikely
nifedipine	No	No
nilutamide	No data	No data
nimodipine	No	No
nitrofurantoin	Yes	No data
nitroglycerin	No	No
nitroprusside	Yes	Yes
nortriptyline	No	No
octreotide	Yes	No data
ofloxacin	Yes	No
olanzapine	No	No
omeprazole	Unlikely	Unlikely
ondansetron	Unlikely	Unlikely
oxazepam	No	Unlikely
oxycodone	No data	No data
paclitaxel	No	Unlikely
pancuronium	No data	No data
pantoprazole	No	No data
paroxetine	No	Unlikely
penicillin	Yes	No
phenobarbital	Yes	Yes
phenytoin	No	No
piperacillin	Yes	No
pravastatin	No	No data
prazepam	No	Unlikely
prazosin	No	No
prednisone	No	No
primidone	Yes	No data
procainamide	Yes	No
promethazine	No	No data
propafenone	No	No
propofol	Unlikely	Unlikely
propoxyphene	No	No
propranolol	No	No
propylthiouracil	No	No data
pseudoephedrine	No	Unlikely
quinapril	No	No
quinidine	No; removed by hemoperfusion	No
quinine	No	No
ramipril	No	No data
ranitidine	No	No
reserpine	No	No
reteplase	No data	No data
rifampin	No	No
risperidone	No data	No data
ritodrine	Yes	Yes
ritonavir	Unlikely	No
rosiglitazone	No	Unlikely
rosuvastatin	No	No data
salsalate	Yes	No
sertraline	No	Unlikely
simvastatin	Unlikely	Unlikely
sotalol	Yes	No data
stavudine	Yes	No data
streptomycin	Yes	Yes
sulbactam	Yes	No
sulfamethoxazole	Yes	No
sulfisoxazole	Yes	Yes
tamoxifen	No data	No data
tazobactam	Yes	No
temazepam	No	Unlikely
terazosin	No	No
tetracycline	No	No
theophylline	Yes	No
thiamine	No	Unlikely
ticarcillin	Yes	No
timolol	No	No
tirofiban	Yes	No data
tobramycin	Yes	Yes
torsemide	No	Unlikely
tramadol	No	No data
trimethoprim	Yes	No
valacyclovir	Yes	No
valproic acid	No	No
valsartan	No	Unlikely
vancomycin	No	No
venlafaxine	No	Unlikely
verapamil	No	No
warfarin	No	No
zalcitabine	No data	No data
ziprasidone	No	Unlikely
zolpidem	No	Unlikely

Identifying life-threatening adverse reactions

Early recognition of a life-threatening adverse drug reaction is a crucial aspect of patient care and safety. This appendix helps you identify life-threatening adverse reactions that are relatively rare or cause symptoms you may not be readily familiar with. Some reactions are potentially lethal from the onset; others can become lethal if they progress.

Acute pancreatitis
Inflammation of the pancreas
Signs and symptoms: sudden onset of epigastric pain, nausea, and vomiting

Acute respiratory distress syndrome (ARDS)
Respiratory insufficiency in which abnormal permeability of the alveolar-capillary membrane causes fluid to fill the alveoli, disrupting gas exchange
Signs and symptoms: dyspnea, tachypnea, and progressive hypoxemia despite oxygen therapy; pulmonary edema

Adrenal suppression
Condition marked by inhibition of one or more of the enzymes essential to adrenocortical hormone production
Signs and symptoms: weakness, fatigue, abdominal pain, appetite and weight loss, dizziness, orthostatic hypotension, increased skin pigmentation

Adynamic ileus
Intestinal obstruction caused by a reduction in intestinal motility
Signs and symptoms: nausea, vomiting, decreased or absent bowel sounds, abdominal distention

Agranulocytopenia
Acute condition caused by deficiencies of neutrophils, basophils, and eosinophils in the blood
Signs and symptoms: chills, fever, headache, malaise, weakness, fatigue

Alkalosis
Increase in blood alkalinity caused by buildup of alkalis or reduction of acids
Signs and symptoms: in metabolic alkalosis—apathy, confusion, stupor (when severe); in respiratory alkalosis—air hunger, muscle twitching, numbness or tingling of extremities or circumoral area

Amyloidosis
Metabolic disorder caused by deposition of protein-containing fibrils in tissues, which may attack the heart and blood vessels, brain, kidneys, liver, spleen, intestines, or endocrine glands
Signs and symptoms: vary with area of invasion

Anaphylactoid shock
Hypersensitivity reaction marked by acute airway obstruction and vascular collapse within minutes of exposure to an antigen
Signs and symptoms: edema, rash, tachycardia, hypotension, respiratory distress, seizures, unconsciousness

Anaphylaxis
Hypersensitivity reaction to an antigen to which the patient has been previously sensitized, causing sudden release of immunologic mediators either locally or throughout the body
Signs and symptoms: urticaria, angioedema, flushing, wheezing, dyspnea, increased mucus production, nausea, vomiting

(continued)

Identifying life-threatening adverse reactions (continued)

Angioedema
Vascular reaction involving deep dermal, submucosal, or subcutaneous tissues in which capillaries become dilated and more permeable; also called angioneurotic edema
Signs and symptoms: edema of skin, mucous membranes, and internal organs; urticaria; giant wheals; respiratory distress

Autoimmune phenomena
Immunologic responses, such as serum sickness, lupus, vasculitis, and hepatitis, associated with development of antibodies (as to a particular drug)
Signs and symptoms: possibly none; or signs and symptoms specific to the particular autoimmune condition

Bone marrow depression
Disruption of healthy blood cell development in the bone marrow (including red and white blood cells and platelets), which impairs or weakens the body's defense against pathogenic organisms, toxins, and irritants
Signs and symptoms: increased susceptibility to infection, fever, weakness

Cardiac tamponade
Condition marked by increased cardiac pressure, which inhibits filling of the heart chambers during diastole
Signs and symptoms: chest pain, weak peripheral pulses, distended neck veins, dyspnea, orthopnea, diaphoresis, anxiety, restlessness, pallor

Cardiomyopathy
Any disease or disorder of the heart that impairs normal cardiac performance
Signs and symptoms: shortness of breath, orthopnea, fatigue, chest pain, syncope

Cardiotoxicity
The quality of being poisonous or harmful to the heart (as with certain drugs)
Signs and symptoms: variable cardiac-related symptoms

Cardiovascular collapse
Sudden loss of effective blood flow to body tissues
Signs and symptoms: hypotension, vasovagal syncope, cardiogenic shock, cardiac arrest

Cerebral ischemia
Temporary lack of arterial or circulatory blood flow to the brain, possibly causing localized tissue death
Signs and symptoms: persistent focal neurologic deficit in the area of distribution of the involved cerebral artery

Chemical arachnoiditis
Inflammation of the arachnoid (middle) layer of the meninges of the brain and spinal cord in response to exposure to a toxic substance
Signs and symptoms: mild nausea or vomiting, headache, fever, neck or back pain and stiffness

Cholesterol embolism
Sudden obstruction of a blood vessel by cholesterol-containing plaques
Signs and symptoms: hypotension, sudden shortness of breath, weak pulse, cyanosis, chest pain, decreased level of consciousness

Disseminated intravascular coagulation
Disorder marked by abnormal activation of coagulation factors in the blood, causing hemostasis, thrombosis, and possibly, organ damage
Signs and symptoms: bleeding (possibly from multiple sites), hematomas, thrombosis, petechiae, ecchymosis, cutaneous oozing

Disulfiram-like reaction
Acute, unpleasant reaction to alcohol ingestion in a patient taking disulfiram (Antabuse) for alcohol aversion therapy
Signs and symptoms: flushing, dyspnea, headache, nausea, copious vomiting, blood pressure fluctuations

Encephalopathy
Generalized dysfunction of the brain
Signs and symptoms: impaired speech, orientation, or cognition; sluggish reaction to stimuli

Eosinophilic pneumonitis
Infiltration of pulmonary alveoli by large numbers of eosinophils and mononuclear cells, causing inflammation
Signs and symptoms: dyspnea, cough, fever, night sweats, pulmonary edema, weight loss

Epileptiform seizures
Sudden, uncontrolled electrical discharge from the cerebral cortex caused by epilepsy
Signs and symptoms: variable; may include a cry, a fall, unconsciousness, overt seizure, amnesia, or incontinence

Erythema multiforme
Hypersensitivity reaction of the skin and mucous membranes; may take a severe multisystemic form
Signs and symptoms: rash, macules, papules, or blisters on the face, palms, and extremities

Fanconi syndrome
Congenital form of anemia caused by excessive amino acids in the blood secondary to renal tubular failure
Signs and symptoms: polyuria; growth impairment; soft, flexible, brittle bones

Granulocytopenia
Abnormal reduction in the number of granulocytes in the blood
Signs and symptoms: increased susceptibility to infection

Heart block
Interference with the normal electrical impulses of the heart, classified by the level of impairment that results (first-, second-, or-third-degree block)
Signs and symptoms: prolonged PR interval, widened QRS interval, and delayed or dropped beats on ECG; other symptoms vary with the degree of heart block and may include dizziness, syncope, shortness of breath, fatigue, and orthostatic hypotension

Hepatomegaly
Liver enlargement
Signs and symptoms: possibly none; or abdominal distention, abdominal pain, and constipation

Hepatotoxicity
Liver inflammation caused by exposure to a toxin or a toxic amount of a substance in the body
Signs and symptoms: jaundice, fatigue, weakness, altered mental status

Hyperkalemia
A condition marked by an excessive amount of potassium in the blood
Signs and symptoms: possibly none; with severe hyperkalemia—muscle weakness, arrhythmias

Hypertensive crisis
Severe blood pressure elevation, usually defined as diastolic pressure higher than 130 mmHg
Signs and symptoms: severe headache, dizziness, light-headedness

Hypertonia
Excessive tension or pressure within a muscle or an artery
Signs and symptoms: muscle pain and spasms

(continued)

Identifying life-threatening adverse reactions (continued)

Impaired myocardial contractility
Decreased contractile ability of the middle layer of the heart muscle wall
Signs and symptoms: shortness of breath, chest pain, edema

Increased intracranial pressure
Increased pressure within the brain, as from increased cerebrospinal fluid pressure or a brain lesion or swelling; also called intracranial hypertension
Signs and symptoms: in infants—bulging fontanel, separated sutures, lethargy, vomiting; in older children and adults—lethargy, vomiting, headache, behavior changes, seizures, neurologic deficits, progressive decrease in level of consciousness

Interstitial pneumonia
Chronic, noninfectious inflammation of the pulmonary alveolar walls
Signs and symptoms: shortness of breath, either with activity or at rest

Ischemic colitis
Inflammation of the colon caused by lack of blood supply to mesenteric arteries of the small intestine
Signs and symptoms: abdominal pain, weight loss

Lactic acidosis
Accumulation of lactic acid in the blood caused by reduced oxygenation and perfusion to tissues, muscles, and major organs
Signs and symptoms: muscle pain, fatigue, hyperventilation, nausea, vomiting, dizziness, light-headedness

Leukocytosis
Abnormal increase in the number of white blood cells (leukocytes) in the blood
Signs and symptoms: fever, hemorrhage

Leukopenia
Abnormal reduction (below 5,000 cells/mm^3) in circulating white blood cells, as from drug-induced impairment of blood cell production
Signs and symptoms: infection, fever, stomatitis, sinusitis

Lupuslike syndrome
A syndrome similar to systemic lupus erythematosus that occurs in response to drug therapy and resolves when the drug is withdrawn
Signs and symptoms: fever; red, scaly, macular skin rash; joint inflammation

Lupus nephritis
Kidney inflammation associated with systemic lupus erythematosus (SLE), marked by deposition of antigen-antibody complexes in the mesangium and basement membrane
Signs and symptoms: hypertension, peripheral edema, proteinuria, renal failure, cardiac decompensation, other symptoms of active SLE (such as fatigue, fever, rash, arthritis, CNS disease)

Megaloblastic anemia
Anemia marked by production and proliferation of megaloblasts (large immature red blood cells) in the bone marrow or circulation
Signs and symptoms: weakness, fatigue, light-headedness, headache, rapid pulse, breathlessness

Metabolic acidosis
Increase in blood acidity caused by buildup of acids or loss of bicarbonate
Signs and symptoms: lethargy, drowsiness, headache, diminished muscle tone and reflexes, hyperventilation, arrhythmias, nausea, vomiting, diarrhea, abdominal pain

Methemoglobinemia
Condition in which a portion of the iron component of hemoglobin has been oxidized to the ferric state, making it incapable of transporting oxygen
Signs and symptoms: cyanosis, dizziness, drowsiness, headache

Neoplasm
Abnormal growth of new tissue, such as a tumor
Signs and symptoms: vary with tumor site

Nephrotoxicity
The quality of causing damage to the kidney (as from a drug); usually leads to increased permeability to proteins, which results in edema and hypoalbuminemia
Signs and symptoms: proteinuria, hematuria, fluid retention

Neuroleptic malignant syndrome
Reaction to a drug that alters the brain's dopamine level or to withdrawal of a drug that increases the dopamine level
Signs and symptoms: sweating, altered mental status, seizures, renal failure

Neutropenia
Abnormal decrease in the level of neutrophils in the blood (usually below 1,500 per μL)
Signs and symptoms: infection, fever, mouth and throat sores

Osmotic nephrosis
Disruption of osmotic pressure in the kidney's renal tubule
Signs and symptoms: fluid retention, edema

Pancytopenia
Deficiency of all cellular elements of the blood, including red blood cells, white blood cells, and platelets
Signs and symptoms: bleeding from the nose and gums, easy bruising, fatigue, shortness of breath

Papilledema
Swelling and inflammation of the optic nerve
Signs and symptoms: severe headache, visual disturbances, blindness

Pericardial effusion
Escape of fluid from blood vessels into the pericardium
Signs and symptoms: hypotension, tachycardia, muffled heart sounds, decreased breath sounds, distended jugular vein, pulsus paradoxus, widened pulse pressure, weak peripheral pulses, pericardial friction rub, tachypnea, edema, cyanosis

Pseudomembranous colitis
Condition in which an inflammatory exudate forms on epithelial tissues of the colon
Signs and symptoms: diarrhea with blood and mucus, abdominal cramps

Pseudotumor cerebri
Benign intracranial hypertension without evidence of a brain tumor
Signs and symptoms: headache, papilledema, elevated cerebrospinal fluid pressure

Pulmonary toxicity
The quality of causing damage to the lungs and alveoli (as from certain drugs)
Signs and symptoms: any respiratory sign or symptom

Renal acidosis
Acidosis caused by accumulation of phosphoric and sulfuric acids in the body, which the kidneys fail to excrete
Signs and symptoms: appetite loss, altered level of consciousness, altered respiratory rate or effort

(continued)

Identifying life-threatening adverse reactions (continued)

Renal failure
Condition marked by a serum creatinine increase of 25% or more, which impairs the kidney's ability to excrete wastes, concentrate urine, and conserve electrolytes
Signs and symptoms: dehydration, fluid overload, altered neurologic status, appetite loss, weight gain, bleeding

Respiratory acidosis
Acidosis resulting from accumulation and retention of carbon dioxide in the lungs
Signs and symptoms: dyspnea, diaphoresis, tremors, decreased reflexes, decreased level of consciousness

Rhabdomyolysis
Acute disorder in which byproducts of skeletal muscle destruction accumulate in the renal tubules, causing renal failure
Signs and symptoms: See "Hyperkalemia" and "Metabolic acidosis."

Salicylate toxicity
Toxic condition caused by overdose of a salicylate, such as aspirin or an aspirin derivative
Signs and symptoms: rapid breathing, irritability, headache, vomiting, and (if extreme) seizures and respiratory failure

Sarcoidosis
Multisystemic disease that causes granulomatous lesions of organs or tissues throughout the body
Signs and symptoms: fatigue, weight loss, shortness of breath, anorexia, skin lesions, cough, skeletal changes (in later stages)

Sepsis
Systemic inflammatory response caused by pathogenic microorganisms or their toxins
Signs and symptoms: tachycardia, fever, rapid breathing, hypothermia, evidence of reduced blood flow to major organs

Serotonin syndrome
Syndrome marked by changes in autonomic, neuromotor, and cognitive-behavioral function, resulting from increased serotonergic stimulation (as from certain drugs)
Signs and symptoms: fever, tremors, myoclonus, diaphoresis, agitation, muscle rigidity, chills, hyperreflexia

Serum sickness
Hypersensitivity reaction to administration of a nonprotein drug
Signs and symptoms: fever, rash, joint pain, edema, lymphadenopathy

Steatosis
Fatty liver degeneration
Signs and symptoms: possibly none; or right upper abdominal quadrant pain, abdominal discomfort, fatigue, malaise

Stevens-Johnson syndrome
Severe allergic reaction marked by severe skin and mucous membrane lesions, most often in response to a drug
Signs and symptoms: respiratory tract infection, fever, sore throat, chills, headache, malaise, vomiting, diarrhea, tachycardia, hypotension, corneal ulcers, conjunctivitis, epistaxis, dysuria, erosive vulvovaginitis, balanitis, seizures, altered level of consciousness, coma

Suicidal ideation
Thoughts of intentionally ending one's life
Signs and symptoms: depressed mood, giving away of possessions, statements indicating a wish to die, risk-taking behavior, alcohol or drug abuse

Sulfone syndrome
Syndrome resulting from sensitivity to the drug dapsone
Signs and symptoms: fever, rash, jaundice, anemia, mucocutaneous pemphigus lesions

Syndrome of inappropriate antidiuretic hormone secretion
Metabolic disturbance marked by an increase in antidiuretic hormone, which causes a decrease in serum sodium concentration
Signs and symptoms: weakness, fatigue, malaise, headache, altered mental status, lethargy, irritability, delirium, psychosis, personality changes, anorexia, nausea, vomiting, thirst, abdominal and muscle cramps

Tardive dyskinesia
Disorder marked by slow, rhythmic involuntary movements of the face, limbs, and torso in patients who have received long-term dopaminergic antagonist therapy
Signs and symptoms: involuntary, repetitive facial grimacing and twisting; tongue protrusion; lip puckering and smacking; chewing or sucking motions; involuntary, snakelike writhing movements (such as wiggling or twisting); excessive blinking; involuntary flexion and extension movements of the fingers and hands

Tetany
Hyperexcitability of nerves and muscles caused by a decrease in extracellular calcium
Signs and symptoms: muscle twitching, cramps, sharp flexion of wrist and ankle joints, seizures

Thrombocytopenia
Abnormal decrease in the number of platelets caused by destruction of erythroid tissue in the bone marrow
Signs and symptoms: purpura, ecchymosis, petechiae, internal hemorrhage, hematuria, abdominal distention, melena

Torsade de pointes
Rapid form of ventricular tachycardia that appears as twisting or shifting QRS complexes on the ECG
Signs and symptoms: pallor, diaphoresis, rapid pulse, low or normal blood pressure, transient or prolonged loss of consciousness

Toxic epidermal necrolysis
Exfoliative skin condition that represents a severe cutaneous reaction (as to a drug, infection, or chemical exposure)
Signs and symptoms: scalded appearance of the skin, skin erosion and redness

Vascular leak syndrome
Leakage of blood from arteries, veins, and capillaries
Signs and symptoms: hypotension, bleeding, petechiae

Vascular thrombosis
Formation or presence of a blood clot in the vascular system
Signs and symptoms: vary with site of clot

Withdrawal phenomena
Physiologic changes caused by discontinuation of a drug or alcohol after prolonged use
Signs and symptoms: vary with type of substance used. In opioid withdrawal—rapid pulse and breathing, runny nose, yawning, restlessness, insomnia, fatigue, pupil dilation, nausea, vomiting, diarrhea, abdominal cramps, weakness, muscle aches, joint pain, hot and cold flushes. In benzodiazepine withdrawal—headache; aches and pains; anxiety; sleep disturbances; feelings of unreality; impaired memory; palpitations; hypersensitivity to noise, light, and touch.

Selected references

American Society of Health-System Pharmacists. ASHP guidelines on handling hazardous drugs. *Am J Health Syst Pharm*. 2006;63(12):1192-1193.

Brunton, L., Lazo, J., and Parker, K. *Goodman & Gilman's The Pharmacological Basis of Therapeutics*, 11th ed. New York: McGraw Hill Professional, 2005.

Drug Facts and Comparisons 2008. Philadelphia, Pa.: Lippincott Williams & Wilkins, 2007.

Drug Information for the Health Care Professional (USP DI Vol 1: Drug Information for the Health Care Professional), 27th ed. Greenwood Village, Colo.: Micromedex Thomson Healthcare, 2007.

Hansten, P.D. *Top 100 Drug Interactions 2007: A Guide to Patient Management*. Edmonds, Wash.: H&H Publications, 2007.

Hansten, P.D., and Horn, J.R. *Drug Interactions Analysis and Management*, 3rd ed. Philadelphia, Pa.: Lippincott Williams & Wilkins, 2008.

The Injectable Drug Reference. Mount Prospect, Ill.: Society of Critical Care Medicine, 2006.

King, J. *King Guide to Parenteral Admixtures 2006*. Napa, Calif.: King Guide Publications, Inc., 2006.

Mosby's Drug Consult 2007, 17th ed. St. Louis, Mo.: 2006.

PDR for Herbal Medicines, 4th ed. Montvale, N.J.: Thomson Healthcare, 2007.

Polovich, M., and Blecher C.S., eds. *Safe Handling of Hazardous Drugs*. Pittsburgh, Pa.: Oncology Nursing Society, 2003.

RxFACTS: Natural Products. St. Louis, Mo.: Facts and Comparisons, 2002.

Shargel, L., Wu-Pong, S., and Yu, A.B. *Applied Biopharmaceutics & Pharmacokinetics*, 5th ed. New York: McGraw-Hill Medical, 2004.

Sweetman, S.C., eds. *Martindale: The Complete Drug Reference*, 35th ed. London: Pharmaceutical Press, 2006.

Trissel, L.A. *Handbook on Injectable Drugs*, 14th ed. Bethesda, Md.: American Society of Hospital Pharmacists, 2007.

2007 Dialysis of Drugs. Verona, Wis.: Nephrology Pharmacy Associates, 2007.

2008 Physician' Desk Reference, 62nd ed. Montvale, N.J.: Thomson Healthcare, 2007.

Walsh, C.T., and Schwartz-Bloom, R.D. *Levine's Pharmacology: Drug Actions and Reactions*, 7th ed. New York: Taylor & Francis Group, 2004.

Online resources

American Regent (injectable drug information): http://www.americanregent.com/.

American Society of Health-System Pharmacists: http://www.ashp.org/ahfs/.

Centers for Disease Control and Prevention (drugs considered hazardous): http://www.cdc.gov/niosh/docs/2004-165/2004-165d.html#o.

DrugPoints System: http://www.micromedex.com/products/drugpoints/.

Drugs.com (patient teaching): http://www.drugs.com/.

Institute for Safe Medication Practices (list of high-alert medications): http://www.ismp.org/Tools/highalertmedications.pdf.

MedlinePlus (medicines): http://www.nlm.nih.gov/medlineplus/medicines.html.

MedlinePlus (patient teaching): http://www.nlm.nih.gov/medlineplus/.

MedWatch (safety information and adverse events reporting program): http://www.fda.gov/medwatch/safety.htm.

Micromedex (Healthcare Series of drug databases): http://www.micromedex.com/products/drugdex/.

MSDS Solutions Center (hazardous drug information): http://msds.com/.

Natural Medicines Comprehensive Database: http://www.naturaldatabase.com.

PubMed: http://pubmed.gov.

RxList (general drug information): http://www.rxlist.com/script/main/hp.asp.

STAT!Ref (online electronic medical library): http://www.statref.com/.

U.S. Department of Labor, Occupational Safety & Health Administration: http://www.osha.gov/dts/osta/otm/otm_vi/otm_vi_2.html.

U.S. Food and Drug Administration (consumer drug information): http://www.fds.gov/cder/drug/DrugSafety/DrugIndex.htm.

U.S. Food and Drug Administration (recalls, market withdrawals, and safety alerts): http://www.fda.gov/opacom/7alerts.html.

U.S. Food and Drug Administration Center for Drug Evaluation and Research: http://www.fda.gov/cder/.

USP DI Volume II (advice for the patient): http://www.usd.edu/library/logins/bin/ipcheck.pl?dbname=u%2Fuspdi.

Index

A

abatacept, 3-4
Abbreviations
common, **S24-S25**
dangerous, **S23**
abciximab, 4-7
Abelcet, 47
Abortion, incomplete, oxytocin for, 487
Abraxane, 491
Access devices, **S10-S15**
Acetadote, 7
Acetaminophen overdose, acetylcysteine for, 7
acetazolamide, 663
Acetylcholine release, atropine for, 84
Acetylcholinesterase insecticide poisoning, atropine for, 84
acetylcysteine, 7-8
Acromegaly, ocreotide for, 471
Actilyse, 27
Actinomycosis, penicillin G potassium for, 507
Activase, 27
Activase rt-PA, 27
Actrapid, 359
Acute coronary syndrome
eptifibatide for, 265
tirofiban for, 613
Acute lymphoblastic leukemia
asparaginase for, 667
clofarabine for, 172
methotrexate for, 418
nelarabine for, 683
pegaspargase for, 684
teniposide injection for, 688
Acute lymphocytic leukemia
cytarabine for, 184, 185
daunorubicin for, 201
Acute myelogenous leukemia, sargramostim for, 579
Acute myeloid leukemia
filgrastim for, 291
gemtuzumab for, 316
idarubicin for, 344
Acute nephrosis, albumin for, 15
Acute nonlymphocytic leukemia
cytarabine for, 184
daunorubicin for, 201
mitoxantrone for, 439
Acute promyelocytic leukemia, arsenic trioxide for, 75
Acute pyelonephritis, levofloxacin for, 389, 390
Acute renal failure, mannitol for, 403
Acute respiratory distress syndrome, 703
acyclovir sodium, 8-11
Adams-Stokes attacks, isoproterenol for, 371
Adenocard, 11
Adenocor, 11
Adenoscan, 11
adenosine, 11-14
Administration rates, **S6**
Adrenal suppression, 703
Adrenocortical insufficiency
cosyntropin for, 671
hydrocortisone for, 331
Adrenocorticoid overmedication
potassium acetate for, 536
potassium chloride for, 538
Adriamycin PFS, 237
Adriamycin RDF, 237
Adrucil, 299
Advate, 61
Adverse reactions, life-threatening, 703-709
Adynamic ileus, 703
agalsidase beta, 663-664
Aggrastat, 612
Agranulocytopenia, 703
AHF, 61-63
albumin (human normal serum), 14-16
Alcohol withdrawal
chlordiazepoxide for, 153
diazepam for, 213
aldesleukin, 16-20
Aldomet, 421, 683
Aldosteronism
potassium acetate for, 536
potassium chloride for, 538
alefacept, 664
alemtuzumab, 664-665
Alfenta, 20
alfentanil hydrochloride, 20-22
Alimta, 503
Alkeran, 407
Allergic dermatoses, diphenhydramine for, 222
Allergic rhinitis, diphenhydramine for, 222
Allergies, methylprednisolone for, 423
Allergy symptoms, diphenhydramine for, 222
allopurinol sodium, 23-25
Alkalosis, 703
Aloprim, 23
Aloxi, 495
Alpha$_1$-antitrypsin deficiency, alpha$_1$-proteinase inhibitor for, 665

Alphanate, 61
AlphaNine SD, 282
alpha$_1$-proteinase inhibitor (human), 665-666
Alpha$_1$-proteinase inhibitor deficiency, alpha$_1$-proteinase inhibitor for, 665
alprostadil, 25-27
alteplase, 27-30
Alti-Acyclovir, 8
Amanta antidote, atropine as, 84
AmBisome, 47
Amevive, 664
Amicar, 39
Amidate, 277
amifostine, 31-33
amikacin sulfate, 33-35
Amikin, 33
amino acid injection, 35-38
amino acids, 35-38
aminocaproic acid, 39-40
aminophylline, 41-44
Aminosyn, 35
Aminosyn-HBC, 35
Aminosyn-RF 5.2%, 35
amiodarone hydrochloride, 44-47
Amnestic
  lorazepam as, 399
  midazolam as, 432
Amphocil, 47
Amphocin, 47
Amphotec, 47
amphotericin B cholesteryl sulfate, 47-54
amphotericin B desoxycholate, 47-54
amphotericin B lipid complex, 47-54
amphotericin B liposome, 47-54
ampicillin sodium, 54-57
ampicillin sodium and tazobactam sodium, 57-59
Ampicin, 54
Amrinone, 355
Amyloidosis, 703
Analgesia
  fentanyl for, 288
  oxymorphone for, 484
  promethazine for, 546
  remifentanil for, 568
  sufentanil for, 595
Anaphylactoid shock, 703
Anaphylaxis, 703
  diphenhydramine for, 222
  epinephrine for, 255
  treatment guidelines for, **S30**
Ancef, 124
Anectine, 591
Anemia
  darbepoetin alfa for, 196
  epoetin alfa for, 260, 261
  folic acid for, 302
Anesthesia
  alfentanil for, 21
  atracurium for, 81
  butorphanol for, 110
  cisatracurium for, 166
  etomidate for, 178
  fentanyl for, 288
  ketamine for, 377
  lidocaine for, 395
  meperidine for, 410
  midazolam for, 432
  nalbuphine for, 454
  pentazocine for, 511
  propofol for, 549
  remifentanil for, 568
  sufentanil for, 594
  thiopental for, 605, 606
  vecuronium for, 638
Anexate, 297
Angioedema, 704
Angina
  abciximab for, 5
  bivalirudin for, 96
  diltiazem for, 220
  eptifibatide for, 265
  nitroglycerin for, 465
Angiomax, 95
anidulafungin, 59-61
Ankylosing spondylitis, infliximab for, 357
Anthrax
  ciprofloxacin for, 163
  doxycycline for, 244
  penicillin G potassium for, 507
Anticholinergic toxicity, physostigmine for, 526
Anticholinesterase agents, blocking effects of, glycopyrrolate for, 323
Anticoagulant overdose, factor IX for, 282
Anticoagulation
  argatroban for, 72
  heparin for, 326
antihemophilic factor, 61-63
antihemophilic factor/von Willebrand factor complex (human, dried, pasteurized), 63-67
anti-inhibitor coagulant complex, 67-69
Antilirium, 526
antithrombin III, human, 69-71
anti-thymocyte globulin (equine) sterile solution, 666-667
anti-thymocyte globulin (rabbit), 666
Antizol, 303
Anxiety
  chlordiazepoxide for, 153
  diazepam for, 213
  lorazepam for, 399
  midazolam for, 432
  oxymorphone for, 484
Anzemet, 229
Apnea, neonatal, aminophylline for, 41

Apnea of prematurity, caffeine citrate for, 111
Apo-Butorphanol, 109
Apo-Cefoxitin, 133
Apo-Chlordiazepoxide, 152
Apo-Cimetidine, 161
Apo-Clindamycin, 169
Appendix, ruptured, pipercillin and tazabactam for, 530
Aquamephyton, 528
Arachnoiditis, chemical, 704
Aralast NP, 665
Aranesp, 195
Aredia, 496
argatroban, 71-74
Arranon, 683
Arrhythmia
  amiodarone for, 45
  digoxin for, 216
  diltiazem for, 220
  edetate for, 676
  esmolol for, 271
  ibutilide for, 342
  lidocaine for, 395
  phenylephrine for, 521
  potassium acetate for, 536
  potassium chloride for, 538
  procainamide for, 541
  propranolol for, 551
  quinidine for, 559
  verapamil for, 640
arsenic trioxide, 74-77
Arterial embolism
  heparin for, 326
  streptokinase for, 589
Arterial thrombosis, streptokinase for, 589
Arthritis. *See also* Gouty arthritis; Rheumatoid arthritis.
  hydrocortisone for, 331
ascorbic acid, 77-78
asparaginase, 667
Aspergillosis
  amphotericin B for, 48
  caspofungin for, 123
  voriconazole for, 650
Astramorph PF, 441
atenolol, 78-80
Atgam, 666
Atherectomy, tirofiban for, 613
Athetosis, diazepam for, 213
AT-III, 69-71
AT-III deficiency, antithrombin III, human for, 70
Ativan, 398
atracurium besylate, 80-84
Atrial fibrillation or flutter
  digoxin for, 216
  diltiazem for, 220
  ibutilide for, 342
  quinidine for, 559
  verapamil for, 640
  warfarin for, 653
atropine sulfate, 84-86
Autoimmune disorders, hydrocortisone for, 331
Autoimmune phenomena, 704
Autoplex-T, 67
Avastin, 93
Avelox, 444
Avirax, 8
Azactam Injection, 88
azathioprine sodium, 668
azithromycin, 86-88
aztreonam, 88-91

B
BabyBIG, 669
Bacteremia
  chloramphenicol for, 151
  daptomycin for, 193
  polymyxin B for, 534
Bacterial meningitis
  ampicillin for, 55
  cefuroxime for, 145
  meropenem for, 412
Bacterial septicemia, imipenem and cilastatin for, 348
Bactocill, 479
Bactrim, 596
basiliximab, 668-669
BCNU, 120
Bebulin VH, 282
Benadryl, 222
BeneFix, 282
Benzodiazepine overdose, flumazenil for, 298
Benzodiazepines, reversing effects of, flumazenil for, 297
benztropine mesylate, 91-93
Beriberi, thiamine for, 604
bevacizumab, 93-95
Bexxar Dosimetric, 622
Bexxar ^{131}I Dosimetric, 622
Bexxar ^{131}I Therapeutic, 622
Bexxar Therapeutic, 622
BiCNU, 120
Big-IV, 669
Biliary colic, atropine for, 84
Biliary tract infection, cefazolin for, 125
Bioclate, 61
Biorphen, 477
bivalirudin, 95-97
Black widow spider bite, calcium gluconate injection, 10% for, 669
Bladder cancer
  cisplatin for, 168
  doxorubicin for, 238
  vinblastine for, 643
Blastomycosis, amphotericin B for, 48
Bleeding, excessive
  aminocaproic acid for, 39
  antihemophilic factor/von Willebrand factor complex for, 64

Bleeding, excessive (continued)
coagulation factor VIIa (recombinant) for, 174
Blenoxane, 97
bleomycin sulfate, 97-100
Blood clotting, preventing, heparin for, 326
Blood levels, monitoring, **S28-S29**
Blood transfusions, sodium chloride for, 586
Bloodstream infection, polymyxin B for, 534
Body surface area
in adults, 695
in children, 696
Bone and joint infection
cefazolin for, 125
cefoxitin for, 133
ceftazidime for, 136
ceftizoxime for, 139
ceftriaxone for, 142
cefuroxime for, 145
ciprofloxacin for, 163
imipenem and cilastatin for, 348
Bone marrow depression, 704
Bone marrow transplantation
fluconazole for, 293
sargramostim for, 579
Bone metastasis
pamidronate for, 497
zoledronic acid for, 658
Boniva IV, 336
bortezomib, 100-102
botulism immune globulin intravenous (human), 669
Botulism, infant, botulism immune globulin intravenous (human) for, 669
Bradycardia, drug-induced, hyoscyamine for, 680
Brain mass, reducing, mannitol for, 403
Brain tumor, carmustine for, 120
BranchAmin 4%, 35
Breast cancer
cyclophosphamide for, 179
dexrazoxane for, 207
docetaxel for, 226
doxorubicin for, 238
epirubicin for, 258
fluorouracil for, 299
gemcitabine for, 312
paclitaxel for, 489
paclitaxel protein-bound particles for, 492
pamidronate for, 497
thiotepa for, 689
trastuzumab for, 629
vinblastine for, 643
Brevibloc, 271
Bronchial secretions, decreasing, atropine for, 84
Bronchitis
levofloxacin for, 389
moxifloxacin for, 444
ofloxacin for, 473
Bronchodilation, epinephrine for, 255
Bronchogenic carcinoma, mechlorethamine for, 405
Bronchospasm
aminophylline for, 41
atropine for, 84
isoproterenol for, 372
bumetanide, 102-104
Bumetanide Injection, 102
Buprenex, 104
buprenorphine hydrochloride, 104-106
Burns
albumin for, 15
ascorbic acid for, 77
Burns (continued)
potassium acetate for, 536
potassium chloride for, 538
Bursitis, methylprednisolone for, 423
Buscopan, 581
Busilvex, 106
busulfan, 106-109
Busulfex, 106
butorphanol tartrate, 109-111

C
Caelyx, 241
Cafcit, 111
caffeine citrate, 111-113
Calciject, 115
Calcijex, 113
calcitrol, 113-115
calcium chloride, 115-117
Calcium deficiencies, calcium gluconate injection, 10% for, 669
Calcium Disodium Versenate, 674
calcium folinate, 386-389
calcium gluconate injection, 10%, 669-670
Calorie replacement, dextrose for, 211
Campath, 664
Campto, 364
Camptosar, 364
Cancidas, 122
Candidemia
anidulafungin for, 60
voriconazole for, 650
Candidiasis
amphotericin B for, 49
anidulafungin for, 60
caspofungin for, 123
fluconazole for, 293
voriconazole for, 650
Capastat Sulfate, 670
capreomycin, 670
carboplatin, 117-119

Cardene IV, 463
Cardiac arrest
epinephrine for, 255
isoproterenol for, 371
norepinephrine for, 470
treatment guidelines for, **S31, S32**
tromethamine for, 631
Cardiac bypass surgery, tromethamine for, 631
Cardiac decompensation, dobutamine for, 224
Cardiac ischemic complications, abciximab for, 5
Cardiac output, low, isoproterenol for, 371
Cardiac rhythm, restoring, epinephrine for, 255
Cardiac surgery
dobutamine as adjunct in, 224
propofol for, 549
Cardiac tamponade, 704
Cardiac valve replacement, warfarin for, 653
Cardiogenic shock
dobutamine for, 224
isoproterenol for, 371
Cardiomyopathy, 704
dexrazoxane for, 207
dobutamine for, 224
Cardiotoxicity, 704
Cardiovascular collapse, 704
Cardiovascular surgery, heparin for, 326
Cardioversion preparation, diazepam for, 213
Cardizem, 219
Carimune NF, 350
carmustine, 120-122
Carnitine deficiency, levocarnitine for, 680
Carnitor, 680
caspofungin acetate, 122-124
Cathflo Activase, 27
cefazolin sodium, 124-127
cefepime hydrochloride, 127-130
Cefizox, 139
cefotaxime sodium, 130-133
cefoxitin sodium, 133-135
ceftazidime, 136-138
ceftizoxime sodium, 139-141
ceftriaxone sodium, 142-144
cefuroxime sodium, 144-147
CellCept Intravenous, 450
Central nervous system depression, drug-induced, doxapram for, 234
Central venous access device, restoring function to, alteplase for, 28
Cerebral ischemia, 704
Cerebral palsy, diazepam for, 213
Cerebrovascular accident, alteplase for, 28
Cerebyx, 678
Ceribidine, 200
Cervical cancer
bleomycin for, 98
topotecan for, 618
Cervical infection, ofloxacin for, 473, 474
Cesarean delivery, cefotaxime for, 130
cetuximab, 147-150
Chemical arachnoiditis, 704
*ChiRho*Stim, 686
Chlamydial infection
doxycycline for, 244
ofloxacin for, 473, 474
chloramphenicol, 150-152
chlordiazepoxide hydrochloride, 152-154
Chloromycetin, 150
chlorothiazide, 154-156
chlorpromazine hydrochloride, 156-159
Choline esters antidote, atropine as, 84
Cholinergic crisis vs. myasthenic crisis, edrophonium for, 251
Cholinergic effects, blocking, glycopyrrolate for, 323
Choriocarcinoma, vinblastine for, 643
Christmas disease, factor IX for, 282
Chromium, 626
Chronic lymphocytic leukemia
alemtuzumab for, 664
immune globulin for, 351
mechlorethamine for, 405
Chronic myelocytic leukemia, mechlorethamine for, 405
Chronic myelogenous leukemia, busulfan for, 107
Chronic pulmonary disease, doxapram for, 233
Chronic renal failure, torsemide for, 620
cidofovir, 159-161
Cidomycin, 318
cimetidine, 161-163
Cipro I.V., 163
ciprofloxacin hydrochloride, 163-165
Ciproxin, 163
Cirrhosis
amino acids for, 37
furosemide for, 305
torsemide for, 620

cisatracurium besylate, 165-167
cisplatin, 167-169
citrovorum factor, 386-389
cladribine, 671
Claforan, 130
Cleocin Phosphate, 169
clindamycin phosphate, 169-172
clofarabine, 172-174
Clolar, 172
Clostridial infection, penicillin G potassium for, 507
Clotting, preventing, heparin for, 326
CMV-IG-IV, 186-189
coagulation factor VIIa (recombinant), 174-175
Coccidioidomycosis, amphotericin B for, 48
codeine phosphate, 175-177
Cogentin, 91
colchicine, 177-179
Colic
  atropine for, 84
  calcium gluconate injection, 10% for, 669
  hyoscyamine for, 679
Colitis
  ischemic, 706
  pseudomembranous, 707
  ulcerative. *See* Ulcerative colitis.
Collagen disorders
  hydrocortisone for, 331
  methylprednisolone for, 423
Colon cancer. *See* Colorectal cancer.
Colorectal cancer
  bevacizumab for, 93
  cetuximab for, 148
  fluorouracil for, 299
Colorectal cancer *(continued)*
  irinotecan for, 365
  leucovorin for, 387
  oxaliplatin for, 482
Colorectal surgery prophylaxis, ertapenem for, 267
Compatibilities, drug, **S2-S5**
Compazine, 543
Continuous-flow centrifugation leukapheresis, hetastarch for, 329
Controlled substances schedule, xiv
Conversions, drug, **S6**
Convulsive therapy, electrically induced, succinylcholine for, 592
Copper, 626
Cordarone, 44
Corlopam, 677
Coronary artery disease
  adenosine for diagnosis of, 12
  dipyridamole for evaluation in, 674
Corticotropin overmedication
  potassium acetate for, 536
  potassium chloride for, 538
Cortrosyn, 671
Corvert, 341
CosmoFer, 367
cosyntropin, 671-672
co-trimoxazole, 596-599
Coumadin, 653
Cramping, calcium gluconate injection, 10% for, 669
Crohn's disease, infliximab for, 357
Crying episodes, atropine for, 84
Cryptococcal meningitis
  amphotericin B for, 49
  fluconazole for, 293
Cryptococcosis, amphotericin B for, 48
crystalline amino acid infusions, 35-38
Cubicin, 193
cyclophosphamide, 179-181
cyclosporine, 181-184
Cyklokapron, 690
Cymevene, 309
Cystitis
  hyoscyamine for, 679
  ofloxacin for, 473
cytarabine, 184-186
cytarabine liposome, 184-186
CytoGam, 186
Cytomegalovirus disease
  cytomegalovirus immune globulin intravenous (human) for, 186
  ganciclovir for, 309
cytomegalovirus immune globulin intravenous (human), 186-189
Cytomegalovirus retinitis
  cidofovir for, 159
  foscarnet for, 678
  ganciclovir for, 309
Cytosar, 184
Cytosar-U, 184
Cytovene, 309
Cytoxan, 179

D

dacarbazine, 189-191
daclizumab, 672
Dalacin, 169
Dantrium Intravenous, 191
dantrolene sodium, 191-193
daptomycin, 193-195
darbepoetin alfa, 195-197
daunorubicin citrate liposome, 197-200

daunorubicin hydrochloride, 200-203
DaunoXome, 197
Dazamide, 663
DDAVP, 205
1-deamino-8-D-arginine vasopressin, 205-206
Deep vein thrombosis, streptokinase for, 589
deferoxamine mesylate, 203-205
Defix, 282
Demadex, 620
Demerol, 409
denileukin diftitox, 672-673
Depacon, 632
DepoCyt, 184
Desferal, 203
desmopressin acetate, 205-206
Detrusor tone, reducing, atropine for, 84
DexFerrum, 367
DexIron, 367
dexmedetomidine hydrochloride, 673
dexrazoxane, 207-209
dextran 40, 209-211
dextran 70, 209-211
dextran 75, 209-211
dextran, high-molecular-weight, 209-211
dextran, low-molecular-weight, 209-211
dextrose, 211-212
d-glucose, 211-212
D.H.E. 45, 673
DHPG, 309-312
Diabetes, hyperosmolar, sodium chloride for, 586
Diabetes insipidus, desmopressin for, 205
Diabetic acidosis
  potassium acetate for, 536
  potassium chloride for, 538
Diabetic gastroparesis, metoclopramide for, 426
Diabetic ketoacidosis, insulin, regular for, 359
Diagnostic procedures
  hyoscyamine for, 680
  ketamine for, 377
Dialysis, effects of, on drug therapy, 700-702
Diarrhea, ocreotide for, 471
Diazemuls, 213
diazepam, 213-215
Diflucan, 293
Digibind, 218
DigiFab, 218
Digitalis toxicity, edetate for, 676
digoxin, 215-218
digoxin immune FAB (ovine), 218-219
Digoxin toxicity, digoxin immune FAB for, 218
dihydroergotamine mesylate, 673-674
Dilantin, 522
Dilaudid, 333
Dilaudid-HP, 333
diltiazem hydrochloride, 219-222
Dilution, drug, sodium chloride for, 586
dimenhydrinate injection, 674
Dinate Injection, 674
diphenhydramine hydrochloride, 222-223
diphenylhydantoin sodium, 522-525
Diphtheria
  erythromycin for, 268
  penicillin G potassium for, 507
Diprivan, 548
dipyridamole, 674
Disseminated intravascular coagulation, 704
Disulfiram-like reaction, 705
Diuresis, mannitol for, 403
Dizziness, dimenhydrinate injection for, 674
Doamix, 663
dobutamine hydrochloride, 223-225
  infusion rates for, **S7**
docetaxel, 225-229
dolasetron mesylate, 229-231
Dolophine, 682
dopamine hydrochloride, 231-233
  infusion rates for, **S8**
Dopram, 233
Dosage calculations, **S6**
doxapram hydrochloride, 233-235
doxercalciferol, 235-237
Doxil, 241
doxorubicin hydrochloride, 237-241
doxorubicin hydrochloride liposomal, 241-244
doxycycline hyclate, 244-246
Doxylar, 244
Dramamine Injection, 674
Dramanate Injection, 674
droperidol, 246-249
drotrecogin alfa (activated), 249-250
Drug compatibilities, **S2-S5**
  with I.V. solutions, 697-699
Drug conversions and calculations, **S6**
Drugs
  administration rates for, **S6**
  diluting, sodium chloride for, 586
  hazardous, **S18, S19-S22**
  high-alert, **S17**

Drugs that look and sound alike, **S26-S27**
Drug therapy, effects of dialysis on, 700-702
Drug toxicity, mannitol for, 403
DTIC, 189
DTIC-Dome, 189
Duodenal ulcer, ranitidine for, 564
Duramorph, 441
Dymenate Injection, 674
Dysparnet, 161
Dyspnea, oxymorphone for, 484

E
Eclampsia, magnesium for, 401
Edema
acetazolamide for, 663
bumetanide for, 103
chlorothiazide for, 155
furosemide for, 305
methylprednisolone for, 423
edetate calcium disodium injection, 674-675
edetate disodium, 676
edrophonium chloride, 251-252
Electrolyte replacement, sodium chloride for, 586
Elitek, 566
Ellence, 257
Eloxitan, 481
Elspar, 667
Embolism. *See also* Pulmonary embolism.
heparin for, 326
streptokinase for, 589
warfarin for, 653
Emphysema, $alpha_1$-proteinase inhibitor for, 665
enalaprilat, 253-255
Encephalitis, herpes simplex, acyclovir for, 9
Encephalopathy, 705
Endocarditis
cefazolin for, 125
daptomycin for, 193
imipenem and cilastatin for, 348
penicillin G potassium for, 507
Endocarditis prophylaxis
ampicillin for, 55
gentamicin for, 319
vancomycin for, 635
Endocrine disorders, methylprednisolone for, 423
Endoscopic retrograde cholangiopancreatography, secretin for, 687
Endoscopy preparation, diazepam for, 213
Endotracheal intubation
alfentanil for, 21
atracurium for, 81
succinylcholine for, 592
vecuronium for, 638
Endoxana, 179
Endrate, 676
Enlon, 251
enoxaparin, 676-677
Enterococcal infection, linezolid for, 397
Eosinophilic pneumonitis, 705
Epileptiform seizures, 705. *See also* Seizures.
epinephrine hydrochloride, 255-257
infusion rates for, **S9**
epirubicin hydrochloride, 257-260
epoetin alfa, 260-262
Epogen, 260
epoprostenol sodium, 262-264
Eposin, 279
Eprex, 260
eptifibatide, 264-266
Eraxis, 59
Erbitux, 147
ertapenem sodium, 266-268
Erysipeloid endocarditis, penicillin G potassium for, 507
Erythema multiforme, 705
Erythrasma, erythromycin for, 268
Erythroblastosis fetalis, albumin for, 15
Erythrocin, 268
Erythrocyte resuspension, albumin for, 15
erythromycin lactobionate, 268-270
esmolol hydrochloride, 271-273
esomeprazole sodium, 273-274
Esophageal cancer, porfimer for, 686
Esophagitis, corrosive, pantoprazole for, 500
Essential hypertension, hydralazine for, 679
estrogens, conjugated, 275-277
Ethylene glycol poisoning, fomepizole injection for, 303
ethylenediamine, 41-44
Ethyol, 31
etomidate, 277-279
Etopophos, 279
etoposide, 279-282
etoposide phosphate, 279-282
Evoltra, 172
Ewing's sarcoma, doxorubicin for, 238
Extrapyramidal disorders, drug-induced, benztropine for, 91
Extravasation, preventing and treating, **S16**
Eye disorders, methylprednisolone for, 423

F

Fabrazyme, 663
Fabry disease, agalsidase beta for, 663
factor VIII, 61-63
factor IX (human), 282-284
factor IX (recombinant), 282-284
factor IX complex (human), 282-284
Factor IX deficiency, factor IX for, 282
Familial periodic paralysis, potassium acetate for, 536
famotidine, 284-286
Fanconi syndrome, 705
Fasturtec, 566
fat emulsions, 286-288
Fatty acid deficiency, fat emulsions for, 286
Febrile neutropenia
- amphotericin B for, 50
- cefepime for, 128
- ciprofloxacin for, 163
- filgrastim for, 291

Feiba VH, 67
fenoldopam mesylate, 677-678
fentanyl citrate, 288-290
Ferrlecit, 587
Fibrazyme, 663
filgrastim, 290-292
Flebogamma, 350
Flolan, 262
Floxin, 473
fluconazole, 293-295
Fluconazole Omega, 293
Fludara, 295
fludarabine phosphate, 295-297
Fluid replacement, sodium chloride for, 586
flumazenil, 297-299
fluorouracil, 299-301
5-fluorouracil, 299-301
Flushing
- I.V. *See* I.V. flushing.
- ocreotide for, 471

folic acid, 301-303
Folic acid antagonist overdose, leucovorin for, 387
folinic acid, 386-389
Folvite, 301
fomepizole injection, 303-304
Fortaz, 136
Fortral, 511
Fortum, 136
foscarnet sodium, 678
Foscavir, 678
fosphenytoin sodium, 678-679
FreAmine, 35
FreAmine-HBC, 35
FreAmine III, 35
5-FU, 299-301
Fungal infection
- amphotericin B for, 50
- voriconazole for, 650

Fungilin, 47
Fungizone Intravenous, 47
furosemide, 304-307
Furoside, 304
Fusospirochetal infection, penicillin G potassium for, 507

G

Galenamet, 161
gallium nitrate, 307-309
Gamimune N, 350
Gammagard Liquid, 350
Gammagard S/D, 350
Gamunex, 350
ganciclovir, 309-312
Ganite, 307
Gastric cancer
- docetaxel for, 226
- doxorubicin for, 238
- fluorouracil for, 299
- mitomycin for, 436

Gastric pH, increasing, ranitidine for, 564
Gastrin secretions, stimulating, secretin for, 687
Gastrinoma, secretin for diagnosis of, 687
Gastroesophageal reflux disease
- esomeprazole for, 273
- famotidine for, 284
- pantoprazole for, 500

Gastrointestinal bleeding, stress-induced, cimetidine for, 161
Gastrointestinal disorders
- hyoscyamine for, 679
- methylprednisolone for, 423

Gastrointestinal infection, ampicillin for, 55
gemcitabine hydrochloride, 312-315
gemtuzumab ozagamicin, 315-318
Gemzar, 312
Genital herpes, acyclovir for, 9
Genital infection, cefazolin for, 125
Genitourinary infection, ertapenem for, 267
gentamicin sulfate, 318-321
Genticin, 318
Gentran 40, 209
Gentran 70, 209
Glaucoma, acetazolamide for, 663
GlucaGen, 321
GlucaGen Diagnostic Kit, 321
glucagon, 321-322
Glucagon Emergency Kit, 321
glycopyrrolate, 322-324
glycopyrronium, 322-324
GM-CSF, 579-581
Gonorrhea
- ampicillin for, 55
- cefotaxime for, 130
- ceftazidime for, 136
- ceftizoxime for, 139

Gonorrhea *(continued)*
ofloxacin for, 473, 474
penicillin G potassium for, 507
Gouty arthritis, colchicine for, 177, 178
granisetron hydrochloride, 324-325
Granulocytopenia, 705
Gynecologic infection
ampicillin and tazobactam for, 57
cefoxitin for, 133
ceftazidime for, 136
ceftizoxime for, 139
cefuroxime for, 145
imipenem and cilastatin for, 348
piperacillin for, 685
ticarcillin and clavulanate potassium for, 608

H

Hairy cell leukemia
cladribine for, 671
pentostatin for, 515
Haverhill fever, penicillin G potassium for, 507
Hazardous I.V. drugs, **S18**
guidelines for, **S19-S22**
Headache, dihydroergotamine for, 674
Head and neck cancer
amifostine for, 31
bleomycin for, 98
cetuximab for, 148
docetaxel for, 226
Head injuries, closed, atropine for, 84
Heart block, 705
hyoscyamine for, 679
isoproterenol for, 371
Heart failure
acetazolamide for, 663
bumetanide for, 103
digoxin for, 216
dobutamine for, 224
furosemide for, 305
Heart failure *(continued)*
inamrinone for, 355
isoproterenol for, 371
milrinone for, 434
nesiritide for, 462
nitroglycerin for, 465
torsemide for, 620
Heart transplantation, cytomegalovirus immune globulin intravenous (human) for, 186
Heart transplant rejection
cyclosporine for preventing, 182
muromonab-CD3 for, 448
Hectoral, 235
HelixateFS, 61
Hematologic disorders
hydrocortisone for, 331
methylprednisolone for, 423
Hemodialysis, sodium chloride for, 586
Hemodynamic imbalance, dopamine for, 231
Hemofil M, 61
Hemophilia
antihemophilic factor for, 61
antihemophilic factor/von Willebrand factor complex for, 64
anti-inhibitor coagulant complex for, 67
coagulation factor VIIa (recombinant) for, 174
desmopressin for, 205
factor IX for, 282
tranexamic acid injection for, 690
Hemorrhage, spontaneous
antihemophilic factor for, 61
Hemorrhage, spontaneous *(continued)*
antihemophilic factor/von Willebrand factor complex for, 64
anti-inhibitor coagulant complex for, 67
Hemorrhagic cystitis, mesna for prevention of, 414
Hemorrhagic episodes, antihemophilic factor/von Willebrand factor complex for, 64
Hepalean, 326
Hepalean Lok, 326
heparin cofactor 1, 69-71
Heparin Leo, 326
Heparin overdose, protamine for, 554
heparin sodium, 326-328
HepatAmine, 35
Hepatic disease, bumetanide for, 103
Hepatic encephalopathy, amino acids for, 37
Hepatic failure, amino acids for, 37
Hepatitis, amino acids for, 37
Hepatomegaly, 705
Hepatotoxicity, 705
HepFlush 10, 326
Hep-Lock, 326
Hep-Lock U/P, 326
Herceptin, 628
Hereditary periodic paralysis, potassium acetate for, 536
Herpes simplex encephalitis, acyclovir for, 9
Herpes simplex virus infection
acyclovir for, 9
foscarnet for, 678
Hespan, 329
hetastarch, 329-330
Hextend, 329

Hiccups, intractable, chlorpromazine for, 157
High-alert drugs, **S17**
Hipfix, 282
Histiocytosis X, vinblastine for, 643
Histoplasmosis
  amphotericin B for, 48
  verteporfin for, 690
HN_2, 405-407
Hodgkin's disease
  bleomycin for, 98
  carmustine for, 120
  cyclophosphamide for, 179
  dacarbazine for, 189
  doxorubicin for, 238
  mechlorethamine for, 405
  thiotepa for, 689
  vinblastine for, 643
Human immunodeficiency virus infection
  daunorubicin citrate liposome for, 198
  zidovudine for, 656
Humate-P, 63
Humulin R, 359
Hyate:C, 61
Hycamtin, 618
hydralazine hydrochloride, 679
Hydrate Injection, 674
Hydration, sodium chloride for, 586
hydrocortisone sodium succinate, 330-333
hydromorphone hydrochloride, 333-336
hyoscine, 679-680
hyoscine hydrobromide, 581-583
hyoscyamine sulfate, 679-680
Hyperadrenocorticism
  potassium acetate for, 536
  potassium chloride for, 538
Hyperbilirubinemia, albumin for, 15
Hypercalcemia
  gallium for, 307
  hydrocortisone for, 331
  pamidronate for, 497
  zoledronic acid for, 658
Hypercalcemic emergency, edetate for, 676
Hyperhidrosis, hyoscyamine for, 679
Hyperkalemia, 705
Hypermotility, colonic, atropine for, 84
Hyperosmolar diabetes, sodium chloride for, 586
Hyperparathyroidism
  doxercalciferol for, 236
  paricalcitol for, 501
Hypersecretory conditions, pathologic
  cimetidine for, 161
  famotidine for, 284
  pantoprazole for, 500
  ranitidine for, 564
Hypersensitivity reaction
  epinephrine for, 255
  promethazine for, 546
Hypertension
  diltiazem for, 220
  enalaprilat for, 253
  esmolol for, 271
  fenoldopam for, 677
  hydralazine for, 679
  labetalol for, 382
  methyldopate for, 421, 683
  nicardipine for, 464
  nitroglycerin for, 465
  torsemide for, 620
Hypertensive crisis, 705
  methyldopate for, 421
  nitroprusside for, 467
Hypertensive episodes, phentolamine for, 684
Hypertonia, 705
  atropine for, 84
Hyperuricemia, rasburicase for, 566
Hypnotic effect, phenobarbital for, 518
Hypocalcemia
  calcitrol for, 113
  calcium chloride for, 116
  calcium gluconate injection, 10% for, 669
Hypocalcemic emergency, calcium chloride for, 115
Hypochloremia, sodium chloride for, 586
Hypogammaglobulinemia, immune globulin for, 351
Hypoglycemia
  dextrose for, 211
  glucagon for, 321
Hypomagnesemia, magnesium for, 400-401
Hyponatremia
  sodium acetate for, 583
  sodium chloride for, 586
Hypophosphatemia, phosphates for, 525
Hypoproteinemia, albumin for, 15
Hypoprothrombinemia, phytonadione for, 529
Hypotension
  dopamine for, 231
  nitroprusside for, 467
  norepinephrine for, 470
  phenylephrine for, 520
Hypotensive emergency, phenylephrine for, 520
Hypothyroidism, levothyroxine for, 681
Hypovolemia
  albumin for, 14
  isoproterenol for, 371
Hypovolemic shock, plasma protein fraction for, 533

I
ibandronate, 336-338
ibritumomab tiuxetan, 338-341
ibutilide fumarate, 341-343
Idamycin PFS, 343
idarubicin hydrochloride, 343-346
Idiopathic thrombocytopenic purpura, immune globulin for, 351
Ifex, 346
Ifex/Mesnex, 346
ifosfamide, 346-348
IGIV, 350-354
Ileus, adynamic, 703
IL-2, 16-20
imipenem and cilastatin sodium, 348-350
immune globulin for I.V. use, human, 350-355
Immunodeficiency, immune globulin for, 351
Imuran, 668
inamrinone lactate, 355-356
Inapsine, 246
Indocin I.V., 680
indomethacin, 680
Infant colic, hyoscyamine for, 679
Infection. *See also specific type.*
  amikacin for, 33
  aztreonam for, 88
  cefotaxime for, 130, 131
  ceftriaxone for, 142
  cefuroxime for, 145
  chloramphenicol for, 151
  clindamycin for, 170
  doxycycline for, 244
  gentamicin for, 319
  imipenem and cilastatin for, 348
Infection *(continued)*
  immune globulin for, 351
  kanamycin for, 374
  linezolid for, 397
  metronidazole for, 430
  nafcillin for, 452
  oxacillin for, 479
  penicillin G potassium for, 507
  piperacillin for, 685
  polymyxin B for, 534
  quinupristin and dalfopristin for, 562
  ticarcillin and clavulanate potassium for, 608
  tobramycin for, 616
  vancomycin for, 635
InFeD, 367
Inflammatory lesions, methylprednisolone for, 423
infliximab, 356-359
Infufer, 367
Infusion rates, **S7**
Infuvite Adult, 446
Infuvite Pediatric, 446
INH poisoning, pyridoxine for, 557
Insecticide poisoning, atropine for, 84
insulin, regular, 359-361
insulin injection, 359-361
Insulin-Toronto, 359
Integrilin, 264
interferon alfa-2b, recombinant, 361-364
interleukin-2, 16-20
Interstitial pneumonia, 706. *See also* Pneumonia.
Intra-abdominal infection
  ampicillin and tazobactam for, 57
  cefepime for, 128
  ceftizoxime for, 139
  ciprofloxacin for, 163
  ertapenem for, 267
Intra-abdominal infection *(continued)*
  imipenem and cilastatin for, 348
  meropenem for, 412
  moxifloxacin for, 444
  piperacillin for, 685
  tigecycline for, 611
Intracranial pressure, increased, 706
Intracranial pressure, reducing
  mannitol for, 403
  thiopental for, 606
Intraocular pressure, reducing, mannitol for, 403
Intron A, 361
Intropin, 231
Invanz, 266
Iodine, 626
irinotecan hydrochloride, 364-366
Iron deficiency, sodium ferric gluconate complex for, 588
Iron-deficiency anemia
  iron dextran for, 367
  iron sucrose for, 369
iron dextran, 367-369
Iron intoxication, deferoxamine for, 203
iron sucrose, 369-371
Isofluorophate antidote, atropine as, 84
Isoniazid poisoning, pyridoxine for, 557
isoproterenol hydrochloride, 371-373
Isoptin, 640
Isuprel, 371
I.V. access devices, **S10-S15**
Iveegam EN, 350
Iveegam Immuno, 350
I.V. flush
  heparin for, 326
  sodium chloride for, 586
I.V. solutions, and drug compatibility, 697-699

J
Joint infection. *See* Bone and joint infection.

K
kanamycin sulfate, 373-376
Kaposi's sarcoma
daunorubicin citrate liposome for, 198
doxorubicin hydrochloride liposomal for, 242
paclitaxel for, 489
vinblastine for, 643
Kawasaki disease, immune globulin for, 351
Kefadim, 136
Kemicetine, 150
Kepivance, 494
Ketalar, 376
ketamine hydrochloride, 376-378
ketorolac tromethamine, 379-381
Kidney transplantation, cytomegalovirus immune globulin intravenous (human) for, 186
Kidney transplant rejection
anti-thymocyte globulin (rabbit) for, 666
muromonab-CD3 for, 448
Kidney transplant rejection, preventing
anti-thymocyte globulin (equine) sterile solution for, 666
azathioprine for, 668
basiliximab for, 668
cyclosporine for, 182
daclizumab for, 672
mycophenolate for, 450
tacrolimus for, 600
Kidrolase, 667
Koate-DVI, 61
Kogenate FS, 61
Kytril, 324

L
labetalol hydrochloride, 381-384
Labor and delivery
butorphanol for, 110
oxymorphone for, 484
oxytocin for, 487
pentazocine for, 511
scopolamine for, 581
Laboratory values, common, 692-694
Lactic acidosis, 706
Lanoxin, 215
Lanoxin Injection Pediatric, 215
Largactil, 156
Lasix, 304
Laughing episodes, atropine for, 84
Lead colic, calcium gluconate injection, 10% for, 669
Lead nephropathy, edetate calcium disodium injection for, 675
Lead poisoining, edetate calcium disodium injection for, 675
LED, 241-244
Legionnares' disease, erythromycin for, 269
Leishmaniasis, amphotericin B for, 49
lepirudin, 384-386
Lesions
inflammatory, methylprednisolone for, 423
osteolytic, pamidronate for, 497
leucovorin calcium, 386-389
Leucovorin rescue, leucovorin for, 387
Leukapheresis, continuous-flow centrifugation, hetastarch for, 329
Leukemia. *See also specific type.*
allopurinol for, 23
cyclophosphamide for, 179
doxorubicin for, 238
vincristine for, 645
Leukine, 579
Leukocytosis, 706
Leukopenia, 706
Leustat, 671
Leustatin, 671
Levaquin, 389
levocarnitine, 680-681
Levo-Dromoran, 392
levofloxacin, 389-392
Levophed, 469
levorphanol tartrate, 392-394
levothyroxine sodium, 681
Levsin, 679
Librium, 152
lidocaine hydrochloride, 394-397
linezolid, 397-398
liothyronine sodium injection, 681-682
liposomal encapsulated doxorubicin, 241-244
Listeria infection, penicillin G potassium for, 507
Litat, 671
Liver transplantation, cytomegalovirus immune globulin intravenous (human) for, 186
Liver transplant rejection, muromonab-CD3 for, 448
Liver transplant rejection, preventing
cyclosporine for, 182

Liver transplant rejection, preventing *(continued)*
mycophenolate for, 450
tacrolimus for, 600
10% LMD, 209-211
Look alike, sound alike drugs, **S26-S27**
Lopressor, 428
lorazepam, 398-400
Lovenox, 676
L-thyroxine, 681
Luminal Sodium, 517
Lung cancer
bevacizumab for, 93
docetaxel for, 226
doxorubicin for, 238
etoposide for, 280
gemcitabine for, 312
paclitaxel for, 489
pemetrexed for, 504
porfimer for, 686
topotecan for, 618
vinblastine for, 643
vinorelbine for, 647
Lung transplantation, cytomegalovirus immune globulin intravenous (human) for, 186
Lupuslike syndrome, 706
Lupus nephritis, 706
Lymphocytic leukemia, fludarabine for, 295
Lymphoma. *See also* Hodgkin's lymphoma; Non-Hodgkin's lymphoma.
allopurinol for, 23
bortezomib for, 100
carmustine for, 120
cyclophosphamide for, 179
denileukin diftitox for, 672
doxorubicin for, 238
nelarabine for, 683
thiotepa for, 689
Lymphosarcoma
mechlorethamine for, 405
methotrexate for, 418
Lysatec rt-PA, 27

M

MabCampath, 664
Macrodex, 209
Macular degeneration, verteporfin for, 690
magnesium sulfate, 400-402
Magnesium sulfate overdose, calcium gluconate injection, 10% for, 669
Malaria, quinidine for, 559
Malignant hyperthermia, dantrolene for, 191
Malignant melanoma
aldesleukin for, 17
dacarbazine for, 189
interferon alfa-2b for, 362
vinblastine for, 643
Malignant pleural mesothelioma, pemetrexed for, 503
Manganese, 626
mannitol, 402-404
Maxipime, 127
Mechanical ventilation
alfentanil for, 21
atracurium for, 81
cisatracurium for, 166
propofol for, 549
succinylcholine for, 592
vecuronium for, 638
mechlorethamine hydrochloride, 405-407
Mefoxin, 133
Megaloblastic anemia, 706
folic acid for, 302
melphalan hydrochloride, 407-409
Meningitis
amphotericin B for, 49
ampicillin for, 55
ceftriaxone for, 142
cefuroxime for, 145
chloramphenicol for, 151
meropenem for, 412
methylprednisolone for, 423
penicillin G potassium for, 507
Meningococcal meningitis, penicillin G potassium for, 507
meperidine hydrochloride, 409-411
meropenem, 412-414
Merrem I.V., 412
Merronem, 412
mesna, 414-415
Mesnex, 414
Mesothelioma, malignant pleural, pemetrexed for, 503
Mestinon, 555
Metabolic acidosis, 706
potassium acetate for, 536
sodium bicarbonate for, 584
tromethamine for, 631
Metabolic alkalosis
potassium chloride for, 538
sodium chloride for, 586
Metalyse, 602
methadone hydrochloride, 682-683
Methanol poisoning, fomepizole injection for, 303
Methemoglobinemia, 707
methocarbamol, 415-417
methotrexate sodium, 417-421
impaired elimination of, leucovorin for, 387

methyldopate hydrochloride, 421-423, 683
methylprednisolone sodium succinate, 423-426
metoclopramide hydrochloride, 426-428
Metoclopramide Omega, 426
metoprolol tartrate, 428-430
Metric conversions, **S6**
metronidazole hydrochloride, 430-431
Microbial infection, imipenem and cilastatin for, 348
midazolam hydrochloride, 431-434
Migraine, dihydroergotamine for, 674
milrinone lactate, 434-435
mitomycin, 436-438
Mitoxana, 346, 438
mitoxantrone hydrochloride, 438-441
Molybdenum, 626
Monarc-M, 61
Monoclate-P, 61
Mononine, 282
morphine sulfate, 441-443
Motion sickness, dimenhydrinate injection for, 674
moxifloxacin hydrochloride, 444-446
Mucositis, oral, palifermin for, 494
Multiple myeloma
  bortezomib for, 100
  carmustine for, 120
  cyclophosphamide for, 179
  melphalan for, 407
  pamidronate for, 497
  zoledronic acid for, 658
Multiple sclerosis
  hydrocortisone for, 331
Multiple sclerosis *(continued)*
  methylprednisolone for, 423
  mitoxantrone for, 439
Multitrace-4 Concentrate, 626
Multitrace-4 Neonatal, 626
Multitrace-4 Pediatric, 626
Multitrace-5 Concentrate, 626
multivitamin infusion, 446-448
muromonab-CD3, 448-450
Muscle cramping, calcium gluconate injection, 10% for, 669
Muscle spasm
  diazepam for, 213
  methocarbamol for, 416
Musculoskeletal conditions
  methocarbamol for, 416
  orphenadrine for, 478
Mustargen, 405
mustine, 405-407
Mutamycin, 436
M.V.I. Adult, 446
M.V.I. Pediatric, 446
Myasthenia gravis, edrophonium for diagnosis of, 251
Myasthenic crisis, pyridostigmine for, 555
Myasthenic crisis vs. cholinergic crisis, edrophonium for, 251
mycophenolate mofetil hydrochloride, 450-452
Mycoplasmal infection, doxycycline for, 244
Mycosis fungoides
  cyclophosphamide for, 179
  mechlorethamine for, 405
  vinblastine for, 643
Myeloid reconstitution, sargramostim for, 579
Mylotarg, 315
Myocardial contractility, impaired, 706
Myocardial infarction
  alteplase for, 27
  atenolol for, 79
  enoxaparin for, 676
  eptifibatide for, 265
  metoprolol for, 428
  nitroglycerin for, 465
  reteplase for, 572
  streptokinase for, 589
  tenecteplase for, 602
  warfarin for, 653
Myocet, 241
Myopia, pathologic, verteporfin for, 690
Myxedema coma
  levothyroxine for, 681
  liothyronine for, 681

N

N-acetylcysteine, 7-8
nafcillin sodium, 452-454
nalbuphine hydrochloride, 454-456
nalmefene hydrochloride, 456-458
naloxone hydrochloride, 458-460
Narcan, 458
Narcoanalysis, thiopental for, 606
Narcosynthesis, thiopental for, 606
Natrecor, 461
Nausea and vomiting
  chlorpromazine for, 157
  dimenhydrinate injection for, 674
  diphenhydramine for, 222
  dolasetron for, 229, 230
  droperidol for, 247
  granisetron for, 325
  metoclopramide for, 426

Nausea and vomiting *(continued)*
ondansetron for, 476
palonosetron for, 495
prochlorperazine for, 544
promethazine for, 546
Navelbine, 647
Nebcin, 615
Neck cancer. *See* Head and neck cancer.
Neisseria meningitidis carriers, rifampin for, 574
nelarabine, 683-684
Nembutal Sodium, 513
Neonatal group B streptococcal disease, ampicillin for, 55
Neoplasm, 707
Neoplastic disease, methylprednisolone for, 423
neostigmine methylsulfate, 460-461
Neo-Synephrine, 520
Neovascularization, subfoveal choroidal, verteporfin for, 690
Nephrosis, osmotic, 707
Nephrotic syndrome, hydrocortisone for, 331
Nephrotoxicity, 707
nesiritide, 461-463
Neupogen, 290
Neuroblastoma
cyclophosphamide for, 179
doxorubicin for, 238
Neuroleptic malignant syndrome, 707
Neurologic procedures, fentanyl for, 288
Neuromuscular blockade, reversing
edrophonium for, 251
hyoscyamine for, 680
neostigmine for, 460
pyridostigmine for, 555
Neurosurgery, propofol for, 549
Neurosyphilis, penicillin G potassium for, 507
Neutropenia, 707
febrile. *See* Febrile neutropenia.
Neutrophil recovery, sargramostim for, 579
Nexium I.V., 273
NiaStase, 174
nicardipine, 463-465
Nimbex, 165
Nipent, 515
Nipride, 467
nitrogen mustard, 405-407
nitroglycerin, 465-467
infusion rates for, **S8**
Nitropress, 467
nitroprusside sodium, 467-469
infusion rates for, **S7**
Non-Hodgkin's lymphoma
bleomycin for, 98
ibritumomab for, 339
rituximab for, 577
tositumomab and iodine[131] tositumomab for, 623
Norcuron, 637
norepinephrine bitartrate, 469-471
Norepinephrine extravasation, phentolamine for, 685
Norflex, 477
Norphyl, 41
Novamine, 35
Novantrone, 438
Novastan, 71
Novolin ge Toronto, 359
Novolin R, 359
Novolin R PenFill, 359
NovoSeven, 174
Nubain, 454
Nutritional supplement, amino acids as, 36, 37

O

ocreotide acetate, 471-473
Octagam, 350
ofloxacin, 473-475
Oliguria, mannitol for, 402, 403
Oncaspar, 684
Oncovin, 644
ondansetron hydrochloride, 475-477
Ontak, 672
Onxol, 488
Opana, 484
Open-heart surgery, fentanyl in, 288
Opioid dependence, methadone for, 682
Opioid depression, reversing, naloxone for, 459
Opioid effects, reversing, nalmefene for, 456
Opioid overdose
nalmefene for, 456
naloxone for, 459
Oral mucositis, palifermin for, 494
Orencia, 3
Organ rejection, preventing
anti-thymocyte globulin (equine) sterile solution for, 666
azathioprine for, 668
basiliximab for, 668
cyclosporine for, 182
daclizumab for, 672
muromonab-CD3 for, 448
mycophenolate for, 450
tacrolimus for, 600
orphenadrine citrate, 477-479
Orthoclone OKT3, 448
Orthopedic procedures, fentanyl for, 288
Osmitrol, 402
Osmotic nephrosis, 707

Osteoarthritis, methylprednisolone for, 423
Osteolytic lesions, pamidronate for, 497
Osteomalacia, calcium gluconate injection, 10% for, 669
Osteoporosis
  ibandronate for, 337
  zoledronic acid for, 658
Osteosarcoma, methotrexate for, 418
Ovarian cancer
  amifostine for, 31
  carboplatin for, 117, 118
  cisplatin for, 168
  cyclophosphamide for, 179
  doxorubicin hydrochloride liposomal for, 242
  gemcitabine for, 312
  paclitaxel for, 489
  thiotepa for, 689
  topotecan for, 618
oxacillin sodium, 479-481
oxaliplatin, 481-484
oxymorphone hydrochloride, 484-486
oxytocin, 486-488

P
paclitaxel, 488-491
paclitaxel protein-bound particles, 491-494
Paget's disease
  pamidronate for, 497
  zoledronic acid for, 658
Pain
  buprenorphine for, 105
  butorphanol for, 110
  codeine for, 176
  hydromorphone for, 334
  ketorolac for, 380
  levorphanol for, 393
  methadone for, 682
  mitoxantrone for, 439
Pain *(continued)*
  morphine for, 442
  nalbuphine for, 454
  oxymorphone for, 484
  pentazocine for, 511
palifermin, 494-495
palonosetron hydrochloride, 495-496
pamidronate disodium, 496-498
Pancreas transplantation, cytomegalovirus immune globulin intravenous (human) for, 186
Pancreatic cancer
  fluorouracil for, 299
  gemcitabine for, 312
  mitomycin for, 436
  streptozocin for, 687
Pancreatic duct, cannulation of, secretin for, 687
Pancreatic dysfunction, secretin for diagnosis of, 686
Pancreatic secretions, stimulating, secretin for, 686
Pancreatitis
  acute, 703
  hyoscyamine for, 679
pancuronium bromide, 498-500
Pancytopenia, 707
pantoprazole sodium, 500-501
Papilledema, 707
Paralysis, periodic
  potassium acetate for, 536
  potassium chloride for, 538
Paraplatin, 117
Paraplatin, AQ, 117
paricalcitol, 501-503
Parkinsonism
  atropine for, 84
  benztropine for, 91
Parkinson's disease, hyoscyamine for, 679
Paroxysmal atrial tachycardia, digoxin for, 216
Paroxysmal supraventricular tachycardia
  adenosine for, 12
  phenylephrine for, 521
  quinidine for, 559
  verapamil for, 640
Parvolex, 7
Pasteurella infection, penicillin G potassium for, 507
Patent ductus arteriosus
  alprostadil for, 26
  indomethacin for, 680
Pavulon, 498
Paxene, 488
pegaspargase, 684
PEG-L-aspargase, 684
Pelvic infection, ertapenem for, 267
Pelvic inflammatory disease
  azithromycin for, 87
  clindamycin for, 170
  erythromycin for, 269
  ofloxacin for, 473
  pipercillin and tazabactam for, 530
pemetrexed, 503-506
Penbritin, 54
penicillin G potassium, 506-509
Penile cancer, bleomycin for, 98
Pentacarinat, 509
Pentam, 509
pentamidine isethionate, 509-511
pentazocine, 511-513
pentobarbital sodium, 513-515
pentostatin, 515-517
Pentothal, 605
Pepcid Injection, 284
Peptic ulcer
  atropine for, 84
  glycopyrrolate for, 323

Percutaneous coronary intervention
abciximab for, 5
argatroban for, 72
eptifibatide for, 265
Percutaneous transluminal coronary angiography, tirofiban for, 613
Pericardial effusion, 707
Peritonitis, pipercillin and tazabactam for, 530
Persantine IV, 674
pethidine hydrochloride, 409-411
Pfizerpen, 506
phenobarbital sodium, 517-520
phentolamine, 684-685
Phentolamine blocking test, 685
phenylephrine hydrochloride, 520-522
infusion rates for, **S9**
phenytoin sodium, 522-525
Pheochromocytoma, phentolamine for diagnosing, 685
Pheochromocytomectomy, phentolamine for, 684
phosphates, 525-526
Photofrin, 686
Phyllocontin, 41
Physostigmine antidote, atropine as, 84
physostigmine salicylate, 526-528
phytomenadione, 528-529
phytonadione, 528-529
Pilocarpine antidote, atropine as, 84
piperacillin sodium, 685-686
piperacillin sodium and tazobactam sodium, 530-532
Pitocin, 486
Plaque psoriasis
alefacept for, 664
infliximab for, 357
Plasmanate, 532
plasma protein fraction, 532-534
Plasma volume expansion
dextran for, 209
hetastarch for, 329
Platinex, 167
Platinol, 167
PMS-Butorphanol, 109
PMS-Deferoxamine, 203
PMS-Neostigmine Methylsulfate, 460
Pneumonitis, eosinophilic, 705
Pneumonia
azithromycin for, 86
cefazolin for, 125
cefepime for, 128
ciprofloxacin for, 163
ertapenem for, 267
hydrocortisone for, 331
levofloxacin for, 389, 390
linezolid for, 397
moxifloxacin for, 444
ofloxacin for, 473
pentamidine for, 510
piperacillin for, 685
pipercillin and tazabactam for, 530
sulfamethoxazole-trimethoprim for, 597
Polycythemia vera, mechlorethamine for, 405
Polygam S/D, 350
Polymicrobial infection, imipenem and cilastatin for, 348
polymyxin B sulfate, 534-536
porfimer, 686
Post-anesthesia care, physostigmine for, 527
Postpartum bleeding, oxytocin for, 487
Post peripheral blood pregenitor cell transplantation, sargramostim for, 579
potassium acetate, 536-538
potassium chloride, 538-540
Potassium depletion
potassium acetate for, 536
potassium chloride for, 538
Precedex, 673
Preeclampsia, magnesium for, 401
Pregnancy risk categories, xiv
Premarin Intravenous, 275
Primary aldosteronism
potassium acetate for, 536
potassium chloride for, 538
Primary pulmonary hypertension, epoprostenol for, 262
Primaxin, 348
procainamide hydrochloride, 540-543
ProcalAmine, 35
prochlorperazine edisylate, 543-545
Procrit, 260
Proctitis, hydrocortisone for, 331
Procytox, 179
Profilnine SD, 282
Prograf, 599
Prolastin, 665
Proleukin, 16
promethazine hydrochloride, 546-548
Pronestyl, 540
Proplex T (heat-treated), 282

propofol, 548-551
propranolol hydrochloride, 551-553
Prostate cancer
  docetaxel for, 226
  mitoxantrone for, 439
Prostatitis
  ciprofloxacin for, 163
  levofloxacin for, 389, 390
  ofloxacin for, 473
Prostigmin, 460
Prostin VR Pediatric, 25
Prosulf, 553
protamine sulfate, 553-555
Protective equipment, **S20**
Prothrombin deficiency, anticoagulant-induced, phytonadione for, 528
Protium, 500
Protonix IV, 500
Pseudomembranous colitis, 707
Pseudotumor cerebri, 707
Psoriasis
  alefacept for, 664
  infliximab for, 357
  methotrexate for, 418
Psoriatic arthritis, infliximab for, 357
Pulmonary disease, doxapram for, 233
Pulmonary edema, furosemide for, 305
Pulmonary embolism
  alteplase for, 28
  heparin for, 326
  streptokinase for, 589
  warfarin for, 653
Pulmonary hypertension, epoprostenol for, 262
Pulmonary toxicity, 707
Pylorospasm, small intestine, atropine for, 84
pyridostigmine bromide, 555-557
Pyridoxine deficiency, pyridoxine for, 557
pyridoxine hydrochloride, 557-558

Q

Quelicin, 591
quinidine gluconate, 558-562
quinupristin and dalfopristin, 562-564

R

Radiologic examination
  glucagon as diagnostic aid for, 321
  metoclopramide for, 426
ranitidine hydrochloride, 564-566
Rapilysin, 572
rasburicase, 566-567
Rat bite fever, penicillin G potassium for, 507
Reclast, 658
Recombinate, 61
Rectal cancer. *See* Colorectal cancer.
ReFacto, 61
Refludan, 384
Reglan, 426
Regonol, 555
Remicade, 356
remifentanil hydrochloride, 568-570
Renal acidosis, 707
Renal cancer
  aldesleukin for, 17
  vinblastine for, 643
Renal colic, hyoscyamine for, 679
Renal disease
  bumetanide for, 103
  furosemide for, 305
Renal failure, 708
  amino acids for, 37
  torsemide for, 620
Renal function, inadequate, mannitol as test dose for, 402
Renal-cell carcinoma, aldesleukin for, 17
RenAmin, 35
ReoPro, 4
Replenine, 282
RespiGam, 570
Respiratory alkalosis, 708
Respiratory depression, doxapram for, 233
Respiratory secretions, inhibiting, hyoscyamine for, 680
respiratory syncytial virus immune globulin intravenous, 570-572
Respiratory system disorders, methylprednisolone for, 423
Respiratory tract infection
  ampicillin for, 54
  cefazolin for, 124
  cefoxitin for, 133
  ceftizoxime for, 139
  ceftriaxone for, 142
  cefuroxime for, 145
  ciprofloxacin for, 163
  erythromycin for, 268
  imipenem and cilastatin for, 348
  respiratory syncytial virus immune globulin intravenous for, 570
Retavase, 572
reteplase, recombinant, 572-574
Retinitis, cytomegaloviris. *See* Cytomegalovirus retinitis.
Retrovir, 656
Revex, 456
Revimune, 231
Rhabdomyolysis, 708
Rheumatic disorder, methylprednisolone for, 423
Rheumatic fever, erythromycin for, 268

Rheumatoid arthritis
abatacept for, 3
azathioprine for, 668
infliximab for, 357
rituximab for, 577
Rhinitis, allergic, hyoscyamine for, 679
Rickets, calcium gluconate injection, 10% for, 669
Rickettsial infection, doxycycline for, 244
Rifadin, 574
rifampicin, 574-576
rifampin, 574-576
Rigidity, hyoscyamine for, 679
Rimacillin, 54
Rimapurinol, 23
Rituxan, 576
Rituxan Mab Thera, 576
rituximab, 576-579
Robaxin, 415
Robinul, 322
Robinul-Neostigmine, 460
Rocephin, 142
Rogitine, 684
Romazicon, 297
RSV-IGIV, 570-572

S

Salicylate toxicity, 708
Salivation
decreasing, atropine for, 84
inhibiting, hyoscyamine for, 680
Sandimmun, 181
Sandimmune, 181
Sandostatin, 471
Sarcoidosis, 708
sargramostim, 579-581
Scalds
potassium acetate for, 536
potassium chloride for, 538
scopolamine hydrobromide, 581-583
Scurvy, ascorbic acid for, 77
SecreFlo, 686
SecreMax, 686
secretin, 686-687
Secretions, respiratory, hyoscyamine for inhibiting, 680
Sedation
dexmedetomidine for, 673
lorazepam for, 399
midazolam for, 432
pentobarbital for, 513
phenobarbital for, 518
promethazine for, 546
propofol for, 549
scopolamine for, 581
sufentanil for, 595
Seizures
diazepam for, 213
fosphenytoin for, 679
magnesium for, 401
pentobarbital for, 513
phenobarbital for, 518
thiopental for, 606
valproate for, 633
Selenium, 626
Sepsis, 708
drotrecogin alfa for, 249
Septicemia
ampicillin for, 55
cefazolin for, 125
cefotaxime for, 131
cefoxitin for, 133
ceftizoxime for, 139
ceftriaxone for, 142
cefuroxime for, 145
imipenem and cilastatin for, 348
piperacillin for, 685
Septic shock, isoproterenol for, 371
Septra, 596
Serotonin syndrome, 708
Serum sickness, 708
Shigellosis, sulfamethoxazole-trimethoprim for, 597
Shock
dopamine for, 231
hetastarch for, 329
phenylephrine for, 520
Simulect, 668
Sinusitis
ciprofloxacin for, 163
levofloxacin for, 389, 390
moxifloxacin for, 444
Sinus tachycardia, esmolol for, 271
Skeletal muscle relaxation
atracurium for, 81
cisatracurium for, 166
pancuronium for, 499
succinylcholine for, 592
vecuronium for, 638
Skin and skin-structure infection
ampicillin for, 54
ampicillin and tazobactam for, 57
cefazolin for, 124
cefoxitin for, 133
ceftazidime for, 136
ceftizoxime for, 139
ceftriaxone for, 142
cefuroxime for, 145
ciprofloxacin for, 163
daptomycin for, 193
ertapenem for, 267
erythromycin for, 268
levofloxacin for, 389, 390
linezolid for, 397
moxifloxacin for, 444
ofloxacin for, 473, 474
piperacillin for, 685
pipercillin and tazabactam for, 530
quinupristin and dalfopristin for, 562
tigecycline for, 611
Skin cancer, bleomycin for, 98
Skin disorder, methylprednisolone for, 423
Skin-structure infection. *See* Skin and skin-structure infection.

Small-bowel intubation, metoclopramide for, 426
SMZ-TMP, 596-599
sodium acetate, 583-584
sodium and potassium phosphates, 525-526
sodium bicarbonate, 584-585
sodium chloride, 586-587
Sodium chloride replacement, sodium chloride for, 586
Sodium depletion, sodium chloride for, 586
Sodium Diuril, 154
sodium ferric gluconate complex, 587-589
Soft-tissue infection
  ampicillin for, 54
  piperacillin for, 685
Solid tumors
  allopurinol for, 23
  doxorubicin for, 238
Solu-Cortef, 330
Solu-Medrol, 423
Solutions, I.V., and drug compatibility, 697-699
Sporotrichosis, amphotericin B for, 49
Stadol, 109
Status asthmaticus, isoproterenol for, 372
Status epilepticus
  diazepam for, 213
  fosphenytoin for, 678
  lorazepam for, 399
  phenobarbital for, 518
  phenytoin for, 522
Steatosis, 708
Stem cells, harvesting, filgrastim for, 291
Stem-cell transplantation, busulfan for, 107
Stevens-Johnson syndrome, 708
Stiff-man syndrome, diazepam for, 213
Stomach cancer. *See* Gastric cancer.
Storzolamide, 663
Streptase, 589
streptokinase, 589-591
streptozocin, 687-688
Stroke, alteplase for, 28
Stupor, levothyroxine for, 681
Subfoveal choroidal neovascularization, verteporfin for, 690
Sublimaze, 288
succinylcholine chloride, 591-594
Sufenta, 594
sufentanil citrate, 594-596
Suicidal ideation, 708
sulfamethoxazole-trimethoprim, 596-599
Sulfone syndrome, 708
Supraventricular tachycardia, esmolol for, 271
Surgery preparation
  lorazepam for, 399
  oxymorphone for, 484
  pentazocine for, 511
  phenobarbital for, 518
Surgical procedures, ketamine for, 377
Surgical prophylaxis
  cefazolin for, 125
  cefotaxime for, 130
  cefoxitin for, 133
  ceftriaxone for, 142
  metronidazole for, 430
Syndrome of inappropriate antiduretic hormone secretion, 709
Synercid, 562
Synthroid, 681
Syntocinon, 486

T
T_3, 681
T_4, 681
Tachyarrhythmia
  digoxin for, 216
  diltiazem for, 220
tacrolimus, 599-602
Talwin, 511
Tardive dyskinesia, 709
Tarivid, 473
Tavanic, 389
Taxol, 488
Taxotere, 225
Tazicef, 136
Tazocin, 530
Temperature conversions, **S6**
tenecteplase, 602-603
teniposide injection, 688-689
Tenormin I.V. Injection, 78
Tensilon, 251
Testicular cancer
  bleomycin for, 98
  cisplatin for, 168
  etoposide for, 280
  ifosfamide for, 346
  vinblastine for, 643
Testosterone overmedication
  potassium acetate for, 536
  potassium chloride for, 538
Tetanus
  chlorpromazine for, 157
  diazepam for, 213
Tetany, 709
  calcium gluconate injection, 10% for, 669
Thallium myocardial perfusion imaging, dipyridamole for, 674
Tham, 631
theophylline, 41-44
Thiamine deficiency, thiamine for, 604
thiamine hydrochloride, 604-605
thiopental sodium, 605-608
Thioplex, 689
thiotepa, 689-690
Thrombate III, 69

Thrombocytopenia, 709
  argatroban for, 72
  lepirudin for, 384
Thrombocytopenic purpura, idiopathic, immune globulin for, 351
Thromboembolic disease, lepirudin for, 384
Thrombosis
  antithrombin III, human for, 70
  argatroban for, 72
  heparin for, 326
  streptokinase for, 589
  warfarin for, 653
Thymoglobulin, 666
Thyroid cancer, doxorubicin for, 238
Thyroid function, reduced, levothyroxine for, 681
ticarcillin disodium and clavulanate potassium/clavulanic acid, 608-610
tigecycline, 610-612
Timentin, 608
tirofiban hydrochloride, 612-615
tissue plasminogen activator, recombinant, 27-30
TNKase, 602
tobramycin sulfate, 615-618
topotecan hydrochloride, 618-620
Toradol, 379
torasemide, 620-622
Torsades de pointes, 709
torsemide, 620-622
tositumomab and iodine^{131} tositumomab, 622-626
Total parenteral nutrition
  amino acids for, 36
  fat emulsions for, 286
  magnesium for, 401
  thiamine for, 604
  trace metals for, 626
Toxic epidermal necrolysis, 709
trace metals, 626-628
Tracheal intubation, succinylcholine for, 592
Tracrium, 80
Trandate, 381
tranexamic acid injection, 690
Tranquilizing effect, scopolamine for, 581
Transplant patients
  anti-thymocyte globulin (equine) sterile solution for, 666
  azathioprine for, 668
  basiliximab for, 668
  cyclosporine for, 182
  cytomegalovirus immune globulin intravenous (human) for, 186
  daclizumab for, 672
  ganciclovir for, 309
  muromonab-CD3 for, 448
  mycophenolate for, 450
  tacrolimus for, 600
trastuzumab, 628-631
Travasol, 35
Tremors, hyoscyamine for, 679
Trichinosis
  hydrocortisone for, 331
  methylprednisolone for, 423
Triiodothyronine Injection, 681
Triostat, 681
Trisenox, 74
tromethamine, 631-632
TrophAmine, 35
Truphylline, 41
Tuberculosis
  capreomycin for, 670
  rifampin for, 574
Tuberculous meningitis, methylprednisolone for, 423
Tygacil, 610

U

Ulcer, intractable, famotidine for, 284
Ulcerative colitis
  hydrocortisone for, 331
  infliximab for, 357
Ultiva, 568
Unasyn, 57
Ureteral colic, atropine for, 84
Urethritis
  ampicillin for, 55
  ofloxacin for, 473, 474
Uric acid levels, elevated, allopurinol for, 23
Urinary tract disorder, atropine for, 84
Urinary tract infection
  amikacin for, 33
  ampicillin for, 55
  cefazolin for, 125
  cefepime for, 127, 128
  cefoxitin for, 133
  ceftazidime for, 136
  ceftizoxime for, 139
  cefuroxime for, 145
  ciprofloxacin for, 163
  imipenem and cilastatin for, 348
  levofloxacin for, 389, 390
  ofloxacin for, 473
  piperacillin for, 685
  polymyxin B for, 534
  sulfamethoxazole-trimethoprim for, 597
  ticarcillin and clavulanate potassium for, 608
Uromitexan, 414
Uterine bleeding, estrogens, conjugated for, 275

V

Valium, 213
valproate sodium, 632-635
Vancocin, 635

vancomycin hydrochloride, 635-637
Varicella zoster infection, acyclovir for, 9
Vasotec IV, 253
Vascular leak syndrome, 709
Vascular thrombosis, 709
VCR, 644-647
vecuronium bromide, 637-639
Velbe, 642
Velcade, 100
Venipuncture, **S10-S15**
Venofer, 369
Venous thrombosis
  heparin for, 326
  warfarin for, 653
Ventricular arrhythmia
  amiodarone for, 45
  edetate for, 676
  procainamide for, 541
VePesid, 279
verapamil hydrochloride, 640-642
verteporfin, 690
Vertigo
  dimenhydrinate injection for, 674
  diphenhydramine for, 222
Vfend I.V., 650
Vibramycin Hyclate, 244
vinblastine sulfate, 642-644
Vincasar PFS, 644
vincristine sulfate, 644-647
vinorelbine tartrate, 647-650
Viraferon, 361
Vistide, 159
Visudyne, 690
Vitamin B_6 dependency syndrome, pyridoxine for, 557
vitamin C, 77-78
Vitamin deficiency, multivitamin infusion for, 446
VLB, 642-644
Voluven, 329
Vomiting. *See* Nausea and vomiting.
von Willebrand disease
  antihemophilic factor/von Willebrand factor complex for, 64
  desmopressin for, 205
voriconazole, 650-652
VP-16-213, 279
Vulvar cancer, bleomycin for, 98
Vumon, 688

W

warfarin sodium, 653-655
Water intake, excessive, sodium chloride for, 586
Water replacement, sodium chloride for, 586
Wernicke's encephalopathy, thiamine for, 604
Wilms' tumor, doxorubicin for, 238
Withdrawal phenomena, 709
Wolff-Parkinson-White syndrome, adenosine for, 12
Wound healing, enhancing, ascorbic acid for, 77

XY

Xerostomia, amifostine for, 31
Xigris, 249
Xylocaine, 394
Xylocard, 394

Z

Zanosar, 687
Zantac, 564
Zavedos, 343
Zemaira, 665
Zemplar, 501
Zenapax, 672
Zevalin, 338
zidovudine, 656-658
Zinacef, 144
Zinc, 626
Zinecard, 207
Zinnat, 144
Zita, 161
Zithromax, 86
Zofran, 475
Zofran Preservative Free, 475
zoledronic acid, 658-660
Zollinger-Ellison syndrome
  cimetidine for, 161
  ranitidine for, 564
Zometa, 658
Zosyn, 530
Zovirax, 8
Zygomycosis, amphotericin B for, 49
Zyvox, 397
Zyvoxam, 397